Everything
You Need to
Know about
Drugs

Everything
You Need to
Know about
Drugs

Springhouse Corporation
Springhouse, PA

Staff

Executive Director
Matthew Cahill

Editorial Director
Patricia Dwyer Schull, RN, MSN

Art Director
John Hubbard

Senior Editor
H. Nancy Holmes

Editors
Marcia Andrews, Margaret Eckman, Kathy E. Goldberg, Catherine E. Harold, Peter H. Johnson, Elizabeth Mauro, Nancy Priff, Doris Weinstock, Patricia A. Wittig

Clinical Project Editors
Patricia Kardish Fischer, RN, BSN; Judith Schilling McCann, RN, MSN

Clinical Editors
Ann M. Barrow, RN, MSN, CCRN; Lori Musolf Neri, RN, MSN; Beverly Ann Tscheschlog, RN

Assistant Acquisitions Editor
Louise Quinn

Copy Editors
Cynthia C. Breuninger (manager), Christine Cunniffe, Mary Durkin, Barbara E. Hodgson, Brenna Mayer, Christina P. Ponczek, Pamela Wingrod

Designers
Lesley Weissman-Cook (book designer), Donald G. Knauss (project manager), Joseph Clark, Mary Ludwicki, Kaaren Mitchel, Mary Stangl

Typography
Diane Paluba (manager), Joyce Rossi Biletz, Phyllis Marron, Valerie Rosenberger

Manufacturing
Deborah Meiris (director), T.A. Landis

Production Coordinator
Margaret A. Rastiello

Editorial Assistants
Carol Caputo, Beverly Lane, Mary Madden, Jeanne Napier

Indexer
Barbara E. Hodgson

The drug selections, dosages, and procedures in this book are based on current clinical recommendations by medical, pharmaceutical, pharmacologic, and nursing authorities. These selections and dosages comply with currently accepted standards; nevertheless, they can't be considered absolute and universal recommendations. For individual application, all recommendations must be considered in light of the reader's medical condition and, before taking new or infrequently used drugs, in light of the latest drug package-insert information. The authors and the publisher disclaim responsibility for any adverse effects resulting directly or indirectly from the suggested recommendations, from any undetected errors, or from the reader's misunderstanding of the text.

Printed in the United States of America
EYNKD-020397

℞ A member of the Reed Elsevier plc group

Library of Congress Cataloging-in-Publishing Data
Everything you need to know about drugs.
   p. cm.
   Includes index.
1. Drugs—Popular works. I. Springhouse Corporation
RM301.15E94 1996
615'.1—dc20   96-16575
ISBN 0-87434-864-1 (alk. paper)   CIP

Contents

Advisory Board

Contributors and Consultants

Douglas R. Allington, PharmD
Clinical Assistant Professor
School of Pharmacy and Allied Health
University of Montana
Missoula

Alan Caspi, PharmD, MBA
Director of Pharmacy
Lenox Hill Hospital
New York

Marlene Ciranowicz, RN, MSN, CDE
Independent Consultant
Dresher, Pa.

Michael R. Cohen, RPh, MS, FASHP
President, Institute for Safe Medication Practices
Warminster, Pa.

Douglas D. DeCarolis, RPh, PharmD
Inpatient Clinical Coordinator
Minneapolis VA Medical Center

Patricia A. Diehl, RN, MA, BSN
Associate Professor of Nursing
Department of Health Restoration
School of Nursing
West Virginia University
Morgantown

Mark J. Ellison, PharmD, FCP, BCPS
Assistant Director, Glaxo Research Institute
Research Triangle Park, N.C.

Mary Beth Gross, PharmD, FASCP
Manager, Pharmacy
Mercy Hospital Medical Center
Associate Professor of Pharmacy
Drake University
Des Moines, Iowa

James R. Hildebrand III, PharmD
Director, Drug Information Center
Associate Professor
Philadelphia College of Pharmacy and Science

Cary E. Johnson, PharmD
Associate Professor of Pharmacy
Clinical Pharmacist, Pediatrics
College of Pharmacy, University of Michigan
Ann Arbor

James A. Koestner, PharmD
Clinical Pharmacist, Trauma
Pharmacy Department
Vanderbilt University Hospital
Nashville, Tenn.

Mark S. Luer, PharmD
Assistant Professor
College of Pharmacy
University of Illinois at Chicago

Mary Y. Ma, PharmD
Antimicrobial Clinical Specialist
VA West Los Angeles Medical Center
Assistant Professor of Clinical Pharmacy
University of California at San Francisco

Denise H. Rhoney, PharmD
Clinical Research Fellow
University of North Carolina at Chapel Hill

Mark S. Roth, RPh, MS
Clinical Coordinator for I.V. Nutrition Support
New York Hospital, Cornell Medical Center
New York

Irving Salit, MD, CM, FRCP(C)
Head, Division of Infectious Diseases
Director, Immunodeficiency Clinic
Toronto Hospital

Donna J. Schroeder, PharmD
Director, Drug Information Analysis Services
Division of Clinical Pharmacy
University of California at San Francisco

J. Michael Spivey, PharmD, BCPS
Assistant Professor of Family Medicine
East Carolina University School of Medicine
Greenville, N.C.

Joseph F. Steiner, RPh, PharmD
Professor of Clinical Pharmacy
School of Human Medicine and Pharmacy
University of Wyoming
Casper

Acknowledgments

We would like to thank the following companies for permission to use photographs of the following drugs in the full-color *Photoguide to Tablets and Capsules*.

Abbott Laboratories
Biaxin®
Depakote®
Depakote® Sprinkle
E.E.S.®
Ery-Tab®
Erythromycin Base Filmtab®
Hytrin®
PCE®

Astra Merck
Prilosec®

Bristol-Myers Squibb Company
BuSpar®
Capoten®
Cefzil®
Duricef®
Estrace®
Pravachol®
Sumycin®
Veetids®

Daniels Pharmaceuticals, Inc.
Levoxyl®

Dupont/Merck
Coumadin®
Percocet®
Sinemet®
Sinemet® CR

Eli Lilly and Company
Axid®
Ceclor®
Darvocet-N® 100
Lorabid®
Prozac®

ESI/Lederle Generics
atenolol

Ethex Corporation
potassium chloride

Forest Pharmaceutical, Inc.
Armour®Thyroid
Lorcet® 10/650

GlaxoWellcome Inc.
Ceftin®
Lanoxin®
Zantac®
Zantac® EFFERdose®
Zovirax®

Goldline Laboratories, Inc.
verapamil hydrochloride

Hoechst Marion Roussel, Inc.
Altace®
Carafate®
Cardizem®
Cardizem® CD
Cardizem® SR®
DiaBeta®
Lasix®
Seldane®
Seldane-D®
Trental®

Hoffman-La Roche, Inc.
Bumex®
Klonopin®
Naprosyn®
Toradol®
Valium®

Janssen Pharmaceutical, Inc.
Hismanal®
Propulsid®

Knoll Pharmaceutical Company
E-Mycin®
ibuprofen®
Synthroid®
Vicodin®
Vicodin ES®

Lederle Laboratories
Maxzide®
Maxzide®-25 mg
Suprax®
Verelan®

Lemmon Company
acetaminophen and codeine (300 mg/30 mg)
Cotrim® DS

MD Pharmaceutical, Inc.
methylphenidate hydrochloride

Merck & Co., Inc.
Mevacor®
Pepcid®
Prinivil®
Vasotec®
Zocor®

Miles, Inc.
Adalat®
Cipro®

Mylan Pharmaceuticals Inc.
propoxyphene napsylate with acetaminophen

Novopharm USA Inc. Division of Novopharm Limited
amoxicillin trihydrate

Ortho/McNeil Pharmaceutical
Floxin®
Tylenol® with Codeine No. 3

Proctor and Gamble Pharmaceuticals
Macrodantin®

Purepac Pharmaceutical Co.
acetaminophen and codeine (300 mg/60 mg)

Rhône-Poulenc Rorer Pharmaceuticals Inc.
Dilacor XR®
Lozol®
Slo-bid® Gyrocaps®

A.H. Robins Company
Micro-K Extencaps®

Roxane Laboratories, Inc.
Roxicet™

Sandoz Pharmaceuticals Corporation
DynaCirc®
Pamelor®

Schein Pharmaceutical, Inc.
nortriptyline hydrochloride

Schering-Plough Corporation
Claritin®
K-Dur®
Theo-Dur®

G.D. Searle & Company
Ambien®
Calan®

SmithKline Beecham Pharmaceuticals
Amoxil®
Augmentin®
Compazine®
Compazine® Spansule®
Dyazide®
Paxil®
Relafen®
Tagamet®
Tagamet® Tiltab®

Solvay Pharmaceuticals, Inc.
Orasone®

The Upjohn Company
Ansaid®
Deltasone®
Glynase®
Halcion®
Micronase®
Motrin®
Ogen®
Provera®
Xanax®

U.S. Pharmaceuticals Group Pfizer Inc.
Cardura®
Glucotrol®
Glucotrol XL™
Norvasc®
Procardia XL®
Zithromax®
Zoloft®

Warner-Lambert Company
Accupril®
Dilantin®
Dilantin® Kapseals®
gemfibrozil
Lopid®
Nitrostat®

Watson Laboratories, Inc.
hydrocodone bitartrate and acetaminophen

Whitby Pharmaceuticals, Inc.
Lortab®

Wyeth-Ayerst Laboratories
Ativan®
Inderal®
Lodine®
Premarin®

Zeneca Pharmaceuticals
Nolvadex®
Tenormin®
Zestril®

Foreword

To most Americans, health care means going to the doctor's office, a trip we make more than 600 million times a year. We receive about 2 billion prescriptions annually, for which we spend an average of $25 apiece at one of more than 65,000 pharmacies. Then we go home and take our medicine. Simple, safe, and easy, right? Wrong.

Incorrect use of drugs accounts for about *5 million* hospital admissions a year. Although doctors, nurses, and pharmacists are reliable sources of drug information, problems occur despite their explanations. First, the information we need to understand is vast and hard to remember. In the doctor's office and the pharmacy, we receive information on our diagnosis and the name of the drug being prescribed. We may also hear why the drug's being given, what it does, and how to take it. What's more, we may be counseled about side effects, cautioned against drinking alcohol or taking other drugs, and advised what to do if we miss a dose. Those of us who are hearing this for the first time are likely to be overwhelmed.

Second, many of us unintentionally cause ourselves problems by stopping a drug too soon because we don't feel better quickly or we don't like the side effects. Third, many of us continue to drink alcohol or take other drugs while using prescription drugs. Most people don't realize that alcohol and everyday products such as cough and cold remedies, aspirin, vitamins, and oral contraceptives can affect the action of other drugs.

But all's not lost. Now, there's easy, understandable, authoritative help at hand. *Everything You Need to Know about Drugs* provides the information you need to take medications safely and wisely. It lists thousands of drugs, of which just 200 account for half of all prescriptions written, so you'll most likely find yours here. This book makes it easy to find information, too. Drugs are listed alphabetically for quick location. For each drug, easy-to-read headings break details down into readily grasped bits that include:
• Why the drug is prescribed and its typical dosages
• How to take the drug
• What to do if you miss a dose

• What to do if you think you've taken an overdose
• Important advice on what to tell your doctor before you start taking any drug
• How the drug works in your body
• Whether you should drive while taking your medication
• Whether a less expensive generic drug is available.

In addition, special information boxes on each page tell you if a drug can cause serious or frequent side effects, and offer tips on how to avoid or relieve them if they occur. Sections in the back of the book address many more topics, such as how to give yourself eardrops and injections, insert a suppository, take your pulse or blood pressure, and treat poisoning. The book also features information on:
• more than 100 alternative therapies
• drugs typically prescribed for common illnesses
• adding fiber to your diet
• cutting down on cholesterol and salt
• increasing (or reducing) potassium in your diet
• choosing a calcium supplement
• avoiding allergy triggers.

Everything You Need to Know about Drugs is the next best thing to talking with your doctor, nurse, or pharmacist. The book can reinforce their directions by providing answers to questions, solutions to problems, and reminders of key facts. It also gives you all you need for an informed discussion with your doctor, nurse, or pharmacist.

Doctors know that some medication-related problems may occur even under ideal circumstances, but that most problems can be prevented. They're working on ways to reduce and prevent medication-related complications and deaths. However, there's something *you* can do on your own right now: Strive to be an informed, educated consumer. And start with a copy of *Everything You Need to Know about Drugs*.

Lawrence M. Brass, M.D.
Associate Professor
Departments of Neurology and Epidemiology &
Public Health
Yale University School of Medicine
New Haven, Conn.

GUIDE TO DRUGS: ACCUPRIL THROUGH ZYLOPRIM

Accupril

Accupril is one of several drugs called angiotensin-converting enzyme (ACE) inhibitors. It prevents the conversion of the hormone angiotensin I to the hormone angiotensin II, which constricts blood vessels. As a result, blood vessels relax and blood pressure decreases.

Why it's prescribed

Doctors prescribe Accupril to reduce high blood pressure or to relieve symptoms of congestive heart failure, such as shortness of breath, fatigue, and swelling in the legs. Accupril comes in tablets. Doctors usually prescribe the following amounts for adults.
▶ **For high blood pressure,** 10 milligrams (mg) each day, adjusted every 2 weeks as needed. Usual dosage is 20, 40, or 80 mg a day as a single dose or divided into two equal doses.
▶ **For heart failure,** at first, 5 mg twice a day if the person is also taking a diuretic (water pill), or 10 mg twice a day if the person isn't taking a diuretic. Dosage is increased weekly. The usual dosage is 20 to 40 mg divided into two equal doses.

How to take Accupril

• Take Accupril exactly as your doctor has directed. Take it 1 hour before or 2 hours after a meal.
• Continue to take Accupril even if you feel well. Stopping suddenly could worsen your condition.

ACCUPRIL'S OTHER NAME

Accupril's generic name is quinapril hydrochloride.

 SIDE EFFECTS

Call your doctor if you have any of these possible drug side effects. Call *immediately* about any labeled "serious."

Serious: swelling of the face, lips, hands, feet, throat, or tongue; difficulty breathing; flaking and itching of the skin, with loss of hair and nails or overgrowth of skin on the palms and soles

Common: headache; irregular heartbeat; dry, persistent, tickling cough; skin sensitivity to sunlight
Tip: To avoid skin reactions, use sunscreen and wear protective clothing when outdoors.

Other: dizziness, light-headedness, fainting, sleepiness, nervousness, depression, palpitations, fast pulse, chest pain, dry mouth, stomach pain, constipation, back pain, feeling of ill health, increased sweating
Tips: Stand up slowly to minimize dizziness. Use caution during exercise and in hot weather. If you faint, stop taking Accupril and call your doctor immediately.

 DRUG INTERACTIONS

Combining certain drugs may alter their action or produce unwanted side effects. Tell your doctor about other drugs you're taking, especially:
• blood pressure drugs
• diuretics (water pills)
• Eskalith
• potassium supplements and salt substitutes containing potassium.

If you miss a dose

Take the missed dose as soon as possible. However, if it's almost time for your next dose, skip the missed dose and take your next dose as scheduled. Don't take a double dose.

If you suspect an overdose

Consult your doctor.

Warnings

• Make sure your doctor knows your medical history. You may not be able to take Accupril if you have kidney or liver disease.

• Don't take Accupril if you are pregnant or think you may be.
• Keep medical appointments. The doctor will check your blood pressure regularly to make sure Accupril is working properly and will also draw blood to measure the amount of potassium in your blood.

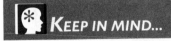 **KEEP IN MIND...**

* Take on empty stomach.
* Stand up slowly to avoid dizziness.
* Call doctor about swelling.

Accutane

Accutane decreases the amount of sebum (the skin's natural lubricant), shrinks the glands that produce sebum, and prevents skin cells from hardening and blocking the flow of sebum.

Why it's prescribed

Doctors prescribe Accutane to help treat severe acne that hasn't improved with other treatments. It comes in capsules. Doctors usually prescribe the following amounts for adults and teenagers.

▶ **For severe acne not responsive to conventional therapy,** dosage depends on body weight, usually half a milligram (0.5 mg) to 2 mg for each 2.2 pounds of body weight divided into two equal doses every day for 15 to 20 weeks.

How to take Accutane

• Take Accutane exactly as your doctor has directed, either with a meal or shortly after.

If you miss a dose

Take the missed dose as soon as possible. However, if it's almost time for your next dose, skip the missed dose and take your next dose as scheduled. Don't take a double dose.

 If you suspect an overdose

Contact your doctor *immediately*. Excessive Accutane can cause

 SIDE EFFECTS

Call your doctor if you have any of these possible drug side effects.

Serious: none reported

Common: pinkeye (eye burning, itching, redness), flaking and cracking of the lips and mouth, rash, dry skin, increased fat levels in the blood; pain in muscles, bones, and joints

Other: headache, fatigue, dry eyes, vision problems, nausea, vomiting, bleeding and inflammation of the gums, anemia (fatigue), peeling of the palms and toes, skin sensitivity to sunlight, thinning hair, increased blood sugar level (increased thirst, hunger, weight loss)

Tips: Perform frequent mouth care using a nonalcoholic mouthwash. Use sunscreen and avoid too much sun when you first start taking Accutane.

 DRUG INTERACTIONS

Combining certain drugs and products may alter drug action or produce unwanted side effects. Tell your doctor about other products you're using, especially:
• alcohol
• preparations that dry the skin, such as medicated soaps, acne preparations that contain skin-peeling agents, alcohol-based products (cosmetics, cologne, shaving products), vitamin A, tetracycline antibiotics.

---

more severe degrees of the drug's side effects, such as headache, vomiting, flushing, and dizziness.

 Warnings

• Make sure your doctor knows your medical history. Some conditions might affect your use of this drug.
• Don't take this drug if you're pregnant or think you may be. Don't take it if you're breast-feeding.
• Accutane is not recommended for children because they're especially prone to its side effects.
• If you have diabetes, Accutane can affect your blood sugar level. If

you notice any change, tell your doctor.
• When you start taking Accutane, your acne may worsen temporarily. If the problem becomes severe, call your doctor.
• Don't donate blood for at least 30 days after you stop taking Accutane.

ACCUTANE'S OTHER NAMES

Accutane's generic name is isotretinoin. A Canadian brand name is Accutane Roche.

KEEP IN MIND...

* Take with or just after meals.
* Avoid sun exposure when starting drug.
* Call doctor about vision problems or burning, itching, or redness of eyes.

Achromycin Ophthalmic

Achromycin Ophthalmic (for eyes) is a tetracycline antibiotic that kills bacteria and stops bacterial growth. It's applied directly to the eyes.

Why it's prescribed

Doctors prescribe Achromycin Ophthalmic to treat eye infections. It comes in eyedrops and an eye ointment. Doctors usually prescribe the following amounts for adults and children.

▶ **For superficial eye infections,** 2 drops instilled in the eye two or four times a day, or more often if infection is severe. Or, a small amount of ointment applied to the eye every 2 to 12 hours.

▶ **For conjunctivitis,** 2 drops in each eye or a small amount of ointment applied to each eye two, three, or four times a day for at least 3 weeks.

▶ **For trachoma,** 2 drops in each eye two, three, or four times a day for at least 3 weeks. Or, a small amount of ointment applied twice a day to each eye for 2 months.

How to use Achromycin Ophthalmic

- Follow your doctor's instructions exactly.
- If you're using the eyedrops, shake the bottle well first.
- Be sure to wash your hands before and after using this drug.
- As you apply the drops or ointment, don't allow the dropper or

ACHROMYCIN OPHTHALMIC'S OTHER NAME

Achromycin Ophthalmic's generic name is tetracycline hydrochloride.

container to touch your eye, the surrounding skin, or any other surface.

- Achromycin Ophthalmic ointment may cause your vision to blur for a few minutes after you apply it.
- Use all the drug prescribed by your doctor, even if your eye seems better after a few days.

If you miss a dose

Apply the missed dose as soon as possible. However, if it's almost time for your next dose, skip the missed dose and apply the next dose as scheduled. Don't apply a double dose.

 If you suspect an overdose

Consult your doctor.

 Warnings

- Make sure your doctor knows your medical history. You may not

be able to use Achromycin Ophthalmic if you have kidney problems or have ever had an allergic reaction to tetracycline.

- Don't use this drug in children younger than age 8; it could stunt their growth or stain their teeth.
- If your symptoms don't go away after a few days or if they become worse, call your doctor.

 KEEP IN MIND...

- Wash hands before and after applying this drug.
- Don't touch tip of dropper to eye or other surface.
- Call doctor about itching or swelling of eyelids or constant burning.

 SIDE EFFECTS

Call your doctor if you have any of these possible drug side effects.

Serious: none reported

Common: none reported

Other: blurred vision (with ointment); eye itching, swelling, or burning; skin inflammation or itching, skin sensitivity to sunlight
Tip: Use sunscreen and limit your exposure to sun.

 DRUG INTERACTIONS

Combining certain drugs and products may alter drug action or produce unwanted side effects. Tell your doctor about other drugs and products you're using, especially:

- Accutane
- medicated cosmetics or cover-ups
- preparations that dry the skin, such as soaps, cleansers, acne preparations, and alcohol-based products (cosmetics, cologne, shaving products).

Achromycin V

Achromycin V is an antibiotic that kills many different types of bacteria by preventing them from reproducing.

Why it's prescribed

Doctors prescribe Achromycin V to help treat infections. It comes in capsules. Doctors usually prescribe the following amounts for adults; children's dosages appear in parentheses.

▶ **For infections caused by sensitive bacteria (including *Rickettsia, Chlamydia, Mycoplasma,* and organisms that cause trachoma),** 1 to 2 grams (g) daily, divided into two to four equal doses. (Children over age 8: 25 to 50 milligrams (mg) for each 2.2 pounds of body weight daily, divided into equal doses and taken every 6 hours.)

▶ **For uncomplicated urethral, cervical, or rectal infections caused by *Chlamydia,*** 500 mg four times a day for at least 7 days.

▶ For brucellosis, 500 mg every 6 hours for 3 weeks, combined with 1 g of streptomycin injected every 12 hours for the 1st week and once a day for the 2nd week.

▶ **For gonorrhea in adults sensitive to penicillin,** initially, 1.5 g, then 500 mg every 6 hours for a total dose of 9 g.

▶ **For syphilis in adults sensitive to penicillin,** a total of 30 to 40 g, divided into equal doses over 10 to 15 days.

ACHROMYCIN V'S OTHER NAMES

Achromycin V's generic name is tetracycline hydrochloride. Other brand names include Panmycin, Robitet, Sumycin; and, in Canada, Apo-Tetra and Novotetra.

 ## SIDE EFFECTS

Call your doctor if you have any of these possible drug side effects. Call *immediately* about any labeled "serious."

Serious: increased pressure on the brain (headache, vomiting, blurred vision)

Common: stomach upset, nausea, diarrhea, kidney changes, permanent discoloration of teeth, enamel defects, delayed bone growth in children under age 8

Other: dizziness, darkened tongue, swollen tongue or mouth, thrush (white, patchy appearance of tongue), trouble swallowing, appetite loss, vomiting, irritation of esophagus, mouth infections, colitis, lesions around anus or genitals, blood problems (sore throat, fever, unusual bruising or bleeding, tarry stools), increased sensitivity to sun, darker skin color, allergic reaction to drug (fever, swelling, hives, rash)

Tips: If dizziness occurs, remember to stand up and climb stairs slowly. When getting out of bed, sit up slowly and dangle your legs over the side of the bed for several minutes before standing. To avoid infections in your mouth, practice excellent oral hygiene while taking Achromycin V. Because this drug may make your skin more sensitive to sunlight, limit your exposure to the sun and wear a sunscreen and protective clothing when you go out.

 ## DRUG AND FOOD INTERACTIONS

Combining certain drugs and foods may alter drug action or produce unwanted side effects. Tell your doctor about your diet and other drugs you're taking, especially:
- anticoagulants (blood thinners) such as Coumadin
- birth control pills
- calcium supplements
- diarrhea drugs containing kaolin, pectin, or bismuth subsalicylate
- Eskalith
- iron supplements such as Feasol
- laxatives and antacids containing aluminum, magnesium, calcium or sodium bicarbonate
- methoxyflurane (a general anesthetic)
- milk and other dairy products
- penicillins
- sodium bicarbonate
- vitamin A.

Continued on next page ▶

How to take Achromycin V

• Take this drug 1 hour before or 2 hours after meals to improve the drug's absorption.
• To help prevent stomach irritation, drink 8 ounces of water with each dose, and take your last dose of the day at least 1 hour before bedtime.
• Don't take Achromycin V with dairy products or iron supplements.
• Sit upright for an hour after you take a dose.
• Take your entire prescription, even if you start to feel better.

If you miss a dose

Take the missed dose as soon as possible, but try to space it as far apart from the next regular dose as you can. Then resume your regular dosing schedule. Don't take two doses at once.

If you suspect an overdose

Consult your doctor.

Warnings

• Make sure your doctor knows your medical history. You may not be able to take Achromycin V if you are overly sensitive to it or have diabetes or liver or kidney problems.
• If you're pregnant or breast-feeding, don't take Achromycin V; it could stain or harm your baby's teeth.
• This drug is not recommended for children under age 8 because it may permanently discolor teeth or slow the growth of their bones.
• Achromycin V may reduce the effectiveness of birth control pills. Use an additional form of birth control while taking this drug.
• Don't use old or expired Achromycin V.

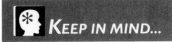

* Take with water 1 hour before or 2 hours after meals.
* Don't take Achromycin V after 4th month of pregnancy.
* Wear a sunscreen outdoors.

Actifed

Actifed combines an antihistamine and a decongestant. The antihistamine reduces the effect of histamine, a natural substance that causes itching, sneezing, runny nose, and watery eyes. The decongestant clears nasal secretions by narrowing nasal blood vessels.

Why it's taken

Actifed is used to relieve sneezing, runny nose, and congestion caused by hay fever and other allergies. It's not recommended for relief of cold symptoms, because it won't cure, prevent, or shorten the course of a cold. You can buy Actifed without a prescription. It comes in tablets, extended-release capsules, caplets, and liquid. The following amounts are usually recommended for adults.
▶ **To relieve symptoms of allergies or hay fever,** 1 tablet (2.5 milligrams [mg]) every 4 to 6 hours. Maximum dosage is 4 tablets (10 mg) a day.

How to take Actifed

• Follow the package directions exactly. Don't increase the dosage or take the drug for longer than recommended.
• Don't crush or chew the tablets.
• Swallow the extended-release capsules whole, or mix the contents with applesauce and swallow without chewing.

SIDE EFFECTS

Call your doctor if you have any of these possible drug side effects. Call *immediately* about any labeled "serious."

Serious: severe tiredness, irregular heartbeat, difficulty breathing, trouble sleeping

Common: drowsiness, thick nasal secretions
Tip: Make sure you know how you react to Actifed before driving or performing other activities that require alertness.

Other: headache, nausea
Tip: If the drug irritates your stomach, take it with food or a full glass (8 ounces) of water.

DRUG INTERACTIONS

Combining certain drugs may alter their action or produce unwanted side effects. Tell your doctor about other drugs you're taking, especially:
• antibiotics, such as erythromycin and clarithromycin
• antifungal drugs, especially Nizoral and Sporanex
• beta blockers, such as Lopressor and Tenormin
• caffeine, diet pills
• MAO inhibitors, such as Nardil and Parnate
• Symmetrel.

If you miss a dose

Take the missed dose as soon as possible. But if it's almost time for your next dose, skip the missed dose and take your next dose as scheduled. Don't take a double dose.

If you suspect an overdose

Contact your doctor *immediately*. Excessive Actifed can cause irregular pulse, nausea, vomiting, fatigue, excitability, dry mouth, dilated pupils, and seizures.

Warnings

• Before taking Actifed, consult your doctor if you have high blood pressure, asthma, diabetes, glaucoma, heart or thyroid disease, or urinary tract problems or if you're pregnant or breast-feeding.
• Children and older adults may be especially prone to Actifed's side effects.
• In people with high blood pressure, Actifed may further increase blood pressure.

KEEP IN MIND...

∗ Consult doctor about high blood pressure before taking.
∗ Swallow capsules whole.
∗ Take with food.

Actigall

Actigall, a natural bile acid used to treat certain types of gallstones, blocks the production of cholesterol in the liver and the absorption of cholesterol from food in the intestine.

Why it's prescribed

Doctors prescribe Actigall to dissolve gallstones made of cholesterol in people who can't or won't undergo surgery. It dissolves only uncalcified gallstones, and works best when these stones are small. Actigall comes in capsules. Doctors usually prescribe the following amounts for adults.

▶ **For dissolving small gallstones,** 8 to 10 milligrams for each 2.2 pounds of body weight orally each day, divided into two or three equal doses.

How to take Actigall

• Take Actigall exactly as your doctor has directed.
• Take it with meals, unless your doctor tells you otherwise.

If you miss a dose

Take the missed dose as soon as you remember, or take a double dose at your next dose.

 If you suspect an overdose

Contact your doctor. Excessive Actigall can cause diarrhea.

ACTIGALL'S OTHER NAME

Actigall's generic name is ursodiol.

 SIDE EFFECTS

Call your doctor if you have any of these possible drug side effects.

Serious: none reported

Common: none reported

Other: headache, fatigue, anxiety, depression, difficulty sleeping, runny nose, nausea, vomiting, stomach upset, metallic taste, abdominal pain, gallbladder inflammation (abdominal pain, indigestion, nausea, vomiting), diarrhea, constipation, mouth sores, gas, cough, rash, dry skin, hives, itching, thinning hair; pain in joints, muscles, or back

DRUG INTERACTIONS

Combining certain drugs may alter their action or produce unwanted side effects. Tell your doctor about other drugs you're taking, especially:
• antacids that contain aluminum, such as Basaljel and ALternaGEL
• drugs to lower cholesterol or fats, such as Questran, Colestid, and Atromid-S
• estrogens or birth control pills.

Warnings

• Make sure your doctor knows your medical history. You may not be able to take Actigall if you've ever had an unusual reaction to similar drugs called bile sequestering agents, such as Questran and Colestid.
• If you're breast-feeding, tell your doctor before you take Actigall.
• Expect the doctor to order liver function tests before you start taking Actigall and after 1 month, after 3 months, and then every 6 months while you're taking it.
• Most people must take Actigall for a long time and must have ultrasound images of the gallbladder taken every 6 months.

• In up to half the people who take Actigall, gallstones come back after 5 years. Before you start taking this drug, discuss with your doctor such alternatives as watchful waiting or surgery to remove your gallbladder.

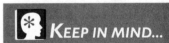 **KEEP IN MIND...**

∗ Take with meals.

∗ Keep appointments for liver function tests and gallbladder ultrasound.

∗ Discuss treatment alternatives (observation, or gallbladder removal).

Actimmune

Actimmune is a man-made version of interferon, which the body produces to help fight infections and kill tumor cells.

Why it's prescribed

Doctors prescribe Actimmune to treat chronic granulomatous disease—the name for a group of inherited diseases that weaken the immune system. It comes in an injectable form. Doctors usually prescribe the following amounts for adults.

▶ **For chronic granulomatous disease,** as prescribed by the doctor. Dosage depends on body size, body surface area, and other individual factors. Doses are usually taken three times a week.

How to take Actimmune

• Refrigerate Actimmune immediately after you obtain it, but don't freeze it. Be careful not to shake vials.

• Inject Actimmune exactly as your doctor has directed. Don't use more or less of it and don't use it more often than directed. Read the patient instruction sheet that comes with each package. Make sure you understand how to prepare and administer the injection, dispose of syringes, and store vials. If you have any questions, check with your doctor.

• If possible, inject the drug at bedtime. Inject it just below the skin

SIDE EFFECTS

Call your doctor if you have any of these possible drug side effects. Call *immediately* about any labeled "serious."

Serious: blood problems (fever of 101° F or higher, cough, sore throat, mouth sores, burning on urination, easy bruising, blood in urine, bleeding from gums, nosebleeds)

Common: flulike symptoms (headache, aching muscles, fever, chills)
Tip: Your doctor may prescribe Tylenol to relieve these temporary symptoms at the start of therapy.

Other: fatigue, confusion, difficulty thinking or concentrating, trouble walking, nausea, vomiting, diarrhea, rash, redness or tenderness at the injection site
Tips: Get extra rest while taking this drug. Rotate the injection site to avoid redness and tenderness.

DRUG INTERACTIONS

Combining certain drugs may alter their action or produce unwanted side effects. Tell your doctor about other drugs you're taking, especially:
• AZT
• drugs that depress the bone marrow, such as Bactrim, Accupril, Vasotec, and Dilantin.

on your upper arm below the shoulder, or on the front of your thigh.
• Each vial is for a single use only. Discard any unused portions of vials and discard vials that have been left at room temperature for more than 12 hours.

If you miss a dose

Don't take the missed dose, and don't take a double dose. Call your doctor for instructions.

If you suspect an overdose

Consult your doctor.

Warnings

• Make sure your doctor knows your medical history. You may not be able to take Actimmune if you have heart disease, a condition affecting your brain or spinal cord, or a history of seizures.

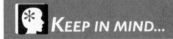
KEEP IN MIND...

∗ Refrigerate drug.

∗ Inject into shoulder or front of thigh.

∗ Call doctor about flulike symptoms.

Acular

Acular is an eye medication that reduces eye inflammation. It's one of many nonsteroidal anti-inflammatory drugs (NSAIDs). NSAIDs are thought to reduce inflammation and pain by inhibiting production of the hormone called prostaglandin and by impeding the action of other body substances.

Why it's prescribed

Doctors prescribe Acular to relieve inflammation and redness of the eye caused by seasonal allergies, or to relieve inflammation after eye surgery. Acular comes in eyedrops. Doctors usually prescribe the following amount for adults.

▶ **For relief of itchy eyes caused by seasonal allergy,** 1 drop in each eye four times a day.

How to use Acular

• Use Acular exactly as directed by your doctor.
• Don't use Acular while wearing soft contact lenses.
• Be sure to wash your hands before and after using this drug.
• Don't touch the tip of the dropper to your eye, the surrounding skin, or any other surface.
• Right after using the drops, press your fingertip gently against the inner corner of your eye next to the bridge of your nose. Hold it there for 1 minute to allow your eye to absorb the drug.
• Your eyes may sting or burn for a short time after instilling the drops. However, this is expected.

ACULAR'S OTHER NAME

Acular's generic name is ketorolac tromethamine.

SIDE EFFECTS

Call your doctor if you have any of these possible drug side effects.

Serious: allergic reaction (red, itching eyes)
Common: brief stinging and burning of the eyes
Tip: This reaction should be temporary. Dab your eyes gently with a tissue; don't rub them.
Other: superficial eye infection or superficial inflammation of the cornea
Tip: Obtain frequent eye exams.

DRUG INTERACTIONS

Combining certain drugs may alter their action or produce unwanted side effects. Tell your doctor about other drugs you're taking, especially:
• anticoagulants (blood thinners) such as Coumadin.

• Store Acular away from heat in a dark, tightly closed container and protect it from freezing.
• Discard the Acular container once you no longer need it. Don't use the drug for any future problems unless your doctor says otherwise.

If you miss a dose

Apply the missed dose as soon as possible. However, if it's almost time for your next dose, skip the missed dose and apply your next dose as scheduled. Don't apply a double dose.

 ### If you suspect an overdose

Instilling too much Acular in your eye probably won't cause problems. However, if you accidentally ingest the eyedrops, drink fluids to dilute them and call your doctor.

Warnings

• Make sure your doctor knows your medical history. You may not be able to use Acular if you've ever had an unusual reaction to aspirin or other NSAIDs, if you've ever had a bleeding disorder, or if you're pregnant or breast-feeding.
• Consult your doctor before using Acular for a child.
• Check with your doctor if your symptoms don't improve or if they get worse.
• To prevent other eye problems from developing, see your doctor regularly for eye examinations.

 ### KEEP IN MIND...

* Wash hands before and after using eyedrops.

* Don't touch tip of dropper to eye or any other surface.

* Expect brief burning and stinging of eyes.

* Don't use while wearing soft contact lenses.

* Don't use leftover drops for future problems without doctor's okay.

Adalat

Adalat is one of several drugs called calcium channel blockers. It blocks calcium from entering the heart muscle, thereby slowing heart contractions, widening the heart's blood vessels, and allowing more oxygen-carrying blood to reach and nourish the heart.

Why it's prescribed

Doctors prescribe Adalat for chest pain or high blood pressure. It comes in extended-release tablets and capsules. Doctors usually prescribe the following amounts for adults.

▶ **For chest pain,** at first, 10 milligrams (mg) three times a day. Usual effective range is 10 to 20 mg three times a day. Some people may require up to 30 mg four times a day. Maximum dosage is 180 mg a day.

▶ **For high blood pressure,** 30 or 60 mg extended-release capsules once a day, adjusted over 7 to 14 days.

How to take Adalat

• Take this drug exactly as your doctor directs. Keep taking it even when you feel well and don't have any chest pain. Don't switch to another brand without consulting your doctor (not all brands have the same effects).

• Swallow tablets or capsules whole. Don't break, crush, or chew

ADALAT'S OTHER NAMES

Adalat's generic name is nifedipine. Other brand names include Adalat CC, Procardia, Procardia XL; and, in Canada, Adalat FT, Adalat P.A., and Nu-Nifed.

SIDE EFFECTS

Call your doctor if you have any of these possible drug side effects.

Serious: none reported

Common: increased chest pain, dizziness, light-headedness, flushing, headache, nausea, heartburn

Tip: Although chest pain is usually temporary, report it to the doctor immediately.

Other: weakness, muscle cramps, fainting, swollen feet or ankles, heart palpitations, stuffy nose, diarrhea, difficulty breathing

DRUG INTERACTIONS

Combining certain drugs may alter their action or produce unwanted side effects. Tell your doctor about other drugs you're taking, especially:
• beta blockers, such as Inderal
• ulcer drugs, such as Tagamet and Zantac.

them. (Don't be alarmed if the empty shell appears in your stool.)
• Don't stop taking Adalat suddenly because your previous problem could return. Your doctor will tell you how to reduce your dosage gradually before stopping.

If you miss a dose

Take the missed dose as soon as possible. However, if it's almost time for your next dose, skip the missed dose and take your next dose as scheduled. Don't take a double dose.

If you suspect an overdose

Contact your doctor *immediately.* Excessive Adalat can cause widening of the blood vessels and low blood pressure, leading to dizziness and weakness.

Warnings

• Make sure your doctor knows your medical history. You may not be able to take Adalat if you have other problems, especially other heart or blood vessel disorders, kidney disease, or liver disease.
• Make sure your doctor knows if you're pregnant or breast-feeding before you begin taking Adalat.
• Follow any special diet or exercise programs the doctor prescribes.
• See your doctor regularly so your progress can be checked.

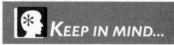
KEEP IN MIND...

* Don't break, crush, or chew tablets or capsules.

* Don't stop taking unless doctor approves.

* Follow special diet and exercise programs.

Adapin

Adapin, a tricyclic antidepressant, elevates mood by increasing levels of the chemicals norepinephrine and serotonin in the brain.

Why it's prescribed

Doctors prescribe Adapin to relieve depression. It comes in capsules. Doctors usually prescribe the following amounts for adults.

▶ **For depression, anxiety, or both,** initially, 50 to 75 milligrams (mg) a day, divided into equal doses and taken throughout the day. Maximum dosage: 300 mg a day.

How to take Adapin

• Don't take any more Adapin than your doctor prescribes. And don't stop taking it abruptly.
• You may open the capsule and sprinkle the drug on food if you have trouble swallowing capsules.

If you miss a dose

Take the missed dose as soon as possible. But if it's almost time for your next dose, skip the missed dose and take your next dose as scheduled. Don't take a double dose.

If you suspect an overdose

Contact your doctor *immediately*. Excessive Adapin can cause agitation, hallucinations, seizures, oversedation, and irregular heartbeat.

ADAPIN'S OTHER NAMES

Adapin's generic name is doxepin hydrochloride. Other brand names include Sinequan; and, in Canada, Novo-Doxepin and Triadapin.

SIDE EFFECTS

Call your doctor if you have any of these possible drug side effects. Call *immediately* about any labeled "serious."

Serious: seizures, heart problems (palpitations, chest pain, rapid heart rate), increased blood pressure (headache, blurred vision)

Common: drowsiness, dizziness, fainting, blurred vision, dry mouth, swollen tongue, constipation, difficulty urinating, sweating
Tips: Avoid activities that require full alertness or coordination until you know how Adapin affects you. Relieve dry mouth with sugarless hard candy or gum. Avoid constipation by adding fluids and fiber-rich foods to your diet.

Other: tremors, weakness, confusion, headache, nervousness, changes in muscle tone or function, ringing in ears, dilated pupils, nausea, vomiting, loss of appetite, intestinal blockage (abdominal pain), sensitivity to sun, allergic reaction (fever, swelling, hives, rash)
Tip: To prevent skin reactions, use a sunscreen, wear protective clothing, and avoid prolonged exposure to intense sunlight.

DRUG INTERACTIONS

Combining certain drugs may alter their action or produce unwanted side effects. Tell your doctor about other drugs you're taking, especially:
• alcohol
• antiarrhythmic drugs, such as Quinaglute Dura-tabs and Rythmol
• antidepressants, such as Elavil, Pamelor, Prozac, and Zoloft
• MAO inhibitors, such as Eldepryl and Nardil
• phenothiazines, such as Thorazine
• Tagamet
• Tolinase

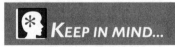 Warnings

• Make sure your doctor knows your medical history. You may not be able to take Adapin if you have glaucoma, difficulty urinating, asthma, blood or intestinal problems, a mental disorder, seizures, an enlarged prostate, an overactive thyroid, or heart, kidney, or liver problems.
• Tell your doctor if you're pregnant or breast-feeding.

• Your doctor will probably decrease your dosage gradually and then have you stop taking Adapin temporarily if you need surgery.

KEEP IN MIND...

∗ Don't stop taking abruptly.
∗ Stand up slowly to avoid dizziness.
∗ Avoid alcohol.

Adipost

Adipost is thought to aid the transmission of nerve impulses to the appetite control center in the brain. The drug has only a temporary effect; it works for the first few weeks of dieting, until new eating and exercise habits are set.

Why it's prescribed

Doctors prescribe Adipost to suppress the appetite. Adipost comes in tablets, capsules, and sustained-release capsules. Doctors usually prescribe the following amounts for adults.

▶ **For short-term use in some types of obesity,** 35 milligrams (mg) two or three times a day. Maximum dosage is 70 mg three times a day, or 1 sustained-release capsule daily.

How to take Adipost

• Take the tablets or capsules 1 hour before meals.
• Take sustained-release capsules 30 to 60 minutes before breakfast. Swallow them whole.
• To avoid withdrawal fatigue and depression, don't stop taking this drug abruptly.

If you miss a dose

Take the missed dose as soon as possible. However, if it's almost time for your next dose, skip the missed dose and take your next dose as scheduled. Don't take a double dose.

ADIPOST'S OTHER NAMES

Adipost's generic name is phendimetrazine tartrate. Other brand names include Anorex SR, Bontril, Obezine, Phenazine, Prelu-2, Trimcaps, and Wehless.

 SIDE EFFECTS

Call your doctor if you have any of these possible drug side effects.

Serious: none reported

Common: nervousness, difficulty sleeping, fast pulse, palpitations
Tip: To avoid sleep problems, take the last dose of the day about 4 to 6 hours before bedtime.

Other: dizziness, tremor, headache, high blood pressure (headache, blurred vision, nosebleeds), blurred vision, dry mouth, nausea, stomach cramps, diarrhea, constipation, pain on urination
Tips: Avoid activities that require you to be alert, such as driving a car, until you know how the drug affects you. To avoid constipation, increase fluids and high-fiber foods in your diet.

 DRUG AND FOOD INTERACTIONS

Combining certain drugs and foods may alter drug action or produce unwanted side effects. Tell your doctor about your diet and other drugs you're taking, especially:
• ammonium chloride
• antacids, Alka-Seltzer
• ascorbic acid (vitamin C)
• caffeine, including nonprescription drugs containing caffeine
• Diamox
• drugs for mental illness, such as Thorazine or Temaril
• Haldol
• MAO inhibitors such as Nardil (discontinue MAO inhibitor 14 days before starting Adipost)
• tricyclic antidepressants such as Elavil.

 If you suspect an overdose

Contact your doctor *immediately.* Excessive Adipost can cause headache, dizziness, fatigue, bluish skin, difficulty breathing, poor coordination, fast pulse, kidney and liver impairment, nausea, vomiting, and coma.

 Warnings

• Make sure your doctor knows your medical history. You may not be able to take Adipost if you have an overactive thyroid, high blood pressure, heart or blood vessel disease, or glaucoma.

KEEP IN MIND...

* Take before meals.
* Don't break, crush, or chew sustained-release capsules.
* Avoid caffeine.

Advil

Advil is a nonsteroidal anti-inflammatory drug (NSAID) that reduces inflammation, pain, and fever, probably by stopping the body from producing substances called prostaglandins.

Why it's taken

Advil is taken to reduce fever and some types of pain with inflammation, such as menstrual pain. You can buy Advil without a prescription. It comes in tablets and a liquid. The following amounts are usually recommended for adults; children's dosages appear in parentheses.

▶ **For mild to moderate pain and menstrual pain**, 200 to 400 milligrams (mg) every 4 to 6 hours as needed.

▶ **For fever**, 200 to 400 mg every 4 to 6 hours, but not more than 1.2 grams a day. (Children ages 6 months to 12 years: if fever is below 102.5 °F, 5 mg for each 2.2 pounds (lb) of body weight every 6 to 8 hours. For higher fevers, 10 mg for each 2.2 lb every 6 to 8 hours, but not more than 40 mg for each 2.2 lb a day.)

How to take Advil

• Follow the package instructions or your doctor's advice. Advil begins to take effect against pain and fever within 30 minutes. Although

ADVIL'S OTHER NAMES

Advil's generic name is ibuprofen. Other brand names include Excedrin-IB, Genpril, Haltran, Ibuprin, Ibuprohm, Ibu-Tab, Medipren, Midol-200, Motrin, Nuprin, Pamprin-IB, Rufen, Trendar; and, in Canada, Apo-Ibuprofen and Novo-Profen.

 SIDE EFFECTS

Call your doctor if you have any of these possible drug side effects. Call *immediately* about any labeled "serious."

Serious: gastrointestinal bleeding (dark or bloody vomit or stools), prolonged bleeding from a cut, wheezing, difficulty breathing, reddened burnlike rash, high blood pressure (headache, blurred vision), decreased urination, yellow-tinged skin and eyes

Common: headache, drowsiness, dizziness, ringing in ears, stomach distress

Tip: Take with meals or milk to avoid nausea.

Other: confusion, hives, sensitivity to sunlight, water retention

 DRUG INTERACTIONS

Combining certain drugs may alter their action or produce unwanted effects. Tell your doctor about other drugs you're taking, especially:
• alcohol, aspirin, corticosteroids such as Decadron and Kenalog
• anticoagulants (blood thinners) such as Coumadin
• lithium
• thiazide diuretics (water pills), such as HydroDIURIL and Vaseretic.

Advil reduces pain at low dosages, anti-inflammatory effects don't occur at dosages below 400 mg four times a day
• If you buy Advil without a prescription, don't take more than 1.2 g a day or take it for more than 3 days.

If you miss a dose

If you're taking Advil on a regular schedule, take the missed dose as soon as possible. However, if it's almost time for your next dose, skip the missed dose and go back to your regular schedule.

If you suspect an overdose

Contact your doctor *immediately.* Excessive Advil may cause dizziness, drowsiness, vomiting, abdominal pain, and difficulty breathing.

Warnings

• You may not be able to take Advil if you have nasal polyps, severe hives, stomach or intestinal disorders (such as an ulcer), high blood pressure, a blood coagulation defect, a drug allergy, or a history of heart, liver, or kidney disease.
• Don't use Advil during pregnancy or while breast-feeding.

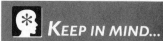 **KEEP IN MIND...**

＊ Take with meals or milk.
＊ Advil won't reduce inflammation at dosages below 400 mg four times a day.
＊ Don't take longer than 3 days.

AeroBid

AeroBid, a cortisone-like drug, prevents certain cells in the lungs and airways from releasing substances that cause asthma symptoms.

Why it's prescribed

Doctors prescribe AeroBid to prevent and treat asthma symptoms. It won't stop an asthma attack already in progress, but it will reduce the frequency and severity of asthma attacks when used regularly. AeroBid comes as an inhalant. Doctors usually prescribe the following amounts for adults and children age 6 and over.

▶ **To prevent asthma in people who require steroids to control symptoms,** 2 inhalations (500 micrograms) twice a day. Maximum dosage is 4 inhalations twice a day, morning and evening.

How to use AeroBid

• Use this drug exactly as the doctor has directed. AeroBid is used with a special inhaler and comes with directions. Read the directions carefully before using.
• Using a spacer device with the inhaler may help to ensure that you inhale the proper dosage. If your doctor recommends this device, follow the doctor's directions or the manufacturer's instructions closely.
• If you're also taking a drug to open your airways (called a bronchodilator), use it several minutes before AeroBid.
• Gently warm the canister to room temperature before using it (for example, by carrying it in a pocket).

AeroBid's other name

AeroBid's generic name is flunisolide.

Side effects

Call your doctor if you have any of these possible drug side effects.

Serious: none reported

Common: none reported

Other: headache, watery eyes, throat irritation, hoarseness, nausea, vomiting, diarrhea, dry mouth, upper respiratory tract infection, cold symptoms; fungal infections of the nose, mouth, and throat

Tips: Check often for symptoms of fungal infections, such as pain when eating or swallowing and creamy white, curdlike patches on the insides of your mouth, nose, and throat. To help prevent such infections, gargle or rinse your mouth with water after each inhaler use. Don't swallow the water.

Drug interactions

Combining certain drugs may alter their action or produce unwanted side effects. Tell your doctor about other drugs you're taking.

• Store the drug between 36° and 86° F.
• Keep the inhaler clean and unobstructed. Wash it with warm water and dry it thoroughly after each use.
• If you've been using AeroBid for a long time, don't stop using it suddenly. Consult your doctor.

If you miss a dose

Take the missed dose as soon as possible. Then take any remaining doses for that day at regularly spaced times.

If you suspect an overdose

Consult your doctor.

Warnings

• Make sure your doctor knows your medical history. You may not be able to use AeroBid if you have a respiratory infection or tuberculosis or are pregnant or breast-feeding.

• Don't use AeroBid to halt an asthma attack already in progress.
• Call your doctor if you experience a period of unusual stress, such as injury, infection, or surgery; if you have symptoms of a mouth, throat, or lung infection; or if your symptoms get worse or don't improve.
• If your child's been taking AeroBid for a long time, be sure to keep periodic follow-up appointments so the doctor can monitor your child's growth and test adrenal gland function.

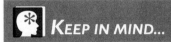
Keep in mind...

*Don't use to stop asthma attack already in progress.

*Wash inhaler with warm water and dry thoroughly after use.

*Gargle or rinse mouth with water after each inhaler use.

Afrin

Afrin is a decongestant applied directly to the mucus lining of the nose. It temporarily relieves stuffy nose and congestion due to colds and allergies by narrowing tiny blood vessels in the nose. This reduces blood flow and congestion in the swollen nasal membranes.

Why it's taken

Afrin is taken to relieve a stuffy nose caused by colds, sinus problems, or allergies. It's available without a prescription and comes in nose drops and nasal spray. Doctors usually prescribe the following amounts for adults and children over age 6; the dosage for younger children follows in parentheses.

▶ **For nasal congestion,** 2 to 3 drops or sprays in each nostril twice a day. (Children ages 2 to 6: 2 to 3 drops of children's strength in each nostril twice a day for no longer than 3 to 5 days.)

How to use Afrin

• If you're treating yourself, read the package instructions carefully.
• If your doctor prescribed this drug or gave you special instruc-

AFRIN'S OTHER NAMES

Afrin's generic name is oxymetazoline hydrochloride. Other brand names include Allerest 12-Hour Nasal, Chlorphed-LA, Coricidin Nasal Mist, Dristan Long Lasting, Duramist Plus, Duration 12-Hour Nasal, 4-Way Long-Acting Nasal, Neo-Synephrine 12 Hour, Nostrilla, Sinarest 12-Hour, and Sinex Long-Acting.

SIDE EFFECTS

Call your doctor if you have any of these possible drug side effects. Call *immediately* about any labeled "serious."

Serious: cardiovascular collapse (life-threatening loss of blood pressure, cardiac arrest)

Common: none reported

Other: headache, drowsiness, dizziness, difficulty sleeping, sedation, palpitations, high blood pressure (headache, blurred vision), return of stuffy nose or nasal irritation (with excessive or long-term use), dry nose and throat, increased nasal discharge, stinging, sneezing
Tips: To minimize dizziness, get up slowly from a sitting or standing position and take care when walking. To relieve dryness in nose and throat, use a cool-mist dehumidifier.

DRUG INTERACTIONS

Combining certain drugs may alter their action or produce unwanted side effects. Tell your doctor about other drugs you're taking.

tions on how to use it, follow those instructions exactly.
• Don't use more Afrin than recommended and don't use it more often than recommended.

If you miss a dose

If you're using Afrin on a regular schedule, take the missed dose right away if you remember within an hour or so. However, if you don't remember until later, skip the missed dose and take your next dose as scheduled.

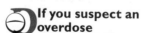

If you suspect an overdose

Contact your doctor *immediately.* Excessive Afrin can cause drowsiness, dizziness, weakness, sweating, slowing down of the nervous system (extreme sleepiness, difficulty waking), high or low blood pressure, slow pulse, extremely slow breathing, coma, and cardiovascu-

lar collapse (life-threatening loss of blood pressure, cardiac arrest).

Warnings

• Before using Afrin, consult your doctor if you have heart disease, high blood pressure, an overactive thyroid, or diabetes.
• Don't share the container because this could spread the infection.

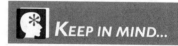

KEEP IN MIND...

*Don't share container.

*Use only as often and as long as directed.

*Get doctor's approval to use if you have heart disease, high blood pressure, overactive thyroid, or diabetes.

AK-Homatropine

AK-Homatropine is one of several drugs called anticholinergics. Applied directly to the eye, it prevents certain nerve impulses from reaching eye muscles. This, in turn, causes the pupils to enlarge.

Why it's prescribed

Doctors prescribe AK-Homatropine to treat such eye conditions as uveitis (inflammation of the uveal tract, which consists of the iris and related structures). They also use it to dilate the pupils before eye examinations and before and after eye surgery. AK-Homatropine comes in eyedrops. Doctors usually prescribe the following amounts for adults and children.
▶ **For uveitis,** 1 to 2 drops in the affected eye every 3 to 4 hours. (Children: use 2% eyedrops only.)

How to use AK-Homatropine

• Use this drug exactly as your doctor directs.
• Wash your hands before and after using the drops.
• To prevent contamination, don't touch the applicator tip to your eye, the surrounding area, or any other surface.
• After using the drops, press your finger against the inner corner of your eye for 1 minute to help your

AK-Homatropine's OTHER NAMES

AK-Homatropine's generic name is homatropine hydrobromide. Other brand names include I-Homatrine, Isopto Homatropine; and, in Canada, Minims-Homatropine.

 SIDE EFFECTS

Call your doctor if you have any of these possible side effects.
Serious: none reported

Common: blurred vision, unusual eye sensitivity to light
Tips: Avoid hazardous activities, such as driving, until your vision clears. Wear dark glasses to protect your eyes from the light.

Other: eye irritation, irritability, confusion, sleepiness, poor coordination, fast pulse, dry mouth, dry skin, flushing, fever
Tip: To relieve dry mouth, use sugarless hard candy or gum.

 DRUG INTERACTIONS

Combining certain drugs may alter their action or produce unwanted side effects. Tell your doctor about other drugs you're taking.

eye absorb the drug by preventing it from draining out.
• Store with the container tightly closed.

If you miss a dose

Apply the missed dose as soon as possible. However, if it's almost time for the next dose, skip the missed dose and apply the next dose as scheduled. Don't apply a double dose.

 If you suspect an overdose

Contact your doctor *immediately.* Excessive AK-Homatropine can cause dry mouth, blurred vision, poor coordination, difficulty speaking, hallucinations, a fast pulse, decreased intestinal activity, and flushed, dry skin.

Warnings

• Make sure your doctor knows your medical history. You may not be able to use AK-Homatropine if you have other problems, such as glaucoma or other eye disorders.
• If you're pregnant or breast-feeding, tell your doctor before you start using AK-Homatropine.
• Older adults, infants, young children, and older children with blond hair and blue eyes may be especially prone to AK-Homatropine's side effects.

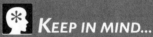 **KEEP IN MIND...**

∗ Wash hands before and after using.

∗ Don't touch applicator tip to eye or other surface.

∗ Avoid driving until vision clears.

∗ Wear dark glasses to protect eyes against light.

Akineton

Akineton is one of several drugs called antidyskinetics. It improves muscle control and reduces stiffness, permitting more normal body movements. Akineton is also used to control severe reactions to such drugs as Serpasil, Navane, and Haldol.

Why it's prescribed

Doctors prescribe Akineton to treat Parkinson's disease or to treat some side effects of other drugs. Akineton comes in tablets. Doctors usually prescribe the following amounts for adults.

▶ **For Parkinson's disease,** 2 milligrams (mg) three or four times a day, up to a maximum of 16 mg a day.

▶ **To treat severe side effects of some other drugs,** 2 mg one to three times a day, depending on severity of symptoms. Usual dose is 2 mg a day.

How to take Akineton

• Take this drug only as your doctor has directed.

• To reduce stomach upset, take it with or immediately after meals, unless the doctor tells you otherwise.

If you miss a dose

Take the missed dose as soon as possible. However, if it's within 2 hours of your next scheduled dose, skip the missed dose and take your next scheduled dose. Don't take a double dose.

 If you suspect an overdose

Contact your doctor *immediately.* Excessive Akineton can cause anxiety, agitation, and restlessness, followed by disorientation, confusion, hallucinations, delusions, anxiety, agitation, restlessness, dilated pupils, and blurred vision. Additional symptoms include dryness of the nose and throat, difficulty swallowing, difficulty urinating, fever, headache, fast pulse, high blood pressure, fast breathing, and hot, dry, flushed skin.

 Warnings

• Make sure your doctor knows your medical history. You may not be able to take Akineton if you've ever had an enlarged prostate, irregular pulse, glaucoma, seizures, or bowel obstruction.

• Older adults may be especially prone to Akineton's side effects.

• Although Akineton will make your muscles less spastic, it also may increase your tremors.

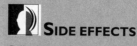 **SIDE EFFECTS**

Call your doctor if you have any of these possible drug side effects.

Serious: none reported

Common: constipation
Tip: Avoid constipation by increasing fluids and high-fiber foods in your diet.

Other: confusion, disorientation, unusual feeling of well-being, restlessness, irritability, incoherence, dizziness, increased tremor, blurred vision, dry mouth, constipation, nausea, vomiting, stomach upset, difficulty urinating, rash, hives

DRUG INTERACTIONS

Combining certain drugs may alter their action or produce unwanted side effects. Tell your doctor about other drugs you're taking, especially:
• antacids (take at least 1 hour after Akineton)
• drugs for psychosis (mental illness)
• Symmetrel (another drug for Parkinson's disease)
• tricyclic antidepressants such as Elavil.

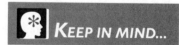 **KEEP IN MIND...**

* Take with or immediately after meals.

* Increase fluid and fiber in diet.

* Don't take within 1 hour of taking an antacid.

AKINETON'S OTHER NAME

Akineton's generic name is biperiden hydrochloride.

Aldactazide

Aldactazide is a combination of two diuretics (water pills). It lowers blood pressure by decreasing excess water in the body.

Why it's prescribed

Doctors prescribe Aldactazide to treat high blood pressure and swelling (edema), mainly of the legs and feet. It comes in tablets. Doctors usually prescribe the following amounts for adults.

▶ **For high blood pressure,** 50 to 100 milligrams (mg) a day.

▶ **For edema,** 25 to 200 mg a day.

How to take Aldactazide

• Take Aldactazide exactly as the doctor has directed. If you take one daily dose, take it in the morning after breakfast. If you take more than one daily dose, take the last dose before 6 p.m. so the need to urinate won't disturb your sleep.

If you miss a dose

Take the missed dose as soon as possible. However, if it's almost time for your next dose, skip the missed dose and take your next dose as scheduled. Don't take a double dose.

 If you suspect an overdose

Contact your doctor *immediately*. Excessive Aldactazide can cause

ALDACTAZIDE'S OTHER NAMES

Aldactazide is a combination of the generic drugs hydrochlorothiazide and spironolactone. Another brand name is Spirozide. A Canadian brand name is Novo-Spirozine.

 SIDE EFFECTS

Call your doctor if you have any of these possible drug side effects. Call *immediately* about any labeled "serious."

Serious: shortness of breath, fever, low back pain, bruising, confusion, irregular heartbeat, bright red tongue, high or low potassium level in the body (dizziness, irregular pulse, muscle cramps)

Common: sensitivity to light
Tip: Protect yourself with sunscreen, hat, and protective clothing when you go outside.

Other: nausea, vomiting, fatigue, dizziness, headache, cough, decreased sex drive
Tips: If Aldactazide causes stomach upset, take it with milk or a meal. Avoid hazardous activities until you know how Aldactazide affects you.

DRUG INTERACTIONS

Combining certain drugs may alter their action or produce unwanted side effects. Tell your doctor about other drugs you're taking, especially:
• blood pressure drugs called ACE inhibitors, such as Capoten and Vasotec
• digoxin
• lithium
• potassium supplements such as K-Dur.

---

low blood pressure (dizziness, fainting).

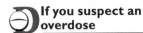 **Warnings**

• Make sure your doctor knows your medical history. You may not be able to take Aldactazide if you are allergic to sulfa drugs, have liver or kidney disease, or have too much potassium in your body.
• If you're pregnant or breast-feeding, check with your doctor before taking Aldactazide. Older adults are especially prone to Aldactazide's side effects.
• Tell your doctor if you're on a special diet, such as one for diabetes.

• Like other diuretics, Aldactazide increases urination and thus can decrease the amount of potassium in your body. Your doctor may ask you to eat more high-potassium foods, such as bananas and citrus fruits, and may prescribe a potassium supplement.

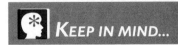 **KEEP IN MIND...**

*Take with milk or meal if drug upsets stomach.

*Eat high-potassium foods.

*Report low-potassium effects.

*Limit sun exposure.

Aldactone

Aldactone is a diuretic (water pill). It helps to lower blood pressure by causing increased urination and boosting the amount of potassium in the body.

Why it's prescribed

Doctors prescribe Aldactone to treat high blood pressure, swelling (edema), potassium deficiency, or a condition called hyperaldosteronism (excess of the hormone aldosterone). It comes in tablets. Doctors usually prescribe the following amounts for adults; children's dosages appear in parentheses.

▶ **For edema,** 25 to 200 milligrams (mg) once a day or divided into equal doses. (Children: 3.3 mg for each 2.2 pounds of body weight once a day or divided into equal doses.)

▶ **For high blood pressure,** 50 to 100 mg once a day or divided into equal doses.

▶ **For deficiency potassium,** 25 to 100 mg each day.

▶ **For hyperaldosteronism,** 100 to 400 mg once a day.

How to take Aldactone

• Take Aldactone exactly as directed. The doctor may want you to take a higher dose of Aldactone at first and then reduce the amount as your body adjusts to the drug.
• If you take a single dose each day, take it in the morning. If you take more than one dose each day, take the last dose by 6 p.m. (unless the

SIDE EFFECTS

Call your doctor if you have any of these possible drug side effects. Call *immediately* about any labeled "serious."

Serious: too much potassium (confusion, irregular heartbeat, nervousness, difficulty breathing, unusual fatigue, weakness of the legs, numbness or tingling in the hands, feet, or lips)

Common: none reported

Other: headache, appetite loss, nausea, diarrhea, hives, dehydration, drowsiness, dry mouth, increased thirst, lack of energy, breast soreness and menstrual disturbances in women
Tip: To avoid nausea, take with food or milk.

DRUG AND FOOD INTERACTIONS

Combining certain drugs and foods may alter drug action or produce unwanted side effects. Tell your doctor about your diet and other drugs you're taking, especially:
• digoxin
• drugs for high blood pressure, such as Capoten and Altace
• Indocin
• potassium-rich foods, such as bananas, carrots, and nonfat dry milk
• potassium supplements and salt substitutes containing potassium.

doctor tells you otherwise) to help prevent the need to urinate from disturbing your sleep.

If you miss a dose

Take the missed dose as soon as possible. However, if it's almost time for your next dose, skip the missed dose and take your next dose as scheduled. Don't take a double dose.

If you suspect an overdose

Contact your doctor *immediately.* Excessive Aldactone can cause dehydration and dangerous electrolyte disturbances (sleepiness, nausea, fatigue, behavior changes, seizures, coma).

Warnings

• Make sure your doctor knows your medical history. You may not be able to take Aldactone if you have diabetes, urinary problems, or kidney or liver disease or if you're pregnant.

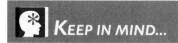

KEEP IN MIND...

*Take with meals or milk.

*Take last dose by 6 p.m.

*Avoid salt substitutes.

*Call doctor about high potassium effects.

Aldomet

Aldomet reduces blood pressure by relaxing blood vessels so blood can pass through them more easily.

Why it's prescribed

Doctors prescribe Aldomet to treat high blood pressure. It comes in tablets and a liquid. Doctors usually prescribe the following amounts for adults.

▶ **For high blood pressure,** 250 milligrams (mg) two to three times a day for the first 48 hours, then increased as needed every 2 days. Dosage may be adjusted if other blood pressure drugs are added or removed. Maintenance dosage is 500 mg to 2 grams (g) a day divided into two to four equal doses. Maximum recommended dosage is 3 g a day.

How to take Aldomet

• Take this drug exactly as your doctor has directed. Don't stop taking it suddenly, even if you think it's not working. Instead, contact your doctor.
• You may take your entire dosage in the evening or at bedtime.

If you miss a dose

Take the missed dose as soon as possible. However, if it's almost time for your next dose, skip the missed dose and take your next dose as scheduled. Don't take a double dose.

ALDOMET'S OTHER NAMES

Aldomet's generic name is methyldopa. Canadian brand names include Apo-Methyldopa, Dopamet, Novomedopa, and Nu-Medopa.

 SIDE EFFECTS

Call your doctor if you have any of these possible drug side effects. Call *immediately* about any labeled "serious."

Serious: hemolytic anemia (fever, chills, back pain), hepatic necrosis (abdominal pain, nausea, vomiting, yellow-tinged skin and eyes)

Common: drowsiness, decreased alertness, slowed thought processes, dizziness, swelling, stuffy nose, dry mouth, fever, weight gain
Tips: Call your doctor immediately if you develop a fever shortly after starting this drug. Avoid potentially hazardous activities until you know how Aldomet affects you. Prevent dizziness by standing up slowly.

Other: headache, weakness, fatigue, uncontrollable movements, nightmares or vivid dreams, depression, slow pulse, chest pain, nausea, vomiting, diarrhea, inflammation of the pancreas (severe abdominal pain, nausea, fever), reversible blood disorders (fatigue, bruising, bleeding), breast swelling or unusual milk production, rash, impotence

 DRUG INTERACTIONS

Combining certain drugs may alter their action or produce unwanted side effects. Tell your doctor about other drugs you're taking, especially:
• amphetamines, Levophed
• Eskalith
• Larodopa
• phenothiazines (drugs for anxiety, nausea and vomiting, or psychosis)
• tricyclic antidepressants such as Elavil.

 If you suspect an overdose

Contact your doctor *immediately*. Excessive Aldomet can cause sleepiness, low blood pressure (dizziness, fatigue), impaired heart functioning (fluttering in chest, dizziness), and coma.

Warnings

• Make sure your doctor knows your medical history. You may not be able to take Aldomet if you have Parkinson's disease, kidney or liver problems, or depression or if you've ever had liver problems when taking Aldomet in the past.
• Older adults may be especially prone to Aldomet's side effects.
• Follow any special diet the doctor prescribes, such as a low-salt diet.

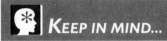 **KEEP IN MIND...**

*Expect to increase dosage gradually at first.

*Call doctor immediately about fever.

*Stand up slowly to avoid dizziness.

Aldoril

Aldoril is a combination of a thiazide diuretic (water pill) and a drug called a sympatholytic. The diuretic decreases excess water in the body by boosting the flow of urine. The sympatholytic relaxes blood vessels to help blood pass through them more easily.

Why it's prescribed

Doctors prescribe Aldoril to treat high blood pressure. It comes in tablets of varying strengths marked Aldoril 15 or 25 (containing 250 mg of methyldopa and 15 or 25 mg respectively of hydrochlorothiazide) or D30 or D50 (containing 500 mg of methyldopa and 30 or 50 mg respectively of hydrochlorothiazide. Doctors usually prescribe the following amounts for adults.

▶ **For high blood pressure,** initially, 1 Aldoril 15 tablet two or three times a day, 1 Aldoril 25 tablet twice a day, or 1 Aldoril D30 or D50 tablet twice a day.

How to take Aldoril

- Take this drug exactly as your doctor has directed. Keep taking it even if you feel well.
- Take Aldoril after breakfast.

If you miss a dose

Take the missed dose as soon as possible. However, if it's almost time for your next dose, skip the missed dose and take your next dose as scheduled. Don't take a double dose.

ALDORIL'S OTHER NAMES

Aldoril is a combination of the generic drugs methyldopa and hydrochlorothiazide.

 SIDE EFFECTS

Call your doctor if you have any of these possible drug side effects. Call *immediately* about any labeled "serious."

Serious: fever, irregular heartbeat, muscle cramps, weak pulse

Common: dizziness, dry mouth, headache, fatigue, increased urination
Tips: These effects may occur at first but should diminish. Prevent dizziness by standing up slowly and taking care when walking. Take your last dose by 6 p.m., unless the doctor tells you otherwise, to prevent increased urination from interrupting your sleep.

Other: anxiety, vivid dreams, sensitivity to light, decreased sex drive, appetite loss, pain or numbness in hands or feet, stuffy nose
Tip: Stay out of direct sunlight, wear sunglasses and protective clothing, and apply a sunblock when you go outdoors.

 DRUG INTERACTIONS

Combining certain drugs may alter their action or produce unwanted side effects. Tell your doctor about other drugs you're taking, especially:
- alcohol
- barbiturates such as phenobarbital
- corticosteroids such as prednisone
- diabetes drugs such as Diabeta
- lithium
- MAO inhibitors, such as Nardil and Parnate
- nonsteroidal anti-inflammatory drugs such as Motrin

 If you suspect an overdose

Contact your doctor *immediately*. Excessive Aldoril can cause low blood pressure (dizziness, fatigue, weakness).

 Warnings

- Make sure your doctor knows your medical history. You may not be able to take Aldoril if you are breast-feeding or have angina, diabetes, kidney or liver disease, lupus, depression, or inflammation of the pancreas.

- Older adults may be especially prone to Aldoril's side effects.
- If you have diabetes, be aware that Aldoril can increase your blood sugar level.
- Follow any prescribed diet, such as a low-salt diet.

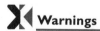 **KEEP IN MIND...**

* Take last dose by 6 p.m.

* Call doctor right away about fever and symptoms of too much potassium loss.

* If diabetic, watch for increased blood sugar.

Aleve

Aleve, a nonsteroidal anti-inflammatory drug (NSAID), probably relieves pain by blocking the body's production of prostaglandin.

Why it's taken

Aleve is taken to treat mild to moderate aches and pains and to reduce fever. You can buy Aleve without a prescription. It comes in film-coated tablets. The following amounts are usually recommended for adults; dosage for older adults appears in parentheses.

▶ **For minor aches and pains and fever,** 1 tablet every 8 to 12 hours, or 2 tablets as a first dose and then 1 tablet 12 hours later. Maximum dose is 3 tablets in 24 hours. (Adults over age 65: 1 tablet every 12 hours.)

How to take Aleve

• If you're treating yourself, follow the package directions carefully.
• Take each dose with a full glass (8 ounces) of water. Stay upright for about 30 minutes afterward.

If you miss a dose

Take the missed dose as soon as possible. However, if it's almost time for your next dose, skip the missed dose and take your next dose as scheduled. Don't take a double dose.

ALEVE'S OTHER NAMES

Aleve's generic name is naproxen sodium. Other brand names include Anaprox; and, in Canada, Apo-Naproxen, Novo-Naprox, and Nu-Naprox.

 SIDE EFFECTS

Call your doctor if you have any of these possible drug side effects. Call *immediately* about any labeled "serious."

Serious: peptic ulcer (nausea, vomiting, heartburn, dark or bloody vomit or stools), blood disorders (bleeding of gums, fatigue, fever, chills), kidney problems (decreased urination), liver problems (nausea, vomiting, yellow-tinged skin and eyes)

Common: headache, drowsiness, dizziness, swelling of the feet or lower legs, ringing in ears, nausea, itching
Tips: Avoid hazardous activities, such as driving a car, until you know how Aleve affects you. Take with food to avoid stomach upset.

Other: confusion, mood changes, palpitations, vision disturbances, painful urination, shortness of breath, hives

 DRUG INTERACTIONS

Combining certain drugs may alter their action or produce unwanted side effects. Tell your doctor about other drugs you're taking, especially:
• alcohol
• aspirin and other anticoagulants (blood thinners) such as Coumadin
• Benemid, Mexate
• diuretics (water pills) and other blood pressure drugs
• oral diabetes drugs
• protein-bound drugs such as Dilantin
• steroids.

 If you suspect an overdose

Contact your doctor *immediately.* Excessive Aleve can cause drowsiness, nausea, and vomiting.

Warnings

• Before taking Aleve, consult your doctor if you have an intestinal disorder or kidney, heart, or blood vessel disease, or you are pregnant.
• Don't take this drug if you're allergic to aspirin.

• Be aware that older adults may be especially prone to stomach upset from Aleve.
• Before giving a urine specimen, tell the lab staff that you're taking Aleve.

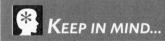 **KEEP IN MIND...**

∗ Take with full glass of water.
∗ Stay upright for 30 minutes.
∗ Don't take if allergic to aspirin.

Alkeran

Alkeran interferes with the growth of cancer cells and eventually destroys those cells.

Why it's prescribed

Doctors prescribe Alkeran to treat a cancer called multiple myeloma or, in women, advanced ovarian cancer tumors that can't be removed surgically. It comes in tablets and an injectable form. Doctors usually prescribe the following amounts for adults.

▶ **For multiple myeloma,** initially 6 milligrams (mg) orally once a day for 2 to 3 weeks; then the drug is stopped for up to 4 weeks or until the person's blood counts stop declining and start to rise again.

▶ **For advanced ovarian cancer,** 0.2 mg for each 2.2 pounds of body weight orally daily for 5 days, repeated every 4 to 6 weeks depending on your blood count.

How to take Alkeran

• Take Alkeran only as directed by your doctor. Take it on an empty stomach, at least 1 hour before or 2 hours after a meal.
• If you're taking Alkeran and other drugs, take each drug at the proper time. Don't mix them.
• Don't stop taking Alkeran without first checking with your doctor. If you vomit shortly after taking a dose, call your doctor immediately for instructions on whether to take the dose again.

If you miss a dose

Don't take the missed dose and don't take a double dose. Instead,

ALKERAN'S OTHER NAMES

Alkeran's generic name is melphalan (also called L-phenylalanine mustard).

 SIDE EFFECTS

Call your doctor if you have any of these possible drug side effects. Call *immediately* about any labeled "serious."

Serious: unusual bleeding or bruising; black, tarry stools; blood in urine or stool; pinpoint red spots on skin; bleeding ulcers of the mouth, rectum, and vagina; lung inflammation (pain on breathing, shortness of breath, cough, fever); infection (fever, chills, sore throat, hoarseness, pain in lower back or side); fever; closing up of throat; swelling of face, lips, neck, hands, and feet

Tips: To reduce the risk of bleeding, be careful when using a razor, toothbrush, or dental floss. Avoid people with infections. Take your temperature daily. Call the doctor immediately if you have an infection.

Common: none reported

Other: skin inflammation, itching, rash, hair loss, kidney stones
Tip: To help prevent kidney problems, drink extra fluids so you'll urinate more.

 DRUG INTERACTIONS

Combining certain drugs may alter their action or produce unwanted side effects. Tell your doctor about other drugs you're taking, especially:
• anticoagulants (blood thinners) such as Coumadin, aspirin
• gout drugs such as Benemid
• drugs that suppress the bone marrow, such as Bactrim, Vasotec, and Dilantin
• vaccines (wait until 3 months after stopping Alkeran).

return to your regular schedule and contact your doctor.

 If you suspect an overdose

Contact your doctor *immediately.* Excessive Alkeran can cause bone marrow suppression (fatigue, bruising, infection) and calcium loss (muscle spasms, irregular pulse, difficulty breathing and swallowing).

 Warnings

• Make sure your doctor knows your medical history. Some conditions may affect your use of this drug.
• Don't take this drug if you're pregnant or think you may be. Avoid pregnancy during therapy.
• Consult your doctor before having any dental work done.

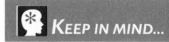 **KEEP IN MIND...**

* Take at least 1 hour before or 2 hours after meal.

* Keep taking even if drug causes nausea and vomiting.

* Avoid aspirin.

Altace

Altace is an angiotensin-converting enzyme (ACE) inhibitor. It blocks the action of a hormone, angiotensin, which constricts blood vessels. This relaxes blood vessels and lowers blood pressure.

Why it's prescribed

Doctors prescribe Altace to treat high blood pressure. It comes in capsules. Doctors usually prescribe the following amounts for adults.
▶ **For high blood pressure,** initially 2.5 milligrams (mg) once a day for people who are not taking a diuretic (water pill); 1.25 mg once a day for people who are taking a diuretic. Dosage is increased as necessary. Maintenance dosage is 2.5 to 20 mg a day as a single dose or divided into several equal doses.

How to take Altace

• Take Altace exactly as your doctor has directed.
• Take it on an empty stomach, at least 1 hour before or 2 hours after a meal.
• Keep taking this drug even if you feel well.

If you miss a dose

Take the missed dose as soon as possible. However, if it's almost time for your next dose, skip the missed dose and take your next dose as scheduled. Don't take a double dose.

 If you suspect an overdose

Contact your doctor immediately. Excessive Altace can cause very low blood pressure (extreme dizziness, weakness, and fatigue; fainting).

ALTACE'S OTHER NAME

Altace's generic name is ramipril.

 SIDE EFFECTS

Call your doctor if you have any of these possible drug side effects. Call *immediately* about any labeled "serious."

Serious: seizures, irregular heartbeats, heart attack (chest pain); swelling of face, lips, hands, feet, throat, and tongue

Common: dry, persistent, tickling cough
Tip: To relieve this symptom, drink more fluids.

Other: headache; dizziness; fatigue; weakness; anxiety; depression; trouble sleeping; loss of reflexes; numbness; tingling; increased sensitivity to pain or touch; tremor; fainting; shortness of breath; difficulty swallowing; increased saliva; nausea; vomiting; stomach pain; appetite loss; constipation; diarrhea; dry mouth; taste disturbance; rash, itching, or inflammation; skin sensitivity to sunlight; increased potassium level (irregular heartbeat, shortness of breath, weakness or heaviness in the legs, numbness or tingling in hands, feet, or lips); increased sweating; weight gain; joint or muscle pain
Tips: Know how Altace affects you before driving. Protect yourself in the sunlight with sunscreen and protective clothing.

 DRUG INTERACTIONS

Combining certain drugs may alter their action or produce unwanted side effects. Tell your doctor about other drugs you're taking, especially:
• diuretics (water pills; stop taking 3 days before starting Altace)
• Eskalith
• insulin and other diabetes drugs
• potassium supplements, salt substitutes containing potassium.

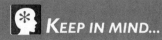 **Warnings**

• Make sure your doctor knows your medical history. Some conditions may affect your use of this drug.
• Don't take this drug if you're pregnant. If you become pregnant while taking it, consult your doctor.
• If you're diabetic, be aware that Altace may cause low blood sugar, especially at first. Report any change to your doctor.
• If you have kidney problems, expect the doctor to closely monitor your kidney function when you first begin taking Altace.

KEEP IN MIND...

* Take at least 1 hour before or 2 hours after meal.
* Keep taking even if you feel well.
* Avoid salt substitutes.

ALternaGEL

A LternaGEL neutralizes excess stomach acid. It also reduces the amount of phosphate in the blood by binding with phosphate in the intestines, producing a substance that's excreted in the stool.

Why it's taken

ALternaGEL is taken to relieve heartburn, sour stomach, acid indigestion, or peptic ulcer; it's also sometimes prescribed for people with kidney failure to help control excessive amounts of phosphate in the blood. You can buy ALternaGEL without a prescription. It comes as an oral suspension. The following amounts are usually recommended for adults.

▶ **As an antacid and to relieve peptic ulcer,** 1 to 2 teaspoons (tsp), taken with milk or water five to six times a day.

▶ **To reduce phosphate in the blood,** 1 to 2 tsp two to four times a day.

How to take ALternaGEL

• If you're treating yourself, follow the instructions on the label. If your doctor has prescribed ALternaGEL, follow any special instructions.

• Take ALternaGEL 1 hour after meals and at bedtime, unless the doctor tells you otherwise.

• Shake the oral suspension well; drink a small amount of milk or water with your dose.

ALternaGEL's OTHER NAMES

ALternaGEL's generic name is aluminum hydroxide. Other brand names include Alu-Cap, Alu-Tab, Amphojel, Basaljel, Dialume, and Nephrox.

 SIDE EFFECTS

Call your doctor if you have any of these possible drug side effects.

Serious: none reported

Common: constipation
Tip: Avoid constipation by increasing fluids and high-fiber foods in your diet. If you become constipated, ask your doctor about using laxatives or stool softeners or alternating this drug with another antacid.

Other: appetite loss, bowel obstruction, abnormally low blood phosphate level (appetite loss, feelings of ill health, muscle weakness)

 DRUG INTERACTIONS

Combining certain drugs may alter their action or produce unwanted side effects. Tell your doctor about other drugs you're taking, especially:
• antibiotic drugs for tuberculosis
• enteric coated drugs, such as Dulcolax, Lanoxin, and Dilantin
• iron supplements
• ulcer drugs such as Tagamet
• phenothiazines (drugs for anxiety, nausea, vomiting or psychosis).

• Don't take ALternaGEL for more than 2 weeks unless the doctor tells you to.

If you miss a dose

If your doctor wants you to take this drug on a regular schedule, take the missed dose as soon as possible. However, if it's almost time for your next dose, skip the missed dose and take your next dose as scheduled. Don't take a double dose.

If you suspect an overdose

Consult your doctor.

Warnings

• Consult your doctor before taking ALternaGEL if you have stomach or lower abdominal pain, cramps, bloating, soreness, nausea, or vomiting.

• If your stomach problem doesn't improve or if it keeps coming back, consult your doctor.

• If you're on a low-salt diet and have been taking large doses of ALternaGEL for a long time, tell your doctor. Each 5 ml of suspension contains 2 to 3 mg of sodium.

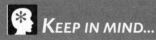 KEEP IN MIND...

* Shake suspension well before measuring.

* Take doses 1 hour after meals and at bedtime.

* Call doctor if stomach problem doesn't improve or keeps coming back or if constipation occurs.

* Don't take longer than 2 weeks.

Alupent

Alupent relaxes muscles in the air passages, helping to ease breathing.

Why it's prescribed

Doctors prescribe Alupent to stop asthma attacks, to treat bronchospasm (difficulty breathing) associated with chronic lung diseases, or to prevent bronchospasm caused by exercise. Alupent comes in tablets, syrup, inhalation aerosol, and inhalation solution. Doctors usually prescribe the following amounts for adults and children.

▶ **To stop asthma attacks in process,** 2 to 3 inhalations, repeated no more often than every 3 to 4 hours. Maximum, 12 inhalations a day. (Children: same as adults.)

▶ **For chronic asthma and bronchospasm,** 20 milligrams (mg) orally every 6 to 8 hours. (Children: 10 to 20 mg orally every 6 to 8 hours.) Or, by nebulizer, adults and children ages 12 and over: 5 to 15 inhalations every 4 hours as needed. (Children ages 6 to 11: 0.1 to 0.2 milliliters of diluted solution every 4 hours as needed.)

How to take Alupent

• Take this drug exactly as the doctor has directed; don't use it more often than recommended.
• Alupent's oral forms take effect in 15 minutes; the inhalation form, in 1 minute; the aerosol nebulizer form, in 5 to 30 minutes.

ALUPENT'S OTHER NAMES

Alupent's generic name is metaproterenol sulfate. Other brand names include Arm-A-Med Metaproterenol, Dey-Dose Metaproterenol, Dey-Lute Metaproterenol, and Metaprel.

SIDE EFFECTS

Call your doctor if you have any of these possible drug side effects. Call *immediately* about any labeled "serious."

Serious: (with excessive use) narrowed airways and cardiac arrest

Common: none reported

Other: nervousness, weakness, drowsiness, tremor, fast pulse, palpitations, high blood pressure (headache, chest pain, dizziness, nosebleeds), vomiting, nausea, bad taste in mouth, dry mouth

DRUG INTERACTIONS

Combining certain drugs may alter their action or produce unwanted side effects. Tell your doctor about other drugs you're taking, especially:
• beta blockers, such as Corgard, Inderal, Lopressor, and Tenormin
• Larodopa.

• If you're using Alupent aerosol plus a steroid aerosol (such as Beclovent, Decadron Respihaler, or AeroBid) or Atrovent aerosol, take Alupent 5 minutes before the other drug (unless your doctor tells you otherwise).

If you miss a dose

If you're using this drug daily, take the missed dose as soon as possible. Take any remaining doses that day at regularly spaced intervals.

 If you suspect an overdose

Contact your doctor *immediately.* Excessive Alupent can cause severe dizziness, light-headedness, headache, chills, fever, nausea, vomiting, muscle cramps, weakness, blurred vision, shortness of breath, and anxiety or restlessness.

Warnings

• Make sure your doctor knows your medical history. You may not be able to take Alupent if you have brain damage, seizures, diabetes, underactive thyroid, or heart or blood vessel disease or if you are pregnant or breast-feeding.
• Don't take Alupent if you have an unusually rapid pulse.
• Older adults may be especially prone to Alupent's side effects.
• If you have diabetes, the doctor may need to adjust the dosage of your diabetes drug.
• Call your doctor right away if you still have trouble breathing after taking a dose or if your condition gets worse.

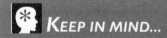 KEEP IN MIND...

* Don't take if you have unusually rapid pulse.
* Use Alupent before other aerosols.
* Call doctor immediately about continued trouble breathing.

Ambien

Ambien is a central nervous system depressant. By interacting with tiny cells called receptors, it slows down the central nervous system and helps to induce sleep.

Why it's prescribed

Doctors prescribe Ambien for insomnia (difficulty falling or staying asleep). Ambien comes in tablets. Doctors usually prescribe the following amounts for adults.

▶ **For short-term treatment of insomnia,** 10 milligrams (mg) immediately before bedtime. Dosage is usually reduced to 5 mg for elderly or ill people and those with liver impairment. Maximum dosage is 10 mg a day.

How to take Ambien

• Take Ambien only as your doctor has directed. Don't take it for more than 10 days without discussing it with your doctor. Persistent insomnia may be a symptom of a medical or psychiatric problem.
• You may take Ambien with or without food. However, taking it on an empty stomach may help it work faster.
• Take Ambien just before you go to bed. It works very quickly to put you to sleep. Don't take Ambien if your schedule doesn't allow you to get a full night's sleep; you may wake up feeling drowsy.
• If you've been taking Ambien for a long time, check with your doctor before you stop taking the drug. The doctor may advise you to reduce the

AMBIEN'S OTHER NAME

Ambien's generic name is zolpidem tartrate.

SIDE EFFECTS

Call your doctor if you have any of these possible drug side effects. Call *immediately* about any labeled "serious."

Serious: hallucinations, abnormal thoughts or behavior

Common: none reported

Other: daytime drowsiness, light-headedness, abnormal dreams, memory loss, dizziness, headache, hangover effect, increased insomnia, palpitations, inflamed sinuses, sore throat, dry mouth, nausea, vomiting, diarrhea, back or chest pain, flulike symptoms, allergic reactions (rash, hives, itching, trouble breathing, facial swelling)

Tip: Don't drive or do anything else that could be dangerous until you know how Ambien affects you.

DRUG INTERACTIONS

Combining certain drugs may alter their action or produce unwanted side effects. Tell your doctor about other drugs you're taking, especially:
• alcohol and drugs that make you relaxed and sleepy, such as cold and allergy medicines, sedatives, tranquilizers, pain relievers, narcotics, barbiturates, seizure drugs, and muscle relaxants.

---

amount you take gradually. For the first few nights after you stop taking Ambien, you may have difficulty sleeping (rebound insomnia).

If you miss a dose

Not applicable because Ambien is taken only as needed.

If you suspect an overdose

Contact your doctor *immediately.* Excessive Ambien can cause severe drowsiness, staggering, and difficulty breathing.

Warnings

• Make sure your doctor knows your medical history. You may not be able to take Ambien if you have

a history of alcohol or drug abuse, liver or kidney disease, chronic lung disease, depression, or sleep apnea (temporary stoppage of breathing during sleep).
• If you're pregnant, tell your doctor before you start taking Ambien.
• Older adults may be especially prone to Ambien's side effects, especially confusion and falling.
• Ambien can be habit-forming if you take too much.

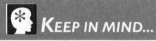

KEEP IN MIND...

* Take just before going to bed.
* Don't take for longer time than prescribed.
* Don't stop taking abruptly.

Amoxil

Amoxil, a penicillin-type antibiotic, destroys the cell walls of invading bacteria.

Why it's prescribed

Doctors prescribe Amoxil to treat bacterial infections. Amoxil comes in chewable tablets, capsules, and an oral suspension. Doctors usually prescribe the following amounts.

▶ **For bacterial infections,** for adults and children weighing 44 pounds (lb) or more, 250 to 500 milligrams (mg) every 8 hours. For children weighing under 44 lb, 20 mg for each 2.2 lb of body weight daily, taken every 8 hours.

▶ **For severe bacterial infections,** 40 mg for each 2.2 lb daily divided into equal doses taken every 8 hours.

How to take Amoxil

• Take this drug exactly as your doctor has directed. Take it on a full or empty stomach at evenly spaced times, day and night.

• Chew or crush the chewable tablets before swallowing. Swallow the capsules whole. Don't break, chew, or crush them.

• Take the liquid form straight or mixed with other liquids. Take it immediately after mixing, and drink all the liquid.

• Finish all of this drug, even if you feel better. If you stop too soon, symptoms may recur.

AMOXIL'S OTHER NAMES

Amoxil's generic name is amoxicillin trihydrate. Other brand names include Larotid, Polymox, Trimox, Wymox; and, in Canada, Apo-Amoxi, Novamoxin, and Nu-Amoxi.

 SIDE EFFECTS

Call your doctor if you have any of these possible drug side effects. Call *immediately* about any labeled "serious."

Serious: fast or irregular breathing, fever, joint pain, light-headedness, allergic reactions (shortness of breath, rash, hives, itching, facial swelling), blood problems (fatigue, bruising, bleeding, chills, weakness)

Common: nausea, diarrhea
Tip: Notify your doctor before taking diarrhea medicine; it may make your diarrhea worse or make it last longer.

Other: vomiting

DRUG INTERACTIONS

Combining certain drugs may alter their action or produce unwanted side effects. Tell your doctor about other drugs you're taking, especially:
• Benemid
• Zyloprim.

If you miss a dose

Take the missed dose as soon as possible. If you take two doses a day and it's almost time for your next dose, space the missed dose and your next dose 5 to 6 hours apart. If you're taking three or more doses a day, space the missed dose and the next dose 2 to 4 hours apart. Then go back to your regular schedule.

 If you suspect an overdose

Contact your doctor *immediately.* Excessive Amoxil can cause muscle pain and spasm, pain in fingertips or toes, and seizures.

Warnings

• Make sure your doctor knows your medical history. You may not be able to take Amoxil if you're allergic to other penicillins or to cephalosporins, Fulvicin, or Cuprimine or if you're pregnant or breast-feeding. (Be sure to carry medical identification that identifies your allergy.) Also, kidney, stomach, or intestinal disease or infectious mononucleosis may increase your risk of side effects from Amoxil.

• If you're diabetic, be aware that Amoxil may cause false test results with some urine sugar tests. Consult your doctor.

• If your symptoms don't improve within a few days or worsen, check with your doctor.

 KEEP IN MIND...

∗ Don't break, chew, or crush capsules.

∗ Take liquid straight or mix with other liquids.

∗ Call doctor if symptoms don't improve or worsen.

Amphojel

Amphojel is an antacid that neutralizes stomach acid through a chemical reaction.

Why it's taken

Amphojel is taken for heartburn, acid indigestion, sour stomach, gastroesophageal reflux (backflow of stomach contents into the esophagus), and too much phosphate in the blood. You can buy Amphojel without a prescription. It comes in tablets and an oral suspension. The following amounts are usually recommended for adults.

▶ **As an antacid,** two 0.3-gram (g) tablets, one 0.6-g tablet, or 2 teaspoons of suspension five or six times a day between meals.

How to take Amphojel

• If you're treating yourself, read the package instructions carefully to find out how much to use and when to use it.
• If your doctor prescribed Amphojel or gave you special instructions on how to use it, follow those instructions exactly.
• Shake the oral suspension well, and take it with a small amount of water or fruit juice.

If you miss a dose

Take the missed dose as soon as possible. However, if it's almost time for your next dose, skip the missed dose and take your next dose as scheduled. Don't take a double dose.

 If you suspect an overdose

Consult your doctor.

AMPHOJEL'S OTHER NAME

Amphojel's generic name is aluminum hydroxide.

 SIDE EFFECTS

Call your doctor if you have any of these possible drug side effects.

Serious: none reported

Common: constipation

Tip: If you become constipated, ask your doctor about using laxatives or stool softeners or alternating Amphojel with a magnesium-containing antacid.

Other: appetite loss, blockage of bowel, too little phosphate in blood (appetite loss, overall feeling of illness, muscle weakness)

DRUG INTERACTIONS

Combining certain drugs may alter their action or produce unwanted side effects. Tell your doctor about other drugs you're taking, especially:
• corticosteroids
• Cuprimine
• Dolobid
• enteric-coated drugs, such as Ecotrin (take at least 1 hour before or after Amphojel)
• iron
• Laniazid, Myambutol
• Lanoxin
• phenothiazines (used for anxiety, nausea and vomiting, or psychosis)
• thyroid hormones
• ulcer drugs such as Tagamet
• Zyloprim.

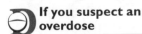 **Warnings**

• Before taking Amphojel, consult your doctor if you have other medical problems, especially kidney disease, or if you're pregnant.
• Don't give this drug to children under age 6.
• Be aware that older adults with bone problems or Alzheimer's disease should not take this drug. It contains aluminum, which may cause their condition to get worse.

• Follow a low-phosphate diet if recommended by your doctor.
• Don't switch to another antacid without consulting your doctor.

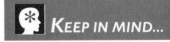 **KEEP IN MIND...**

∗ Shake oral suspension well, and take with water or fruit juice.

∗ Don't switch antacid brands without checking with doctor.

∗ To avoid constipation, increase fluids and fiber in diet.

Anadrol-50

Anadrol-50 is an anabolic steroid, related to the male sex hormone testosterone. Anabolic steroids help rebuild tissues, assisting the body to recover from the effects of severe illness, injury, or infection.

Why it's prescribed

Doctors prescribe Anadrol-50 to treat aplastic anemia. It comes in tablets. Doctors usually prescribe the following amounts for adults and children.

▶ **For aplastic anemia,** 1 to 5 milligrams for each 2.2 pounds of body weight once a day.

How to take Anadrol-50

• Take Anadrol-50 exactly as your doctor has directed. If stomach upset occurs, take it with food.

If you miss a dose

Don't take a double dose. Adjust your schedule as follows:
• If you take one dose a day, take the missed dose as soon as possible. However, if you don't remember it until the next day, skip the missed dose and take your next scheduled dose.
• If you take more than one dose a day, take the missed dose as soon as possible. However, if it's almost time for your next dose, skip the missed dose and take your next dose as scheduled.

If you suspect an overdose

Consult your doctor.

ANADROL-50'S OTHER NAMES

Anadrol-50's generic name is oxymetholone. A Canadian brand name is Anapolon 50.

SIDE EFFECTS

Call your doctor if you have any of these possible drug side effects. Call *immediately* about any labeled "serious."

Serious: liver cell tumors (yellow-tinged skin and eyes, easy bruising or bleeding), excess calcium in blood (nausea, vomiting, tiredness)

Common: unusual body hair growth; oily skin or hair; excessive sweating; nervousness; moodiness; impotence; deepening voice; hair loss; vaginal burning, itching, dryness; changes in menstrual cycle

Other: nausea, vomiting, diarrhea, constipation, appetite change, irritable bladder, muscle cramps, acne, hoarseness, enlarged clitoris, male-pattern baldness, more frequent erections, enlarged penis and breasts, shrinking of testicles

DRUG INTERACTIONS

Combining certain drugs may alter their action or produce unwanted side effects. Tell your doctor about other drugs you're taking, especially:
• anticoagulants (blood thinners) such as Coumadin
• diabetes drugs, including insulin
• drugs that can damage the liver such as Tylenol.

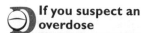 Warnings

• Make sure your doctor knows your medical history. You may not be able to take Anadrol-50 if you have diabetes, epilepsy, migraine, or heart, kidney, or liver disease.
• Don't take this drug if you're pregnant or breast-feeding. Use an effective, nonhormonal birth-control method when taking Anadrol-50.
• Be aware that Anadrol-50 may cause children to stop growing, may cause boys to develop too fast sexually, and may lead to male-like changes in girls. Children should have X-rays of wrist bones taken to evaluate bone maturation before starting this drug.

• Anadrol-50 may cause male-like changes in adult women, which may persist even after the drug is stopped.
• For this drug to work properly, you must eat a diet high in protein and calories. Consult your doctor for dietary recommendations.
• If you're diabetic, this drug may affect your blood sugar level. Tell your doctor if you notice a change.

KEEP IN MIND...

* Take with food or meals if stomach upset occurs.

* Eat high-protein, high-calorie diet.

* Call doctor about yellow-tinged skin and eyes and urination changes.

Anafranil

Anafranil is one of several drugs called tricyclic antidepressants. It's thought to act by increasing the amounts of certain beneficial chemicals in the brain.

Why it's prescribed

Doctors prescribe Anafranil to treat obsessive-compulsive disorder. Anafranil comes in capsules. Doctors usually prescribe the following amounts for adults; children's dosages appear in parentheses.

▶ **For obsessive-compulsive disorder,** initially 25 milligrams (mg) a day, divided into several equal doses, gradually increased to 100 mg daily during first 2 weeks. Then, dosage is increased to maximum of 250 mg a day divided into several equal doses as needed. (Children and teenagers: initially 25 mg a day divided into several equal doses, gradually increased to daily maximum of 3 mg for each 2.2 pounds of body weight a day or 200 mg a day, whichever is smaller.)

How to take Anafranil

• Take this drug exactly as the doctor has directed. You'll probably be instructed to take it with meals. After the correct amount is established, your doctor may tell you to take your entire daily dose at bedtime to avoid daytime sleepiness.
• You may not notice the drug's full effect for 2 weeks or longer.
• Don't stop taking this drug suddenly because doing so may cause nausea and headache.

ANAFRANIL'S OTHER NAME

Anafranil's generic name is clomipramine hydrochloride.

 ## SIDE EFFECTS

Call your doctor if you have any of these possible drug side effects. Call *immediately* about any labeled "serious."

Serious: seizures, blood problems (fatigue, infections, bruising, bleeding), suicidal thoughts
Tips: To avoid infection, stay away from people who are ill or have an infection. If fatigue is a problem, avoid strenuous physical activity.

Common: unusual sleepiness, tremor, dizziness, nervousness, muscle spasms, abnormal vision, dry mouth, constipation, nausea, appetite change, difficulty urinating, inability to ejaculate, sweating, altered sex drive
Tips: Avoid activities that require you to be fully alert until you know how the drug affects you. To relieve dry mouth, use sugarless candy or gum or a saliva substitute. If you become constipated, drink more fluids and increase the amount of high-fiber foods in your diet.

Other: headache, trouble sleeping, weakness, aggressiveness, palpitations, fast pulse, middle ear infection in children, laryngitis, runny nose, diarrhea, stomach pain, painful menstruation, impotence, rash, dry skin, itching, skin sensitivity to sunlight, muscle pain, weight gain
Tip: Use sunblock, wear protective clothing, and avoid prolonged exposure to strong sunlight.

 ## DRUG INTERACTIONS

Combining certain drugs may alter their action or produce unwanted side effects. Tell your doctor about other drugs you're taking, especially:
• alcohol and other drugs that make you relaxed and sleepy, such as cold and allergy medicine, sedatives, tranquilizers, pain medication, seizure drugs, and muscle relaxants
• Catapres
• MAO inhibitors such as Nardil (stop taking at least 2 weeks before starting Anafranil)
• Primatene Mist, Bronkaid Mist
• Ritalin
• Tagamet.

• Store Anafranil at room temperature in a dry spot — not in the bathroom, near the kitchen sink, or in another damp place. Heat and moisture can cause the drug to deteriorate.

If you miss a dose

Don't take a double dose. Adjust your schedule as follows:
• If you take several doses a day, take the missed dose as soon as possible. However, if it's almost time

Continued on next page ▶

for your next dose, skip the missed dose and take your next dose as scheduled.

• If you take one daily dose at bedtime, don't take the missed dose in the morning because it may cause disturbing side effects during waking hours. Instead, check with your doctor.

If you suspect an overdose

Contact your doctor *immediately*. Excessive Anafranil can cause a slow pulse, low blood pressure (dizziness, weakness), irritability, drowsiness, lack of awareness, increased reflexes, and fever.

Warnings

• Make sure your doctor knows your medical history. You may not be able to take Anafranil if you have a history of seizures, brain damage, urine retention, glaucoma, an overactive thyroid, an adrenal tumor, or heart, kidney, or liver disease or if you've recently had a heart attack.

• If you're pregnant or breast-feeding, tell your doctor before you start taking Anafranil.

• Anafranil is not recommended for children under age 10.

• Be aware that children and older adults may be especially prone to Anafranil's side effects.

• If you're diabetic, this drug may affect your blood sugar levels.

• Be aware that Anafranil can provoke suicidal thoughts and increase the risk of suicide. Let your family and friends know about this possible side effect. You'll probably receive a prescription for only a small amount of the drug so that your doctor can monitor you for this side effect.

• Avoid drinking alcohol while you're taking Anafranil. Alcohol can increase the possibility of experiencing the side effects of this drug.

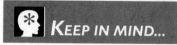

KEEP IN MIND...

* Take with meals.
* Don't stop taking abruptly.
* If diabetic, watch for change in blood sugar level.
* Avoid alcohol.

Anaprox

Anaprox, a nonsteroidal anti-inflammatory drug (NSAID), relieves pain probably by blocking the body's production of prostaglandin.

Why it's prescribed

Doctors prescribe Anaprox to treat mild to moderate pain. Anaprox comes in film-coated tablets. Doctors usually prescribe the following amounts.

▶ **For rheumatoid arthritis or osteoarthritis,** 275 to 500 milligrams (mg) twice a day.

▶ **For juvenile arthritis in children,** 10 mg for each 2.2 pounds of body weight twice a day.

▶ **For acute gout attack,** initially, 825 mg, followed by 275 mg every 8 hours until attack subsides.

▶ **For mild to moderate pain,** 550 mg initially, followed by 275 mg every 6 to 8 hours, as needed; or 550 mg every 12 hours. Maximum dosage is 1,375 mg a day.

How to take Anaprox

• Take this drug exactly as your doctor directs.
• Take each dose with a full glass (8 ounces) of water. Stay upright for about 30 minutes afterward.
• This drug starts to relieve pain within 1 hour and starts to relieve arthritis symptoms within 14 days. Pain relief lasts about 7 hours.

If you miss a dose

Take the missed dose as soon as possible. However, if it's almost time for your next dose, skip the missed dose and take your next dose as scheduled. Don't take a double dose.

 If you suspect an overdose

Contact your doctor *immediately*. Excessive Anaprox can cause drowsiness, nausea, and vomiting.

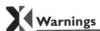 **Warnings**

• Before taking Anaprox, consult your doctor if you have an intestinal disorder or kidney, heart, or blood vessel disease.
• Don't take this drug if you're allergic to aspirin.

• If you're pregnant, check with your doctor before taking this drug.
• Be aware that older adults may be prone to stomach upset.
• Don't take Anaprox and Aleve at the same time.

ANAPROX'S OTHER NAMES

Anaprox's generic name is naproxen sodium. Other brand names include Aleve; and, in Canada, Apo-Naproxen, Novo-Naprox, and Nu-Naprox.

 SIDE EFFECTS

Call your doctor if you have any of these possible drug side effects. Call *immediately* about any labeled "serious."

Serious: peptic ulcer (nausea, vomiting, heartburn, dark or bloody vomit or stools), blood disorders (bleeding gums, fatigue, fever, chills), kidney problems (decreased urination), liver problems (nausea, vomiting, yellow-tinged skin and eyes)

Common: headache, drowsiness, dizziness, swelling of feet or lower legs, ringing in ears, nausea, itching
Tip: Take doses with food to avoid stomach upset.

Other: confusion, mood changes, palpitations, vision disturbances, painful urination, prolonged bleeding from wounds, shortness of breath, hives

 DRUG INTERACTIONS

Combining certain drugs may alter their action or produce unwanted side effects. Tell your doctor about other drugs you're taking, especially:
• alcohol
• aspirin and other anticoagulants (blood thinners) such as Coumadin
• Benemid, Mexate
• diuretics (water pills) and other blood pressure drugs
• oral diabetes drugs
• protein-bound drugs such as Dilantin
• steroids.

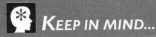 **KEEP IN MIND...**

* Take with full glass of water.
* Stay upright for 30 minutes.
* Don't take Anaprox and Aleve at the same time.

Anavar

Anavar is an anabolic steroid related to the male sex hormone testosterone. It helps to rebuild tissues weakened by serious illness or injury.

Why it's prescribed

Doctors prescribe Anavar to aid recovery from severe illness, injury, or infection. Anavar comes in tablets. Doctors usually prescribe the following amounts for adults; children's dosages are in parentheses.
▶ **To combat the effects of steroid drugs, osteoporosis, or prolonged immobility,** 2.5 milligrams (mg) two to four times a day, up to 20 mg a day. (Children: 0.25 mg for each 2.2 pounds of body weight each day.)

How to take Anavar

• Take this drug only as directed by your doctor.

If you miss a dose

Take the missed dose as soon as possible. But if it's almost time for your next dose, skip the missed dose and take your next dose as scheduled. Don't take a double dose.

If you suspect an overdose

Consult your doctor.

Warnings

• Make sure your doctor knows your medical history. You may not be able to take Anavar if you have epilepsy, migraines, or heart, liver, or kidney disease.

ANAVAR'S OTHER NAMES

Anavar's generic name is oxandrolone. Another brand name is Oxandrin.

SIDE EFFECTS

Call your doctor if you have any of these possible drug side effects. Call *immediately* about any labeled "serious."

Serious: liver tumors (yellow-tinged skin and eyes, easy bruising or bleeding), excess calcium (nighttime urination, increased thirst, constipation)

Common: weight gain, ankle swelling, unusual body hair growth, oily skin or hair, flushing, excessive sweating, moodiness, decreased breast size; vaginal burning, itching, dryness; changes in menstrual cycle, acne
Tips: Your doctor may advise you to restrict your salt intake or may prescribe water pills to treat swelling. For vaginal dryness, a vaginal moisturizer, K-Y Gel, is available without a prescription.

Other: nausea, vomiting, diarrhea, muscle spasms, constipation, appetite change, irritable bladder (frequent urination in small amounts), hoarseness, enlarged clitoris, changes in sex drive, male-pattern baldness; more frequent erections, enlarged penis and breasts, shrinking of testicles, impotence, inflammation of the sperm ducts (extreme tenderness, swelling in groin and scrotum)
Tips: Take doses with food to avoid nausea. Drink more fluids and eat more high-fiber foods to avoid constipation.

DRUG INTERACTIONS

Combining certain drugs may alter their action or produce unwanted side effects. Tell your doctor about other drugs you're taking, especially:
• anticoagulants (blood thinners) such as Coumadin
• diabetes drugs, including insulin
• drugs that damage the liver such as Tylenol.

• Don't take this drug if you're pregnant or breast-feeding. Use an effective, nonhormonal birth control method while taking Anavar.
• Anavar may cause children to stop growing, may cause boys to develop too fast sexually, and may lead to male-like changes in girls. Children should have X-rays of wrist bones taken to evaluate bone growth before starting this drug.
• Anavar may cause male-like changes in women, which may persist even after the drug is stopped.

• For Anavar to work properly, you must eat a high-protein, high-calorie diet.
• If you're diabetic, be aware that this drug may affect your blood sugar level.

KEEP IN MIND...

* Take with food or meals.
* Eat high-protein, high-calorie diet.
* Call doctor if menstrual irregularities occur.

Android

Android, a male hormone, stimulates normal development in men whose bodies produce too little hormone.

Why it's prescribed

Doctors prescribe Android to replace male hormones when the body can't produce enough or to treat breast cancer in women. It comes in tablets, buccal tablets, and capsules. Doctors usually prescribe the following amounts for adults.

▶ **For males with slow growth and sexual development,** 10 to 50 milligrams (mg) orally, or 5 to 25 mg buccal tablets daily.

▶ **For failure of the testicles to descend in postpubertal males,** 30 mg orally or 15 mg buccal tablets daily.

▶ **For breast cancer in postmenopausal women,** 50 to 200 mg orally, or 25 to 100 mg buccally daily.

How to take Android

• Take Android only as your doctor has directed.

• Place a buccal tablet between your cheek and gum and wait for it to dissolve (30 to 60 minutes). Don't swallow it whole, drink, eat, chew, smoke, or swallow excessively until you can no longer taste it. Then brush your teeth or rinse your mouth to help prevent tooth decay or mouth irritation. Place the tablet in a different spot in your cheek with each dose.

If you miss a dose

Take the missed dose as soon as possible. However, if it's almost time

ANDROID'S OTHER NAMES

Android's generic name is methyltestosterone. Other brand names include Oreton Methyl, Testred, and Virilon.

 SIDE EFFECTS

Call your doctor if you have any of these possible drug side effects. Call *immediately* about any labeled "serious."

Serious: liver problems (yellow-tinged skin and eyes, bruising, bleeding), excess calcium (nighttime urination, increased thirst, constipation)

Common: unusual body hair growth, weight gain, decrease in breast size, oily skin or hair, flushing, sweating, moodiness, menstrual irregularities, vaginal burning, itching, or dryness
Tip: Report unusual weight gain to the doctor.

Other: acne, muscle cramps or spasms, swelling, irritation of lining of mouth (with buccal tablets), nausea, vomiting, diarrhea, constipation, appetite change, difficulty urinating, hoarseness, enlarged clitoris, altered sex drive, male-pattern baldness, frequent erections, enlarged penis and breasts, shrinking of testicles, impotence, inflammation of sperm ducts (extreme tenderness, swelling in groin and scrotum)
Tip: Take the regular tablets or capsules with food to reduce stomach upset.

 DRUG INTERACTIONS

Combining certain drugs may alter their action or produce unwanted side effects. Tell your doctor about other drugs you're taking, especially:
• anticoagulants (blood thinners) such as Coumadin
• diabetes drugs, including insulin
• drugs that can cause liver damage such as Tylenol.

for your next dose, skip the missed dose and take your next dose as scheduled. Don't take a double dose.

 If you suspect an overdose

Consult your doctor.

 Warnings

• Make sure your doctor knows your medical history. You may not be able to take Android if you have heart, liver, or kidney disease.
• Don't take this drug if you're pregnant or breast-feeding. Use nonhormonal birth control while taking Android.

• Android may cause children to stop growing, boys to develop too fast sexually, and male-like changes in girls. Children should have X-rays of wrist bones taken to evaluate bone growth.
• To help Android work properly, eat a high-calorie, high-protein diet.

KEEP IN MIND...

* Take regular tablets or capsules with food.
* Let buccal tablets dissolve between cheek and gum.
* Eat high-calorie, high-protein diet.

Ansaid

Ansaid is a nonsteroidal anti-inflammatory drug (NSAID). NSAIDs are thought to reduce inflammation and pain by inhibiting production of a hormone called prostaglandin.

Why it's prescribed

Doctors prescribe Ansaid to relieve the inflammation, swelling, stiffness, and joint pain of arthritis. Ansaid comes in tablets and (in Canada) extended-release tablets. Doctors usually prescribe the following amounts for adults.

▶ **For rheumatic arthritis or osteoarthritis,** 200 to 300 milligrams a day divided into two or three equal doses.

How to take Ansaid

• Take exactly as directed. Take the tablets in the evening with food or an antacid plus a full glass (8 ounces) of water. Stay upright for 15 to 30 minutes after taking Ansaid.

If you miss a dose

If the missed dose is only 1 or 2 hours overdue, take it as soon as possible. If more time has elapsed, skip the missed dose and take your next dose as scheduled.

 If you suspect an overdose

Contact your doctor *immediately*. Excessive Ansaid can cause lethargy, coma, slow breathing, and stomach pain.

ANSAID'S OTHER NAMES

Ansaid's generic name is flurbiprofen. Canadian brand names include Apo-Flurbiprofen, Froben, and Novo-Flurproten.

 ## SIDE EFFECTS

Call your doctor if you have any of these possible drug side effects. Call *immediately* about any labeled "serious."

Serious: congestive heart failure (shortness of breath), bleeding in the digestive tract (blood in vomit or stools), kidney damage (low back pain, blood in urine), blood disorders (easy bruising or bleeding, chills, fever, fatigue)

Common: headache, dizziness, swelling, diarrhea, nausea, burning or pain on urination
Tip: Until you know how you react to Ansaid, don't drive or perform activities that require you to be totally alert.

Other: anxiety, trouble sleeping, tremor, memory loss, weakness, drowsiness, depression, high blood pressure (headache, blurred vision), asthma, runny nose, ringing in ears, vision changes, constipation, gas, vomiting, yellow-tinged skin and eyes, rash, weight changes
Tip: To avoid constipation, drink more fluids and eat more high-fiber foods.

 ## DRUG INTERACTIONS

Combining certain drugs may alter their action or produce unwanted side effects. Tell your doctor about other drugs you're taking, especially:
• alcohol
• anticoagulants (blood thinners) such as Coumadin
• aspirin or Tylenol
• diuretics (water pills)
• Mexate.

Warnings

• Make sure the doctor knows about any other medical conditions you have. They may affect your use of this drug.
• Consult your doctor if you're breast-feeding or become pregnant while taking Ansaid.
• Older adults may be especially prone to Ansaid's side effects.
• Schedule regular medical check-ups so your doctor can monitor your progress and check for unwanted side effects.

• Before having a dental or surgical procedure, tell the dentist or doctor that you're taking Ansaid.

 ## KEEP IN MIND...

* Take with food or antacid plus full glass of water.

* Stay upright for 15 to 30 minutes after taking.

* Report shortness of breath, blood in vomit or stool, or fainting.

Antabuse

Antabuse increases the amount of a substance called acetaldehyde in the body. This causes a highly unpleasant reaction when any alcohol is ingested.

Why it's prescribed

Doctors prescribe Antabuse to help treat chronic alcoholism. It comes in tablets. Doctors usually prescribe the following amounts for adults.

▶ **To help manage chronic alcoholism,** 250 to 500 milligrams (mg) a day for 1 to 2 weeks. Dosage may be reduced to 125 to 500 mg a day until self-control is achieved.

How to take Antabuse

• Take Antabuse only as your doctor has directed. You'll probably be instructed to take it each morning. However, if it makes you drowsy, ask your doctor if you may take it at bedtime.

• Before taking the first dose, make sure you haven't had any alcoholic beverages or alcohol-containing product or drug for 12 hours.

If you miss a dose

Take the missed dose as soon as possible. However, if it's almost time for your next dose, skip the missed dose and take your next dose as scheduled. Don't take a double dose.

If you suspect an overdose

Contact your doctor *immediately*. Excessive Antabuse can cause stomach upset, vomiting, drowsi-

ANTABUSE'S OTHER NAME

Antabuse's generic name is disulfiram.

SIDE EFFECTS

Call your doctor if you have any of these possible drug side effects. Call *immediately* about any labeled "serious."

Serious: alcohol reaction (from use of alcohol while taking Antabuse), causing blurred vision, chest pain, confusion, dizziness or fainting, fast pulse, flushing or redness of the face, sweating, nausea, vomiting, headache, difficulty breathing, weakness

Common: none reported

Other: drowsiness, headache, fatigue, delirium, depression, eye pain or tenderness, vision changes, metallic or garlic taste, impotence, skin irritation, acne; pain, numbness, tingling, or weakness in hands or feet

DRUG AND FOOD INTERACTIONS

Combining certain drugs, foods, and products may alter drug action or produce unwanted side effects. Consult your doctor about the following items:

• alcohol and alcohol-containing foods or other products, such as tonics, elixirs, sauces, vinegars, cough syrups, and mouthwashes
• anticoagulants (blood thinners) such as Coumadin
• anti-infective drugs, such as Flagyl, Laniazid, and Spectrobid
• drugs that make you relaxed and sleepy, such as barbiturates, sedatives, narcotics, and seizure drugs such as Dilantin
• tricyclic antidepressants, especially Elavil.

ness, extreme sleepiness, hallucinations, speech impairment, poor coordination, and coma.

Warnings

• Make sure your doctor knows your medical history. You may not be able to take Antabuse if you've ever had heart problems, diabetes, underactive thyroid, seizures, or a kidney or liver problem or if you are pregnant.

• Don't drink any alcohol, even small amounts, while taking Antabuse and for 14 days after you stop; it could make you very ill.

• Alcohol is found in many products besides beverages. Read the ingredients list on product labels.

• Avoid breathing fumes of alcohol-containing products or applying them to your skin because your body may absorb the alcohol.

• Carry an identification card stating that you're using Antabuse.

KEEP IN MIND...

* Wait 12 hours after last alcohol intake before first dose.

* Don't drink alcohol or use alcohol-containing products.

* Check for alcohol in ingredients on product labels.

Antiminth

Antiminth is used to treat worm infections, such as pinworms or roundworms. It paralyzes the worms, which are then eliminated in the stool.

Why it's prescribed

Doctors prescribe Antiminth for pinworm and roundworm infections. Antiminth comes in tablets (Canada only) and an oral suspension. Doctors usually prescribe the following amounts for adults and children over age 2.

▶ **For roundworm or pinworm,** 11 milligrams for each 2.2 pounds of body weight given as a single dose. Maximum dosage is 1 gram. For pinworm, dosage is repeated in 2 weeks.

How to take Antiminth

• Take this drug exactly as your doctor directs. You may take it with food, milk, or fruit juice.
• If you're taking the oral suspension, use a specially marked measuring spoon, not a household teaspoon, to measure each dose accurately. Shake the suspension well before pouring your dose.
• Keep taking Antiminth for the full time prescribed.

If you miss a dose

Not applicable for single doses. If you miss a repeat dose for pinworm, take it as soon as possible.

ANTIMINTH'S OTHER NAMES

Antiminth's generic name is pyrantel pamoate. Other brand names include Reese's Pinworm Medicine and, in Canada, Combantrin.

 SIDE EFFECTS

Call your doctor if you have any of these possible drug side effects.
Serious: none reported
Common: none reported
Other: headache, dizziness, drowsiness, difficulty sleeping, appetite loss, nausea, vomiting, stomach pains, cramps, diarrhea, spasms of the rectum, rash, fever, weakness
Tip: Until you know how Antiminth affects you, don't drive or do anything else that requires you to be fully alert.

 DRUG INTERACTIONS

Combining certain drugs may alter their action or produce unwanted side effects. Tell your doctor about other drugs you're taking, especially:
• Entacyl (another drug for pinworm and roundworm infection).

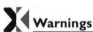 **If you suspect an overdose**

Consult your doctor.

Warnings

• Make sure your doctor knows your medical history. You may not be able to take Antiminth if you have severe malnutrition, anemia, or a liver disorder.
• If your symptoms don't improve within a few days or if they get worse, consult your doctor.
• To avoid reinfection and spread of the infection to others, practice good personal hygiene, especially good hand-washing technique. Wash the area around your rectum daily, and change your underclothes and bedding every day. Be sure to wash your hands and clean your fingernails before meals and after bowel movements. Until your infection clears up, don't prepare food for others.
• If you're taking Antiminth for pinworms, be aware that pinworms pass easily from person to person. Therefore, the doctor may recommend that all members of your household be treated at the same time to prevent the risk of spreading the infection.

 KEEP IN MIND...

* Shake suspension well before pouring.

* Call doctor if symptoms don't improve within a few days.

* Don't drive until you know how you react to drug.

* Practice good personal hygiene.

Antivert

Antivert is an antihistamine that acts on the brain to prevent or treat motion sickness, nausea, and vomiting.

Why it's prescribed

Doctors prescribe Antivert to prevent or treat nausea, vomiting, and dizziness resulting from motion sickness or to treat dizziness caused by certain medical problems. Antivert comes in regular tablets, chewable tablets, and capsules. Doctors usually prescribe the following amounts for adults.

▶ **For motion sickness,** 25 to 50 milligrams (mg) 1 hour before travel, repeated every travel day during the trip.

▶ **For vertigo,** 25 to 100 mg a day in divided doses.

How to take Antivert

• Another brand of meclizine (Bonine) is available without a prescription. If you're treating yourself, follow the label instructions carefully.
• If your doctor prescribed the drug, follow the doctor's instructions exactly.
• If you're using Antivert for motion sickness, take it 1 hour before starting your trip and continue to take it regularly every travel day during the trip.
• Antivert takes effect in about 1 hour; its effect lasts 8 to 24 hours.

If you miss a dose

Take the missed dose as soon as possible. However, if it's almost time

ANTIVERT'S OTHER NAMES

Antivert's generic name is meclizine hydrochloride. Other brand names include Bonine, D-Vert, Meni-D, Ru-Vert M; and, in Canada, Bonamine.

 SIDE EFFECTS

Call your doctor if you have any of these possible drug side effects.

Serious: none reported

Common: drowsiness, stomach irritation, vomiting
Tips: Avoid potentially hazardous activities, such as driving, until you know how Antivert affects you. Call the doctor if drowsiness persists or becomes bothersome. If Antivert causes stomach irritation, take it with food or a glass of milk or water. If you vomit a lot, be sure to drink plenty of fluids to prevent dehydration.

Other: fatigue, blurred vision, dry mouth
Tips: To relieve dry mouth, try using sugarless gum or hard candy or ice chips. If the condition lasts more than 2 weeks, see your doctor or dentist.

 DRUG INTERACTIONS

Combining certain drugs may alter their action or produce unwanted side effects. Tell your doctor about other drugs you're taking, especially:
• alcohol and other drugs that make you relaxed and sleepy, such as sedatives (Xanax and Valium) and cold and allergy medicines such as Benadryl.

for your next dose, skip the missed dose and take your next dose as scheduled. Don't take a double dose.

 If you suspect an overdose

Contact your doctor *immediately.* Excessive Antivert can cause you to feel overly excited or agitated, then drowsy. Severe overdose can cause seizures, hallucinations, and stoppage of breathing.

Warnings

• Make sure your doctor knows your medical history. You may not be able to take Antivert if you have other medical problems; if you're allergic to similar drugs, such as Bucladin-S, Marezine, or Dramamine; or if you have narrow-angle glaucoma, asthma, an enlarged prostate, or a blockage of the genitourinary or digestive tract.
• If you're pregnant or breast-feeding, check with your doctor before taking Antivert.

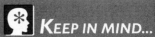 **KEEP IN MIND...**

* Take with food, milk, or water if stomach upset occurs.

* Take 1 hour before starting trip and every travel day during trip.

* Avoid alcohol and other sedatives.

* Call doctor if drowsiness persists.

Anturane

Anturane removes excess uric acid, which causes gout, from the body. Although it doesn't cure gout, it may help prevent attacks.

Why it's prescribed

Doctors prescribe Anturane to treat gout. It comes in tablets and capsules. Doctors usually prescribe the following amounts for adults.

▶ **For intermittent or chronic gout,** 200 to 400 milligrams (mg) twice a day for the first week, then 400 mg twice a day. Maximum dosage is 800 mg a day.

How to take Anturane

• Take this drug exactly as your doctor has directed to prevent attacks.

If you miss a dose

Take the missed dose as soon as possible. However, if it's almost time for your next dose, skip the missed dose and take your next dose as scheduled. Don't take a double dose.

 If you suspect an overdose

Contact your doctor *immediately.* Excessive Anturane may cause nausea, vomiting, stomach pain, clumsiness or unsteadiness, labored breathing, seizures, and coma.

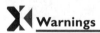 **Warnings**

• Make sure your doctor knows your medical history. You may not

ANTURANE'S OTHER NAMES

Anturane's generic name is sulfinpyrazone. A Canadian brand name is Anturan.

 SIDE EFFECTS

Call your doctor if you have any of these possible drug side effects. Call *immediately* about any labeled "serious."

Serious: blood problems (fever, chills, bleeding gums, nosebleeds, blood in urine)

Common: nausea, stomach upset, kidney stones

Tips: Take with food if drug upsets your stomach. If this doesn't help, take it with an antacid. If you still have stomach upset, call your doctor. Increase fluid intake to prevent kidney stones.

Other: dizziness, ringing in ears, stomach pain, blood loss, rash

 DRUG INTERACTIONS

Combining certain drugs may alter their action or produce unwanted side effects. Tell your doctor about other drugs you're taking, especially:
• anticoagulants (blood thinners) such as Coumadin
• aspirin and other salicylates, including Pepto-Bismol (may trigger gout attack)
• Benemid
• diabetes drugs (except insulin).

be able to take Anturane if you have a stomach ulcer or other stomach or bowel problems or if you are pregnant.

• Be aware that Anturane won't relieve a gout attack that has already started.

• When you first start taking Anturane, it may increase the amount of uric acid in your kidneys, leading to kidney stones. To help prevent this, the doctor may advise you to drink at least 10 to 12 full glasses (8 ounces each) of fluids daily or may prescribe an additional drug to make your urine less acidic.

• Anturane may make your gout attacks more frequent, severe, and prolonged for 6 to 12 months after you start taking it. For this reason, the doctor may also prescribe certain other drugs for the first 3 to 6 months.

• Avoid foods that are high in purine (anchovies, liver, sardines, kidneys, sweetbreads, peas, and lentils), because they may contribute to gout.

• Expect the doctor to order periodic blood and kidney function tests.

 KEEP IN MIND...

* Increase fluid intake when starting drug.
* Take with food or antacid if drug upsets stomach.
* Don't use to relieve gout attack in progress.
* Avoid high-purine foods.

Apresoline is thought to act by widening the blood vessels, which reduces blood pressure, helps to improve heart function, and increases blood flow to the brain and kidneys.

Why it's prescribed

Doctors prescribe Apresoline to lower blood pressure or to treat heart failure. Apresoline comes in tablets. It's also available in an injectible form. Doctors usually prescribe the following amounts for adults.

▶ **For high blood pressure,** initially, 10 milligrams (mg) orally four times a day, gradually increased to 50 mg four times a day as needed. Maximum recommended dosage is 200 mg a day, but some people may need 300 to 400 mg a day.

How to take Apresoline

• Take Apresoline exactly as your doctor has directed. Take it at the same times each day, preferably mealtimes.

• Keep taking this drug for as long as the doctor has ordered, even after you begin to feel better.

• If your doctor instructs you to take your blood pressure at home, follow the doctor's directions closely and report any change.

If you miss a dose

Take the missed dose as soon as possible. However, if it's almost time

APRESOLINE'S OTHER NAMES

Apresoline's generic name is hydralazine hydrochloride. A Canadian brand name is Novo-Hylazin.

 SIDE EFFECTS

Call your doctor if you have any of these possible drug side effects. Call *immediately* about any labeled "serious."

Serious: lupus-like syndrome (fast pulse, palpitations)

Common: headache, chest pain, salt retention (weight gain, swelling in legs), nausea, vomiting, diarrhea, appetite loss, stomach pain, rash, nosebleeds, blood in urine or stool, fatigue

Tip: Headache, nausea, vomiting, diarrhea, and loss of appetite may go away as your body adjusts to the drug.

Other: numbness, tingling, pain, or weakness in hands or feet; dizziness; irregular pulse; rash; blood problems (chills, fever)

Tips: To minimize dizziness, rise slowly from a sitting or lying position. Occasionally, Apresoline causes an irregular pulse; this usually stops 2 to 4 hours after taking a dose. If it doesn't, call your doctor immediately.

 DRUG INTERACTIONS

Combining certain drugs may alter their action or produce unwanted side effects. Tell your doctor about other drugs you're taking, especially:
• MAO inhibitors such as Marplan
• Proglycem.

for your next dose, skip the missed dose and take your next dose as scheduled. Don't take a double dose.

 If you suspect an overdose

Contact your doctor *immediately*. Excessive Apresoline can cause very low blood pressure (extreme dizziness or weakness), fast or irregular pulse, headache, flushed skin, and shock (weak pulse, moist or pale skin, trouble breathing and awakening).

 Warnings

• Make sure your doctor knows your medical history. You may not be able to take Apresoline if you

have kidney, heart, or blood vessel disease (such as stroke).

• If you're pregnant or think you may be, check with your doctor before taking Apresoline.

• Older adults may be especially prone to Apresoline's side effects.

• Follow a low-salt diet if your doctor has prescribed one.

 KEEP IN MIND...

∗ Take at mealtimes, if possible.

∗ Continue taking even if you begin to feel better.

∗ Don't drive until you know how drug affects you.

AquaMEPHYTON

AquaMEPHYTON is vitamin K. It promotes the formation of prothrombin, a substance that's necessary for blood clotting.

Why it's prescribed

Doctors prescribe AquaMEPHYTON to correct a low level of prothrombin in the body. AquaMEPHYTON comes in tablets; it's also available in an injectable form. Doctors usually prescribe the following amounts for adults; children's dosages appear in parentheses.

▶ **For low prothrombin,** 2 to 25 milligrams (mg) orally daily. (Children: 5 to 10 mg orally daily. Infants: 2 mg orally daily.)

▶ **For low prothrombin due to blood thinners,** 2.5 to 10 mg, repeated in 12 to 48 hours, as needed, based on laboratory test results.

How to take AquaMEPHYTON

• Take AquaMEPHYTON only as your doctor directs. Don't use this drug more often than prescribed.

If you miss a dose

Take the missed dose as soon as possible, and report it to your doctor. Don't take a double dose.

AquaMEPHYTON's OTHER NAMES

AquaMEPHYTON's generic name is phytonadione, or vitamin K1. Other brand names are Konakion and Mephyton.

 SIDE EFFECTS

Call your doctor if you have any of these possible drug side effects. Call *immediately* about any labeled "serious."

Serious: bronchospasm (wheezing, shortness of breath), severe allergic reaction (swelling of face, throat, and vocal cords)

Common: dizziness
Tip: Prevent dizziness by standing up slowly and taking care while walking.

Other: nausea, vomiting, seizurelike movements, abdominal cramps, sweating

 DRUG AND FOOD INTERACTIONS

Combining certain drugs and foods may alter drug action or produce unwanted side effects. Tell your doctor about your diet and other drugs you're taking, especially:
• anticoagulants (blood thinners) such as Coumadin
• Aquasol E
• green leafy vegetables, fish, pork, beef liver, and tomatoes
• mineral oil
• Questran.

If you suspect an overdose

Contact your doctor *immediately*. Excessive AquaMEPHYTON can cause yellow-tinged skin and eyes, nausea, vomiting, and extreme fatigue.

 Warnings

• Make sure your doctor knows your medical history. You may not be able to take AquaMEPHYTON if you have a drug allergy, G6PD deficiency, or liver problems.
• Make sure your doctor knows if you're pregnant or breast-feeding before you begin taking AquaMEPHYTON.

• See your doctor to have regular blood tests to adjust dose of AquaMEPHYTON.
• Before you have dental work done, tell your dentist that you're taking AquaMEPHYTON.

KEEP IN MIND...

* Notify doctor of missed dose.
* Don't increase foods high in vitamin K.
* Tell your doctors and dentist that you're taking AquaMEPHYTON.
* Keep appointments for regular blood tests.

Aquasol A

Aquasol A is vitamin A (retinol). Vitamin A is an essential vitamin, necessary for normal bone growth and healthy eyes and skin.

Why it's prescribed

Doctors prescribe Aquasol A for vitamin A deficiency. It comes in capsules, an oral solution, and an injectable form. Doctors usually prescribe the following doses; children's dosages appear in parentheses.

▶ **For severe vitamin A deficiency,** 100,000 to 500,000 International Units (IU) orally for three days, followed by 50,000 IU orally for 2 weeks; then 10,000 to 20,000 IU orally for 2 months. (Children: varied dosages by injection.)

▶ **To prevent recurrence of vitamin A deficiency,** adequate diet and RDA vitamin A supplements. (Children ages 1 to 8: 5,000 to 10,000 IU orally daily for 2 months, then adequate diet and RDA vitamin A supplements.)

How to take Aquasol A

• Take Aquasol A only as recommended by your doctor, dietician, or nutritionist.
• Oral solutions can be dropped into the mouth or mixed with food or fruit juice.

If you miss a dose

If you miss a dose for 1 or more days, there's no cause for concern

---

AQUASOL A'S OTHER NAMES

Aquasol A's generic name is retinol. Another brand name is Vitamin A.

SIDE EFFECTS

Call your doctor if you have any of these possible drug side effects. Call *immediately* about any labeled "serious."

Serious: bulging fontanel (soft spot on top of head) in infants, headache, double vision, severe headache, confusion or unusual excitement, seizures, severe vomiting, yellow-tinged skin, bleeding of gums, peeling of skin, especially on lips and palms

Common: fatigue, nausea, vomiting

Other: bone or joint pain; irritability; nighttime urination; discoloration of feet, palms of hands, or skin around nose and lips; appetite loss; hair loss; slow bone growth

DRUG INTERACTIONS

Combining certain drugs may alter their action or produce unwanted side effects. Tell your doctor about other drugs you're taking, especially:
• Accutane
• antibiotics, such as Achromycin and Myciguent
• anticholesterol drugs, such as Questran and Colestid
• birth control pills
• calcium supplements, multivitamins
• mineral oil.

---

since it takes some time for your body to become seriously low in vitamins. Resume your regular schedule. Don't take a double dose.

If you suspect an overdose

Contact your doctor *immediately.* Excessive Aquasol A can cause bleeding gums, bulging soft spot on top of infant's head, confusion, excitement, dizziness, drowsiness, double vision, and severe headache.

Warnings

• Make sure your doctor knows your medical history. You may not be able to take Aquasol A if you have malabsorption syndrome, chronic alcoholism, liver disease, kidney disease, or a sensitivity to vitamin A or if you're pregnant or breast-feeding.
• Older adults and young children may be especially prone to vitamin-A overdose.

KEEP IN MIND...

∗ Don't exceed recommended dose.

∗ Mix oral solution with juice or food.

∗ Don't start new drugs without asking doctor.

Aquasol E

Aquasol E is a vitamin E supplement. It helps to correct vitamin E deficiency in people whose bodies don't absorb fat properly. The body needs vitamin E to protect cell membranes.

Why it's prescribed

Doctors prescribe Aquasol E for people at risk for vitamin E deficiency due to surgical removal of the stomach or certain disorders of the bowel, liver, or pancreas. You can buy Aquasol E without a prescription. It comes in capsules and oral solution (for children). The following amounts are usually recommended.

▶ **Recommended daily allowance** (the amount most healthy people need to stay in good health):
• Children age 3 and under: 5 to 10 international units (IU)
• Children ages 4 to 10: 11.7 IU
• Males age 11 and over: 16.7 IU
• Females age 11 and over: 13 IU
• Pregnant women: 16.7 IU
• Breast-feeding women: 18 to 20 IU.

▶ **For vitamin E deficiency in premature infants and people with impaired fat absorption (cystic fibrosis) or biliary atresia,** 60 to 70 IU daily. Maximum daily dose is 300 IU. (Premature infants: 5 IU daily. Full-term infants: 5 IU per

AQUASOL E'S OTHER NAMES

Aquasol E's generic name is vitamin E (also known as d-alpha tocopherol acetate). Other brand names include Amino-Opti-E, E-200 I.U. Softgels, E-400 I.U., E-Complex-600, E-Vitamin Succinate, and Vita Plus E.

SIDE EFFECTS

Call your doctor if you have any of these possible drug side effects. Call *immediately* about any labeled "serious."

Serious: (in high doses) easy bleeding and bruising, blood clots (shortness of breath, chest pain, pain in legs, anxiety)

Common: none reported

Other: (in high doses) blurred vision, diarrhea, nausea, vomiting, dizziness, headache, fatigue

DRUG INTERACTIONS

Combining certain drugs may alter their action or produce unwanted side effects. Tell your doctor about other drugs you're taking, especially:
• anticoagulants (blood thinners) such as Coumadin
• AquaMEPHYTON
• Questran
• mineral oil (such as in some laxatives).

quart of formula. Children: 1 IU for each 2.2 pounds of body weight daily.)

How to take Aquasol E

• If you're taking this supplement without a prescription, follow any precautions on the label. If the doctor has prescribed it, follow the doctor's directions exactly.
• Swallow the capsules whole; don't open them.
• Drop the liquid directly into the child's mouth or mix it with fruit juice, cereal, or another food.
• Don't take more than the recommended daily amount. Taking more than 400 units daily for a long time may cause other harmful effects, such as bruising, bleeding, and blurred vision.
• Store Aqyasol E in a tightly closed, light-resistant container to prevent deterioration of the drug.

If you miss a dose

If your doctor has advised you to take Aquasol E, try to remember to take it daily. Otherwise, don't worry if you miss a few days; it takes some time for your body to become seriously deficient in vitamins.

If you suspect an overdose

Contact your doctor *immediately*. Excessive Aquasol E may cause high blood pressure (headache, swelling of legs, visual disturbances).

Warnings

• Make sure your doctor knows your medical history. You may not be able to take Aquasol E if you have bleeding, because Aquasol E could make this condition worse.

- If you're pregnant or breast-feeding, take this and other dietary supplements only as recommended by your doctor. Taking excessive amounts could harm you or your baby.
- If your baby is using an unfortified formula, ask your doctor whether you should give the baby vitamin supplements.

- If your diet is high in polyunsaturated fats, your vitamin E requirement may be higher. Your doctor may recommend that you eat more foods that are high in vitamin E. These foods include green leafy vegetables, vegetable oil, nuts, wheat germ, eggs, meat, liver, dairy products, and cereal.
- Many people take vitamin E for its antioxidant properties, believing that it may help prevent cancer and other conditions. These effects are unproven; talk to your doctor before taking it on your own. Taking very large amounts of Aquasol E could cause a blood clot in a vein.

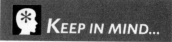 **KEEP IN MIND...**

* Don't open capsules.
* Drop liquid directly into mouth or mix with food or beverage.
* Don't take more than prescribed or recommended daily amount.
* Immediately report signs of bruising or bleeding (blood in urine or stools, nosebleeds).

Aralen Phosphate

Aralen is used to prevent or treat malaria. Researchers think it binds to and alters the genes of the parasites that cause malaria.

Why it's prescribed

Doctors prescribe Aralen Phosphate to prevent malaria and to treat acute malaria attacks. Aralen Phosphate comes in tablets. It's also available in an injectable form. Doctors usually prescribe the following amounts for adults; children's dosages are in parentheses.

▶ **To treat malaria,** 2 tablets, then 1 tablet in 6 to 8 hours, followed by 1 tablet a day for the next 2 days. (Children: initially 10 mg for each 2.2 pounds [lb] of body weight orally, then 5 mg for each 2.2 lb at 6, 24, and 48 hours. Dosage should not exceed 10 mg for each 2.2 lb in 24 hours.)

▶ **To prevent malaria,** 1 tablet a week (Children: 5 mg a week) begun 2 weeks before probable exposure and continued for 4 to 6 weeks afterward.

How to take Aralen Phosphate

• Take Aralen Phosphate exactly as your doctor has directed.
• Take this drug immediately before or after meals.
• If you're using it once a week, take it on the same day each week. If you're taking two daily doses, take with breakfast and dinner.
• If you're using Aralen Phosphate to treat malaria, keep taking it for the full time prescribed, even if you begin to feel better.

ARALEN PHOSPHATE'S OTHER NAME

Aralen Phosphate's generic name is chloroquine phosphate.

 SIDE EFFECTS

Call your doctor if you have any of these possible drug side effects. Call *immediately* about any labeled "serious."

Serious: blood problems (bleeding gums, nosebleeds, fatigue, weakness)

Common: blurred vision
Tip: Be sure to have occasional eye examinations.

Other: headache, fatigue, irritability, nightmares, seizures, dizziness, low blood pressure (dizziness, weakness, fatigue), ringing in ears, appetite loss, stomach cramps, diarrhea, nausea, vomiting, mouth sores, itching, skin problems
Tip: Avoid excessive sun exposure.

 DRUG INTERACTIONS

Combining certain drugs may alter their action or produce unwanted side effects. Tell your doctor about other drugs you're taking, especially:
• ALternaGEL, Basaljel, Kaopectate, Milk of Magnesia, Riopan (take 1 or 2 hours before or after Aralen)
• Tagamet.

If you miss a dose

Adjust your schedule as follows:
• If you take one dose every 7 days, take the missed dose as soon as possible; then return to your regular schedule.
• If you take one dose a day, take the missed dose as soon as possible. If you don't remember until the next day, skip the missed dose and take your next dose as scheduled.
• If you take more than one dose a day, take the missed dose right away if you remember within an hour. If you don't remember until later, skip the missed dose and take your next dose as scheduled.

 If you suspect an overdose

Contact your doctor *immediately.* Excessive Aralen Phosphate can cause headache, drowsiness, vision disturbances, cardiovascular collapse (loss of blood pressure, ineffective heart pumping), seizures, and respiratory failure.

 Warnings

• Make sure your doctor knows your medical history. You may not be able to take Aralen Phosphate if you have liver disease, alcoholism, G6PD deficiency, or psoriasis.
• Children should avoid long-term use of Aralen Phosphate; they're extremely susceptible to this drug's toxic effects.

KEEP IN MIND...

* Take before or after meals.
* Take on regular schedule for full time prescribed.
* Avoid sun exposure.

Aristocort

Aristocort is a cortisone-like drug used to relieve inflammation, swelling, redness, itching, and allergic reactions.

Why it's prescribed

Doctors prescribe Aristocort as an adrenal gland hormone replacement in treating Addison's disease, to reduce inflammation, or to suppress the immune system. It comes in tablets and a syrup. Doctors usually prescribe the following amounts for adults; children's dosages are in parentheses.

▶ **For severe inflammation or to induce immunosuppression,** 4 to 60 milligrams (mg) a day in a single dose or divided into equal doses. (Children: 416 micrograms [mcg] to 1.7 mg for each 2.2 pounds [lb] of body weight a day in a single dose or divided into equal doses.)

▶ **For Addison's disease or adrenal insufficiency,** 4 to 12 mg a day in a single dose or divided into equal doses. (Children: 117 mcg for each 2.2 lb a day in a single dose or divided into equal doses.)

How to take Aristocort

• Take this drug exactly as your doctor has directed.
• Keep Aristocort syrup in the refrigerator; don't freeze it.
• If you're taking one dose a day, take it in the morning.
• Don't stop taking this drug abruptly or without your doctor's approval.

ARISTOCORT'S OTHER NAMES

Aristocort's generic name is triamcinolone. Other brand names are Kenacort; and, in Canada, Ledercort.

 ## SIDE EFFECTS

Call your doctor if you have any of these possible drug side effects. Call *immediately* about any labeled "serious."

Serious: congestive heart failure (shortness of breath), high blood pressure (headache, swelling of legs)

Common: unusual feeling of well-being, trouble sleeping, stomach ulcers, fatigue, muscle weakness, joint pain, fever, nausea, dizziness, fainting
Tips: To improve your sleeping, take your last dose several hours before bedtime. To reduce stomach irritation, take with food.

Other: uncharacteristic behavior, cataracts, glaucoma, appetite increase, delayed wound healing, skin eruptions, osteoporosis, abnormal hair growth, infections, high blood sugar level (increased urination, thirst, and hunger), growth suppression (in children)
Tips: Call your doctor if your wounds or cuts seem to heal slowly. If you're on long-term therapy, call if you notice sudden weight gain.

 ## DRUG INTERACTIONS

Combining certain drugs may alter their action or produce unwanted side effects. Tell your doctor about other drugs you're taking, especially:
• anticoagulants (blood thinners) such as Coumadin
• aspirin, Indocin, Advil, and other nonsteroidal anti-inflammatory drugs (NSAIDs)
• barbiturates such as Solfoton
• Dilantin
• Diuril, HydroDIURIL
• Rifadin
• skin-test antigens (delay skin testing until you've completed Aristocort therapy)
• vaccines and toxoids (get doctor's approval before immunizations).

If you miss a dose

Adjust your schedule as follows:
• If you take one dose a day, take the missed dose as soon as possible; then take your next dose as scheduled.
• If you take several doses a day, take the missed dose as soon as possible; then resume your regular schedule. If you don't remember until the next dose is due, take a double dose.

 ## If you suspect an overdose

Contact your doctor *immediately*. Excessive Aristocort can cause muscle weakness, a round "moon" face, fat pads on your face or trunk, swelling, or osteoporosis (bone deterioration).

Continued on next page ▶

X Warnings

• Make sure your doctor knows your medical history. You may not be able to take Aristocort if you've ever had stomach ulcers, kidney disease, high blood pressure, osteoporosis, diabetes, underactive thyroid, cirrhosis, ulcerative colitis, blood clot, seizures, myasthenia gravis, heart failure, tuberculosis, herpes of the eye, or emotional instability.

• If you're pregnant or breast-feeding, check with your doctor before you start taking Aristocort.
• Be aware that this drug may make older adults more prone to osteoporosis.
• If you're diabetic, be aware that this drug may increase your insulin requirements.
• Carry medical identification stating that you're using Aristocort.

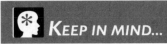

KEEP IN MIND...

* Don't stop taking abruptly or without doctor's consent.
* Avoid contact with people who are ill.
* Call doctor about slow wound healing.
* Carry medical identification stating that you're using Aristocort.

Armour Thyroid

Armour Thyroid stimulates the metabolism in all body tissues. Without thyroid hormone, metabolism slows down and becomes sluggish.

Why it's prescribed

Doctors prescribe Armour Thyroid when the body's thyroid gland isn't producing enough or any thyroid hormone. This drug comes in tablets. Doctors usually prescribe the following amounts.

▶ **For mild hypothyroidism in adults,** initially, 60 milligrams (mg) a day, increased by 60 mg every 30 days until desired response occurs. Usual maintenance dosage, 60 to 180 mg a day as a single dose.

▶ **For severe hypothyroidism in adults and congenital or severe hypothyroidism in children,** initially, 15 mg a day, increased by 30 mg a day after 2 weeks and to 60 mg a day 2 weeks later. After 2 months, dosage increased to 120 mg a day as needed for 2 months, then increased to 180 mg a day as needed.

How to take Armour Thyroid

• Take your dose at the same time each day, preferably before breakfast, to maintain constant hormone levels and to avoid insomnia.

If you miss a dose

Take the missed dose as soon as possible. However, if it's almost time

ARMOUR THYROID'S OTHER NAMES

Armour Thyroid's generic name is thyroid USP (desiccated). Other brand names include Thyrar, Thyroid Strong, Thyroid USP Enseals, and Westhroid.

 SIDE EFFECTS

Call your doctor if you have any of these possible drug side effects. Call *immediately* about any labeled "serious."

Serious: changes in heart rhythm (rapid heartbeat), increased blood pressure (headache, blurred vision), cardiac collapse (severe low blood pressure, extreme dizziness and fainting)

Common: nervousness, insomnia, fever, vomiting

Other: twitching, infection, chest pain, diarrhea, abdominal cramps, weight loss, heat intolerance, sweating, menstrual irregularities

 DRUG INTERACTIONS

Combining certain drugs may alter their action or produce unwanted side effects. Tell your doctor about other drugs you're taking, especially:
• anticoagulants (blood thinners) such as Coumadin
• cholestyramine (Questran)
• epinephrine and related drugs, such as Primatene Mist
• insulin and oral diabetes drugs, such as Diabeta and Micronase.

for your next dose, skip the missed dose and take your next dose as scheduled. Don't take a double dose.

 If you suspect an overdose

Contact your doctor *immediately*. Excessive Armour Thyroid can cause agitation, nervousness, palpitations, tremors, sweating, and chest pain.

✕ Warnings

• Make sure your doctor knows your medical history. You may not be able to take Armour Thyroid if your hypothyroidism follows a recent heart attack or if you have untreated severe hypothyroidism, uncorrected adrenal insufficiency, angina, high blood pressure, heart or blood vessel disease, lung disease, diabetes, or kidney problems.

• Tell the doctor that you're taking Armour Thyroid before having any thyroid function tests.
• Don't change brands.

✱ KEEP IN MIND...

∗ Take at same time each day, preferably before breakfast.

∗ Don't store in a warm, humid area.

∗ Call doctor immediately about any chest pain, palpitations, sweating, nervousness, shortness of breath, rapid heartbeat, or unusual bruising or bleeding.

Artane

Artane is a muscle-affecting drug used to treat Parkinson's disease. By improving muscle control and reducing stiffness, it allows more normal movements.

Why it's prescribed

Doctors prescribe Artane to help manage symptoms of Parkinson's disease or to control severe reactions to certain drugs. Artane comes in tablets, sustained-release capsules, and elixir. Doctors usually prescribe the following amounts for adults.

▶ **For all forms of parkinsonism and drug-induced parkinsonism and as a supplement to Larodopa in managing parkinsonism,** 1 milligram (mg) on the first day, 2 mg on the second day; then increased by 2 mg every 3 to 5 days until total of 6 to 10 mg a day is given.

How to take Artane

- Take this drug exactly as your doctor has directed. If you're taking the tablets or elixir, the doctor may instruct you to take three daily doses with meals, or four daily doses (with the last dose taken before bedtime), or may switch you to sustained-release capsules taken twice daily.
- Some people develop a tolerance to Artane. If this happens, the doctor may need to increase the amount you take.

ARTANE'S OTHER NAMES

Artane's generic name is trihexyphenidyl hydrochloride. Other brand names include Trihexane, Trihexy-2, Trihexy-5; and, in Canada, Aparkane, Apo-Trihex, and Novohexyldyl.

 SIDE EFFECTS

Call your doctor if you have any of these possible drug side effects.

Serious: none reported

Common: dry mouth
Tip: To relieve dry mouth, use cool drinks, ice chips, or sugarless gum or hard candy.

Other: nervousness, dizziness, headache, restlessness, hallucinations, unusual feeling of well-being, memory loss, fast pulse, blurred vision, constipation, nausea, difficulty urinating
Tips: Avoid activities that require alertness until you know how Artane affects you. Call your doctor if you start to have trouble urinating.

 DRUG INTERACTIONS

Combining certain drugs may alter their action or produce unwanted side effects. Tell your doctor about other drugs you're taking, especially:
- Symmetrel.

If you miss a dose

Take the missed dose as soon as possible. However, if it's within 2 hours of your next dose, skip the missed dose and take your next dose as scheduled.

 If you suspect an overdose

Contact your doctor *immediately.* Excessive Artane may cause agitation, restlessness, disorientation, confusion, hallucinations, delusions, anxiety, blurred vision, dry mucous membranes, difficulty swallowing, increased body temperature, headache, fast pulse and breathing, high blood pressure (headache), and flushed, dry, hot skin.

Warnings

- Make sure your doctor knows your medical history. You may not be able to take Artane if you've ever had an enlarged prostate, blockage in the urinary or digestive tract, glaucoma, or a heart, kidney, or liver disorder.
- Tell your doctor if you are pregnant or breast-feeding.
- Be aware that children and older adults may be especially prone to Artane's side effects.

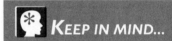 **KEEP IN MIND...**

* Avoid activities that require alertness until you know how drug affects you.

* Relieve dry mouth with cool drinks, ice chips, or sugarless gum or candy.

* Call doctor about trouble urinating.

Asacol

Asacol reduces inflammation and other symptoms of bowel disease. Researchers think it works by inhibiting the production of the hormone prostaglandin in the bowel.

Why it's prescribed

Doctors prescribe Asacol to treat inflammatory bowel diseases such as ulcerative colitis. It comes in tablets. Doctors usually prescribe the following amounts for adults.
▶ **For ulcerative colitis, inflammation of the rectum and anus, or inflammation of the rectum and sigmoid colon,** two 400-milligram tablets three times a day.

How to take Asacol

• Be sure to swallow tablets whole.
• Take Asacol with a full (8-ounce) glass of water before meals and at bedtime.
• Take Asacol only as your doctor directs.
• Keep taking Asacol for the full treatment time prescribed by your doctor, even if you feel better within several days. Don't skip any doses.

If you miss a dose

If you remember the same night, take the missed dose as soon as possible. If you don't remember until the

ASACOL'S OTHER NAMES

Asacol's generic name is mesalamine. Other brand names include Pentasa and Rowasa.

 SIDE EFFECTS

Call your doctor if you have any of these possible drug side effects. Call *immediately* about any labeled "serious."

Serious: rash, wheezing, itching, hives, fever, severe headache, pancolitis (severe pain, cramping, bloody diarrhea), chest pain, shortness of breath, yellow-tinged skin and eyes

Common: stomach pain and cramps

Other: headache, dizziness, fatigue, hair loss, gas, diarrhea, nausea, allergic reaction (itching, rash, hives), wheezing, appetite loss, unusual tiredness

Tip: Mild headache and stomach discomfort usually go away as your body adjusts to the drug. Check with your doctor if they persist or become bothersome.

 DRUG INTERACTIONS

Combining certain drugs may alter their action or produce unwanted side effects. Tell your doctor about other drugs you're taking, especially:
• lactulose
• omeprazole
• salicylates such as aspirin
• sulfasalazine

next morning, skip the missed dose and resume your regular schedule.

 If you suspect an overdose

Consult your doctor.

 Warnings

• Make sure your doctor knows your medical history. You may not be able to take Asacol if you are allergic to aspirin or have kidney disease.
• Have regular medical checkups so the doctor can evaluate your progress.

 KEEP IN MIND...

* Take before meals and at bedtime.
* Swallow tablets whole with 8-ounce glass of water.
* Keep taking for full treatment time prescribed.
* Don't skip any doses.
* Expect headache and stomach discomfort to be temporary.

Ascorbicap

Ascorbicap is vitamin C (ascorbic acid). Vitamin C is necessary for cell activity and growth.

Why it's taken

Ascorbicap is taken for vitamin C deficiency (scurvy), burns, and wound healing and before stomach surgery. Ascorbicap and other brands of vitamin C are available without a prescription in tablets, effervescent tablets, sugar-free tablets, time-released tablets and capsules, liquid, solution, syrup, and an injectable form. By prescription, Ascorbicap comes in tablets, extended-release capsules, caplets, and liquid. The following doses are usually recommended; children's dosages appear in parentheses.

▶ **For scurvy,** 100 to 500 milligrams (mg) a day orally, then a maintenance dosage of 50 mg a day. (Children: 100 to 300 mg a day orally, then a maintenance dosage of 35 mg a day. Infants: 50 to 100 mg a day orally.)

▶ **For poor nutrition,** 45 to 60 mg a day orally. (Children and infants: at least 35 to 40 mg a day orally.)

▶ **For burns, wounds, and prolonged healing,** 200 to 500 mg a day orally. (Children: 100 to 200 mg a day orally.)

▶ **Before stomach surgery,** 1 gram daily for 4 to 7 days.

How to take Ascorbicap

• Take Ascorbicap only as recommended by your doctor, dietician, or nutritionist.

• Drop oral solutions into your mouth or mix with food.
• Completely dissolve effervescent tablets in water, and then drink all of the liquid.

If you miss a dose

Take the missed dose as soon as possible. But if it's almost time for your next dose, skip the missed dose and take your next dose as scheduled. Don't take a double dose.

 If you suspect an overdose

Consult your doctor.

 Warnings

• Before taking Ascorbicap, consult your doctor if you have an aspirin allergy, asthma, diabetes, kidney problems, or drug or alcohol addiction.
• If you're breast-feeding, check with your doctor before you begin taking Ascorbicap.
• Older adults and infants may be especially prone to Ascorbicap's side effects.

 SIDE EFFECTS

Call your doctor if you have any of these possible drug side effects.

Serious: none noted

Common: fatigue, insomnia, diarrhea, heartburn, nausea and vomiting
Tip: Be cautious when driving or operating machinery due to the potential for fatigue.

Others: headache, tooth erosion, kidney stones
Tip: Increase fluid intake to avoid kidney stones.

 DRUG INTERACTIONS

Combining certain drugs may alter their action or produce unwanted side effects. Tell your doctor about other drugs you're taking, especially:
• amphetamines such as in many diet pills
• anticoagulants (blood thinners) such as Coumadin
• aspirin and aspiring-containing products
• birth control pills
• iron pills such as Feosol
• sulfa drugs such as Bactrim
• tobacco (smokers may need higher Ascorbicap dosage)
• tricyclic antidepressants, such as Elavil and Pamelor.

 KEEP IN MIND...

* Take only as directed.
* Mix oral solutions with food or liquids.
* Smokers may need more Ascorbicap than nonsmokers.

Asendin

Asendin, a tricyclic antidepressant, is thought to ease depression by altering the activity of certain chemicals in the brain.

Why it's prescribed

Doctors prescribe Asendin to treat depression. Asendin comes in tablets. Doctors usually prescribe the following amounts for adults.

▶ **For depression,** initially 50 milligrams (mg) two or three times a day, increased to 100 mg two or three times a day on the 3rd day if tolerated.

How to take Asendin

• Take Asendin exactly as directed.
• Take it with food, unless your doctor tells you otherwise.
• When effective dosage is established, entire dosage may be taken at bedtime.

If you miss a dose

Adjust your schedule as follows:
• If you usually take one dose a day at bedtime, call your doctor for instructions. Don't take the missed dose in the morning because it may cause disturbing side effects during the day.
• If you take more than one dose a day, take the missed dose as soon as possible. However, if it's almost time for your next dose, skip the missed dose and take your next dose as scheduled. Don't take a double dose.

ASENDIN'S OTHER NAME

Asendin's generic name is amoxapine.

SIDE EFFECTS

Call your doctor if you have any of these possible drug side effects. Call *immediately* about any labeled "serious."

Serious: seizures; fever with fast pulse, fast breathing, and sweating; allergic reaction (swelling, rash, fever)

Common: drowsiness, dizziness, blurred vision, dry mouth, constipation
Tips: Until you know how Asendin affects you, don't drive or perform other activities that require you to be alert. To prevent dizziness, stand up slowly. To relieve dry mouth, use sugarless gum or hard candy, ice chips, or a saliva substitute.

Other: weakness, confusion, headache, nervousness, ringing in ears, sensitivity to sunlight.
Tip: Avoid direct sunlight if possible. Wear protective clothing and use a sunblock with a skin protection factor (SPF) of 15 or higher.

DRUG INTERACTIONS

Combining certain drugs may alter their action or produce unwanted side effects. Tell your doctor about other drugs you're taking, especially:
• alcohol
• antidepressants, called MAO inhibitors, such as Nardil
• barbiturates (found in some sleeping pills and seizure drugs)
• epinephrine
• Ritalin
• Tagamet.

If you suspect an overdose

Contact your doctor *immediately*. Excessive Asendin can cause agitation, confusion, hallucinations, fever, and seizures.

Warnings

• Make sure your doctor knows your medical history. You may not be able to take Asendin if you're breast-feeding or if you become pregnant while taking this drug.

• Be aware that children and older adults may be vulnerable to Asendin's side effects.
• If you have diabetes, be aware that this drug may affect your blood sugar level.

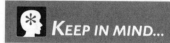

KEEP IN MIND...

* Take with food.
* Stand up slowly to avoid dizziness.
* Don't drive until you know how drug affects you.

Aspirin

Aspirin is one of several drugs called salicylates. Researchers suspect that it works to relieve pain and inflammation by preventing the body from producing hormones called prostaglandins. Aspirin reduces fever by widening blood vessels in the skin, which helps heat to leave the body more rapidly.

Why it's taken

Aspirin is taken for mild pain or fever, rheumatoid arthritis, osteoarthritis, and other inflammatory conditions. Doctors also prescribe it to lessen the chance of heart attack, stroke, or other problems that may occur when blood clots block a blood vessel. Aspirin is a nonprescription drug that comes in capsules, tablets, chewable tablets, chewing gum tablets, delayed-release (enteric-coated) tablets, extended-release tablets, and suppositories. The following amounts are recommended for adults; children's dosages appear in parentheses, except for juvenile rheumatoid arthritis.

▶ **For rheumatoid arthritis, osteoarthritis, or other inflammatory**

SIDE EFFECTS

Call your doctor if you have any of these possible drug side effects. Call *immediately* about any labeled "serious."

Serious: Reye's syndrome (vomiting, extreme fatigue, agitation, confusion), allergic reaction (trouble breathing; wheezing; flushing, redness, or other changes in skin color; hives; itching; swelling of eyelids, face, or lips)

Common: ringing in ears, nausea, vomiting, stomach upset, rash
Tips: Call your doctor immediately about ringing in the ears; this indicates too much aspirin. To avoid stomach upset, take your doses after meals or with food (except for enteric-coated tablets and suppositories).

Other: bruising

DRUG INTERACTIONS

Combining certain drugs may alter their action or produce unwanted side effects. Tell your doctor about other drugs you're taking, especially:
- alcohol (may cause stomach problems)
- antacids in high doses
- anticoagulants (blood thinners) such as Coumadin
- Anturane
- Benemid
- beta blockers (for high blood pressure or chest pain), such as Corgard, Inderal, Lopressor, and Tenormin
- corticosteroids, steroids
- diabetes drugs (except insulin)
- drugs used to acidify the urine (such as ammonium chloride)
- Mexate
- other nonsteroidal anti-inflammatory drugs (NSAIDs) for pain relief such as Advil.

conditions, initially 2.4 to 3.6 grams (g) orally each day divided into several equal doses spaced 4 to 6 hours apart. Maintenance dosage is 3.6 to 5.4 g each day divided into equal doses.

▶ **For juvenile rheumatoid arthritis,** children weighing 55 pounds (lb) or less: 60 to 90 milligrams (mg) for each 2.2 lb of body weight orally each day divided into equal doses spaced 4 to 6 hours apart. Children weighing more than 55

lb: 2.4 to 3.6 g orally each day divided into equal doses.

▶ **For mild pain or fever,** 325 to 650 mg orally or rectally every 4 hours as needed. (Children over age 11: same as adults. Children ages 2 to 11: 6.5 mg for each 2.2 lb of body weight each day orally or rectally divided into four to six equal doses.)

▶ **To help prevent blood clotting,** 1.3 g orally each day divided into two to four equal doses.

▶ **To lower the risk of heart attack in people with a history of heart attack or unstable angina,** 160 to 325 mg orally each day.

How to take aspirin

• If you're treating yourself, follow the package instructions carefully.

• If your doctor prescribed aspirin or gave you special instructions on how to use it, follow those instructions exactly. Don't use more of it or use it more often than recommended.

• Take the tablets and capsules with a full glass (8 ounces) of water. To prevent irritation that may lead to trouble swallowing, stay upright for 15 to 30 minutes after taking aspirin.

• Chewable tablets can be chewed, dissolved in liquid, crushed, or swallowed whole. Enteric-coated tablets must be swallowed whole. Check with your pharmacist about how to take extended-release tablets; some can be broken (but not crushed); others must be swallowed whole.

• If you're using a suppository and it's too soft to insert, chill it in the refrigerator for 30 minutes or run cold water over the foil wrapper.

• If you're taking aspirin to prevent heart attack, stroke, or other problems caused by blood clots, take only the amount ordered. Talk to your doctor if you need extra medication to relieve pain or fever; the doctor may not want you to take extra aspirin.

• Don't use any aspirin product if it has a strong, vinegar-like odor. This odor means the drug is breaking down and is no longer effective.

If you miss a dose

If you're taking aspirin regularly and you miss a dose, take the missed dose as soon as possible. However, if it's almost time for your next dose, skip the missed dose and take your next dose as scheduled. Don't take a double dose.

If you suspect an overdose

Call your doctor *immediately* if you experience ringing in your ears or hearing loss; this may indicate that you have too much aspirin in your system (aspirin toxicity).

Warnings

• Make sure your doctor knows your medical history. Other conditions may affect your use of aspirin.

• Don't take aspirin if you're in the last trimester of pregnancy, unless your doctor directs you to.

• Don't give aspirin to children or teenagers who have fever or other symptoms of a viral infection; it puts them at risk for a serious disorder called Reye's syndrome.

• Older adults may be especially prone to aspirin's side effects.

• Don't take aspirin to reduce your chance of heart attack or stroke unless your doctor advises you to. The drug has blood-thinning properties that may increase your chance of serious bleeding.

• Check the labels of all nonprescription and prescription drugs and skin products (shampoo, for example) for aspirin, other salicylates, or salicylic acid. Count these products as part of your total aspirin dosage for the day to avoid overdose. Pepto-Bismol is an example of a commonly used nonprescription drug that contains salicylates.

• Don't take aspirin for 5 days before surgery (including dental surgery) unless your doctor or dentist tells you to. It may cause bleeding problems.

• Don't use the chewable forms of aspirin for 7 days after having your tonsils removed, a tooth pulled, or other dental or mouth surgery.

• Don't place aspirin directly on a tooth or gum surface because it may cause a burn and erode the tooth enamel.

• See your doctor at regular intervals if you're taking aspirin for more than 10 days (5 days for children) or if you're taking large amounts.

• Call the doctor if you're taking aspirin to relieve pain and the pain lasts for more than 10 days (5 days for children) or gets worse, if new symptoms occur, or if redness or swelling occurs.

• Consult your doctor if you're taking aspirin to reduce a fever and the fever lasts more than 3 days, returns, or gets worse; if new symptoms occur; or if redness or swelling occurs.

• If you're taking aspirin for a sore throat and your throat is very painful or if the pain lasts more than 2 days or occurs with or is followed by fever, headache, rash, nausea, or vomiting, you should also notify your doctor.

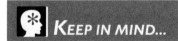 **KEEP IN MIND...**

∗ Take after meals or with food (except for enteric-coated tablets and suppositories).

∗ Take tablets and capsules with full glass of water.

∗ Swallow enteric-coated tablets whole.

∗ Don't give to children or teenagers with viral symptoms.

∗ Call doctor if pain or fever persists or worsens.

Atarax

Atarax is believed to induce calm and relieve anxiety by suppressing certain activity in the nervous system. It also inhibits the effects of histamine, a substance produced by the body that causes sneezing, itching, runny nose, and additional symptoms of colds, hay fever, and other allergies.

Why it's prescribed

Doctors prescribe Atarax to help control anxiety and stress, to relieve itching caused by allergies, or to treat nausea and vomiting. Atarax comes in tablets, capsules, syrup, and an oral liquid. It's also available in an injectable form. Doctors usually prescribe the following amounts for adults; children's dosages are in parentheses.

▶ **For anxiety,** 50 to 100 milligrams (mg) orally four times a day. (Children under age 6: 50 mg orally daily divided into three or four equal doses. Children age 6 and over: 50 to 100 mg orally daily divided into equal doses.)

▶ **For itching due to allergies,** 25 mg orally three or four times a day. (Children under age 6: 50 mg orally daily divided into three or four equal doses. Children age 6 and over: 50 to 100 mg orally daily divided into equal doses.)

ATARAX'S OTHER NAMES

Atarax's generic name is hydroxyzine hydrochloride. Other brand names include Anxanil, Atozine, Hydroxacen, Hyzine-50, Quiess, Vistaject-25, Vistaject-50, Vistaril, Vistazine 50; and, in Canada, Apo-Hydroxyzine, Multipax, and Novohydroxyzin.

 SIDE EFFECTS

Call your doctor if you have any of these possible drug side effects.

Serious: none reported

Common: drowsiness, dry mouth, stomach upset

Tips: Make sure you know how you react to Atarax before you perform activities that require you to be totally alert. To relieve dry mouth, use sugarless hard candy or gum, ice chips, mouthwash, or a saliva substitute. To reduce stomach upset, take your doses with food, water, or milk.

Other: involuntary muscle movements

 DRUG INTERACTIONS

Combining certain drugs may alter their action or produce unwanted side effects. Tell your doctor about other drugs you're taking, especially:

• alcohol (can cause drug overdose)

• other drugs that make you relaxed and sleepy, such as sleeping pills and tranquilizers.

How to take Atarax

• Take this drug exactly as directed by your doctor.

If you miss a dose

Take the missed dose as soon as possible. However, if it's almost time for your next regular dose, skip the missed dose and take your next dose as scheduled. Don't take a double dose.

 If you suspect an overdose

Contact your doctor *immediately*. Excessive Atarax may cause seizures, clumsiness, drowsiness, difficulty breathing, mouth dryness, and hallucinations.

 Warnings

• Make sure your doctor knows your medical history. If you're pregnant or think you may be, check with your doctor before you start taking Atarax.

• Don't take Atarax if you're breast-feeding.

• Children and older adults are especially prone to Atarax's side effects.

• Atarax may cover up symptoms of appendicitis or drug overdose. If you develop symptoms of appendicitis (such as stomach pain, cramping, or tenderness) or if you think you may have taken an overdose of another drug, tell your doctor you're taking Atarax.

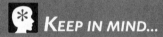 **KEEP IN MIND...**

∗ Take with food, water, or milk.

∗ Don't drink alcoholic beverages while on Atarax.

∗ Avoid driving until you know how drug affects you.

Ativan

Ativan is one of several drugs called benzodiazepines. It acts directly on the brain to reduce anxiety, treat seizures, relieve insomnia, and induce relaxation or sedation.

Why it's prescribed

Doctors prescribe Ativan to treat anxiety, tension, agitation, irritability, and insomnia (difficulty sleeping). In the hospital, it may be given as premedication before surgery. Ativan comes in regular tablets, sublingual tablets (placed under the tongue), and an oral solution. It's also available in an injectable form. Doctors usually prescribe the following amounts for adults.

▶ **For anxiety,** 2 to 6 milligrams (mg) orally a day divided into equal doses. Maximum dosage is 10 mg a day.

▶ **For insomnia due to anxiety,** 2 to 4 mg orally at bedtime.

How to take Ativan

• Check the label carefully and take only the amount prescribed. Don't take Ativan longer than directed. Extended use may cause drug dependence and withdrawal symptoms.
• Don't stop taking Ativan without your doctor's approval.

If you miss a dose

If you're only an hour off schedule, take the missed dose right away. If

ATIVAN'S OTHER NAMES

Ativan's generic name is lorazepam. Canadian brand names include Apo-Lorazepam, Novolorazem, and Nu-Loraz.

 SIDE EFFECTS

Call your doctor if you have any of these possible drug side effects. Call *immediately* about any labeled "serious."

Serious: extreme agitation (after stopping suddenly in people who are physically dependent on the drug)

Common: drowsiness, lack of energy, hangover
Tip: Avoid potentially hazardous activities, such as driving a car, until you know how Ativan affects you.

Other: fainting, restlessness, visual disturbances, dry mouth

 DRUG INTERACTIONS

Combining certain drugs may alter their action or produce unwanted side effects. Tell your doctor about other drugs you're taking, especially:
• alcohol and other drugs that make you relaxed and sleepy, such as sleeping pills and tranquilizers
• digoxin
• tobacco.

you don't remember it within an hour, skip the missed dose and take your next dose as scheduled. Don't take a double dose.

 If you suspect an overdose

Contact your doctor *immediately*. Excessive Ativan can cause confusion, staggering, slurred speech, extreme drowsiness, and weakness.

 Warnings

• Make sure your doctor knows your medical history. You may not be able to take Ativan if you have a history of psychosis (mental illness), myasthenia gravis, Parkinson's disease, respiratory or liver problems, drug addiction, or drug abuse.

• Don't take Ativan if you have glaucoma.
• If you're pregnant or breast-feeding, tell your doctor before you start taking Ativan.
• Be aware that older adults are especially likely to become dizzy, drowsy, light-headed, clumsy, and less alert when taking Ativan.

KEEP IN MIND...

∗ Avoid driving until you know how drug affects you.

∗ Take only as long as directed.

∗ Don't stop taking without doctor's approval.

Atromid-S

Atromid-S is used to reduce the amount of fatty substances, such as cholesterol and triglycerides, in the blood. It seems to interfere with the body's ability to make blood fats and to speed the removal of fats from the body. This effect may help prevent heart attacks and other problems that can occur when fatty substances clog the blood vessels.

Why it's prescribed

Doctors prescribe Atromid-S to lower the levels of cholesterol and triglycerides in the blood. It comes in capsules. Doctors usually prescribe the following amounts for adults.

▶ **To reduce high levels of fats in the blood,** 2 grams a day divided into two to four equal doses. (Some people may respond to lower doses.)

How to take Atromid-S

• Take this drug exactly as your doctor has prescribed.
• Don't break, chew, or crush the capsules; swallow them whole.
• Don't stop taking Atromid-S abruptly; check with your doctor.

If you miss a dose

Take the missed dose as soon as possible. However, if it's almost time for your next dose, skip the missed dose and take your next dose as scheduled. Don't take a double dose.

ATROMID-S'S OTHER NAMES

Atromid-S's generic name is clofibrate. Canadian brand names include Claripex and Novofibrate.

 SIDE EFFECTS

Call your doctor if you have any of these possible drug side effects. Call *immediately* about any labeled "serious."

Serious: irregular heartbeat, kidney failure (decreased urination, itching, confusion), blood problems (fever, chills, fatigue, infection)

Common: nausea, diarrhea, vomiting, stomach upset, weight gain
Tip: Take with food or right after meals to avoid stomach upset.

Other: fatigue, weakness, mouth sores, gas, rash, itching
Tips: Try to get extra rest while on this drug. Perform frequent mouth care with a nonalcoholic rinse.

 DRUG INTERACTIONS

Combining certain drugs may alter their action or produce unwanted side effects. Tell your doctor about other drugs you're taking, especially:
• anticoagulants (blood thinners) such as Coumadin
• Benemid
• birth control pills
• Lasix
• oral diabetes drugs
• other drugs that lower blood fats, such as Mevacor, Pravachol, and Zocor
• Rifadin.

 If you suspect an overdose

Consult your doctor.

Warnings

• Make sure your doctor knows your medical history. You may not be able to take Atromid-S if you have kidney or liver disease or peptic ulcers.
• If you're pregnant or think you may be, check with your doctor before you start taking this drug.
• Don't use Atromid-S if you're breast-feeding; it can cause unwanted side effects in your baby.
• Don't give this drug to children under age 2; they need cholesterol for normal development.

• Have your blood cholesterol and triglyceride levels measured regularly.
• When you stop using Atromid-S, your blood fat levels may rise again. To prevent this, your doctor may recommend a special diet.

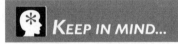 **KEEP IN MIND...**

* Don't break, chew, or crush capsules.
* Take with food.
* Don't stop taking abruptly.
* Have blood fat levels measured regularly.

Atrovent

Atrovent is a bronchodilator — a drug that widens narrowed breathing passages and increases the flow of air into the lungs.

Why it's prescribed

Doctors prescribe Atrovent to reduce coughing, wheezing, shortness of breath, and troubled breathing resulting from lung disease or seasonal allergies. Atrovent comes in an inhaler, a solution for a nebulizer, and a nasal spray. Doctors usually prescribe the following amounts for adults; children's dosages appear in parentheses.

▶ **For closing up of the throat associated with lung disease,** 1 to 2 inhalations four times a day. Additional inhalations may be needed. Total inhalations shouldn't exceed 12 in 24 hours. Or 250 to 500 micrograms (mcg) of inhalation solution dissolved in normal saline solution and taken by nebulizer every 4 to 6 hours. (Children ages 5 to 12: 125 to 250 mcg of nebulizer solution dissolved in normal saline solution, taken by nebulizer every 4 to 6 hours.)

▶ **For seasonal allergy,** 2 sprays in each nostril twice a day, increased to three or four times a day if needed. Maximum dosage is 8 sprays in each nostril daily.

How to use Atrovent

• Use this drug exactly as directed by your doctor.
• Using a spacer device with the inhaler may help to ensure that you inhale the proper dosage. If your

ATROVENT'S OTHER NAME

Atrovent's generic name is ipratropium bromide.

SIDE EFFECTS

Call your doctor if you have any of these possible drug side effects.

Serious: none reported

Common: none reported

Other: nervousness, dizziness, headache, cough, nausea, dry mouth, rash

Tip: If Atrovent causes dry mouth, use sugarless hard candy or gum or a saliva substitute.

DRUG INTERACTIONS

Combining certain drugs may alter their action or produce unwanted side effects. Tell your doctor about other drugs you're taking, especially:
• anticholinergics, such as Darbid and Pro-Banthine
• Opticrom.

doctor recommends this device, follow the doctor's directions or the manufacturer's instructions closely.
• If you're also using a steroid inhaler, use Atrovent first; then wait about 5 minutes before using the steroid.
• If you're using Atrovent inhalation to treat acute asthma attacks, you must use it only in a nebulizer in combination with other prescribed drug.

If you miss a dose

Take the missed dose as soon as possible. However, if it's almost time for your next dose, skip the missed dose and take your next dose as scheduled. Don't take a double dose.

 If you suspect an overdose

Consult your doctor.

 Warnings

• Make sure your doctor knows your medical history. You may not be able to take Atrovent if you have other problems, especially closed-angle glaucoma, an enlarged prostate, or obstruction of the bladder neck.
• Don't use Atrovent if you're allergic to soyalecithin or related food products, such as soybeans and peanuts.
• Avoid accidentally spraying Atrovent into your eyes because this may blur your vision briefly.

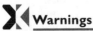 **KEEP IN MIND...**

* Use spacer device if recommended.

* Wait 5 minutes before using any steroid inhaler.

* Use sugarless hard candy or gum or saliva substitute to relieve dry mouth.

Augmentin

Augmentin is a combination antibiotic. It acts by destroying the cell walls of bacteria, which eventually kills the bacteria or prevents their growth.

Why it's prescribed

Doctors prescribe Augmentin to treat certain bacterial infections. Augmentin comes in chewable tablets, film-coated tablets, and an oral suspension. Doctors usually prescribe the following amounts for adults; children's dosages appear in parentheses.

▶ **For lower respiratory infections, middle ear infections, sinus inflammation, skin infections, and urinary tract infections,** 250 milligrams (mg) every 8 hours. For more severe infections, 500 mg every 8 hours. (Children: 20 to 40 mg for each 2.2 pounds of body weight each day divided into equal doses taken every 8 hours.)

How to take Augmentin

• Take this drug exactly as directed. Keep taking Augmentin, even after you begin to feel better.
• You may take Augmentin on a full or an empty stomach.
• Crush or chew the chewable tablets well before swallowing.
• To measure the oral suspension, use a specially marked measuring spoon, not a household teaspoon.

AUGMENTIN'S OTHER NAMES

Augmentin is a combination of the generic drugs amoxicillin and clavulanate potassium. A Canadian brand name is Clavulin.

 SIDE EFFECTS

Call your doctor if you have any of these possible drug side effects. Call *immediately* about any labeled "serious."

Serious: allergic reaction (difficulty breathing, itching, rash, hives, wheezing), blood disorders such as anemia (weakness, fatigue)

Common: nausea, diarrhea
Tips: Call the doctor if nausea or diarrhea persists or becomes severe. Don't take diarrhea drug without checking with your doctor.

Other: vomiting

DRUG INTERACTIONS

Combining certain drugs may alter their action or produce unwanted side effects. Tell your doctor about other drugs you're taking, especially:
• drugs for gout, such as Zyloprim and Benemid.

If you miss a dose

Take the missed dose as soon as possible. However, if it's almost time for your next dose and you usually take two doses a day, space the missed dose and the next one 5 to 6 hours apart. If you take three or more doses a day, space the missed dose and the next one 2 to 4 hours apart. Then go back to your regular schedule. Don't take a double dose.

If you suspect an overdose

Contact your doctor *immediately.* Excessive Augmentin can cause seizures or unusual sensitivity of the nervous system and muscles (muscle pain, twitching).

Warnings

• Make sure your doctor knows your medical history. You may not be able to take Augmentin if you have other problems, especially kidney, stomach, or intestinal disease or infectious mononucleosis.
• Tell your doctor if you're allergic to other penicillins or cephalosporins, Fulvicin, or Cuprimine. Make sure that you carry medical identification that describes your allergy.
• If you're breast-feeding, discuss with your doctor whether you should take Augmentin.
• If you have diabetes and test your urine for sugar, be aware that this drug may cause false results with some urine sugar tests. Call your doctor before changing your diet or the dosage of your diabetes drug.

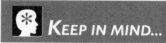 **KEEP IN MIND...**

∗ Chew or crush chewable tablets well before swallowing.
∗ Take at evenly spaced times.
∗ Finish entire amount prescribed.

Axid

Axid reduces the amount of acid produced by the stomach, helping to treat stomach and intestinal ulcers and to prevent ulcers from recurring.

Why it's prescribed

Doctors prescribe Axid to treat peptic ulcers or to prevent their return. They may also prescribe it to treat gastroesophageal reflux, a condition in which the stomach's contents flow backward into the esophagus. Axid comes in capsules. Doctors usually prescribe the following amounts for adults.

▶ **For active duodenal ulcers,** 300 milligrams (mg) each day at bedtime, or 150 mg twice a day.

▶ **As maintenance therapy for duodenal ulcers,** 150 mg each day.

▶ **For benign gastric ulcers,** 150 mg twice a day or 300 mg for 8 weeks.

▶ **For gastroesophageal reflux,** 150 mg twice a day.

How to take Axid

• Follow your doctor's instructions exactly.

• If you're taking one capsule daily, take it at bedtime, unless your doctor gives you other instructions.

• If you're taking two capsules, take one in the morning and one at bedtime.

• Continue to take the drug even after you begin to feel better. If you stop too soon, your ulcer may not heal completely.

If you miss a dose

Take the missed dose as soon as possible. However, if it's almost time for your next dose, skip the missed dose and take your next dose as

AXID'S OTHER NAME

Axid's generic name is nizatidine.

 ## SIDE EFFECTS

Call your doctor if you have any of these possible drug side effects. Call *immediately* about any labeled "serious."

Serious: thrombocytopenia (bruising and bleeding), severe skin inflammation

Common: sleepiness, excessive sweating
Tip: Talk to your doctor if sleepiness or sweating is excessive or persistent.

Other: irregular heartbeats, rash, hives, fever

 ## DRUG AND FOOD INTERACTIONS

Combining certain drugs and foods may alter drug action or produce unwanted side effects. Tell your doctor about your diet and other drugs you're taking, especially:

• antacids (wait 30 minutes to 1 hour before taking Axid)
• aspirin
• Carafate
• drugs that can affect the bone marrow, such as Amphotericin B and cancer drugs, such as Cisplatin and Methotrexate
• Nizoral
• tobacco (stop smoking or wait until after day's last dose)
• tomato-based, mixed-vegetable juices such as V8 Juice

scheduled. Don't take a double dose.

 ## If you suspect an overdose

Contact your doctor *immediately.* Excessive Axid can cause excessive tear production, increased saliva production, vomiting, and diarrhea.

Warnings

• Make sure your doctor knows your medical history. You may not be able to take Axid if you have other medical problems, especially kidney or liver disease or an allergy to this or other drugs.

• If you're pregnant or breast-feeding, check with your doctor before you start taking Axid.

• Be aware that older adults may be especially prone to Axid's side effects.

• Avoid foods and other substances that irritate your stomach, such as alcohol, carbonated soft drinks, and citrus products.

 ## KEEP IN MIND...

∗ Keep taking even after you begin to feel better.

∗ Don't smoke while using drug.

∗ Avoid tomato-based, mixed-vegetable juices.

∗ After taking antacid, wait 30 minutes to 1 hour before taking Axid.

Azactam

Azactam is a new type of antibiotic called a monobactam. It eliminates infection by destroying bacterial cell walls. This eventually kills the bacteria or prevents bacterial growth.

Why it's prescribed

Doctors prescribe Azactam to treat bacterial infections. Azactam comes in a vial and must be given by intramuscular injection. It's also available in an intravenous form. Doctors usually prescribe the following amounts for adults.

▶ **For certain infections of the urinary tract, lower respiratory tract, female reproductive tract, blood, skin, or abdomen or for surgical infections,** 500 milligrams to 2 grams (g) every 8 to 12 hours.

▶ **For severe, total-body infections** or life-threatening infections, 2 g every 6 to 8 hours. Maximum dosage is 8 g a day.

How to take Azactam

• Azactam is typically administered by a visiting nurse.
• The drug is injected deeply into a large muscle mass, such as the upper outside part of the buttock or the outside area of the thigh.
• For this drug to be most effective, it must be administered at evenly spaced times.

AZACTAM'S OTHER NAME

Azactam's generic name is aztreonam.

• Keep a record of where the drug was injected each time so that injection sites can be rotated.
• To help clear up your infection completely, the nurse will be sure to administer all of the drug prescribed.

If you miss a dose

Consult your doctor.

 ### If you suspect an overdose

Consult your doctor.

 Warnings

• Make sure your doctor knows your medical history. You may not be able to take Azactam if you're allergic to penicillin or cephalosporin or if you have other problems, especially liver or kidney disease.

 SIDE EFFECTS

Call your doctor if you have any of these possible drug side effects. Call *immediately* about any labeled "serious."

Serious: seizures, allergic reaction (difficulty breathing; wheezing; tightness in the chest; difficulty swallowing; hives; rash; itching; pain, swelling, or redness at the injection site)

Common: weakness, low blood pressure (dizziness)

Other: headache, difficulty sleeping, confusion, diarrhea, nausea, vomiting, tingling of fingers or toes, nasal congestion, ringing in the ears, double vision, sweating

Tip: Talk to your doctor if diarrhea or vomiting is persistent or severe.

 DRUG INTERACTIONS

Combining certain drugs may alter their action or produce unwanted side effects. Tell your doctor about other drugs you're taking, especially:
• Benemid
• Lasix
• other drugs used to treat infection.

 KEEP IN MIND...

* Inject deeply into large muscle mass.

* Administer at evenly spaced times.

* Take entire amount prescribed.

Azelex

Azelex is used to treat acne. This drug works by fighting the tiny organisms that accompany acne flare-ups.

Why it's prescribed

Doctors prescribe Azelex to treat acne eruptions. Azelex comes in a cream. Doctors usually prescribe the following amounts for adults.

▶ **For mild to moderate acne**, a thin film applied twice a day, in the morning and evening. Frequency may be reduced to once a day for a person who's sensitive to the drug. The length of time Azelex is prescribed varies depending on the severity of the acne; however, most people improve within 4 weeks.

How to use Azelex

• Use Azelex only as your doctor directs, for the full prescribed treatment period.
• Thoroughly wash and pat dry the affected skin areas before applying Azelex.
• Apply a thin film of Azelex, massaging it gently and thoroughly into affected areas.
• Keep Azelex away from your mouth, eyes, and other mucous membranes. If it gets in your eyes, rinse them with large amounts of water; check with your doctor if eye irritation persists.
• Don't use airtight dressings or wrappings over treated areas.

AZELEX'S OTHER NAME

Azelex's generic name is azelaic acid cream.

• Wash your hands well after applying Azelex.

If you miss a dose

Apply the missed dose as soon as possible. However, if it's almost time for your next dose, skip the missed dose and go back to your regular schedule. Don't apply a double dose.

 If you suspect an overdose

Consult your doctor. Although overdose of Azelex has not been reported, the most likely symptoms would be redness, rash, burning, or itching.

 Warnings

• Make sure your doctor knows your medical history. You may not be able to use Azelex if you're allergic to other drugs.
• Make sure your doctor knows if you're pregnant or breast-feeding before you begin using Azelex.
• Don't give Azelex to children under age 12 without your doctor's consent.

 SIDE EFFECTS

Call your doctor if you have any of these possible drug side effects. Call *immediately* about side effects labeled "serious."

Serious: severe skin irritation (peeling), worsening asthma (difficulty breathing, shortness of breath)

Common: burning, stinging, itching, tingling
Tip: Temporary irritation may occur if you apply Azelex to broken or inflamed skin, especially at the beginning of treatment. Call your doctor about persistent or severe irritation.

Other: reddening, rash, dry skin, skin color changes (especially in a dark complexion)
Tip: Call your doctor about any color changes.

 DRUG INTERACTIONS

Combining certain drugs may alter their action or produce unwanted side effects. Tell your doctor about other drugs you're taking.

 KEEP IN MIND...

* Use morning and evening.
* Wash and dry area first.
* Wash hands after applying.
* Don't use on children under age 12.
* Report skin color changes.

Azmacort

Azmacort eases breathing by preventing cells in the lungs and airways from releasing substances that cause asthma symptoms. Azmacort is meant to prevent an asthma attack; it won't relieve one.

Why it's prescribed

Doctors prescribe Azmacort to prevent symptoms of asthma in people with asthma who are dependent on steroids. Azmacort comes as an inhalation aerosol. Doctors usually prescribe the following amounts for adults; children's dosages appear in parentheses.

▶ **For steroid-dependent asthma,** 2 inhalations three to four times a day. Maximum dosage is 16 inhalations a day. (Children ages 6 to 12: 1 to 2 inhalations three to four times a day. Maximum dosage is 12 inhalations a day.)

How to use Azmacort

• Use this drug exactly as directed. Take it every day in regularly spaced doses.
• Carefully follow the directions that come with the inhaler.
• Using a spacer device with the inhaler may help to ensure that you inhale the right amount. If your doctor recommends this device, follow the directions given.
• If you're also using a bronchodilator, use it several minutes before Azmacort.
• Keep the inhaler clean and unobstructed. Wash it with warm water

AZMACORT'S OTHER NAME

Azmacort's generic name is triamcinolone acetonide.

 SIDE EFFECTS

Call your doctor if you have any of these possible drug side effects.

Serious: none reported

Common: fungal infections of the mouth (pain when eating or swallowing; creamy white, curdlike patches on the inside of your mouth, nose, or throat)

Tip: To help prevent fungal infections, gargle or rinse your mouth with water after each inhaler use. Don't swallow the water.

Other: hoarseness, cough, dryness or irritation of the nose, throat, tongue, or mouth

 DRUG INTERACTIONS

Combining certain drugs may alter their action or produce unwanted side effects. Tell your doctor about other drugs you're taking.

and dry it thoroughly after each use.
• Call your doctor if the drug starts to lose its effectiveness; the doctor may need to change the dosage.
• Don't stop using this drug suddenly. Your doctor may want you to gradually reduce the amount you're taking.

If you miss a dose

Take the missed dose as soon as possible. Then take any remaining doses for that day at regularly spaced times. Don't take a double dose.

 If you suspect an overdose

Consult your doctor.

X Warning

• Make sure your doctor knows your medical history. Other medical conditions may affect your use of Azmacort.
• Don't use Azmacort if you have tuberculosis, an untreated infec-

tion, or a herpes infection of the eye.
• If you're breast-feeding, consult your doctor before you start taking this drug.
• If you've recently switched to Azmacort from an oral steroid, the doctor may advise you to switch back to the oral steroid during periods of stress or severe asthma attacks.
• Don't use this drug to halt an asthma attack already in progress.
• Carry medical identification indicating your need for additional steroids during stress.

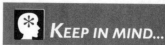 **KEEP IN MIND...**

* Don't use to halt asthma attack already in progress.

* Use spacer device to ensure proper dosage.

* Gargle or rinse mouth with water after each inhaler use.

* Don't stop taking suddenly.

Azulfidine

Azulfidine is a sulfa drug that kills bacteria and some fungi in the bowel.

Why it's prescribed

Doctors prescribe Azulfidine to treat inflammatory bowel disease. Azulfidine comes in tablets and an oral suspension. Doctors usually prescribe the following amounts for adults and children.

▶ **For ulcerative colitis or Crohn's disease,** initially 3 to 4 grams (g) each day divided into equal doses; usual maintenance dosage is 1.5 to 2 g each day divided into equal doses spaced 6 hours apart. (Children over age 2: initially, 40 to 60 milligrams [mg] for each 2.2 pounds [lb] of body weight each day, divided into three or four equal doses, then 30 mg for each 2.2 lb a day, divided into four equal doses.)

How to take Azulfidine

• Take this drug exactly as your doctor has directed.
• Take the entire amount prescribed, even if you soon feel better.

If you miss a dose

Take the missed dose as soon as possible. But if it's almost time for your next dose, skip the missed dose and take your next dose as scheduled. Don't take a double dose.

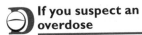

If you suspect an overdose

Contact your doctor *immediately*. Excessive Azulfidine can cause diz-ziness, drowsiness, headache, appetite loss, abdominal pain, nausea, vomiting, unconsciousness, and death.

AZULFIDINE'S OTHER NAME

Azulfidine's generic name is sulfasalazine.

SIDE EFFECTS

Call your doctor if you have any of these possible drug side effects. Call *immediately* about any labeled "serious."

Serious: seizures, kidney damage (low back pain, inability to urinate), flaking around mouth, skin blistering, anemia (fatigue, weakness), allergic reaction (hives, itching, hair loss, swelling around eyes), fever, chills

Common: nausea, vomiting, diarrhea, yellow-orange urine or skin
Tips: Take with food to avoid nausea. Urine and skin discoloration will disappear after you've finished this prescription.

Other: headache, depression, abdominal pain, appetite loss, sensitivity to light, crystals in the urine
Tips: To help prevent crystals in the urine, take each dose with a full (8-ounce) glass of water and drink several more glasses of water during the day. Protect yourself from sunlight with sunscreen and protective clothing.

DRUG INTERACTIONS

Combining certain drugs may alter their action or produce unwanted side effects. Tell your doctor about other drugs you're taking, especially:

• anticoagulants (blood thinners) such as Coumadin
• birth control pills
• digoxin
• drugs used to treat infection
• folic acid, iron
• oral diabetes drugs.

Warnings

• Make sure your doctor knows your medical history. You may not be able to take Azulfidine if you have anemia, kidney or liver disease, severe allergies, asthma, G6PD deficiency, a blockage of the urinary or digestive tract, a blood disorder, porphyria, or an allergic reaction to aspirin, a sulfa drug, a diuretic (water pill, such as Lasix), or drugs for diabetes or glaucoma.
• Don't take this drug if you're pregnant or breast-feeding.

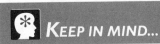

KEEP IN MIND...

* Take each dose with full glass of water after meals.

* Take entire amount prescribed.

* Expect yellow-orange-tinged urine or skin.

Bactrim

Bactrim is a sulfonamide antibiotic. It eliminates infections by interfering with invading bacteria.

Why it's prescribed

Doctors prescribe Bactrim to treat bronchitis, middle ear infections, traveler's diarrhea, urinary tract infections, and *Pneumocystis carinii* pneumonia (common in people with AIDS). Bactrim comes in tablets and an oral suspension. It's also available in an injectable form. Doctors usually prescribe the following amounts for adults; children's dosages are in parentheses.

▶ **For urinary tract infections and chronic bronchitis and ear infections,** 2 tablets every 12 hours for 10 days. (Children age 2 months and over: 1 to 4 teaspoons [tsp] depending on body weight.)

▶ **For chronic urinary tract infections,** ½ or 1 tablet once a day or three times a week for 3 to 6 months.

▶ **For traveler's diarrhea,** 2 tablets every 12 hours for 5 days.

▶ **For *Pneumocystis carinii* pneumonia,** 2½ to 5 tablets every 6 hours. (Children age 2 months and over: 1 to 5 tsp every 6 hours.)

How to take Bactrim

• Take this drug exactly as directed.

SIDE EFFECTS

Call your doctor if you have any of these possible drug side effects. Call *immediately* about any labeled "serious."

Serious: allergic reaction (wheezing, hives, difficulty breathing, fever, sore throat, joint pain, blood problems (weakness, fatigue, shortness of breath, headache, easy bruising), severe skin inflammation

Common: nausea, vomiting, diarrhea
Tips: Take your doses with food to avoid nausea. Notify your doctor if diarrhea gets worse; you may be able to take a diarrhea drug.

Other: headache, seizures, fatigue, difficulty sleeping, appetite loss, itching, yellow-tinged skin and eyes, crystals in the urine (kidney stones)
Tip: To prevent kidney stones, drink extra water.

DRUG INTERACTIONS

Combining certain drugs may alter their action or produce unwanted side effects. Tell your doctor about other drugs you're taking, especially:
• anticoagulants (blood thinners) such as Coumadin
• birth control pills
• Dilantin
• oral diabetes drugs
• vitamin C.

• Take tablets or the oral suspension with a full glass (8 ounces) of water.

• If you have trouble swallowing the tablets, you may crush them and take with water or mix with soft food such as applesauce or pudding.

• If you're taking the oral suspension, shake the bottle well first. Use a specially marked spoon or dropper, not a household teaspoon, to measure the correct dose.

• Keep taking Bactrim even after you begin to feel better.

• The doctor may adjust your dose if you have or develop kidney failure (decreased urine output) while you're taking Bactrim.

If you miss a dose

Take the missed dose as soon as possible. However, if it's almost time for your next dose, adjust your schedule as follows:

• If you're taking two doses a day, space the skipped dose and the next dose 6 hours apart. Then resume your regular schedule.

• If you're taking three or more doses a day, space the skipped dose and the next dose 2 to 4 hours apart. Then resume your regular schedule.

If you suspect an overdose

Contact your doctor *immediately*. Excessive Bactrim can cause depression, appetite loss, yellow-tinged skin and eyes, headache, nausea, vomiting, diarrhea, and facial swelling.

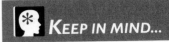 ### Warnings

• Make sure your doctor knows your medical history. You may not be able to take Bactrim if you're allergic to other sulfa drugs or if you have other problems, especially kidney or liver problems, porphyria, severe allergies, asthma, or AIDS.

• If you're pregnant or breast-feeding, consult your doctor before you start taking Bactrim.
• Bactrim isn't recommended for infants under age 2 months.
• Be aware that older adults may be more prone to Bactrim's side effects.
• If you have diabetes, you may need to change urine sugar testing procedures while taking Bactrim.

KEEP IN MIND...

* Take tablets or oral suspension with full glass of water.
* Tablets may be crushed and taken with water.
* Keep taking drug even after you feel better.
* Drink extra water.

Bactroban

Bactroban is a non-penicillin antibiotic that's applied to the skin to treat bacterial infections. It eliminates skin infections by inhibiting bacteria from synthesizing essential substances. This eventually kills bacteria or prevents their growth.

Why it's prescribed

Doctors prescribe Bactroban to treat bacterial infections of the skin, such as impetigo. In Canada, you can buy Bactroban without a prescription. Bactroban comes in an ointment. Doctors usually prescribe the following amounts for adults and children.

▶ **For impetigo,** a small amount applied to affected areas two to three times a day for 1 to 2 weeks.

How to use Bactroban

• If you're treating yourself, read the package instructions carefully to find out how much to use and when to use it.
• If your doctor prescribed this drug or gave you special instructions on how to use it, follow those instructions exactly.
• Before applying Bactroban, clean the affected area with soap and water and dry it thoroughly. Then apply a small amount of the ointment and rub it in gently. You can cover the treated area with a gauze dressing if you wish.

 BACTROBAN'S OTHER NAME

Bactroban's generic name is mupirocin.

 SIDE EFFECTS

Call your doctor if you have any of these possible drug side effects. Call *immediately* about any labeled "serious."

Serious: other infections caused by bacteria that Bactroban doesn't kill, kidney problems (decreased urination, confusion)

Common: none reported

Other: burning, stinging, itching, rash
Tips: These side effects usually go away over time. Check with your doctor if they persist or become bothersome.

DRUG INTERACTIONS

Combining certain drugs may alter their action or produce unwanted side effects. Tell your doctor about other drugs you're taking.

• Keep this drug out of your eyes. If you do get some in your eyes, flush your eyes with water.
• To make sure your infection heals completely, continue to use Bactroban for the full treatment time prescribed, even if your symptoms disappear. Don't skip any doses. However, don't use this ointment longer than the doctor prescribes or the package instructions recommend.

If you miss a dose

Apply the missed dose as soon as possible. However, if it's almost time for your next dose, skip the missed dose and apply your next dose as scheduled.

 If you suspect an overdose

Consult your doctor.

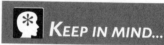 **Warnings**

• Tell your doctor if you're pregnant or breast-feeding before you start taking Bactroban.
• Don't use Bactroban on burns or large open wounds. The drug could be absorbed into your body and cause kidney problems.
• Call your doctor or pharmacist if your condition doesn't improve within 3 to 5 days or if it gets worse.

KEEP IN MIND...

* Apply small amount of ointment and rub in gently.
* Use for full treatment time prescribed.
* Call doctor about burning, stinging, itching, or rash.

Basaljel

Basaljel is an antacid that neutralizes stomach acid through a chemical reaction.

Why it's taken

Basaljel is taken for heartburn, acid indigestion, sour stomach, gastroesophageal reflux (backflow of stomach contents into the esophagus), and too much phosphate in the blood. You can buy Basaljel without a prescription. It comes in tablets, capsules, and an oral suspension. The following amounts are usually recommended for adults.

▶ **As an antacid,** 2 teaspoons of suspension or 1 to 2 tablets or capsules every 2 hours as needed. Maximum dosage is 24 capsules, tablets, or teaspoons a day.

▶ **To prevent formation of kidney stones,** 2 to 3 tablespoons of suspension or 2 to 6 tablets or capsules 1 hour after meals and at bedtime.

How to take Basaljel

• If you're treating yourself, read the package instructions carefully. If your doctor prescribed Basaljel or gave you special instructions on how to use it, follow the special directions.

• Shake the oral suspension well and take it with a small amount of water or fruit juice.

If you miss a dose

Take the missed dose as soon as possible. However, if it's almost time for your next dose, skip the missed dose and take your next dose as scheduled. Don't take a double dose.

BASALJEL'S OTHER NAME

Basaljel's generic name is aluminum carbonate.

 SIDE EFFECTS

Call your doctor if you have any of these possible drug side effects.

Serious: none reported

Common: constipation
Tip: If constipation occurs, ask your doctor about using laxatives or stool softeners or alternating Basaljel with a magnesium-containing antacid.

Other: appetite loss, bowel blockage, too little phosphate in the blood (appetite loss, overall feeling of illness, muscle weakness)

 DRUG INTERACTIONS

Combining certain drugs may alter their action or produce unwanted side effects. Tell your doctor about other drugs you're taking, especially:
• Cuprimine
• digoxin
• Dolobid
• enteric-coated drugs such as Ecotrin (take at least 1 hour before or after Basaljel)
• iron
• Laniazid, Myambutol
• phenothiazines (used for anxiety, nausea and vomiting, or psychosis)
• steroids
• thyroid drugs
• ulcer drugs
• Zyloprim.

 If you suspect an overdose

Consult your doctor.

 Warnings

• Make sure your doctor knows your medical history. You may not be able to take Basaljel if you have kidney disease or are pregnant.
• Don't give this drug to children under age 6.
• Older adults with bone problems or Alzheimer's disease should not take this drug. It contains aluminum, which may cause their condition to get worse.

• Follow a low-phosphate diet if the doctor recommends it.
• If you're taking Basaljel to prevent kidney stones, drink plenty of fluids.
• Don't switch to another antacid without consulting your doctor.

KEEP IN MIND...

* Shake oral suspension well, and take with water or juice.

* Take 1 hour after meals and at bedtime or as ordered.

* Drink plenty of fluids.

Beconase AQ

Beconase AQ eases breathing by reducing inflammation of the mucous membrane that lines the insides of the nose.

Why it's prescribed

Doctors prescribe Beconase AQ to relieve stuffy nose and irritation caused by hay fever, allergies, and nasal problems or to prevent nasal polyps from returning after surgical removal. Beconase AQ comes in nasal aerosol, nasal spray, and oral inhalant. Doctors usually prescribe the following amounts for adults and children over age 12; amounts for younger children appear in parentheses.

▶ **To relieve allergy symptoms or to prevent recurrence of nasal polyps after surgery,** 1 or 2 sprays (nasal form) in each nostril two, three, or four times a day.

▶ **To prevent asthma attacks,** 2 to 4 inhalations (oral form only) three or four times a day. Maximum dosage is 20 inhalations a day. (Children ages 6 to 12: 1 to 2 inhalations three or four times a day. Maximum dosage is 10 inhalations a day.)

How to use Beconase AQ

• Before using this drug, read the directions that come with the container. Follow them exactly.
• For this drug to work, you must use it every day at regular intervals as your doctor prescribes. Up to 4 weeks may pass before you feel the drug's full effects.

BECONASE AQ'S OTHER NAMES

Beconase AQ's generic name is beclomethasone dipropionate. Another brand name is Vancenase.

SIDE EFFECTS

Call your doctor if you have any of these possible drug side effects.

Serious: none reported

Common: mild nasal burning and stinging (with nasal form)
Tip: Use good nasal and oral hygiene.

Other: headache, stuffy nose, sneezing, nosebleeds, watery eyes, nausea, vomiting (with nasal form); hoarseness, fungal infections of the mouth or throat, throat irritation, dry mouth (with oral form)
Tip: If you suspect a fungal infection, notify your doctor.

DRUG INTERACTIONS

Combining certain drugs may alter their action or produce unwanted side effects. Tell your doctor about other drugs you're taking.

If you miss a dose

Take the missed dose as soon as possible. However, if it's almost time for your next dose, skip the missed dose and take your next dose as scheduled. Don't take a double dose.

If you suspect an overdose

Consult your doctor.

Warnings

• Make sure your doctor knows your medical history. Tell your doctor if you've recently had nasal surgery or an injury to your nose or if you have other medical conditions, especially lung disease, such as tuberculosis; an infection of the mouth, nose, sinuses, throat, or lungs; a herpes infection of the eye; or any untreated infection.
• If you're breast-feeding, tell your doctor before you start using Beconase AQ.
• If you're using the nasal form of Beconase AQ for more than a few weeks, see your doctor regularly. Call the doctor if you develop

symptoms of a nasal, sinus, or throat infection.
• For the oral form, consult your doctor if you have an asthma attack that doesn't improve after you take a bronchodilator; if signs of mouth, throat, or lung infection occur; if your symptoms don't improve; or if your condition worsens.
• Before surgery (including dental surgery) or emergency treatment, tell the doctor or dentist that you're taking Beconase AQ.
• Carry medical identification stating that you're taking Beconase AQ.

KEEP IN MIND...

* Take daily at regular intervals.
* Carry medical identification stating that you're taking Beconase AQ.
* Before surgery, tell doctor or dentist that you're taking Beconase AQ.

Benadryl

Benadryl inhibits histamine, a body substance that causes itching, sneezing, runny nose, and watery eyes.

Why it's taken

Benadryl is taken to relieve stuffy nose, hay fever symptoms, nonproductive cough, difficulty sleeping, and motion sickness. It's also used to reduce tremors and stiffness in Parkinson's disease. You can buy Benadryl without a prescription. It comes in tablets, capsules, elixir, syrup, and an injectable form. The following amounts are usually recommended for adults; children's dosages appear in parentheses.

▶ **For runny nose, allergy symptoms, motion sickness, and Parkinson's disease,** 25 to 50 milligrams (mg) orally three or four times a day. (Children age 12 and over: same as adults. Children under age 12: 5 mg for each 2.2 pounds of body weight orally each day.)

▶ **As a nighttime sleep aid,** 50 mg orally at bedtime.

▶ **For a nonproductive cough,** 25 mg orally every 4 to 6 hours, but no more than 150 mg a day. (Children ages 6 to 12: 12.5 mg orally every 4 to 6 hours, but no more than 75 mg a day. Children ages 2 to 6: 6.25 mg orally every 4 to 6 hours, but no more than 25 mg a day.)

BENADRYL'S OTHER NAMES

Benadryl's generic name is diphenhydramine hydrochloride. Other brand names include AllerMax, Banophen, Beldin, Belix, Bena-D, Benahist, Nordryl, and Phendry.

SIDE EFFECTS

Call your doctor if you have any of these possible drug side effects.

Serious: none reported

Common: drowsiness, nausea, dry mouth
Tips: Make sure you know how you react to this drug before you drive or perform other tasks that require you to be fully alert. To reduce nausea, take doses with food, milk, or water.

Other: confusion, headache, palpitations, stuffy nose, hives

DRUG INTERACTIONS

Combining certain drugs may alter their action or produce unwanted side effects. Tell your doctor about other drugs you're taking, especially:
• alcohol and other drugs that make you and relaxed and sleepy, such as narcotic painkillers and tranquilizers
• MAO inhibitors such as Nardil.

How to take Benadryl

• If you're treating yourself, follow the directions on the label. If the doctor prescribed this drug, follow any special directions.
• Benadryl begins to take effect within 15 minutes.
• If you're taking Benadryl to prevent motion sickness, take it at least 1 to 2 hours before traveling.

If you miss a dose

If you're taking this drug regularly and you miss a dose, take the missed dose as soon as possible. However, if it's almost time for your next dose, skip the missed dose and take your next dose as scheduled. Don't take a double dose.

If you suspect an overdose

Contact your doctor *immediately.* Excessive Benadryl can cause drowsiness, seizures, coma, and stoppage of breathing.

Warnings

• Make sure your doctor knows your medical history. You may not be able to take Benadryl if you have asthma, glaucoma, a bladder disorder, heart disease, high blood pressure, or an overactive thyroid or if you're pregnant or breast-feeding.
• Children and older adults are especially prone to Benadryl's side effects.
• Benadryl can hide signs of aspirin overdose, such as ringing in the ears.

KEEP IN MIND...

* Take at least 1 to 2 hours before traveling.
* Don't drive until you know how drug affects you.
* Take with food, milk, or water.

Benemid

Benemid eliminates excess uric acid, a cause of gout.

Why it's prescribed

Doctors prescribe Benemid to treat gout or to help antibiotics work better. It comes in tablets. Doctors usually prescribe the following amounts for adults; children's dosages are in parentheses.

▶ **For gout,** 250 milligrams (mg) twice a day for the first week, then 500 mg twice a day, to a maximum of 2 grams a day.

▶ **To help penicillin fight infection,** 500 mg four times a day. (Children weighing over 110 pounds [lb]: same as adults. Children weighing 110 lb or less: initially, 25 mg for each 2.2 lb of body weight, then 40 mg for each 2.2 lb of body weight a day divided into four equal doses.)

How to take Benemid

• Take this drug exactly as the doctor has directed.

If you miss a dose

If you're taking this drug regularly, take the missed dose as soon as possible. However, if it's almost time for your next dose, skip the missed dose and take your next dose as scheduled. Don't take a double dose.

 If you suspect an overdose

Contact your doctor *immediately*. Excessive Benemid can cause nau-

BENEMID'S OTHER NAMES

Benemid's generic name is probenecid. Other brand names include Probalan; and, in Canada, Benuryl.

 SIDE EFFECTS

Call your doctor if you have any of these possible drug side effects. Call *immediately* about any labeled "serious."

Serious: hemolytic anemia (fever, chills, stomach pain)

Common: headache, stomach upset
Tip: Take Benemid with milk, food, or an antacid.

Other: dizziness, appetite loss, vomiting, sore gums, frequent urination, skin inflammation, itching, fever, kidney stones
Tip: At first, Benemid will increase the amount of uric acid in your kidneys, putting you at risk for kidney stones. Your doctor will tell you to drink at least 10 full (8-ounce) glasses of fluid daily or will prescribe another drug to help prevent kidney problems.

 DRUG AND FOOD INTERACTIONS

Combining certain drugs and foods may alter drug action or produce unwanted side effects. Tell your doctor about your diet and other drugs you're taking, especially:
• alcohol
• foods high in purine, such as anchovies, liver, sardines, kidneys, peas, and lentils
• Indocin
• Mexate
• oral diabetes drugs
• salicylates such as aspirin (can trigger gout).

sea, copious vomiting, seizures, stupor, and coma.

 Warnings

• Make sure your doctor knows your medical history. You may not be able to take Benemid if you have a peptic ulcer, a kidney disorder, or a blood disorder.
• If you're diabetic, be aware that Benemid may cause false-positive results on sugar tests.
• Don't use this drug to stop an acute gout attack.

• Benemid may cause more severe attacks of gout for the first 6 to 12 months that you take it. For this reason, the doctor may prescribe an anti-inflammatory drug for the first 3 to 6 months.

KEEP IN MIND...

∗ Drink at least 10 full glasses of fluid daily.

∗ Don't take to stop acute gout attack.

∗ Avoid aspirin and alcohol.

Bentyl

Bentyl relieves spasms, especially of the bowels, stomach, and bladder.

Why it's prescribed

Doctors prescribe Bentyl to relieve digestive cramps or spasms. Bentyl comes in tablets, capsules, and a syrup. It's also available in an injectable form. Doctors usually prescribe the following amounts for adults; children's dosages appear in parentheses.

▶ **For irritable bowel syndrome and certain other digestive disorders,** initially 20 milligrams (mg) orally four times a day, increased to 40 mg four times a day. (Children age 2 and older: 10 mg orally three or four times a day. Children ages 6 months to 2 years: 5 to 10 mg orally three or four times a day.)

How to take Bentyl

• Follow your doctor's directions exactly.
• Take Bentyl 30 minutes to 1 hour before meals, unless your doctor instructs you otherwise.
• Swallow Bentyl capsules whole.
• Check with your doctor before you stop using Bentyl; the doctor may want you to reduce the amount you take gradually.

If you miss a dose

Take the missed dose as soon as possible. However, if it's almost time for your next dose, skip the missed dose and take your next dose as scheduled. Don't take a double dose.

 If you suspect an overdose

Contact your doctor *immediately*. Excessive Bentyl can cause mental changes, flushed skin, and fast pulse.

 Warnings

• Make sure your doctor knows your medical history. You may not be able to take Bentyl if you have digestive, heart, liver, or kidney disease; glaucoma; an overactive thyroid; or urinary problems or if you're pregnant or breast-feeding.
• Older adults may be especially prone to Bentyl's side effects.

BENTYL'S OTHER NAMES

Bentyl's generic name is dicyclomine hydrochloride. Other brand names include Antispas, A-Spas, Di-Spaz, Or-Tyl, Spasmoject; and, in Canada, Bentylol, Formulex, and Lomine.

 ## SIDE EFFECTS

Call your doctor if you have any of these possible drug side effects.

Serious: none reported

Common: headache, dizziness, palpitations, constipation, dry mouth, difficulty urinating
Tip: To relieve dry mouth, use sugarless hard candy or gum, ice chips, or a saliva substitute.

Other: decreased sweating, drowsiness, nervousness, confusion, fast pulse, blurred vision, nausea, vomiting
Tip: Because you may not sweat as much while taking Bentyl, your body temperature may increase. Hot baths, saunas, and exercise will make you dizzy or faint.

 ## DRUG INTERACTIONS

Combining certain drugs may alter their action or produce unwanted side effects. Tell your doctor about other drugs you're taking, especially:
• antacids (take 2 to 3 hours before or after taking Bentyl)
• antihistamines such as Benadryl
• Demerol
• Doriden
• drugs for irregular heart rhythms, such as Cardioquin, Norpace, and Procan
• drugs for Parkinson's disease such as Symmetrel
• Nizoral
• tricyclic antidepressants.

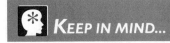 KEEP IN MIND...

* Take 30 minutes to 1 hour before meals.

* Swallow capsules whole.

* Avoid hot baths.

Benylin DM

B enylin DM is a cough suppressant that helps to relieve coughs caused by colds or the flu. It works by directly affecting the part of the brain that controls coughing.

Why it's prescribed

Doctors prescribe Benylin DM to relieve a nonproductive (dry) cough. You can also buy Benylin DM without a prescription. It comes in an extended-release liquid, lozenges, and a solution. Doctors usually prescribe the following amounts.

▶ **For nonproductive cough,** 10 to 20 milligrams (mg) every 4 hours, or 30 mg every 6 to 8 hours. Or, 60 mg of the extended-release liquid twice a day. Maximum dosage is 120 mg a day.
• Children age 12 and older: same as adults.
• Children ages 6 to 12: 5 to 10 mg every 4 hours, or 15 mg every 6 to 8 hours. Or, 30 mg of the extended-release liquid twice a day. Maximum dosage is 60 mg a day.
• Children ages 2 to 6: 2.5 to 5 mg every 4 hours, or 7.5 mg every 6 to 8 hours. Or, 15 mg of the extended-release liquid twice a day. Maximum dosage is 30 mg a day.
• Children under age 2: dosage must be individualized.

BENYLIN DM's OTHER NAMES

Benylin DM's generic name is dextromethorphan hydrobromide. Other brand names include Children's Hold, DM Syrup, Hold, Mediquell, Pertussin Cough Suppressant, Robitussin Pediatric, St. Joseph Cough Suppression for Children, and Vicks Formula 44 Pediatric Formula.

 SIDE EFFECTS

Call your doctor if you have any of these possible drug side effects.
Serious: none reported
Common: none reported
Other: drowsiness, dizziness, nausea, vomiting, stomach pain
Tip: Until you know how Benylin DM affects you, don't drive or perform other activities that require you to be totally alert.

 DRUG INTERACTIONS

Combining certain drugs may alter their action or produce unwanted side effects. Tell your doctor about other drugs you're taking, especially:
• MAO inhibitors such as Nardil (wait 2 weeks before starting and after stopping Benylin DM).

How to take Benylin DM

• If you're treating yourself, read the label instructions carefully to find out how much to take and how often to take it.
• If your doctor prescribed the drug or gave you special instructions on how to use it, follow those instructions.

If you miss a dose

If you're taking Benylin DM regularly, take the missed dose as soon as possible. However, if it's almost time for your next dose, skip the missed dose and take your next dose as scheduled.

 If you suspect an overdose

Contact your doctor *immediately.* Excessive Benylin DM can cause nausea, vomiting, drowsiness, dizziness, blurred vision, uncontrollable eye movements, shallow breathing, inability to urinate, stupor, and coma.

 Warnings

• Make sure your doctor knows your medical history. You may not be able to take Benylin if you're allergic to aspirin or you have asthma or liver disease.
• Don't take Benylin DM if you have a lot of mucus or phlegm with your cough or if you have a chronic cough due to asthma, emphysema, or smoking,
• If your cough doesn't improve after 7 days or if you have a rash, high fever, or persistent headache with the cough, call your doctor.

✳ KEEP IN MIND...

* Call doctor if cough doesn't improve after 7 days.
* Don't take to relieve chronic cough due to asthma, emphysema, or smoking.
* Don't drive until you know how drug affects you.

Betagan

Betagan reduces pressure within the eye by decreasing the production of eye fluids and possibly by speeding removal of fluids through the eye.

Why it's prescribed

Doctors prescribe Betagan to treat chronic open-angle glaucoma and to reduce high intraocular pressure (pressure within the eye). Betagan comes in eyedrops. Doctors usually prescribe the following amounts for adults.

▶ **For chronic open-angle glaucoma and high pressure within the eye,** 1 to 2 drops in eye once or twice a day.

How to use Betagan

• Use this drug exactly as directed by the doctor.
• Wash your hands before and after instilling the drops.
• Don't touch the dropper to your eye, the surrounding skin, or any other surface.

If you miss a dose

Don't apply a double dose. Adjust your schedule as follows:
• If you use one dose a day, apply the missed dose as soon as possible. However if you don't remember until the next day, skip the missed dose and apply your next dose as scheduled.
• If you use more than one dose a day, apply the missed dose as soon as possible. However, if it's almost time for your next dose, skip the missed dose and apply your next dose as scheduled.

BETAGAN'S OTHER NAME

Betagan's generic name is levobunolol hydrochloride.

 SIDE EFFECTS

Call your doctor if you have any of these possible drug side effects. Call *immediately* about any labeled "serious."

Serious: asthma attack (in people with a history of asthma), heart failure (weakness, shortness of breath)

Common: stinging and burning of eyes, low blood pressure (weakness, dizziness), slow pulse, fainting
Tip: You may experience stinging and burning right after you use the drops, but it should be only temporary. Dab your eyes with a tissue, but don't rub them.

Other: headache, dizziness, depression, nausea, hives

 DRUG INTERACTIONS

Combining certain drugs may alter their action or produce unwanted side effects. Tell your doctor about other drugs you're taking, especially:
• catecholamine-depleting drugs such as Serpasil
• Daranide, Diamox, Neptazane
• drugs that constrict the pupils, such as Propine Sterile Ophthalmic Solution and Bronkaid Mist
• oral beta blockers (often used to reduce blood pressure), such as Inderal and Lopressor.

 If you suspect an overdose

Contact your doctor *immediately.* Excessive Betagan can cause extreme low blood pressure (weakness, dizziness), slow pulse, closing up of the throat, and heart failure (weakness, shortness of breath).

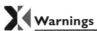 **Warnings**

• Make sure your doctor knows your medical history. You may not be able to use Betagan if you have other problems, especially chronic bronchitis, emphysema, or other lung disease; diabetes; heart or blood vessel disease; an overactive thyroid; or myasthenia gravis.

• If you're pregnant, tell your doctor before you start taking Betagan.
• Be aware that infants and older adults may be especially prone to Betagan's side effects.
• If you're diabetic, be aware that Betagan may cover up some symptoms of low blood sugar, such as trembling and a fast pulse.

 KEEP IN MIND...

* Don't use more often than ordered.
* Wash hands before and after instilling.
* Don't touch dropper to eye or surrounding area.

Betapace

Betapace suppresses an irregular heartbeat by decreasing the heart rate and reducing the heart's need for blood and oxygen. It also lowers blood pressure.

Why it's prescribed

Doctors prescribe Betapace to help steady an irregular heartbeat, to reduce high blood pressure, or to treat chest pain. Betapace comes in tablets. Doctors usually prescribe the following amounts for adults.

▶ **For life-threatening irregular heartbeats,** 80 milligrams (mg) twice a day at first, increased every 2 to 3 days as needed and tolerated; most people respond to a daily dosage of 160 to 320 mg.

▶ **For high blood pressure or chest pain,** 80 mg twice a day, increased weekly in 80-mg increments taken twice a day as needed and tolerated.

How to take Betapace

• Carefully follow your doctor's instructions and the label directions.
• Take Betapace on an empty stomach 1 hour before or 2 hours after a meal.
• Be sure to take all of the drug, even if you feel well. Don't stop taking it suddenly.

If you miss a dose

Take the missed dose as soon as possible. However, if it's almost time for your next dose, skip the missed dose and take your next dose as scheduled. Don't take a double dose.

BETAPACE'S OTHER NAMES

Betapace's generic name is sotalol. A Canadian brand name is Sotacor.

 SIDE EFFECTS

Call your doctor if you have any of these possible drug side effects. Call *immediately* about any labeled "serious."

Serious: irregular heartbeats, congestive heart failure (shortness of breath, chest pain, anxiety), heart block (fatigue, dizziness, fainting), closing up of the throat

Common: headache, dizziness, weakness, fatigue, slow pulse, nausea, difficulty breathing

Tip: If any of these side effects persists or becomes severe, call your doctor.

Other: none reported

 DRUG INTERACTIONS

Combining certain drugs may alter their action or produce unwanted side effects. Tell your doctor about other drugs you're taking, especially:
• calcium channel blockers such as Calan
• drugs used to lower blood pressure
• other drugs used to steady the heartbeat

 If you suspect an overdose

Contact your doctor *immediately.* Excessive Betapace can cause a slow pulse, heart failure (weakness, shortness of breath), low blood pressure (weakness, dizziness), closing up of the throat, and high blood sugar (nausea, headache, weakness).

 Warnings

• Make sure your doctor knows your medical history. You may not be able to take Betapace if you have other heart problems such as congestive heart failure, asthma, kidney problems, or diabetes.
• Tell your doctor if you're pregnant or breast-feeding.

• If you're diabetic, be aware that Betapace may increase your blood sugar level. If you're taking insulin or an oral diabetes drug, the dosage of these drugs may need to be adjusted. Betapace may also mask symptoms of low blood sugar.
• Your doctor will probably want to check your blood regularly (especially if you take a diuretic, or water pill) to make sure that the levels of minerals and salts (electrolytes) in your blood remain normal.

KEEP IN MIND...

∗ Take on empty stomach 1 hour before or 2 hours after meal.

∗ Keep taking even if you feel well.

∗ Don't stop taking suddenly.

Betaseron

Betaseron is a naturally occurring protein that modifies the immune response by interacting with receptors on cell surfaces.

Why it's prescribed

Doctors prescribe Betaseron to reduce the frequency of flareups in people with the relapsing-remitting form of multiple sclerosis. Betaseron comes in a powder for injection. Doctors usually prescribe the following amounts for adults.
▶ **To reduce the frequency of flareups in people with relapsing-remitting multiple sclerosis,** 8 million international units (0.25 milligrams) injected just under the skin every other day.

How to take Betaseron

• Follow your doctor's instructions and the label directions to prepare the solution and self-administer the injection.
• Take this drug at the same time each day. Inject it immediately after you prepare it.
• Inject the preparation just under the skin (subcutaneously) of the shoulder muscle or the front of the thigh muscle.
• Rotate the injection site to reduce pain, inflammation, and other side effects at the injection site.
• Dispose of syringes and needles in an appropriate puncture-proof container.
• Refrigerate the drug or reconstituted product (up to 3 hours) at 36° to 46° F. Don't freeze it.

BETASERON'S OTHER NAME

Betaseron's generic name is recombinant interferon beta-1b.

 SIDE EFFECTS

Call your doctor if you have any of these possible drug side effects. Call *immediately* about any labeled "serious."

Serious: suicidal feelings or tendencies, blood problems (flulike symptoms, fever, chills, overall feelings of illness)
Tip: Alert your family and friends to the possibility of suicidal feelings in addition to notifying your doctor if any actually occur.

Common: menstrual abnormalities, pain and inflammation at injection site, swollen glands
Tips: Take Betaseron at bedtime to help reduce flulike symptoms. Rotate the injection site to avoid pain and inflammation. Avoid people who are sick or have an infection.

Other: depression, anxiety, confusion, headache, dizziness, sore throat, diarrhea, constipation, difficulty breathing, sensitivity to sunlight
Tips: Call your doctor if you experience mood swings, lack of interest in daily activities, or severe depression. Avoid prolonged exposure to sunlight or sunlamps. Wear protective clothing and use sunscreen.

 DRUG INTERACTIONS

Combining certain drugs may alter their action or produce unwanted side effects. Tell your doctor about any other drugs you're taking.

If you miss a dose

Take the missed dose as soon as possible. However, if it's almost time for your next dose, skip the missed dose and take your next dose as scheduled. Don't take a double dose.

 If you suspect an overdose

Consult your doctor.

 Warnings

• Make sure your doctor knows your medical history. Other medical conditions, such as seizures, heart disease, or irregular heartbeats, may affect your use of this drug.
• If you're pregnant, tell your doctor before you start taking Betaseron. If you get pregnant during therapy, notify the doctor and stop taking the drug. This drug can cause a spontaneous abortion.
• Keep follow-up doctor appointments and obtain periodic lab tests as ordered so your doctor can check your progress.

KEEP IN MIND...

∗ Take at same time each day.
∗ To reduce mild flulike symptoms, take at bedtime.
∗ Rotate injection site.
∗ Be aware of suicidal feelings.
∗ Protect eyes and skin from sun.

Betoptic

Betoptic reduces pressure within the eye by decreasing the production of eye fluids and possibly by speeding removal of fluids through the eye.

Why it's prescribed

Doctors prescribe Betoptic to treat chronic open-angle glaucoma and to lower intraocular pressure (pressure within the eye). Betoptic comes in an ophthalmic solution and an ophthalmic suspension. Doctors usually prescribe the following amounts for adults.

▶ **For chronic open-angle glaucoma and high pressure within the eye,** 1 or 2 drops of 0.5% solution or 0.25% suspension twice a day.

How to use Betoptic

• Use this drug exactly as your doctor has directed. Don't use more of it and don't use it more often than ordered; otherwise, your body may absorb too much of the drug, increasing the chance of side effects.
• Wash your hands before and after using the drug.
• Shake the suspension well before using.
• Don't touch the dropper to your eye, the surrounding skin, or any other surface.

If you miss a dose

Don't apply a double dose. Adjust your schedule as follows:
• If you use one dose a day, apply the missed dose as soon as possible. However if you don't remember until the next day, skip the missed

BETOPTIC'S OTHER NAME

Betoptic's generic name is betaxolol hydrochloride.

dose and apply your next dose as scheduled.
• If you use more than one dose a day, apply the missed dose as soon as possible. However, if it's almost time for your next dose, skip the missed dose and apply your next dose as scheduled.

If you suspect an overdose

Contact your doctor *immediately.* Excessive Betoptic can cause double vision, slow pulse, extremely low blood pressure (dizziness, weakness), fatigue, sleepiness, seizures, nausea, vomiting, diarrhea, hallucinations, headache, and coma.

SIDE EFFECTS

Call your doctor if you have any of these possible drug side effects.
Serious: none reported
Common: stinging of eyes
Tip: You may experience stinging right after you use the drops, but this should be only temporary. Dab your eyes with a tissue, but don't rub them.
Other: difficulty sleeping, confusion, occasional tearing of the eyes, unusual sensitivity to light
Tip: If this drug makes your eyes unusually sensitive to light, wear dark glasses.

DRUG INTERACTIONS

Combining certain drugs may alter their action or produce unwanted side effects. Tell your doctor about other drugs you're taking, especially:
• calcium channel blockers such as Calan
• Crystodigin, Lanoxin
• diabetes drugs, including insulin
• epinephrine eye preparations such as Glaucon
• beta blockers, such as Corgard and Tenormin
• phenothiazines (used for anxiety, nausea and vomiting, or psychosis)
• Serpasil.

Warnings

• Make sure your doctor knows your medical history. You may not be able to use Betoptic if you have other problems, especially a heart or lung problem, diabetes, or an overactive thyroid.

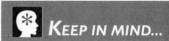 KEEP IN MIND...

* Wash hands before and after using.
* Don't touch dropper to eye or surrounding area.
* Wear dark glasses if eyes become sensitive to light.

Biaxin

Biaxin is one of several antibiotics called macrolides. It stops bacteria from producing proteins, which eventually kills the bacteria or prevents their growth.

Why it's prescribed

Doctors prescribe Biaxin to treat bacterial infections of various parts of the body, including acute flare-ups of chronic bronchitis, certain types of pneumonia, some skin infections, and acute middle ear infections. Biaxin comes in tablets and oral suspension. Doctors usually prescribe the following amounts for adults; children's dosages appear in parentheses (except for middle ear infections).

▶ **For acute sore throat, tonsillitis, or uncomplicated skin and skin-structure infections,** 250 mg every 12 hours for 10 days. (Children: 15 mg for each 2.2 pounds [lb] of body weight a day, divided into equal doses spaced 12 hours apart for 10 days.)

▶ **For acute sinusitis of the upper jaw,** 500 mg every 12 hours for 14 days. (Children: 15 mg for each 2.2 lb a day, divided into equal doses spaced 12 hours apart for 10 days.)

▶ **For acute flare-ups of chronic bronchitis,** 250 to 500 mg every 12 hours for 7 to 14 days.

▶ **For acute middle ear infection in children,** 15 mg for each 2.2 lb a day, divided into equal doses spaced 12 hours apart for 10 days.

BIAXIN'S OTHER NAME

Biaxin's generic name is clarithromycin.

SIDE EFFECTS

Call your doctor if you have any of these possible drug side effects.

Serious: none reported

Common: diarrhea, nausea, abnormal taste

Tip: These side effects should go away as your body adjusts to the drug. However, check with your doctor if they persist or become bothersome.

Other: headache, upset stomach, abdominal pain

DRUG INTERACTIONS

Combining certain drugs may alter their action or produce unwanted side effects. Tell your doctor about other drugs you're taking, especially:
- anticoagulants (blood thinners) such as Coumadin
- Seldane
- Tegretol
- Theo-Dur.

How to take Biaxin

- Take this drug exactly as directed by your doctor. You may take it either with meals or on an empty stomach.
- Take all of the drug prescribed, even if you begin to feel better.

If you miss a dose

Take the missed dose as soon as possible. However, if it's almost time for your next dose, skip the missed dose and take your next dose as scheduled. Don't take a double dose.

If you suspect an overdose

Consult your doctor.

Warnings

- Make sure your doctor knows your medical history. You may not be able to take Biaxin if you have other problems, especially liver or kidney problems.
- If you're pregnant or breast-feeding, tell your doctor before you start taking Biaxin.

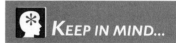

KEEP IN MIND...

* Take either with or without food.
* Finish entire prescription.
* Call doctor about unusual bleeding or bruising.

Bicillin L-A

Bicillin L-A is a penicillin-type antibiotic used to fight infection. It destroys the cell walls of the invading bacteria, eventually killing the bacteria or preventing their growth.

Why it's prescribed

Doctors prescribe Bicillin L-A to treat bacterial infections and to prevent rheumatic fever or a kidney disease called glomerular nephritis. Bicillin L-A comes in an injectable form. Doctors usually prescribe the following amounts.

▶ **For upper respiratory infections,** 1.2 million units into the muscle (intramuscularly [I.M.]) once a day. (Children weighing more than 59 pounds [lb]: 900,000 units I.M. once a day. Children weighing 59 lb or less: 300,000 to 600,000 units I.M. once a day.)

▶ **For syphilis of less than 1 year's duration or for exposure to syphilis,** 2.4 million units I.M. in a single dose.

▶ **For syphilis of more than 1 year's duration,** 2.4 million units I.M. at 7-day intervals for three doses.

▶ **For congenital syphilis in children under age 2,** 50,000 units for each 2.2 lb of body weight I.M. as a single dose.

▶ **To prevent rheumatic fever or glomerular nephritis,** 1.2 million units I.M. once a month, or 600,000 units twice a month.

BICILLIN L-A'S OTHER NAMES

Bicillin L-A's generic name is penicillin G benzathine. Another brand name is Permapen.

 SIDE EFFECTS

Call your doctor if you have any of these possible drug side effects. Call *immediately* about any labeled "serious."

Serious: seizures, allergic reaction (difficulty breathing, light-headedness, rash, hives, itching, wheezing), bloody or decreased amount of urine, unusual bleeding or bruising

Common: diarrhea, stomach cramps, fever, joint pain, sore throat

Other: sensitivity or pain in fingers and toes, bleeding or bruising, infection; pain and redness, especially on leg

 DRUG INTERACTIONS

Combining certain drugs may alter their action or produce unwanted side effects. Tell your doctor about other drugs you're taking, especially:

- Benemid
- Colestid
- Garamycin, Amikin, Kantrex, Myciguent, Netromycin, streptomycin
- Midamor, Aldactone, Dyrenium.

How to take Bicillin L-A

- A nurse or doctor administers Bicillin L-A. It's injected deep into the muscle of the upper outer section of the buttock.

If you miss a dose

If you're scheduled to receive more than one injection and have missed a dose, arrange to receive it as soon as possible.

 If you suspect an overdose

Contact your doctor *immediately.* Excessive Bicillin can cause seizures and unusual sensitivity of the muscles and nerves (hand or leg cramping or tingling).

 Warnings

- Make sure your doctor knows your medical history. You may not be able to take Bicillin L-A if you're allergic to penicillin or if you have asthma, a bleeding disorder, mononucleosis, or a kidney, stomach, or intestinal disease.

- If you're breast-feeding, check with your doctor before you start taking Bicillin L-A.

- If you're allergic to penicillin, you should carry medical identification stating this.

KEEP IN MIND...

∗ Immediately report allergic reaction.

∗ Report serious side effects immediately.

∗ Keep appointments for follow-up injections.

Biltricide

Biltricide is one of several anthelmintics — drugs used to treat fluke (worm) infections. It works by causing spastic paralysis of the worm's muscles, which eventually leads to disintegration.

Why it's prescribed

Doctors prescribe Biltricide to treat the blood for fluke infections (which are also called snail fever, schistosomiasis, or bilharziasis). Biltricide comes in tablets. Doctors usually prescribe the following amounts for adults and children age 4 and older.

▶ **For infection caused by the** *Schistosoma* **fluke (schistosomiasis),** 20 milligrams (mg) for each 2.2 pounds (lb) of body weight three times a day as a 1-day treatment. Let 4 to 6 hours elapse between doses.

▶ **For Chinese liver fluke infection (clonorchiasis),** 25 mg for each 2.2 lb of body weight three times a day as a 1-day treatment.

How to take Biltricide

• Take this drug only as directed by your doctor.

• Don't chew the tablets; their bitter taste may cause you to vomit or gag. Instead, swallow tablets whole with a small amount of liquid during meals.

BILTRICIDE'S OTHER NAME

Biltricide's generic name is praziquantel.

SIDE EFFECTS

Call your doctor if you have any of these possible drug side effects. Call *immediately* about any labeled "serious."

Serious: extreme fatigue, liver problems (nausea, vomiting, yellow-tinged skin and eyes)

Common: drowsiness, overall feeling of illness
Tip: Avoid hazardous activities, such as driving or operating machinery, on the day of treatment and the day after.

Other: dizziness, fever, headache, abdominal discomfort, nausea, hives, sweating

DRUG INTERACTIONS

Combining certain drugs may alter their action or produce unwanted side effects. Tell your doctor about other drugs you're taking, especially:
• steroids.

• Take this drug for the full time of treatment to help clear up your infection completely.

If you miss a dose

Take the missed dose as soon as possible. However, if it's almost time for your next dose, skip the missed dose and take your next dose as scheduled.

If you suspect an overdose

Consult your doctor.

 Warnings

• Make sure your doctor knows your medical history. You may not be able to take Biltricide if you have other medical problems, especially liver disease.

• Don't take this drug if you have worm cysts in your eyes because doing so could cause permanent eye damage.

• If you're breast-feeding, stop on the day you begin taking Biltricide. Don't restart breast-feeding until 72 hours after you complete the treatment. During this time, squeeze out your breast milk with a pump and discard it.

 KEEP IN MIND...

* Swallow tablets whole with liquid during meals.

* Take for full time of treatment.

* Don't breast-feed during treatment or for 72 hours afterward.

Bleph-10

Bleph-10 is an infection-fighting eye medication. It works against bacteria by interfering with the way the bacteria use folic acid.

Why it's prescribed

Doctors prescribe Bleph-10 to treat certain eye infections. Bleph-10 comes in eyedrops and an eye ointment. Doctors usually prescribe the following amounts for adults and children.

▶ **For serious inflammation or ulcers of the cornea, trachoma, and chlamydial infection of the eye,** 1 to 2 drops of 10% solution instilled into the lower eyelid every 2 to 3 hours during the day, or 1 to 2 drops of 15% solution instilled every 1 to 2 hours initially. The interval between doses is increased as the eye condition responds. Or a small amount of 10% ointment applied to the eyelid four times a day and at bedtime. Ointment may be used at night along with drops during the day.

How to use Bleph-10

• Use Bleph-10 exactly as directed by your doctor. Be sure to use all of the drug prescribed, even if your symptoms improve after a few days.
• Wash your hands before and after using this drug.

BLEPH-10'S OTHER NAMES

Bleph-10's generic name is sulfacetamide sodium 10%. Other brand names include Cetamide, Sodium Sulamyd, and Sulf-10.

 ## SIDE EFFECTS

Call your doctor if you have any of these possible drug side effects. Call *immediately* about any labeled "serious."

Serious: Stevens-Johnson syndrome (dry, scaly, red rash on hands, face, and feet; fever; sore throat; muscle pain), allergic reaction (constant eyelid swelling, itching, and burning; rash; blisters in mouth or on eyelids; skin redness and peeling)

Common: pain on instilling eyedrops
Tip: Dab your eyes with a tissue, but don't rub them.

Other: slowed healing of corneal wounds (with ointment), headache or brow pain, sensitivity to light, infection
Tip: To protect your eyes, wear sunglasses in bright light.

 ## DRUG INTERACTIONS

Combining certain drugs may alter their action or produce unwanted side effects. Tell your doctor about other drugs you're taking, especially:
• Garamycin eye medications
• local anesthetics, products containing PABA (wait 30 minutes to 1 hour before using Bleph-10)
• silver eye preparations such as silver nitrate.

• Expect your eyes to sting or blur for a few minutes after you apply the drops or ointment.

If you miss a dose

Take the missed dose as soon as possible. However, if it's almost time for your next dose, skip the missed dose and take your next dose as scheduled.

 ## If you suspect an overdose

Consult your doctor.

 ## Warnings

• Make sure your doctor knows your medical history. You may not be able to take Bleph-10 if you are allergic to any type of sulfa medication.
• Don't share this eye medication with anyone. If someone in your family develops the same symptoms you have, call your doctor.

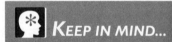 ## KEEP IN MIND...

∗ Wash hands before and after using.

∗ Use entire amount prescribed.

∗ Expect brief stinging or burning of eyes.

∗ Don't share drug with anyone.

Blinx is an eye medication that works by preventing the growth of fungi and bacteria.

Why it's prescribed

Doctors prescribe Blinx to wash the eye after certain procedures. You can also buy Blinx without a prescription. It comes in an eye ointment and eyedrops. Doctors usually prescribe the following amounts for adults.

▶ **For irrigation of the eye,** 1 to 2 eyedrops into the affected eye up to four times a day, or small amount of ointment applied once or twice a day.

How to use Blinx

- If you're treating yourself, read the package instructions carefully.
- If your doctor prescribed this drug or gave you special instructions on how to use it, follow those instructions exactly.
- Wash your hands before and after using this drug.
- Don't use Blinx if the solution is cloudy or discolored.
- To use Blinx as an eyewash, fill the eyecup half full. Then apply the cup tightly to the affected eye and tilt your head backward. Open your eye wide and rotate the eyeball to thoroughly wash the eye.

BLINX'S OTHER NAMES

Blinx's generic name is boric acid. Another brand name is Collyrium.

SIDE EFFECTS

Call your doctor if you have any of these possible drug side effects. Call *immediately* about side effects labeled "serious."

Serious: eye pain or redness, vision changes

Common: none reported

Other: none reported

DRUG INTERACTIONS

Combining certain drugs may alter their action or produce unwanted side effects. Tell your doctor about other drugs you're taking, especially:
- Herplex
- Liquifilm.

- Don't touch the tip of the solution container to any other surface.

If you miss a dose

Consult your doctor.

If you suspect an overdose

Contact your doctor *immediately.* Excessive Blinx can cause low blood pressure (dizziness, weakness), shock (severe dizziness, severe weakness), restlessness, weakness, seizures, nausea, vomiting, diarrhea, absence of urination, increased or decreased body temperature, and rash.

Warnings

- Make sure your doctor knows your medical history. Don't use Blinx if you have a lacerated or torn eye, a scratched cornea, or a cut in your eye.
- Don't share this drug with anyone else because this could spread infection.
- Don't use Blinx while wearing soft contact lenses.
- Be aware that Blinx is toxic if absorbed from abraded skin or wounds.

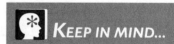

KEEP IN MIND...

∗Wash hands before and after using.

∗Don't touch tip of solution container to any other surface.

∗Don't use while wearing soft contact lenses.

Blocadren

Blocadren decreases the heart's oxygen needs and prevents narrowing of arteries.

Why it's prescribed

Doctors prescribe Blocadren to control high blood pressure and to help prevent heart attacks and migraine headaches. It comes in tablets. Doctors usually prescribe the following amounts for adults.

▶ **For high blood pressure,** initially 10 milligrams (mg) twice a day. Usual maintenance dosage is 20 to 40 mg a day. Maximum dosage is 60 mg a day.

▶ **As long-term therapy after a heart attack,** 10 mg twice a day.

▶ **To prevent migraine headache,** 20 mg as a single dose or divided into two equal doses a day, increased as needed, to a maximum of 30 mg a day.

How to take Blocadren

• Take this drug exactly as directed by your doctor.

• Don't stop taking Blocadren suddenly because this could cause a heart attack. Your doctor may want you to reduce the amount you take gradually.

If you miss a dose

Take the missed dose as soon as possible. However, if it's within 4 hours of your next dose, skip the missed dose and take your next dose as scheduled. Don't take a double dose.

BLOCADREN'S OTHER NAMES

Blocadren's generic name is timolol maleate. Another brand name is Apo-Timol.

 SIDE EFFECTS

Call your doctor if you have any of these possible drug side effects. Call *immediately* about any labeled "serious."

Serious: closing up of the throat (difficulty breathing), congestive heart failure (shortness of breath, fatigue)

Common: slow pulse, low blood pressure (dizziness, weakness), difficulty breathing, sensitivity to cold

Tips: Until you know how Blocadren affects you, avoid activities that require you to be totally alert. Avoid prolonged exposure to cold.

Other: fatigue, lethargy, vivid dreams, nausea, vomiting, diarrhea, difficulty breathing, rash, fever

 DRUG INTERACTIONS

Combining certain drugs may alter their action or produce unwanted side effects. Tell your doctor about other drugs you're taking, especially:

• allergy shots (may cause serious reaction)
• Cardizem, Calan
• Crystodigin, Lanoxin
• diabetes drugs, including insulin
• Indocin.

 If you suspect an overdose

Contact your doctor *immediately*. Excessive Blocadren can cause severe low blood pressure (severe dizziness, severe weakness, fainting), fast pulse, heart failure (shortness of breath), and closing up of the throat (difficulty breathing).

Warnings

• Make sure your doctor knows your medical history. You may not be able to take Blocadren if you have heart, liver, kidney, or lung disease; diabetes; or an overactive thyroid or if you're pregnant or breast-feeding.

• Be aware that older adults may be especially prone to Blocadren's side effects.

• If you're diabetic, be aware that Blocadren may cause your blood sugar level to rise and may mask symptoms of low blood sugar.

• If you're taking Blocadren to treat high blood pressure, learn how to measure your blood pressure.

• Before having surgery (including dental surgery) or emergency treatment, tell the doctor or dentist that you're taking Blocadren.

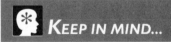 **KEEP IN MIND...**

* Don't stop taking suddenly.
* Don't drive until you know how drug affects you.
* Avoid exposure to cold.

Brethine

Brethine is a bronchodilator. It works by relaxing smooth muscle in the airways, which increases the flow of air in the breathing passages and lungs. This relieves the cough, wheezing, shortness of breath, and difficulty breathing associated with certain respiratory conditions.

Why it's prescribed

Doctors prescribe Brethine to help treat breathing problems related to such conditions as asthma and chronic bronchitis. Brethine comes in tablets and an aerosol inhaler. It's also available in an injectable form. Doctors usually prescribe the following amounts for adults and children over age 11.

▶ **For closing up of the throat (bronchospasm) in people with asthma and chronic bronchitis,** 2 inhalations 60 seconds apart, repeated every 4 to 6 hours; or 5 milligrams (mg) tablets for adults and 2.5 mg for children over age 11 every 8 hours.

How to take Brethine

• Take this drug exactly as directed by your doctor.
• If you're taking Brethine by aerosol inhaler, never take more than two puffs in a row.
• Brethine takes effect 5 to 30 minutes after inhalation and 1 to 2 hours after an oral dose.

BRETHINE'S OTHER NAMES

Brethine's generic name is terbutaline sulfate. Another brand name is Bricanyl.

SIDE EFFECTS

Call your doctor if you have any of these possible drug side effects. Call *immediately* about any labeled "serious."

Serious: closing up of throat (with long-term use)

Common: nervousness, tremor, headache

Other: drowsiness, sweating, palpitations, fast pulse, dryness and irritation of nose and throat (with aerosol form), vomiting, nausea
Tip: Practice good oral and nasal hygiene.

DRUG INTERACTIONS

Combining certain drugs may alter their action or produce unwanted side effects. Tell your doctor about other drugs you're taking, especially:
• beta blockers such as Inderal
• Crystodigin, Lanoxin, Larodopa
• drugs that stimulate the nervous system, such as caffeine, Bronkaid, and Catapres
• MAO inhibitors such as Nardil.

If you miss a dose

If you're using Brethine regularly, take the missed dose as soon as possible. Then take remaining doses that day at regularly spaced intervals. Don't take a double dose.

 ## If you suspect an overdose

Contact your doctor *immediately.* Excessive Brethine can cause an irregular heartbeat, seizures, nausea, and vomiting.

Warnings

• Make sure your doctor knows your medical history. You may not be able to take Brethine if you have other problems, especially a history of seizures, brain damage, diabetes, mental illness, heart disease, high

blood pressure, an overactive thyroid, or Parkinson's disease.
• If you're breast-feeding, tell your doctor before you start taking Brethine.
• If your wheezing gets worse or your breathing becomes more troubled after you take Brethine, stop the drug and call your doctor *immediately.*

 ## KEEP IN MIND...

* Never use inhaler more than twice in a row.

* Call doctor about bothersome nervousness, tremor, or headache.

* Stop drug and call doctor *immediately* if wheezing gets worse or breathing becomes more difficult after using drug.

Bronkometer

Bronkometer relaxes smooth muscle in the airways, which increases the flow of air in the breathing passages and lungs. This relieves the cough, wheezing, shortness of breath, and difficulty breathing associated with certain respiratory conditions.

Why it's prescribed

Doctors prescribe Bronkometer to relieve the symptoms of asthma, bronchitis, and emphysema and to prevent wheezing and troubled breathing triggered by exercise. Bronkometer comes as an inhaler. Doctors usually prescribe the following amounts for adults.

▶ **For bronchial asthma or closing up of the throat (bronchospasm) due to bronchitis or emphysema,** 1 to 2 inhalations, or more if needed.

How to use Bronkometer

• Use Bronkometer exactly as your doctor has prescribed. Don't take more of it than ordered; overuse can cause serious side effects or make the drug less effective.
• Don't use this drug if it's cloudy or discolored.
• If you're taking a second inhaled drug along with Bronkometer, take Bronkometer first and wait 5 minutes before taking the other drug.
• This drug takes effect in 1 to 6 minutes.

BRONKOMETER'S OTHER NAME

Bronkometer's generic name is isoetharine mesylate.

SIDE EFFECTS

Call your doctor if you have any of these possible drug side effects.

Serious: allergic reaction (blue skin, severe dizziness, rash, constant facial flushing, swelling of face or eyelids, increased difficulty breathing)

Common: tremor, headache, rapid pounding heartbeat
Tip: These side effects should disappear after you use the drug for a while. If they don't, tell your doctor.

Other: excitement, fast pulse, changes in blood pressure, nausea, vomiting

DRUG AND FOOD INTERACTIONS

Combining certain drugs and foods may alter drug action or produce unwanted side effects. Tell your doctor about your diet and other drugs you're taking, especially:
• beta blockers such as Inderal
• caffeine-containing foods and drinks, such as coffee, tea, cola, and chocolate
• epinephrine and other sympathomimetic drugs, such as Allerest and Sudafed
• Lanoxin, Crystodigin, Larodopa.

If you miss a dose

Take the missed dose as soon as possible. Then space out the day's remaining doses evenly. Don't take a double dose.

If you suspect an overdose

Contact your doctor *immediately.* Excessive Bronkometer can cause chest pain, seizures, chills, fever, severe muscle cramps, nausea, vomiting, fast or slow pulse, shortness of breath, and severe trembling or weakness.

Warnings

• Make sure your doctor knows your medical history. You may not be able to use Bronkometer if you have an overactive thyroid, high blood pressure, or heart disease.

• If you're pregnant or think you may be or if you're breast-feeding, check with your doctor before you start taking Bronkometer.
• Seek emergency care if your skin turns blue and you experience severe dizziness, a rash, continuous facial flushing, swelling of your face or eyelids, or increased difficulty breathing.
• If your breathing isn't easier after using Bronkometer, call your doctor immediately.

KEEP IN MIND...

∗ Don't use more often than prescribed.

∗ Don't use if cloudy or discolored.

∗ Avoid caffeine.

Bucladin-S Softab

Bucladin-S Softab is an antihistamine used to prevent motion sickness. Researchers suspect that it works by affecting certain structures in the inner ear.

Why it's prescribed

Doctors prescribe Bucladin-S Softab to prevent nausea, vomiting, and dizziness due to motion sickness and to treat vertigo. Bucladin-S Softab comes in chewable tablets. Doctors usually prescribe the following amounts for adults.

▶ **To prevent motion sickness,** 50 milligrams (mg) at least ½ hour before beginning travel, repeated after 4 to 6 hours if needed.

▶ **For vertigo,** 50 mg one to three times a day. Maintenance dosage is 50 mg twice a day.

How to take Bucladin-S Softab

• Take this drug exactly as your doctor has directed. Place the tablets in your mouth, and let them dissolve without water, chew them, or swallow them whole.

• Don't stop taking this drug suddenly after using it for a long time. Your symptoms could return.

If you miss a dose

If you must take this drug regularly, take the missed dose as soon as pos-

sible. However, if it's almost time for your next dose, skip the missed dose and take your next dose as scheduled.

 If you suspect an overdose

Contact your doctor *immediately*. Excessive Bucladin-S Softab can cause sedation, difficulty sleeping, hallucinations, reduced alertness, tremors, stoppage of breathing, and severe heart and blood vessel problems.

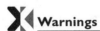 **Warnings**

• Make sure your doctor knows your medical history. You may not be able to take Bucladin-S Softab if you have heart failure, an enlarged

prostate, glaucoma, or blockage of the bowel or urinary tract.

• If you're breast-feeding, be aware that Bucladin-S Softab may reduce your flow of breast milk.

• Children and older adults may be especially prone to certain side effects, such as dryness of the mouth, nose, and throat.

 SIDE EFFECTS

Call your doctor if you have any of these possible drug side effects.

Serious: none reported

Common: drowsiness
Tip: Avoid driving and other activities that require alertness until you know how Bucladin-S Softab affects you.

Other: headache, dizziness, jitters, blurred vision, dry mouth, inability to urinate
Tip: To relieve dry mouth, use sugarless gum or candy, ice chips, or a saliva substitute.

 DRUG INTERACTIONS

Combining certain drugs may alter their action or produce unwanted side effects. Tell your doctor about other drugs you're taking, especially:
• alcohol and other drugs that make you relaxed and sleepy, such as tranquilizers, sedatives, and narcotic pain relievers.

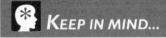 **KEEP IN MIND...**

∗ Let tablets dissolve in mouth, chew, or swallow whole.

∗ Avoid alcohol.

∗ Avoid driving until drug effect known.

∗ Don't stop taking this drug suddenly.

BUCLADIN-S SOFTAB'S OTHER NAME

Bucladin-S Softab's generic name is buclizine hydrochloride.

Bumex

Bumex is a diuretic (water pill). It increases the flow of urine, helping to rid the body of excess water.

Why it's prescribed

Doctors prescribe Bumex to stimulate urination and reduce the amount of water in the body. This may help to improve the condition of people with heart failure or kidney or liver disease. Bumex comes in tablets and an injectable form. Doctors usually prescribe the following amounts for adults.

▶ **To reduce swelling (edema) in congestive heart failure or liver or kidney disease,** 0.5 to 2 milligrams (mg) orally once a day. If needed, second and third doses may be taken at 4- to 5-hour intervals. Maximum dosage is 10 mg a day.

How to take Bumex

• Take this drug exactly as the doctor has prescribed.

If you miss a dose

Take the missed dose as soon as possible. However, if it's almost time for your next dose, skip the missed dose and take your next dose as scheduled. Don't take a double dose.

If you suspect an overdose

Contact your doctor *immediately*. Excessive Bumex can severely deplete your electrolytes (salts) and fluid, possibly causing circulatory

BUMEX'S OTHER NAME

Bumex's generic name is bumetanide.

 SIDE EFFECTS

Call your doctor if you have any of these possible drug side effects.

Serious: none reported

Common: none reported

Other: dizziness, headache, dehydration, temporary deafness, nausea, more frequent or nighttime urination, rash, muscle pain and tenderness, too little sodium, calcium, or magnesium in the body (difficulty waking, poor reflexes, muscle spasms, trouble swallowing)

Tips: To minimize dizziness, get up slowly from a bed or chair. So that the urge to urinate doesn't interrupt your sleep, take Bumex before 6 p.m., unless the doctor tells you differently. To prevent excessive water and potassium loss, call your doctor if you experience persistent vomiting or diarrhea with another illness. To replace lost potassuium, eat foods and drinks containing potassium (for example, citrus fruits and orange juice) or take a potassium supplement.

 DRUG INTERACTIONS

Combining certain drugs may alter their action or produce unwanted side effects. Tell your doctor about other drugs you're taking, especially:

• antibiotics
• Benemid
• blood pressure drugs
• Crystodigin, Lanoxin
• Eskalith, Lithobid
• other diuretics (water pills) such as Lasix
• pain relievers, such as Indocin and Tylenol
• Zaroxylin.

---

system collapse (extremely low blood pressure, severe fatigue and weakness, stoppage of the heart).

Warnings

• Make sure your doctor knows your medical history. Other conditions may affect your use of this drug.
• If you become pregnant while taking Bumex, tell your doctor.

• Be aware that older adults are especially prone to Bumex's side effects.
• If you're a diabetic, be aware that Bumex may increase your blood sugar level.

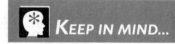 **KEEP IN MIND...**

* Take before 6 p.m.
* Get adequate potassium in your diet.
* Stand up slowly.

BuSpar

BuSpar is a tranquilizer used to reduce anxiety and suppress aggressive behavior. Exactly how it works is unknown.

Why it's prescribed

Doctors prescribe BuSpar to relieve symptoms of anxiety. It comes in tablets. Doctors usually prescribe the following amounts for adults.

▶ **For anxiety disorders or short-term relief of anxiety,** 5 milligrams (mg) three times a day. Dosage is increased by 5 mg every 3 days. Usual maintenance dosage is 20 to 30 mg a day divided into equal doses. Total dosage should not exceed 60 mg a day.

How to take BuSpar

• Take this drug exactly as your doctor has prescribed.
• Be aware that you may not feel BuSpar's full effect until you've taken it for 1 or 2 weeks. In the meantime, continue to take your doses regularly. Don't increase the amount you're taking, thinking that the drug is ineffective.

If you miss a dose

Take the missed dose as soon as possible. However, if it's almost time for your next dose, skip the missed dose and take your next dose as scheduled. Don't take a double dose.

BuSpar's other name

BuSpar's generic name is buspirone hydrochloride.

 SIDE EFFECTS

Call your doctor if you have any of these possible drug side effects.

Serious: none reported

Common: dizziness, drowsiness
Tips: Avoid driving and other activities that require you to be alert and well coordinated until you know how BuSpar affects you. If dizziness or drowsiness persists or gets worse, call your doctor.

Other: nervousness, difficulty sleeping, headache, dry mouth, nausea, diarrhea, fatigue
Tips: If you experience nausea, take your doses with food to buffer the drug's effect on the stomach. To relieve dry mouth, try sugarless hard candy or gum or a saliva substitute, if necessary. Also practice good and frequent oral hygiene.

 DRUG INTERACTIONS

Combining certain drugs may alter their action or produce unwanted side effects. Tell your doctor about other drugs you're taking, especially:
• alcohol and other drugs that make you relaxed or sleepy, such as tranquilizers, narcotics, sleeping pills, sedatives, and cold and allergy medicines.

 If you suspect an overdose

Contact your doctor *immediately*. Excessive BuSpar can cause severe dizziness, drowsiness, unusually small pupils, nausea, and vomiting.

 Warnings

• Make sure your doctor knows your medical history. You may not be able to take BuSpar if you have other problems, especially a history of drug abuse or dependency or kidney or liver disease.
• If you're pregnant or breast-feeding, tell your doctor before you start taking BuSpar.

• If you're taking this drug regularly for a long time, schedule regular checkups so the doctor can monitor your progress and check for side effects.

KEEP IN MIND...

* Drug's full effect may take 1 to 2 weeks to appear.

* Call doctor if drowsiness or dizziness persists or gets worse.

* Avoid driving until you know how drug affects you.

Cafergot

Cafergot contains caffeine and ergotamine. Ergotamine narrows the blood vessels, and caffeine helps the ergotamine to work better and faster.

Why it's prescribed

Doctors prescribe Cafergot to prevent migraine, cluster, and vascular headaches. It comes in tablets and suppositories. Doctors usually prescribe the following amounts for adults.

▶ **To prevent migraine, cluster, or vascular headache,** 2 tablets or 1 suppository at the first sign (aura) of headache. The maximum amount for a single headache attack is 6 tablets or 2 suppositories. For more than one headache attack per week, the maximum weekly amount is 10 tablets or 6 suppositories.

How to take Cafergot

• Take this drug exactly as your doctor has prescribed.
• For best results, take Cafergot at the first sign of a headache. Rest in a dark, quiet room.
• If you frequently experience nausea and vomiting with your headaches, use the suppositories rather than the oral tablets.
• If the suppository is too soft, moisten it with cold water before inserting it.
• Don't take more than 6 tablets or 2 suppositories for a single headache attack, or more than 10 tablets or 6 suppositories in a week.

CAFERGOT'S OTHER NAMES

Cafergot is a combination of the generic drugs ergotamine and caffeine. Another brand name is Wigraine.

SIDE EFFECTS

Call your doctor if you have any of these possible drug side effects. Call *immediately* about any labeled "serious."

Serious: numbness, blistering, discoloration, or tingling in toes or fingers; weakness; chest pain; fast or slow pulse; swelling or itching; vision change

Common: diarrhea, dizziness, drowsiness
Tip: Prevent dizziness by standing up slowly and taking care when walking.

Other: nausea, vomiting, rectal ulcers

DRUG INTERACTIONS

Combining certain drugs may alter their action or produce unwanted side effects. Tell your doctor about other drugs you're taking, especially:
• alcohol
• beta blockers such as Inderal
• nicotine.

• If you've been using Cafergot regularly, don't stop taking it abruptly. Doing so may increase the frequency and duration of headaches. Your doctor may want you to reduce the amount you take gradually.

If you miss a dose

Not applicable because Cafergot is taken only as needed.

If you suspect an overdose

Contact your doctor *immediately.* Excessive Cafergot can cause drowsiness, tingling or numbness in your hands or feet, high blood pressure (headache, blurred vision), or low blood pressure (dizziness, weakness).

Warnings

• Make sure your doctor knows your medical history. You may not be able to take Cafergot if you have other problems, especially high blood pressure or diseases of the blood vessels, kidney, or liver.
• If you're pregnant or breast-feeding, don't take this drug.
• Older adults may be especially prone to Cafergot's side effects.
• Use Cafergot only for migraine, cluster, or vascular headaches. It won't relieve the symptoms of tension headaches.

KEEP IN MIND...

* Take at first sign of headache.
* Rest in dark, quiet room for 2 hours after taking.
* Don't stop taking abruptly after regular use.
* Avoid alcohol.

Calan

Calan blocks calcium from entering the heart muscle, thereby slowing the heartbeat. It also widens blood vessels, allowing more oxygen-carrying blood to nourish the heart.

Why it's prescribed

Doctors prescribe Calan for chest pain, fast or irregular heartbeats, or high blood pressure. Calan comes in immediate-release tablets, extended-release tablets, and extended-release capsules. It's also available in an injectable form. Doctors usually prescribe the following amounts for adults.

▶ **For chest pain and irregular heartbeat,** 80 to 120 milligrams (mg) orally three times a day, increased weekly as necessary. Some people may require up to 480 mg a day.

▶ **For high blood pressure,** 240 mg in an extended-release tablet orally once a day in the morning; if response isn't adequate, another ½ tablet in the evening or 1 tablet every 12 hours. Or, 80 mg in an immediate-release tablet three times a day.

How to take Calan

• Take Calan only as your doctor directs. If you're taking an extended-release tablet, swallow it whole, without crushing or chewing it.

CALAN'S OTHER NAMES

Calan's generic names are verapamil and verapamil hydrochloride. Other brand names include Calan SR (slow-release), Isoptin, Isoptin SR, Verelan; and, in Canada, Apo-Verap, Novo-Veramil, and Nu-Verap.

SIDE EFFECTS

Call your doctor if you have any of these possible drug side effects. Call *immediately* about any labeled "serious."

Serious: shortness of breath, difficulty breathing except when upright, wheezing, palpitations, irregular heartbeats, swollen legs, pale or bluish skin

Common: constipation, dizziness
Tips: Avoid constipation by increasing fluids and high-fiber foods in your diet. Prevent dizziness by standing up slowly and taking care when walking.

Other: fatigue, headache, slow pulse, nausea
Tips: Get extra rest. Take your doses with food to avoid nausea, although food may decrease your body's ability to absorb the extended-release forms, requiring a change in the amount you take.

DRUG INTERACTIONS

Combining certain drugs may alter their action or produce unwanted side effects. Tell your doctor about other drugs you're taking, especially:
• heart drugs (except nitroglycerin as needed for chest pain)
• drugs for high blood pressure, seizures, tuberculosis, or glaucoma
• Eskalith, Lithobid.

• Take your drug even if you feel well. Stopping suddenly could worsen your condition.

If you miss a dose

Take the missed dose as soon as possible. However, if it's almost time for your next dose, skip the missed dose and take your next dose as scheduled. Don't take a double dose.

If you suspect an overdose

Contact your doctor *immediately.* Excessive Calan can cause extreme low blood pressure (severe dizziness and weakness), heart attack (chest pain, shortness of breath), and sudden death.

 Warnings

• Make sure your doctor knows your medical history. You may not be able to take Calan if you have another heart or blood vessel disorder or kidney or liver disease.
• If you're pregnant or breast-feeding, tell your doctor before you begin taking Calan.

 KEEP IN MIND...

∗ Take with food.

∗ Don't crush or chew extended-release capsules or tablets.

∗ Increase fluids and fiber in diet.

Calciferol

Calciferol, a form of vitamin D, helps the body to absorb and use calcium and phosphate and helps to regulate the body's calcium balance.

Why it's prescribed

Doctors prescribe Calciferol to treat lack of vitamin D and disorders in which calcium isn't used properly by the body. Calciferol comes in tablets, capsules, and oral liquid. It's also available in an injectable form. Doctors usually prescribe the following amounts for adults; children's dosages appear in parentheses.

▶ **For vitamin D-dependent rickets,** 250 micrograms (mcg) to 1.5 milligrams (mg) orally a day. (Children: 75 to 125 mcg daily.)
▶ **For vitamin D-resistant rickets,** 250 mcg to 1.5 mg orally a day. (Children: 1 to 2 mg orally a day, increased as needed.)
▶ **For rickets caused by seizure drugs,** 50 mcg to 1.25 mg orally each day.
▶ **To correct osteomalacia (softening of the bones) in adults with severe vitamin D deficiency and intestinal disorders,** 250 mcg injected into the muscle daily.
▶ **For seizures,** 50 to 1.25 mcg orally a day.

How to take Calciferol

• Take Calciferol exactly as your doctor has directed. Don't take

CALCIFEROL'S OTHER NAMES

Calciferol's generic name is ergocalciferol. Other brand names include Deltalin Gelseals, Drisdol; and, in Canada, Radiostol.

SIDE EFFECTS

Call your doctor if you have any of these possible drug side effects. Call *immediately* about any labeled "serious." (Side effects usually occur only with overdose.)

Serious: seizures, calcium deposits in soft tissues, impaired kidney function (decreased amount of urine), too much calcium in the blood (increased thirst, increased urination, constipation, vomiting, difficulty waking)

Common: none reported

Other: headache, dizziness, weakness, sleepiness, strange behavior, runny nose, pinkeye, eye sensitivity to light, ringing in ears, appetite loss, nausea, vomiting, constipation, diarrhea, dry mouth, metallic taste, excessive urination, itching, bone and muscle pain, weight loss
Tips: Use sunglasses when in bright light. Take care when driving or operating machinery. Increase fluids and high-fiber foods. Use frequent mouth care.

DRUG INTERACTIONS

Combining certain drugs may alter their action or produce unwanted side effects. Tell your doctor about other drugs you're taking, especially:
• Barbita, Dilantin
• corticosteroids
• dietary supplements containing vitamin D, calcium, or phosphorus
• Diuril, HydroDIURIL
• Lanoxin, Crystodigin
• Milk of Magnesia and other magnesium-containing antacids
• mineral oil
• Questran.

more of it than ordered; too much vitamin D can be toxic.
• Swallow tablets whole; don't crush or chew them.

If you miss a dose

Adjust your schedule as follows:
• If you're taking one dose every other day, take the missed dose as soon as possible. If you don't remember it until the next day, take it at that time. Then skip one day and return to your regular schedule. Don't take a double dose.

• If you're taking one or more doses a day, take the missed dose as soon as possible. However, if you don't remember until the next day, skip the missed dose and take your next dose as scheduled. Don't take a double dose.

 ## If you suspect an overdose

Contact your doctor *immediately.* Excessive Calciferol can cause too much phosphate in the blood (seizures, cramps, decreased feeling in fingers and toes), too much calcium in the blood and urine (increased thirst and urination, constipation, vomiting, difficulty waking), and heart or kidney failure.

Warnings

• Make sure your doctor knows your medical history. You may not be able to take Calciferol if you have other problems, especially a kidney, heart, or blood vessel disorder.

• If you're pregnant or breast-feeding, tell your doctor before you begin taking Calciferol.

• Be aware that infants may be particularly sensitive to Calciferol's side effects.

• If you're on a high dose of Calciferol, expect the doctor to order periodic blood tests to check the amount of calcium, potassium, and other substances in your body.

• If you have too little phosphate in your body (hypophosphatemia), the doctor may put you on a special diet.

• Your doctor may ask you to increase calcium in your diet. Foods that are high in calcium include dairy products, such as milk, cheese, and yogurt.

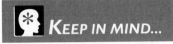

KEEP IN MIND...

∗ Don't increase dosage.

∗ Don't take other preparations containing vitamin D, calcium, or phosphorus.

∗ Call doctor about dry mouth, nausea, vomiting, metallic taste, and constipation.

Calderol

Calderol is a form of vitamin D that stimulates the absorption of calcium from the digestive tract and helps calcium to move from the bones to the bloodstream.

Why it's prescribed

Doctors prescribe Calderol to treat diseases in which calcium is not used properly by the body or to treat bone disease in people with kidney disease who are undergoing kidney dialysis. Calderol comes in capsules. Doctors usually prescribe the following amounts for adults.

▶ **For bone disease in people with chronic kidney failure,** initially 300 to 350 micrograms once a week, increased at 4-week intervals if necessary.

How to take Calderol

• Take this drug exactly as your doctor tells you.
• Because the dosage is different from person to person, don't change the amount or frequency.

If you miss a dose

Take the missed dose as soon as you remember. This day will become your new day of the week that you take your weekly dose.

If you suspect an overdose

Contact your doctor immediately. Excessive Calderol can cause too much calcium in the blood (increased thirst and urination, constipation,

CALDEROL'S OTHER NAME

Calderol's generic name is calcifediol.

 SIDE EFFECTS

Call your doctor if you have any of these possible drug side effects. Call *immediately* about any labeled "serious."

Serious: high blood pressure (headache, blurred vision)

Common: none reported

Other: headache, sleepiness, pinkeye, skin sensitivity to sunlight, runny nose, nausea, vomiting, diarrhea, constipation, metallic taste, dry mouth, appetite loss, weight loss, abnormally large amount of urine, weakness, bone and muscle pain

Tips: Use sunglasses to protect your eyes in strong sunlight. If you experience nausea, take your doses with food to buffer the drug's effect on your stomach. To avoid constipation, drink more liquids and eat more high-fiber foods. Perform frequent mouth care.

✕ DRUG INTERACTIONS

Combining certain drugs may alter their action or produce unwanted side effects. Tell your doctor about other drugs you're taking, especially:
• Colestid, Questran
• corticosteroids
• Crystodigin, Lanoxin
• magnesium-containing antacids such as Milk of Magnesia
• other vitamin D-like preparations such as Calciferol.

vomiting, difficulty waking). More severe degrees of overdose can cause heart and kidney failure.

✕ Warnings

• Make sure your doctor knows your medical history. You may not be able to take Calderol if you have other problems, especially a kidney disorder or heart or blood vessel problems.
• If you're pregnant or breast-feeding, tell your doctor before you begin taking Calderol.
• Expect the doctor to order periodic blood tests (every week at first) to measure the amount of calcium in your blood.

• Try to include calcium-rich foods in your daily diet. Good sources of calcium include collards, turnip greens, broccoli, dried beans, sardines, salmon, tofu, and dairy products. Choose low-fat dairy products because they're lower in cholesterol.

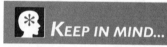 KEEP IN MIND...

∗ Include calcium-rich foods in daily diet.

∗ Choose low-fat dairy products.

∗ Expect to have periodic blood tests.

Capoten

Capoten relaxes blood vessels, thus lowering blood pressure. Capoten also helps to avoid weakening of the heart after a heart attack.

Why it's prescribed

Doctors prescribe Capoten to reduce blood pressure, to treat congestive heart failure, or to treat kidney problems in diabetics who use insulin. Capoten comes in tablets. Doctors usually prescribe the following amounts for adults.

▶ **For high blood pressure,** 25 milligrams (mg) two or three times a day at first, increased to 50 mg two or three times a day as needed after 1 to 2 weeks. Maximum dosage is 450 mg a day.

▶ **For congestive heart failure,** 6.25 to 12.5 mg three times a day at first, increased gradually to 50 mg three times a day as needed. Maximum dosage is 450 mg a day.

▶ **For kidney problems,** 25 mg three times a day.

How to take Capoten

• Carefully follow the label directions and your doctor's instructions.
• Take Capoten 1 hour before meals unless your doctor tells you otherwise.
• Don't stop taking this drug, even if you feel better.

If you miss a dose

Take the missed dose as soon as possible. However, if it's almost time

CAPOTEN'S OTHER NAMES

Capoten's generic name is captopril. Canadian brand names include Apo-Capto and Syn-Captopril.

 SIDE EFFECTS

Call your doctor if you have any of these possible drug side effects. Call *immediately* about any labeled "serious."

Serious: kidney failure (little or no urine), blood problems (fatigue, fever, chills, bruising or bleeding, infection), fast pulse, low blood pressure (dizziness, weakness)

Common: bad taste in mouth, dry cough, hives, rash

Other: fainting; chest pain; appetite loss; frequent urination; itching; fever; swelling of face, hands, and feet; too much potassium in the blood (anxiety, weakness, dizziness)

Tips: Tell your doctor if you experience dizziness, light-headedness, or fainting after taking Capoten for a few days or after heavy sweating, which depletes body water and lowers blood pressure. Avoid becoming overheated.

 DRUG INTERACTIONS

Combining certain drugs may alter their action or produce unwanted side effects. Tell your doctor about other drugs you're taking, especially:
• Aldactone, Dyrenium, Midamor
• antacids (take at least 2 hours before or after Capoten)
• Crystodigin, Lanoxin
• diabetes drugs, including insulin
• diuretics (water pills) and other blood pressure drugs
• Eskalith
• nonsteroidal anti-inflammatory drugs (NSAIDs) such as Advil
• potassium supplements.

for your next dose, skip the missed dose and take your next dose as scheduled. Don't take a double dose.

 If you suspect an overdose

Contact your doctor *immediately.* Excessive Capoten can cause severe low blood pressure (weakness, dizziness).

 Warnings

• Make sure your doctor knows your medical history. Other conditions may affect drug use.

• If you become pregnant or are breast-feeding, tell your doctor.
• Call your doctor promptly if you become sick while taking Capoten.

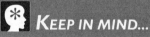 **KEEP IN MIND...**

* Take 1 hour before meals.
* Don't stop taking without doctor's approval.
* Follow any prescribed special diet.

Capozide

Capozide is a combination of a diuretic (water pill) and captopril, a drug that's used to reduce high blood pressure. Capozide relaxes blood vessels and decreases the amount of blood to the heart. When the heart has less blood to circulate, it doesn't have to work as hard, which leads to a decreased risk of heart attack or stroke.

Why it's prescribed

Doctors prescribe Capozide to treat high blood pressure. It's available in tablets of varying strengths: Capozide 25/15 contains 25 milligrams (mg) of captopril and 15 mg of the diuretic hydrochlorothiazide (HCTZ); Capozide 25/25 contains 25 mg of each; Capozide 50/15 contains 50 mg of captopril and 15 mg of HCTZ; and Capozide 50/25 contains 50 mg of captopril and 25 mg of HCTZ. Doctors usually prescribe the following amount for adults.

▶ **For high blood pressure,** 1 tablet Capozide 25/15 daily, adjusted as needed (dosage differs from person to person).

How to take Capozide

• Take Capozide exactly as your doctor has prescribed. Don't increase the dose or frequency without consulting your doctor.
• Take Capozide 1 hour before a meal.

CAPOZIDE'S OTHER NAMES

Capozide combines two generic drugs: captopril and hydrochlorothiazide.

 SIDE EFFECTS

Call your doctor if you have any of these possible drug side effects. Call *immediately* about any labeled "serious."

Serious: angioedema (swelling of face, tongue, vocal cords), low blood pressure (dizziness, weakness), abdominal pain, chest pain, fast pulse

Common: dizziness, loss of taste, rash
Tip: Prevent dizziness by standing up slowly and taking care while walking.

Other: flushing, cough, nausea, vomiting, infection (fever, cough, sore throat), skin sensitivity to sun, too much potassium (fast pulse, nausea, diarrhea, abdominal cramps, decreased urination)
Tip: Report symptoms of infection and high potassium to your doctor.

 DRUG INTERACTIONS

Combining certain drugs may alter their action or produce unwanted side effects. Tell your doctor about other drugs you're taking, especially:
• alcohol
• anticoagulants (blood thinners) such as Coumadin
• Digoxin
• insulin, oral diabetes drugs such as Micronase
• lithium
• MAO inhibitors, such as Nardil and Parnate
• nonsteroidal anti-inflammatory medications such as Advil
• steroids such as prednisone.

• No matter how many doses you take each day, make sure to take your last dose at least several hours before bedtime to prevent the need to urinate from disrupting your sleep. The diuretic in Capozide will increase the amount and frequency of urination.
• You may not feel Capozide's effects until 6 to 8 weeks after starting the drug.

If you miss a dose

Take the missed dose as soon as possible. However, if it's almost time for your next dose, skip the missed dose and take your next dose as scheduled. Don't take a double a dose.

 If you suspect an overdose

Contact your doctor *immediately.* Excessive Capozide can cause low blood pressure (dizziness, weakness, fainting) and low electrolytes (palpitations, weakness, nausea, vomiting, confusion).

Capozide (continued)

✗ Warnings

• Make sure your doctor knows your medical history. You may not be able to take Capozide if you have angioedema or kidney problems.

• If you're pregnant or breast feeding, check with your doctor before taking Capozide.
• Older adults may be especially prone to Capozide's side effects.

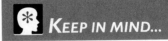

KEEP IN MIND...

* Take 1 hour before a meal.
* Take last daily dose at least several hours before bedtime.
* Rise slowly to prevent dizziness.
* Report facial swelling, abdominal or chest pain, or rash.
* Protect skin from sun.

Carafate

Carafate is used to treat peptic (duodenal) ulcers. It works by forming a barrier over the ulcer, which protects the ulcer from stomach acid and thus allows it to heal.

Why it's prescribed

Doctors prescribe Carafate to prevent and treat a type of peptic ulcer called a duodenal ulcer. It comes in tablets. Doctors usually prescribe the following amounts for adults.

▶ **For short-term (up to 8 weeks) treatment of duodenal ulcers,** 1 gram (g) four times a day.

▶ **As maintenance therapy for duodenal ulcers,** 1 g two times a day.

How to take Carafate

• Take this drug only as your doctor has directed.

• Carafate works best on an empty stomach; take it with water only, 1 hour before meals and at bedtime.

• If you have difficulty swallowing, try placing the tablet in an ounce of water. Let the tablet sit in the water at room temperature until it dissolves. Then drink the fluid.

• Keep taking this drug for as long as your doctor has prescribed, even after you've begun to feel better.

If you miss a dose

Take the missed dose as soon as possible. However, if it's almost time

CARAFATE'S OTHER NAMES

Carafate's generic name is sucralfate. A Canadian brand name is Sulcrate.

 SIDE EFFECTS

Call your doctor if you have any of these possible drug side effects.

Serious: none reported

Common: constipation
Tips: To avoid constipation, drink plenty of fluids and eat more high-fiber foods. If you do become constipated, call your doctor, who may prescribe a laxative.

Other: dizziness, sleepiness, nausea, stomach upset, diarrhea; formation of bezoar, a ball of hair and vegetable fiber in the intestine (abdominal pain and cramps)

 DRUG INTERACTIONS

Combining certain drugs may alter their action or produce unwanted side effects. Tell your doctor about other drugs you're taking, especially:
• aspirin
• antacids (take at least a half hour before or after Carafate)
• Tagamet, Zantac, Cipro, Lanoxin, Noroxin, Dilantin, tetracycline, Theo-Dur (take at least 2 hours before or after Carafate).

for your next dose, skip the missed dose and take your next dose as scheduled. Don't take a double dose.

 If you suspect an overdose

Consult your doctor.

 Warnings

• Make sure your doctor knows your medical history. You may not be able to take Carafate if you have other problems, especially if you've had kidney failure or a bowel obstruction.

• If you're pregnant or breast-feeding, check with your doctor before you start taking this drug.

• Avoid activities that could worsen your ulcer. For example, don't smoke because smoking increases the production of stomach acid. Also, don't drink alcoholic beverages, take aspirin, or eat foods that irritate your stomach.

KEEP IN MIND...

* Take with water 1 hour before meals and at bedtime.

* Take at least a half hour apart from antacid.

* Don't smoke, drink alcoholic beverages, take aspirin, or eat foods that irritate stomach.

Cardene

Cardene blocks calcium from entering the heart muscle, thereby slowing heart contractions. It also widens the heart's blood vessels, allowing more oxygen-carrying blood to reach and nourish the heart.

Why it's prescribed

Doctors prescribe Cardene for chest pain or high blood pressure. Cardene comes in immediate-release capsules and sustained-release capsules. It's also available in an injectable form. Doctors usually prescribe the following amounts for adults.

▶ **For chest pain,** initially 20 milligrams (mg) orally three times a day (immediate-release capsule only). Dosage is adjusted every 3 days according to the person's response.

▶ **For high blood pressure,** initially 20 to 40 mg orally three times a day (immediate-release capsule) or 30 mg twice a day (sustained-release capsule).

How to take Cardene

• Take this drug only as your doctor has prescribed.
• Keep taking Cardene even if you feel well.
• If you've been taking Cardene regularly for several weeks, don't suddenly stop taking it. Your doctor may want you to reduce the amount you take gradually.

If you miss a dose

Take the missed dose as soon as possible. However, if it's almost time

CARDENE'S OTHER NAME

Cardene's generic name is nicardipine.

 SIDE EFFECTS

Call your doctor if you have any of these possible drug side effects. Call *immediately* about any labeled "serious."

Serious: chest pain, fast pulse

Common: dizziness, headache, drowsiness, weakness, swelling of the lower legs, palpitations, tingling, numbness
Tips: Avoid hazardous activities until you know how this drug affects you. To prevent dizziness, stand up slowly and take care when walking.

Other: nausea, stomach upset, dry mouth, rash
Tips: Some people experience more frequent, severe, or long-lasting chest pain when they start taking Cardene or when the dosage is changed. Call your doctor immediately if chest pain occurs. Take with food to avoid stomach upset.

 DRUG INTERACTIONS

Combining certain drugs may alter their action or produce unwanted side effects. Tell your doctor about other drugs you're taking, especially:
• beta blockers (for chest pain or high blood pressure)
• blood pressure drugs
• Sandimmune
• Tagamet
• Theo-Dur.

for your next dose, skip the missed dose and take your next dose as scheduled. Don't take a double dose.

 If you suspect an overdose

Contact your doctor *immediately.* Excessive Cardene can cause low blood pressure (dizziness, weakness), slow pulse, drowsiness, confusion, and slurred speech.

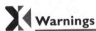 **Warnings**

• Make sure your doctor knows your medical history. You may not be able to take Cardene if you have other heart or blood vessel problems or a liver or kidney disorder.

• If you're pregnant, tell your doctor before you start taking Cardene.
• Be aware that older adults may be especially prone to Cardene's side effects.
• If your doctor instructs you to take your blood pressure at home, report any change.
• Follow any prescribed special diet, such as a low-salt diet.

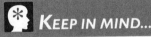 **KEEP IN MIND...**

∗ Don't stop taking suddenly.
∗ Follow any special diet.
∗ Call doctor immediately about chest pain.

Cardizem SR

Cardizem SR blocks calcium from entering the heart muscle, thereby slowing heart contractions. The drug also widens the heart's blood vessels, allowing more oxygen-carrying blood to reach and nourish the heart.

Why it's prescribed

Doctors prescribe Cardizem SR to relieve and control chest pain (angina), to reduce high blood pressure, and to correct irregular heartbeats. Cardizem SR comes in sustained-release and extended-release capsules. It's also available in an injectable form. Doctors usually prescribe the following amounts for adults.

▶ **For chest pain,** 60 to 120 milligrams (mg) of Cardizem SR orally three or four times a day before meals and at bedtime. Dosage is increased gradually to maximum of 360 mg per day divided into equal doses.

▶ **For high blood pressure,** 60 to 120 mg of Cardizem SR orally twice a day, adjusted as necessary.

How to take Cardizem SR

• Take this drug exactly as your doctor has prescribed.
• Don't crush or chew the capsules; swallow them whole.
• If you've been taking Cardizem SR regularly, don't suddenly stop taking it. Your doctor may want you to reduce the amount you take gradually.

CARDIZEM SR'S OTHER NAMES

Cardizem SR's generic name is diltiazem. Other brand names include Dilacor XR.

 SIDE EFFECTS

Call your doctor if you have any of these possible drug side effects. Call *immediately* about any labeled "serious."

Serious: irregular heartbeat, heart failure (shortness of breath, fatigue)

Common: headache, fatigue, drowsiness, swelling of the feet and ankles, nausea, constipation, rash, sudden weight gain (more than 3 pounds in 1 week)
Tip: Weigh yourself each week and record your weight.

Other: dizziness, weakness, nervousness, depression, difficulty sleeping, confusion, flushing, slow pulse, vomiting, diarrhea, excessive or nighttime urination, itching, skin sensitivity to sunlight
Tips: Avoid hazardous activities until you know how this drug affects you. Take your last dose several hours before bedtime to avoid having nighttime urination disrupt your sleep. Wear protective clothing and sunscreen outdoors.

 DRUG INTERACTIONS

Combining certain drugs may alter their action or produce unwanted side effects. Tell your doctor about other drugs you're taking, especially:
• beta blockers (for high blood pressure or chest pain)
• Lanoxin
• Sandimmune
• Tagamet.

If you miss a dose

Take the missed dose as soon as possible. However, if it's almost time for your next dose, skip the missed dose and take your next dose as scheduled. Don't take a double dose.

If you suspect an overdose

Contact your doctor *immediately.* Excessive Cardizem SR can cause heart block (shortness of breath) and low blood pressure (fatigue, dizziness, weakness, fainting).

Warnings

• Make sure your doctor knows your medical history. You may not be able to take Cardizem SR if you have other medical problems, especially other heart conditions or a liver or kidney disorder.
• If you're pregnant or breast-feeding, check with your doctor before you start taking this drug.
• Older adults may be especially prone to Cardizem SR's side effects.

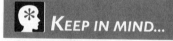 **KEEP IN MIND...**

∗ Swallow capsules whole.
∗ Weigh yourself weekly and record your weight.
∗ Don't stop drug suddenly.

Cardura

Cardura is one of several drugs called alpha blockers. It lowers high blood pressure by relaxing blood vessels, which allows blood to pass through the vessels more easily.

Why it's prescribed

Doctors prescribe Cardura to treat high blood pressure. Cardura comes in tablets. Doctors usually prescribe the following amounts for adults.

▶ **For high blood pressure,** initially 1 milligram (mg) each day. After drug's effect on blood pressure is determined 2 to 6 hours and 24 hours after first dose, dosage may be increased gradually (every 2 weeks) to 2 mg a day. If necessary, dose increased to 4 mg a day, then 8 mg. Maximum dosage is 16 mg a day.

How to take Cardura

• Take this drug exactly as your doctor has prescribed.

If you miss a dose

Take the missed dose as soon as possible. However, if it's almost time for your next dose, skip the missed dose and take your next dose as scheduled. Don't take a double dose.

If you suspect an overdose

Contact your doctor immediately. Excessive Cardura can cause extremely low blood pressure (severe weakness and dizziness, fatigue).

CARDURA'S OTHER NAME

Cardura's generic name is doxazosin mesylate.

 ## SIDE EFFECTS

Call your doctor if you have any of these possible drug side effects. Call *immediately* about any labeled "serious."

Serious: irregular heartbeat

Common: dizziness

Tips: Stand up slowly to minimize dizziness. Usually, this effect diminishes after the first dose, but it may recur if you stop taking the drug for a few days or if the amount you're taking is changed. If the problem persists or becomes severe, tell your doctor.

Other: headache, vertigo, sleepiness, drowsiness, weakness, swelling, palpitations, fast pulse, pain and tingling in fingers or toes, nausea, vomiting, diarrhea, constipation, rash, itching, runny nose, muscle or joint pain, muscle weakness

Tips: Make sure you know how you react to Cardura before you drive or perform other activities that could be dangerous if you're not fully alert. Call your doctor if you develop a rash or muscle or joint pain.

 ## DRUG INTERACTIONS

Combining certain drugs may alter their action or produce unwanted side effects. Tell your doctor about other drugs you're taking.

Warnings

• Make sure your doctor knows your medical history. You may not be able to take Cardura if you have other medical problems, especially liver disease.

• If you're pregnant or breast-feeding, check with your doctor before taking this drug.

• Don't take Cardura with other blood pressure drugs unless your doctor directs you to do so. Taking this combination of drugs may cause dangerously low blood pressure, possibly leading to loss of consciousness.

• Your doctor may teach you how to take your blood pressure at home. If so, check your blood pressure at regular intervals and call your doctor if you detect significant changes.

• Keep medical appointments. You'll need to see your doctor at least every 2 weeks until your dosage is set properly, then at regular intervals so your progress can be checked.

KEEP IN MIND...

* Don't take with other blood pressure drugs.

* Take blood pressure at home if instructed.

* Call doctor about rash, muscle or joint pain, or irregular heartbeat.

Carnitor helps carry fatty acids into the body's cells. There, the fatty acids are used to produce energy.

Why it's prescribed

Doctors prescribe Carnitor to treat deficiencies of carnitine (a B vitamin). Carnitor comes in tablets and an oral liquid. It's also available in an injectable form. Doctors usually prescribe the following amounts for adults; children's dosages appear in parentheses.

▶ **For carnitine deficiency,** 990 milligrams (mg) orally two or three times a day. Or, 10 to 30 milliliters (ml) (1 to 3 grams [g]) of oral liquid each day. The amount given depends on how the patient responds; more may be given. (Children: 50 to 100 mg for each 2.2 pounds of body weight orally a day, divided into equal doses; maximum dosage is 3 g per day.)

▶ **As dietary supplement for kidney patients,** 500 to 750 mg orally each day.

How to take Carnitor

• Take Carnitor only as your doctor directs.
• If you're taking the oral liquid, you may mix it with other liquids to mask the taste.
• Drink oral liquid slowly to minimize stomach upset. If stomach up-

CARNITOR'S OTHER NAME

Carnitor's generic name is levocarnitine.

SIDE EFFECTS

Call your doctor if you have any of these possible drug side effects.

Serious: none reported

Common: nausea, vomiting, cramps, diarrhea
Tips: Drink oral liquid slowly to avoid these side effects. Take during or after meals to avoid nausea.

Other: body odor
Tip: Remember to wash frequently to avoid body odor.

DRUG INTERACTIONS

Combining certain drugs may alter their action or produce unwanted side effects. Tell your doctor about other drugs you're taking, especially:
• Depakote
• D,L-carnitine (vitamin B_T) supplements.

---

set persists, the doctor may reduce your dosage.
• Space doses throughout the day (every 3 to 4 hours) during or after meals.

If you miss a dose

Take the next dose as soon as possible. However, if it's almost time for your next dose, skip the missed dose and go back to your regular schedule. Don't take a double dose.

 If you suspect an overdose

Consult your doctor. Excessive Carnitor may cause diarrhea.

 Warnings

• Make sure your doctor knows your medical history. Other medi-

cal conditions may affect your use of Carnitor.
• If you're pregnant or breast-feeding, tell your doctor before you begin taking Carnitor.
• Don't share Carnitor with others (some people have used it to improve athletic performance).
• Be sure to keep all scheduled follow-up appointments. Your doctor will probably want to check your blood levels of certain substances.

KEEP IN MIND...

* Take oral liquid slowly.
* Avoid vitamin B_T supplements.
* Don't share Carnitor with others.

Cartrol

Cartrol is one of several drugs that reduce high blood pressure. Although its action is not fully known, Cartrol slows the heart rate and increases the force of each contraction.

Why it's prescribed

Doctors prescribe Cartrol to treat high blood pressure or impaired kidney activity that leads to high blood pressure. Cartrol comes in tablets. Doctors usually prescribe the following amounts for adults.

▶ **For high blood pressure,** 2.5 milligrams (mg) orally once a day, gradually increased to 5 to 10 mg a day as needed.

▶ **For high blood pressure in people with impaired kidney function,** the usual dose of Cartrol given at 24-, 48-, or 72-hour intervals, depending on the results of blood tests.

How to take Cartrol

• Take Cartrol only as your doctor directs, at the same time each day.
• Continue to take Cartrol for the entire time prescribed, even if you feel better.
• You may have to take this drug for the rest of your life to keep your blood pressure down.

If you miss a dose

It's important to take each dose of Cartrol, especially when taking only one dose a day. If you miss a dose, take it as soon as possible.

CARTROL'S OTHER NAME

Cartrol's generic name is carteolol hydrochloride.

 SIDE EFFECTS

Call your doctor if you have any of these possible drug side effects. Call *immediately* about any labeled "serious."

Serious: conduction disturbances of the heart (weakness, dizziness, fainting)

Common: weakness, muscle cramps

Other: exhaustion, tiredness, fatigue, sleepiness

 DRUG INTERACTIONS

Combining certain drugs may alter their action or produce unwanted side effects. Tell your doctor about other drugs you're taking, especially:
• calcium channel blockers, such as Cardizem and Procardia
• catecholamine-depleting drugs or Serpalan
• digitalis glycosides such as Digoxin
• general anesthetics
• insulin or oral diabetes drugs, such as Diabeta and Micronase (doctor will adjust dosage as necessary).

However, if it's within 8 hours of your next dose, skip the missed dose and go back to your regular schedule. Don't take a double dose.

 If you suspect an overdose

Contact your doctor *immediately.* Signs of a possible overdose (in the order in which they may occur) include slow heartbeat, severe dizziness or fainting, fast or irregular heartbeat, difficulty breathing, bluish-colored fingernails or palms, and seizures.

Warnings

• Make sure your doctor knows your medical history. You may not be able to take Cartrol if you have bronchial asthma, heart disease, a blood vessel disorder, or thyroid disease. Also, Cartrol can worsen congestive heart failure, producing shortness of breath or difficulty breathing, unusually fast heartbeat, cough, or fatigue when you exert yourself.
• If you're pregnant or breast-feeding, tell your doctor before you begin taking Cartrol.
• Follow your doctor's recommendations for weight control and diet; for example, your doctor may prescribe a low-salt diet.

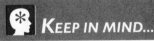 **KEEP IN MIND...**

* Take at same time each day.
* Follow any special diet.
* Finish entire amount prescribed.
* Report difficulty breathing, fast heartbeat, cough, or fatigue on exertion.

Cataflam

Cataflam is a nonsteroidal anti-inflammatory drug (NSAID). It reduces inflammation, pain, and fever, possibly by curbing the body's production of chemicals known as prostaglandins.

Why it's prescribed

Doctors prescribe Cataflam to treat arthritis, painful menstruation, and other types of pain. It comes in immediate-release, enteric-coated, and slow-release tablets and in suppositories. Doctors usually prescribe the following amounts for adults.

▶ **For osteoarthritis and rheumatoid arthritis,** 100 to 150 milligrams (mg) orally divided into two or three equal doses a day.

▶ **For ankylosing spondylitis,** 25 mg orally four times a day and 25 mg at bedtime, if necessary.

▶ **For pain and primary dysmenorrhea,** 50 mg of immediate-release tablets every 8 hours, to a maximum of 150 to 200 mg a day.

How to take Cataflam

• Take Cataflam only as your doctor directs.
• Don't crush, break, or chew enteric-coated tablets.

If you miss a dose

Take the missed dose as soon as possible. However, if it's almost time for your next dose, skip the missed dose and go back to your regular schedule. Don't take a double dose.

CATAFLAM'S OTHER NAME

Cataflam's generic name is diclofenac potassium.

 ## SIDE EFFECTS

Call your doctor if you have any of these possible drug side effects. Call *immediately* about any labeled "serious."

Serious: gastrointestinal bleeding (blood in stools or vomit), nephrotic syndrome (swelling, decreased urine output), liver problems (nausea, fatigue, itching, skin discoloration), Stevens-Johnson syndrome (burnlike rash), allergic reaction (hives, difficulty breathing), congestive heart failure (swelling in legs, shortness of breath), high blood pressure (headache, blurred vision)

Common: headache, ringing in ears, abdominal pain or cramps, constipation, diarrhea, indigestion, nausea, fluid retention
Tip: To minimize nausea, take Cataflam with milk or meals.

Other: anxiety, depression, dizziness, drowsiness, insomnia, irritability, jerking movements, migraine, swelling, blurred vision, eye pain, night blindness, abdominal distention, gas, peptic ulcer, appetite change, asthma, itching, hair loss, sensitivity to sunlight, changes in blood sugar, back, leg, or joint pain

 ## DRUG INTERACTIONS

Combining certain drugs may alter their action or produce unwanted side effects. Tell your doctor about other drugs you're taking, especially:
• anticoagulants (blood thinners) such as Coumadin
• aspirin
• Eskalith, Lanoxin, Mexate, Sandimmune
• HydroDIURIL and potassium-sparing diuretics (water pills)
• insulin or oral diabetes drugs.

If you suspect an overdose

Consult your doctor.

 ## Warnings

• Make sure your doctor knows your medical history. You may not be able to take this drug if you have a liver or kidney disorder, heart disease, high blood pressure, asthma, allergies to aspirin or other NSAIDs, or peptic ulcer disease.
• Don't use Cataflam during the last trimester of pregnancy or while breast-feeding.

• Older people and those taking diuretics (water pills) should use Cataflam cautiously because it may increase potassium in the blood, causing palpitations, and confusion.

KEEP IN MIND...

* Don't take during late pregnancy.
* Take with milk or meals.
* Don't crush, break, or chew enteric-coated tablets.

Catapres

Catapres relaxes blood vessels so that blood passes through them more easily, thus decreasing blood pressure.

Why it's prescribed

Doctors prescribe Catapres to treat high blood pressure. It comes in tablets and a skin patch. Doctors usually prescribe the following amounts for adults.

▶ **For high blood pressure,** 0.1 milligram (mg) orally twice a day, increased by 0.1 to 0.2 mg a day on a weekly basis. Or, a skin patch is applied once every 7 days.

How to take Catapres

• Take Catapres tablets at the same times each day; take your last dose immediately before bedtime.
• If you're using Catapres skin patches, read the instructions that come with the patches.
• Apply the patch to a clean, dry, hairless area of intact skin on your upper arm or chest.
• Change the patch and its placement every 7 days or as often as your doctor directs.
• Keep the skin patch on while showering, bathing, and swimming.
• Even if you feel well, continue to take Catapres exactly as directed; stopping the drug abruptly may cause severe high blood pressure.

If you miss a dose

Take the missed dose as soon as possible. If you miss changing the skin patch for 3 or more days, check with your doctor right away. If you go too long without Catapres, your blood pressure may increase dangerously.

If you suspect an overdose

Contact your doctor *immediately*. Excessive Catapres can cause difficulty breathing, dizziness, faintness, pinpoint pupils, slow heartbeat, tiredness, or weakness.

Warnings

• Make sure your doctor knows your medical history. You may not be able to take Catapres if you have heart or kidney disease or if you're allergic to adhesive.
• If you're pregnant or breastfeeding, check with your doctor before taking this drug.

SIDE EFFECTS

Call your doctor if you have any of these possible drug side effects. Call *immediately* about any labeled "serious."

Serious: severe headache, visual changes, dizziness, fainting, difficulty breathing, unusual tiredness

Common: drowsiness, constipation, dry mouth; itching or rash (with skin patch)
Tip: Become familiar with your reaction to Catapres before you drive, use machines, or perform other hazardous activities that require alertness.

Other: depression, fatigue, nervousness, headache, vivid dreams, low blood pressure (dizziness, weakness), slow heartbeat, nausea, vomiting, inability to urinate, impotence, swollen legs or feet, pale or cold fingertips or toes, insomnia
Tip: To protect fingers and toes, wear warm socks and gloves when out in cold weather.

DRUG INTERACTIONS

Combining certain drugs may alter their action or produce unwanted side effects. Tell your doctor about other drugs you're taking, especially:
• alcohol
• antidepressants, including MAO inhibitors, such as Eldepryl and Parnate
• beta blockers such as Inderal
• sleeping pills, such as Halcion, and tranquilizers, such as Xanax.

CATAPRES'S OTHER NAMES

Catapres's generic name is clonidine hydrochloride; the skin patch's generic name is clonidine. A Canadian brand name is Dixarit.

KEEP IN MIND...

* Take tablets at same times each day.
* Change patch and its placement every week.
* Don't stop taking abruptly.

Ceclor

Ceclor is an antibiotic that kills or stops the growth of bacteria.

Why it's prescribed

Doctors prescribe Ceclor to treat skin, inner ear, urinary tract, or respiratory system infections. It comes in capsules and oral liquid. Doctors usually prescribe the following amounts for adults; children's dosages appear in parentheses.

▶ **For respiratory, urinary, skin, throat, ear, and other infections caused by bacteria,** 250 to 500 milligrams (mg) orally every 8 hours; up to 500 to 1,000 mg every 8 hours for severe infection. (Children, 20 mg for each 2.2 pounds (lb) of body weight orally a day divided into equal doses taken every 8 hours. For more serious infections, 40 mg for each 2.2 lb a day, not to exceed 1 gram a day.)

How to take Ceclor

• Take Ceclor only as your doctor prescribes; take at evenly spaced intervals over 24 hours.
• If you're taking the liquid, shake the bottle well. Then use a medicine dropper or a measuring spoon to pour each dose accurately.
• Take the entire amount of Ceclor as your doctor directs, even if you feel better after a few days. If you stop taking it too soon, your infection may return.
• Ceclor, kept in the refrigerator, is good for 14 days.

If you miss a dose

Don't take a double dose. Adjust your schedule as follows; then resume your normal schedule.

CECLOR'S OTHER NAME

Ceclor's generic name is cefaclor.

SIDE EFFECTS

Call your doctor if you have any of these possible drug side effects. Call *immediately* about any labeled "serious."

Serious: allergic reaction (rash, hives, fever, joint pain), severe diarrhea

Common: mild diarrhea, nausea, rash

Tips: If symptoms persist or worsen, call your doctor. For mild diarrhea, take a diarrhea drug containing kaolin or attapulgite (Kaopectate or Diasorb) but no other type (they may increase or prolong diarrhea).

Other: dizziness, headache, sleepiness, uneasiness, vomiting, appetite and weight loss, upset stomach, abdominal cramps, mouth sores, blood in urine, vaginal itching and discharge, blood problems (unusual tiredness or weakness), fever, liver problems (yellow-tinged skin and eyes)

Tip: If Ceclor upsets your stomach, take it with food.

DRUG INTERACTIONS

Combining certain drugs may alter their action or produce unwanted side effects. Tell your doctor about other drugs you're taking, especially:
• chloramphenicol
• Probalan.

• If you're taking one dose a day, separate the missed dose and the next scheduled dose by 10 to 12 hours.
• If you're taking two doses a day, space the missed dose and the next dose 5 to 6 hours apart.
• If you're taking three or more doses a day, space the missed dose and the next dose 2 to 4 hours apart.

If you suspect an overdose

Contact your doctor *immediately*. Signs of an overdose may include muscle spasms or seizures.

Warnings

• Make sure your doctor knows your medical history. You may not be able to take Ceclor if you have kidney or liver problems, an allergy to penicillin, or other allergies.
• If you're breast-feeding, consult your doctor before using Ceclor.
• If you have diabetes, Ceclor may affect the results on urine glucose tests. Check with your doctor before changing your diet or the dosage of your diabetes drug.

KEEP IN MIND...

* Take in evenly spaced doses around the clock.
* Take with meals.
* Finish the entire amount prescribed.
* Report rash to the doctor.

CeeNU

CeeNU is a drug that's used to treat some cancers. It works by interfering with the growth of cancer cells and destroying them.

Why it's prescribed

Doctors prescribe CeeNU for the treatment of brain tumors and Hodgkin's disease. It comes in capsules. Doctors usually prescribe the following amounts for adults and children.

▶ **For brain tumors or Hodgkin's disease,** dosage depends on the patient's size. Dosage is reduced over time as treatment progresses and blood cell production in the body improves.

How to take CeeNU

• Take CeeNU orally as a single dose every 6 weeks.
• Take CeeNU 2 to 4 hours after a meal to improve absorption of the drug.

If you miss a dose

Consult your doctor.

If you suspect an overdose

Contact your doctor *immediately*. Signs and symptoms of overdose may include nausea, vomiting, and bone marrow suppression (fever, sore throat, fatigue, bruising, and bleeding).

CeeNU's other name

CeeNU's generic name is lomustine.

SIDE EFFECTS

Call your doctor if you have any of these possible drug side effects. Call *immediately* about any labeled "serious."

Serious: blood problems (fatigue, fever, bleeding, bruising), kidney problems (decreased urine, fatigue, lethargy)

Common: nausea, vomiting
Tip: Take a nausea-reducing product before taking CeeNU, as your doctor directs.

Other: inflamed mouth lining (pain, redness)
Tip: Rinse your mouth frequently with a nonalcoholic mouthwash or warm salt water.

DRUG INTERACTIONS

Combining certain drugs may alter their action or produce unwanted side effects. Tell your doctor about other drugs you're taking, especially:
• alcohol
• anticoagulants (blood thinners) such as Coumadin
• aspirin
• other drugs that suppress blood cell production.

Warnings

• Make sure your doctor knows your medical history. You may not be able to take CeeNU if you have other problems, especially chickenpox, shingles, infection, kidney disease, or lung disease.
• If you're breast-feeding, stop while taking CeeNU; the drug may be toxic to the infant.
• If you are overly sensitive to CeeNU, your doctor may change your course of treatment.
• Avoid becoming pregnant while taking CeeNU.
• Both women and men who are taking CeeNU should discuss the risk of sterility or birth defects with their doctors.

• Watch for signs of infection (fever, sore throat, fatigue) and bleeding (easy bruising, nosebleeds, bleeding gums, black or tarry stools). Check your temperature daily.
• Be sure to keep all scheduled follow-up appointments. Your doctor may want to check blood levels of certain substances.

KEEP IN MIND...

∗ Take on an empty stomach.
∗ Don't take aspirin.
∗ Watch for signs of infection or bleeding.
∗ Stop breast-feeding and prevent pregnancy.

Ceftin

Ceftin is an antibiotic that's used to treat bacterial infections. It works by killing or stopping the growth of bacteria.

Why it's prescribed

Doctors prescribe Ceftin for many types of bacterial infections. It comes in tablets and an oral suspension. Doctors usually prescribe the following amounts for adults; children's dosages are in parentheses.

▶ **For throat infections, tonsillitis, and less serious urinary, respiratory, and skin infections,** 250 milligrams (mg) every 12 hours; up to 500 mg every 12 hours for severe infections. (Children ages 3 months to 12 years: 125 mg of Ceftin orally every 12 hours.)

▶ **For uncomplicated urinary tract infections,** 250 mg every 12 hours; up to 500 mg every 12 hours for severe infections.

▶ **For ear infections (otitis media),** 250 mg twice a day. (Children: 30 milligrams for each 2.2 pounds of body weight a day, divided into two equal doses, for 10 days.)

How to take Ceftin

• Take Ceftin only as your doctor directs.
• Take the tablets with food. Don't crush them. If you can't swallow the tablet whole, take the oral suspension.
• Kept refrigerated, the oral suspension is good for 10 days.
• Take all of the drug in your prescription, even if you're feeling bet-

CEFTIN'S OTHER NAME

Ceftin's generic name is cefuroxime axetil.

 SIDE EFFECTS

Call your doctor if you have any of these possible drug side effects. Call *immediately* about any labeled "serious."

Serious: blood problems (fatigue, bruising, bleeding, fever, chills, infection), severe allergic reaction (difficulty breathing, rash, itchy skin), infectious diarrhea, restlessness, pale skin, appetite loss

Common: hives

Other: headache, uneasiness, numbness or tingling, dizziness, nausea, appetite and weight loss, vomiting, inflamed tongue, abdominal cramps, painful defecating or urinating, anal or genital itching, yeast infection, liver disorders (abdominal pain, yellow-tinged skin and eyes)

 DRUG INTERACTIONS

Combining certain drugs may alter their action or produce unwanted side effects. Tell your doctor about other drugs you're taking, especially:
• alcohol
• diuretics (water pills)
• Probalan.

ter. Don't stop taking Ceftin suddenly.

If you miss a dose

Take the missed dose as soon as you remember; take the next dose 5 to 6 hours later. Then resume your normal schedule. Don't take a double dose.

 If you suspect an overdose

Contact your doctor *immediately.* Excessive Ceftin may cause seizures.

 Warnings

• Make sure your doctor knows your medical history. You may not be able to take Ceftin if you're allergic to any antibiotics or if you have other medical problems, particularly kidney disease.

• If you're pregnant or breast-feeding, consult your doctor before taking Ceftin.
• While taking Ceftin, check with your doctor before taking diarrhea drugs; they may increase or prolong diarrhea.
• Check with your doctor before taking any new drugs or if you develop new medical problems.
• If your symptoms persist or worsen, call your doctor.

 KEEP IN MIND...

∗ Take with food.
∗ Don't drink alcohol.
∗ Ask doctor before taking drugs for diarrhea.
∗ Finish entire amount prescribed.

Cefzil

Cefzil is an antibiotic that's used to treat bacterial infections. It works by killing or stopping the growth of bacteria.

Why it's prescribed

Doctors prescribe Cefzil to treat infections that are caused by bacteria. It comes in tablets and oral liquid. Doctors usually prescribe the following amounts.

▶ **For strep throat or tonsillitis in adults and children age 13 and older,** 500 milligrams (mg) a day for at least 10 days.

▶ **For middle ear infection in infants and children ages 6 months to 12 years,** 15 mg for each 2.2 pounds of body weight every 12 hours for 10 days.

▶ **For bacterial bronchitis in adults and children age 13 and older,** 500 mg every 12 hours for 10 days.

▶ **For uncomplicated skin infections in adults and children age 13 and older,** 250 mg twice a day, or 500 mg once or twice a day.

How to take Cefzil

• Take Cefzil only as your doctor directs in evenly spaced doses.
• Shake the oral liquid well before measuring your dose.
• Store Cefzil safely in the refrigerator; discard unused portion after 14 days.
• Take all of the drug as prescribed, even after you begin to feel better.

If you miss a dose

Take the missed dose as soon as possible. However, if it's almost time

CEFZIL'S OTHER NAME

Cefzil's generic name is cefprozil.

SIDE EFFECTS

Call your doctor if you have any of these possible drug side effects. Call *immediately* about any labeled "serious."

Serious: severe allergic reaction (difficulty breathing, hives, itching)

Common: diarrhea, nausea

Tip: Mild diarrhea and nausea may go away as your body adjusts to the drug. If diarrhea and nausea persist or get worse, contact the doctor.

Other: dizziness, hyperactivity, headache, nervousness, sleeplessness, vomiting, abdominal pain, abnormal blood test results, genital itching or irritation, liver problem (yellow-tinged skin and eyes), rashes or hives, increased infection

DRUG INTERACTIONS

Combining certain drugs may alter their action or produce unwanted side effects. Tell your doctor about other drugs you're taking, especially:
• aminoglycosides, such as Gentamycin and Tobramycin
• Probalan.

---

for your next dose, skip the missed dose and go back to your regular schedule. Don't take a double dose.

If you suspect an overdose

Contact your doctor *immediately*. Signs and symptoms of overdose may include severe nausea, vomiting, and diarrhea.

Warnings

• Make sure your doctor knows your medical history. Don't take Cefzil if you're allergic to this or other antibiotics, such as penicillin. If you have kidney, liver, or intestinal problems, your dosage of Cefzil may need to be adjusted.
• If you're pregnant or breast-feeding, consult your doctor before taking Cefzil.

• If you're on hemodialysis, take Cefzil after a treatment session because hemodialysis removes this drug.
• If you're diabetic, be aware that Cefzil can cause false positive readings on urine sugar tests. Check with your doctor; you may need to change the way you check your sugar level.

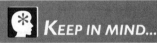

*Don't take if allergic to penicillin.
* Take at evenly spaced intervals.
* Shake oral liquid before taking.
* Finish entire prescription.
* Take after hemodialysis.

Celontin

Celontin is used to control seizures in epilepsy. It works by regulating brain and nervous system activities so that seizures are reduced.

Why it's prescribed

Doctors prescribe Celontin to treat epilepsy. It comes in capsules and an oral liquid. Doctors usually prescribe the following amounts for adults and children.

▶ **To control seizures,** 300 milligrams (mg) a day, increased by 300 mg a day at weekly intervals as needed to maximum daily dosage of 1.2 grams.

How to take Celontin

• Take Celontin only as your doctor directs, usually every day in regularly spaced doses.
• Never stop taking Celontin abruptly; this may cause seizures. Your doctor will want to slowly decrease the dosage.
• Keep this drug away from heat. Don't use capsules that have melted.

If you miss a dose

Take the missed dose as soon as possible. However, if it's almost time for your next dose, skip the missed dose and go back to your regular schedule. Don't take a double dose.

 If you suspect an overdose

Contact your doctor *immediately*. Excessive Celontin can cause nau-

CELONTIN'S OTHER NAME

Celontin's generic name is methsuximide.

 SIDE EFFECTS

Call your doctor if you have any of these possible drug side effects. Call *immediately* about any labeled "serious."

Serious: blood problems (fatigue, infections, bleeding, bruising)

Common: drowsiness, dizziness, nausea, vomiting, drastic appetite and weight loss, unsteadiness on feet

Tips: Avoid driving or other activities that require alertness until you know how Celontin affects you. To help relieve dizziness, sit up or stand up slowly; when getting out of bed, sit up and dangle your legs over the side of the bed for several minutes before standing; and don't climb stairs too quickly. Take your doses with food or milk to avoid stomach upset.

Other: irritability, nervousness, headache, sleeplessness, confusion, depression, aggression, blurred vision, sensitivity to light, swollen eyes, diarrhea, weight loss, abdominal pain, rash, itching, hives

 DRUG INTERACTIONS

Combining certain drugs may alter their action or produce unwanted side effects. Tell your doctor about other drugs you're taking, especially:
• alcohol and other drugs that slow down the central nervous system
• antidepressants, such as Marplan, Pamelor, Sinequan, and Tofranil
• folic acid
• Haldol
• other seizure drugs, such as Dilantin and Solfoton.

---

sea, vomiting, sleepiness, and slowed breathing.

 Warnings

• Make sure your doctor knows your medical history. You shouldn't take Celontin if you're overly sensitive or allergic to this or other seizure drugs. You may not be able to take Celontin if you have liver or kidney problems.
• Notify your doctor if you're pregnant or breast-feeding before you start taking Celontin.

KEEP IN MIND...

* Take every day in evenly spaced doses.
* Take with food or milk.
* Never stop taking abruptly.
* Avoid alcohol.

Centrax

Centrax is a drug that's taken to reduce feelings of nervousness or tension. It works by regulating brain and nervous system activities.

Why it's prescribed

Doctors prescribe Centrax to treat anxiety. It comes in tablets and capsules. Doctors usually prescribe the following amounts for adults.
▶ **For anxiety,** 20 to 60 milligrams (mg) a day, divided into equal doses. Or, 20 to 40 mg at bedtime.

How to take Centrax

• Take Centrax only as your doctor directs.
• To avoid experiencing withdrawal symptoms, don't stop taking Centrax abruptly. Consult your doctor, who may want to decrease your dosage gradually.

If you miss a dose

Take the missed dose right away if you remember it within 1 hour. If more than 1 hour has passed, skip the missed dose and resume your regular schedule. Don't take a double dose.

 If you suspect an overdose

Contact your doctor *immediately.* Signs and symptoms of overdose may include extreme tiredness, difficulty breathing, and slurred speech.

CENTRAX'S OTHER NAME

Centrax's generic name is prazepam.

 SIDE EFFECTS

Call your doctor if you have any of these possible drug side effects.

Serious: none reported

Common: drowsiness, lethargy, hangover
Tip: Avoid activities that require alertness or coordination until you know how Centrax affects you.

Other: dizziness, loss of muscle control, fainting, light-headedness, dry mouth, nausea, vomiting, abdominal discomfort, rash

 DRUG INTERACTIONS

Combining certain drugs may alter their action or produce unwanted side effects. Tell your doctor about other drugs you're taking, especially:
• alcohol or other drugs that slow down the central nervous system
• antihistamines, such as Benedryl and Actifed
• barbiturates such as Solfoton
• digoxin
• MAO inhibitors, such as Eldepryl and Parnate
• narcotics
• Sinemet
• Tagamet
• tobacco.

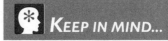 **Warnings**

• Make sure your doctor knows your medical history. Other medical conditions may affect your use of this drug.
• Don't take Centrax if you're allergic to this drug or have glaucoma. Talk to your doctor.
• Don't take Centrax if you're pregnant, especially during the first trimester.
• Don't use this drug in children under age 18.
• Be aware that older adults or adults with kidney or liver disorders may need a lower dosage of Centrax.

• Be aware that abuse and addiction may occur with this drug.
• Be sure to keep all scheduled follow-up appointments. Your doctor may want to check your blood levels of certain substances.

KEEP IN MIND...

* Don't take if you have glaucoma.
* Don't take double doses.
* Don't stop taking abruptly.
* Avoid alcohol.
* Avoid driving or dangerous activities.

Ceredase

Ceredase is a drug that's used to control Gaucher's disease. This disease occurs when a person lacks a substance that enables the body to convert fats to energy. Left untreated, Gaucher's disease can lead to serious blood, liver, bone, or spleen problems. Ceredase helps the body process fats in a more normal way; it does not cure the disease, however. Lifelong use of Ceredase may be needed to control the condition.

Why it's prescribed

Doctors prescribe Ceredase to help control Gaucher's disease. It comes only in an injectable form. Doctors usually prescribe the following amounts for adults and children.

▶ **For Gaucher's disease,** intravenous dosage depends on the patient's weight. At first, Ceredase may be given up to three times a week or at intervals of 1 to 4 weeks. Once desired response is reached, dosage may be reduced and given once every 3 to 6 months.

How to take Ceredase

• A health care professional will administer doses of Ceredase to you.
• Follow your doctor's directions for receiving Ceredase.
• The doctor will monitor and adjust the amount you're given and your schedule as needed.

CEREDASE'S OTHER NAME

Ceredase's generic name is alglucerase.

SIDE EFFECTS

Call your doctor if you have any of these possible drug side effects. Call *immediately* about any labeled "serious."

Serious: allergic reaction (itching, flushing, hives, facial swelling, difficulty breathing, chest pain)

Common: none reported

Other: abdominal discomfort, nausea, vomiting, chills, slight fever, fatigue, hot flashes, headache, mouth sores, swelling of legs or arms, diarrhea, change in menstrual cycle, discomfort, burning, swelling at injection site

DRUG INTERACTIONS

Combining certain drugs may alter their action or produce unwanted side effects. Tell your doctor about other drugs you're taking.

If you miss a dose

No information available. Consult your doctor.

If you suspect an overdose

Consult your doctor.

Warnings

• Make sure your doctor knows your medical history. You may not be able to take this drug if you have other medical problems, especially prostate cancer or prior allergic reactions to human chorionic gonadotropin hormone (hCG); your dosage may need to be adjusted.
• If you're pregnant or breast-feeding, tell your doctor before you begin receiving Ceredase.
• Discuss the symptoms of hypersensitivity to Ceredase with your doctor. If you have allergies, pretreatment with antihistamines may be required.

• Because Ceredase is made from human tissue, it's possible (although unlikely) that diseases caused by viruses could be passed on through the drug; the tissue is tested for hepatitis and human immunodeficiency virus (HIV) before being used. Discuss any concerns with your doctor.
• Discuss the risks and benefits of therapy with your doctor before you begin receiving Ceredase.
• If Ceredase treatment is stopped, symptoms of Gaucher's disease are likely to return.

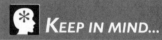

* May need to take for the rest of your life.

* Take antihistamines before Ceredase as directed.

* Discuss progress with doctor regularly.

Cerezyme

Cerezyme is a drug that's used to control Gaucher's disease. This disease occurs when a person lacks a substance that enables the body to convert fats to energy. Left untreated, Gaucher's disease can lead to serious blood, liver, bone, or spleen problems. Cerezyme helps the body process fats in a more normal way; it does not cure the disease, however. Lifelong use of Cerezyme may be needed to control the condition.

Why it's prescribed

Doctors prescribe Cerezyme to help control Gaucher's disease. It comes only in an injectable form. Doctors usually prescribe the following amounts for both adults and children.

▶ **For Gaucher's disease,** intravenous dosage depends on the patient's weight. Frequency of dosing typically is once every 2 weeks but may range from three times weekly to once monthly, depending on severity of the disease. Once desired response is established, dosage may be reduced and given at 3- to 6-month intervals.

How to take Cerezyme

• A health care professional will administer doses of Cerezyme to you.

CEREZYME'S OTHER NAME

Cerezyme's generic name is imiglucerase.

 SIDE EFFECTS

Call your doctor if you have any of these possible drug side effects. Call *immediately* about any labeled "serious."

Serious: allergic reaction (itching, flushing, hives, facial swelling, difficulty breathing, chest pain, nausea)

Common: none reported

Other: headache, dizziness, mild low blood pressure, abdominal discomfort, decreased urinary frequency, rash, fatigue, hot flashes, mouth sores, swelling of legs or arms, diarrhea, change in menstrual cycle
Tip: To help relieve dizziness, sit up, stand up, and climb stairs slowly. When getting out of bed, first sit up and dangle your legs over the side of the bed for several minutes before standing up.

 DRUG INTERACTIONS

Combining certain drugs may alter their action or produce unwanted side effects. Tell your doctor about other drugs you're taking.

• Follow your doctor's directions for receiving Cerezyme.
• The doctor will monitor and adjust the amount you're given and your schedule as needed.

If you miss a dose

No information available. Consult your doctor.

 If you suspect an overdose

Consult your doctor.

Warnings

• Make sure your doctor knows your medical history. Other medical conditions may affect your use of Cerezyme.
• If you're pregnant or breast-feeding, tell your doctor before you begin receiving Cerezyme.

• Make sure your doctor knows about prior allergic reactions to this or other drugs, especially Ceredase.
• For the most beneficial effects, be sure to keep all appointments to receive Cerezyme regularly.

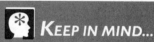 **KEEP IN MIND...**

* May require lifelong use.

* Discuss progress with doctor.

* Sit, stand, and climb stairs slowly to avoid dizziness.

* Attend all treatment sessions.

Cerumenex

Cerumenex is a substance that softens and helps remove accumulated earwax.

Why it's prescribed

Doctors prescribe Cerumenex to help soften and flush away accumulated earwax. It comes as a liquid solution to be placed in the ear. Doctors usually prescribe the following for adults.

▶ **To remove earwax,** apply enough to fill the ear canal.

How to use Cerumenex

• Use Cerumenex only as your doctor directs.
• If allergy is suspected, test first by placing 1 drop of Cerumenex on your inner forearm; cover with a small bandage and leave in place for 24 hours. If any reaction (redness, swelling) occurs, don't use Cerumenex.
• Tilt the head 45 degrees to the side with the ear you're flushing pointing up toward the ceiling. Pull up and back on the ear to straighten the ear canal and help the Cerumenex reach the ear wax.
• Fill the ear canal with Cerumenex. Avoid getting the drug on the skin outside the ear. If contact does occur, wash the skin well with soap and water.
• Take care not to touch the applicator tip to the ear canal, the surrounding skin, or any other surface.
• Moisten cotton plug with Cerumenex before placing in ear.

CERUMENEX'S OTHER NAME

Cerumenex's generic name is triethanolamine polypeptide oleate-condensate.

SIDE EFFECTS

Call your doctor if you have any of these possible drug side effects. Call *immediately* about any labeled "serious."

Serious: skin irritation (skin ulcers, burning)

Common: none reported

Other: ear redness or itching; inflammation with possible oozing, weeping, or crusting; burning; pain
Tip: If side effects occur, stop using Cerumenex and contact the doctor immediately.

DRUG INTERACTIONS

Combining certain drugs may alter their action or produce unwanted side effects. Tell your doctor about other drugs you're taking.

Leave cotton in place for 15 to 30 minutes, but no longer. Then flush ear gently with warm water, using a rubber bulb syringe.
• You may repeat the dose one time if wax remains in the ear.
• Don't use the drops more often than prescribed.
• Use Cerumenex only in the ears.
• Keep the container tightly closed and away from moisture.

If you miss a dose

No information available. Consult your doctor.

If you suspect an overdose

Contact your doctor *immediately*. Signs of overdose may include severe vomiting and diarrhea.

Warnings

• Make sure your doctor knows your medical history. Other medical conditions may affect your use of Cerumenex.

• You shouldn't use Cerumenex if you have a punctured eardrum or an infection of the middle or outer ear.
• If you're pregnant or breast-feeding, consult your doctor before using Cerumenex.
• Cerumenex is not recommended for children.

KEEP IN MIND...

* Don't use if you have a punctured eardrum or ear infection.
* Use only in ears.
* Pull up and back on ear to straighten ear canal.
* Don't use more often than recommended.
* Flush ears gently.

Chenix

Chenix dissolves gallstones that are formed from cholesterol.

Why it's prescribed

Doctors prescribe Chenix to treat gallstones that are composed only of cholesterol. It works best on small gallstones. Chenix is used in patients who don't need to have their gallbladders removed or who must avoid surgery for other reasons. It comes in tablets. Doctors usually prescribe the following amounts for adults.

▶ **To dissolve gallstones without surgery,** 250 milligrams (mg) twice a day for the first 2 weeks followed, as tolerated, by weekly increases of 250 mg a day, up to 13 to 16 mg for each 2.2 pounds of body weight a day for up to 24 months.

How to take Chenix

• Take Chenix only as your doctor directs. Therapy may last up to 18 months.

If you miss a dose

Take the missed dose as soon as possible. However, if it's almost time for your next dose, skip the missed dose and go back to your regular schedule. Don't take a double dose.

 If you suspect an overdose

Contact your doctor *immediately*. Signs of overdose may include severe diarrhea.

CHENIX'S OTHER NAME

Chenix's generic name is chenodiol.

 SIDE EFFECTS

Call your doctor if you have any of these possible drug side effects. Call *immediately* about any labeled "serious."

Serious: liver problems (nausea, vomiting, yellow-tinged skin and eyes)

Common: diarrhea

Tips: Report diarrhea to your doctor and follow dosage instructions carefully. Your doctor may prescribe diarrhea drugs and reduce Chenix dosage until diarrhea subsides. Increase the amount of fluids you drink to avoid dehydration that may occur with diarrhea.

Other: cramps, heartburn, constipation, nausea, vomiting, drastic appetite and weight loss

Tip: Take your doses with food to avoid nausea.

DRUG INTERACTIONS

Combining certain drugs may alter their action or produce unwanted side effects. Tell your doctor about other drugs you're taking, especially:
• antacids containing aluminum
• Atromid-S
• birth control pills
• Colestid
• estrogens
• Questran.

Warnings

• Make sure your doctor knows your medical history. You may not be able to take Chenix if you have any liver disorder, blood vessel disease, disease of the pancreas, or other medical problem. You may need another course of treatment or surgery.
• Tell your doctor about past allergic reactions to this or other drugs.
• Chenix is not recommended during pregnancy. If you're pregnant or breast-feeding, your doctor may recommend another treatment for gallstones.

• Immediately report worsening symptoms, such as sudden chest pain, nausea, and vomiting.
• Report diarrhea; it may mean that your dose needs to be adjusted.
• Attend all scheduled follow-up appointments so the doctor can check your progress.

 KEEP IN MIND...

∗ Take only as directed.
∗ Don't take during pregnancy.
∗ Report worsening symptoms.

Chibroxin

Chibroxin is an antibiotic that's used to treat bacterial infections of the eye. It works by destroying the bacteria or preventing them from reproducing.

Why it's prescribed

Doctors prescribe Chibroxin to treat conjunctivitis, an infection of the eye that's caused by bacteria. The drug comes in eyedrops. Doctors usually prescribe the following amounts for adults and children over age 1.

▶ **For conjunctivitis caused by certain bacteria,** 1 or 2 drops in the affected eye four times a day for up to 7 days. If condition warrants, 2 drops may be applied every 2 hours during the waking hours of the first day of treatment.

How to use Chibroxin

• Use Chibroxin only as your doctor directs.
• Wash your hands before and after applying Chibroxin.
• Clean crusted material from the eye area before applying Chibroxin.
• Don't touch the tip of the tube or dropper to your eye or the surrounding area.

If you miss a dose

Apply the missed dose as soon as possible. However, if it's almost time for your next dose, skip the

CHIBROXIN'S OTHER NAMES

Chibroxin's generic name is norfloxacin. A Canadian brand name is Noroxin.

 SIDE EFFECTS

Call your doctor if you have any of these possible drug side effects.

Serious: none reported

Common: none reported

Other: local burning or discomfort, itching, blood or fluid accumulation in the eye and eyelid membranes, light sensitivity, allergic reaction (rash)
Tips: To protect eyes, wear sunglasses. Stop using Chibroxin and call your doctor at the first sign of an allergic reaction.

DRUG INTERACTIONS

Combining certain drugs may alter their action or produce unwanted side effects. Tell your doctor about other drugs you're taking, especially:
• anticoagulants (blood thinners) such as Coumadin
• caffeine
• cyclosporine
• theophylline.

missed dose and continue with your regular schedule. Don't apply a double dose.

 If you suspect an overdose

Consult your doctor.

Warnings

• Make sure your doctor knows your medical history. You may not be able to use Chibroxin if you're allergic to this or similar antibiotics.
• Chibroxin isn't recommended during pregnancy or breast-feeding because possible side effects aren't fully known.
• Don't share eye medications, washcloths, or towels with family members. If anyone develops the same symptoms, notify the doctor.

• Be aware that prolonged use may promote growth of other infection-causing organisms, including fungi.

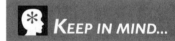 **KEEP IN MIND...**

* Wash hands before and after using.

* Don't touch eye with tip of tube or dropper.

* Don't share drug, washcloths, or towels.

* Stop taking if rash or other reaction occurs.

* Don't take longer than recommended.

Chloromycetin

Chloromycetin is an antibiotic that kills or prevents the growth of bacteria.

Why it's prescribed

Doctors prescribe Chloromycetin to treat infections that are caused by several types of bacteria. The drug comes in capsules and oral liquid. It's also available in an injectable form. Doctors usually prescribe the following amounts for adults and children.

▶ **For meningitis, salmonella food poisoning, and other bacterial infections,** 50 to 100 milligrams (mg) for each 2.2 pounds (lb) of body weight orally a day, divided into equal doses taken every 6 hours. Maximum dosage is 100 mg for each 2.2 lb a day.

How to take Chloromycetin

• Take Chloromycetin only as your doctor directs.
• Store the capsules away from warm or damp places, which may cause them to break down; keep the oral liquid from freezing.
• Take capsules with a full glass (8 ounces) of water on an empty stomach, 1 hour before or 2 hours after a meal. Don't open the capsule; it has an unpleasant taste.

If you miss a dose

Take the missed dose as soon as possible. However, if it's almost time for your next dose, adjust your schedule as follows:

CHLOROMYCETIN'S OTHER NAMES

Chloromycetin's generic name is chloramphenicol. A brand name in Canada is Novochlorocap.

 SIDE EFFECTS

Call your doctor if you have any of these possible drug side effects. Call *immediately* about any labeled "serious."

Serious: anemia, severe allergic reaction (fever, rash, itching, restlessness, difficulty swallowing or breathing), gray baby syndrome (bloated stomach, gray skin tone, extreme sleepiness, difficulty breathing)

Common: blood disorder (fatigue, fever, infection, bleeding, bruising)

Other: headache, mild depression, confusion, inflamed tongue and mouth, poor vision, nausea, vomiting, diarrhea, intestinal problem, infections from other organisms, jaundice

 DRUG INTERACTIONS

Combining certain drugs may alter their action or produce unwanted side effects. Tell your doctor about other drugs you're taking, especially:
• anticoagulants (blood thinners) such as Coumadin
• iron supplements, vitamin B_{12}, folic acid
• oral diabetes drugs, such as Diabinese and Orinase
• seizure drugs, such as Dilantin and Solfoton.

• If you take two doses a day, space the missed dose and the next dose 5 to 6 hours apart. Then resume your normal schedule.
• If you take three or more doses a day, space the missed dose and the next dose 2 to 4 hours apart. Then resume your normal schedule.

 If you suspect an overdose

Call your doctor *immediately*. Excessive Chloromycetin can cause nausea, vomiting, and diarrhea.

Warnings

• Make sure your doctor knows your medical history. You may not be able to take Chloromycetin if

you have liver or kidney problems or blood disorders or if you use other drugs that affect bone marrow or cause blood disorders.
• Pregnant women should not take Chloromycetin within 1 or 2 weeks of delivery date. Don't take while breast-feeding.
• If you don't notice improvement in a few days or if your symptoms worsen, notify your doctor.

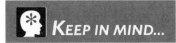 **KEEP IN MIND...**

∗ Take with water on empty stomach.

∗ Don't take in late pregnancy or if breast-feeding.

∗ Store capsules away from warmth or dampness.

Chloromycetin eardrops

C hloromycetin eardrops is an antibiotic that's used to treat bacterial infections of the ear. It works by killing or inhibiting bacteria.

Why it's prescribed

Doctors prescribe Chloromycetin eardrops to treat infections of the outer ear canal. It comes in eardrops. Doctors usually prescribe the following amounts for adults and children.

▶ **For external ear canal infection,** 2 to 3 drops into ear canal three to four times a day.

How to use Chloromycetin eardrops

• Use Chloromycetin eardrops only as your doctor directs.
• Wash your hands before and after using the drug.
• To apply the eardrops, lie down or tilt your head so the infected ear is up. Gently pull your earlobe up and back (down and forward for children) to straighten the ear canal; then squeeze the drops into the ear canal.
• To avoid reinfection, don't touch your ear with the medicine dropper.
• Keep your head tilted for 1 to 2 minutes. Then put a sterile cotton

CHLOROMYCETIN EARDROPS'S OTHER NAMES

Chloromycetin eardrops's generic name is chloramphenicol. A Canadian brand name is Sopamycetin.

SIDE EFFECTS

Call your doctor if you have any of these possible drug side effects.

Serious: none reported

Common: none reported

Other: ear itching or burning, sore throat, itching, hives, rash, angioedema (face, tongue, and throat swelling), other infections not affected by Chloromycetin
Tip: Report sore throat to doctor.

DRUG INTERACTIONS

Combining certain drugs may alter their action or produce unwanted side effects. Tell your doctor about other drugs you're taking.

ball into your ear opening to hold the drug in.

If you miss a dose

Take the missed dose as soon as possible. However, if it's almost time for your next dose, skip the missed dose and follow your regular schedule. Don't apply a double dose.

 If you suspect an overdose

Consult your doctor.

Warnings

• Make sure your doctor knows your medical history. If you have a punctured eardrum, you'll need a different treatment.
• Make sure your doctor knows about prior allergic reactions to this or other drugs.
• Tell your doctor if you're pregnant or breast-feeding before you take this drug.

• Don't share this drug with anyone; use separate washcloths and towels to prevent spreading the infection.
• Watch for signs of reinfection by an organism that isn't affected by Chloromycetin eardrops; these signs include continued pain, inflammation, or fever.
• Avoid prolonged use of Chloromycetin eardrops.

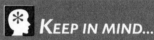

* Don't take if you have a punctured eardrum.

* Wash hands before and after using.

* Don't share drug, washcloths, or towels.

* Report sore throat to doctor.

* Report pain, inflammation, or fever.

Chlor-Trimeton prevents the body's allergic response (although it won't reverse a response that's already in progress). The drug works by stopping the effects of histamine, a body substance that causes itching, sneezing, runny nose, and other allergy symptoms.

Why it's prescribed

Doctors prescribe Chlor-Trimeton to treat hay fever and other allergies. You can buy Chlor-Trimeton without a prescription. It comes in tablets, chewable tablets, timed-release tablets and capsules, and syrup. It's also available in an injectable form. Doctors usually prescribe the following amounts for adults and children over age 12.
▶ **For allergy symptoms,** 4 milligrams (mg) orally every 4 to 6 hours, maximum of 24 mg a day.

How to take Chlor-Trimeton

• Take Chlor-Trimeton only as your doctor or package instructions direct.
• Don't break, chew, or crush timed-release tablets or capsules.
• Chlor-Trimeton takes effect in 15 to 60 minutes, and the effect lasts for up to 24 hours.

CHLOR-TRIMETON'S OTHER NAMES

Chlor-Trimeton's generic name is chlorpheniramine. Other brand names include Aller-Chlor, Chlo-Amine, Chlor-100, Chlorate, Chlor-Niramine, Chlor-Pro, Chlorspan-12, Chlortab, Genallerate, Pfeiffer's Allergy, Phenetron, Pyranistan, Telachlor, Teldrin, Trymegen; and, in Canada, Chlor-Tripolon.

 SIDE EFFECTS

Call your doctor if you have any of these possible drug side effects.

Serious: none reported

Common: jittery feeling, drowsiness (especially elderly patients), dry mouth
Tips: Avoid driving or other activities requiring alertness until you know how the drug affects you. If symptoms persist or worsen, tell your doctor. Relieve dry mouth with ice chips or sugarless gum or hard candy.

Other: sleepiness, excitability (in children), low blood pressure (dizziness, weakness), palpitations, stomach upset, inability to urinate, chest congestion, rash, hives
Tip: Take your doses with food or a full glass (8 ounces) of milk or water to reduce upset stomach.

DRUG INTERACTIONS

Combining certain drugs may alter their action or produce unwanted side effects. Tell your doctor about other drugs you're taking, especially:
• alcohol and other drugs that slow down the central nervous system (some allergy and cold remedies, drugs for seizures, pain relievers)
• antidepressants (called MAO inhibitors) such as Marplan
• aspirin in high doses.

If you miss a dose

Take the missed dose as soon as possible. However, if it's almost time for your next dose, skip the missed dose and take your next dose at the regular time. Don't take a double dose.

 If you suspect an overdose

Contact your doctor *immediately*. Excessive Chlor-Trimeton can cause extreme tiredness, seizures, flushed skin, nausea, vomiting, and diarrhea.

Warnings

• Make sure your doctor knows your medical history. You may not be able to take Chlor-Trimeton if you have asthma.

• If you're breast-feeding, tell your doctor before taking this drug.
• Don't give this drug to children under age 12 unless directed by doctor.
• Before undergoing allergy skin tests, tell the doctor that you're taking Chlor-Trimeton; it may affect test results. Stop taking the drug 4 days before the tests.

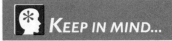 **KEEP IN MIND...**

* Don't break, crush, or chew timed-release forms.
* Take with food or liquid.
* Stop drug 4 days before allergy skin tests.

Choledyl

Choledyl relaxes the muscles of the airways and blood vessels, causing them to enlarge. This makes breathing easier.

Why it's prescribed

Doctors prescribe Choledyl to help treat bronchial asthma, chronic bronchitis, and emphysema. It comes in immediate-release, extended-release, and delayed-release tablets; elixir; and syrup. Doctors usually prescribe the following amounts for adults; children's dosages appear in parentheses.

▶ **For acute bronchial asthma, chronic bronchitis, and emphysema,** 4.7 milligrams (mg) for each 2.2 pounds (lb) of body weight every 8 hours for nonsmokers; same dose every 6 hours for smokers. (Children ages 9 to 16: 4.7 mg for each 2.2 lb every 6 hours. Children ages 1 to 9: 6.2 mg for each 2.2 lb, every 6 hours.) After a certain daily maintenance dosage is established, 1 sustained-action tablet every 12 hours may be substituted.

How to take Choledyl

- Take Choledyl only as your doctor directs.
- Take after meals and at bedtime.
- Don't chew, crush, or dissolve tablets.
- Store this drug at room temperature; protect tablets from moisture and elixir from light.

CHOLEDYL'S OTHER NAMES

Choledyl's generic name is oxtriphylline. In Canada, brand names include Apo-Oxtriphylline and Novotriphyl.

 SIDE EFFECTS

Call your doctor if you have any of these possible drug side effects.

Serious: none reported

Common: restlessness, dizziness, insomnia, seizures, palpitations, fast heart rate , nausea, vomiting, anorexia
Tip: Report these symptoms; they may indicate overstimulation of the nervous system.

Other: headache, light-headedness, muscle twitching, flushing, bitter aftertaste, stomach upset, heavy feeling in stomach, rapid breathing, hives

 DRUG INTERACTIONS

Combining certain drugs may alter their action or produce unwanted side effects. Tell your doctor about other drugs you're taking, especially:
- barbiturates, such as Solfoton, Dilantin, Rifadin, and Tegretol
- beta blockers, such as Inderal and Lopressor
- ephedrine nasal spray such as Bronkaid
- Eskalith
- influenza virus vaccine, macrolide antibiotics (such as E-Mycin), Tagamet, birth control pills, quinolone antibiotics (such as Cipro)
- tobacco
- Zyloprim in high doses.

If you miss a dose

Take the missed dose as soon as you remember. However, if it's almost time for your next dose, skip the missed dose and take your next dose at the regular time. Don't take a double dose.

 ## If you suspect an overdose

Contact your doctor *immediately.* Excessive Choledyl can cause nausea, vomiting, insomnia, seizures, fast heart rate, and breathing difficulties.

Warnings

- Make sure your doctor knows your medical history. You may not be able to take Choledyl if you smoke or have an ulcer, glaucoma, diabetes, or heart, kidney, or liver problems.
- Make sure your doctor knows if you're overly sensitive to caffeine or other substances.
- Tell your doctor if you're pregnant or breast-feeding.

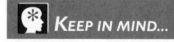 **KEEP IN MIND...**

* Take after meals and at bedtime.

* Don't chew, crush, or dissolve tablets.

* Store at room temperature; protect from light and moisture.

Chronulac

Chronulac is a laxative. It works by drawing moisture into the colon from surrounding tissues in the body. This helps stimulate bowel action.

Why it's prescribed

Doctors prescribe Chronulac to relieve constipation and to help treat patients with severe liver disease. In some cases, it's used to reduce the amount of ammonia in the blood. Chronulac comes in a syrup. Doctors usually prescribe the following amounts for adults.

▶ **For constipation,** 10 to 20 grams (g) or 15 to 30 milliliters (ml) a day.

▶ **For severe liver disease,** at first, 20 to 30 g or 30 to 45 ml three or four times a day, until two or three soft stools are produced daily. Usual dosage is 60 to 100 g a day, divided into equal doses. Or, 200 g (300 ml) diluted as an enema every 4 to 6 hours as needed.

How to take Chronulac

• Take Chronulac only as your doctor directs.
• Take each dose of Chronulac in or with a full glass (8 ounces) of cold water or fruit juice; drink a second glass of water by itself as your doctor directs.
• To cut Chronulac's sweet taste, dilute with water or fruit juice or give with food.

CHRONULAC'S OTHER NAMES

Chronulac's generic name is lactulose. Other brand names include Cephulac, Cholac, Chronulac, Constilac, Duphalac, Enulose, Generlac, Portalac; and, in Canada, Lactulax.

SIDE EFFECTS

Call your doctor if you have any of these possible drug side effects.

Serious: none reported

Common: none reported

Other: abdominal cramps, belching, diarrhea, bloating, gas, dehydration

DRUG INTERACTIONS

Combining certain drugs may alter their action or produce unwanted side effects. Tell your doctor about other drugs you're taking, especially:
• antacids
• antibiotics
• oral neomycin.

• Chronulac takes effect in 24 to 48 hours.
• Store at room temperature, don't freeze, and store away from heat and moisture. Store securely out of children's reach.

If you miss a dose

Take the missed dose as soon as possible. However, if it's almost time for your next dose, skip the missed dose and take your next dose at the regular time. Don't take a double dose.

If you suspect an overdose

Consult your doctor.

Warnings

• Make sure your doctor knows your medical history. You may not be able to take Chronulac if you are allergic to laxatives or other drugs or substances, have diabetes, or are pregnant or breast-feeding.
• Don't use this or any laxative if you have symptoms of appendicitis or an inflamed bowel; these in-

clude lower abdominal or stomach pain, bloating, cramping, soreness, nausea, or vomiting. Instead, call your doctor *immediately.*
• Don't give this or any laxative to a child under age 6 unless your doctor prescribes it.
• If you notice a sudden change in your bowel habits or function that lasts longer than 2 weeks or that returns periodically, contact your doctor before taking Chronulac.
• Chronulac contains large amounts of carbohydrates, sodium, and sugar; if you're on a low-calorie, low-salt, or low-sugar diet, check with your doctor or pharmacist before taking Chronulac.
• Follow your doctor's directions to replace fluid loss.

KEEP IN MIND...

* Keep away from children.
* Take with water or juice.
* Works in 24 to 48 hours.
* Store at room temperature.

Cibacalcin

C ibacalcin is used to treat conditions that lead to bone loss. It works by halting the mineral loss and physical breakdown of bone.

Why it's prescribed

Doctors prescribe Cibacalcin to treat bone loss due to Paget's disease. It's available only in an injectable form. Doctors usually prescribe the following amounts for adults.
▶ **For Paget's disease,** 0.5 milligrams (mg) under the skin. Maintenance dose is 0.25 mg a day or every other day.

How to take Cibacalcin

• Take Cibacalcin only as your doctor directs.
• Take it at bedtime, if possible, to minimize nausea and vomiting.
• Your face may flush and feel warm soon after your injection; this effect usually lasts about 1 hour.

If you miss a dose

Take the missed dose as soon as possible. However, if it's almost time for your next dose, skip the missed dose and go back to your regular schedule. Don't take a double dose.

 If you suspect an overdose

Contact your doctor *immediately*. Excessive Cibacalcin can cause nausea and vomiting.

CIBACALCIN'S OTHER NAMES

Cibacalcin's generic name is calcitonin (human). The generic name of a similar drug, Miacalcin, is calcitonin (salmon).

 ## SIDE EFFECTS

Call your doctor if you have any of these possible drug side effects. Call *immediately* about any labeled "serious."

Serious: severe allergic reaction (swelling, difficulty breathing, skin rash or hives)

Common: headache, nausea, inflammation at injection site

Other: unusual taste, diarrhea, drastic appetite and weight loss, facial flushing; hand swelling, tingling, and tenderness; hypercalcemia relapse (bone pain, kidney stones, increased urination, vomiting, thirst, constipation, lethargy, slowed heart rate, muscle weakness, fracture, strange behavior, coma), low calcium level (lockjaw), high blood sugar (increased thirst and urination, weight loss)

 ## DRUG INTERACTIONS

Combining certain drugs may alter their action or produce unwanted side effects. Tell your doctor about other drugs you're taking, especially:
• calcium-containing preparations, including some antacids such as Tums
• vitamin D, including supplements such as Calderol.

 ## Warnings

• Make sure your doctor knows your medical history. You may not be able to take Cibacalcin if you're allergic to it, to similar drugs, or to proteins.
• Tell your doctor if you're pregnant or breast-feeding before you begin taking Cibacalcin.
• Your doctor may request blood or urine tests periodically to monitor your progress while you're taking Cibacalcin.
• If your symptoms subside after 6 months, treatment may be cancelled until they return.

• If the drug loses its effectiveness, increased dosages are of no value.

 ## KEEP IN MIND...

* Consult doctor before taking drug if you wish to breast-feed.
* Take only as directed, preferably at bedtime.
* Facial flushing may occur.
* If drug loses its effectiveness, increasing the dosage is of no value.
* Keep doctor appointments to monitor progress during treatment.

Ciloxan

 C iloxan is used to treat eye infections that are caused by certain types of bacteria. Ciloxan works by killing or stopping the increase of bacteria.

Why it's prescribed

Doctors prescribe Ciloxan to treat eye infections such as conjunctivitis. It comes as eyedrops. Doctors usually prescribe the following amounts for adults and children over age 12.

▶ **For eye sores (corneal ulcers),** 2 drops in the affected eye every 15 minutes for the first 6 hours, then 2 drops every 30 minutes for the rest of day 1. On day 2, 2 drops hourly. On days 3 to 14, 2 drops every 4 hours.

▶ **For bacterial conjunctivitis,** 1 or 2 drops in the affected eye as directed every 2 hours, while awake, for the first 2 days; then 1 or 2 drops every 4 hours, while awake, for the next 5 days.

How to use Ciloxan

• Use Ciloxan only as your doctor directs.
• Wash your hands before and after applying the eyedrops.
• Clean discharge from the eye area before using the eyedrops.
• Don't touch the tip of the dropper to the eye or to the area surrounding the eye.
• After using the drops, apply light finger pressure to the eye area, as directed, for 1 minute.

 SIDE EFFECTS

Call your doctor if you have any of these possible drug side effects. Call *immediately* about any labeled "serious."

Serious: allergic reaction (itching, redness around the eye and inside eyelid)

Common: burning or discomfort, crusting or scales, feeling that something is in the eye, white crystalline precipitate (in the superficial portion of the corneal defect in patients with corneal ulcers)

Other: none reported

 DRUG INTERACTIONS

Combining certain drugs may alter their action or produce unwanted side effects. Tell your doctor about other drugs you're taking.

CILOXAN'S OTHER NAME

Ciloxan's generic name is ciprofloxacin hydrochloride.

• Store eyedrops at room temperature, away from heat and light.
• Treatment may continue past 14 days if needed.

If you miss a dose

Apply the missed dose as soon as possible. However, if it's nearly time for your next application, skip the missed dose and return to your regular schedule. Don't apply a double dose.

If you suspect an overdose

If you apply too many eyedrops, flush your eye with warm water, and call your doctor. Don't repeat the dose.

Warnings

• Make sure your doctor knows your medical history. You may not be able to use Ciloxan if you're allergic to this or other antibiotics.

• Make sure your doctor knows if you're pregnant or breast-feeding before you start using Ciloxan.
• Don't share eye medications, washcloths, or towels with other people. If family members develop the same symptoms, tell your doctor right away.
• Prolonged use may cause other organisms, such as fungi, to spread.

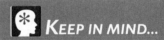 **KEEP IN MIND...**

∗ Wash crust from eyes before using drops.

∗ Don't touch dropper to eye or other surface.

∗ Don't share eye medications, washcloths, or towels.

∗ Call doctor about itching and rash.

Cinobac

Cinobac is used to prevent and treat urinary tract infections. It works by killing the microscopic organisms that cause infection.

Why it's prescribed

Doctors prescribe Cinobac to treat urinary tract infections. You can buy Cinobac without a perscription. It comes in capsules. Doctors usually prescribe the following amounts for adults and children over age 12.

▶ **For urinary tract infections,** 1 gram each day, divided into two to four equal doses, for 7 to 14 days.

How to take Cinobac

• Take Cinobac only as your doctor directs.
• Take your doses at evenly spaced times, day and night, to keep a constant amount of Cinobac in your body.
• To prevent the infection from coming back, continue taking this drug for the full time of treatment, even if you start to feel better.

If you miss a dose

Take the missed dose as soon as possible. But if it's almost time for your next dose, adjust your schedule as follows:
• If you're taking two doses a day, space the missed dose and the next dose 5 to 6 hours apart. Then resume your regular schedule.
• If taking three or more doses a day, space the missed dose and the

CINOBAC'S OTHER NAME

Cinobac's generic name is cinoxacin.

SIDE EFFECTS

Call your doctor if you have any of these possible drug side effects. Call *immediately* about any labeled "serious."

Serious: seizures

Common: dizziness, headache, nausea, vomiting, abdominal pain
Tips: Check with your doctor if side effects persist or become severe. Make sure you know how you react to Cinobac before you drive, use machines, or perform other hazardous activities that require alertness. Take Cinobac with meals or snacks to decrease stomach upset.

Other: drowsiness, insomnia, ringing in the ears, diarrhea, distorted taste, rash, hives, itching, sensitivity to sunlight
Tip: Avoid bright sunlight and wear sunblock.

DRUG INTERACTIONS

Combining certain drugs may alter their action or produce unwanted side effects. Tell your doctor about other drugs you're taking, especially:
• caffeine
• oral anticoagulants (blood thinners) such as Coumadin
• Probalan
• theophylline.

---

next dose 2 to 4 hours apart. Then resume your regular schedule.

If you suspect an overdose

Contact your doctor *immediately.* Signs and symptoms of Cinobac overdose include nausea, vomiting, diarrhea, and abdominal pain.

Warnings

• Make sure your doctor knows your medical history. You may not be able to take Cinobac if you have other medical problems, especially kidney or liver disease. Make sure the doctor knows if you're allergic to this or similar drugs.
• Tell your doctor if you're pregnant or breast-feeding before you take Cinobac.

• Don't give Cinobac to children under age 12 unless directed by your doctor; it may interfere with bone development.
• If your symptoms don't improve within a few days or if they get worse, check with your doctor.

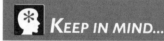

KEEP IN MIND...

* Take at evenly spaced intervals, day and night.
* Take with food.
* Avoid bright sunlight.
* Finish entire amount prescribed.
* Don't give drug to children under age 12.

Cipro

Cipro is a drug that's used to fight bacterial infections. It works by killing the bacteria.

Why it's prescribed

Doctors prescribe Cipro to treat various bacterial infections. It comes in tablets. It's also available in an injectable form. Doctors usually prescribe the following amounts for adults.

▶ **For mild to moderate urinary tract infections,** 250 milligrams (mg) orally every 12 hours.

▶ **For severe or complicated urinary tract infections; mild to moderate bone and joint, respiratory, or skin infections; or infectious diarrhea,** 500 mg orally every 12 hours.

▶ **For severe or complicated bone or joint, respiratory, or skin and skin-structure infections,** 750 mg orally every 12 hours.

▶ **For uncomplicated gonorrhea,** 250 mg orally in a single dose.

How to take Cipro

• Take Cipro only as your doctor directs.
• Take each dose with a full glass (8 ounces) of water, preferably 2 hours after a meal.
• Take Cipro at evenly spaced times, day and night.
• To stop your symptoms from coming back, take Cipro for the entire time it's prescribed.

If you miss a dose

Take the missed dose as soon as possible. But if it's almost time for your next dose, skip the missed dose and

CIPRO'S OTHER NAME

Cipro's generic name is ciprofloxacin.

 SIDE EFFECTS

Call your doctor if you have any of these possible drug side effects. Call *immediately* about any labeled "serious."

Serious: seizures, heart attack (chest pain, shortness of breath)

Common: nausea, diarrhea, rash, sensitivity to sunlight, dizziness, drowsiness

Tips: Avoid direct sunlight to prevent light-sensitivity reactions. Avoid tasks that require alertness, such as driving, until you know how the drug affects you. Take Cipro 2 hours after meals to avoid nausea.

Other: headache; restlessness; shakiness; light-headedness; confusion; hallucinations; burning, tingling, or other sensations; vomiting; abdominal pain or discomfort; oral yeast infection; kidney stones; kidney inflammation (flank pain); joint or back pain; achiness; neck or chest pain

 DRUG INTERACTIONS

Combining certain drugs may alter their action or produce unwanted side effects. Tell your doctor about other drugs you're taking, especially:
• antacids with magnesium hydroxide or aluminum hydroxide, Carafate (ulcer drug)
• caffeine
• iron supplements or vitamin supplements with iron (take 2 hours before or after Cipro)
• Probalan
• Theo-Dur.

take your next dose on schedule. Don't take a double dose.

 If you suspect an overdose

Consult your doctor.

 Warnings

• Make sure your doctor knows your medical history. You may not be able to take Cipro if you have a drug allergy or a disorder that might cause seizures. If you have a kidney disorder, your doctor may adjust your dosage.
• Don't take Cipro if you're pregnant. Stop breast-feeding while taking this drug.

• Drink several extra glasses of water every day while taking this drug to help to prevent kidney stones.
• If your symptoms don't improve or become worse within a few days, check with your doctor.

KEEP IN MIND...

* Take with full glass (8 ounces) of water.

* Take at evenly spaced times, day and night.

* Drink extra water daily.

Citroma

Citroma is a laxative that works by drawing water into the bowel from surrounding body tissues. It's one of several salt-based laxatives.

Why it's taken

Citroma is taken to treat constipation and to empty a person's bowel before surgery. You can buy Citroma without a prescription. It comes in an oral liquid. The following amounts are usually taken.

▶ **For constipation or to empty bowel before surgery,** adults and children age 12 and older, 11 to 25 grams (g) a day as a single dose or divided. (Children ages 6 to 12: 5.5 to 12.5 g a day as a single dose or divided; children ages 2 to 6: 2.7 to 6.25 g a day as a single dose or divided into equal doses.)

How to take Citroma

• Chill liquid or pour it over ice before taking to improve the taste.
• Time your use of Citroma so that its results don't interfere with your activities or sleep. Citroma produces a watery stool in 3 to 6 hours.
• Shake the liquid well; take it with a large amount of water when used as laxative.
• Store at room temperature, away from heat and moisture; prevent liquid from freezing.

If you miss a dose

No information available. Consult your doctor.

SIDE EFFECTS

Call your doctor if you have any of these possible drug side effects.

Serious: none reported

Common: abdominal cramping, nausea, diarrhea
Tip: Increase the amount of fluids you drink to avoid dehydration that can occur with diarrhea.

Other: laxative dependence with long-term or excessive use, fluid and salt imbalance with daily use

DRUG INTERACTIONS

Combining certain drugs may alter their action or produce unwanted side effects. Tell your doctor about other drugs you're taking, especially:
• all oral drugs (separate administration times, as your doctor directs).

If you suspect an overdose

Consult your doctor.

Warnings

• Make sure your doctor knows your medical history. Don't take Citroma if you have abdominal pain, nausea, vomiting, or other symptoms of appendicitis; acute surgical abdomen (abdominal distension, tenderness, rigidity; fever); heart disease; late pregnancy; fecal impaction, rectal fissures, or rectal bleeding; blocked or perforated intestine; or kidney disease.
• If you're pregnant or breastfeeding, make sure you tell your doctor before you begin taking Citroma.
• Citroma is for short-term use only; chronic overuse may cause dependence and can lead to damaged nerves, muscles, intestines, and bowel.

• Be aware that Citroma is a powerful laxative. Citroma's results may be quicker and more pronounced than you expect.
• Make sure that your fluid intake, exercise, and diet are adequate; discuss these with your doctor. If fiber is recommended, add bran and cereals, whole grains, fresh fruit, and vegetables to your diet.
• If you use Citroma often or for a long time, your doctor may want to check your blood levels of magnesium frequently. Be sure to keep all follow-up appointments.

KEEP IN MIND...

∗ Chill liquid before taking.

∗ Shake liquid well and take with water.

∗ Store liquid at room temperature.

∗ Avoid long-term use.

∗ Add dietary fiber as doctor advises.

Citrucel

Citrucel is a laxative that absorbs water and expands to increase the bulk and moisture content of the stools. This encourages bowel activity and elimination.

Why it's taken

Citrucel is taken to treat chronic constipation. Your doctor may tell you to take Citrucel for other reasons; it's useful for debilitated people and those with postpartum constipation, irritable bowel syndrome, and other intestinal disorders and to treat laxative abuse and to empty the colon before barium enema examinations. You can buy Citrucel without a prescription. It comes in powder and tablets. The following amounts are usually recommended for adults; children's dosages are in parentheses.

▶ **For chronic constipation,** 1 to 3 heaping tablespoons of powder in 8 ounces (240 milliliters [ml]) of cold water one to three times a day; or 4 to 12 tablets one to three times a day. (Children ages 6 to 12: 1 to 1½ level tablespoons in 4 ounces of cold water one to three times a day, or 4 to 5 tablets one to three times a day.)

How to take Citrucel

- Follow the package directions exactly.
- Don't take the powder dry or chew the tablets.
- Take powdered Citrucel with at least 8 ounces of water or a pleas-

CITRUCEL'S OTHER NAMES

Citrucel's generic name is methylcellulose. Another brand name is Cologel.

SIDE EFFECTS

Call your doctor if you have any of these possible drug side effects. Call *immediately* about any labeled "serious."

Serious: intestinal obstruction (abdominal cramps and pain)

Common: nausea
Tip: Take with a pleasant tasting liquid to avoid nausea.

Other: vomiting, diarrhea, laxative dependence
Tip: If you develop diarrhea, increase the amount of liquids you drink to avoid dehydration that can occur with diarrhea.

DRUG INTERACTIONS

Combining certain drugs may alter their action or produce unwanted side effects. Tell your doctor about other drugs you're taking.

ant-tasting liquid to mask grittiness. Children ages 6 to 12 should take Citrucel with at least 4 ounces of liquid.
- Citrucel takes effect in 12 to 24 hours. Peak effects may not occur for up to 3 days.

If you miss a dose

Take the missed dose as soon as possible. But if it's almost time for your next dose, skip the missed dose and take your next dose on schedule. Don't take a double dose.

 If you suspect an overdose

Consult your doctor.

 Warnings

- Make sure your doctor knows your medical history. Other medical conditions may affect your use of Citrucel.
- Don't take Citrucel or any laxative if you have abdominal pain, nausea, vomiting, or other symptoms of appendicitis or acute surgical abdomen (abdominal distension, pain, and rigidity; fever) or if you have intestinal blockage or ulceration, disabling adhesions (abdominal pain), or difficulty swallowing.
- Make sure your doctor knows if you're pregnant or breast-feeding before you begin taking Citrucel.
- Your doctor may recommend an adequate diet, fluids, and exercise before taking a laxative for constipation; bran, other cereals, fresh fruit, and vegetables are frequently recommended sources of fiber.
- Take any other drugs at least 1 hour before or after taking Citrucel.

KEEP IN MIND...

* Take with lots of fluid.
* Expect effect in 12 to 24 hours.
* Take other drugs 1 hour before or after Citrucel.

Claritin

C laritin is a type of drug, called an antihistamine, that's used to treat allergic reactions such as hay fever. It works by blocking the effects of histamines in the body. Histamines, produced by the body, cause itching, sneezing, runny nose, and watery eyes.

Why it's prescribed

Doctors prescribe Claritin to treat the seasonal allergy syndrome called hay fever. It comes in tablets and long-acting, extended-release tablets (Claritin-D). Doctors usually prescribe the following amounts for adults and children over age 12.

▶ **For hay fever,** 10 milligrams (mg) each day. For patients with liver failure, 10 mg every other day.

How to take Claritin

• Take Claritin only as your doctor directs.
• Take it once a day, at least 2 hours after a meal, and don't eat for at least 1 hour.
• Don't increase or decrease the amount you take without first talking to your doctor.
• Claritin takes effect in 1 hour, and effects last for at least 24 hours.

If you miss a dose

Take the missed dose as soon as possible. But if it's almost time for your next dose, skip the missed dose and

CLARITIN'S OTHER NAME

Claritin's generic name is loratadine.

SIDE EFFECTS

Call your doctor if you have any of these possible drug side effects. Call *immediately* about any labeled "serious."

Serious: seizures, irregular heartbeat, severe allergic reaction (face and throat swelling, difficulty breathing), liver problems (nausea, vomiting, yellow-tinged skin and eyes)

Common: heartburn, abdominal discomfort

Other: headache, sleepiness, fatigue, dry mouth, anxiety, depression, heartburn, itching, dry skin, hair loss, breast enlargement, swelling of arms and legs
Tip: To relieve dry mouth and skin, use a cool-mist humidifier.

DRUG INTERACTIONS

Combining certain drugs may alter their action or produce unwanted side effects. Tell your doctor about other drugs you're taking, especially:
• allergy skin tests (stop taking Claritin 4 days before tests)
• E-Mycin.

---

take your next dose on schedule. Don't take a double dose.

If you suspect an overdose

Contact your doctor *immediately.* Signs and symptoms of Claritin overdose may include sleepiness, fast heart rate, and headache.

Warnings

• Make sure your doctor knows your medical history. You may not be able to take Claritin if you're allergic or overly sensitive to this or other antihistamines or if you have any liver or kidney impairment.
• Check with your doctor before taking Claritin if you're pregnant or breast-feeding.

• Children under age 12 should not use Claritin unless a doctor orders.
• If symptoms persist or worsen, contact your doctor.
• Stop taking Claritin 4 days before you're scheduled for allergy skin tests so that test results are accurate. Tell the doctor that you've been taking Claritin.

KEEP IN MIND...

* Take once a day.
* Take 2 hours after food; don't eat for 1 hour.
* Stop drug 4 days before allergy tests.
* Takes effect in 1 hour; lasts 24 hours.

Clearasil

Clearasil is an acne medication that works by killing bacteria and blackheads on the skin's surface.

Why it's prescribed

Doctors prescribe Clearasil to treat acne. You can buy Clearasil without a prescription. It comes in cream, gel, liquid cleanser, lotion, and bar soap. Doctors usually prescribe the following amounts for adults and children.

▶ For acne, a small amount applied one to three times a day, depending on the person's tolerance level and how well the drug is working.

How to use Clearasil

• Use as your doctor directs. You may need to start with a milder version of this drug and change to 10% strength after 3 to 4 weeks as your tolerance increases.
• Wash your face thoroughly 20 to 30 minutes before applying Clearasil.
• If you have fair skin or live in a very dry climate, begin with one application a day.
• Don't use near your eyes, on mucous membranes, or on sensitive or highly inflamed skin. Protect your

CLEARASIL'S OTHER NAMES

Clearasil's generic name is benzoyl peroxide. Other brand names are Acne-Aid, Acne-10, Ben-Aqua 5, Benoxyl, Benzac W Wash, Clear By Design, Cuticura Acne, Del Aqua, Desquam-X, Fostex, Loroxide, Oxal 10, Oxy 10, PanOxyl, Persa-Gel, Vanoxide, Xerac BP5, and Zeroxin.

SIDE EFFECTS

Call your doctor if you have any of these possible drug side effects.

Serious: none reported

Common: none reported

Other: stinging on application, warmth, painful irritation, itching, pimples, rash, bleaching of hair or clothing

Tip: If painful irritation or pimples develop, stop using the drug and notify your doctor.

DRUG INTERACTIONS

Combining certain drugs and products may alter drug action or produce unwanted side effects. Tell your doctor about other drugs you're taking and products you're using, especially:

• abrasives
• alcohol-containing products, such as cosmetics, aftershave, and cologne.
• medical soaps and cleansers
• other acne treatments and peeling agents.

hair and clothing to avoid possible bleaching.
• Stop using temporarily if dryness, redness, and peeling occur 3 to 4 days after starting treatment. Check with your doctor to find out when to start using it again.

If you miss a dose

Apply the missed dose as soon as possible. Then resume your regular schedule.

If you suspect an overdose

Consult your doctor.

Warnings

• Make sure your doctor knows your medical history. Don't use

Clearasil if you're allergic to it or to any ingredient in it.
• If you're pregnant or breast-feeding, contact your doctor before using this drug.

KEEP IN MIND...

* Wash face 20 to 30 minutes before using drug.
* Don't use near eyes or on very sensitive skin.
* Stop using if dryness, redness, and peeling occur.
* Call doctor if painful irritation occurs.
* May bleach hair or clothing.

Cleocin

Cleocin is used to treat infections caused by some types of bacteria. It works by killing the bacteria.

Why it's prescribed

Doctors prescribe Cleocin to treat bacterial infections. It comes in capsules. It's also available in an injectable form. Doctors usually prescribe the following amounts for adults; children's dosages appear in parentheses.

▶ **For bacterial infections,** 150 to 450 milligrams (mg) orally every 6 hours. (Children older than age 1 month: 8 to 20 mg for each 2.2 pounds [lb] of body weight orally a day, divided into equal doses given every 6 to 8 hours.)

How to take Cleocin

• Take Cleocin only as your doctor directs.
• Take your doses at evenly spaced times, day and night, to keep a constant amount of the drug in your blood.
• Take capsules with a full glass (8 ounces) of water or with meals to prevent throat irritation.
• Store this drug at room temperature in a tightly closed container. Keep it away from heat.
• Take Cleocin for the full course of treatment. Stopping too soon might allow your infection to return.

If you miss a dose

Take the missed dose as soon as possible. But if it's almost time for your

CLEOCIN'S OTHER NAME

Cleocin's generic name is clindamycin hydrochloride.

 SIDE EFFECTS

Call your doctor if you have any of these possible drug side effects. Call *immediately* about any labeled "serious."

Serious: severe, bloody diarrhea; abdominal pain with vomiting; black, tarry, or bloody stools; allergic reaction (chest tightness, wheezing, hives, itching, rash); blood problems (bruising, bleeding, fever, chills, increased infection)

Common: nausea, diarrhea, difficulty swallowing
Tips: Take your doses with meals and a full glass of water to avoid nausea and difficulty swallowing. If diarrhea develops, check with your doctor before taking any nonprescription diarrhea drugs.

Other: severe heartburn, gas, drastic weight loss, bitter taste

 DRUG INTERACTIONS

Combining certain drugs may alter their action or produce unwanted side effects. Tell your doctor about other drugs you're taking, especially:
• E-Mycin and other antibiotics
• kaolin (in some diarrhea drugs).

next dose (and you take three or more doses a day), space the missed dose and the next dose 2 to 4 hours apart. Then go back to your regular schedule. Don't take a double dose.

 If you suspect an overdose

Consult your doctor.

Warnings

• Make sure your doctor knows your medical history. You may not be able to take Cleocin if you have other medical problems, especially diseases of the liver, kidney, stomach, or intestines; asthma; or allergies.
• If you're pregnant or breastfeeding, inform your doctor before taking this drug.

• Notify your doctor if your symptoms don't improve in a few days or if they get worse.

 KEEP IN MIND...

∗ Take capsules with water or food.

∗ Store at room temperature.

∗ Finish entire amount prescribed.

∗ Call doctor if symptoms don't improve or get worse.

∗ Call doctor before taking any diarrhea drugs.

Clinoril

Clinoril inhibits production of prostaglandins, the chemicals that cause inflammation and pain.

Why it's prescribed

Doctors prescribe Clinoril to treat the pain and inflammation caused by arthritis. It comes in tablets. Doctors usually prescribe the following amounts for adults.

▶ **For long-term forms of arthritis,** at first, 150 milligrams (mg) twice a day, increased to 200 mg twice a day as needed.

▶ **For short-term forms of arthritis,** 200 mg twice a day for 7 to 14 days.

How to take Clinoril

• Follow your doctor's instructions exactly.

• To help prevent stomach upset, take each dose with milk, food, or antacids. Don't lie down for 15 to 30 minutes after taking the drug.

If you miss a dose

Take the missed dose as soon as you remember. But if it's almost time for your next dose, skip the missed dose and take your next dose as scheduled. Don't take a double dose.

 If you suspect an overdose

Contact your doctor *immediately.* Excessive Clinoril can cause dizziness, drowsiness, vomiting, headache, decreased wakefulness, numbness, and abdominal pain.

CLINORIL'S OTHER NAMES

Clinoril's generic name is sulindac. Canadian brand names include Apo-Sulin and Novo-Sundac.

 SIDE EFFECTS

Call your doctor if you have any of these possible drug side effects. Call *immediately* about any labeled "serious."

Serious: stomach pain or burning; bloody or black, tarry stools; bruising, bleeding; vision changes; swelling of face, feet, or lower legs; nausea; peptic ulcer; inflamed pancreas (abdominal pain, vomiting); nephrotic syndrome (body swelling); kidney failure (decreased urine); aplastic anemia; Stevens-Johnson syndrome (red, burnlike rash); allergic reaction (swelling of face, tongue, or throat; difficulty breathing)

Common: heartburn, rash
Tip: Take with milk, food, or antacid to avoid heartburn.

Other: headache, nervousness, mental disturbances, low blood pressure (dizziness, weakness), ringing in ears, rash, itching, fever
Tip: Avoid driving or other hazardous activities that require mental alertness until you're familiar with the effects of this drug.

 DRUG INTERACTIONS

Combining certain drugs may alter their action or produce unwanted side effects. Tell your doctor about other drugs you're taking, especially:
• aspirin or anticoagulants (blood thinners) such as Coumadin
• Benemid
• Dolobid
• drugs for seizures, thyroid problems, or inflammation
• Mexate, Sandimmune
• sulfonamides (Bactrim), any oral diabetes drugs (Micronase).

 Warnings

• Make sure your doctor knows your medical history. You may not be able to take Clinoril if you have a history of gastrointestinal bleeding, liver or kidney disease, asthma, heart disease, high blood pressure, or fluid retention.

• Tell your doctor if aspirin or another anti-inflammatory drug has ever caused you to have difficulty breathing or chest tightness.

• Make sure your doctor knows if you're pregnant or breast-feeding before you take Clinoril.

• This drug can hide the symptoms of an infection. If you have diabetes, inspect your feet carefully.

 KEEP IN MIND...

∗ Take with milk, food, or an antacid.

∗ Remain upright for 15 to 30 minutes after taking.

∗ Don't take with aspirin.

Clomid

Clomid is used to induce ovulation in some women who are having difficulty becoming pregnant. It works by stimulating the release of hormones that bring about ovulation and prepare the body for pregnancy.

Why it's prescribed

Doctors prescribe Clomid to induce ovulation in the treatment of infertility. Clomid comes in tablets. Doctors usually prescribe the following amounts for adults.

▶ **To induce ovulation,** 50 to 100 milligrams (mg) once a day for 5 days, starting any time; or 50 to 100 mg once a day for 5 days, starting on day 5 of menstrual cycle (1st day of menstrual flow is day 1). Repeat until conception occurs or until three courses of treatment are completed.

How to take Clomid

• Take Clomid only as your doctor directs. Ovulation usually occurs 4 to 10 days after the last day of treatment, but individual times vary.

If you miss a dose

Take the missed dose as soon as possible. If you remember the missed dose at the time of your next scheduled dose, take both doses together. If you miss more than one dose, check with your doctor.

CLOMID'S OTHER NAMES

Clomid's generic name is clomiphene citrate. Other brand names include Milophene and Serophene.

 SIDE EFFECTS

Call your doctor if you have any of these possible drug side effects. Call *immediately* about any labeled "serious."

Serious: blurry vision or other vision problem, bloating, stomach or pelvic pain, sudden shortness of breath.

Common: hot flashes, breast discomfort, high blood sugar (increased thirst, hunger, weight loss)
Tip: These side effects may go away as your body adjusts to the drug.

Other: headache, restlessness, insomnia, dizziness, light-headedness, depression, fatigue, tension, high blood pressure (headache, blurred vision), nausea, vomiting, increased appetite, weight gain, increased urination, temporarily enlarged ovaries and ovarian cysts, hives, rash, other skin allergy, temporary hair loss
Tip: Avoid hazardous activities, such as driving or operating machinery, until you're familiar with this drug's effects.

 DRUG INTERACTIONS

Combining certain drugs may alter their action or produce unwanted side effects. Tell your doctor about other drugs you're taking.

If you suspect an overdose

Consult your doctor.

Warnings

• Make sure your doctor knows your medical history. You may not be able to take Clomid if you have any bleeding disorder, ovarian cyst, liver disorder, thyroid or adrenal gland problem, or any other medical condition; also discuss allergies to drugs, foods, preservatives, or other substances.
• Stop taking the drug and contact the doctor immediately if you think you're pregnant, to avoid possible birth defects in the fetus.
• Multiple births may occur with this drug. Chance of multiple births increases with higher doses.

• Make sure you discuss all the risks and benefits of taking this drug with your doctor.
• Measure and chart your body temperature as your doctor directs to determine when ovulation occurs.

 KEEP IN MIND...

* Chart temperature carefully.
* Ovulation may occur 4 to 10 days after treatment.
* Don't take after pregnancy begins.
* Multiple births can occur.
* Report vision problems.
* Repeat treatment up to three times.

Cloxapen

Cloxapen is a penicillin, a type of antibiotic used to treat bacterial infections. It stops bacteria from multiplying, especially those that resist other penicillins.

Why it's prescribed

Doctors prescribe Cloxapen to treat bacterial infections known as staph infections. Cloxapen comes in capsules. Doctors usually prescribe the following amounts for adults; children's dosages appear in parentheses.

▶ **For staph infections,** 250 to 500 milligrams (mg) every 6 hours. (Children weighing more than 44 pounds [lb]: same dosage as adults. Children weighing 44 lb or less: 50 to 100 mg for each 2.2 pounds of body weight each day, divided into equal doses given every 6 hours.)

How to take Cloxapen

- Take Cloxapen only as directed.
- Don't break, chew, or crush the capsules before swallowing.
- Take each dose with a full glass (8 ounces) of water on an empty stomach, either 1 hour before or 2 hours after meals. Don't take with fruit juice or sodas; they may stop Cloxapen from working.
- Take the full amount prescribed, even after you start to feel better.
- Discard any leftover drug.

If you miss a dose

Take the missed dose as soon as possible. But if it's almost time for your next dose, adjust your schedule as follows:

- If you take two doses a day, space the missed dose and the next dose 5 to 6 hours apart. Then resume your regular schedule.
- If you take three or more doses a day, space the missed dose and the next dose 2 to 4 hours apart. Then resume your regular schedule.

 If you suspect an overdose

Contact your doctor *immediately*. Excessive Cloxapen may cause seizures.

CLOXAPEN'S OTHER NAMES

Cloxapen's generic name is cloxacillin sodium. Other brand names include Tegopen; and, in Canada, Apo-Cloxi, Novo-Cloxin, Nu-Cloxi, and Orbenin.

 Warnings

- Make sure your doctor knows your medical history. You may not be able to take Cloxapen if you're allergic to penicillin or other antibiotics or if you have kidney disease, mononucleosis, or stomach and intestinal problems.

 SIDE EFFECTS

Call your doctor if you have any of these possible drug side effects. Call *immediately* about any labeled "serious."

Serious: allergic reaction (difficulty breathing, rash, hives, itching, wheezing), liver problems (yellow-tinged skin and eyes), blood problems (bleeding, bruising, fever, chills, increased infection, fatigue)

Common: nausea, heartburn, diarrhea

Tip: Don't take any diarrhea drugs without first checking with your doctor; some drugs can make your diarrhea worse.

Other: vomiting, other infection

DRUG INTERACTIONS

Combining certain drugs may alter their action or produce unwanted side effects. Tell your doctor about other drugs you're taking, especially:
- other antibiotics (take at least 1 hour after Cloxapen or as directed)
- Probalan.

- If you're pregnant or breastfeeding, check with your doctor before taking Cloxapen.
- If you become allergic to Cloxapen, carry medical identification that indicates this.
- Tell your doctor that you're taking Cloxapen before you have medical tests.
- Older adults and ill or infection-prone people are more susceptible to other infections when taking large doses and prolonged therapy of Cloxapen.

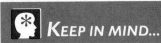 KEEP IN MIND...

* Don't break, chew, or crush capsules.
* Take with water, on an empty stomach, 1 hour before or 2 hours after meals.
* Don't take with juice or soda.

Clozaril

C lozaril works by interfering with certain chemical activities in the body.

Why it's prescribed

Doctors prescribe Clozaril to treat schizophrenia in people who are not helped by other treatments. It comes in tablets. Doctors usually prescribe the following amounts for adults.

▶ **For schizophrenia,** at first, 12.5 milligrams (mg) once or twice a day, increased by 25 to 50 mg a day to a total of 300 to 450 mg a day at the end of 2 weeks. Further dosage increases should not occur more than once or twice a week and should not exceed 100 mg. Maximum daily dosage is 900 mg.

How to take Clozaril

• Take Clozaril only as your doctor directs.
• If you must stop taking Clozaril, it's usually withdrawn gradually. However, your doctor may stop treatment suddenly if necessary; watch for returning symptoms and tell the doctor about them.

If you miss a dose

Take the missed dose as soon as possible. However, if it's almost time for your next dose, skip the missed dose and continue with your regular schedule. Don't take a double dose.

 If you suspect an overdose

Contact your doctor *immediately*. Excessive Clozaril can cause dizzi-

CLOZARIL'S OTHER NAME

Clozaril's generic name is clozapine.

 SIDE EFFECTS

Call your doctor if you have any of these possible drug side effects. Call *immediately* about any labeled "serious."

Serious: seizures, chest pain, severe blood problems (chills, fever, increased infection)

Common: drowsiness, sedation, fast heartbeat, low blood pressure (dizziness, weakness), high blood pressure (headache, blurred vision), dry mouth, constipation, excessive salivation
Tips: Stand up slowly to avoid dizziness. While taking this drug, avoid driving and other hazardous activities that require alertness and coordination. Use ice chips or sugarless candy or gum to relieve dry mouth.

Other: fainting, headache, tremor, disturbed sleep or nightmares, restlessness, confusion, slurred speech, depression, anxiety, nausea, vomiting, heartburn, constipation, urination problems, abnormal ejaculation, fever, weight gain, decreased, increased, or lack of muscle tone. *After abrupt withdrawal:* sudden return of psychotic symptoms

 DRUG INTERACTIONS

Combining certain drugs may alter their action or produce unwanted side effects. Tell your doctor about other drugs you're taking, especially:
• alcohol and all nonprescription drugs
• anticoagulants (blood thinners) such as Coumadin
• Digoxin and drugs to treat high blood pressure.

ness or fainting; drowsiness; fast, slow, or irregular heartbeat; hallucinations; heavy salivation; slow, irregular, or troubled breathing; and nervousness.

 Warnings

• Make sure your doctor knows your medical history. You may not be able to take Clozaril if you have kidney, liver, prostate, or heart disease; glaucoma; epilepsy; an immune system disorder; or bone marrow suppression.
• Make sure your doctor knows if you're pregnant or breast-feeding before you begin taking Clozaril.

• Clozaril is available only through a special monitoring program that requires weekly blood tests; attend all treatment sessions and be sure to report flulike symptoms and signs of infection to your doctor immediately.

KEEP IN MIND...

* Attend all scheduled testing sessions.
* Use ice or sugarless candy or gum for dry mouth.
* Avoid driving.

Cogentin

Cogentin is a drug that's used to treat Parkinson's disease. Cogentin helps relieve the symptoms of Parkinson's disease and drug-induced Parkinson-like symptoms by affecting nervous system activity.

Why it's prescribed

Doctors prescribe Cogentin for Parkinson's disease and for drug-induced involuntary movement disorders. It comes in tablets. It's also available in an injectable form. Doctors usually prescribe the following amounts for adults.

▶ **For drug-induced involuntary movement disorders,** 1 to 4 milligrams (mg) orally once or twice a day.

▶ **For acute dystonic reaction,** 1 to 2 mg by injection, followed by 1 to 2 mg orally twice a day to prevent recurrence.

▶ **For Parkinson's disease,** 0.5 to 6 mg orally once a day. Initial dose of 0.5 to 1 mg is increased by 0.5 mg every 5 to 6 days. Dosage is adjusted for individual needs.

How to take Cogentin

• Take Cogentin only as your doctor directs.
• If you take a single daily dose, take it at bedtime.
• To reduce stomach upset, take Cogentin with meals or a snack.
• Don't stop taking Cogentin abruptly. Check with your doctor, who may tell you to gradually reduce the dosage.

COGENTIN'S OTHER NAMES

Cogentin's generic name is benztropine mesylate. Canadian brand names include Apo-Benztropine, Bensylate, and PMS Benztropine.

 ## SIDE EFFECTS

Call your doctor if you have any of these possible drug side effects. Call immediately about any labeled "serious."

Serious: heart palpitations, rapid or slow heartbeat

Common: constipation
Tip: To relieve constipation, drink more fluids and eat high-fiber foods.

Other: disorientation, restlessness, irritability, hallucinations, headache, sleepiness, depression, muscular weakness, flushing, dilated pupils, blurred vision, eye sensitivity to light, difficulty swallowing, dry mouth, nausea, vomiting, heartburn, urinary hesitancy or retention, increased body temperature, decreased sweating
Tips: Limit activities during hot weather. Wear sunglasses to protect eyes from light.

 ## DRUG INTERACTIONS

Combining certain drugs may alter their action or produce unwanted side effects. Tell your doctor about other drugs you're taking, especially:
• phenothiazines such as Thorazine
• Symmetrel
• tricyclic antidepressants, such as Elavil and Pamelor.

If you miss a dose

Take the missed dose as soon as you remember. But if you remember within 2 hours of your next scheduled dose, skip the missed dose and resume your normal schedule. Don't take a double dose.

 ## If you suspect an overdose

Contact your doctor *immediately.* Signs of overdose include clumsiness, drowsiness, fast heartbeat, trouble breathing, flushed skin, seizures, and unconsciousness.

Warnings

• Make sure your doctor knows your medical history. You may not be able to take Cogentin if you're allergic to this drug or its components or if you have glaucoma.
• Tell your doctor if you're pregnant or breast-feeding before taking Cogentin.
• Be aware that children and older adults may be especially prone to Cogentin's side effects.
• Have regular checkups, especially during the first few months of taking Cogentin, so your doctor can adjust your dosage as needed.

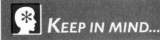 KEEP IN MIND...

∗ Take with meals or snack.
∗ Limit activities in hot weather.
∗ Relieve dry mouth with ice, liquids, or candy.

Cognex

ognex improves the thinking ability of people with Alzheimer's disease by allowing the buildup of a certain chemical in the brain.

Why it's prescribed

Doctors prescribe Cognex to relieve — but not cure or stop — some symptoms of Alzheimer's disease that affect the person's thinking ability. It comes in capsules. Doctors usually prescribe the following amounts for adults.

▶ **For mild to moderate dementia in Alzheimer's disease,** at first, 10 milligrams (mg) four times a day. After 6 weeks, dosage may be increased to 20 mg four times a day, depending on tolerance and other factors. After 6 weeks, dosage may increase to 30 mg four times a day; then after another 6 weeks, to 40 mg four times a day.

How to take Cognex

• Take Cognex only as your doctor directs.
• Take Cognex at least 1 hour after eating. If stomach upset is a problem, you can take Cognex with meals but this may reduce blood levels of the drug, requiring a dosage increase.
• Don't stop taking Cognex suddenly. This could make your symptoms worse.

If you miss a dose

Take the missed dose as soon as you remember. However, if it's within 2 hours of your next dose, skip the missed dose and go back to your

COGNEX'S OTHER NAME

Cognex's generic name is tacrine.

 SIDE EFFECTS

Call your doctor if you have any of the following possible drug side effects.

Serious: none reported

Common: increased urination, elevated blood enzyme levels
Tips: Empty your bladder regularly if this drug causes frequent urination; an adult incontinence pad may be helpful. Your doctor will probably order occasional blood tests to check your blood enzyme levels.

Other: drastic appetite and weight loss, agitation, weakness, muscle aches or pain, small hemorrhages under the skin (bruising or pinpoint red spots), nausea, vomiting, diarrhea, heartburn, loose stools, changes in stool color, jaundice, hallucinations, coldlike symptoms (runny nose, coughing), respiratory or urinary infection, flushing, rash, chest or back pain
Tip: Call your doctor if any of these side effects persists or becomes severe.

 DRUG INTERACTIONS

Combining certain drugs may alter their action or produce unwanted side effects. Tell your doctor about other drugs you're taking, especially:
• anticholinergics, such as Atropisol and Cogentin
• cholinergic drugs such as Urecholine
• cholinesterase inhibitors such as Prostigmin
• muscle relaxants, such as Flexeril and Valium
• Tagamet
• Theo-Dur.

regular schedule. Don't take a double dose.

 If you suspect an overdose

Contact your doctor *immediately.* Excessive Cognex can cause enlarged pupils, irregular breathing, fast and weak pulse, nausea, vomiting, muscle weakness, sweating, and excess salivation.

 Warnings

• Make sure your doctor knows your medical history. You may not be able to take Cognex if you're allergic to similar drugs, if you've had a drug-related form of jaundice, or if you have sinus problems, heart disease, peptic ulcers, liver or kidney disease, asthma, prostate or urinary problems, intestinal problems, or seizures.

KEEP IN MIND...

* Improves thinking ability.
* Take all doses on time for best effect.
* Take between meals if possible.
* Don't stop drug suddenly.

Colace

Colace, a laxative, works by allowing liquid contents of the bowel to enter and soften stools.

Why it's taken

Colace is taken to prevent constipation from developing, not for treating existing constipation. It's recommended for people who shouldn't strain during defecation, such as those recovering from heart or rectal surgery, and for women with constipation after childbirth. You can buy Colace without a prescription. It comes in tablets, capsules, an oral solution, and syrup. The following amounts are usually recommended for adults and children over age 12; younger children's dosages appear in parentheses.

▶ **To soften stools,** 50 to 200 milligrams (mg) once a day until bowel movements are normal. (Children under age 3: 10 to 40 mg once a day. Children ages 3 to 6: 20 to 60 mg once a day. Children ages 6 to 12: 40 to 120 mg orally once a day.)

How to take Colace

• Carefully read the package directions before taking your first dose.
• Mix liquid forms in milk, fruit juice, or infant formula.

COLACE'S OTHER NAMES

Colace's generic name is docusate sodium. Other brand names are Afko-Lube, Diocto, Dioeze, Diosuccin, Dio-Sul, Disonate, Di-Sosul, DOK, Doss, Doxinate, D-S-S, Duosol, Genasoft, Laxinate 100, Modane Soft, Molatoc, Pro-Sof, Regulax SS, Regulex, Regutol, Stulex, and Therevac.

 SIDE EFFECTS

Call your doctor if you have any of these possible drug side effects. Call *immediately* about any labeled "serious."

Serious: severe cramping
Tip: Stop taking Colace and call your doctor.

Common: diarrhea, mild abdominal cramping

Other: throat irritation, laxative dependence
Tip: If these symptoms persist or become severe, call your doctor.

 DRUG INTERACTIONS

Combining certain drugs may alter their action or produce unwanted side effects. Tell your doctor about other drugs you're taking, especially:
• mineral oil
• other drugs (take at least 2 hours before or after Colace).

• Store at room temperature and protect liquid from light.
• Colace usually takes effect within 24 to 72 hours after taking.
• Use Colace only occasionally, for no longer than 1 week at a time without your doctor's knowledge, even if you're still constipated.

If you miss a dose

Consult your doctor or pharmacist.

 If you suspect an overdose

Consult your doctor.

Warnings

• Make sure your doctor knows your medical history. Colace is not recommended for people who are sensitive to the drug or for those with intestinal obstruction, abdominal pain, vomiting or other signs of appendicitis, fecal impaction, or acute surgical abdomen (abdominal pain, distension, rigidity, tenderness; fever).

• If you're pregnant, check with your doctor before taking Colace.
• Don't give Colace to children under age 6 unless it's prescribed by a doctor.
• Before taking for constipation, discuss your need for adequate fluid intake, exercise, and diet with your doctor.
• Drink at least 6 to 8 glasses of water or other liquids daily.
• Be aware that overuse of Colace can make you dependent on it. In severe cases, overuse of laxatives can damage the nerves, muscles, and other tissues of the bowel.

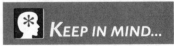 **KEEP IN MIND...**

∗ Get enough fluids, exercise, and dietary fiber.
∗ Mask taste with milk, fruit juice, or formula.
∗ Don't take with mineral oil.

Cold remedies

Cold remedies containing aspirin or Tylenol decrease fever, muscle soreness, and headaches. Remedies with antihistamines have a drying effect to relieve runny nose and watery eyes; those with decongestants reduce stuffiness. Cough medicines may contain a cough suppressant, an expectorant, or both.

Why they're taken

Cold remedies are taken for temporary relief from common cold symptoms. They're available without a prescription. They come in tablets, capsules, powders, liquids, syrups, nasal sprays, and drops.

How to take cold remedies

• Take cold remedies only as your doctor and the package instructions direct. Never exceed the recommended dose.
• To avoid side effects, take only one cold remedy at a time.

If you miss a dose

Take the missed dose as soon as possible. However, if it's almost time for your next dose, skip the missed dose and take the next dose at the regularly scheduled time. Don't take a double dose.

COMMON COLD REMEDIES

Some common cold remedies include Actifed Cold and Sinus, Benadryl Allergy/Cold, Bromafed, Dimetane, Robitussin, Sudafed Cold and Cough, Triaminic, and Tylenol Cold Multisymptom Formula.

 ## SIDE EFFECTS

Call your doctor if you have any of these possible drug side effects. Call *immediately* about any labeled "serious."

Serious: palpitations (fluttering in chest), fast heart rate, severe allergic reaction (swollen face and throat, difficulty breathing)

Common: drowsiness, excitement, dry mouth and skin, headache, dizziness, nausea

Tips: Avoid activities that require alertness, such as driving or using power tools, until you know how the drug affects you. Take with food to relieve nausea. Drink more fluids to help relieve dry mouth and skin.

Other: many drug side effects possible from different cold remedies; read package label or insert for full listing

 ## DRUG INTERACTIONS

Combining certain drugs may alter their action or produce unwanted side effects. Tell your doctor about other drugs you're taking, especially:
• all prescription drugs
• diet pills with the stimulant phenylpropanolamine.

 ## If you suspect an overdose

Consult your doctor.

Warnings

• Before taking any cold remedy, consult your doctor if you're pregnant or breast-feeding.
• To prevent stuffiness from continuing after your cold goes away, don't overuse the nasal spray.
• Use a cough suppressant if you have a dry, hacking cough. Use an expectorant if your cough brings up mucus. Also, drink plenty of fluids to make your mucus easier to cough up.
• If you use a decongestant, take only the amount directed because it can raise your blood pressure. Check decongestant labels for phenylpropanolamine, a stimulant and diet pill ingredient that can produce unwanted side effects, such as slowed breathing and decreased level of wakefulness.
• Many liquid forms of drugs contain alcohol to dissolve the other ingredients and caffeine to neutralize the effects of alcohol or antihistamines. Avoid these if you can't tolerate them.

 ## KEEP IN MIND...

* Take the correct remedy for your symptoms.
* Don't suppress a productive cough.
* Watch for drowsiness and take precautions.

Colestid

Colestid combines with bile acid to form a substance that's excreted from the body. The liver then makes new bile acid from cholesterol in the blood, thus reducing cholesterol levels.

Why it's prescribed

Doctors prescribe Colestid to reduce blood cholesterol levels. Colestid comes in tablets and in powder and granule forms. Doctors usually prescribe the following amounts for adults.

▶ **For high cholesterol,** 5 to 30 grams once a day or divided into equal doses.

How to take Colestid

• Take Colestid only as your doctor directs.
• To make Colestid more palatable, mix and refrigerate the next day's dose the previous evening.
• To avoid choking, never take Colestid powder or granules in their dry form. Instead, add the proper amount of Colestid to at least 3 ounces of your favorite drink.
• Stir until the drug becomes a uniform suspension. Then drink the solution.
• After drinking all the liquid, rinse the glass with a little more liquid and drink that also, to make sure you get all of the drug.
• Don't stop taking Colestid without first checking with your doctor. Your cholesterol level might go up again, but the diet recommended by your doctor helps prevent this.

COLESTID'S OTHER NAME

Colestid's generic name is colestipol hydrochloride.

 SIDE EFFECTS

Call your doctor if you have any of these possible drug side effects. Call *immediately* about any labeled "serious."

Serious: intestinal obstruction (increased abdominal pain and cramping), blood acid disorder (fast breathing, confusion)

Common: constipation
Tip: Drink plenty of fluids and eat fiber-rich foods, such as fruits, vegetables, and whole-grain cereals.

Other: headache, dizziness, gas, nausea, vomiting, fatty stools, hemorrhoids, rash, irritated tongue and anal area, deficiency of vitamins A, D, E, K, and folic acid (fatigue, decreased bone and tooth growth, increased infection, dry skin, bleeding)

 DRUG INTERACTIONS

Combining certain drugs may alter their action or produce unwanted side effects. Tell your doctor about other drugs you're taking, especially:
• any oral drug
• digitalis glycosides such as Lanoxin
• oral diabetes drugs.

If you miss a dose

Take the missed dose as soon as possible. However, if it's almost time for your next dose, skip the missed dose and follow your regular schedule. Don't take a double dose.

 If you suspect an overdose

Consult your doctor.

Warnings

• Make sure your doctor knows your medical history. You may not be able to take Colestid if you have problems involving your kidneys, liver, gallbladder, stomach, or intestines.
• If you're pregnant, check with the doctor before taking this drug.

• Be aware that older adults may be especially sensitive to Colestid's side effects.
• For Colestid to work properly, follow your doctor's recommendations for diet, weight control, exercise, and smoking cessation.
• If severe constipation develops, decrease the dosage or add a stool softener, as directed by your doctor. Eat a diet high in fiber and fluids.
• See your doctor regularly to check your cholesterol level.

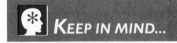 **KEEP IN MIND...**

∗ Don't take dry; mix with food or drinks.

∗ See doctor regularly for cholesterol checks.

∗ Watch for signs of vitamin deficiency.

Colsalide

Colsalide is used to treat gout, a type of arthritis that affects the blood and joints. Colsalide works by reducing pain and inflammation in joints. This drug has no effect on nongouty arthritis.

Why it's prescribed

Doctors prescribe Colsalide for preventing attacks of gout and for long-term gout treatment. Colsalide comes in tablets and sugar-coated granules. It's also available in an injectable form. Doctors usually prescribe the following amounts for adults.

▶ **To prevent gout attacks or for long-term gout treatment,** 0.5 or 0.6 milligrams (mg) orally once a day — every day for people who have more than one attack a year, 1 to 4 days a week for people who have an attack less than once a year. In severe cases, 1 to 1.8 mg a day.

▶ **To prevent gout attacks in people undergoing surgery,** 0.5 to 0.6 mg orally three times a day, 3 days before and 3 days after surgery.

▶ **For attacks of gout and gouty arthritis,** at first, 0.5 to 1.2 mg orally, then 0.5 or 0.6 mg every 1 to 2 hours until pain is relieved; nausea, vomiting, or diarrhea occurs; or the maximum dosage of 10 mg is reached.

How to take Colsalide

• Take Colsalide only as your doctor directs. It begins to take effect within 12 hours.

COLSALIDE'S OTHER NAMES

Colsalide's generic name is colchicine. A Canadian brand name is Novocolchicine.

SIDE EFFECTS

Call your doctor if you have any of these possible drug side effects. Call *immediately* about any labeled "serious."

Serious: blood disorders (fatigue, infection, fever, chills)

Common: nausea, vomiting, abdominal pain, diarrhea
Tip: To avoid nausea, take this drug with food.

Other: nerve disorder, hives, rash, hair loss

DRUG INTERACTIONS

Combining certain drugs may alter their action or produce unwanted side effects. Tell your doctor about other drugs you're taking, especially:
• alcoholic beverages and products that contain alcohol
• Butazone
• diuretics (water pills), called loop diuretics, such as Lasix
• vitamin B_{12}.

• Store in a tightly closed, light-resistant container.
• Stop taking Colsalide as soon as gout pain is relieved or at the first sign of a stomach problem, as ordered.

If you miss a dose

Take the missed dose as soon as possible. However, if it's almost time for your next dose, skip the missed dose and follow your regular schedule. Don't take a double dose.

If you suspect an overdose

Contact your doctor immediately. Excessive Colsalide can cause nausea or other digestive system problems, extremely low blood pressure (dizziness, weakness), blood in urine, decreased urination, muscle weakness, paralysis, delirium, seizures, and death.

X Warnings

• Make sure your doctor knows your medical history. You may not be able to take Colsalide if you have any heart, kidney, liver, or intestinal problems.
• Make sure your doctor knows if you're pregnant or breast-feeding before you begin taking Colsalide. To avoid birth defects, don't take during pregnancy.

KEEP IN MIND...

∗ Take with meals.
∗ Stop taking as soon as pain is relieved or stomach upset occurs.
∗ Don't take when pregnant.
∗ Avoid alcohol.
∗ Store carefully; drug is toxic.

Compazine

Compazine is used to relieve or prevent nausea and vomiting. It's also used to manage some psychiatric problems. Compazine works by suppressing chemical reactions in the nerves and brain that bring about nausea and vomiting.

Why it's prescribed

Doctors prescribe Compazine to treat or prevent severe nausea and vomiting and to help control some symptoms of psychotic disorders. Compazine comes in tablets, sustained-release capsules, suppositories, and syrup. It's also available in an injectable form. Doctors usually prescribe the following amounts for adults; children's dosages appear in parentheses.

▶ **For nausea control before surgery,** by injection 1 to 2 hours before anesthesia, repeated once in 30 minutes, if necessary.

▶ **For severe nausea and vomiting,** 5 to 10 milligrams (mg) orally three or four times a day; 15 mg sustained-release capsules orally on arising; 10 mg sustained-release capsules orally every 12 hours; or 25 mg by suppository twice a day. (Children weighing 20 to 29 pounds: 2.5 mg orally or by suppository once or twice a day. Maximum dosage is 7.5 mg a day; control is usually obtained with one dose. Children 30 to 39 pounds: 2.5 mg orally or by suppository two or

COMPAZINE'S OTHER NAMES

Compazine's generic name is prochlorperazine. Other brand names include Stemetil; and, in Canada, PMS Prochlorperazine and Prorazin.

SIDE EFFECTS

Call your doctor if you have any of these possible drug side effects. Call *immediately* about any labeled "serious."

Serious: tardive dyskinesia (involuntary muscle movements), neuroleptic malignant syndrome (rigid muscles, fever, rapid heart rate, confusion), chills, headache, extreme tiredness, skin problems, severe infection, blurred vision, blood disorders (fatigue, bleeding, bruising, increased infection), difficulty urinating, uncontrolled movements of mouth, tongue, or other area
Tips: To reduce risk of infection, avoid people with infections. Use a soft toothbrush, and avoid increased activity.

Common: liver problem (nausea, vomiting, yellow-tinged skin and eyes), eye sensitivity to sunlight, dizziness, dry mouth, constipation
Tips: Stay out of bright sunlight or wear protective clothing and sunblock. Make sure you know how Compazine affects you before you drive a car or perform other hazardous activities.

Other: drowsiness, dark urine, menstrual irregularities, inhibited ejaculation, allergic reaction (rash, itching, fever, swelling), male breast enlargement, weight gain, increased appetite

DRUG INTERACTIONS

Combining certain drugs may alter their action or produce unwanted side effects. Tell your doctor about other drugs you're taking, especially:
• adrenergic blockers, such as Inderal and Lopressor
• alcohol and other drugs that slow down the central nervous system (tranquilizers, sleeping pills, cold and flu remedies)
• antacids (take 2 hours before or after Compazine)
• anticholinergics (antidepressants and drugs for Parkinson's disease)
• barbiturates such as Solfoton
• Dilantin
• diuretics (water pills), such as Vaseretic and HydroDIURIL.

three times a day. Maximum dosage is 10 mg a day; control is usually obtained with one dose. Children 40 to 87 pounds: 2.5 mg orally or by suppository three times a day; or 5 mg orally or by suppository twice a day. Maximum dosage is 15 mg a day; control is usually obtained with one dose.)

▶ **For symptoms of psychotic disorders,** 5 to 10 mg orally three or four times a day. (Children ages 2 to 12, 2.5 mg orally or by suppository two or three times a day, but not more than 10 mg on day 1. Dosage increased gradually to recommended maximum if necessary. Children ages 2 to 5, maximum daily dosage is 25 mg; children ages 6 to 12, maximum daily dosage is 25 mg.)

Continued on next page ▶

Compazine (continued)

▶ **To manage symptoms of severe psychoses,** initial treatment by injection. Oral form may be used after symptoms are controlled.

▶ **For nonpsychotic anxiety,** by injection every 3 to 4 hours; or 5 to 10 mg orally three or four times a day. Or, 15-mg sustained-release capsule once a day or 10-mg sustained-release capsule every 12 hours.

How to take Compazine

• Take Compazine only as your doctor directs.
• Swallow sustained-release capsules whole; don't crush, break, or chew them.
• Dilute oral liquid with juice, milk, coffee, soda, tea, water, or soup, or mix with pudding.
• To prevent skin allergy, avoid getting liquid concentrate on hands or clothing.
• Compazine takes effect 30 to 40 minutes after oral use or 60 minutes after suppository use, and it lasts 3 to 4 hours (regular-release, suppository) or 10 to 12 hours (sustained-release capsules).
• Store in a light-resistant container. Slight yellowing does not affect potency, but discard extremely discolored solutions.

If you miss a dose

Adjust your dosage as follows:
• If you take one dose a day, take the missed dose as soon as possible. But if you don't remember the missed dose until the next day, skip it and go back to your regular schedule.
• If you take more than one dose a day, take the missed dose within 1 hour; if more time lapses, skip it and take your next dose on schedule. Don't take a double dose.

If you suspect an overdose

Contact your doctor *immediately*. Do not induce vomiting. Signs and symptoms of Compazine overdose may include unarousable sleep, uncontrolled muscle movements, seizures, high or low body temperature, and agitation.

✗ Warnings

• Make sure your doctor knows your medical history. You may not be able to take Compazine if you have heart or blood disease, glaucoma, seizure disorders, Parkinson's disease, or kidney or liver problems.
• If you're pregnant or breast-feeding, check with your doctor before taking Compazine.
• Compazine is not recommended for people who are overly sensitive to this drug or for children under age 2.
• Don't give Compazine to children with acute illnesses, such as chickenpox, measles, or dehydration. These conditions increase the risk of developing neuroleptic malignant syndrome.
• Compazine is used cautiously in patients who have been exposed to extreme heat and in children with acute illness.
• Be aware that children and older adults are especially prone to Compazine's side effects.
• Use Compazine only when vomiting can't be controlled by other measures or when only a few doses are required. If more than four doses are needed in 24 hours, notify the doctor.
• Don't drink alcoholic beverages while taking Compazine.
• Don't use Compazine for motion sickness; it's ineffective for this.
• Be aware that Compazine may affect the way the body regulates heat and cold.
• In people who are tested for phenylketonuria, Compazine may result in a false-positive test.

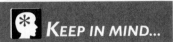

* Use for short-term only.
* Don't use for motion sickness.
* Don't crush, break, or chew sustained-release capsules.
* Discard extremely discolored liquid.
* Avoid direct sunlight.

Cordarone

Cordarone regulates nerve impulses that make the heart beat.

Why it's prescribed

Doctors prescribe Cordarone to correct irregular heartbeats. It comes in tablets. It's also available in an injectable form. Doctors usually prescribe the following amounts for adults.

▶ **For irregular heartbeat,** 800 to 1,600 milligrams (mg) orally a day for 1 to 3 weeks until improvement occurs, then 650 to 800 mg a day orally for 1 month, then 200 to 600 mg orally a day.

How to take Cordarone

• Take Cordarone only as your doctor directs.
• Divide initial large oral dose into three equal doses and take with meals to decrease the chance of stomach upset. Maintenance dosage may be taken once a day or may be divided into two equal doses taken with meals.

If you miss a dose

Skip the missed dose completely and go back to your regular schedule. If you miss two or more doses in a row, check with your doctor.

 If you suspect an overdose

Contact your doctor *immediately.* Excessive Cordarone can cause slow heart rate, dizziness, and fatigue.

CORDARONE'S OTHER NAME

Cordarone's generic name is amiodarone hydrochloride.

 SIDE EFFECTS

Call your doctor if you have any of these possible drug side effects. Call *immediately* about any labeled "serious."

Serious: irregular heartbeat, congestive heart failure (difficulty breathing, chest pain), liver problems (nausea, vomiting, yellow-tinged skin and eyes), thyroid problems (fast or slow heartbeat, excitement, sluggishness)

Common: uneasiness, fatigue, vision problems, nausea, vomiting, skin sensitivity to sunlight (possibly for several months after stopping drug) *Tip:* Wear protective clothing and use sunblock.

Other: numb or tingling fingers and toes, jerking muscle movements, dizziness, headache, muscle weakness, constipation, blue-gray skin tone, male breast enlargement

DRUG INTERACTIONS

Combining certain drugs may alter their action or produce unwanted side effects. Tell your doctor about other drugs you're taking, especially:
• anticoagulants (blood thinners) such as Coumadin
• Dilantin
• heart drugs (Cardioquin, Cardizem, Lopressor, Pronestyl, Tambocor)
• Theo-Dur.

Warnings

• Make sure your doctor knows your medical history. You may not be able to take Cordarone if you have a slow, irregular heart rate or heart, lung, or thyroid disease; if you have a pacemaker; or if you use other antiarrhythmics.
• Make sure your doctor knows if you're breast-feeding or if you become pregnant while taking Cordarone.
• Be aware that older adults may be more prone to Cordarone's side effects and are more likely than younger adults to develop thyroid problems.
• Side effects are more common at high doses but are usually reversible within 4 months of stopping Cordarone.
• See your doctor regularly to make sure the drug is working properly.
• Before surgery, dental work, or emergency treatment, tell the doctor or dentist that you're taking Cordarone.
• Carry medical identification stating that you're taking Cordarone.

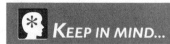 KEEP IN MIND...

* Take with meals.
* Avoid direct sunlight.
* Takes effect within 1 to 3 weeks.

Cordran

Cordran relieves inflammation and itching.

Why it's prescribed

Doctors prescribe Cordran to treat various types of skin irritation, such as itching, swelling, and redness. Cordran comes in cream, lotion, ointment, and tape. Doctors usually prescribe the following amounts for adults and children.
▶ **For skin inflammation,** a small amount of cream, lotion, or ointment applied two or three times a day, or tape applied every 12 to 24 hours.

How to use Cordran

• Apply Cordran only as directed.
• Wash your hands before and after applying Cordran.
• Gently wash the affected area before applying Cordran. To prevent skin damage, rub Cordran in gently, leaving a thin coat.
• Before applying tape, shave or clip hair to allow good contact with skin and easy removal. Allow skin to dry for 1 hour. Don't use tape on moist areas or on skin folds or creases.
• Replace tape every 12 hours. Cut tape with scissors; don't tear it.
• Keep Cordran away from the eyes, mucous membranes, and ear canals. If the drug gets in your eyes, flush them with lots of water.
• Don't bandage or wrap the area being treated unless your doctor directs you to do so. If you're told to use an airtight covering, don't leave it in place longer than 16

CORDRAN'S OTHER NAMES

Cordran's generic name is flurandrenolide. Other brand names include Cordran SP; and, in Canada, Drenison.

 SIDE EFFECTS

Call your doctor if you have any of these possible drug side effects. Call *immediately* about any labeled "serious."

Serious: increased heart rate, decreased blood pressure (dizziness, weakness), shock

Common: fever; discolored, scarred, or infected skin; skin irritation or ulceration; hypersensitivity; infection
Tip: If skin irritation occurs, notify the doctor and remove any dressing.

Other: burning, itching, dryness, redness, pimplelike eruptions, rash and inflammation, decreased skin color, boils (with tape), Cushing's syndrome (fatigue, weight loss, swelling, increased hair growth, increased thirst and hunger), high blood sugar, sugar in urine

DRUG INTERACTIONS

Combining certain drugs may alter their action or produce unwanted side effects. Tell your doctor about other drugs you're taking, especially:
• antibiotics
• antifungal drugs.

---

hours each day, and don't use it on infected or moist, runny areas.
• If your skin is irritated by adhesive material, hold the dressing in place with gauze, elastic bandages, stockings, or a stockinette.
• When using Cordran on a child's diaper area, don't use tight-fitting diapers or plastic pants.

If you miss a dose

Apply the missed dose as soon as possible. But if it's almost time for your next dose, skip the missed dose and apply the next scheduled dose. Don't apply a double dose.

 If you suspect an overdose

Consult your doctor.

 Warnings

• Make sure your doctor knows your medical history. You may not

---

be able to use Cordran if you have allergies or other medical problems.
• Tell your doctor right away if you become pregnant while using Cordran.
• Don't apply Cordran to your breasts before breast-feeding.
• Children and adolescents using this drug should have frequent medical checkups because it can affect growth.
• Older adults may be especially susceptible to Cordran's side effects.

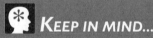 **KEEP IN MIND...**

∗ Wash hands before and after using.
∗ Clean skin before applying.
∗ Bandage only if doctor directs.

Corgard

Corgard reduces the heart's need for oxygen, which decreases heart rate and blood pressure.

Why it's prescribed

Doctors prescribe Corgard to treat angina (chest pain) or high blood pressure. Corgard comes in tablets. Doctors usually prescribe the following amounts for adults.

▶ **For chest pain,** 40 milligrams (mg) once a day at first, increased in 40- to 80-mg increments until optimum response occurs. Usual maintenance dosage range is 40 to 240 mg a day.

▶ **For high blood pressure,** 40 mg once a day at first, increased in 40- to 80-mg increments until optimum response occurs. Usual maintenance dosage range is 40 to 320 mg a day. Dosages of 640 mg are necessary in rare cases.

How to take Corgard

• Take Corgard only as your doctor directs, even when you're feeling well.
• Check your pulse rate before each dose as your doctor directs. If your pulse is slower than your usual rate, don't take the dose; call your doctor.
• Your doctor may increase the amount you take gradually to find the amount that causes the best response.
• Don't stop taking Corgard abruptly without discussing with your doctor; it can make symptoms worse. The amount you take should be reduced gradually over 1 to 2 weeks.

CORGARD'S OTHER NAMES

Corgard's generic name is nadolol. A Canadian brand name is Syn-Nadolol.

SIDE EFFECTS

Call your doctor if you have any of these possible drug side effects. Call *immediately* about any labeled "serious."

Serious: wheezing, difficulty breathing, confusion, hallucinations, slow or irregular heartbeat, cold feet or hands, swollen feet or ankles

Common: dizziness, drowsiness

Tips: Some mild side effects (such as drowsiness) go away over time as your body adjusts to the drug. Avoid hazardous activities, such as driving, while taking Corgard. Take care when standing to avoid dizziness.

Other: fatigue, lethargy, nausea, vomiting, diarrhea, rash, fever

DRUG INTERACTIONS

Combining certain drugs may alter their action or produce unwanted side effects. Tell your doctor about other drugs you're taking, especially:
• aspirin and other nonsteroidal anti-inflammatory drugs (NSAIDs) such as Motrin
• drugs for high blood pressure
• epinephrine
• heart drugs such as Digoxin
• insulin, oral diabetes drugs such as Diabinase and Macronase.

If you miss a dose

Take the missed dose right away if you remember within an hour or so. However, if it's within 8 hours of your next dose, skip the missed dose and resume your regular schedule. Don't take a double dose.

If you suspect an overdose

Contact your doctor *immediately*. Excessive Corgard can cause dizziness, fatigue, shortness of breath, wheezing, and slow heart rate.

Warnings

• Make sure your doctor knows your medical history. You may not be able to take Corgard if you have heart or blood vessel disease, diabetes, kidney disease, liver disease, depression, asthma, hay fever, hives, bronchitis, emphysema, slow heartbeat, or an overactive thyroid.
• If you're pregnant or breast-feeding, check with your doctor before taking Corgard.
• Be aware that older adults may be especially sensitive to the side effects of this drug.

KEEP IN MIND...

* Take pulse before each dose.
* Keep taking even if feeling well.
* Don't stop taking abruptly.
* Don't take double doses.

Cortaid

Cortaid relieves itching, redness, swelling, and discomfort of various skin problems.

Why it's used

Doctors recommend Cortaid for skin inflammation due to allergy or other skin problems. You can buy Cortaid without a prescription. It comes in an aerosol, cream, gel, lotion, ointment, rectal foam, and topical solution. The following amounts are usually recommended for adults and children.

▶ **For skin and scalp inflammation,** small amount of cream, gel, lotion, ointment, or topical solution applied one to four times a day. Or, aerosol sprayed onto affected area one to four times a day. When condition is controlled, dosage is reduced to one to three times a week as needed.

▶ **For inflamed rectum,** 1 applicatorful of rectal foam once or twice a day for 2 to 3 weeks, then every other day as needed.

CORTAID'S OTHER NAMES

Cortaid's generic name is hydrocortisone. Other brand names include Acticort, Aeroseb-HC, Bactine, CaldeCORT, Carmol-HC, Cetacort, Cortef, Cortenema, Cortinal, Cortizone, Cortril, Delacort, Dermacort, Dermolate, Dermtex HC, Durel-Cort, Ecosone, Hycortole, Hydrocortex, HydroTex, Hytone, Maso-Cort, Microcort, Nutracort, Orabase-HCA, Penecort, Proctocort, Rocort, and T/Scalp.

SIDE EFFECTS

Call your doctor if you have any of these possible drug side effects.

Serious: none reported

Common: fever, inflammation, blisters, burning, itching, pain, pus, discoloration
Tip: If you experience any of the above skin reactions, remove any airtight (occlusive) dressing and contact your doctor.

Other: irritation, dryness, redness, folliculitis (inflammation at site of hair growth), Cushing's syndrome (fatigue, weight loss, swelling, increased hair growth, increased thirst, hunger), high blood sugar

DRUG INTERACTIONS

Combining certain drugs may alter their action or produce unwanted side effects. Tell your doctor about other drugs you're taking, especially:
- antibiotics
- antifungal drugs.

How to use Cortaid

- Use Cortaid only as your doctor directs.
- Wash your hands before and after using Cortaid. Gently wash affected skin before applying Cortaid.
- To prevent skin damage, rub it in gently, leaving a thin coat. To apply Cortaid to the scalp or hairy areas, part the hair and apply directly to the skin.
- Don't use Cortaid on eyes or mucous membranes or in ear canals; the drug may be used safely on the face, groin, and armpits and under breasts.
- When using the aerosol form near the face, cover your eyes and avoid inhaling the spray.
- If you're allergic to the tape's adhesive, hold the dressing in place with gauze, elastic bandages, stockings, or stockinette.

- Leave the dressing in place no longer than 16 hours each day.
- Avoid using plastic pants or tight-fitting diapers on treated areas in young children.
- To prevent recurrence, continue treatment for a few days after your skin clears up.
- Don't use Cortaid more often or for a longer time than your doctor has instructed.

If you miss a dose

Apply the missed dose as soon as possible. But if it's almost time for your next regular dose, skip the missed dose and apply the next dose as scheduled. Don't apply a double dose.

If you suspect an overdose

Consult your doctor.

 **Warnings**

• Make sure your doctor knows your medical history. You may not be able to use Cortaid if you're allergic to this product or to any drugs or foods.

• If you're pregnant or breast-feeding, check with your doctor before using Cortaid.

• Don't use Cortaid on a child under age 2 without a doctor's order.

• Be aware that children, adolescents, and older adults are especially prone to the drug's side effects.

• Over-absorption of this drug into the body is likely with airtight (occlusive) dressings or long-term treatment.

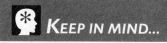 **KEEP IN MIND...**

* Wash affected skin before applying drug.

* Don't use with antifungals or antibiotics.

* Watch for signs of skin irritation or infection.

Cortisporin

Cortisporin combines an infection-fighting antibiotic that kills bacteria and an anti-inflammatory that decreases swelling within the ear.

Why it's prescribed

Doctors prescribe Cortisporin to treat ear infections and other problems of the ear canal. It comes in eardrops. Doctors usually prescribe the following amounts for adults; children's dosages appear in parentheses.

▶ **For ear canal infections,** 4 drops in the ear three or four times a day. (Children: 3 drops in the ear three or four times a day.)

▶ **For mastoid cavity infections,** 4 or 5 drops in the ear every 6 to 8 hours.

How to use Cortisporin

• Use Cortisporin only as your doctor directs.

• Wash your hands before and after applying the drops.

• Before using Cortisporin, warm the eardrops to body temperature (98.6° F) by holding the bottle in your hand for a few minutes. Don't heat the bottle on the stove or in the microwave; the drug won't work if it gets too warm.

• To insert the eardrops, lie down or tilt your head so the infected ear is up. Gently pull your earlobe up

CORTISPORIN'S OTHER NAMES

Cortisporin is a combination of neomycin, polymyxin B, and hydrocortisone. Other brand names include AK-Spore HC Otic, LazerSporin-C, Octicir, Ortega Otic-M, Otocort, Otoreid-HC, and Pediotic.

 SIDE EFFECTS

Call your doctor if you have any of these possible drug side effects. Call immediately about any labeled "serious."

Serious: irritation around ear (redness, swelling, pain)

Common: none reported

Other: none reported

 DRUG INTERACTIONS

Combining certain drugs may alter their action or produce unwanted side effects. Tell your doctor about other drugs you're taking.

and back (down and forward for children) to straighten the ear canal; then squeeze the drops into the canal.

• Don't touch your ear with the medicine dropper, to avoid reinfection.

• Keep your head tilted for 1 to 2 minutes. Then put a sterile cotton ball into your ear opening to hold the drug in.

• Use the entire amount of Cortisporin that's prescribed, even after you feel better, to prevent the infection from returning. But don't use it for longer than 10 days without your doctor's approval.

If you miss a dose

Apply the missed dose as soon as you remember unless it's almost time for your next regular dose. If so, skip the missed dose and go back to your regular schedule.

 If you suspect an overdose

Consult your doctor.

 Warnings

• Make sure your doctor knows your medical history. You may not be able to use Cortisporin if you have other ear problems, such as a punctured eardrum; you may need a different prescription.

• Make sure your doctor knows if you're allergic to any drugs, especially antibiotics such as Garamycin, streptomycin, or Nebcin or if you're pregnant or breast-feeding.

• If your symptoms last longer than 1 week or become worse, call your doctor.

KEEP IN MIND...

* Don't use if eardrum is punctured.

* Warm drops only in hands.

* Don't touch ear with dropper.

* Don't use for longer than 10 days.

* Report persistent pain or other symptoms.

Cotrim

Cotrim is an antibiotic that eliminates infections by interfering with invading bacteria.

Why it's prescribed

Doctors prescribe Cotrim to treat bronchitis, middle ear infections, traveler's diarrhea, urinary tract infections, and *Pneumocystis carinii* pneumonia (common in people with AIDS). Cotrim comes in tablets and a liquid. Doctors usually prescribe the following amounts for adults; children's dosages appear in parentheses.

▶ **For urinary tract infections, chronic bronchitis, and ear infections,** 2 tablets every 12 hours for 10 days. (Children over age 2 months: 1 to 4 teaspoons [tsp], depending on body weight.)

▶ **For chronic urinary tract infections,** ½ or 1 tablet once a day or three times a week for 3 to 6 months.

▶ **For traveler's diarrhea,** 2 tablets every 12 hours for 5 days.

▶ **For *Pneumocystis carinii* pneumonia,** 2½ to 5 tablets every 6 hours. (Children age 2 months and over: 1 to 5 tsp every 6 hours.)

How to take Cotrim

• Take this drug exactly as directed, with a full glass of water.
• If you have trouble swallowing tablets, you may crush them.
• To take the liquid, shake it first. Measure doses with a specially marked spoon or dropper.

COTRIM'S OTHER NAMES

Cotrim's generic name is cotrimoxazole (sometimes called sulfamethoxazole-trimethoprim). Other brand names include Bactrim, Septra, SMZ-TMP, Sulfamethoprim, Uroplus; and, in Canada, Apo-Sulfatrim, Novotrimel, and Roubac.

SIDE EFFECTS

Call your doctor if you have any of these possible drug side effects. Call *immediately* about any labeled "serious."

Serious: allergic reaction (wheezing, hives, difficulty breathing), fever, sore throat, joint pain, blood problems (weakness, fatigue, shortness of breath, easy bruising), severe skin inflammation

Common: nausea, vomiting, diarrhea
Tip: Take your doses with food to avoid nausea.

Other: headache, seizures, fatigue, difficulty sleeping, appetite loss, itching, yellow-tinged skin and eyes, kidney stones (severe flank pain, difficulty urinating, blood in urine)
Tip: To prevent kidney stones, drink extra water.

DRUG INTERACTIONS

Combining certain drugs may alter their action or produce unwanted side effects. Tell your doctor about other drugs you're taking, especially:
• anticoagulants (blood thinners) such as Coumadin
• birth control pills
• Dilantin
• oral diabetes drugs
• vitamin C.

• Keep taking Cotrim even after you begin to feel better.

If you miss a dose

Take the missed dose as soon as possible. However, if it's almost time for your next dose, adjust your schedule as follows; then resume your regular schedule.
• If you're taking two doses a day, space the skipped dose and the next dose 6 hours apart.
• If you're taking three or more doses a day, space the skipped dose and the next dose 2 to 4 hours apart.

If you suspect an overdose

Contact your doctor *immediately.* Excessive Cotrim can cause depression, appetite loss, yellowish skin and eyes, headache, nausea, vomiting, diarrhea, and facial swelling.

Warnings

• Make sure your doctor knows your medical history. You may not be able to take Cotrim if you are allergic to other sulfa drugs, are pregnant or breast-feeding, or have kidney or liver problems, porphyria, severe allergies, asthma, or AIDS.

KEEP IN MIND...

* Take with full glass of water.
* May crush tablets.
* Keep taking drug even after you feel better.

Coumadin

Coumadin is an anticoagulant (blood thinner). It helps treat certain heart, lung, and blood vessel disorders. Coumadin reduces the blood's clotting tendency, to help prevent dangerous clots from blocking veins and arteries and causing heart attack or stroke.

Why it's prescribed

Doctors prescribe Coumadin to prevent blood clots in patients with heart, lung, and blood vessel disorders. It comes in tablets. Doctors usually prescribe the following amounts for adults.

▶ **To prevent blood clots,** 10 to 15 milligrams (mg) for 2 to 4 days, then based on response. Usual long-term dosage to maintain the correct amount of the drug in the body is 2 to 10 mg once a day.

How to take Coumadin

• Take Coumadin only as your doctor directs. Don't take more or less than prescribed, and don't take it more often or longer than directed.
• Take Coumadin at the same time each day.

If you miss a dose

Take the missed dose as soon as possible. Then go back to your regular schedule. If you miss an entire day's dosage, don't take the missed dose at all. Never take a double dose; this may cause bleeding.

COUMADIN'S OTHER NAMES

Coumadin's generic name is warfarin sodium. Other brand names include Sofarin; and, in Canada, Warfilone.

 SIDE EFFECTS

Call your doctor if you have any of these possible drug side effects. Call *immediately* about any labeled "serious."

Serious: hemorrhage with excessive dosage (feeling that something is wrong, fast heartbeat, dizziness, feeling cold, extreme weakness, pale skin), severe infection, pain or swelling in joints or stomach, unusual backaches, diarrhea, constipation, headache, bleeding gums, bruises or purplish marks on skin, nosebleeds, heavy bleeding or oozing from cuts or wounds, excessive or unexpected menstrual bleeding, blood in urine or sputum, vomit that looks like coffee grounds, bloody or black tarry stools, allergic reaction (fever, rash)
Tip: Notify your doctor at once if you have any signs of bleeding.

Common: none reported

Other: drastic appetite and weight loss, nausea, vomiting, cramps, mouth sores, liver problems (yellow-tinged skin and eyes, nausea), hives, hair loss
Tip: Take Coumadin with food to prevent nausea.

 DRUG AND FOOD INTERACTIONS

Combining certain drugs may alter their action or produce unwanted side effects. Tell your doctor about other drugs you're taking, especially:
• alcohol
• anabolic steroids, corticosteroids
• Antabuse
• antiarrhythmics, such as Cordarone and Quinaglute Dura-tabs
• antibiotics and antifungals, such as Achromycin, Bactrim, Cipro, E-Mycin, Flagyl, Keflex, Monistat, Rifadin, Tapazole, and Unipen
• Anturane, heparin
• Atromid-S, Mevacor
• barbiturates, tricyclic antidepressants (Elavil), sedatives
• Carafate, Tagamet
• Danocrine, Nolvadex
• diuretics, such as Aldactone, Edecrin, and HydroDIURIL
• flu shot
• nonsteroidal anti-inflammatory agents (NSAIDs) such as Motrin
• oral birth-control pills with estrogen
• Tegretol
• thyroid medications such as PTU
• Trental
• Tylenol
• vitamin E, vitamin K, calcium (including foods that contain these vitamins or minerals).

Coumadin (continued)

If you suspect an overdose

Contact your doctor *immediately*. Excessive Coumadin can cause bruising, bleeding gums, blood in stools or urine, or nosebleeds.

Warnings

• Make sure your doctor knows your medical history. You may not be able to take Coumadin if you have a bleeding tendency; any drainage tubes; ulcers or other intestinal or stomach problems; heart, liver, or kidney disease; high blood pressure or blood disorders; or vitamin K deficiency. Also, make sure your doctor knows if you've undergone recent eye, brain, or spinal cord surgery.

• Make sure your doctor knows if you're pregnant or breast-feeding before you begin taking Coumadin. Discuss the need to delay pregnancy while taking Coumadin to avoid harming yourself or the baby.

• Coumadin is not recommended for children under age 18.

• To reduce the risk of injuring yourself while taking Coumadin, always wear shoes, place a nonskid mat in your bathtub, shave with an electric razor, and use a soft toothbrush. Check with your doctor before beginning any strenuous exercise programs, and avoid risky activities, such as roughhousing with children and pets.

• Keep all appointments for follow-up blood tests. If test results show that your blood isn't clotting correctly, your doctor may decrease the amount of Coumadin you take.

• Be sure to let other doctors and your dentist know that you're taking Coumadin; wear a medical identification tag that lets others know you're a Coumadin user.

• Ask your doctor how to handle mild pain, such as headache or back pain. You'll probably be told to use Tylenol. Don't use aspirin or Motrin.

• Tell your doctor if menstruation is heavier than usual; your dosage may need to be changed.

• Don't change your diet without talking to your doctor. Doing so could affect your Coumadin dosage.

• Eat the same daily amount of leafy green vegetables, which contain vitamin K. Eating different amounts daily could change Coumadin's effect.

• Read all food labels. Foods and supplements that contain vitamin K can interfere with how well Coumadin works.

• Ask your doctor to provide you with an educational guide about Coumadin.

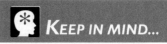

* Take at same time each day.
* Don't use aspirin or Motrin.
* Don't take double doses.
* Take precautions against bleeding.

Creon

Creon is used to treat a digestive problem in which the body doesn't produce a substance it needs to digest starches, fats, and proteins. Creon replaces the missing substance, enabling the body to digest these foods.

Why it's prescribed

Doctors prescribe Creon to treat digestive disorders due to enzyme insufficiency in diseases such as cystic fibrosis. You can also buy Creon without a prescription. Creon comes in tablets and capsules. The following amounts are usually recommended for adults and children over age 6; younger children's dosages appear in parentheses.

▶ **For enzyme-insufficient digestive disorders,** dosage varies with condition being treated. Initially, 2 to 4 tablets; dosage varies according to individual's personal diet and digestive activity. (Children under age 6: 1 to 2 tablets.)

How to take Creon

• Take Creon only as your doctor directs. If you buy Creon without a prescription, read the package label or insert and follow the directions carefully.
• Take Creon with meals.
• Don't crush or chew delayed-release tablets or capsules. However, capsules containing enteric-coated microspheres (check the la-

bel) may be opened and the contents sprinkled on a small amount of soft food or applesauce.
• Creon's effects last for 1 to 2 hours.
• Store Creon in an airtight container at room temperature.

If you miss a dose

Take the missed dose as soon as possible. However, if it's almost time for your next dose, skip the missed dose and go back to your regular schedule. Don't take a double dose.

 If you suspect an overdose

Contact your doctor *immediately*. Signs of a Creon overdose include clumsiness or staggering, confusion (especially in older people), dizziness, fever, facial flushing, hallucinations, trouble breathing, slow or fast heartbeat, nervousness, restlessness, or irritability.

✕ Warnings

• Make sure your doctor knows your medical history. You may not

be able to take Creon if you're overly sensitive to this drug or have any allergies or a pancreas disorder.
• Before taking Creon, tell your doctor if you're pregnant or breastfeeding.
• Follow your doctor's directions for getting the right balance of fat, protein, and starch in your diet.
• Tell your doctor about your progress with treatment; fewer bowel movements and improved stool consistency are signs that treatment is working.

SIDE EFFECTS

Call your doctor if you have any of these possible drug side effects.

Serious: none reported

Common: none reported

Other: nausea, diarrhea (with high doses); excess uric acid in the blood, with high doses (painful, swollen joints; fever; chills)
Tip: If diarrhea occurs, drink more liquids and ask your doctor about taking an diarrhea drug.

◪ DRUG INTERACTIONS

Combining certain drugs may alter their action or produce unwanted side effects. Tell your doctor about other drugs you're taking, especially:
• antacids.

CREON'S OTHER NAMES

Creon's generic name is pancreatin. Other brand names include Dizymes Tablets, Donnazyme, Entozyme, Hi-Vegi-Lip Tablets, Pancreatin, and Pancrezyme 4X Tablets.

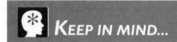 KEEP IN MIND...

* Take Creon with meals.
* Effective for 1 to 2 hours.
* Don't crush or chew delayed-release forms.
* Don't take antacids.
* Balance fat, protein, and starch in diet.

Cyclocort

Cyclocort relieves the itching, redness, swelling, and discomfort of skin problems.

Why it's prescribed

Doctors prescribe Cyclocort for skin inflammation and irritation due to allergy or other skin problems. Cyclocort comes in cream, lotion, and ointment. Doctors usually prescribe the following amounts for adults and children.

▶ **For skin inflammation,** a light film applied to affected area two or three times a day.

How to use Cyclocort

- Use Cyclocort only as your doctor directs.
- Gently wash the affected skin before applying.
- To prevent skin damage, rub in gently, leaving a thin coat. Part hair and apply directly to skin when treating hairy sites.
- Avoid getting Cyclocort near eyes or mucous membranes. Do not use on face, armpits, groin, in ear canals, or under breasts without your doctor's consent.
- If your doctor tells you to use an airtight dressing, apply it as directed. Don't leave it in place longer than 16 hours a day or use it on infected, moist, or seeping skin.
- If you're sensitive to tape adhesive, hold dressings in place with gauze, elastic bandages, or stockings.
- Change dressings as your doctor directs.
- Avoid using plastic pants or tight-fitting diapers on treated areas in young children. Children may ab-

 SIDE EFFECTS

Call your doctor if you have any of these possible drug side effects. Call *immediately* about any labeled "serious."

Serious: hypothalamic-pituitary-adrenal (HPA) axis suppression (weight gain, moonlike face, increased infections)

Common: other infections (fever, inflammation or warmth in affected area), overly moist or mushy tissue, fever, discoloration, streaky scarring, heat rash (with airtight dressings)
Tip: Stop using the drug and notify the doctor if any of these occurs.

Other: burning, itching, irritation, dryness, redness, acnelike eruptions or pimples, inflamed hair follicles, flaking or itching around the mouth, loss of skin color, hairiness, rash, Cushing's syndrome (fatigue, impotence, edema, hair growth), high blood sugar (increased hunger, thirst, or urination)
Tip: Stop using the drug and call the doctor if any of these occurs.

 DRUG INTERACTIONS

Combining certain drugs may alter their action or produce unwanted side effects. Tell your doctor about other drugs you're taking, especially:
- antibiotics
- antifungal drugs.

CYCLOCORT'S OTHER NAME

Cyclocort's generic name is amcinonide.

sorb larger amounts of the drug and be more prone to overdose.
- Keep using Cyclocort for a few days after your condition clears up to make sure it doesn't come back.

If you miss a dose

Apply the missed dose as soon as possible. However, if it's almost time for your next dose, skip the missed dose and go back to your regular schedule. Don't apply a double dose.

 If you suspect an overdose

Consult your doctor.

 Warnings

- Make sure your doctor knows your medical history. You may not

be able to use Cyclocort if you're allergic to other drugs or are pregnant or breast-feeding.
- Side effects are more likely with use of airtight dressings, prolonged treatment, or use on extensive body surface.

 KEEP IN MIND...

* Apply a thin film.
* Don't use on face, armpits or groin, in ear canals, or under breasts.
* Use dressings only as directed.
* Stop using and call doctor if symptoms worsen.

Cyclogyl

Cyclogyl is an eye medication that's used to enlarge, or dilate, the pupil before eye exams or other procedures. It works by relaxing the muscle that normally closes the pupil in response to bright light.

Why it's prescribed

Doctors prescribe Cyclogyl for medical procedures, such as eye exams, that require completely dilated pupils. Cyclogyl comes in eyedrops. Doctors usually prescribe the following amounts for adults; children's dosages appear in parentheses.

▶ **To dilate the pupils,** 1 or 2 drops in each eye followed by 1 or 2 drops in 5 to 10 minutes, if needed. (Children: 1 drop in each eye, followed by 1 drop in 5 to 10 minutes, if necessary.)

How to use Cyclogyl

• Use Cyclogyl only as your doctor directs.
• Wash your hands before and after using Cyclogyl eyedrops.
• To avoid contamination, don't touch the tip of the dropper to your eye, the surrounding skin, or any other surface when applying drops.
• Tilt your head back and pull the lower eyelid away from the eye. Drop the drug into this space.

CYCLOGYL'S OTHER NAMES

Cyclogyl's generic name is cyclopentolate hydrochloride. Other brand names include Ak-Pentolate; and, in Canada, Minims Cyclopentolate.

 ## SIDE EFFECTS

Call your doctor if you have any of these possible drug side effects. Call *immediately* about any labeled "serious."

Serious: seizures

Common: blurred vision, eye sensitivity to sunlight
Tips: Don't drive or operate machinery until blurriness goes away. Protect your eyes with dark glasses.

Other: irritability, confusion, drowsiness, hallucinations, clumsiness, behavior problems in children, rapid heartbeat, stinging on applying, eye dryness, inability to urinate, dry skin, flushing, fever, contact dermatitis in eye and conjunctivitis (eye redness and discharge)

 ## DRUG INTERACTIONS

Combining certain drugs may alter their action or produce unwanted side effects. Tell your doctor about other drugs you're taking, especially:
• belladonna alkaloids such as atropine sulfate
• glaucoma drugs such as Isopto Carpine
• Miostat
• Ocusert Pilo.

• Cyclogyl may sting your eyes at first.
• Close your eyes and press gently on the inside corners of the eyelids for a minute to prevent tears from washing away the drops.
• Your pupils will begin to dilate rapidly, with peak effects occurring in 30 to 60 minutes. Effects last for 1 day or less.

If you miss a dose

Not applicable because Cyclogyl is used as needed.

 ### If you suspect an overdose

Contact your doctor *immediately.* Signs and symptoms of Cyclogyl overdose may include flushing, dry skin, delerium, fast heart rate, dizziness, and decreased respiratory rate.

 ## Warnings

• Make sure your doctor knows your medical history. You may not be able to use Cyclogyl if you have glaucoma or pressure in the eye or an allergy to this or any other drug.

KEEP IN MIND...

* Don't touch dropper to eye or any other surface.

* Stings at first; causes blurry vision.

* Effect lasts 1 day or less.

* Wear dark glasses to protect eyes.

Cylert

Cylert stimulates nerve activity in the brain to improve concentration and decrease restlessness.

Why it's prescribed

Doctors prescribe Cylert to treat attention deficit hyperactivity disorder in children. It comes in tablets and chewable tablets. Doctors usually prescribe the following amounts for children age 6 and older.

▶ **For attention deficit hyperactivity disorder,** at first, 37.5 milligrams (mg) in the morning, increased by 18.75 mg weekly as needed. Effective dosage range is 56.25 to 75 mg a day; maximum dosage is 112.5 mg a day.

How to take Cylert

• Use Cylert only as your doctor directs; don't change the dosage without the doctor's approval.
• Give to the child at least 6 hours before bedtime to avoid sleeping problems.
• Chewable tablets must not be swallowed whole; make sure the child chews before swallowing.
• Cylert is part of a total treatment program that includes social, educational, and psychological treatment. Improvement with Cylert may take 3 or 4 weeks to occur.
• To avoid severe depression, don't stop giving your child Cylert suddenly. Talk to your doctor about stopping gradually by taking smaller doses.

If you miss a dose

Give your child the missed dose as soon as possible. However, if you

---

CYLERT'S OTHER NAME

Cylert's generic name is pemoline.

 SIDE EFFECTS

Call your doctor if you have any of these possible drug side effects. Call *immediately* about any labeled "serious."

Serious: seizures

Common: uncontrolled movements or sounds, rapid heartbeat
Tip: Try resting to reduce rapid heartbeat; if heartbeat doesn't slow down, call your doctor.

Other: sleeplessness, twitching or other uncontrolled motion, irritability, depression, dizziness, headache, hallucinations, drastic appetite and weight loss, stomach pain, nausea, diarrhea, rash, jaundice (yellow-tinged skin and eyes)
Tip: If dizziness occurs or alertness is affected, make sure your child is safe before riding a bicycle or performing other hazardous activities.

 DRUG INTERACTIONS

Combining certain drugs may alter their action or produce unwanted side effects. Tell your doctor about other drugs you're taking, especially:
• insulin and oral diabetes drugs.

---

don't remember until the next day, skip the missed dose and go back to the regular schedule. Don't give a double dose.

If you suspect an overdose

Contact your doctor *immediately*. Signs and symptoms of overdose include agitation, confusion, seizures, fast heartbeat, hallucinations, headache, high blood pressure (headache, blurred vision), fever with sweating, enlarged pupils, muscle trembling, restlessness, eye tics, and vomiting.

✖ Warnings

• Make sure your child's doctor knows his or her medical history. Your child may not be able to take Cylert if he or she has a kidney or liver problem, severe mental illness, or a drug allergy.

• Cylert may precipitate a condition called Tourette syndrome in children. Report any signs, such as uncontrolled movement or sounds, especially when Cylert is first used.
• Cylert may become habit-forming if too much is taken; it has a greater potential for abuse and dependence than previously thought. Some signs of dependence are a strong desire to increase the dose or depression, weakness, or other unusual behavior when the drug is stopped.

 KEEP IN MIND...

* Don't give near bedtime.
* Don't swallow chewable tablets whole.
* Keep follow-up appointments.
* Don't stop taking abruptly.

CytoGam

CytoGam is used to prevent or treat illness when a patient's immune system is impaired (suppressed) and can't fight certain diseases on its own. CytoGam works by replacing the patient's missing disease-fighting substances.

Why it's prescribed

Doctors prescribe CytoGam to prevent or treat certain illnesses in a patient whose immune system is suppressed — for example, after kidney transplant. It's available only in an injectable form. Doctors usually prescribe the following amounts for adults.

▶ **To prevent disease after kidney transplant,** 150 milligrams (mg) for each 2.2 pounds (lb) of body weight by injection within 72 hours of transplant operation; then 100 mg for each 2.2 lb by injection every 2 weeks after transplant for 8 weeks; then 50 mg for each 2.2 lb at 12 and 16 weeks after transplant.

How to take CytoGam

• A health care professional will administer CytoGam to you.
• CytoGam is given by intravenous injection only. Follow your doctor's directions for receiving treatment.

 SIDE EFFECTS

Call your doctor if you have any of these possible drug side effects. Call *immediately* about any labeled "serious."

Serious: severe allergic reaction (difficulty breathing, dizziness, fainting), low blood pressure (dizziness, weakness)

Common: none reported
Tip: If either side effect occurs, your doctor will stop the injections.

Other: nausea, vomiting, wheezing, flushing, chills, muscle cramps, back pain, fever
Tip: Report if any of these side effects occur while the drug is being given.

 DRUG INTERACTIONS

Combining certain drugs may alter their action or produce unwanted side effects. Tell your doctor about other drugs you're taking, especially:
• live-virus vaccines (delay for at least 3 months).

CytoGam's other name

CytoGam's generic name is cytomegalovirus immune globulin, intravenous (CMV-IGIV).

If you miss a dose

If you miss a scheduled injection, reschedule it as soon as possible. Check with your doctor about any scheduling problems.

 If you suspect an overdose

Contact your doctor *immediately.* Signs of overdose include chest tightness, chills, dizziness, fever, nausea, red face, sweating, unusual tiredness or weakness, and vomiting.

 Warnings

• Make sure your doctor knows your medical history. You may not be able to receive CytoGam if you are allergic to other immune system drugs, have other immune system or heart problems, or are on any special diet.
• Before you begin receiving CytoGam, tell your doctor if you're pregnant or breast-feeding.
• Be aware that during the treatment, a nurse will check your blood pressure, heart rate, and temperature frequently.

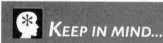 **KEEP IN MIND...**

* Given only by injection.
* Follow treatment directions; expect nurse to check often.
* Delay live-virus vaccinations.

Cytomel

Cytomel increases the body's oxygen supply and speeds up the body's energy production process. It increases the body's metabolism, which is a function of the thyroid gland.

Why it's prescribed

Doctors prescribe Cytomel for underactive thyroid, goiter, and other thyroid problems. It comes in tablets. Doctors usually prescribe the following amounts.

▶ **For underactive thyroid in children,** 5 micrograms (mcg) each day, increased by 5 mcg every 3 to 4 days until desired response is achieved.

▶ **For advanced underactive thyroid (myxdema),** at first, 5 mcg once a day, increased by 5 to 10 mcg every 1 or 2 weeks until daily dosage reaches 25 mcg. Then increased by 12.5 to 25 mcg a day every 1 to 2 weeks.

▶ **For goiter,** at first, 5 mcg each day; may be increased by 5 to 10 mcg a day every 1 to 2 weeks until daily dosage reaches 25 mcg. Then increased by 12.5 to 25 mcg a day every 1 to 2 weeks.

▶ **For thyroid hormone replacement,** at first, 25 mcg each day, increased by 12.5 to 25 mcg every 1 to 2 weeks until desired response occurs.

▶ **For test to determine thyroid problem,** 75 to 100 mcg once a day for 7 days.

How to take Cytomel

• Take Cytomel only as your doctor directs.

CYTOMEL'S OTHER NAMES

Cytomel's generic name is liothyronine sodium. Another brand name is Cyronine.

SIDE EFFECTS

Call your doctor if you have any of these possible drug side effects. Call *immediately* about any labeled "serious."

Serious: chest pain, difficulty breathing, rapid or irregular heartbeat, increased blood pressure (headache, blurred vision), unusual bleeding or bruising

Common: nervousness, sleeplessness, shakiness, headache, diarrhea
Tip: Don't drive or perform other activities that require alertness and coordination until you know how Cytomel affects you.

Other: abdominal cramps, vomiting, weight loss, heat intolerance, heavy sweating, irregular menstruation, bone problem in children

DRUG INTERACTIONS

Combining certain drugs may alter their action or produce unwanted side effects. Tell your doctor about other drugs you're taking, especially:

• Colestid, Questran (separate doses by 4 to 5 hours)
• epinephrine such as in Bronkaid
• insulin and oral diabetes drugs
• oral anticoagulants (blood thinners) such as Coumadin.

• Take Cytomel in the morning to prevent sleeplessness at night.
• Take Cytomel at the same time each day.
• Don't change the drug brand.
• Cytomel's effects may not be noticeable for several weeks.

If you miss a dose

Take the missed dose as soon as possible. But if it's almost time for your next dose, skip the missed dose and go back to your regular dosing schedule. If you miss two or more doses in a row, call your doctor for directions. Don't take a double dose.

 ## If you suspect an overdose

Contact your doctor *immediately.* Excessive Cytomel can cause chest pain, palpitations, sweating, and nervousness.

Warnings

• Make sure your doctor knows your medical history. You may not be able to take Cytomel if you're overly sensitive to this or other drugs, if you're pregnant, or if you have diabetes, high blood pressure, other thyroid or adrenal problems, or a kidney, lung, or heart problem.
• Stop taking Cytomel 7 to 10 days before thyroid tests.

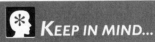 KEEP IN MIND...

∗ Take at same time each day.

∗ Effects seen within several weeks.

∗ Don't change brands.

Cytotec is a drug that's used to prevent stomach ulcers when a patient is taking nonsteroidal anti-inflammatory drugs (NSAIDs) such as Motrin for long-term therapy. Cytotec works by replacing certain substances in the body that are lost when NSAIDs are used.

Why it's prescribed

Doctors prescribe Cytotec to prevent stomach ulcers in patients who are taking aspirin or other NSAIDs. It comes in tablets. Doctors usually prescribe the following amounts for adults.

▶ **To prevent ulcers,** 200 micrograms (mcg) four times a day. If dosage isn't tolerated, decreased to 100 mcg four times a day.

How to take Cytotec

• Take Cytotec only as your doctor directs.
• For best effect and to decrease the risk of diarrhea, take Cytotec with or after meals and at bedtime.
• If you're a premenopausal woman, begin taking Cytotec on the 2nd or 3rd day of your menstrual period.
• Keep taking Cytotec for the full time of treatment, even if you start to feel better, but don't take it for more than 4 weeks without your doctor's consent.

CYTOTEC'S OTHER NAME

Cytotec's generic name is misoprostol.

SIDE EFFECTS

Call your doctor if you have any of these possible drug side effects.

Serious: none reported

Common: diarrhea, abdominal pain
Tip: These symptoms usually go away as your body adjusts to the drug; check with your doctor if they persist or worsen.

Other: headache, nausea, gas, heartburn, vomiting, constipation, menstrual change or problem

DRUG INTERACTIONS

Combining certain drugs may alter their action or produce unwanted side effects. Tell your doctor about other drugs you're taking, especially:
• antacids containing magnesium such as Riopan
• tobacco.

If you miss a dose

Take the missed dose as soon as possible. However, if it's almost time for your next regular dose, skip the missed dose and go back to your regular schedule. Never take a double dose.

If you suspect an overdose

Contact your doctor *immediately.* Signs and symptoms of Cytotec overdose may include nausea, vomiting, and diarrhea.

 Warnings

• Make sure your doctor knows your medical history. You may not be able to take Cytotec if you have a blood vessel disease or have had uncontrolled seizures.
• Don't take this drug if you're pregnant; it may cause miscarriage,

often with potentially life-threatening bleeding. Ask your doctor about effective birth control methods to use during treatment.
• If you're breast-feeding, check with your doctor before using Cytotec.
• Cytotec is not recommended for children under age 18.
• Don't take Cytotec if you have a known allergy to other NSAIDs.

 KEEP IN MIND...

* Don't take while pregnant.
* Take at mealtimes and bedtime.
* Don't take for more than 4 weeks.
* Avoid antacids with magnesium.

Cytovene

Cytovene is used to treat infections caused by viruses. It works by disabling the virus so that it can't spread.

Why it's prescribed

Doctors prescribe Cytovene to prevent or treat — but not cure — an eye infection called cytomegalovirus (CMV) in patients with weakened immune systems, including those with AIDS and some transplant patients. It comes in capsules. It's also available in an injectable form. Doctors usually prescribe the following amounts for adults.

▶ **For CMV eye infections,** 1,000 milligrams orally three times a day. Dosage is adjusted for patients with poor kidney function.

How to take Cytovene

• Take Cytovene only as your doctor directs.
• Take each dose with food.
• Take Cytovene on a regular schedule to maintain the right amount of the drug in the body.

If you miss a dose

Take the missed dose as soon as possible. However, if it's almost time for your next regular dose, skip the missed dose and go back to your regular schedule. Never take a double dose.

 If you suspect an overdose

Contact your doctor *immediately*. Excessive Cytovene can cause nau-

---

CYTOVENE'S OTHER NAME

Cytovene's generic name is ganciclovir.

 SIDE EFFECTS

Call your doctor if you have any of these possible drug side effects. Call *immediately* about any labeled "serious."

Serious: seizures, thrombocytopenia (bleeding, bruising)

Common: agranulocytosis (increased risk of infection)
Tip: To reduce infection risk, avoid people who are sick or infected.

Other: strange dreams, confusion, incoordination, dizziness, headache, behavior changes, irregular heartbeat, high blood pressure (headache, blurred vision), low blood pressure (dizziness, weakness), nausea, vomiting, diarrhea, appetite and weight loss, detached retina, liver problems (yellow-tinged skin and eyes, unusual tiredness); inflammation, pain, and throbbing at injection site

 DRUG INTERACTIONS

Combining certain drugs may alter their action or produce unwanted side effects. Tell your doctor about other drugs you're taking, especially:
• cancer drugs
• corticosteroids such as Decadron
• immunosuppressants, such as Immuran and Sandimmune
• Probalan
• Retrovir (AZT).

---

sea, vomiting, diarrhea, fever, chills, and sore throat.

 Warnings

• Make sure your doctor knows your medical history. You may not be able to take Cytovene if you have a kidney problem or are allergic to this or other drugs.
• Make sure your doctor knows if you're pregnant or breast-feeding before you begin taking Cytovene. Both men and women should use effective birth control methods and condoms during treatment and for at least 90 days afterward.
• Follow your doctor's advice about drinking enough fluids.
• Attend all follow-up appointments so that your doctor can check for any

blood problems that might be caused by this drug. Have regular eye exams, too, to check for sight loss.
• To avoid bleeding, follow your doctor's tooth and gum care advice, wear shoes when walking, and avoid contact sports.

KEEP IN MIND...

∗ Take with food at regular intervals.
∗ Drink plenty of fluids.
∗ Finish entire amount prescribed.
∗ Get regular eye exams.
∗ Avoid bleeding risks.

Cytoxan

Cytoxan fights cancer by affecting the growth of cancer cells.

Why it's prescribed

Doctors prescribe Cytoxan to treat cancer of the breast, head, neck, prostate, lung, and ovary. It's also used to treat Hodgkin's disease and other blood-related cancers, as well as kidney disease. It comes in tablets. It's also available in an injectable form. Doctors usually prescribe the following amounts.
▶ **For cancer,** 1 to 5 milligrams (mg) for each 2.2 pounds (lb) of body weight orally once a day.
▶ **For kidney disease characterized by swelling in children,** 2.5 to 3 mg for each 2.2 lb orally once a day for 60 to 90 days.

How to take Cytoxan

• Take Cytoxan only as your doctor directs.
• Take doses with meals or in the morning.

If you miss a dose

Don't take the missed dose at all and don't double your next dose. Instead, skip the missed dose and then go back to your regular schedule.

 ## If you suspect an overdose

Contact your doctor *immediately.* Excessive Cytoxan can cause hair loss, nausea, vomiting, and increased susceptibility to infection.

CYTOXAN'S OTHER NAMES

Cytoxan's generic name is cyclophosphamide. Other brand names include Neosar; and, in Canada, Procytox.

 ## SIDE EFFECTS

Call your doctor if you have any of these possible drug side effects. Call *immediately* about any labeled "serious."

Serious: heart or lung damage, blood problems (bleeding, bruising, fatigue, increased infection), allergic reaction (swelling of face and throat, difficulty breathing)

Common: nausea, vomiting, hair loss
Tips: To avoid nausea, take drug with or after meals. Be aware that hair loss is usually temporary.

Other: appetite and weight loss, mouth sores, other cancers, menstrual problems, decreased sex drive, pain in joints, decreased level of awareness, seizures, fast heart rate

 ## DRUG INTERACTIONS

Combining certain drugs may alter their action or produce unwanted side effects. Tell your doctor about other drugs you're taking, especially:
• aspirin
• barbiturates such as Solfoton
• Chloromycetin
• corticosteroids such as Decadron
• Lanoxin.

 ## Warnings

• Make sure your doctor knows your medical history. You may not be able to take Cytoxan if you have blood problems, kidney or liver disease, chickenpox, shingles, thyroid problems, or drug allergies or if you've recently undergone radiation or chemotherapy.
• Tell your doctor if you're pregnant; Cytoxan may cause birth defects. Use effective birth control methods while taking Cytoxan and for 4 months after stopping the drug.
• Stop breast-feeding while taking Cytoxan to avoid possible harm to the infant.
• To avoid urinary problems, use the bathroom every 1 to 2 hours and drink at least 3 quarts of water every day.
• If cystitis occurs (abdominal and flank pain, painful urination, blood in urine), stop taking Cytoxan and tell your doctor.
• Watch for signs of infection (fever, sore throat, fatigue) and bleeding (easy bruising, nosebleeds, bleeding gums, bloody stools) and report them to your doctor. Check your temperature every day.

 ## KEEP IN MIND...

* Prevent pregnancy while taking.
* Take with food or in morning.
* Check temperature every day.

Dacriose

Dacriose is a liquid solution that's used to clear debris from the eyes.

Why it's used

Dacriose is used whenever there's a need to wash the eye surface or to clear irritating particles from the eye. You can buy Dacriose without a prescription. It comes in eye-drops. The following amount is usually recommended for adults and children.

▶ **To clean the eye,** flush each eye with 1 to 2 drops three or four times a day, or as needed.

How to use Dacriose

- Read the package label or insert, and follow the instructions carefully.
- Check the expiration date before using.
- Wash your hands before and after using the eyedrops.
- Avoid touching the tip of the dropper to your eye, the surrounding area, or any other surface.
- Flush the affected eye as needed, pressing the sides of the bottle to control the rate of flow. Turn your head from side to side so the drug coats the entire eye.
- Store Dacriose in a tightly closed, light-resistant container.
- To prevent spreading infections, don't share Dacriose with anyone else.

If you miss a dose

Apply the missed dose as soon as possible. However, if it's almost time for your next dose, skip the missed dose and go back to your regular schedule. Don't apply a double dose.

 If you suspect an overdose

Consult your doctor.

 Warnings

- Make sure your doctor knows your medical history. You may not be able to use Dacriose if you're overly sensitive to this drug or any other drug or substance.
- Don't use Dacriose as a saline solution for rinsing and soaking contact lenses.
- If you experience eye pain, changes in vision, or continued redness or irritation of the eye, contact your doctor.
- Don't use the solution if it becomes cloudy or changes color.

DACRIOSE'S OTHER NAMES

Dacriose is an eye irrigation solution. Other brand names include Eye-Stream, I-Lite Eye Drops, Lauro Eye Wash, Lavoptik Eye Wash, and Murine Eye Drops.

 SIDE EFFECTS

Call your doctor if you have any of these possible drug side effects.

Serious: none reported

Common: none reported

Other: allergic reaction to the solution (eye redness or tearing)

DRUG INTERACTIONS

Combining certain drugs may alter their action or produce unwanted side effects. Tell your doctor about other drugs you're using, especially:
- polyvinyl alcohol (found in contact lens solutions).

 KEEP IN MIND...

- Wash hands before and after using.
- Don't touch dropper to eye or any surface.
- Tilt head to spread solution.
- Don't share drug with anyone.
- Avoid polyvinyl alcohol (found in contact lens solutions).

Dalmane

Dalmane induces sleep by slowing down certain nerve and brain activities.

Why it's prescribed

Doctors prescribe Dalmane to treat insomnia. It comes in capsules. Doctors usually prescribe the following amounts for adults.

▶ **For insomnia,** 15 to 30 milligrams, repeated once if needed.

How to take Dalmane

• Take Dalmane only as your doctor directs; overuse can lead to dependence.

• Take at bedtime. Dalmane works best within 30 minutes to 1 hour after taking it. Keep taking Dalmane as your doctor directs, even if it doesn't help you sleep the first night; it's more effective on the second, third, and fourth nights of use.

• Don't stop taking Dalmane suddenly because this can cause unpleasant withdrawal symptoms. Your doctor will probably want to reduce your dosage gradually.

If you miss a dose

If you're taking Dalmane regularly for a specific condition, take the missed dose if you remember it within an hour or so. However, if it's almost time for your next dose, skip the missed dose and go back to your regular schedule. Don't take a double dose.

DALMANE'S OTHER NAMES

Dalmane's generic name is flurazepam hydrochloride. Other brand names include Durapam; and, in Canada, Apo-Flurazepam, Novoflupam, and Somnol.

 ## SIDE EFFECTS

Call your doctor if you have any of these possible drug side effects. Call *immediately* about any labeled "serious."

Serious: slowed breathing

Common: daytime sleepiness, dizziness, uncoordination, headache
Tip: Don't drive or perform activities requiring alertness until you know how the drug affects you.

Other: confusion, nausea, vomiting, heartburn, liver problems (yellow-tinged skin and eyes, unusual tiredness)

 ## DRUG INTERACTIONS

Combining certain drugs may alter their action or produce unwanted side effects. Tell your doctor about other drugs you're taking, especially:
• alcoholic beverages, drugs that make you relaxed or sleepy, such as many allergy and cold remedies, narcotic pain relievers, muscle relaxants, sleeping pills, and seizure drugs
• Antabuse
• birth control pills
• Dilantin
• INH
• Rifadin
• Tagamet
• tobacco.

 ### If you suspect an overdose

Contact your doctor *immediately.* Overdose may be especially dangerous in children. Excessive Dalmane can cause confusion, drowsiness, slow heartbeat, difficulty breathing, slow reactions, slurred speech, and staggering.

 ### Warnings

• Make sure your doctor knows your medical history, especially if you have liver, kidney, or lung problems; depression; suicidal tendencies or a history of drug abuse; or drug allergies or if you're pregnant or breast-feeding.

• Be aware that children and older adults are especially prone to Dalmane's side effects.

• See your doctor regularly to monitor your progress.

• Make sure your doctor and dentist know that you're taking Dalmane before you undergo any medical or dental tests or procedures.

 ### KEEP IN MIND...

* Take at bedtime.

* Don't increase dose or use long-term.

* Don't stop taking suddenly.

Danocrine

Danocrine is used to treat many medical problems, such as endometriosis, in which tissue like the lining of the uterus grows elsewhere in the body; breast cysts; and an inherited condition called angioedema, which causes swelling of the arms, legs, throat, windpipe, bowels, or sexual organs. Danocrine works by suppressing estrogen in the body and increasing proteins that destroy bacteria. Estrogen suppression helps to treat endometriosis and breast cysts. Protein increase works against symptoms of angioedema.

Why it's prescribed

Doctors prescribe Danocrine to treat endometriosis and breast cysts and to prevent angioedema. The drug comes in capsules. Doctors usually prescribe the following amounts for adults.

▶ **For mild endometriosis,** at first, 100 to 200 milligrams (mg) twice a day. Later dosage is based on how well the person responds.

▶ **For moderate to severe endometriosis,** 400 mg twice a day for 3 to 6 months or up to 9 months.

▶ **For cystic breast disease,** 100 to 400 mg each day, divided into two equal doses, for 2 to 6 months.

▶ **To prevent angioedema,** 200 mg two or three times a day until the desired response is reached. Then

DANOCRINE'S OTHER NAMES

Danocrine's generic name is danazol. A Canadian brand name is Cyclomen.

 SIDE EFFECTS

Call your doctor if you have any of these possible drug side effects. Call immediately about any labeled "serious."

Serious: thrombocytopenia (bruising, bleeding), liver problems (yellow-tinged skin and eyes, confusion)

Common: masculine effects in women (weight gain, hairiness, decrease in breast size, oily skin or hair), flushing, excess sweating, vaginitis (itching, dryness, burning), vaginal bleeding, nervousness, menstrual irregularities, emotional instability

Other: clitoral enlargement, changed sex drive, hoarse or deeper voice, dizziness, headache, sleep problem, fatigue, tremor, irritability, excitation, lethargy, depression, chills, numb fingers and toes, high blood pressure (headache, blurred vision), stomach irritation, nausea, vomiting, diarrhea, constipation, change in appetite, muscle cramps, prostate enlargement, prostate cancer, increased skin sensitivity to sunlight

Tips: Stop taking Danocrine and talk to your doctor at the first sign of hormone-related, masculinizing side effects, such as deepening of the voice; some may not be reversible even after stopping treatment. To protect skin from sunlight, stay out of the sun whenever possible, especially between the hours of 10 a.m. and 3 p.m. Use a sunblock and wear protective clothing, including a hat and sunglasses.

 DRUG INTERACTIONS

Combining certain drugs may alter their action or produce unwanted side effects. Tell your doctor about other drugs you're taking.

dosage is decreased by half every 1 to 3 months.

How to take Danocrine

• Take Danocrine only as your doctor directs, for the full time prescribed.

• Don't increase or decrease the dosage without talking to your doctor first. Remember that the number of doses you take each day, the time allowed between doses, and the length of time you take this drug depend on your specific medical problem.

• Store Danocrine away from heat and direct light. Don't keep this drug in the bathroom, near the

kitchen sink, or in other damp places because heat and moisture can cause it to deteriorate.

• Pain relief for breast cysts begins within 1 month; times vary for relief of other problems.

• Your doctor may suggest periodic dosage decreases or gradual withdrawal from Danocrine.

If you miss a dose

Take the missed dose as soon as possible. However, if it's almost time for your next dose, skip the missed dose and take your next dose on schedule. Don't take a double dose.

Continued on next page ▶

If you suspect an overdose

Consult your doctor.

Warnings

• Make sure your doctor knows your medical history. You may not be able to take Danocrine if you have abnormal vaginal bleeding or bleeding gums; kidney, liver, or heart problems; diabetes; or epilepsy or are prone to seizures or migraines.

• Danocrine is not recommended during pregnancy. Make sure your doctor knows if you're pregnant or breast-feeding before you begin taking Danocrine. This drug may cause masculine changes in female babies. The doctor may ask you to take an early pregnancy test immediately before you start treatment with Danocrine.

• While taking Danocrine, use a nonhormonal birth-control method, such as a diaphragm or condoms; don't use birth control pills.

• Be aware that in older men, Danocrine may increase the risk of prostate enlargement or prostate cancer.

• If you have diabetes, be aware that Danocrine may affect your blood sugar levels. Call your doctor if you notice any change in the results of your blood or urine tests.

• Follow your doctor's recommendations for eating foods that are high in calories and protein while you're taking Danocrine.

• Get regular checkups to make sure that Danocrine doesn't cause unwanted side effects.

• If you're taking Danocrine for breast cysts, follow your doctor's directions for examining your breasts regularly. Call the doctor immediately if a breast lump enlarges or if there are any changes in how your breasts feel. Be aware that for 50% of women, breast cysts return within 1 year after treatment with Danocrine stops.

• Wear only cotton underwear and wash after intercourse, to decrease the risk of vaginal infection.

• Be aware that your menstrual period may be irregular or absent while you're taking Danocrine. If your period doesn't begin within 60 to 90 days after you stop taking this drug, check with your doctor.

KEEP IN MIND...

* Don't take during pregnancy.

* Don't use birth control pills; use a nonhormonal contraceptive, such as condoms or a diaphragm.

* Eat a high-calorie, protein-rich diet.

* Examine breasts regularly.

* Wear cotton underwear.

* Report masculinizing side effects.

Dantrium

Dantrium helps relieve muscle spasms, cramping, and tightness caused by multiple sclerosis, cerebral palsy, stroke, and other conditions. The drug works by relaxing muscles.

Why it's prescribed

Doctors prescribe Dantrium to relieve muscle-related symptoms (such as spasms and cramps) in conditions such as multiple sclerosis, cerebral palsy, stroke, and spinal cord injury. They also sometimes prescribe Dantrium before surgery to prevent or manage malignant hyperthermia crisis, a rare condition that occurs after anesthesia and causes high fever and muscle contractions. Dantrium relieves symptoms but doesn't cure the underlying condition. It comes in capsules and is also available in an injectable form. Doctors usually prescribe the following amounts for adults; children's dosages appear in parentheses.

▶ **For muscle spasms and symptoms of severe chronic disorders,** 25 milligrams (mg) orally once a day, increased gradually by 25 mg at a time, up to 100 mg two to four times a day, to a maximum of 400 mg a day. (Children: 0.5 mg for each 2.2 pounds (lb) of body weight orally twice a day; increased to three times a day, then four times a day. Dosage increased as needed by 0.5 mg for each 2.2 lb daily to 3 mg for each 2.2 lb two to four times a day. Maximum dosage is 100 mg four times a day.)

DANTRIUM'S OTHER NAME

Dantrium's generic name is dantrolene sodium.

 SIDE EFFECTS

Call your doctor if you have any of these possible drug side effects. Call *immediately* about any labeled "serious."

Serious: seizures, hepatitis (yellow-tinged skin and eyes, fever, itchiness), allergic reaction (fever, severe diarrhea, severe weakness, rash, itching, hives), fluid in lungs (difficulty breathing), unusual bleeding, blood in urine or stools

Common: muscle weakness, drowsiness, dizziness, headache
Tip: Make sure you know how Dantrium affects you before you drive, use machines, or perform other activities that could be dangerous if you're not alert.

Other: confusion, nervousness, uneasiness, insomnia, hallucinations, rapid or irregular heartbeat, blood pressure changes, watery eyes, double vision, weight loss, constipation, cramping, difficulty swallowing, metallic taste, frequent urination or incontinence, difficulty achieving erection, eczema flare-up, skin sensitivity to sunlight, abnormal hair growth, drooling, sweating, muscle pain, chills, fever
Tips: Tell your doctor about any abdominal discomfort or digestive problems immediately. Use sunblock and wear protective clothing outdoors, including a hat and sunglasses. Stay out of the sun, especially between the hours of 10 a.m. and 3 p.m.

 DRUG INTERACTIONS

Combining certain drugs may alter their action or produce unwanted side effects. Tell your doctor about other drugs you're taking, especially:
- alcohol
- Aldomet
- anabolic steroids, such as Anabolin, Anadrol, Anavar, Diolban, and Maxibolin
- Antabuse
- Cordarone
- drugs that make you relaxed or sleepy, such as sleeping pills, tranquilizers, muscle relaxants, narcotic pain relievers, and many cold, flu, and allergy remedies
- gold salts
- male hormones
- Tylenol.

▶ **To prevent or manage malignant hyperthermia crisis before surgery,** 4 to 8 mg for each 2.2 lb orally a day, divided into three or four equal doses, for 1 or 2 days before surgery. Final dose is administered 3 to 4 hours before surgery.

Continued on next page ▶

Dantrium (continued)

▶ **To prevent recurrence of malignant hyperthermia crisis,** 4 to 8 mg for each 2.2 lb daily, divided into four equal doses, for up to 3 days after crisis.

How to take Dantrium

• Take Dantrium only as your doctor directs. For best effect, take the daily total divided into four equal doses.
• Take capsules with milk or meals to prevent upset stomach.
• If you have trouble swallowing the capsules, empty the number of capsules needed for one dose into a small amount of fruit juice or other liquid; stir gently to mix the powder with the liquid; then drink it right away. Rinse the glass with a little more liquid and drink that too to make sure you've taken the entire dose.
• The doctor may reduce your dosage depending on your response to this drug.
• Store Dantrium away from heat and direct light. Don't keep it in the bathroom, near the kitchen sink, or in another damp place because heat and moisture can cause the drug to deteriorate.

If you miss a dose

Take the missed dose right away if you remember within 1 hour or so. Then go back to your regular schedule. If more than 1 hour has lapsed, skip the missed dose and take your next dose on schedule. Don't take a double dose.

 ## If you suspect an overdose

Contact your doctor immediately. Excessive Dantrium can cause nausea, vomiting, decreased wakefulness, and slowed breathing.

 ## Warnings

• Make sure your doctor knows your medical history. You may not be able to take Dantrium if you have other medical problems, especially heart, lung, or liver disease or a condition that causes spasms. To determine the condition of your liver, your doctor may ask you to have liver function studies performed before you start taking Dantrium.
• Be aware that liver toxicity (hepatitis) is more likely to occur in women over age 35, people taking other drugs along with Dantrium, and people taking 400 mg or more of Dantrium a day.
• Be especially careful to avoid choking when eating; some people may have trouble swallowing when taking Dantrium.
• Because Dantrium will enhance the effects of alcohol, be sure to avoid alcoholic beverages while you're taking this drug.
• See your doctor for regular checkups, especially with long-term use. Your doctor may want you to have regular blood tests to check for unwanted side effects of the drug.
• Follow your doctor's recommendations for getting rest and physical therapy.

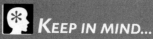 ## KEEP IN MIND...

* Take with milk or meals or mixed in liquid.
* Be careful not to choke.
* Avoid alcohol.
* Protect yourself from sunlight.
* Have regular checkups and blood tests.

Daraprim

Daraprim is used to treat infections — such as malaria — that are caused by one-celled animals called protozoa. Daraprim works by killing protozoa that invade the body.

Why it's prescribed

Doctors prescribe Daraprim to treat malaria in travelers and a disease (called toxoplasmosis) that's caused by protozoa found in raw meat and cat feces. This drug may be prescribed along with one or more additional drugs. Daraprim comes in tablets. Doctors usually prescribe the following amounts for adults; children's dosages appear in parentheses.

▶ **For preventing and stopping the spread of malaria,** 25 milligrams (mg) once a week. (Children over age 10: same as adults. Children ages 4 to 10: 12.5 mg once a week. Children under age 4: 6.25 mg once a week.) Continued in all age-groups 6 to 10 weeks after leaving infestation areas.

▶ **For malaria attack,** 25 mg Daraprim once a day for 2 days. Daraprim isn't recommended alone in nonimmune persons; if it must be used alone in partially immune persons, 50 mg daily for 2 days. (Children over age 10: same as adults. Children ages 4 to 10: 25 mg for 2 days.)

▶ **For toxoplasmosis,** at first, 50 to 75 mg once a day for 1 to 3 weeks, along with 1 to 4 grams (g) of

DARAPRIM'S OTHER NAME

Daraprim's generic name is pyrimethamine.

SIDE EFFECTS

Call your doctor if you have any of these possible drug side effects. Call *immediately* about any labeled "serious."

Serious: seizures, severe blood problems (fatigue, bleeding, bruising, dizziness, sore throat, other signs of infection), severe skin problem such as Stevens-Johnson syndrome (red, burnlike rash), fever, yellow-tinged skin and eyes, burning and tingling of tongue

Common: change or loss of taste, appetite loss, nausea, vomiting, diarrhea, light-headedness
Tip: To reduce nausea and vomiting, take doses with meals or snacks.

Other: abnormal skin pigmentation, dry mouth, insomnia, fatigue, depression

DRUG INTERACTIONS

Combining certain drugs may alter their action or produce unwanted side effects. Tell your doctor about other drugs you're taking, especially:
• drugs that suppress bone marrow, such as Colchicine and Doxorubicin
• seizure drugs such as Depakote and Dilantin
• sulfa drugs, such as Bactrim.

Microsulfon once a day, then 25 mg once a day for 4 to 5 weeks along with 1 g Microsulfon every 6 hours. (Children: 1 mg for each 2.2 pounds [lb] of body weight, but not more than 100 mg a day, divided into two equal doses for 2 to 4 days; then 0.5 mg for each 2.2 lb daily for 4 weeks, along with 100 mg Microsulfon for each 2.2 lb a day, divided into equal doses taken every 6 hours.

How to take Daraprim

• Take Daraprim only as your doctor directs.
• Take with meals to minimize stomach distress.

If you miss a dose

Take the missed dose as soon as possible. However, if it's almost time for your next dose, skip the missed dose and go back to your regular schedule. Don't take a double dose.

If you suspect an overdose

Contact your doctor *immediately.* Excessive Daraprim can cause bruising, bleeding, vomiting, and seizures.

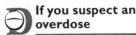
Continued on next page ▶

✕ Warnings

• Make sure your doctor knows your medical history. You may not be able to take Daraprim if you have a drug allergy, anemia or other blood disorder, liver problems, or seizures or are breast-feeding.

• Keep this drug out of children's reach. Children and infants are extremely prone to Daraprim's side effects.

• Your doctor will want to check your blood regularly. Be sure to keep all follow-up appointments.

• Check with your doctor before having dental work done. Be sure to tell your dentist that you're taking Daraprim.

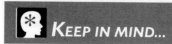

KEEP IN MIND...

* Take with meals.

* Call doctor before dental work.

* Report any rash, bleeding, skin problems, or infection.

* Keep follow-up appointments for blood tests.

Darvocet-N 100 is a combination drug prescribed for relief of pain when nonprescription pain relievers are ineffective. Darvocet-N 100 contains a narcotic. Although the complete action of the drug is unknown, it seems to block pain impulses from reaching the brain, leading to pain relief.

Why it's prescribed

Darvocet-N 100 is prescribed for mild pain relief with or without fever. It comes in tablets. Doctors usually prescribe the following amounts for adults.

▶ **For mild pain relief,** 1 tablet every 4 hours as needed. Maximum recommended dosage is 6 tablets in 24 hours.

How to take Darvocet-N 100

• Take Darvocet-N 100 exactly as prescribed by your doctor. Don't increase the amount or frequency without speaking to your doctor first.
• Store the drug at room temperature and away from heat, light, and moisture.

DARVOCET-N 100's OTHER NAMES

Darvocet-N 100 is a combination of two generic drugs: acetaminophen and propoxyphene. Other brand names include Dolene-AP-65, Doxapap-N, D-Rex 65, E-Lor, Genagesic, Pro Pox with APAP, Propacet 100, and Wygesic. This drug also comes as Darvocet-N 50, containing half the amount of acetaminophen and propoxyphene.

SIDE EFFECTS

Call your doctor if you have any of these possible drug side effects. Call *immediately* about any labeled "serious."

Serious: decreased and shallow breathing, extreme tiredness, physical and psychological dependence, seizures, cold clammy skin, shortness of breath, slow heartbeat

Common: dizziness, nausea, vomiting, drowsiness
Tips: When lying or sitting, get up slowly to avoid dizziness. Take with food to avoid nausea. Avoid driving or other activities that require alertness until you know how Darvocet-N 100 affects you.

Other: constipation, inability to urinate
Tip: Increase fluids to avoid constipation.

DRUG INTERACTIONS

Combining certain drugs may alter their action or produce unwanted side effects. Tell your doctor about other drugs you're taking, especially:
• acetaminophen and products containing acetaminophen (can cause liver damage)
• alcohol
• antidepressants, such as Eldepryl, Pamelor, and Parnate
• tranquilizers, such as Ativan and Xanax.

If you miss a dose

Not applicable because Darvocet-N 100 is taken as needed.

If you suspect an overdose

Contact your doctor *immediately.* Excessive Darvocet-N 100 can cause shallow, slow breathing; deep sleep; and slow or difficult waking.

Warnings

• Make sure your doctor knows your medical history. Don't take Darvocet-N 100 if you have a history of depression, suicidal thoughts, or drug addiction. As a narcotic pain reliever, it can depress your mood and become habit-forming.

• If you're pregnant or breast-feeding, tell your doctor before taking Darvocet-N 100.
• Don't take this drug if you're allergic to Tylenol.
• Be aware that older adults may be especially prone to this drug's side effects.

KEEP IN MIND...

* Take only as prescribed.
* Avoid alcohol and acetaminophen.
* Can cause drowsiness.
* Can be habit-forming.

Darvon

Darvon appears to change both the brain's perception of and response to pain.

Why it's prescribed

Doctors prescribe Darvon to relieve pain from dental work and surgery. It comes in tablets, capsules, and an oral liquid. Doctors usually prescribe the following amounts for adults.

▶ **For mild to moderate pain,** 65 milligrams (mg) every 4 hours as needed, to a maximum dosage of 390 mg a day.

How to take Darvon

- Take Darvon only as your doctor directs.
- Darvon begins to take effect within 15 to 60 minutes; its effect lasts 4 to 6 hours.
- Don't take more than the recommended dosage. Taking Darvon longer than recommended or increasing the dosage without the doctor's consent can make the drug habit-forming.
- Don't stop taking Darvon suddenly. Your doctor may want to reduce your dosage gradually.

If you miss a dose

Take the missed dose as soon as you remember. However, if it's almost time for your next dose, skip the miss-

 SIDE EFFECTS

Call your doctor if you have any of these possible drug side effects. Call *immediately* about any labeled "serious."

Serious: slowed breathing

Common: dizziness, sleepiness, nausea, vomiting
Tips: Don't drive or perform other hazardous activities that require mental alertness until you're completely familiar with Darvon's effects on you. Call your doctor if dizziness persists or becomes bothersome. Take doses with food or milk to minimize stomach upset.

Other: headache, unusual excitement or happiness, sleeplessness, constipation, physical and psychological dependence
Tip: To avoid constipation, drink more fluids and eat more high-fiber foods.

 DRUG INTERACTIONS

Combining certain drugs may alter their action or produce unwanted side effects. Tell your doctor about other drugs you're taking, especially:
- alcohol and other drugs that slow your nervous system, such as sleeping pills, tranquilizers, muscle relaxants, narcotic pain relievers, and many cold, flu, and allergy remedies
- anticoagulants (blood thinners) such as Coumadin
- Tegretol.

ed dose and go back to your regular schedule. Don't take a double dose.

 If you suspect an overdose

Contact your doctor *immediately.* Severe reactions, such as decreased respirations, and coma may result if you take too much Darvon or combine it with other drugs. Other signs of a Darvon overdose may include dizziness, shortness of breath, and seizures.

Warnings

- Because Darvon may worsen certain medical conditions, make sure your doctor knows if you have

heart, liver, lung, or kidney disease; asthma; a seizure disorder; emotional instability; or a history of drug or alcohol abuse.
- If you're pregnant or breast-feeding, check with your doctor before taking Darvon.
- Be aware that older adults may be especially prone to Darvon's side effects.

 KEEP IN MIND...

- Take with food or milk.
- Avoid alcohol.
- Don't stop taking suddenly.

DARVON'S OTHER NAMES

Darvon's generic name is propoxyphene hydrochloride. Other brand names are Dolene; and, in Canada, Novopropoxyn. The generic name of a similar drug, Darvon-N, is propoxyphene napsylate. The brand name in Canada is Daloxene.

Daypro

Daypro is used to relieve inflammation, swelling, and pain caused by arthritis. Daypro doesn't cure arthritis, and it works to relieve symptoms only as long as it's taken.

Why it's prescribed

Doctors prescribe Daypro to treat arthritis pain and other arthritis symptoms. It comes in caplets. Doctors usually prescribe the following amounts for adults.

▶ **For osteoarthritis or rheumatoid arthritis,** at first, 1,200 milligrams (mg) a day. Then, the smallest dosage that's effective to minimize side effects. People with a small build or those with mild symptoms may require only 600 mg a day. Maximum dosage is 1,800 mg or 26 mg for each 2.2 pounds of body weight, whichever is lower, divided into equal doses.

How to take Daypro

• Take Daypro only as your doctor directs. It may take 2 to 4 weeks for the drug's full effect to occur.
• For best absorption, take Daypro 30 minutes before or 2 hours after meals. If stomach upset occurs, Daypro may be taken with milk or meals.
• Don't take more often or in greater doses than recommended; overuse may lead to unwanted side effects, especially in older adults.

If you miss a dose

Take the missed dose as soon as possible. However, if it's almost time

DAYPRO'S OTHER NAME

Daypro's generic name is oxaprozin.

 SIDE EFFECTS

Call your doctor if you have any of these possible drug side effects. Call *immediately* about any labeled "serious."

Serious: severe bleeding in digestive system (bloody or tarry stools), ringing in ears, vision changes
Tip: Report vision or hearing problems immediately.

Common: nausea, heartburn, diarrhea, constipation, rash
Tip: To avoid nausea and heartburn, take drug with milk or meals.

Other: depression, sleeping problems, confusion, stomach pain or distress, weight loss, gas, vomiting, frequent or infrequent urination, liver problems, skin sensitivity to sunlight
Tip: To protect skin, use a sunblock, wear protective clothing, and avoid exposure to direct sunlight.

 DRUG INTERACTIONS

Combining certain drugs may alter their action or produce unwanted side effects. Tell your doctor about other drugs you're taking, especially:
• alcohol
• aspirin
• blood pressure drugs
• corticosteroids
• diuretics (water pills)
• methotrexate
• oral anticoagulants (blood thinners) such as Coumadin.

for your next dose, skip the missed dose and go back to your regular schedule. Don't take a double dose.

 If you suspect an overdose

Contact your doctor *immediately.* Signs and symptoms of Daypro overdose may include drowsiness, nausea, vomiting, and abdominal pain.

Warnings

• Make sure your doctor knows your medical history. You may not be able to take Daypro if you are overly sensitive to this or other

drugs, including aspirin; have nasal polyps or ulcers; or have liver, kidney, or heart disease or conditions that cause you to retain water.
• Tell your doctor if you're pregnant before you take Daypro.

 KEEP IN MIND...

* Results may take 2 to 4 weeks.
* Take between meals if possible.
* Protect yourself from direct sunlight.
* Don't take more than recommended.

DDAVP

DDAVP is a hormone-based drug that decreases the flow rate of urine.

Why it's prescribed

Doctors prescribe DDAVP to reduce nighttime urination in children age 6 and over. It comes in a nasal spray and an injectable form. Doctors usually prescribe the following amounts.

▶ **For bed-wetting in children age 6 and over,** at first, 20 micrograms (mcg) of nasal spray at bedtime. Maximum recommended dosage is 40 mcg a day.

How to use DDAVP

• Use DDAVP only as your child's doctor directs.

• Before using the spray, have your child gently blow his or her nose to clear the nasal passages. Measure the dose carefully, and tell the child to inhale the drug into the nostrils as the doctor directs.

• DDAVP begins to take effect within 1 hour and lasts for 8 to 12 hours.

If you miss a dose

Don't give your child a double dose. Adjust schedule as follows:

• If your child takes one dose a day, give him or her the missed dose as soon as possible. Then go back to the regular schedule. If you don't remember until the next day, skip the missed dose and go back to the regular schedule.

• If your child takes more than one dose a day, give him or her the

SIDE EFFECTS

Call your doctor if you have any of these possible drug side effects.

Serious: none reported

Common: headache, runny nose

Other: slight increase in blood pressure (with high doses), nasal congestion, inflamed nasal lining, nausea, abdominal cramps, flushed skin

Tip: For a mild headache, the child may take aspirin or Tylenol unless the doctor gives you other instructions.

DRUG INTERACTIONS

Combining certain drugs may alter their action or produce unwanted side effects. Tell your doctor about other drugs you're taking, especially:
• alcohol
• Atromid-S
• Bronkaid
• Declomycin
• Eskalith.

missed dose as soon as possible. Then go back to the regular schedule. However, if it's almost time for the next dose, skip the missed dose and give the next dose on schedule.

If you suspect an overdose

Contact the doctor *immediately*. Excessive DDAVP can cause drowsiness, headache, confusion, no urine output, and weight gain.

Warnings

• Make sure your child's doctor knows his or her medical history. Your child may not be able to use DDAVP if he or she is overly sensitive to this or other drugs or has von Willebrand's disease, hemophilia A, heart disease, blood vessel disease, high blood pressure, other conditions such as cystic fibrosis, or a stuffy nose caused by a cold or an allergy.

• Nasal congestion, allergic nasal problems, or upper respiratory infections may impair drug absorption. Report congestion or breathing difficulties to the doctor; your child may need a dosage adjustment.

• Follow the doctor's recommendations for fluid intake to avoid side effects.

• Have your child wear a medical identification tag or bracelet to let others know he or she is using DDAVP.

KEEP IN MIND...

* Gently blow nose before using nasal solution.

* Report congestion or trouble breathing.

* Limit fluid intake.

DDAVP'S OTHER NAMES

DDAVP's generic name is desmopressin acetate. Another brand name is Stimate.

Debrox

Debrox is a solution that helps soften and remove accumulated earwax. It works by breaking the earwax into globules that can be flushed away.

Why it's used

Debrox is used to treat impacted earwax. You can buy Debrox without a prescription. It comes in eardrops. The following amounts are usually recommended for adults and children over age 12.

▶ **To remove earwax,** 5 to 10 drops into ear canal twice a day.

How to use Debrox

• Use Debrox only as your doctor directs, especially for children under age 12. Read the package label or insert carefully before using.

• Avoid touching the dropper to the ear or any other surface to prevent contamination.

• To instill ear drops, pull auricle up and back.

• Allow the solution to remain in the ear for 15 to 30 minutes; then, using a rubber bulb syringe, gently flush the ear with warm water.

• Don't use Debrox for more than 4 days unless your doctor directs.

DEBROX'S OTHER NAMES

Debrox's generic name is carbamide peroxide. Other brand names include Auro Ear Drops and Murine Ear Drops.

 SIDE EFFECTS

Call your doctor if you have any of these possible drug side effects. Call *immediately* about any labeled "serious."

Serious: inflammation or irritation

Common: none reported

Other: bleaching of skin
Tip: Wash affected area twice with soap and water to minimize bleaching.

 DRUG INTERACTIONS

Combining certain drugs may alter their action or produce unwanted side effects. Tell your doctor about other drugs you're taking.

If you miss a dose

Apply the missed dose as soon as possible. However, if it's almost time for your next dose, skip the missed dose and go back to your regular schedule.

 If you suspect an overdose

Contact your doctor *immediately* if Debrox is swallowed. Symptoms include burning in the mouth or throat and an enlarged abdomen.

❌ **Warnings**

• Make sure your doctor knows your medical history. Don't use Debrox if you have an injured or punctured eardrum or if you have ear drainage or discharge, pain, or rash.

• If you're pregnant or breast-feeding, tell your doctor before you begin using Debrox.

• Don't let children under age 12 administer Debrox to themselves.

• Don't use Debrox to treat swimmer's ear.

• Call your doctor if redness, pain, or swelling persists.

 KEEP IN MIND...

∗ Don't use if eardrum is punctured.

∗ Don't touch dropper to the ear.

∗ Flush ear with warm water after 15 to 30 minutes.

∗ Report persistent redness, pain, or swelling.

Decadron

Decadron in its oral form is used to treat the symptoms of allergic reactions and a variety of other skin problems as well as asthma, arthritis, tumors, and other conditions. It's also used as part of a diagnostic test for a hormonal problem called Cushing's syndrome (adrenal gland overproduction). Decadron decreases inflammation, stimulates bone marrow growth, and helps the body process protein, fat, and carbohydrates.

Why it's prescribed

Doctors prescribe oral Decadron to treat the swelling, inflammation, and itching of allergic reactions; for tumors; and as a diagnostic test for Cushing's syndrome. Decadron comes in tablets, an oral solution, and an elixir. It's also available in an injectable form. Doctors usually prescribe the following amounts for adults.

▶ **For inflammation, allergic reactions, and tumors,** 0.75 to 9 milligrams (mg) orally a day.

▶ **For Cushing's syndrome test,** after first testing without oral Decadron, 0.5 mg orally every 6 hours for 48 hours; then, urine collected for the next two 24-hour periods and tested.

DECADRON'S OTHER NAMES

Oral Decadron's generic name is dexamethasone. Other brand names include Dexamethasone Intensol, Dexone, Hexadrol, Mymethasone; and, in Canada, Deronil and Dexasone.

 SIDE EFFECTS

Call your doctor if you have any of these possible drug side effects. Call *immediately* about any labeled "serious."

Serious: congestive heart failure (difficulty breathing), acute adrenal problem (muscle weakness, joint pain, fever, nausea, dizziness, fainting)

Common: feeling of well-being, sleeplessness, stomach ulcers
Tip: Take Decadron with food to prevent stomach irritation.

Other: strange behavior, increased pressure in head (headache, vision changes), high blood pressure (headache, blurred vision), swelling, cataracts, glaucoma, increased appetite, inflamed pancreas (abdominal pain, nausea, vomiting), slow wound healing, acne, osteoporosis, hairiness, infections, gas, poor growth in children
Tip: To detect any eye problems, you may want to have your eyes examined by an eye doctor before you start taking oral Decadron and during your treatment if you're going to be taking this drug long-term.

 DRUG INTERACTIONS

Combining certain drugs may alter their action or produce unwanted side effects. Tell your doctor about other drugs you're taking, especially:
• anticoagulants (blood thinners) such as Coumadin
• aspirin and other nonsteroidal anti-inflammatory drugs (NSAIDs)
• barbiturates such as Solfoton
• Dilantin
• potassium-depleting drugs such as thiazide diuretics (water pills)
• Rifadin
• skin-test antigens, toxoids, and vaccines (delay until after Decadron treatment ends).

How to take Decadron

• Take Decadron only as your doctor directs. Don't take it more often or for a longer period than prescribed.
• If you take a single daily dose, take it in the morning for best results.
• Store oral Decadron away from heat and direct light. Don't keep it in the bathroom, near the kitchen sink, or in another damp place because heat and moisture can cause the drug to deteriorate.

• Don't stop taking Decadron suddenly. Check with your doctor first. You may need to reduce the amount you take gradually to prevent serious — even fatal — side effects.

If you miss a dose

Take the missed dose as soon as possible. Then take any remaining doses for that day at regularly spaced intervals. However, if it's almost time for your next dose, skip the missed dose and take the next dose on schedule. Don't take a double dose.

If you suspect an overdose

Contact your doctor *immediately*. Excessive Decadron can cause infections, muscle weakness, and osteoporosis.

Warnings

• Make sure your doctor knows your medical history. You may not be able to take Decadron if you're overly sensitive to this or other drugs or their components (such as sulfite preservatives); if you're prone to emotional swings or pyschotic tendencies; or if you have a fungal infection such as *Candida*, an ulcer or other condition that affects the digestive system, bone or muscle-related diseases, diabetes, seizures, tuberculosis, herpes that affects the eyes, or liver, kidney, heart, thyroid, or blood-related problems.

• If you're pregnant or breast-feeding, check with your doctor before taking Decadron.

• Be aware that older patients taking Decadron long-term may be more prone to osteoporosis.

• Be aware that long-term use of oral Decadron can lower your resistance to infections and make them harder to treat. Report any signs of infection, such as sore throat, fever, sneezing, or coughing.

• Before surgery or dental work, make sure the doctor or dentist knows that you're taking oral Decadron.

• Take vitamin D or calcium supplements as your doctor directs.

• If you're taking oral Decadron over a long period of time, your doctor may ask you to follow a diet that's low in salt, rich in potassium, or both. Follow any special diet directions.

• With long-term use, follow your doctor's recommendations about exercise or physical therapy. Have regular eye exams and medical checkups.

• Notify the doctor if your condition returns or worsens after any change in the amount you take or after you've stopped taking this drug.

• Carry medical identification telling others that you're using oral Decadron and that you may need more of the drug during an emergency, a severe asthma attack or other illness, or unusual stress.

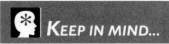

KEEP IN MIND...

* Take with food.

* Take single doses in morning.

* Don't stop taking suddenly; death can result.

* Have regular eye exams and checkups.

* Take vitamin D or calcium as directed.

* Carry medical identification.

Decadron Phosphate (for eyes)

Decadron Phosphate (for eyes) stimulates the production of certain enzymes that decrease inflammation.

Why it's prescribed

Doctors prescribe Decadron Phosphate to relieve redness, inflammation, and other eye problems resulting from eye irritation, allergy, or injury. It comes in eyedrops and an ointment. Doctors usually prescribe the following amounts for adults and children.

▶ **For inflammations of eye and eye area, burns, injury by objects in the eye, and conjunctivitis due to allergy,** 1 to 2 drops in the eye four to six times a day or a $\frac{1}{2}$- to 1-inch ribbon of ointment applied into the space inside the lower lid three or four times a day. In severe cases, drops may be used hourly. As condition improves, dosage is reduced to twice a day, then once a day. Treatment may last several weeks.

How to use Decadron Phosphate (for eyes)

- Use this drug only as your doctor directs.
- Shake liquid drops before using.
- Wash your hands before and after using this drug.
- To avoid contamination, don't touch the applicator tip to any surface, including your eye.

DECADRON PHOSPHATE'S OTHER NAMES

Decadron Phosphate's generic name is dexamethasone sodium phosphate. Another brand name is Maxidex Ophthalmic Suspension.

 SIDE EFFECTS

Call your doctor if you have any of these possible drug side effects. Call *immediately* about any labeled "serious."

Serious: vision changes (decreased acuity, clouding, decreased field of vision)

Common: none reported

Other: increased pressure in eyeball (eye pain, blurred vision), thinning of cornea (clear covering over front of eyeball), poor corneal wound healing, viral or fungal corneal infection, corneal ulcer

 DRUG INTERACTIONS

Combining certain drugs may alter their action or produce unwanted side effects. Tell your doctor about other drugs you're taking.

- After using the drops, close your eyes for 1 to 2 minutes so the drug can be absorbed.
- Once your eye infection is cured, discard any leftover drug.

If you miss a dose

Apply the drug as soon as possible. Then apply any remaining doses for that day at regularly spaced intervals. But if it's almost time for your next application, skip the missed dose and go back to your regular schedule. Don't apply a double dose.

 If you suspect an overdose

Contact your doctor *immediately.* Excessive use can cause worsening glaucoma; cataracts; vision defects; burning, stinging, redness, or watering of eyes; and other side effects affecting the entire body.

 Warnings

- Make sure your doctor knows your medical history. You may not be able to use Decadron Phosphate if you're allergic to any drug or if you have glaucoma, herpes, fungal or viral diseases of the eye, infected eye abrasions, or other conditions that affect the eyes.
- If you're pregnant or breast-feeding, check with your doctor before you begin using this drug.
- Don't share your drug, towels, or washcloths with others. If a family member has the same symptoms, call the doctor.
- Don't rub or scratch the area around your eye while using this drug.

 KEEP IN MIND...

- * Keep eyes closed for 1 or 2 minutes to absorb drug.
- * Don't share drug, towels, or washcloths.
- * Report any vision changes.

Decadron Phosphate (for skin)

Decadron Phosphate in its topical (skin) form is used to treat skin and scalp problems. It works by decreasing inflammation, itching, redness, and irritation.

Why it's prescribed

Doctors prescribe topical Decadron Phosphate for inflammation, itching, and other symptoms of problems that affect the skin and scalp. It comes in an aerosol, a gel, and a cream. Doctors usually prescribe the following amounts for adults.

▶ **For skin and scalp inflammation,** a small amount of cream, gel, or aerosol applied three or four times a day.

How to use Decadron Phosphate (for skin)

• Use topical Decadron Phosphate only as your doctor directs.
• Wash your hands before and after applying Decadron. Then wash and dry the affected area.
• If you're using the aerosol on your scalp, first shampoo and dry your hair. Then gently shake the aerosol can and begin to apply the aerosol to your dry scalp. Holding the can upright, slide the applicator tube under your hair so that it touches your scalp. Spray while moving tube to all affected areas, keeping the tube under the hair and in contact with the scalp throughout each spray, which should take about 2 seconds. Spot-spray poorly covered areas by slid-

SIDE EFFECTS

Call your doctor if you have any of these possible drug side effects. Call *immediately* about any labeled "serious."

Serious: high blood pressure (headache, blurred vision), moon face, weight gain

Common: skin breakdown, infection (redness, oozing, pain), scarring, heat rash (with airtight dressings)
Tip: Check with your doctor if you develop a rash, itching, burning, dryness, or signs of infection.

Other: burning, itching, irritation, dryness, inflamed hair follicles, hairiness, acne, inflammation around mouth, allergic reaction (rash, hives, swelling), loss of skin color

DRUG INTERACTIONS

Combining certain drugs may alter their action or produce unwanted side effects. Tell your doctor about other drugs you're taking, especially:
• antifungal drugs and antibiotics (don't use Decadron until the doctor says the infection is controlled).

ing the applicator tube through the hair to the scalp, then pressing and immediately releasing the spray button. Don't massage the drug into the scalp or spray it on your forehead.
• If you're using the gel or cream, gently wash and dry the affected skin first. Then apply a thin coat of the drug to the affected area. Rub the gel or cream in gently to avoid injuring your skin. If you're treating a hairy area, part the hair and apply the drug directly to the skin.
• If you're using the aerosol on your skin, begin by gently washing and drying the affected area. Shake the can well; then spray as you move the nozzle over the affected area. The spray contains alcohol, which may irritate or sting open sores. To avoid freezing skin tissue, don't spray longer than 3 seconds or from closer than 6 inches.

• Don't apply any form of this drug to or near the eyes, nose, mouth, or open sores.
• Don't wrap the treated area with a bandage or other tight dressing without your doctor's consent.
• If you're using topical Decadron to treat diaper rash in a young child, don't cover the treated area with a tight-fitting diaper or plastic pants; this could cause too much drug absorption.
• If the doctor orders an airtight wrap (such as plastic wrap), don't leave it in place longer than 16 hours each day. Don't use an airtight dressing on infected or moist, runny areas.
• If your skin is irritated by adhesives (due to allergy), hold dressings in place with gauze, elastic bandages, stockings, or a stockinette.

DECADRON PHOSPHATE'S OTHER NAME

Decadron Phosphate's generic name is dexamethasone sodium phosphate.

Continued on next page ▶

• Change dressings as your doctor directs; stop using Decadron and the dressing and call the doctor if you develop scarring or streaking, skin death, or fever or other signs of infection.

• Continue using Decadron for a few days after your skin clears to prevent the problem from coming back.

• Be sure to store Decadron away from heat and direct light to prevent the drug from deteriorating.

If you miss a dose

Apply the drug as soon as possible. But if it's almost time for your next application, skip the missed dose and apply the next one on schedule.

If you suspect an overdose

Consult your doctor.

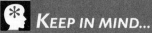

Warnings

• Make sure your doctor knows your medical history. You may not be able to use topical Decadron if you're allergic to it or to other drugs, if you have poor circulation, or if you've recently had chicken-pox or an infection.

• Tell your doctor if you're pregnant or breast-feeding before you begin using topical Decadron.

• Unwanted absorption into the body is more likely to occur with airtight dressings (used more than 16 hours a day), prolonged treatment, or extensive body-surface treatment.

• Keep all appointments for follow-up visits so your doctor can check your progress and detect side effects early.

• Notify your doctor if your symptoms return or worsen after you've decreased the dosage or stopped using the drug.

KEEP IN MIND...

* Use aerosol on dry scalp after shampooing; don't rub it in.

* Keep drug away from eyes, mouth, nose, and open sores.

* Don't spray longer than 3 seconds or from closer than 6 inches.

* Use a bandage or dressing only if doctor tells you to.

* Don't use tight diapers or plastic pants over treated area.

* Don't use with antifungal or antibiotic drugs.

Declomycin

Declomycin is an antibiotic that's used to treat bacterial infections. It works by killing the invading organisms.

Why it's prescribed

Doctors prescribe Declomycin to treat infections such as pneumonia and gonorrhea. It comes in tablets and capsules. Doctors usually prescribe the following amounts for adults; children's dosages appear in parentheses.

▶ **For bacterial or protozoal infections,** 150 milligrams (mg) every 6 hours or 300 mg every 12 hours. (Children over age 8: 6 to 12 mg for each 2.2 pounds of body weight a day, divided into equal doses taken every 6 to 12 hours.)

▶ **For gonorrhea,** first, 600 mg; then 300 mg every 12 hours for 4 days.

How to take Declomycin

• Take Declomycin only as your doctor directs.
• Take each dose with a full glass (8 ounces) of water, at least 1 hour before or 2 hours after meals.
• To prevent heartburn, take it at least 1 hour before bedtime.
• Don't sit or lie down for 90 seconds after taking a dose.
• Take the amount prescribed to prevent reinfection.

If you miss a dose

Take the missed dose as soon as possible. But if it's almost time for your next dose, skip the missed dose and

DECLOMYCIN'S OTHER NAME

Declomycin's generic name is demeclocycline hydrochloride.

 SIDE EFFECTS

Call your doctor if you have any of these possible drug side effects. Call *immediately* about any labeled "serious."

Serious: increased pressure in head (headache, vision changes), severe anemia (fatigue), allergic reactions (swelling of throat and face, difficulty breathing)

Common: nausea, vomiting, diarrhea, rash, sensitivity to sun, hives
Tip: Avoid direct sunlight and wear protective clothing and a sunblock.

Other: inflammation around heart (fever, pain, dry cough, fluttering in chest), drastic appetite and weight loss, anal or genital inflammation, diabetes insipidus (weakness, increased thirst and urination)

 DRUG AND FOOD INTERACTIONS

Combining certain drugs and certain foods may alter drug action or produce unwanted side effects. Tell your doctor about your diet and other drugs you're taking, especially:

• antacids or laxatives containing aluminum, magnesium, or calcium; diarrhea drugs; food, milk, and dairy products (take 1 hour before or 2 hours after Declomycin)
• birth control pills
• iron products such as Feosol, zinc (take 2 hours before Declomycin)
• oral anticoagulants (blood thinners) such as Coumadin
• penicillins such as Megacillin.

go back to your regular schedule. Don't take a double dose.

 If you suspect an overdose

Contact your doctor *immediately.* Signs and symptoms of a Declomycin overdose may include nausea, vomiting, and diarrhea.

Warnings

• Make sure your doctor knows your medical history. You may not be able to take Declomycin if you're allergic to tetracyclines, if you have poor kidney or liver function, or if you're in the last half of pregnancy.

• While you're taking Declomycin, don't use birth control pills. Switch to a nonhormonal form of birth control.

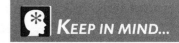 **KEEP IN MIND...**

* Don't take with milk, food, antacids, or iron.

* Take at least 1 hour before bedtime.

* Avoid sunlight and wear protective clothing.

Delta-Cortef

Delta-Cortef decreases inflammation by suppressing the immune response and increasing blood cell production.

Why it's prescribed

Doctors prescribe Delta-Cortef to help treat inflammation, immune system problems, and colitis. Delta-Cortef comes in tablets and syrup. Doctors usually prescribe the following amounts for adults.

▶ **For severe inflammation or immunosuppression,** 2.5 to 15 milligrams two to four times a day.

How to take Delta-Cortef

• Take Delta-Cortef only as your doctor directs.
• To reduce stomach upset, take it with food when possible.
• After long-term treatment, follow your doctor's directions for gradually reducing your dosage.

If you miss a dose

Adjust your schedule as follows:
• If you usually take one dose a day, take the missed dose as soon as possible; then go back to your regular schedule. If you don't remember until the next day, skip the missed dose and resume your normal schedule.
• If you usually take several doses a day, take the missed dose as soon as possible. However, if it's almost time for your next dose, double the next dose.

DELTA-CORTEF'S OTHER NAMES

Delta-Cortef's generic name is prednisolone. Other brand names include Prelone and, in Canada, Novo Prednisolone.

 SIDE EFFECTS

Call your doctor if you have any of these possible drug side effects. Call *immediately* about any labeled "serious."

Serious: severe hormonal disorder following stress (from infection, surgery, or trauma), such as adrenal gland insufficiency (fatigue, muscle weakness, joint pain, fever, appetite and weight loss, nausea, difficulty breathing, dizziness, fainting) or Cushing's syndrome (sudden weight gain or swelling)

Common: unrealistic feeling of well-being, insomnia, stomach ulcer

Other: strange behavior, false brain tumor (headache, vision changes), high blood pressure (headache, blurred vision), cataracts, glaucoma, stomach irritation, increased appetite, inflamed pancreas (abdominal pain, nausea, vomiting), delayed wound healing, acne, osteoporosis, hairiness, infections
Tip: Tell your doctor if skin wounds are healing unusually slowly.

 DRUG INTERACTIONS

Combining certain drugs may alter their action or produce unwanted side effects. Tell your doctor about other drugs you're taking, especially:
• aspirin and other nonsteroidal anti-inflammatory drugs (NSAIDs)
• Dilantin, Rifampin
• oral anticoagulants (blood thinners) such as Coumadin
• potassium-depleting drugs such as thiazide diuretics (water pills)
• skin-test antigens (delay skin testing until Delta-Cortef therapy ends).

 If you suspect an overdose

Contact your doctor. Excessive Delta-Cortef may cause infections and muscle weakness.

 Warnings

• Make sure your doctor knows your medical history. You may not be able to take Delta-Cortef if you're allergic to this drug; if you have diabetes, tuberculosis, a fungal infection, herpes, an ulcer, digestive problems, or a heart, liver, lung, kidney, bone, muscle, blood, or thyroid disorder; or if you're prone to seizures or psychotic tendencies.
• With long-term treatment, follow your doctor's directions regarding exercise or physical therapy and vitamin D or calcium supplements.
• Carry a card identifying your drug needs.

KEEP IN MIND...

* Take with food.
* Don't stop taking abruptly.
* Carry a medical identification card.

Deltasone

Deltasone is used to relieve severe inflammation in many diseases. It decreases inflammation, mainly by regulating the body's immune system.

Why it's prescribed

Doctors prescribe Deltasone to help treat many diseases that involve a poor immune response or severe inflammation, such as flare-ups of multiple sclerosis, ulcerative colitis, acute leukemia, blood disorders, tuberculosis, arthritis, lupus, Stevens-Johnson syndrome, asthma, and allergic drug reactions. The drug comes in tablets, a liquid, and a syrup. Doctors usually prescribe the following amounts for adults.

▶ **For severe inflammation or immunosuppression,** 2.5 to 15 milligrams (mg) each day, divided into equal doses. Once appropriate drug level in body is reached, maintenance dose is given once a day or every other day. Dosage must be individualized.

▶ **For multiple sclerosis flare-up,** 200 mg once a day for 1 week; then 80 mg every other day for 1 month.

▶ **For other diseases listed above,** dosage is individualized.

How to take Deltasone

• Take Deltasone only as your doctor directs — no more or less and for no longer.

• To prevent stomach upset, take with food.

DELTASONE'S OTHER NAMES

Deltasone's generic name is prednisone. Other brand names include Liquid Pred, Meticorten, Orasone, Panasol, Prednicen-M, Prednisone Intensol, Sterapred; and, in Canada, Apo-Prednisone, Novo-Prednisone, and Winpred.

SIDE EFFECTS

Call your doctor if you have any of these possible drug side effects. Call *immediately* about any labeled "serious."

Serious: bloody or black, tarry stools; severe hormonal problem following stress (from infection, surgery, or trauma) or abrupt withdrawal after long-term use, such as Cushing's syndrome (weight gain, swelling) or adrenal gland insufficiency (fatigue, muscle weakness, joint pain, fever, weight loss, nausea, difficulty breathing, dizziness, fainting); low potassium level (dizziness, tiredness, weakness, leg cramps, nausea, stomach upset); high blood sugar (frequent urination, thirst); and after abrupt withdrawal, increased inflammation, fatigue, weakness, pain, fever, dizziness, lethargy, depression, fainting, low blood pressure (dizziness, weakness), difficulty breathing, appetite and weight loss, low blood sugar (tremor, clammy skin, irritability)

Tip: Weigh yourself daily and report sudden weight gain to the doctor; this could indicate a hormonal disorder.

Common: unrealistic feeling of well-being, sleeplessness, stomach ulcer

Other: false brain tumor (headache, vision changes), high blood pressure (headache, blurred vision), cataracts, glaucoma, stomach irritation, increased appetite, inflamed pancreas (nausea, vomiting, abdominal pain), delayed wound healing, acne, muscle weakness, osteoporosis, hairiness, infections, poor growth in young children

Tips: Tell your doctor if a skin wound seems to be healing slowly. Talk with your doctor about having an eye exam before starting treatment with Deltasone. This will make it easier to detect any vision changes that may occur while taking the drug.

DRUG INTERACTIONS

Combining certain drugs may alter their action or produce unwanted side effects. Tell your doctor about other drugs you're taking, especially:

• aspirin, Indocin, and other nonsteroidal anti-inflammatory drugs (NSAIDs)

• barbiturates (sedatives), Dilantin, Rifadin, and other drugs for seizures or tuberculosis

• oral anticoagulants (blood thinners) such as Coumadin

• skin-test antigens, toxoids, and vaccines (delay skin testing until Deltasone treatment ends)

• thiazide diuretics (water pills), such as HydroDIURIL and Vaseretic, and other drugs that cause potassium loss

• For better results and less toxicity, take a once-daily dose in the morning.

• Don't stop taking this drug suddenly; doing so could be fatal. If

Continued on next page ▶

you plan to stop using Deltasone, check with your doctor so your dosage can be reduced gradually.

If you miss a dose

Adjust your schedule as follows:
• If you take one dose every other day, take the missed dose as soon as possible if you remember it the same morning. If not, wait and take it the next morning. Then skip a day and resume your regular schedule.
• If you take one dose a day, take the missed dose as soon as possible. If you don't remember until the next day, skip the missed dose and take your next dose on schedule. Don't take a double dose.
• If you take several doses a day, take the missed dose as soon as possible; then go back to your regular schedule. If you don't remember until your next dose is due, double the next dose.

If you suspect an overdose

Contact your doctor *immediately*. Excessive Deltasone can cause muscle weakness, osteoporosis, decreased ability to fight stress, weight gain, and moonlike face.

Warnings

• Make sure your doctor knows your medical history. You may not be able to take Deltasone if you are sensitive to this drug; if you have a fungal infection, an ulcer, kidney or liver disease, high blood pressure, osteoporosis, diabetes, a thyroid problem, diverticulitis, ulcerative colitis, blood clot, seizures, muscle weakness, congestive heart failure, tuberculosis, or herpes eye infection; if you've recently had abdominal surgery; or if you have a history of emotional instability or psychotic tendencies.

• If you're pregnant or breast-feeding, check with your doctor before taking Deltasone.
• Be aware that steroid use in children may suppress growth and maturation.
• Be aware that older adults may be more susceptible to osteoporosis from chronic use of Deltasone.
• If you're diabetic, you may need increased insulin while taking Deltasone; check your blood sugar levels carefully.
• Store this drug away from heat and direct light. For example, don't store it in the bathroom, near the kitchen sink, or in any other damp area. Heat and moisture may cause the drug to break down and lose its effectiveness.
• Take steps to protect yourself from infection, and take your temperature frequently. Deltasone may worsen an infection or hide its symptoms.
• Follow a low-sodium diet that's high in potassium and protein, as your doctor directs. Also follow doctor's orders regarding exercise or physical therapy and vitamin D or calcium supplements.
• Before you have medical tests, tell the doctor you're taking Deltasone.
• With long-term treatment, schedule regular eye exams and follow-up trips to the doctor to check your progress.
• Carry a medical identification card that lets others know about your need for this drug.

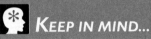

KEEP IN MIND...

* Take with food — preferably once a day in morning.

* Never stop taking suddenly; doing so can be fatal.

* Follow doctor's diet and exercise directions.

* Carry a medical identification card.

Demadex

Demadex is a diuretic (water pill) that helps rid the body of excess water and minerals.

Why it's prescribed

Doctors prescribe Demadex to treat high blood pressure and for heart, kidney, or liver disorders that cause the body to retain water. The drug comes in tablets. It's also available in an injectable form. Doctors usually prescribe the following amounts for adults.

▶ **For congestive heart failure and chronic kidney failure,** at first, 10 to 20 milligrams (mg) orally once a day. If response is poor, dose is doubled until response is good. Maximum dosage is 200 mg a day.

▶ **For liver disease,** at first, 5 to 10 mg orally once a day. If response is poor, dose is doubled until response is good. Maximum dosage is 40 mg a day.

▶ **For high blood pressure,** at first, 5 mg orally a day, increased to 10 mg if needed and tolerated. If response is still poor in 4 to 6 weeks, another drug is added.

How to take Demadex

• Take Demadex only as your doctor directs.

If you miss a dose

Take the missed dose as soon as possible. However, if it's almost time for your next dose, skip the missed

DEMADEX'S OTHER NAME

Demadex's generic name is torsemide.

 SIDE EFFECTS

Call your doctor if you have any of these possible drug side effects. Call *immediately* about any labeled "serious."

Serious: heart trouble, chest pain

Common: diarrhea, constipation, nausea, excessive urination
Tip: Take drug in the morning to avoid nighttime urination.

Other: dizziness, headache, nervousness, insomnia, swelling, stuffy or runny nose, cough, sore throat, heartburn, weakness, pain, low potassium level (muscle weakness, cramps)
Tip: Stand up slowly to avoid dizziness.

DRUG INTERACTIONS

Combining certain drugs may alter their action or produce unwanted side effects. Tell your doctor about other drugs you're taking, especially:
• Aldactone, Edecrin
• aminoglycosides, such as Nebcin and Myciguent
• aspirin and other nonsteroidal anti-inflammatory drugs (NSAIDs)
• Benemid
• Eskalith, Lithobid
• Lanoxin
• Questran (take at least 3 hours before or after Demadex).

dose and take your regular dose as scheduled. Don't take a double dose.

 If you suspect an overdose

Contact your doctor *immediately*. Signs and symptoms of a Demadex overdose may include dizziness, dry skin and mouth, and fluttering in the chest.

Warnings

• Make sure your doctor knows your medical history. You may not be able to take Demadex if you are overly sensitive to this or a similar drug, have liver or kidney disease, or are pregnant or breast-feeding.

• This drug can cause excessive urination and water loss; it's used cautiously in older people and others who are prone to this problem.

• Follow your doctor's recommendations for a high-potassium diet. Foods rich in potassium include citrus fruits, tomatoes, and bananas.

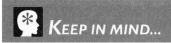 **KEEP IN MIND...**

* Take dose in morning.

* Eat more citrus fruits, tomatoes, bananas, dates, and apricots.

* Report muscle weakness or cramps.

Demerol

Demerol is a narcotic that's used to relieve pain. It works by changing how the brain perceives and responds to pain.

Why it's prescribed

Doctors prescribe Demerol to treat moderate to severe pain. It comes in tablets and a banana-flavored syrup. Doctors usually prescribe the following amounts for adults; children's dosages appear in parentheses.

▶ **For moderate to severe pain,** 50 to 150 milligrams (mg) every 3 to 4 hours, as needed. (Children: 1.1 to 1.76 mg for each 2.2 pounds of body weight every 3 to 4 hours. Maximum dosage is 100 mg every 4 hours, as needed.)

How to take Demerol

• Take Demerol only as your doctor directs.
• Take Demerol syrup with a full glass (8 ounces) of water to avoid mouth and throat numbness.
• Demerol begins to take effect about 15 minutes after an oral dose. Effects last 2 to 4 hours.
• After taking Demerol regularly for several weeks or more, don't stop taking it suddenly because this could cause side effects from withdrawal. Check with your doctor for instructions on stopping the drug gradually.
• Don't share Demerol with others who may need pain relief.

If you miss a dose

Take the missed dose as soon as possible. However, if it's almost time for your next dose, skip the missed dose and take your regular dose as scheduled. Don't take a double dose.

SIDE EFFECTS

Call your doctor if you have any of these possible drug side effects. Call *immediately* about any labeled "serious."

Serious: seizures, (with high doses) slow or troubled breathing, persistent nausea or vomiting, low blood pressure (weakness, dizziness), irregular heartbeat

Common: light-headedness, sweating, sleepiness or drowsiness, clouded senses, unreasonable feeling of well-being, nausea, vomiting, constipation, inability to urinate, muscle twitching
Tips: Avoid driving and other hazardous activities that require mental alertness until you're familiar with Demerol's effects on you. For constipation, your doctor may recommend a laxative or stool softener.

Other: unreasonable excitement, tremor, dizziness, diarrhea, hallucinations, vision difficulties, dry mouth, flushing of face, itching, rash
Tip: To relieve dry mouth, try sucking on sugarless candy or ice chips or chewing sugarless gum.

DRUG INTERACTIONS

Combining certain drugs may alter their action or produce unwanted side effects. Tell your doctor about other drugs you're taking, especially:
• alcohol and other drugs that slow down the central nervous system, such as sleeping pills, sedatives, some antihistamines, general anesthetics, hypnotics, other narcotic pain relievers (morphine), and phenothiazines (Thorazine)
  • aminophylline
  • antidepressants called MAO inhibitors, such as Parnate, and tricyclic antidepressants such as Elavil
  • Dilantin
  • heparin
  • methicillin
  • sodium bicarbonate (baking soda)
  • sulfonamides (Bactrim).

If you suspect an overdose

Contact your doctor *immediately*. Signs of overdose include cold clammy skin, confusion, seizures, severe dizziness or drowsiness, low blood pressure, nervousness or restlessness, pinpoint pupils, slow heartbeat, slow or troubled breathing, and severe weakness.

Warnings

• Make sure your doctor knows your medical history. You may not be able to take Demerol if you are

DEMEROL'S OTHER NAME

Demerol's generic name is meperidine hydrochloride.

overly sensitive to this or other drugs or have received drugs called MAO inhibitors, such as Parnate, within the past 14 days. Make sure the doctor knows if you have a head injury or other condition that causes extra pressure on the brain, asthma or another breathing problem, irregular heartbeat, glaucoma, seizures, abdominal problems, liver or kidney disease, underactive thyroid, Addison's disease, narrowing of the urethra, prostate problems, a drug abuse problem, or an addiction.

• Demerol may be used by some patients who are allergic to morphine.

• If you're pregnant or breast-feeding, check with your doctor before taking Demerol.

• Demerol should not be given to infants under age 6 months.

• Be aware that children and older adults are especially prone to Demerol's side effects.

• Demerol is not recommended for chronic pain because it accumulates in the body with long-term use and often becomes toxic, especially in patients with poor kidney function.

• When taking Demerol after surgery, follow instructions for turning, coughing, and deep breathing to prevent collapsed lung.

• Demerol should not be given to infants under age 6 months.

• Your doctor may want to alternate Demerol with a nonnarcotic pain reliever, such as aspirin, Tylenol, or Motrin. Doing this may improve your pain control while lowering the dose of narcotic.

• Be aware that Demerol can cause drug dependence and has the potential for abuse.

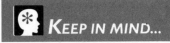

KEEP IN MIND...

* Never take a double dose.

* Take syrup with full glass of water to avoid numbness.

* Not recommended for chronic pain; can be toxic.

* Don't stop taking suddenly; may be fatal.

Demulen

Demulen is a birth control pill. It prevents pregnancy by intefering with ovulation, stopping sperm movement, and preventing fertilized eggs from attaching in the uterus.

Why it's prescribed

Doctors prescribe Demulen to prevent pregnancy. It comes in tablets. Doctors usually prescribe the following amounts for adults.

▶ **For contraception,** one-phase pills: 1 tablet once a day, beginning on day 5 of menstrual cycle (1st day of menstrual flow is day 1). With 20- and 21-tablet packages, new dosing cycle begins 7 days after last tablet is taken. With 28-tablet packages, dosage is 1 tablet a day without interruption. Two-phase pills: 1 color tablet each day for 10 days; then next color tablet for 11 days. Three-phase pills: 1 tablet each day as specified by the brand.

How to take Demulen

• Take Demulen only as your doctor directs.
• Take tablets at the same time each day; take at night to avoid nausea and headaches.
• Use an additional method of birth control, such as condoms or a diaphragm with spermicide, for the first week of birth-control pill use, as directed.

SIDE EFFECTS

Call your doctor if you have any of these possible drug side effects. Call *immediately* about any labeled "serious."

Serious: blood clots (numbness, stiffness, or pain in legs or buttocks; chest pain), severe skin reaction, high blood pressure (headache, blurred vision)

Common: headache, dizziness, nausea, vomiting, diarrhea, breast tenderness, breakthrough bleeding
Tip: These side effects are common at first; they should diminish after 3 to 6 months.

Other: depression, lethargy, migraine, bloating, swelling, visual disturbances (blind spots, blurriness, or flashing lights), worsening vision, intolerance of contact lenses, vomiting, diarrhea, constipation, weight loss or gain, cervical secretions, vaginal yeast infection, menstrual changes, rash, acne, oily skin, darkening skin color, breast changes, change in blood sugar level (weakness; increased thirst, hunger, and urination), sex drive change, abdominal cramps, bloating, pain or discomfort, skin sensitivity to sunlight
Tips: Immediately report to the doctor abdominal pain; numbness, stiffness, or pain in the legs. Weigh yourself at least twice a week during treatment, and report any sudden weight gain. Avoid ultraviolet light or prolonged exposure to sunlight.

DRUG INTERACTIONS

Combining certain drugs may alter their action or produce unwanted side effects. Tell your doctor about other drugs you're taking, especially:
• corticosteroids such as Decadron
• Dantrium and other drugs that may harm the liver
• Nolvadex, Parlodel, Sandimmune
• oral anticoagulants (blood thinners) such as Coumadin
• Rifadin, Solfoton, Tegretol
• tobacco.

DEMULEN'S OTHER NAMES

The generic name for Demulen is ethinyl estradiol and desogestrel. Other brand names of the one-phase form are Desogen and Ortho-Cept.

If you miss a dose

Missed doses in midcycle greatly increase the chance of pregnancy. Adjust your schedule as follows:
• If you miss 1 tablet, take it as soon as you remember or take 2 tablets the next day; then continue your regular schedule.

• If you miss 2 consecutive days, take 2 tablets a day for 2 days; then resume your normal schedule. Use an additional method of birth control for 7 days.
• If you miss 3 or more days, discard the remaining tablets in the

monthly package and use a different birth control method.

If your next menstrual period doesn't begin on time, check with your doctor to rule out pregnancy before starting a new dosing cycle. If your menstrual period begins, start a new dosing cycle 7 days after you took the last tablet.

If you suspect an overdose

Consult your doctor.

Warnings

• Make sure your doctor knows your medical history. You may not be able to take Demulen if you have a blood clotting disorder, blood vessel or heart disease, blood clots in eyes (double vision), migraine headaches, seizures, asthma, known or suspected breast cancer or other cancer, kidney or liver disease, vaginal bleeding, or a history of jaundice with pregnancy or earlier use of birth control pills.
• Stop taking the pills and call your doctor if you think you may be pregnant; don't take them if you're breast-feeding.

• Birth control pills may help protect you from cancer of the ovaries or uterus, and they don't appear to increase the risk of breast cancer. However, they may increase the risk of cervical cancer.
• The hormones in birth control pills may affect treatment for diabetes. Follow your doctor's directions.
• The three-phase form of Demulen may cause fewer side effects, such as breakthrough bleeding and spotting.
• Examine breasts monthly as directed.
• Stop taking birth control pills at least 1 week before surgery to decrease risk of blood clots. Use another method of birth control at this time as your doctor directs.
• Check with your doctor about how soon you may attempt pregnancy after stopping hormonal birth control. Many doctors recommend that women not become pregnant within 2 months after stopping drug; pregnancy may be hard to achieve soon after drug is discontinued.
• If you're on prolonged therapy (5 years or longer), your doctor may advise you to stop using Demulen and use other birth control methods.

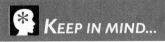

* Take at same time each day.
* Many side effects go away after 3 to 6 months.
* Stop taking pills and call doctor if you think you may be pregnant.
* Avoid ultraviolet light and bright sunlight.
* Examine breasts monthly.

Depakene is an anticonvulsant — a drug that's used to control seizures in disorders such as epilepsy. Depakene works by regulating nerve impulses in the brain.

Why it's prescribed

Doctors prescribe Depakene to help control seizures. It comes in capsules and syrup. Doctors usually prescribe the following amounts for adults and children.

▶ **For seizures,** at first, 15 milligrams (mg) for each 2.2 pounds (lb) of body weight daily, increased every week by 5 to 10 mg for each 2.2 lb daily, up to maximum of 60 mg for each 2.2 lb daily.

How to take Depakene

• Take Depakene only as your doctor directs.
• Swallow capsules whole, without breaking or chewing them, to avoid irritating the mouth.
• To avoid upset stomach, take Depakene with food or water; don't take it with milk.
• Mix the syrup with food or a beverage.
• Don't stop taking Depakene abruptly; seizures could result.

If you miss a dose

Take the missed dose as soon as possible. But if you don't remember until the next day, skip the missed dose and take your next dose as scheduled. Don't take a double dose.

DEPAKENE'S OTHER NAME

Depakene's generic names are valproic acid (capsules) and sodium valproate (syrup).

 SIDE EFFECTS

Call your doctor if you have any of these possible drug side effects. Call *immediately* about any labeled "serious."

Serious: unusual bleeding or bruising, extreme drowsiness or weakness, yellow-tinged eyes or skin, trembling, fever, inflammation of pancreas (abdominal pain, nausea, vomiting)

Common: sleepiness, nausea, vomiting, indigestion, diarrhea, abdominal cramps

Tip: Avoid driving and other activities that require mental alertness until you know how Depakene affects you.

Other: emotional upset, depression, strange behavior, hyperactivity, muscle weakness, tremor, constipation, appetite change, weight gain or loss, hair loss

 DRUG INTERACTIONS

Combining certain drugs may alter their action or produce unwanted side effects. Tell your doctor about other drugs you're taking, especially:
• alcohol
• antacids, aspirin, Tagamet
• anticoagulants (blood thinners) such as Coumadin
• birth control pills or estrogen supplements
• blood pressure drugs such as Aldomet
• other seizure drugs such as Dilantin.

If you suspect an overdose

Contact your doctor *immediately*. Excessive Depakene can cause difficulty breathing and deep coma.

 Warnings

• Make sure your doctor knows your medical history. You may not be able to take Depakene if you're overly sensitive to it or you have any liver problems.
• If you're pregnant or breast-feeding, don't take this drug until you talk with your doctor.
• People at high risk for developing liver problems while taking this drug are those with metabolic or psychological disorders, those who are taking more than one seizure drug, and children under age 2.
• Don't take the syrup if you're on a low-salt diet.
• If tremors occur, your doctor may reduce your dosage.

KEEP IN MIND...

∗ Take with food or water, not with milk.
∗ Don't take syrup if on low-salt diet.
∗ Don't stop taking suddenly.

Depakote

Depakote is an anticonvulsant — a drug that's used to control seizures in disorders such as epilepsy. It's thought to increase nerve impulses in the central nervous system.

Why it's prescribed

Doctors prescribe Depakote to help control seizures. It comes in enteric-coated tablets and in capsules. Doctors usually prescribe the following amounts for adults and children.

▶ **For seizures,** at first, 15 milligrams (mg) for each 2.2 pounds (lb) of body weight once a day, increased by 5 to 10 mg for each 2.2 lb a day at weekly intervals, up to maximum of 60 mg for each 2.2 lb a day.

How to take Depakote

• Take Depakote only as your doctor directs.
• Swallow tablets or capsules whole, without breaking or chewing them, to avoid irritating the mouth and throat.
• To avoid upset stomach, take Depakote with food or water; don't take it with milk.
• Don't stop taking Depakote abruptly; seizures could result.

If you miss a dose

Take the missed dose as soon as possible. But if you don't remember until the next day, skip the missed dose and take your next dose as scheduled. Don't take a double dose.

DEPAKOTE'S OTHER NAME

Depakote's generic name is divalproex sodium.

 SIDE EFFECTS

Call your doctor if you have any of these possible drug side effects. Call *immediately* about any labeled "serious."

Serious: inflamed pancreas (abdominal pain, nausea, vomiting), liver toxicity (unusual bleeding or bruising, extreme drowsiness or weakness, appetite loss, vomiting, yellow-tinged eyes and skin, trembling, fever)

Common: sleepiness, nausea, indigestion
Tip: Avoid driving and other activities that require mental alertness until you know how Depakote affects you.

Other: emotional upset, depression, strange behavior, hyperactivity, muscle weakness, tremor, diarrhea, abdominal cramps, constipation, appetite change, weight gain or loss, hair loss

 DRUG INTERACTIONS

Combining certain drugs may alter their action or produce unwanted side effects. Tell your doctor about other drugs you're taking, especially:
• alcohol
• antacids, aspirin, Tagamet, Thorazine
• anticoagulants (blood thinners) such as Coumadin
• birth control pills and estrogen supplements
• blood pressure drugs such as Aldomet
• other seizure drugs such as Dilantin.

 If you suspect an overdose

Contact your doctor *immediately*. Excessive Depakote can cause seizures and difficulty breathing.

Warnings

• Make sure your doctor knows your medical history. You may not be able to take Depakote if you're overly sensitive to it or you have any liver problems.
• If you're pregnant or breast-feeding, don't take this drug until you talk with your doctor.

• People at high risk for developing liver problems while taking this drug are those with metabolic or psychological disorders, those who are taking more than one seizure drug, and children under age 2.
• If tremors occur, your doctor may reduce your dosage.

 KEEP IN MIND...

∗ Swallow tablets or capsules whole.

∗ Take with food or water, not with milk.

∗ Don't stop taking suddenly.

DES

DES is used to replace estrogen, a female hormone that regulates sexual development and the menstrual cycle in women. DES helps to relieve postmenopausal symptoms, such as as hot flashes, sweating, chills, faintness, and dizziness. DES also affects cells and other hormones in the body to help fight certain cancers.

Why it's prescribed

Doctors prescribe DES to provide additional estrogen when needed (as in menopause) and to treat symptoms of prostate cancer in men and breast cancer in men and postmenopausal women. DES comes in tablets and enteric-coated tablets. It's also available in an injectable form. Doctors usually prescribe the following amounts for adults.

▶ **For prostate cancer,** at first, 1 to 3 milligrams (mg) orally once a day; may be reduced to 1 mg a day. Then increased up to 200 mg or more as needed three times a day.

▶ **For advanced breast cancer in men and postmenopausal women,** 15 mg orally once a day.

How to take DES

• Take DES only as your doctor directs.

• Take it with or right after meals to avoid stomach upset.

• Don't crush, break, or chew enteric-coated tablets, which are

SIDE EFFECTS

Call your doctor if you have any of these possible drug side effects. Call *immediately* about any labeled "serious."

Serious: stroke, heart attack (chest or arm pain); blood clots (shortness of breath; abdominal pain; pain, numbness, or stiffness in arms, legs, or buttocks; pressure or pain in chest), vaginal bleeding or discharge, breast lumps, yellow-tinged eyes and skin, dark urine, light-colored stools; severe headache; visual disturbances, such as blind spots, flashing lights, or blurriness; sudden weight gain; swelling of hands or feet

Common: nausea, diarrhea, headache, dizziness, tiredness
Tips: Take DES with meals to reduce nausea. Be aware of how DES affects you before driving or operating machinery.

Other: high blood pressure (headache, blurred vision), decreased urination, vomiting, bloating, constipation, excessive thirst, weight changes, appetite changes, inflamed pancreas (nausea, vomiting, abdominal pain), loss of sex drive, hives, skin changes, hairiness or hair loss; (in men) breast enlargement, testicular wasting, impotence; (in women) menstrual irregularities, breast tenderness or enlargement
Tip: To avoid constipation, increase fluids and high-fiber foods in your diet.

DRUG INTERACTIONS

Combining certain drugs may alter their action or produce unwanted side effects. Tell your doctor about other drugs you're taking, especially:

• corticosteroids such as Decadron
• Nolvadex
• oral anticoagulants (blood thinners) such as Coumadin
• Parlodel
• Rifadin, Solfoton, Tegretol
• Sandimmune.

meant to dissolve only after reaching the intestine.

If you miss a dose

Take the missed dose as soon as possible. However, if it's almost time for your next dose, skip the missed dose and go back to your regular schedule. Don't take a double dose.

 ## If you suspect an overdose

Contact your doctor *immediately.* Excessive DES can cause nausea, vomiting, abdominal cramps, diarrhea, and weight loss.

DES's OTHER NAMES

DES's generic name is diethylstilbestrol (also known as stilboestrol). A Canadian brand name is Honvol.

Warnings

• Make sure your doctor knows your medical history. You may not be able to take DES if you have depression, bone disease, migraines, seizures, diabetes, artery disease, or heart, liver, or kidney problems.

• DES is not recommended for people with blood-clotting problems, estrogen-dependent tumors, or undiagnosed abnormal genital bleeding or for men with breast cancer (except when cancer has spread).

• DES is not recommended during pregnancy. Drastic genital changes may occur in children of women taking this drug during pregnancy. Female children have a higher-than-normal risk of developing cervical and vaginal cancer. Male children may be more prone to testicular tumors or cysts and infertility.

• If you have diabetes, be aware that DES may raise your blood sugar levels. Tell your doctor if you notice a change in your test results so your diabetes drug dosage can be adjusted.

• Be sure to have a thorough physical exam before beginning long-term DES treatment and yearly checkups thereafter.

• To help prevent blood clots, stop taking DES at least one month before prolonged immobilization — such as after knee or hip surgery — which can cause a clotting problem.

• Perform breast self-examination monthly, as your doctor directs.

• Don't share DES with anyone else; this may be dangerous for the other person whose health and body composition are different from yours.

• Notify your doctor if your menopausal symptoms (such as hot flashes, sweating, chills, faintness, and dizziness) don't improve.

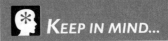

KEEP IN MIND...

* Don't take during pregnancy.

* Take with or right after meals.

* Swallow enteric-coated tablets whole.

* Don't share DES.

* Perform monthly breast self-exams.

Desenex

Desenex is used to fight fungal infections that affect the skin. It works by killing the fungus.

Why it's used

Desenex is used to treat various fungal infections of the skin, such as athlete's foot. You can buy it without a prescription. Desenex comes in cream, ointment, aerosol, and powder. The following amounts are usually recommended.

▶ **For athlete's foot and similar fungal infections,** apply twice a day to thoroughly clean skin. Treat infection in crotch area for 2 weeks; treat athlete's foot or fungal infection of smooth skin for 4 weeks.

How to use Desenex

• Use Desenex only as your doctor and the package label direct. Aerosols are best for hairy areas; powders for moist areas such as skin folds. Ointment or cream should be used at night; powder may be used during the day.

• Apply cream generously to affected area and surrounding skin; rub in well.

• Don't use cream on pus-covered sores or badly broken skin. Don't apply it around or in your eyes, mouth, or nose.

DESENEX'S OTHER NAMES

Desenex is a combination of undecylenic acid and zinc undecylenate. Other brand names include Cruex and Quinsana Plus.

SIDE EFFECTS

Call your doctor if you have any of these possible drug side effects.

Serious: none reported

Common: none reported

Other: skin irritation

DRUG INTERACTIONS

Combining certain drugs may alter their action or produce unwanted side effects. Tell your doctor about other drugs you're taking.

• Sprinkle powder on the feet, between toes, and in socks and shoes to control athlete's foot.

• Store powder form away from warm or damp places.

• Use Desenex for the entire recommended treatment period, even if your condition seems to improve. To keep your infection from coming back, continue using Desenex for 2 more weeks after burning, itching, and other symptoms subside.

If you miss a dose

Apply the missed dose as soon as possible. Then go back to your regular schedule. Don't apply a double dose.

 If you suspect an overdose

Consult your doctor.

 Warnings

• Desenex is not recommended for people who are overly sensitive to this drug. Consult your doctor if you think you may be.

• Don't use Desenex on children under age 2 unless your doctor directs.

• Don't use Desenex to treat fungal infections of the nails.

• If your skin problem doesn't improve within 4 weeks or becomes worse, check with your doctor.

• To help prevent reinfection after treatment ends, use powder form of drug each day after bathing and careful drying.

KEEP IN MIND...

* Use powder on skin folds and other moist areas.

* Don't use cream on badly broken skin.

* Store powder away from warm, damp places.

* Complete entire treatment.

* Continue using Desenex for 2 weeks after symptoms subside.

Desoxyn

Desoxyn helps increase attention span and decrease restlessness.

Why it's prescribed

Doctors prescribe Desoxyn to treat attention deficit hyperactivity disorder (ADHD) in children and for short-term use as a diet aid for obese adults. It comes in tablets and sustained-release tablets. Doctors usually prescribe the following amounts.

▶ **For ADHD in children age 6 and older,** 2.5 to 5 milligrams (mg) once or twice a day, increased by 5 mg a week, as needed.

▶ **For obesity,** 2.5 to 5 mg two or three times a day, 30 minutes before meals; or 10 to 15 mg of sustained-release tablets once a day.

How to take Desoxyn

• Take Desoxyn only as directed. Effects last for up to 24 hours.
• Don't crush sustained-release tablets; swallow them whole.

If you miss a dose

Don't take a double dose. Adjust your schedule as follows:
• If you take one dose a day, take the missed dose as soon as possible, but not less than 6 hours before bedtime to avoid trouble sleeping. If you don't remember the missed dose until the next day, skip it and go back to your regular schedule.
• If you take two or three doses a day and you remember an hour or so after the missed dose, take the dose right away. If you don't remember until later, skip it and go back to your regular schedule.

DESOXYN'S OTHER NAME

Desoxyn's generic name is methamphetamine hydrochloride.

 SIDE EFFECTS

Call your doctor if you have any of these possible drug side effects. Call *immediately* about any labeled "serious."

Serious: racing, irregular, or pounding heartbeat

Common: nervousness, insomnia, talkativeness
Tip: To avoid insomnia, take Desoxyn in the morning or at least 6 hours before bedtime.

Other: irritability, overexcitability, tremor, high blood pressure (headache, blurred vision), low blood pressure (dizziness, weakness), large pupils, dry mouth, metallic taste, nausea, vomiting, abdominal cramps, diarrhea, constipation, appetite and weight loss, impotence, hives, changed sex drive
Tips: Avoid activities that require alertness or good coordination until you know how you react to this drug. To relieve dry mouth, use sugarless candy or gum or ice chips.

 DRUG INTERACTIONS

Combining certain drugs may alter their action or produce unwanted side effects. Tell your doctor about other drugs you're taking, especially:
• ammonium chloride, vitamin C
• antacids, Diamox, sodium bicarbonate
• caffeine
• Haldol
• insulin and oral diabetes drugs
• MAO inhibitors such as Parnate (don't use within 14 days before or after Desoxyn)
• phenothiazines, such as Phenergan and Thorazine
• tricyclic antidepressants, such as Elavil and Pamelor.

 If you suspect an overdose

Contact your doctor *immediately*. Excessive Desoxyn can cause fatigue, confusion, aggressiveness, nausea, vomiting, and diarrhea.

Warnings

• Make sure your doctor knows your medical history. You may not be able to take Desoxyn if you have high blood pressure, an overactive thyroid, heart or lung disease, glaucoma, drug allergies, or a history of drug abuse or if you're pregnant or breast-feeding.
• If you're diabetic, monitor your blood sugar levels carefully.

 KEEP IN MIND...

∗ Take at least 6 hours before bedtime.
∗ Swallow tablets whole.
∗ Don't take a double dose.

Desyrel

Desyrel relieves depression and anxiety by inhibiting serotonin, a chemical that's important for sleep and sensory perception.

Why it's prescribed

Doctors prescribe Desyrel to treat depression and anxiety. It comes in tablets. Doctors usually prescribe the following amounts for adults.

▶ **For depression,** initially, 150 milligrams (mg) a day divided into equal doses, increased by 50 mg a day every 3 to 4 days as needed. Average dosage is 150 to 400 mg a day. Maximum daily dosage is 600 mg.

How to take Desyrel

• Take Desyrel only as your doctor directs.
• Desyrel may not take effect for 2 to 4 weeks; don't take more than your doctor has prescribed.
• Take Desyrel after a meal or light snack. This will help your body absorb the drug and will reduce your risk of dizziness or upset stomach.
• Don't stop taking Desyrel without first talking with your doctor.

If you miss a dose

Take the missed dose as soon as possible. However, if it's less than 4 hours until your next dose, skip the missed dose and take your next dose on schedule. Don't take a double dose.

DESYREL'S OTHER NAMES

Desyrel's generic name is trazodone hydrochloride. Other brand names are Trazon and Trialodine.

 ## SIDE EFFECTS

Call your doctor if you have any of these possible drug side effects. Call *immediately* about any labeled "serious."

Serious: irregular heartbeat, heart attack (arm or chest pain), congestive heart failure (shortness of breath), stroke (weakness, slurred speech), painful erection (possibly leading to impotence)
Tip: Stop taking this drug and call your doctor at once if you develop a painful, inappropriate erection; this condition may require surgery.

Common: drowsiness, dizziness
Tip: Avoid driving and other activities that require alertness and coordination until you know how Desyrel affects you; drowsiness and dizziness usually subside after the first few weeks.

Other: nervousness, fatigue, confusion, tremors, weakness, anger, vivid dreams, light-headedness on standing, fast or slow heartbeat, blurred vision, ringing in ears, dry mouth, distorted sense of taste, constipation, nausea, vomiting, appetite and weight loss, urine retention, rash, hives, profuse sweating

 ## DRUG INTERACTIONS

Combining certain drugs may alter their action or produce unwanted side effects. Tell your doctor about other drugs you're taking, especially:
• alcohol and other drugs that slow down the central nervous system, such as drugs for colds or allergies, sleeping pills, narcotic pain relievers, muscle relaxants, and certain anesthetics
• antidepressants
• blood pressure drugs such as Catapres
• Digoxin
• Dilantin.

 ### If you suspect an overdose

Contact your doctor *immediately*. Symptoms of overdose include drowsiness, loss of muscle coordination, nausea, and vomiting.

 ### Warnings

• Make sure your doctor knows your medical history. You may not be able to take Desyrel if you are overly sensitive to this drug; have suicidal thoughts or heart, liver, or kidney disease; or are recovering from a heart attack.
• If you're pregnant or breast-feeding, don't take Desyrel until you talk with your doctor.

 ### KEEP IN MIND...

∗ Take after a meal or snack.
∗ Don't stop taking abruptly.
∗ Don't take when pregnant or breast-feeding.

Dexedrine

Dexedrine is an amphetamine and one of a group of drugs called central nervous system stimulants. These drugs are used to treat attention deficit hyperactivity disorder (ADHD) and certain other disorders. Dexedrine helps improve attention span and decrease restlessness in people who are overactive, easily distracted, and emotionally unstable. It appears to have a calming effect for unknown reasons. Dexedrine is given as part of a program that includes medical, social, educational, and psychological treatments.

Why it's prescribed

Doctors prescribe Dexedrine to treat ADHD and narcolepsy (a sleeping disorder) and for short-term treatment of some types of obesity. Dexedrine comes in tablets and sustained-release capsules. Doctors usually prescribe the following amounts for adults; children's dosages appear in parentheses, except for ADHD.

▶ **For ADHD,** children age 6 and older: 5 milligrams (mg) once or twice a day, increased by 5 mg a week, as needed. Rarely, dosage may exceed a total of 40 mg a day. Children ages 3 to 5: 2.5 mg a day, increased by 2.5 mg a week, as needed.

DEXEDRINE'S OTHER NAMES

Dexedrine's generic name is dextroamphetamine sulfate. Other brand names include Dexedrine Spansule, Oxydess II, Robese, and Spancap 1.

SIDE EFFECTS

Call your doctor if you have any of these possible drug side effects.

Serious: none reported

Common: restlessness, sleeplessness, racing or pounding heartbeat
Tip: Take at least 6 hours before bedtime to avoid sleeplessness at night.

Other: tremor, dizziness, headache, chills, overstimulation, depression, high blood pressure (headache, blurred vision), dry mouth, unpleasant taste, diarrhea, constipation, appetite and weight loss, hives, low sex drive, impotence
Tips: Avoid driving and other activities that require alertness or coordination until you're familiar with the drug's side effects. Use sugarless gum or candy and perform frequent mouth care to relieve dry mouth and unpleasant taste.

DRUG AND FOOD INTERACTIONS

Combining certain drugs and foods may alter drug action or produce unwanted side effects. Tell your doctor about your diet and other drugs you're taking, especially:
- adrenergic blockers such as Lopressor
- ammonium chloride, fruit juices, vitamin C
- antacids, citrate, Diamox, sodium bicarbonate
- antihistamines
- antipsychotics such as Thorazine
- caffeine
- Dilantin, Solfoton
- insulin and oral diabetes drugs
- MAO inhibitors such as Marplan (don't use within 14 days before or after Dexedrine)
- tricyclic antidepressants such as Elavil.

▶ **For narcolepsy,** 5 to 60 mg a day, divided into equal doses. (Children: 5 to 10 mg a day, increased by 5 to 10 mg per week, as needed.

▶ **For obesity,** 5 to 30 mg a day, divided into equal doses of 5 to 10 mg. Or, one 10- or 15-mg sustained-release capsule a day. (Children over age 12: same as adults.)

How to take Dexedrine

- Take Dexedrine only as your doctor directs.
- Take it at least 6 hours before bedtime to avoid sleep interference.
- For obesity, take Dexedrine tablets 30 to 60 minutes before meals; take sustained-release capsules as a single dose in the morning.

Continued on next page ▶

• For children age 12 and older taking Dexedrine for narcolepsy, give the first dose when the child wakes up and additional doses at intervals of 4 to 6 hours.

If you miss a dose

Don't take a double dose. Adjust your schedule as follows:

• If you take one dose a day, take the missed dose as soon as possible, but not less than 6 hours before bedtime to avoid trouble sleeping. If you don't remember the missed dose until the next day, skip it and go back to your regular schedule.

• If you usually take two or three doses a day and you remember within an hour or so of the missed dose, take the dose right away. However, if you don't remember until later, skip it and go back to your regular schedule.

If you suspect an overdose

Contact your doctor *immediately*. Signs and symptoms of Dexedrine overdose may include tremor, confusion, fatigue, vomiting, diarrhea, and palpitations.

Warnings

• Make sure your doctor knows your medical history. You may not be able to take Dexedrine if you're overly sensitive to this or similar drugs; if you've been treated with an MAO inhibitor (a type of antidepressant) in the last 2 weeks; or if you have an overactive thyroid, moderate to severe high blood pressure, hardening of the arteries or other heart or blood vessel disease, glaucoma, motion and vocal tics, Tourette syndrome, or a history of drug abuse.

• This drug is used cautiously in people who are agitated.

• Before you start taking Dexedrine, tell your doctor if you're pregnant or breast-feeding.

• Dexedrine isn't recommended as a primary treatment for obesity. Be aware that some states prohibit its use as a weight-loss aid.

• If you develop a tolerance to Dexedrine's appetite-suppressant effects, call your doctor.

• Fatigue may result as the drug's effects wear off. Don't take more Dexedrine to prevent fatigue; instead, get more rest.

KEEP IN MIND...

* Take at least 6 hours before bedtime.

* For obesity, take 30 to 60 minutes before meals.

* Avoid caffeine.

D.H.E. 45

D.H.E. 45 is used to treat and prevent severe, throbbing headaches, such as migraine and cluster headaches. The drug works by constricting blood vessels that carry blood to the head, thus reducing throbbing.

Why it's prescribed

Doctors prescribe D.H.E. 45 for severe, throbbing headaches only; it has no effect on other types of pain. This drug is available only in an injectable form. Doctors usually prescribe the following amounts for adults.

▶ **For migraine headache,** 1 milligram (mg) injected every 1 to 2 hours, as needed, up to a total of 3 mg per attack. Maximum weekly dosage is 6 mg.

How to take D.H.E. 45

• Take D.H.E. 45 only as your doctor directs.
• D.H.E. 45 works best when used at the first sign of a migraine; lie down and relax in a quiet, darkened room after receiving the injection.
• The drug begins to take effect within 15 to 30 minutes.

If you miss a dose

Consult your doctor.

 If you suspect an overdose

Call your doctor *immediately*. Signs of overdose include seizures, diar-

D.H.E. 45'S OTHER NAMES

D.H.E. 45's generic name is dihydroergotamine mesylate. A Canadian brand name is Dihydroergotamine-Sandoz.

 SIDE EFFECTS

Call your doctor if you have any of these possible drug side effects. Call *immediately* about any labeled "serious."

Serious: high blood pressure (headache, blurred vision), rapid or slow heart rate, chest pain

Common: none reported

Other: dizziness, numbness and tingling in fingers and toes, cold hands or feet, nausea, vomiting, itching, weakness in legs, muscle pain, water retention

Tips: Report coldness in your arms and legs or tingling in your fingers and toes right away. Severe blood vessel constriction can cause tissue damage. Your doctor may give you a blood vessel–dilating drug to counter this effect.

 DRUG INTERACTIONS

Combining certain drugs may alter their action or produce unwanted side effects. Tell your doctor about other drugs you're taking, especially:
• erythromycin
• Inderal and other heart drugs called beta blockers
• insulin.

rhea, nausea, vomiting, stomach pain or bloating, dizziness, drowsiness, weakness, fast or slow heartbeat, severe headache, difficulty in moving bowels, shortness of breath, and excitability.

 Warnings

• Make sure your doctor knows your medical history. You may not be able to take D.H.E. 45 if you're overly sensitive to this or similar drugs or if you have a blood vessel disorder, high blood pressure, an infection, or heart, liver, or kidney dysfunction.
• If you're pregnant or breast-feeding, inform your doctor before using this drug.

• Avoid prolonged use of D.H.E. 45; it may lose its effectiveness or become habit-forming.
• Headaches may get worse when this drug is stopped; if this happens, check with your doctor.
• Examine underlying causes of stress, which may bring on headaches.

 KEEP IN MIND...

* Don't take during pregnancy.
* Use at first sign of migraine.
* Relax in dark, quiet place after injection.
* Report coldness or tingling in arms and legs.
* Avoid prolonged use.

Diabinese

Diabinese is used to treat symptoms of diabetes. It regulates insulin in the body to lower blood sugar levels for people with "sugar" diabetes (diabetes mellitus).

Why it's prescribed

Doctors prescribe Diabinese to treat uncomplicated type II diabetes; the drug relieves symptoms but doesn't cure the disease. Diabinese comes in tablets. Doctors usually prescribe the following amounts for adults; dosages for older adults appears in parentheses.

▶ **To lower blood sugar,** 250 milligrams (mg) once a day, increased by 50 to 125 mg after 5 to 7 days, then every 3 to 5 days, if needed, to a maximum of 750 mg a day. Mild diabetes may respond well to dosages of 100 mg or less a day. (Adults over age 65: at first, 100 to 125 mg each day, increased as described above.)

▶ **To change from insulin to oral treatment,** if insulin dosage is less than 40 units a day, insulin is stopped and Diabinese therapy started as above. If insulin dosage is 40 units or more a day, Diabinese therapy is started as above along with half of normal insulin dosage; insulin dosage reduced further according to person's response.

How to take Diabinese

• Take Diabinese only as your doctor directs. Don't change your dose

DIABINESE'S OTHER NAMES

Diabinese's generic name is chlorpropamide. Other brand names include Glucamide; and, in Canada, Apo-Chlorpropamide and Novopropamide.

SIDE EFFECTS

Call your doctor if you have any of these possible drug side effects. Call *immediately* about any labeled "serious."

Serious: prolonged low blood sugar levels (cool pale skin, difficulty concentrating, shakiness, headache, cold sweats, feelings of anxiety), blood problems (bruising, bleeding, fatigue, fever, chills, increased risk of infection), syndrome of inappropriate antidiuretic hormone caused by increased water retention (decreased urination, confusion, sleepiness). *Tips:* Avoid people who are ill or infected; also avoid strenuous physical activity.

Common: diarrhea, hunger, weight loss

Other: heartburn, nausea, vomiting, tea-colored urine, allergic reaction (rash, itching), facial flushing, skin sensitivity to sunlight, jaundice (yellow-tinged skin and eyes)
Tips: To prevent facial flushing, avoid alcohol and products containing alcohol, even in very small amounts. Limit your exposure to the sun.

DRUG INTERACTIONS

Combining certain drugs may alter their action or produce unwanted side effects. Tell your doctor about other drugs you're taking, especially:
• alcohol
• anabolic steroids and corticosteroids
• anticoagulants (blood thinners) such as Coumadin
• aspirin and aspirin-containing cough, cold, and appetite-control drugs
• blood pressure drugs, such as Catapres, Inderal, and Ismelin
• Chloromycetin
• diuretics (water pills), such as HydroDIURIL and Vaseretic
• MAO inhibitors such as Marplan
• Rifadin
• sulfa drugs such as Bactrim.

or take this drug more often than prescribed without consulting your doctor.
• The drug begins to take effect within 1 hour, and effects last up to 60 hours.
• Take a daily dose with breakfast; if stomach upset occurs, divide the daily amount into two equal doses and take them with your morning and evening meals.

If you miss a dose

Take the missed dose as soon as possible. But if it's within 2 hours of your next dose, skip the missed dose and take the next one on schedule. Don't take a double dose.

If you suspect an overdose

Contact your doctor *immediately*. Signs of overdose include clumsiness or unsteadiness; extreme drowsiness; dry mouth, nose, or throat; fast heartbeat; hallucinations; mood or mental changes; seizures; shortness of breath or trouble breathing; trouble sleeping; and warm, dry, flushed skin.

Warnings

• Make sure your doctor knows your medical history. You may not be able to take Diabinese if you're allergic to this drug or if you have liver or kidney problems or porphyria.

• Diabinese is not recommended for treating type I (insulin-dependent) diabetes, diabetes that can be controlled well by diet, or type II (non-insulin-dependent) diabetes with complications (diabetic coma, major surgery, severe infections, or severe trauma).

• Don't use Diabinese if you're breast-feeding; also, make sure your doctor knows if you're pregnant before taking this drug.

• Be aware that older adults may be especially prone to Diabinese's side effects.

• Don't drink alcoholic beverages while taking Diabinese. Even a small amount can cause facial flushing, dizziness, headache, and slowed breathing.

• If you transfer to Diabinese from another oral drug, usually no transition period is needed. However, some patients require hospitalization during transition from insulin therapy to an oral drug so that they can be monitored frequently.

• For best results, follow your doctor's directions for diet, weight loss, exercise, personal hygiene, and infection prevention; your special diet is the most important part of controlling your diabetes.

• Inform your doctor immediately if you notice decreased urination or bloody urine.

• Make sure you know how to check your blood sugar level and what to do about high and low results; don't change your dosage without your doctor's consent.

• Be aware that side effects, especially low blood sugar levels, may be more frequent or severe than with other drugs because the drug's effects last longer.

• Carry candy or another sugar source that your doctor recommends to treat mild low blood sugar levels. Severe episodes may require hospital treatment. If your blood sugar level drops too low, eat or drink something sugary, such as glucose tablets or fruit juice. If you don't feel better within 15 minutes, eat or drink some more sugary food and call your doctor right away.

• Carry medical identification that lets others know you have diabetes.

 ## KEEP IN MIND...

* Carry candy or other sugary snack to treat mild low blood sugar.

* Follow doctor's orders for diet, weight loss, exercise, hygiene, and infection prevention.

* Don't change drug dosage on your own.

* Avoid alcohol.

* Carry medical identification.

Dialose

Dialose is a laxative that softens stools by drawing liquid into the stools.

Why it's taken

Dialose is taken to prevent constipation. It's especially helpful for people who shouldn't strain during defecation, such as those recovering from heart or rectal surgery or those with constipation after childbirth. You can buy Dialose without a prescription. It comes in capsules, tablets, oral liquid, and syrup. The following amounts are usually recommended for adults and children over age 12; younger children's dosages appear in parentheses.

▶ **To soften stools,** 50 to 500 milligrams (mg) once a day until bowel movements are normal. (Children ages 6 to 12: 40 to 120 mg once a day. Children ages 3 to 6: 20 to 60 mg once a day.

How to take Dialose

• Take Dialose only as your doctor directs. If you bought Dialose without a prescription, read the package directions carefully before taking your first dose.
• Dialose usually begins to take effect within 24 to 72 hours.
• Mix liquid Dialose in milk or fruit juice to mask bitter taste.

DIALOSE'S OTHER NAMES

Dialose's generic name is docusate sodium. Other brand names include Afko-Lube, Colace, Diocto, Dioeze, Diosuccin, Dio-Sul, DOK, Doss, D-S-S, Duosol, Laxinate 100, Modane Soft, Molatoc, Pro-Sof, Regulax SS, Regutol, Stulex, and Therevac.

SIDE EFFECTS

Call your doctor if you have any of these possible drug side effects.

Serious: none reported

Common: mild abdominal cramping
Tip: Stop taking drug and call doctor if cramping becomes severe.

Other: throat irritation, diarrhea, laxative dependence
Tip: Consult your doctor if you can't maintain normal bowel habits without Dialose for 2 weeks.

DRUG INTERACTIONS

Combining certain drugs may alter their action or produce unwanted side effects. Tell your doctor about other drugs you're taking, especially:
• mineral oil
• other oral drugs (take at least 2 hours before or after Dialose).

If you miss a dose

Consult your doctor.

If you suspect an overdose

Consult your doctor.

Warnings

• Make sure your doctor knows your medical history. You may not be able to take Dialose if you're overly sensitive to it. Don't use Dialose if you have an intestinal blockage, fecal impaction, or symptoms of appendicitis or inflamed bowel, such as stomach or lower abdominal pain, cramping, bloating, nausea, or vomiting.
• If you're pregnant, check with your doctor before taking Dialose.
• Before taking for constipation, follow your doctor's advice about getting adequate fluids and exercise; adding high-fiber foods, such as bran and fresh fruit and vegeta-

bles, to your diet; and drinking at least six 8-ounce glasses of water or other liquids a day to help soften stools.
• Use Dialose only occasionally; don't use it for more than 1 week without checking with your doctor. Overuse may make you dependent on laxatives.
• If you notice a sudden change in your bowel habits that lasts longer than 2 weeks or that keeps coming back, check with your doctor to find the cause of your problem before it becomes more serious.

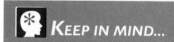

* Drug begins to take effect within 24 to 72 hours.
* Drink plenty of fluids.
* Don't use for more than 1 week.

Diamox

Diamox helps the kidneys excrete water and certain minerals and affects other body functions, such as blood flow and breathing. Diamox also lowers pressure in the eye by decreasing the amount of fluid there.

Why it's prescribed

Doctors prescribe Diamox to help control glaucoma, certain types of seizures, congestive heart failure (heart failure with water retention), and mountain sickness (increased heart and breathing rate, fatigue, headache, nausea). Diamox comes in tablets and extended-release capsules. It also comes in an injectable form. Doctors usually prescribe the following amounts for adults.

▶ **For some types of glaucoma,** 250 milligrams (mg) orally every 4 hours or 250 mg orally twice a day for short-term therapy.

▶ **For congestive heart failure,** 250 to 375 mg orally each day in the morning.

▶ **For some types of chronic glaucoma and before glaucoma surgery,** 250 mg to 1 gram (g) orally each day, divided into equal doses and taken four times a day, or 500 mg extended-release capsules orally twice a day.

▶ **For seizures in adults and children,** 8 to 30 mg for each 2.2 pounds of body weight orally each

 SIDE EFFECTS

Call your doctor if you have any of these possible drug side effects. Call *immediately* about any labeled "serious."

Serious: bloody urine, seizures, aplastic anemia (excessive fatigue, rapid breathing, change in mental status, low white blood cell count), severe allergic reaction (difficulty breathing, facial and throat swelling)
Tips: Check with the doctor as soon as possible if you develop signs of infection, such as a fever or sore throat. Avoid people who are ill or have an infection.

Common: none reported

Other: drowsiness, tingling or other strange sensations, confusion, transient vision change, nausea, vomiting, appetite and weight loss, altered taste, increased thirst and urination, itching
Tip: Avoid driving and other activities that require alertness and coordination until you know how this drug affects you.

 DRUG INTERACTIONS

Combining certain drugs may alter their action or produce unwanted side effects. Tell your doctor about other drugs you're taking, especially:
- amphetamines, such as "speed" and diet pills
- anticholinergics such as atropine sulfate
- aspirin and aspirin-containing products
- Hiprex
- Inversine
- Quinaglute Dura-tabs.

DIAMOX'S OTHER NAMES

Diamox's generic name is acetazolamide. Other brand names include Dazamide; and, in Canada, Acetazolam and Apo-Acetazolamide.

day, divided into equal doses and usually given with other anticonvulsants. Optimum dosage range for adults is 375 mg to 1 g a day.

▶ **For mountain sickness,** 500 to 1,000 mg a day divided into equal doses and taken every 8 to 12 hours, or 500 mg in extended-release capsules twice a day.

How to take Diamox

- Take Diamox only as your doctor directs.
- Take Diamox with food or milk to avoid upset stomach.
- If you have difficulty swallowing tablets, mix a tablet in 2 teaspoons each of hot water and honey or syr-

up. If you have trouble swallowing capsules, call the doctor; the pharmacist may make a suspension of the drug in a flavored syrup.

- To avoid sleep disruption from increased urination, take your dose in the morning with breakfast if you take a single daily dose. If you take it more than once a day, take the last dose no later than 6 p.m. unless the doctor tells you otherwise.
- Take only the amount of drug the doctor ordered. If you think you need more, check with your doctor.

Continued on next page ▶

- If you're taking Diamox to control seizures, don't suddenly stop taking it.
- If you're taking Diamox for mountain sickness, start taking it 24 to 48 hours before ascent and continue taking it for 48 hours while at high altitude.
- Store Diamox at room temperature.

If you miss a dose

Take the missed dose as soon as you remember. But if it's almost time for your next dose, skip the missed dose and take the next dose at the regular time. Don't take a double dose.

If you suspect an overdose

Consult your doctor.

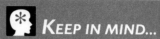 Warnings

- Make sure your doctor knows your medical history. You may not be able to take Diamox if you have Addison's disease, diabetes, gout, or kidney, liver, or lung disease.
- Diamox is not recommended for children, for people who are overly sensitive to it, for those on long-term glaucoma therapy, or for those who have kidney or liver dysfunction, adrenal gland failure, or blood problems.
- If you become pregnant while taking Diamox, notify your doctor.
- Be aware that older adults are prone to excessive water loss with use of Diamox.
- Follow your doctor's advice to follow a high-potassium diet by eating such foods as bananas, potatoes, and orange juice or, if ordered, by taking a potassium supplement. Don't change your diet without checking with your doctor first.

KEEP IN MIND...

* Take with food or milk.
* Take last dose before 6 p.m. to avoid sleep disruption.
* Follow high-potassium diet.
* In seizure treatment, don't stop taking abruptly.
* Report signs of infection, such as fever or sore throat, at once.

Diapid

Diapid is a hormone used to treat diabetes insipidus ("water" diabetes). It helps prevent and control frequent urination, thirst, and water loss.

Why it's prescribed

Doctors prescribe Diapid to treat the symptoms of diabetes insipidus. Diapid comes in a nasal spray. Doctors usually prescribe the following amounts for adults and children.

▶ **For diabetes insipidus,** 1 or 2 sprays in either or both nostrils four times a day and an additional dose at bedtime, if needed, to prevent urination at night. If usual dosage is inadequate, frequency is increased rather than number of sprays.

How to use Diapid

• Use Diapid only as your doctor directs.
• Before using Diapid, gently blow your nose to clear your nasal passages.
• To deliver a uniform, well-diffused spray, hold the bottle and your head upright.
• Use Diapid only on the surface of the nose lining; don't inhale the spray. Inhaling the spray can cause tightness in chest, coughing, and temporary breathing difficulty.
• This drug begins to take effect within 1 hour, and the effects last for 3 to 4 hours.

If you miss a dose

Take the missed dose as soon as possible. However, if it's almost time for your next dose, skip the missed dose and go back to your regular schedule. Don't take a double dose.

DIAPID'S OTHER NAME

Diapid's generic name is lypressin.

SIDE EFFECTS

Call your doctor if you have any of these possible drug side effects. Call *immediately* about any labeled "serious."

Serious: difficulty breathing, swollen face and tongue

Common: headache, dizziness, nasal congestion or ulceration

Other: irritation or itching of nasal passages, runny nose, inflamed eye membranes, heartburn (from excess spray dripping into throat), abdominal cramps, frequent bowel movements

Tip: Ask your doctor about using an antacid or a diarrhea drug if your symptoms become severe.

DRUG INTERACTIONS

Combining certain drugs may alter their action or produce unwanted side effects. Tell your doctor about other drugs you're taking, especially:
• alcohol
• Declomycin
• epinephrine, found in bronchodilators such as Bronkaid
• Eskalith
• heparin.

If you suspect an overdose

Contact your doctor *immediately*. Signs and symptoms of a Diapid overdose include confusion, temporary fluid retention (decreased urination), headache, drowsiness, and weight gain.

Warnings

• Make sure your doctor knows your medical history. You may not be able to use Diapid if you're allergic to this or similar drugs. Diapid should be used cautiously in people with heart or blood vessel disease or high blood pressure.
• Make sure your doctor knows if you are pregnant or breast-feeding before you begin taking Diapid.

• Diapid is especially useful if diabetes insipidus is unresponsive to other treatment or if other diabetes drugs cause side effects.
• Check with your doctor if you have nasal congestion, allergic stuffy or runny nose, or an upper airway infection. These may reduce drug absorption and require larger doses or additional treatment.
• Carry medical identification that tells others about your condition and need for this drug.

 KEEP IN MIND...

∗ Use at bedtime to avoid sleep interruption.

∗ Takes effect within 1 hour; lasts 3 to 4 hours.

∗ Carry medical identification.

Didronel

Didronel stops calcium loss from bones and thus stops bone breakdown.

Why it's prescribed

Doctors prescribe Didronel to treat a bone-weakening disease called Paget's disease and excess calcium in the blood (hypercalcemia). It's also used to prevent abnormal bone growth after hip replacement or spinal surgery. Didronel comes in tablets. It's also available in an injectable form. Doctors usually prescribe the following amounts for adults.

▶ **For Paget's disease,** 5 to 10 milligrams (mg) for each 2.2 pounds (lb) of body weight orally each day, taken for no more than 6 months. Or 11 to 20 mg for each 2.2 lb of body weight orally each day, taken for no more than 3 months. Maximum dosage is 20 mg for each 2.2 lb orally a day.

▶ **For spinal cord injury,** 20 mg for each 2.2 lb of body weight orally once a day for 2 weeks, then 10 mg for each 2.2 lb once a day for 10 weeks.

▶ **For hip replacement surgery,** 20 mg for each 2.2 lb orally once a day for 1 month before total hip replacement and for 3 months afterward.

▶ **For hypercalcemia (cancer-related),** by injection daily for 3 consecutive days, then 20 mg for each 2.2 lb of body weight orally once a day for 30 days. Maximum treatment time is 90 days.

DIDRONEL'S OTHER NAME

Didronel's generic name is etidronate disodium.

SIDE EFFECTS

Call your doctor if you have any of these possible drug side effects.

Serious: none reported

Common: tiredness, muscle spasm

Other: (at high dosages) diarrhea, frequent bowel movements, nausea, bone pain, other pain, increased risk of fracture (especially of thigh bone)

Tip: Ask your doctor about taking a drug for diarrhea if this problem becomes severe.

DRUG INTERACTIONS

Combining certain drugs may alter their action or produce unwanted side effects. Tell your doctor about other drugs you're taking, especially:

• antacids, minerals, vitamins (take 2 hours before or after Didronel).

How to take Didronel

• Take Didronel only as your doctor directs.

• Take it with water or juice 2 hours before a meal. Don't take it with food, milk, or antacids, which may cause poor absorption of the drug.

• Don't eat for 2 hours after taking a dose.

If you miss a dose

Take the missed dose as soon as possible. However, if it's almost time for your next dose, skip the missed dose and go back to your regular schedule. Don't take a double dose.

 If you suspect an overdose

Contact your doctor *immediately.* Signs and symptoms of Didronel overdose may include diarrhea, nausea, muscle spasm, difficulty swallowing, and palpitations.

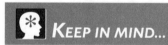 **Warnings**

• Make sure your doctor knows your medical history. You may not be able to take Didronel if you have poor kidney function.

• Tell your doctor if you're pregnant or breast-feeding before you begin taking Didronel.

• Follow your doctor's recommendations for eating a diet that's high in calcium and vitamin D, which are found especially in dairy products.

KEEP IN MIND...

∗ Take with water or juice, not with food, milk, or antacids.

∗ Don't eat for 2 hours after taking.

∗ Increase dairy products in diet.

Diflucan

Diflucan kills two types of infection-causing fungus.

Why it's prescribed

Doctors prescribe Diflucan to treat fungal infections. It comes in tablets and in a powder for mixing with liquids. It's also available in an injectable form. Doctors usually prescribe the following amounts for adults.

▶ **For throat infection,** 1st-day dose of 200 milligrams (mg) orally, followed by 100 mg once a day for at least 2 weeks.

▶ **For infection of esophagus,** 1st-day dose of 200 mg orally, followed by 100 mg once a day. Maximum dosage is 400 mg a day. Treatment continues for at least 3 weeks and for 2 weeks after symptoms resolve.

▶ **For infection throughout body,** 1st-day dose of 400 mg orally, followed by 200 mg once a day. Treatment continues for at least 4 weeks and for 2 weeks after symptoms resolve.

▶ **For meningitis,** 1st-day dose of 400 mg orally, followed by 200 mg once a day. Higher doses may be used. Treatment should continue for 10 to 12 weeks after infection clears.

How to take Diflucan

• Take Diflucan only as your doctor directs.

• To help clear up your infection completely, take Diflucan for the full course of treatment, even if your symptoms improve. A fungal infection may require many months of treatment.

DIFLUCAN'S OTHER NAME

Diflucan's generic name is fluconazole.

 SIDE EFFECTS

Call your doctor if you have any of these possible drug side effects. Call *immediately* about any labeled "serious."

Serious: easy bruising or bleeding, liver toxicity (yellow-tinged skin and eyes), Stevens-Johnson syndrome (red, burnlike rash), fever, sore throat

Common: nausea, headache, dizziness

Tip: Nausea may subside as your body adjusts to Diflucan; check with your doctor if nausea persists or gets worse.

Other: vomiting, abdominal pain, diarrhea, rash

 DRUG INTERACTIONS

Combining certain drugs may alter their action or produce unwanted side effects. Tell your doctor about other drugs you're taking, especially:

• Coumadin
• Depakene, Laniazid
• Dilantin, Sandimmune
• oral diabetes drugs, such as Orinase, Micronase, and Glucotrol
• Rifadin.

If you miss a dose

Take the missed dose as soon as you remember. But if it's almost time for your next dose, skip the missed dose and take your next dose as scheduled. Don't take a double dose.

 If you suspect an overdose

Consult your doctor.

 Warnings

• Make sure your doctor knows your medical history. You may not be able to take Diflucan if you have drug allergies or kidney or liver disease or if you're pregnant or breast-feeding.

• Be aware that people with AIDS are more prone to Diflucan's side effects.

• The safety and effectiveness of this drug in children have not been established.

• Keep appointments for regular follow-up exams; your doctor will monitor your progress and check for unwanted side effects.

• Check with your doctor if your symptoms don't disappear within a few weeks or if you feel worse.

KEEP IN MIND...

* Take full amount prescribed, even if you feel better.

* Side effects more likely in people with AIDS.

* Not usually given to children.

Dilacor XR

Dilacor XR blocks calcium from entering the heart muscle, thereby slowing heart contractions. The drug also widens the heart's blood vessels, allowing more oxygen-carrying blood to reach and nourish the heart.

Why it's prescribed

Doctors prescribe Dilacor XR to relieve and control chest pain (angina), to reduce high blood pressure, and to correct irregular heartbeats. Dilacor XR comes in extended-release capsules. It's also available in an injectable form. Doctors usually prescribe the following amounts for adults.

▶ **For chest pain,** 120 milligrams (mg) orally once a day, increased gradually to maximum of 480 mg a day.

▶ **For high blood pressure,** 180 or 240 mg orally once a day, adjusted as necessary.

How to take Dilacor XR

- Take this drug exactly as your doctor has prescribed.
- Don't crush or chew the capsules; swallow them whole.
- If you've been taking Dilacor XR regularly, don't suddenly stop taking it. Your doctor may want you to reduce your dosage gradually.

If you miss a dose

Take the missed dose as soon as possible. However, if it's almost time

---

DILACOR XR'S OTHER NAMES

Dilacor XR's generic name is diltiazem. Another brand name is Cardizem SR.

 SIDE EFFECTS

Call your doctor if you have any of these possible drug side effects. Call *immediately* about any labeled "serious."

Serious: irregular heartbeat, heart failure (shortness of breath, wheezing)

Common: headache, fatigue, drowsiness, swelling of feet and ankles, nausea, constipation, rash, sudden weight gain (more than 3 pounds in 1 week)
Tip: Weigh yourself each week and record your weight.

Other: dizziness, weakness, nervousness, depression, difficulty sleeping, confusion, flushing, slow pulse, vomiting, diarrhea, excessive or nighttime urination, itching, skin sensitivity to sunlight
Tips: Avoid hazardous activities until you know how this drug affects you. Wear protective clothing and sunscreen outdoors.

 DRUG INTERACTIONS

Combining certain drugs may alter their action or produce unwanted side effects. Tell your doctor about other drugs you're taking, especially:
- beta blockers (for high blood pressure or chest pain)
- Lanoxin
- Sandimmune
- Tagamet.

---

for your next dose, skip the missed dose and take your next dose as scheduled. Don't take a double dose.

 If you suspect an overdose

Contact your doctor *immediately.* Excessive Dilacor XR can cause heart block (shortness of breath) and low blood pressure (fatigue, dizziness, fainting).

 Warnings

- Make sure your doctor knows your medical history. You may not be able to take Dilacor XR if you have other medical problems, especially other heart conditions or a liver or kidney disorder.

- If you're pregnant or breast-feeding, check with your doctor before you start taking this drug.
- Be aware that older adults may be especially prone to Dilacor XR's side effects.

 KEEP IN MIND...

* Swallow capsules whole.
* Keep taking even if no symptoms occur.
* Don't stop drug suddenly.

Dilantin

Dilantin is a seizure drug that works by regulating nerve impulses to the brain.

Why it's prescribed

Doctors prescribe Dilantin to prevent and reduce seizures in epilepsy and other conditions. It may also be used in the treatment of certain nerve and muscle disorders. Dilantin comes in tablets, extended-release capsules, and a liquid suspension. It's also available in an injectable form. Doctors usually prescribe the following amounts for adults; children's dosages appear in parentheses.

▶ **To control seizures,** dosage varies, depending on the individual. At first, 100 milligrams (mg) orally three times a day, increased by 100 mg every 2 to 4 weeks until desired response is obtained. Usual dosage range is 300 to 600 mg a day. Or, if person is stabilized with extended-release capsules, 300 mg extended-release capsule once a day. (Children: 5 mg for each 2.2 pounds (lb) of body weight or 250 mg for each square meter (m2) of body area orally, divided into two or three equal doses a day. Maximum daily dosage is 300 mg.)

▶ **For epilepsy,** first dose by injection, followed by regular doses of 100 mg orally or by injection every 6 to 8 hours. (Children: first dose by injection followed by regular doses based on child's needs.)

DILANTIN'S OTHER NAMES

Dilantin's generic name is phenytoin. The generic name for Dilantin extended-release capsules is phenytoin sodium.

 SIDE EFFECTS

Call your doctor if you have any of these possible drug side effects. Call *immediately* about any labeled "serious."

Serious: blood disorders (fatigue, unusual bleeding or bruising, fever, chills, infection), burnlike rash, skin problems, palpitations, difficulty breathing, extreme weakness, ill feeling
Tips: Avoid people who are ill or have infections; also avoid strenuous physical activity.

Common: uncoordination, slurred speech, confusion, nausea, vomiting, hairiness, blurred or double vision, jerking eye movements, enlarged gums (especially in children)
Tips: Make sure you know how you react to Dilantin before you drive or perform other potentially hazardous activities. Have your teeth professionally cleaned every 3 months.

Other: dizziness, sleeplessness, nervousness, twitching, headache, low blood pressure (dizziness, weakness), rash, pain, sensitivity to sunlight, high blood sugar (frequent thirst and urination), softening of bones
Tips: If you develop a rash, stop taking Dilantin and check with your doctor. Depending on the type of rash, you may resume Dilantin after it clears. If the rash reappears, treatment should stop.

 DRUG INTERACTIONS

Combining certain drugs may alter their action or produce unwanted side effects. Tell your doctor about other drugs you're taking, especially:
- alcohol
- Antabuse
- antiarrhythmics such as Cordarone
- antibiotics, such as Bactrim, Chloromycetin, and Seromycin
- anticoagulants (blood thinners) such as Coumadin
- antihistamines
- aspirin
- Decadron
- Depakene
- flu shots
- folic acid
- ulcer drugs such as Tagamet
- Valium.

How to take Dilantin

- Take Dilantin only as your doctor directs, in the dosage that your doctor orders.

- Remember to take Dilantin every day to maintain a steady level of the drug in your blood and thus prevent seizures.

Continued on next page ▶

- Take Dilantin with or after meals to reduce stomach upset.
- If you're taking the capsules, be sure to swallow them whole; don't open or crush them.
- If you're taking the liquid suspension, read the label carefully. Shake the suspension well before each dose. Use a specially marked measuring spoon (not a household teaspoon) to measure your dose.
- Dilantin capsules are the only oral form that can be given once a day. Toxic levels may result if any other brand or form is given once a day.
- Don't stop taking Dilantin suddenly because seizures may worsen.
- Don't change brands or dosage forms once your treatment is established.
- Store Dilantin in a light-resistant container and away from moisture.

If you miss a dose

Don't take a double dose. Adjust your schedule as follows:
- If you take one dose a day, take the missed dose as soon as possible. But if you don't remember until the next day, skip it and take your next dose on schedule.
- If you take more than one dose a day, take the missed dose as soon as possible. However, if it's less than 4 hours until your next dose, skip the missed dose and take your next dose on schedule.

If you suspect an overdose

Contact your doctor *immediately*. Excessive Dilantin can cause drowsiness, nausea, vomiting, tremor, slurred speech, low blood pressure (dizziness, weakness), and slowed breathing.

Warnings

- Make sure your doctor knows your medical history. You may not be able to take Dilantin if you're overly sensitive to this or similar drugs or if you have heart, lung, liver, or kidney disease; low blood pressure; diabetes; porphyria; an irregular heartbeat; or Adams-Stokes syndrome.
- If you're pregnant or breast-feeding, check with your doctor before taking this drug. Dosages usually increase during pregnancy.
- Be aware that older people are more prone to Dilantin's side effects and thus may require lower dosages.
- If you have diabetes, Dilantin may affect the results of blood and urine sugar tests. Be sure to test carefully.
- Be aware that Dilantin may color urine pink, red, or reddish brown.
- Be aware that heavy alcohol use while taking Dilantin may diminish the drug's benefits.
- Avoid getting Dilantin on clothing because it may stain.
- Maintain good oral hygiene and see your dentist frequently while taking Dilantin.
- Wear a medical identification tag or bracelet stating that you take Dilantin.
- Keep all scheduled doctor's appointments so the doctor can monitor the amount of Dilantin in your blood.

KEEP IN MIND...

* Take with or after meals.
* Use special measuring spoon for liquid.
* Swallow capsules whole; don't open or crush them.
* Shake suspension before taking.
* Don't stop taking suddenly.
* Don't change brands or dosages.

Dilaudid

Dilaudid is a narcotic that alters the way the brain perceives and responds to pain. This brain-centered effect also reduces the urge to cough.

Why it's prescribed

Doctors prescribe Dilaudid to relieve moderate to severe pain or to help stop a cough. The drug comes in tablets, syrup, and suppositories. It's also available in an injectable form. Doctors usually prescribe the following amounts for adults.

▶ **To relieve pain,** 2 to 4 milligrams (mg) as tablets orally every 4 to 6 hours as needed. Or 2 to 4 mg of the drug injected just under the skin every 4 to 6 hours. Or a 3-mg rectal suppository inserted every 6 to 8 hours.

▶ **To stop a cough,** 1 teaspoon (5 milliliters) of syrup every 3 to 4 hours.

How to take Dilaudid

• Take only as much Dilaudid as your doctor prescribes. Taking too much could lead to dependency and raise your risk of overdose.
• If you take Dilaudid regularly for several weeks or more, don't stop the drug abruptly. Your doctor may want to decrease your dosage gradually to minimize side effects.

If you miss a dose

Take the missed dose as soon as possible. However, if it's almost time for your next dose, skip the missed dose and take your next dose as scheduled. Don't take a double dose.

DILAUDID'S OTHER NAME

Dilaudid's generic name is hydromorphone hydrochloride.

SIDE EFFECTS

Call your doctor if you have any of these possible drug side effects. Call *immediately* about any labeled "serious."

Serious: seizures (with large doses), slow or weak breathing, asthma-like attacks

Common: confusion, drowsiness, sedation, euphoria, low blood pressure (dizziness, weakness), nausea, vomiting, constipation, inability to urinate
Tips: Side effects may go away as your body adjusts to the drug; if they continue, tell your doctor. Don't stand up quickly, drive, or perform other activities requiring alertness until you know how you respond to this drug. To help prevent or relieve constipation, drink plenty of fluids and eat high-fiber foods.

Other: addiction, dizziness, abnormally slow heartbeat, blurred or double vision, uncontrollable eye movements

DRUG INTERACTIONS

Combining certain drugs may alter their action or produce unwanted side effects. Tell your doctor about other drugs you're taking, especially:
• alcohol and other drugs that slow down the central nervous system, such as narcotic pain relievers, sedatives, tranquilizers, cold and allergy drugs, anesthetics, and certain antidepressants
• Tagamet.

If you suspect an overdose

Contact your doctor *immediately*. Excessive Dilaudid can cause confusion, very small pupils, severe drowsiness or dizziness, slow or troubled breathing, slow heartbeat, extreme nervousness or restlessness, severe weakness, and seizures.

Warnings

• Make sure your doctor knows your medical history. You may not be able to take Dilaudid if you're allergic to codeine or morphine or if you have kidney, liver, or lung disease; seizures; or a head injury.

• If you're pregnant or think you may be, check with your doctor before taking this drug.
• Children and older adults are especially sensitive to this drug.
• Dilaudid may either worsen or conceal gallbladder pain.

 KEEP IN MIND...

∗ Avoid alcohol, sedatives, and tranquilizers.

∗ Don't stop drug suddenly after steady use.

∗ Tell the doctor if you think you're pregnant.

∗ Take no more than prescribed amount.

Dimetapp

Dimetapp is a combination of two drugs that reduce nasal secretions and prevent histamine reactions, which cause allergy symptoms.

Why it's taken

Dimetapp is taken to relieve a stuffy or runny nose and watery eyes due to colds or allergies such as hay fever. However, it won't cure or shorten the course of a cold. You can buy Dimetapp without a prescription. It comes in tablets, gel capsules, elixir, and extended-release tablets. The following amounts are usually recommended for adults; children's dosages appear in parentheses.

▶ **For cold and allergy symptoms,** 4 milligrams (mg) (1 tablet or 2 teaspoons [tsp] elixir) every 4 hours. (Children ages 6 to 12: 2 mg [½ tablet or 1 tsp elixir] every 4 to 6 hours.)

How to take Dimetapp

• When treating yourself, follow the label directions carefully. Take Dimetapp with food, milk, or water to prevent stomach upset.
• Swallow tablets or extended-release tablets whole; don't break, crush, or chew them.

DIMETAPP'S OTHER NAMES

Dimetapp consists of two generic drugs: brompheniramine and phenylpropanolamine hydrochloride. Other brand names include Bromaline, Bromanate, Bromaphed, Bromatapp, Dimaphen, E.N.T., Genatap, Myphetapp, Pseudo-Chlor, and Vick's DayQuil 4-hour Allergy Relief.

 SIDE EFFECTS

Call your doctor if you have any of these possible drug side effects. Call *immediately* about any labeled "serious."

Serious: exhaustion, irregular heartbeat, difficulty breathing, dry mouth, flushed skin, hallucinations, seizures, mood changes, chest tightness, bruising or bleeding, difficulty sleeping

Common: thick phlegm, drowsiness
Tip: To help loosen phlegm, drink lots of fluids, especially water.

Other: headache, blurred vision, difficulty urinating, appetite loss, nightmares, restlessness, nausea

 DRUG INTERACTIONS

Combining certain drugs may alter their action or produce unwanted side effects. Tell your doctor about other drugs you're taking, especially:
• alcohol and other drugs that slow down the central nervous system, such as cold and allergy drugs, pain relievers, and seizure drugs
• antibiotics, such as Biaxin and Ery-Tab
• antifungal drugs, such as Nizoral and Sporanex
• antiviral drugs such as Symmetrel
• caffeine (diet pills).

If you miss a dose

Take the missed dose as soon as possible. But if it's almost time for your next dose, skip the missed dose and take your next dose as scheduled. Don't take a double dose.

 If you suspect an overdose

Contact your doctor *immediately.* Excessive Dimetapp can cause difficulty breathing, severe drowsiness or excitability, dilated pupils, persistent headache, and seizures.

 Warnings

• Consult your doctor before taking Dimetapp if you have asthma, allergic reactions to antihistamines, heart or blood vessel disease, high blood pressure, glaucoma, diabetes, an overactive thyroid, or urinary tract problems or if you're pregnant or breast-feeding.
• Young children and older adults may be more prone to Dimetapp's side effects.

 KEEP IN MIND...

✴ Take with food or liquid to reduce stomach upset.

✴ Don't crush or chew tablets, capsules, or extended-release tablets.

✴ Drink water to loosen phlegm.

Dipentum

Dipentum is an anti-inflammatory pain reliever that's chemically related to aspirin. It works in the colon (large intestine) to suppress chemical reactions that lead to inflammation in the intestinal lining.

Why it's prescribed

Doctors prescribe Dipentum for people with ulcerative colitis who are unable to take the sulfa drug Azulfidine. It comes in capsules. Doctors usually prescribe the following amount for adults.

▶ **For ulcerative colitis,** 500 milligrams by mouth, twice a day with meals.

How to take Dipentum

• Take Dipentum only as your doctor directs.
• Take it with food and in evenly divided doses to minimize diarrhea.
• Keep taking this drug for the full time prescribed, even if you feel better.

If you miss a dose

Take the missed dose as soon as possible. However, if it's almost time for your next dose, skip the missed dose and take your next dose as scheduled. Don't take a double dose.

 If you suspect an overdose

Contact your doctor *immediately*. Excessive Dipentum can cause diarrhea and a decreased ability to move and function properly.

DIPENTUM'S OTHER NAME

Dipentum's generic name is olsalazine sodium.

 SIDE EFFECTS

Call your doctor if you have any of these possible drug side effects. Call *immediately* about any labeled "serious."

Serious: diarrhea
Tip: Tell your doctor if you develop diarrhea; this problem seems to be related to dosage, but it's hard to distinguish from worsening colitis.

Common: none reported

Other: headache, depression, vertigo, dizziness, nausea, abdominal pain, heartburn, rash, itching, joint pain, skin sensitivity to sunlight, bleeding in digestive tract (bloody stools), bruising
Tips: If you feel dizzy or if you're not fully alert, don't drive or perform other hazardous activities. Protect yourself from the sun by wearing light-colored clothing and a sunblock.

DRUG INTERACTIONS

Combining certain drugs may alter their action or produce unwanted side effects. Tell your doctor about other drugs you're taking, especially:
• aspirin
• Coumadin.

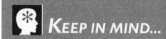 **Warnings**

• Make sure your doctor knows your medical history. You may not be able to take Dipentum if you're allergic to aspirin or other salicylate-type drugs or if you've had kidney problems.
• Make sure your doctor knows if you're pregnant or breastfeeding before you begin taking Dipentum.
• Your doctor may want to check your progress regularly, especially if you need to take the drug for a long time. Dipentum may cause blood problems such as anemia.

KEEP IN MIND...

* Don't take Dipentum if you're allergic to aspirin.

* Take with food in evenly divided doses.

* Report diarrhea to doctor.

* Have regular checkups if taking drug for long period.

* Protect yourself from sunlight with light clothing and sunblock.

* Don't drive if you feel dizzy or if you're not fully alert.

Diquinol

Diquinol is an iodine derivative that kills certain amoebas, microscopic parasites that infect the lining of the intestine.

Why it's prescribed

Doctors prescribe Diquinol to treat amebiasis, an intestinal infection cause by parasites. It comes in tablets. Doctors usually prescribe the following amounts for adults; children's dosages appear in parentheses.

▶ **For intestinal infection,** 630 to 650 milligrams (mg) three times a day, after meals, for 20 days. Total dosage shouldn't exceed 2 grams a day. (Children: 30 to 40 mg for each 2.2 pounds of body weight a day, divided into two or three equal doses each day for 20 days.)

How to take Diquinol

- Follow your doctor's directions.
- If you have trouble swallowing, crush the tablets and mix them with soft food, such as applesauce or chocolate syrup.
- Take all of the drug prescribed; don't stop early.
- Once you've completed a 20-day treatment, don't take additional doses of the drug for 2 to 3 weeks.

If you miss a dose

Take the missed dose as soon as possible. However, if it's almost time for your next dose, skip the missed dose and take your next dose as scheduled. Don't take a double dose.

DIQUINOL'S OTHER NAMES

Diquinol's generic name is iodoquinol. Other brand names include Yodoquinol, Yodoxin; and, in Canada, Diodoquin.

 SIDE EFFECTS

Call your doctor if you have any of these possible drug side effects. Call *immediately* about any labeled "serious."

Serious: fever, exhaustion, rash, bleeding ulcers of rectum, vagina, and mouth

Common: nerve damage in feet, hands, or eyes

Other: widespread nerve damage (related to dosage), pinprick or crawling sensations, weakness, vertigo, malaise, headache, agitation, memory loss, lack of muscle coordination, vision loss, appetite loss, nausea, vomiting, abdominal cramps, diarrhea, constipation, heartburn, stomach pain, anal irritation and itching, hives or boils, discoloration of hair and nails, hair loss, enlarged thyroid, fever, chills

Tip: You may experience diarrhea for the first 2 or 3 days of therapy; tell your doctor if it continues.

 DRUG INTERACTIONS

Combining certain drugs may alter their action or produce unwanted side effects. Tell your doctor about other drugs you're taking.

If you suspect an overdose

Consult your doctor.

Warnings

- Make sure your doctor knows your medical history. You may not be able to take Diquinol if you have liver or kidney disease, changes in optic (eye) nerves, or thyroid disease or if you're allergic to iodine (in which case, Diquinol can cause liver damage).
- Because Diquinol can affect your eyes, you may need to see your eye doctor several times during treatment.
- Diquinol may interfere with thyroid function tests for up to 6 months after you stop taking it.

- To help prevent reinfection, practice good personal hygiene. Always wash your hands thoroughly, and don't prepare food for other people until your stool tests show no more parasites.

 KEEP IN MIND...

* Take entire amount prescribed.
* If you can't swallow the tablets, you may mix them with applesauce or chocolate syrup.
* Visit your eye doctor regularly during therapy.
* Practice excellent hygiene and wash your hands thoroughly while taking this drug.

Ditropan

Ditropan relieves spasms in the bladder by increasing the bladder's capacity and providing pain relief.

Why it's prescribed

Doctors prescribe Ditropan for bladder spasms. It comes in tablets and a liquid. Doctors usually prescribe the following amounts for adults; children's dosages appear in parentheses.

▶ **For bladder spasms,** 5 milligrams (mg) two to four times a day. (Children over age 5: 5 mg two or three times a day.)

How to take Ditropan

• Take Ditropan only as prescribed by your doctor. Your doctor may want you to stop taking it periodically to evaluate whether you still need it.

• Ditropan usually takes effect in 30 to 60 minutes, and relief lasts for 6 to 10 hours.

If you miss a dose

Take the missed dose as soon as possible. But if it's almost time for your next dose, skip the missed dose and take your next dose as scheduled. Don't take a double dose.

If you suspect an overdose

Contact your doctor *immediately.* Excessive Ditropan can cause head-ache, restlessness, flushing, low blood pressure (dizziness, weakness), and slowed breathing.

DITROPAN'S OTHER NAME

Ditropan's generic name is oxybutynin chloride.

SIDE EFFECTS

Call your doctor if you have any of these possible drug side effects. Call *immediately* about any labeled "serious."

Serious: palpitations, fast pulse

Common: constipation, dry mouth and skin, blurred vision, decreased urination, dizziness, drowsiness
Tips: Avoid constipation by increasing fluids and high-fiber foods in your diet. Prevent dizziness by standing slowly and taking care when walking. Be careful driving and operating machinery until you know how this drug affects you.

Other: insomnia, impotence, decreased sweating, fever, decreased production of breast milk
Tip: Avoid strenuous activities in hot weather to avoid becoming overheated from decreased ability to sweat.

DRUG INTERACTIONS

Combining certain drugs may alter their action or produce unwanted side effects. Tell your doctor about other drugs you're taking.

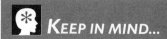

Warnings

• Make sure your doctor knows your medical history. You may not be able to take Ditropan if you have myasthenia gravis, glaucoma, colitis, intestinal obstruction, an overactive thyroid, high blood pressure (headache, blurred vision), an irregular heartbeat, or an enlarged prostate.

• Tell your doctor if you're pregnant or breast-feeding before taking Ditropan.

• Be aware that older adults may be especially prone to Ditropan's side effects.

KEEP IN MIND...

* Take only as directed.

* Avoid becoming overheated in hot weather.

* Don't drive or perform other hazardous activities until you know how this drug affects you.

* Increase fluids and high-fiber foods to prevent constipation.

* Relief lasts 6 to 10 hours

Diulo

Diulo is a diuretic (water pill). It helps the body get rid of excess sodium and water by increasing urination.

Why it's prescribed

Doctors prescribe Diulo to treat high blood pressure and swelling in the lower legs due to heart failure or kidney disease. Diulo comes in tablets. Doctors usually prescribe the following amounts for adults.
▶ **For swelling,** 5 to 20 milligrams (mg) a day.
▶ **For high blood pressure,** 2.5 to 5 mg a day.

How to take Diulo

• Take this drug exactly as your doctor orders. Take only the prescribed amount. Keep taking it, even if you feel well.
• Take it in the morning to avoid nighttime urination.

If you miss a dose

Take the missed dose as soon as possible. However, if it's almost time for your next dose, skip the missed dose and take your next dose as scheduled. Don't take a double dose.

If you suspect an overdose

Contact your doctor *immediately*. Excessive Diulo can cause upset stomach, increased urination, extreme tiredness, and coma.

DIULO'S OTHER NAMES

Diulo's generic name is metolazone. Other brand names include Mykrox and Zaroxolyn.

SIDE EFFECTS

Call your doctor if you have any of these possible drug side effects. Call *immediately* about any labeled "serious."

Serious: severe blood problems (fever, chills, rash, hives, unusual bleeding or bruising, bloody urine, or black, tarry stools), liver problems (confusion, yellow-tinged skin and eyes)

Common: fatigue, low blood pressure (dizziness, weakness), nausea
Tip: To reduce dizziness, avoid sudden posture changes and rise slowly.

Other: dehydration, appetite loss, vomiting, inflamed pancreas, nighttime or frequent urination, skin sensitivity to sun, gout, swelling, allergic reaction (swelling of tobgue or throat, rash, itching), increased thirst, irregular heartbeat, muscle pain or cramps, unusual weakness
Tips: Wear a sunscreen, a hat, and protective clothing outdoors.

DRUG INTERACTIONS

Combining certain drugs may alter their action or produce unwanted side effects. Tell your doctor about other drugs you're taking, especially:
• Advil, Indocin, and other nonsteroidal anti-inflammatory drugs
• alcohol and other drugs that make you feel relaxed or sleepy, such as tranquilizers, sleeping pills, barbiturates, and narcotic pain relievers
• asthma drugs
• Colestid
• Eskalith, Lithobid
• Lanoxin
• Questran

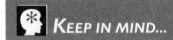 Warnings

• Make sure your doctor knows your medical history. You may not be able to take Diulo if you're allergic to it or if you have diabetes, gout, lupus, an inflamed pancreas, or heart, blood vessel, kidney, or liver disease.
• Tell your doctor right away if you think you're pregnant or if you plan to breast-feed.
• Older adults may be especially prone to Diulo's side effects. They also may lose too much potassium when taking this drug.
• If you're diabetic, be aware that this drug may increase your blood sugar level.

KEEP IN MIND...

* Take exactly as directed.
* Take in morning to avoid nighttime urination.
* Follow low-salt, high-potassium diet if prescribed.

Diuril

iuril is a type of diuretic (water pill). It reduces excess water and sodium by increasing urine production.

Why it's prescribed

Doctors prescribe Diuril to help control high blood pressure, to reduce leg and ankle swelling, and to increase urine production in children with heart disease. It comes in tablets, an oral liquid, and an injectable form. Doctors usually prescribe the following amounts.

▶ **For ankle swelling and high blood pressure in adults,** 500 milligrams (mg) to 2 grams (g) per day orally as one dose or divided into two equal doses.

▶ **To increase urine production** in children, ages 2 to 12: 1 g a day orally as one dose or divided into two equal doses; children under age 2: 10 to 30 mg for each 2.2 pounds of body weight orally each day as one dose or divided into two equal doses.

How to take Diuril

• Follow the dosage instructions carefully.
• If you're taking more than one dose a day, schedule the last dose no later than 6 p.m., unless your doctor directs otherwise, to avoid nighttime urination.
• Take the oral forms with food.
• If you're taking the liquid form, shake the bottle well.

If you miss a dose

Take the missed dose as soon as possible. But if it's almost time for your

SIDE EFFECTS

Call your doctor if you have any of these possible drug side effects. Call *immediately* about any labeled "serious."

Serious: blood disorders (chills, fever, signs of infection, fatigue)

Common: jitteriness, muscle cramps, numbness and tingling, weakness, fatigue, increased urination and thirst, sensitivity to sunlight

Other: dehydration, dizziness, appetite loss, nausea, pancreatitis (abdominal pain, severe vomiting), nighttime urination, dermatitis, rash, impotence, allergic reactions, potassium deficiency (increased thirst and urination, difficulty awakening), blood sugar changes, gout

Tips: Stand up slowly to avoid dizziness. To prevent complications related to fluid and potassium loss, the doctor may recommend eating potassium-rich foods (such as citrus fruits and bananas) or taking a potassium supplement.

DRUG INTERACTIONS

Combining certain drugs may alter their action or produce unwanted side effects. Tell your doctor about other drugs you're taking, especially:
• alcohol
• certain heart drugs such as Lanoxin
• Colestid, Questran
• Eskalith
• narcotics, such as codeine and morphine
• nonsteroidal anti-inflammatory drugs, such as Advil and Motrin
• Solfoton.

next dose, skip the missed dose and take your next dose as scheduled. Don't take a double dose.

 If you suspect an overdose

Contact your doctor *immediately.* Excessive Diuril can cause fluid and potassium loss (dizziness, lethargy, possibly coma).

 Warnings

• Make sure your doctor knows your medical history. You may not be able to take Diuril if you're allergic to sulfa drugs or if you have dia-

betes, gout, lupus, pancreatitis, or kidney or liver disease.
• If your doctor prescribes a low-salt diet, follow it closely.

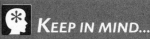 **KEEP IN MIND...**

* Take last dose before 6 p.m. to avoid nighttime urination.
* Stand up slowly to avoid dizziness.
* Follow a high-potassium diet, if prescribed.

DIURIL'S OTHER NAMES

Diuril's generic name is chlorothiazide. Another brand name is Diurigen.

Dolobid

Dolobid is a nonsteroidal anti-inflammatory drug (NSAID) that's used to relieve pain and inflammation. This drug is in the same class as aspirin and Tylenol.

Why it's prescribed

Doctors prescribe Dolobid to relieve mild to moderate pain, stiffness, and joint swelling associated with osteoarthritis or rheumatoid arthritis. It comes in tablets. Doctors usually prescribe the following amounts for adults.

▶ **For joint pain, swelling, and stiffness,** in adults age 65 and under, 500 to 1,000 milligrams (mg) a day, divided into two equal doses, usually every 12 hours. Maximum dosage is 1,500 mg a day.

▶ **For joint pain, swelling, and stiffness,** in adults over age 65, start with half the usual dose.

How to take Dolobid

• Take Dolobid with an antacid or with food and a full (8-ounce) glass of water or milk.
• Don't crush or break the tablets; swallow them whole.
• To prevent irritation of the esophagus, don't lie down for 15 to 30 minutes after taking your dose.

If you miss a dose

Take the missed dose as soon as possible. However, if it's almost time for your next dose, skip the missed dose and take your next dose as scheduled. Don't take a double dose.

DOLOBID'S OTHER NAME

Dolobid's generic name is diflunisal.

SIDE EFFECTS

Call your doctor if you have any of these possible drug side effects. Call *immediately* about any labeled "serious."

Serious: severe stomach or abdominal pain; black, tarry stools; vomiting of blood or material that looks like coffee grounds; bruising or a rash of small red dots

Common: dizziness, headache, ringing in ears, nausea, stomach pain or discomfort, diarrhea, rash
Tip: Make sure you know how you react to this drug before you drive or perform other tasks that require you to be fully alert.

Other: visual disturbances, sleepiness, insomnia, vomiting, constipation, gas, kidney problems, blood in urine, itchiness, sweating, mouth inflammation, dry mucous membranes

DRUG INTERACTIONS

Combining certain drugs may alter their action or produce unwanted side effects. Tell your doctor about other drugs you're taking, especially:
• alcohol
• antacids
• anticoagulants (blood thinners) such as Coumadin
• aspirin, Tylenol, and other aspirin-related drugs
• Rheumatrex
• Sandimmune.

If you suspect an overdose

Contact your doctor *immediately.* Excessive Dolobid can cause drowsiness, nausea, vomiting, hyperventilation, rapid heart rate, sweating, ringing in your ears, disorientation, stupor, and possibly coma.

Warnings

• Make sure your doctor knows your medical history. You may not be able to take Dolobid if you're allergic to any drugs or have other medical problems, especially ulcers, a heart condition, or kidney disease.

• If you're pregnant or breast-feeding, take Dolobid only with your doctor's approval.
• Be aware that older adults are more prone to Dolobid's side effects.
• Before having surgery (including dental surgery), tell the doctor or dentist that you're taking Dolobid.

KEEP IN MIND...

* Take with an antacid or food and full glass of water or milk.

* Swallow tablets whole.

* Call doctor about severe stomach pain or tarry stools.

Dolophine

Dolophine is a narcotic that alters the way the brain perceives and responds to pain.

Why it's prescribed

Doctors prescribe Dolophine to lessen severe, chronic pain and to treat narcotic withdrawal. It comes in tablets and a liquid. Doctors usually prescribe the following amounts for adults.

▶ **For severe pain,** 2.5 to 10 milligrams (mg) every 3 to 4 hours as needed.

▶ **For narcotic withdrawal,** 15 to 40 mg a day at first, adjusted for each individual. The usual dosage ranges from 20 to 120 mg a day. Daily dosages greater than 120 mg require special state and federal approval.

How to take Dolophine

• Dissolve tablets in about 4 ounces of juice or a powdered citrus drink before taking.

• Dilute the liquid form in at least 3 ounces of water.

• If you have severe pain, you'll need to take Dolophine around the clock for best results. Over time, you may need a higher dose to achieve the same pain relief.

• If you're being treated for narcotic withdrawal, your doctor may prescribe an additional drug if you need pain relief.

If you miss a dose

Take the missed dose as soon as possible. However, if it's almost time for your next dose, skip the missed

DOLOPHINE'S OTHER NAMES

Dolophine's generic name is methadone hydrochloride. Another brand name is Methadose.

 SIDE EFFECTS

Call your doctor if you have any of these possible drug side effects. Call *immediately* about any labeled "serious."

Serious: seizures (with large doses), slow breathing

Common: extreme sleepiness, confusion, euphoria, low blood pressure (dizziness, weakness), nausea, vomiting, constipation, inability to urinate

Tip: Drink plenty of fluids and eat fiber-rich foods to minimize constipation; use a laxative or stool softener if necessary.

Other: dizziness, light-headedness, insomnia, involuntary twitching or jerking, slow heart rate, visual disturbances, decreased sex drive, intestinal blockage, physical dependence

Tip: Stand and walk slowly, and avoid driving or other activities that require full alertness until you know how Dolophine affects you.

 DRUG INTERACTIONS

Combining certain drugs may alter their action or produce unwanted side effects. Tell your doctor about other drugs you're taking, especially:

• alcohol
• Dilantin
• Rifadin
• sedatives
• tranquilizers such as Valium
• tricyclic antidepressants, such as Elavil and Sinequan.

dose and take your next dose as scheduled. Don't take a double dose.

 If you suspect an overdose

Contact your doctor *immediately.* Excessive Dolophine can cause your breathing and heart rate to become too slow, possibly leading to cardiac arrest. Pinpoint-size pupils are one sign of overdose.

 Warnings

• Make sure your doctor knows your medical history. You may not be able to take Dolophine if you've had problems with your stomach,

liver, or kidneys; an underactive thyroid; an enlarged prostate; head injury; asthma or other respiratory conditions; or Addison's disease.

• Be aware that Dolophine has a cumulative effect; extreme sleepiness can occur after repeated doses.

KEEP IN MIND...

∗ Increase fluids and fiber in diet.

∗ Take drug around the clock for severe, chronic pain.

∗ Be aware of drug's potential for causing extreme sleepiness.

Domeboro eardrops

Domeboro eardrops inhibit or destroy bacteria and fungi in the ear canal by creating an environment that's too acidic for those organisms. It also reduces inflammation and itching.

Why it's prescribed

Doctors prescribe Domeboro eardrops for infections in the external ear canal or to reduce the risk of getting swimmer's ear. The drug comes as eardrops. Doctors usually prescribe the following amounts for adults and children.

▶ **For infection in external ear canal,** 4 to 6 drops into the ear canal three or four times a day. Or a saturated wick inserted for first 24 hours; treatment is continued with drops.

▶ **To prevent swimmer's ear,** 2 drops in each ear twice a day.

How to use Domeboro eardrops

• Use this drug exactly as your doctor has directed.
• Wash your hands thoroughly and then check your medication. (If it's discolored or contains sediment, notify your doctor and have your prescription refilled.)
• Warm the eardrops by holding the bottle in your hands for 2 minutes. Then open it.
• Fill the dropper with solution; then place the open bottle and dropper within easy reach.

DOMEBORO'S OTHER NAMES

Domeboro Eardrops's generic name is acetic acid. Another brand name is VōSol Otic.

SIDE EFFECTS

Call your doctor if you have any of these possible drug side effects.

Serious: none reported

Common: none reported

Other: ear irritation or itching, hives, worsening infection if the organisms aren't killed by Domeboro Eardrops

DRUG INTERACTIONS

Combining certain drugs may alter their action or produce unwanted side effects. Tell your doctor about other drugs you're taking.

• Lie on your side with your "bad ear" up.
• To straighten your ear canal, gently pull the top of your ear (auricle) upward and backward. (In children, pull the auricle downward and backward to straighten the ear canal.)
• Position the dropper above your ear, and release 1 drop into the ear canal. To prevent reinfection, don't touch the dropper to your ear. Wait until you feel the drop in your ear before releasing remaining drops. Finally, to keep drops from running out of your ear, remain on your side for about 10 minutes. (For a child, release drops into the ear canal; then massage the area in front of the ear. Ask the child to tell you when he or she no longer feels the drug moving around; then let go of the ear.)
• You may plug the ear canal with a piece of cotton moistened with eardrops.

If you miss a dose

Take the missed dose as soon as possible. But if it's almost time for your next dose, skip the missed dose and take your next dose as scheduled. Don't take a double dose.

If you suspect an overdose

Contact your doctor *immediately* if you swallow these eardrops.

Warnings

• Make sure your doctor knows your medical history. You may not be able to use Domeboro eardrops if you have a punctured eardrum.
• Avoid drug contact with eyes or mucous membranes. If you spill any on your skin, wash the affected area twice with soap and water.

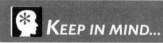

KEEP IN MIND...

* Don't swallow this drug or get it on skin or eyes.

* Give eardrops to children differently than to adults.

* Avoid touching the dropper to your ear.

Donnatal

Donnatal is a combination of drugs that decrease stomach cramps and suppress gastric acid secretion. It also acts as a mild sedative.

Why it's prescribed

Doctors prescribe Donnatal to relieve symptoms of irritable bowel syndrome, acute enterocolitis, and duodenal ulcers. It comes in tablets, extended-release tablets, capsules, and an elixir. Doctors usually prescribe the following amounts for adults; children's dosages appear in parentheses.

▶ **To relieve cramps from stomach and intestinal spasms,** 1 or 2 tablets or capsules or 1 to 2 teaspoons of elixir three to four times a day. (Children weighing up to 10 pounds [lb], 0.5 milliliter [ml] every 4 hours; children weighing 10 to 20 lb, 1 ml every 4 hours; children weighing 20 to 30 lb, 1.5 ml every 4 hours; children weighing 30 to 50 lb, ½ teaspoon every 4 hours; children weighing 50 to 75 lb, ¾ teaspoon every 4 hours; children weighing 75 to 100 lb, 1 teaspoon every 4 hours.)

DONNATAL'S OTHER NAMES

Donnatal is a combination of four generic drugs: phenobarbital, hyoscyamine sulfate, scopolamine hydrobromide, and atropine sulfate. Other brand names include Barbidonna, Barophen, Bellalphen, Donnamor, Donnapine, Hyosophen, Kinesed, Relaxadon, Spaslin, Spasmolin, Spasmophen, Spasquid, and Susano.

SIDE EFFECTS

Call your doctor if you have any of these possible drug side effects. Call *immediately* about any labeled "serious."

Serious: allergic reaction (hives, difficulty breathing, swelling of face and throat, increased heart rate, palpitations)

Common: constipation, dry mouth and skin, dizziness, drowsiness

Other: vision problems, difficult urination, nausea, vomiting, weakness, loss of taste, headache, sleeplessness, decreased sweating

Tips: Call your doctor if these symptoms persist or become worse. Make sure you know how you respond to this drug before you drive or perform other activities requiring alertness. Avoid becoming overheated because reduced sweating can increase your body temperature.

DRUG INTERACTIONS

Combining certain drugs may alter their action or produce unwanted side effects. Tell your doctor about other drugs you're taking.

How to take Donnatal

• Carefully follow the label directions.

• Unless your doctor gives you other instructions, take the drug 30 to 60 minutes before meals.

If you miss a dose

Take the missed dose as soon as possible. However, if it's almost time for your next dose, skip the missed dose and take your next dose as scheduled. Don't take a double dose.

 ### If you suspect an overdose

Contact your doctor *immediately.* Excessive Donnatal can cause headache, vomiting, nausea, blurred vision, dry skin and mouth, and confusion.

Warnings

• Make sure your doctor knows your medical history. You may not be able to take Donnatal if you have a nerve disorder, liver or kidney disease, an overactive thyroid gland, heart disease, or high blood pressure.

• If you're pregnant or breast-feeding, check with your doctor before taking this drug.

• Older adults are especially prone to Donnatal's side effects.

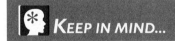

* Never take a double dose.

* Avoid becoming overheated.

* Take drug 30 to 60 minutes before meals.

Dopar

Dopar improves muscle control in conditions caused by a decrease in dopamine, which transmits nerve impulses.

Why it's prescribed

Doctors prescribe Dopar to treat Parkinson's disease or parkinson-type symptoms caused by injury. The drug comes in tablets and capsules. Doctors usually prescribe the following amounts for adults and children over 12.

▶ **For Parkinson's disease or parkinson-type symptoms,** initially 0.5 to 1 gram (g) daily, divided into two or more equal doses. Dosage should be increased by no more than 0.75 g per day, every 3 to 7 days.

How to take Dopar

• Take no more than your doctor prescribes.
• If you have trouble swallowing tablets, crush them and mix them with applesauce.
• Protect Dopar from heat, light, and moisture. If it darkens, don't take it.
• Dopar may not take effect for several weeks. If you don't think the drug is working, don't stop taking it; call your doctor.

If you miss a dose

Take the missed dose as soon as possible. However, if your next scheduled dose is within 2 hours, skip the missed dose and resume your regular schedule. Don't take a double dose.

DOPAR'S OTHER NAMES

Dopar's generic name is levodopa. Another brand name is Larodopa.

SIDE EFFECTS

Call your doctor if you have any of these possible drug side effects. Call *immediately* about any labeled "serious."

Serious: depression or mood changes, unusual or uncontrolled movements, difficult urination, light-headedness or dizziness, irregular heartbeat, severe nausea or vomiting, eyelid spasms, shortness of breath

Common: red or black sweat and urine

Other: fatigue, anxiety, confusion, constipation, insomnia, aggressive behavior, disturbing dreams, euphoria, flushing, blurred vision, increased salivation, dry mouth, bitter taste, gas, stomach upset, sexual changes (increased sex drive, painful erections), liver damage
Tip: To avoid constipation, increase fluids and fiber in your diet.

DRUG AND FOOD INTERACTIONS

Combining certain drugs and foods may alter drug action or produce unwanted side effects. Tell your doctor about your diet and other drugs you're taking, especially:
• antacids, Reglan
• decongestants, asthma drugs, and other stimulants
• Dilantin
• drugs for depression called MAO inhibitors, certain other drugs for mental illness
• foods high in protein or vitamin B_6 (such as avocados, bacon, liver, peas, pork, or tuna)
• Matulane.

If you suspect an overdose

Contact your doctor *immediately.* Excessive Dopar can cause muscle and eyelid twitching, palpitations, or an irregular heartbeat.

Warnings

• Make sure your doctor knows your medical history. You may not be able to take Dopar if you have severe heart, kidney, liver, or lung problems; peptic ulcer; a mental illness; irregular heartbeat; or endocrine disease.

• If you're breast-feeding, tell your doctor before taking Dopar.
• If you have diabetes, the doctor may need to adjust your dosage of insulin or other diabetes drugs. You may also need to switch to another type of urine sugar test.

KEEP IN MIND...

* Avoid foods high in protein and vitamin B_6.

* Your urine and sweat may turn red or black.

* Don't take Dopar if it has darkened.

Doral

Doral is a tranquilizer that acts on the part of the brain responsible for inducing sleep.

Why it's prescribed

Doctors prescribe Doral to relieve sleeplessness. It comes in tablets. Doctors usually prescribe the following amounts for adults.

▶ **For sleeplessness,** 15 milligrams (mg) at bedtime. Older adults may need only 7.5 mg.

How to take Doral

• Follow your doctor's orders. You may be able to take a lower dosage; especially in older people, the doctor may decrease the dosage after 2 days of therapy.
• Take Doral at bedtime.
• If you feel that the drug isn't effective enough, don't increase the amount you take. Tell your doctor.
• If you take Doral for more than 6 weeks in a row, don't suddenly stop taking it; withdrawal symptoms may develop. Talk to your doctor about gradually reducing the dosage.

If you miss a dose

Take the missed dose as soon as possible. However, if it's almost time for your next dose, skip the missed dose and wait until your next bedtime to take another. Don't take a double dose.

DORAL'S OTHER NAME

Doral's generic name is quazepam.

 ## SIDE EFFECTS

Call your doctor if you have any of these possible drug side effects.

Serious: none reported

Common: fatigue, dizziness, daytime drowsiness, headache
Tip: Avoid activities that require coordination and alertness until you see how Doral affects you.

Other: none reported

 ## DRUG INTERACTIONS

Combining certain drugs may alter their action or produce unwanted side effects. Tell your doctor about other drugs you're taking, especially:
• alcohol (don't drink within 24 hours of taking Doral)
• cold and allergy drugs
• narcotics such as morphine
• seizure drugs
• tranquilizers, such as Ativan and Valium.

 ### If you suspect an overdose

Contact your doctor *immediately*. Excessive Doral can cause profound sleepiness, confusion, or even coma.

 ### Warnings

• Make sure your doctor knows your medical history. You may not be able to take Doral if you're overly sensitive to certain tranquilizers; if you have a condition called sleep apnea; if you have liver, kidney, or lung problems; or if you have a history of depression, suicide attempts, or drug abuse.
• Don't take this drug if you're pregnant or breast-feeding. Tell your doctor immediately if you think you might be pregnant.
• Older adults may be especially sensitive to Doral's side effects.
• Doral is not recommended for children under age 18.

KEEP IN MIND...

∗ Don't take this drug while pregnant.
∗ Don't drink alcohol within 24 hours of taking Doral.
∗ Be aware of potential for drowsiness.
∗ Don't increase dosage on your own; call doctor if dosage seems inadequate.

Doryx

Doryx is an antibiotic that kills bacteria by preventing them from reproducing.

Why it's prescribed

Doctors prescribe Doryx to treat bacterial infections, such as urinary tract infections (urethritis), gonorrhea, syphilis, and others. It comes in capsules. Doctors usually prescribe the following amounts for adults; children's dosages appear in parentheses.

▶ **For urethritis, gonorrhea, or** *Chlamydia* **infections,** 100 milligrams (mg) twice a day for 7 to 10 days.

▶ **For syphilis,** 300 mg a day, divided into equal doses, for at least 10 days.

▶ **For other bacterial infections,** 100 mg every 12 hours for the first day, and then 100 mg once a day or 50 mg every 12 hours for 7 to 10 days. (Children weighing 100 pounds (lb) or more: same as adults. Children over age 8 and weighing less than 100 lb: 2 mg for each lb of body weight divided into equal doses and taken every 12 hours for the first day, and then 1 mg per lb once a day or divided into equal doses every 12 hours.

How to take Doryx

• Take this drug exactly as your doctor orders. Take your dose with food, milk, or a full glass (8 ounces)

DORYX'S OTHER NAMES

Doryx's generic name is doxycycline hyclate. Other brand names include Apo-Doxy, Doxy-Caps, Monodox, Vibramycin; and, in Canada, Doxycin, Novodoxylin, and Vibra-Tabs.

 SIDE EFFECTS

Call your doctor if you have any of these possible drug side effects. Call *immediately* about any labeled "serious."

Serious: chest pain, increased pressure in head (confusion, sleepiness, headache), allergic reaction (severe headache, vision changes, hives, itching), anaphylactic shock (swelling, wheezing, difficulty breathing)

Common: stomach upset, nausea, diarrhea, sensitivity to sun, darker skin color
Tips: Limit your exposure to the sun. When you do go outdoors, wear a sunscreen, a hat, and protective clothing. Check with your doctor if the symptoms persist or become severe.

Other: sore throat, irritated tongue, trouble swallowing, loss of appetite, vomiting, fungal infection in the mouth, colitis, inflamed anus or genitals, tooth defects or discoloration, other infections, blood clots
Tips: Practice excellent oral hygiene during treatment. Call your doctor if you develop spots or patches in your mouth.

 DRUG INTERACTIONS

Combining certain drugs may alter their action or produce unwanted side effects. Tell your doctor about other drugs you're taking, especially:
• alcohol
• antacids (including sodium bicarbonate [baking soda])
• anticoagulants (blood thinners) such as Coumadin
• birth control pills (use additional birth control method while taking Doryx)
• diarrhea drugs
• iron supplements
• laxatives containing aluminum, magnesium, or calcium
• penicillin
• seizure drugs, such as Solfoton and Tegretal.

of water to prevent irritation of your esophagus or stomach.
• Don't take capsules within 1 hour of bedtime to avoid heartburn.
• Continue to take this drug even if you start to feel better after a few days. Stopping too soon may allow your infection to return.
• Store this drug away from heat and direct light. Don't keep it in the bathroom, near the kitchen sink, or in other damp places. Heat

or moisture could cause the drug to break down.
• If this drug has changed color, tastes or looks different, has become outdated, or has been stored incorrectly, don't use it; it could cause serious side effects. Discard the bottle and obtain a fresh supply.

If you miss a dose

Take the missed dose as soon as possible. But if it's almost time for your next dose, adjust your schedule as follows:

• If you take one dose a day, space the missed dose and the next dose 10 to 12 hours apart; then resume your regular schedule. Don't take a double dose.

• If you take two doses a day, space the missed dose and the next dose 5 to 6 hours apart; then resume your regular schedule. Don't take a double dose.

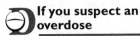

If you suspect an overdose

Contact your doctor *immediately*. Excessive Doryx can cause nausea and vomiting.

✕ Warnings

• Make sure your doctor knows your medical history. You may not be able to take Doryx if you're allergic to it or to other antibiotics (especially tetracyclines) or if you have liver or kidney problems.

• If you're pregnant or breast-feeding, check with your doctor before taking this drug. Doryx could stain your baby's teeth.

• Don't give this drug to children under age 8 because it can stain their teeth and slow down bone growth.

• Because Doryx can interfere with the effectiveness of birth control pills, also use a nonhormonal form of birth control, such as a diaphragm or condoms, while you're taking this drug.

• If you have a job where you're exposed to the sun for long periods of time, notify your doctor, who may prescribe a different antibiotic.

• If you're a diabetic, be aware that Doryx can produce false-positive readings on certain urine sugar tests. Your doctor may instruct you to measure your sugar another way.

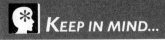

KEEP IN MIND...

* Take with food, milk, or water.

* Use extra form of birth control if you take birth control pills.

* Don't drink alcohol while taking this drug.

* Store drug away from heat, light, and moisture.

Dramamine

Dramamine relieves nausea and vomiting, probably by depressing the part of the brain that's responsible for vomiting.

Why it's taken

Dramamine is taken to relieve nausea and vomiting and to prevent or treat motion sickness. You can buy Dramamine without a prescription. It comes in tablets, chewable tablets, capsules, and syrup. The following amounts are usually recommended for adults; children's dosages appear in parentheses.

▶ **To prevent and treat motion sickness,** 50 to 100 milligrams (mg) every 4 to 6 hours. Maximum dosage is 400 mg in 24 hours. (Children over age 12: same as adults. Children ages 6 to 12: 25 to 50 mg every 6 to 8 hours. Maximum dosage is 150 mg in 24 hours. Children ages 2 to 6: 12.5 to 25 mg every 6 to 8 hours. Maximum dosage is 75 mg in 24 hours.)

How to take Dramamine

• If you're treating yourself, follow the directions on the label. To prevent motion sickness, take this drug at least 30 minutes before traveling.
• Take it with food, milk, or water to reduce stomach upset.

If you miss a dose

Take the missed dose as soon as possible. But if it's almost time for your

next dose, skip the missed dose and take your next dose as scheduled. Don't take a double dose.

If you suspect an overdose

Contact your doctor *immediately.* Excessive Dramamine can cause confusion, flushed skin, dilated pupils, decreased breathing rate, insomnia, seizures, and stomach upset.

Warnings

• You may not be able to take Dramamine if you have glaucoma, asthma, an enlarged prostate, or a seizure disorder. Consult your doctor.

SIDE EFFECTS

Call your doctor if you have any of these possible drug side effects.

Serious: none reported

Common: drowsiness
Tip: Avoid activities that require coordination or full alertness.

Other: occasional headache, palpitations, blurred vision, incoordination, dry mouth, low blood pressure (dizziness, weakness), ringing in ears
Tip: If your mouth feels dry, try using sugarless hard candy or gum.

DRUG INTERACTIONS

Combining certain drugs may alter their action or produce unwanted side effects. Tell your doctor about other drugs you're taking, especially:
• alcohol and other drugs that slow down the central nervous system, such as narcotic pain relievers, sedatives, tranquilizers, cold and allergy drugs, and certain antidepressants
• antibiotics, such as Garamycin and Vancocin
• aspirin
• barbiturates such as Solfoton
• cisplatin
• diuretics (water pills) such as Lasix
• skin tests for allergies
• Theo-Dur.

• If you're pregnant or breast-feeding, check with your doctor before using Dramamine.
• Children and older adults are especially sensitive to this drug's side effects.

KEEP IN MIND...

* Take with food or fluids to reduce stomach irritation.

* For motion sickness, take at least 30 minutes before travel.

* Dramamine may make you drowsy.

DRAMAMINE'S OTHER NAMES

Dramamine's generic name is dimenhydrinate. Other brand names include Calm X, Dimetabs, Dramoject; and, in Canada, Gravol, Nauseatol, and Travamine.

Dulcolax

Dulcolax is a laxative that increases the amount of fluid in the intestines, thus helping to expel solid wastes.

Why it's taken

Dulcolax is taken to relieve constipation; it's also prescribed by doctors to empty the bowel before examinations, childbirth, or surgery. You can buy Dulcolax without a prescription. It comes in tablets, enema, powder (for rectal solution), and suppositories. The following amounts are usually recommended for adults; children's dosages appear in parentheses.

▶ **For chronic constipation, before rectal or bowel examination, childbirth, or surgery,** 10 to 15 milligrams (mg) by mouth in the evening or before breakfast. Dosage may be up to 30 mg, if needed. By rectum, dosage is typically 10 mg for evacuation before examination or surgery. (Children over age 12: same as adults. Children ages 6 to 12: 5 mg by mouth or rectum at bedtime or before breakfast.)

How to take Dulcolax

• If you're treating yourself, follow the package directions exactly.
• Take the tablet on an empty stomach for rapid effect. Because tablets are specially coated to prevent stomach irritation, don't chew, crush, or take them within

SIDE EFFECTS

Call your doctor if you have any of these possible drug side effects. Call *immediately* about any labeled "serious."

Serious: severe stomach pain, laxative dependence

Common: abdominal cramps, diarrhea, burning sensation in rectum (with suppositories)

Other: muscle weakness, nausea, vomiting, diarrhea; rectal bleeding, pain, burning, or itching
Tips: Tell your doctor if you notice rectal bleeding, pain, burning, itching, or other irritation you didn't have before using this drug.

DRUG AND FOOD INTERACTIONS

Combining certain drugs and foods may alter their action or produce unwanted side effects. Tell your doctor about your diet and about other drugs you're taking, especially:
• antacids, milk (don't use within 2 hours before or after taking Dulcolax).

an hour of drinking milk or taking antacids.
• If you're using a suppository and it's too soft to insert, chill it for 30 minutes.
• To help relieve constipation, drink six to eight 8-ounce glasses of liquid daily, eat fiber-rich foods, and get appropriate exercise.

If you miss a dose

Take the missed dose as soon as possible. However, if it's almost time for your next dose, skip the missed dose and take your next dose as scheduled.

 ## If you suspect an overdose

Contact your doctor *immediately*. Excessive Dulcolax can damage bowel structures, foster dependence, and cause weakness, poor coordination, and dizziness.

 ## Warnings

• Consult your doctor before using Dulcolax if you have other medical problems, such as pain in the stomach or lower abdomen, cramping, bloating, nausea, or vomiting.
• Never use Dulcolax for more than 1 week unless your doctor prescribes it.
• Don't give Dulcolax to children under age 6 unless prescribed by a doctor.

KEEP IN MIND...

* Call your doctor about severe stomach pain.
* Take tablets whole; don't chew.
* Increase fiber and fluids in diet.

Duotrate

Duotrate is used to prevent chest pain (angina). Duotrate works by widening the blood vessels, reducing the heart's oxygen needs, and increasing blood flow throughout the heart.

Why it's prescribed

Doctors prescribe Duotrate to prevent angina. (It's not meant to relieve an angina attack in progress.) It comes in extended-release capsules; other brands of this drug come in tablets (Pentylan, Peritrate) and extended-release tablets (Peritrate SA). Doctors usually prescribe the following amounts for adults.

▶ **To prevent angina,** 10 to 20 milligrams (mg) three or four times a day, increased gradually as needed to 40 mg four times a day; or 30 to 80 mg extended-release form twice a day.

How to take Duotrate

• Take this drug exactly as your doctor directs. Take it with a full glass (8 ounces) of water 1 hour before or 2 hours after meals.
• Swallow the extended-release forms whole. Don't crush or chew them.
• You may take an extra dose before anticipated stress or at bedtime if you're sometimes awakened by chest pain.
• Don't stop taking this drug suddenly because this could cause a serious heart problem. Call your doctor, who will tell you how to gradually reduce the amount you take.

DUOTRATE'S OTHER NAMES

Duotrate's generic name is pentaerythritol tetranitrate. Other brand names include Pentylan, Peritrate, P.E.T.N.; and, in Canada, Peritrate SA and Peritrate Forte.

 SIDE EFFECTS

Call your doctor if you have any of these possible drug side effects.

Serious: none reported

Common: headache (may be throbbing), dizziness (especially when standing up)

Tips: Take aspirin or Tylenol for headache. Call your doctor if headache is persistent or severe. To help prevent dizziness, exercise cautiously, stand up slowly, and use stairs carefully.

Other: weakness, fast pulse, flushing, palpitations, fainting, nausea, vomiting, rash

 DRUG INTERACTIONS

Combining certain drugs may alter their action or produce unwanted effects. Tell your doctor about other drugs you're taking, especially:
• alcohol
• blood pressure drugs, such as Cardizem, Corgard, Lopressor, and nitroglycerin
• Ergostat
• phenothiazines, such as Phenergan and Thorazine.

If you miss a dose

Take the missed dose as soon as possible. But if it's within 2 hours of your next dose (or within 6 hours if you take a sustained-release form), skip the missed dose and take your next dose as scheduled. Don't take a double dose.

If you suspect an overdose

Contact your doctor *immediately.* Excessive Duotrate can cause dizziness, weakness, palpitations, throbbing headache, vision problems, flushed skin, sweating, nausea, vomiting, abdominal pains, bloody diarrhea, difficulty breathing, slow pulse, heart disturbances, confusion, fever, paralysis, and seizures.

Warnings

• Make sure your doctor knows your medical history. You may not be able to take Duotrate if you have glaucoma, kidney or liver disease, or severe anemia, or if you've recently had a heart attack or stroke.

Don't take Duotrate to stop an angina attack in progress.

KEEP IN MIND...

∗ Take with full glass of water.
∗ Don't crush or chew extended-release forms.
∗ Don't use to stop angina attack in progress.
∗ Don't stop taking suddenly.

Duragesic

Duragesic is a narcotic that alters the way the brain perceives and responds to pain.

Why it's prescribed

Doctors prescribe Duragesic to help relieve chronic pain that can't be relieved by milder drugs. It comes in skin patches designed to release 25 micrograms (mcg), 50 mcg, 75 mcg, or 100 mcg of the drug per hour. Doctors usually prescribe the following amounts for adults.

▶ **For management of chronic pain,** 1 patch applied to the upper torso on an area of skin that is not irritated and has not been treated with radiation. Therapy usually starts at 25 mcg per hour; dosage can be adjusted as needed and tolerated.

How to use Duragesic

• Apply a new patch to a new site on your skin every 72 hours or as ordered by your doctor.
• Be sure the skin at each site is clean and dry. Hold the new patch in place for 10 to 20 seconds to make sure it stays on.
• Dispose of the old patch by folding it in half, sticky side in, and flushing it down the toilet.
• Don't change dosage or stop using Duragesic suddenly. Doing so may cause withdrawal symptoms. Consult your doctor, who will change or reduce your dosage gradually.

If you miss a dose

If you don't apply a new patch when scheduled, do so as soon as

DURAGESIC'S OTHER NAME

Duragesic's generic name is fentanyl.

 SIDE EFFECTS

Call your doctor if you have any of these possible drug side effects. Call *immediately* about any labeled "serious."

Serious: seizures (with high doses), very slow or weak breathing

Common: confusion, drowsiness, lethargy, euphoria, low blood pressure (dizziness, weakness), constipation, urine retention, itching
Tip: Don't drive or perform activities requiring alertness until you know how Duragesic affects you.

Other: dizziness, slow heart rate, nausea, vomiting, intestinal blockage, skin reaction at the patch site, rigid muscles, physical dependence

 DRUG INTERACTIONS

Combining certain drugs may alter their action or produce unwanted side effects. Tell your doctor about other drugs you're taking, especially:
• alcohol and other drugs that slow down the central nervous system, such as cold and allergy drugs, muscle relaxants, narcotic pain relievers, sedatives, seizure drugs, sleeping pills, tranquilizers, and certain antidepressants.

you can. Don't apply more than one patch at a time. Doing so may cause serious side effects.

 If you suspect an overdose

Contact your doctor *immediately.* Excessive Duragesic can cause your breathing and heart rate to become too slow. Pinpoint-size pupils are one sign of an overdose.

 Warnings

• Make sure your doctor knows your medical history. You may not be able to use Duragesic if you have a head injury, respiratory problems, liver or kidney disease, or an abnormal heart rhythm.
• If you're pregnant or breast-feeding, consult your doctor before you start using Duragesic.

• Young children and older adults are especially prone to Duragesic's side effects.
• High temperature, from fever or hot weather, can increase absorption of Duragesic and may require a dosage adjustment. Tell your doctor if you develop a fever or plan to spend time in a hot climate.

KEEP IN MIND...

∗ Apply each patch according to directions.

∗ Don't change dosage on your own or stop using drug abruptly after steady use.

∗ Avoid alcohol, sedatives, and tranquilizers.

Duricef

Duricef is an antibiotic drug that's related to penicillin. It kills bacteria by damaging their cell walls.

Why it's prescribed

Doctors prescribe Duricef for certain types of urinary tract infections, skin and soft-tissue infections, and strep throat. It comes in tablets, capsules, and an oral liquid. Doctors usually prescribe the following amounts for adults; children's dosages appear in parentheses.

▶ **For urinary tract infections caused by certain organisms, skin and soft tissue infections, and streptococcal pharyngitis,** 500 milligrams (mg) to 2 grams once or twice a day, depending on the infection being treated. (Children: 30 mg for each 2.2 pounds of body weight daily, divided into two equal doses.)

How to take Duricef

- Take Duricef at the same time each day to maintain consistent levels of the drug in your body.
- Take the drug with food or milk to reduce stomach upset.
- Take all the drug, exactly as prescribed, even after you feel better.
- If the drug expires before you've finished the entire prescription, discard it and see your doctor to obtain a new prescription because the expired drug may not work properly.
- Keep the unused drug away from dampness, heat, and light to keep it from deteriorating.

DURICEF'S OTHER NAMES

Duricef's generic name is cefadroxil monohydrate. Another brand name is Ultracef.

 ## SIDE EFFECTS

Call your doctor if you have any of these possible drug side effects. Call *immediately* about any labeled "serious."

Serious: severe allergic reaction (difficulty breathing, very low blood pressure, extreme dizziness and weakness), antibiotic-associated colitis (blood or mucus in diarrhea after taking this drug))

Common: diarrhea, stomach upset, rash
Tip: Take the drug with food to avoid stomach upset.

Other: dizziness, headache, malaise, appetite loss, vomiting, abdominal cramps, irritation of anus or genitals, anemia, allergic reaction (swelling of tongue or throat, rash, itching), shortness of breath

 ## DRUG INTERACTIONS

Combining certain drugs may alter their action or produce unwanted side effects. Tell your doctor about other drugs you're taking, especially:
- antibiotics, such as carbenicillin (injection) and ticarcillin
- anticoagulants (blood thinners) such as Coumadin
- Benemid
- seizure drugs, such as Depakote and Depakene.

If you miss a dose

Take the missed dose as soon as possible. However, if it's almost time for your next dose, skip the missed dose and take your next dose as scheduled. Don't take a double dose.

 ## If you suspect an overdose

Contact your doctor *immediately.* Excessive Duricef can cause seizures.

 ## Warnings

- Make sure your doctor knows your medical history. You may not be able to take Duricef if you're allergic to penicillin, food additives or dyes, or certain foods; if you've had stomach or intestinal disease (especially colitis); or if you have kidney problems.
- If you take large doses or need prolonged therapy, you may be at risk for other types of infection. Notify your doctor if you experience unusual symptoms.

 ## KEEP IN MIND...

- Take drug at same time every day.
- Take with food or milk to reduce stomach upset.
- Finish entire amount prescribed.
- Call doctor if you develop signs of allergic reaction.

Dyazide

Dyazide is a combination of two diuretics (water pills) that cause the body to lose water and sodium through the kidneys. The reduced fluid level reduces the heart's workload.

Why it's prescribed

Doctors prescribe Dyazide to control blood pressure. It comes in capsules. Doctors usually prescribe the following amounts for adults.

▶ **For reducing high blood pressure,** 1 to 2 capsules a day.

How to take Dyazide

• Take this drug exactly as prescribed.

• If you're taking one dose a day, take it in the morning after breakfast.

• If you're taking more than one dose a day, take your last dose before 6 p.m. so the need to urinate won't disturb your sleep.

If you miss a dose

Take the missed dose as soon as possible. However, if it's almost time for your next dose, skip the missed dose and take your next dose as scheduled. Don't take a double dose.

If you suspect an overdose

Contact your doctor *immediately.* Excessive Dyazide can cause low blood pressure (dizziness, fainting) and low potassium levels (irregular

DYAZIDE'S OTHER NAMES

Dyazide is a combination of two generic drugs: hydrochlorothiazide and triamterene. Another brand name is Maxzide.

SIDE EFFECTS

Call your doctor if you have any of these possible drug side effects. Call *immediately* about any labeled "serious."

Serious: shortness of breath, confusion, fever, chills, low back pain, stomach pain, joint pain, sore throat, black stools, easy bleeding or bruising, irregular heartbeat, allergic reaction (hives, swelling in throat, difficulty breathing)
Tip: If you feel like your throat is closing and you have trouble breathing, stop taking this drug and get emergency care *at once.*

Common: skin sensitivity to sunlight
Tip: Use a sunblock to protect skin against sunlight.

Other: nausea, vomiting, fatigue, dizziness, headache
Tips: To minimize nausea, take Dyazide with milk or food. Stand up slowly to avoid dizziness.

DRUG INTERACTIONS

Combining certain drugs may alter their action or produce unwanted side effects. Tell your doctor about other drugs you're taking, especially:
• angiotensin-converting enzyme (ACE) inhibitors, such as Capoten and Vasotec
• Lanoxin
• Lithobid
• other diuretics (water pills) such as Lasix
• potassium supplements
• Sandimmune.

heartbeat, weakness, nausea, vomiting, or confusion).

Warnings

• Make sure your doctor knows your medical history. You may not be able to take Dyazide if you have liver or kidney disease, diabetes, or too much potassium in your blood.
• If you're pregnant or breast-feeding, check with your doctor before taking this drug.
• Older adults may be especially prone to Dyazide's side effects.
• Because this drug may decrease your body's potassium level, your

doctor may instruct you to eat foods high in potassium (such as bananas, apricots, and orange juice), take a potassium supplement, and cut down on salt.

KEEP IN MIND...

* Take exactly as prescribed.
* Take with food or milk to reduce nausea.
* Use a sunblock.
* Eat potassium-rich foods if directed by doctor.

Dymelor

Dymelor lowers blood sugar levels probably by stimulating the pancreas to release insulin while reducing the liver's sugar production.

Why it's prescribed

Doctors prescribe Dymelor along with diet therapy to help control blood sugar levels in people with non-insulin-dependent (type II) diabetes. The drug comes in tablets. Doctors usually prescribe the following amounts for adults.

▶ **To reduce blood sugar in type II diabetes,** initially 250 milligrams (mg) each day before breakfast. Dosage may be increased by 250 to 500 mg after 5 to 7 days, as needed. Maximum recommended dosage is 1.5 grams a day, divided into two or three equal doses taken before meals.

▶ **To replace insulin therapy in type II diabetes,** 250 mg before breakfast if the insulin dosage was less than 20 units a day. Dymelor dosage may be increased over time as described above. If the insulin dosage was 20 to 40 units a day, Dymelor therapy usually starts with 250 mg before breakfast. The insulin dosage is then reduced by 25% to 30% daily or insulin is taken every other day, depending on the person's response to Dymelor.

How to take Dymelor

• Carefully follow the label directions. Take the exact amount your doctor ordered.

DYMELOR'S OTHER NAMES

Dymelor's generic name is acetohexamide. A brand name in Canada is Dimelor.

 ## SIDE EFFECTS

Call your doctor if you have any of these possible drug side effects. Call *immediately* about any labeled "serious."

Serious: very low blood sugar (cool pale skin, difficulty concentrating, shakiness, headache, cold sweats, anxiety), allergic reaction (severe diarrhea, hives, bruising, bleeding, chills, fever), liver problems (yellow-tinged skin and eyes, light-colored stools)
Tips: Carry candy or other simple sugars to treat mild episodes of low blood sugar. Severe episodes may require hospital treatment.

Common: skin sensitivity to sunlight
Tip: Use a sunblock and wear protective clothing and sunglasses while outside.

Other: nausea, heartburn, vomiting, mild drowsiness, headache, dizziness, diarrhea, constipation, appetite changes, stomach pain, fullness, or discomfort.
Tip: Side effects may subside as your body adjusts to the drug. If they persist, consult your doctor.

 ## DRUG INTERACTIONS

Combining certain drugs may alter their action or produce unwanted side effects. Tell your doctor about other drugs you're taking, especially:
• alcohol (except in small quantities)
• antibiotics such as Chloromycetin, sulfa drugs such as Bactrim
• anticoagulants (blood thinners) such as Coumadin
• antidepressants
• aspirin and similar products
• certain diuretics (water pills)
• glucagon
• heart drugs called beta blockers, such as Inderal and Lopressor
• nonprescription drugs for colds, coughs, hay fever, or appetite control
• steroids.

• Take this drug at the same time each day: before breakfast (if you take one dose a day) or before meals (if you take two or more doses a day).
• Don't change the amount you take without your doctor's consent.

If you miss a dose

Take the missed dose as soon as possible. However, if it's almost time for your next dose, skip the missed dose and take your next dose as scheduled. Don't take a double dose.

 ### If you suspect an overdose

Contact your doctor *immediately.* Excessive Dymelor may cause your blood sugar to drop too low, especially if you delay or miss a meal or snack, exercise more than usual, or drink a significant amount of alcohol.

Warnings

• Follow your special meal plan carefully. Diet is critical to controlling your diabetes and is necessary for the drug to work.

• Test the sugar level in your blood or urine as directed by your doctor, and learn to recognize symptoms of low blood sugar: cool pale skin, difficulty concentrating, shakiness, headache, cold sweats, and anxiety. Call your doctor if your blood sugar level drops and you have any of these symptoms. Because Dymelor's effects may last for days, you'll be especially prone to low blood sugar.

• Don't take any other drugs — especially nonprescription drugs for colds, coughs, asthma, hay fever, or appetite control — unless approved by your doctor.

• Carry some form of medical identification that reveals your diabetes and lists the drugs you take.

• During periods of increased stress, such as infection, fever, surgery, or trauma, you may require insulin therapy.

• Be aware that Dymelor relieves symptoms; it doesn't cure your disease.

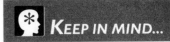

KEEP IN MIND...

* Don't change dosage without doctor's permission.

* Know how to recognize and respond to low blood sugar.

* Drink only small amounts of alcohol.

* Follow your diet carefully.

Dynabac

Dynabac fights disease-causing bacteria by preventing them from growing and spreading.

Why it's prescribed

Doctors prescribe Dynabac to treat bronchitis, some types of pneumonia (such as Legionnaire's disease), uncomplicated skin infections, and tonsillitis or other throat infections (such as strep throat). It comes in tablets. Doctors usually prescribe the following amounts for adults and children age 12 and older.

▶ **For bronchitis and skin infections,** 500 milligrams (mg) for 7 days.

▶ **For pneumonia,** 500 mg for 14 days.

▶ **For throat infections,** 500 mg for 10 days.

How to take Dynabac

• Take Dynabac only as your doctor directs.

• Take it with food or within 1 hour after eating to improve its absorption in the body.

• Don't cut, chew, or crush tablets before swallowing them.

• Take the full amount prescribed, even after you begin to feel better. This will help keep your infection from coming back.

If you miss a dose

Take the missed dose as soon as possible. However, if it's almost time for your next dose, skip the missed dose and go back to your regular dosing schedule. Don't take a double dose.

DYNABAC'S OTHER NAMES

Dynabac's generic name is dirithromycin.

 SIDE EFFECTS

Call your doctor if you have any of these possible drug side effects. Call *immediately* about side effects labeled "serious."

Serious: blood problems (fatigue, bleeding, bruising, fever, chills, infection)

Common: abdominal pain, nausea, diarrhea, headache
Tip: Take with food to avoid nausea.

Other: dizziness, spinning sensation, sleeplessness, vomiting, indigestion, digestive disorder, gas, cough, difficulty breathing, rash, itching, hives, pain, weakness, dehydration
Tip: Drink extra fluids to avoid dehydration.

 DRUG INTERACTIONS

Combining certain drugs may alter their action or produce unwanted side effects. Tell your doctor about other drugs you're taking, especially:
• allergy drugs, such as Hismanal and Seldane
• antacids
• antiarrhythmics, such as Lanoxin and Norpace
• anticoagulants (blood thinners) such as Coumadin
• Cafergot
• Halcion
• Mevacor
• Parlodil
• Sandimmune
• seizure drugs, such as Depakene, Dilantin, and Tegretol
• Theo-Dur.

If you suspect an overdose

Contact your doctor. Although no overdose of Dynabac has been reported, the most likely signs and symptoms would be nausea, vomiting, heartburn, and diarrhea.

 Warnings

• Make sure your doctor knows your medical history. You may not be able to take Dynabac if you have any drug allergies, especially to antibiotics, or if you have a blood or liver disorder.

• Tell your doctor if you're pregnant or breast-feeding before you begin taking Dynabac.

• Don't give Dynabac to children under age 12 without a doctor's consent.

 KEEP IN MIND...

* Take with food.

* Don't cut, chew or crush tablets.

* Finish entire prescription.

* Not for children under age 12.

DynaCirc

DynaCirc is one of several heart drugs called calcium channel blockers. It blocks calcium from traveling across muscle cells, which causes blood vessels to dilate slightly. By dilating blood vessels, DynaCirc reduces the amount of pressure exerted against them by the circulating blood.

Why it's prescribed

Doctors prescribe DynaCirc to reduce high blood pressure. The drug comes in capsules. Doctors usually prescribe the following amounts for adults.

▶ **To reduce high blood pressure,** initially 2.5 milligrams (mg) by mouth twice daily, alone or with a diuretic (water pill). After 2 to 4 weeks, dosage may be increased, probably to 5 mg twice a day. If necessary, daily dosage may be further increased by 5 mg every 2 to 4 weeks, to a maximum dosage of 20 mg a day.

How to take DynaCirc

• Follow the doctor's dosage instructions carefully.
• If you're taking a diuretic (water pill) with DynaCirc, take your last dose several hours before bedtime, so the need to urinate won't disturb your sleep.

DYNACIRC'S OTHER NAME

DynaCirc's generic name is isradipine.

 SIDE EFFECTS

Call your doctor if you have any of these possible drug side effects. Call *immediately* about any labeled "serious."

Serious: heart attack (pain in chest that may radiate to an arm, irregular heartbeat, shortness of breath, apprehension)

Common: dizziness, irregular or rapid heartbeat, low blood pressure (dizziness, fainting), frequent urination, shortness of breath, constipation

Tips: Stand up slowly to avoid dizziness. Notify your doctor if you develop an irregular heartbeat, pronounced dizziness, or constipation.

Other: swelling of hands or feet, flushing, nausea, diarrhea, rash

 DRUG INTERACTIONS

Combining certain drugs may alter their action or produce unwanted side effects. Tell your doctor about other drugs you're taking, especially:
• heart drugs called beta blockers, such as Inderal and Lopressor.

If you miss a dose

Take the missed dose as soon as possible. However, if it's almost time for your next dose, skip the missed dose and take your next dose as scheduled. Don't take a double dose.

 If you suspect an overdose

Contact your doctor *immediately.* Excessive DynaCirc can cause very low blood pressure (dizziness, fainting).

 Warnings

• Make sure your doctor knows your medical history. You may not be able to take DynaCirc if you have congestive heart failure and are taking a heart drug called a beta blocker.
• Visit your doctor regularly to have your blood pressure checked.
• Before undergoing surgery, be sure to tell the anesthetist that you're taking a calcium channel blocker.

 KEEP IN MIND...

∗ Follow dosage instructions carefully.

∗ Stand up slowly to avoid dizziness.

∗ Expect more frequent urination.

∗ Have your blood pressure checked routinely.

Dynapen°

Dynapen is an antibiotic related to penicillin that works especially well against penicillin-resistant bacteria.

Why it's prescribed

Dynapen is prescribed to treat bacterial infections, especially certain Staphylococcus (staph) infections. It comes in capsules and an oral liquid. Doctors usually prescribe the following amounts for adults; children's dosages appear in parentheses.

▶ **For bacterial infections,** 166 to 666 milligrams (mg) every 6 hours, for a total dosage of 1 to 4 grams a day. (Children: 25 to 50 mg for each 2.2 pounds (lb) of body weight a day, divided into equal doses given every 6 hours. Serious infections may require 75 to 100 mg for each 2.2 lb a day.)

How to take Dynapen

• Don't break, chew, or crush the capsules — swallow them whole. If you're taking the liquid, use a dropper or specially marked measuring spoon (not a household teaspoon) to measure each dose accurately.
• Take this drug with a full glass (8 ounces) of water on an empty stomach, either 1 to 2 hours before or 2 to 3 hours after meals, unless otherwise directed by your doctor.
• Take all of this drug, even if you start to feel better. Stopping too soon may allow your infection to return.

DYNAPEN'S OTHER NAMES

Dynapen's generic name is dicloxacillin sodium. Other brand names include Dycill and Pathocil.

SIDE EFFECTS

Call your doctor if you have any of these possible drug side effects. Call *immediately* about any labeled "serious."

Serious: severe diarrhea, allergic reaction (difficulty breathing, rash, hives, wheezing)
Tips: If you develop mild diarrhea, you may take a drug to treat it (such as Kaopectate) that contains a type of finely dispersed clay (kaolin or attapulgite). For severe diarrhea, check with your doctor before taking any diarrhea drug; it could prolong or worsen your diarrhea.

Common: stomach upset, gas
Tip: Take the drug with a full glass of water to reduce stomach upset.

Other: heartburn, vomiting

DRUG INTERACTIONS

Combining certain drugs may alter their action or produce unwanted side effects. Tell your doctor about other drugs you're taking, especially:
• Probalan, a drug for gout
• Probenecid.

If you miss a dose

Take the missed dose as soon as possible. However, don't take a double dose. If it's almost time for your next dose, adjust your dosage schedule as follows; then resume your regular schedule.
• If you take two doses a day, space the missed dose and the next dose 5 to 6 hours apart.
• If you take three or more doses a day, space the missed dose and the next dose 2 to 4 hours apart. Then resume your regular schedule.

 ## If you suspect an overdose

Contact your doctor *immediately.* Excessive Dynapen can cause seizures.

 ## Warnings

• Make sure your doctor knows your medical history. You may not be able to take Dynapen if you have a history of kidney problems, if you have mononucleosis, or if you're allergic to penicillin-type antibiotics.
• Tell the doctor that you're taking Dynapen before you have medical tests because this drug could alter the results.

KEEP IN MIND...

∗Don't crush or chew capsules.
∗Take with water on empty stomach.
∗Contact the doctor if you develop severe diarrhea.

Dyrenium

Dyrenium is a diuretic (water pill), a drug that helps reduce the amount of water in the body. This drug is called a potassium-sparing diuretic because it doesn't cause the body to lose potassium.

Why it's prescribed

Doctors prescribe Dyrenium to reduce leg and ankle swelling (edema) caused by too much fluid in the body. It comes in tablets or, in Canada, in capsules. Doctors usually prescribe the following amounts for adults.

▶ For edema, initially 100 milligrams (mg) twice a day after meals, adjusted as needed. Total dosage should not be more than 300 mg a day.

How to take Dyrenium

• If you take one dose a day, take it in the morning after breakfast. If you take more than one dose a day, take the last dose no later than 6 p.m. to prevent the need to urinate from disturbing your sleep.
• Take after meals or with food or milk to minimize nausea.

If you miss a dose

Take the missed dose as soon as possible. However, if it's almost time for your next dose, skip the missed dose and take your next dose as scheduled. Don't take a double dose.

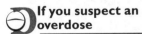 **If you suspect an overdose**

Contact your doctor *immediately*. Excessive Dyrenium can cause de-

---

DYRENIUM'S OTHER NAME

Dyrenium's generic name is triamterene.

 SIDE EFFECTS

Call your doctor if you have any of these possible drug side effects. Call *immediately* about any labeled "serious."

Serious: too much potassium in your system (confusion or nervousness; irregular heartbeat; numbness or tingling in hands, feet, or lips; difficulty breathing; unusual tiredness or weakness; weakness or heaviness in legs), anaphylactic shock (extremely low blood pressure, extreme dizziness, fainting, difficulty breathing)

Common: frequent urination, dizziness, weakness, fatigue
Tip: To minimize dizziness, change positions and stand up slowly.

Other: headache, low blood pressure (dizziness, weakness), dry mouth, nausea, vomiting, diarrhea, sensitivity to sunlight, rash, muscle cramps, kidney problems (reduced urination), jaundice (yellow-tinged skin and eyes)
Tip: Avoid direct sunlight, wear protective clothing, and use a sunblock.

 DRUG AND FOOD INTERACTIONS

Combining certain drugs and certain foods may alter drug action or produce unwanted side effects. Tell your doctor about your diet and other drugs you're taking, especially:
• blood pressure drugs
• Eskalith, Lithobid
• Lanoxin
• nonsteroidal anti-inflammatory drugs (NSAIDs) such as Motrin
• potassium supplements and potassium-rich foods, salt substitutes
• Quinaglute Dura-Tabs
• Symmetrel.

---

hydration and high potassium levels (confusion, nervousness, irregular heartbeat, numbness, difficulty breathing, weakness).

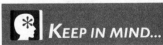 **Warnings**

• Make sure your doctor knows your medical history. You may not be able to take Dyrenium if you have diabetes, kidney or liver disease, gout, menstrual problems, or enlarged breasts.
• Your doctor may tell you to weigh yourself daily and measure how much fluid you drink and how much urine you produce. Take a written record to doctor visits.

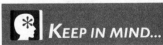 **KEEP IN MIND...**

∗Take after meals or with food or milk.

∗Record daily weight, urine produced, and fluid intake, if ordered.

∗Stand up slowly to avoid dizziness.

Econopred eyedrops

Econopred eyedrops, a type of steroid, help reduce inflammation in the eyes.

Why it's prescribed

Doctors prescribe Econopred eyedrops to reduce inflammation in the front part of the eye, especially the mucous membranes under the eyelids and in the cornea. Doctors usually prescribe the following amounts for adults and children.

▶ **For reducing eye inflammation,** 1 to 2 drops placed in the eye four to six times a day. If the condition is severe, use hourly, tapering off as the doctor specifies and inflammation subsides.

How to use Econopred eyedrops

• Shake the bottle before using the eyedrops. Close the container tightly after use.
• Wash your hands before and after applying the eyedrops.
• To avoid contaminating the eyedrops, be careful not to touch the dropper to your eye or the surrounding skin.
• After applying the drops, press your finger against each tear duct for 1 minute to keep the drug from going into your tear ducts.

ECONOPRED'S OTHER NAMES

Econopred's generic name is prednisolone acetate. Other brand names for these eyedrops include Pred Forte and Pred Mild Ophthalmic.

 SIDE EFFECTS

Call your doctor if you have any of these possible drug side effects. Call *immediately* about any labeled "serious."

Serious: increased pressure in eye (headache, eye pain), various problems affecting cornea; with excessive or long-term use, worsened glaucoma, cataracts, visual problems, possible body-wide effects

Common: burning, stinging when applying the eyedrops
Tip: Pat — don't rub — your eye with a clean tissue.

Other: watery eyes

 DRUG INTERACTIONS

Combining certain drugs may alter their action or produce unwanted side effects. Tell your doctor about other drugs you're taking.

If you miss a dose

Take the missed dose as soon as possible. However, if it's almost time for your next dose, skip the missed dose and take your next dose as scheduled. Don't apply a double dose.

If you suspect an overdose

Consult your doctor.

Warnings

• Make sure your doctor knows your medical history. You may not be able to use Econopred eyedrops if you have an untreated bacterial eye infection or other eye disorder, herpes, or other viral or fungal diseases.
• You may not be able to wear contact lenses while using this drug. Check with your eye doctor.

• If you're on long-term treatment, you may need frequent tests to check the pressure inside your eye.
• Never use leftover eyedrops for a new eye inflammation.
• To avoid spreading the infection, don't share eyedrops, washcloths, or towels. If someone else in your family develops symptoms like yours, call the doctor.

KEEP IN MIND...

* Avoid touching the dropper to your eye.
* Press a finger against each tear duct for 1 minute after using drops.
* Don't wear contact lenses without doctor's permission.
* Don't share eyedrops.

Effexor

Effexor is an antidepressant that works primarily by maintaining levels of the mood-altering chemicals serotonin and norepinephrine in the brain.

Why it's prescribed

Doctors prescribe Effexor to relieve depression. It comes in tablets. Doctors usually prescribe the following amounts for adults.

▶ **To relieve depression,** initially, 75 milligrams (mg) divided into two or three equal doses. The dosage may be increased as needed by 75 mg a day every 4 or more days. For moderate depression, the maximum dosage is usually 225 mg a day. For severe depression, dosage may be as high as 375 mg a day.

How to take Effexor

• Take this drug exactly as prescribed; don't increase the dosage unless your doctor tells you to.
• Take Effexor with food.
• If you've been taking Effexor for 6 weeks or more, don't stop abruptly. Your doctor will taper your dosage gradually.

If you miss a dose

Take the missed dose as soon as possible. However, if it's almost time for your next dose, skip the missed dose and take your next dose as scheduled. Don't take a double dose.

> ### EFFEXOR'S OTHER NAME
>
> Effexor's generic name is venlafaxine hydrochloride.

SIDE EFFECTS

Call your doctor if you have any of these possible drug side effects.

Serious: none reported

Other: headache, sleepiness, dizziness, nervousness, insomnia, nausea, constipation, dry mouth

Tips: Prevent dizziness by standing up slowly and taking care when walking. Avoid constipation by increasing fluids and fiber-rich foods in your diet.

Other: anxiety, high blood pressure (headache, blurred vision), vomiting, abnormal ejaculation, impotence, tremor, sweating, weight loss, lack of strength or energy

DRUG INTERACTIONS

Combining certain drugs may alter their action or produce unwanted side effects. Tell your doctor about other drugs you're taking, especially:
• alcohol
• antidepressants called MAO inhibitors, such as Elavil, Pamelor, and Tofranil
• nonprescription drugs.

If you suspect an overdose

Contact your doctor *immediately*. Excessive Effexor can cause sleepiness, seizures, and possibly abnormalities in heart rate.

Warnings

• Make sure your doctor knows your medical history. You may not be able to take the full dosage of Effexor if you have kidney or certain metabolic problems or a history of mania or seizures.
• Make sure your doctor knows if you're pregnant or breast-feeding before you begin taking Effexor.

Tell the doctor if you intend to become pregnant.
• Because Effexor may lead to increases in blood pressure, especially in higher doses, your doctor may want to check your blood pressure routinely.

KEEP IN MIND...

* Take with food.
* Don't stop taking drug abruptly after long-term use.
* Don't increase your dosage unless your doctor tells you to.
* Have blood pressure checked as doctor orders.

Elase

E lase combines two drugs: fibrinolysin, which attacks the components of blood clots, and desoxyribonuclease, which attacks DNA. Together, they clean debris from wound surfaces and promote healing.

Why it's prescribed

Doctors prescribe Elase for cleaning inflamed and infected wounds, such as burns, surgical wounds, circumcisions, and episiotomies. It's also used to treat vaginal inflammation from cervicitis and vaginitis. Elase comes in an ointment. Doctors usually prescribe the following amounts.

▶ **To dissolve debris from inflamed or infected wounds,** in adults and children, a small amount applied three times a day.

▶ **For mild to moderate cervicitis or vaginitis,** in adults, 5 milliliters inserted by vaginal applicator once a day at bedtime for 5 days or until the tube is empty.

How to use Elase

• Take the drug exactly as prescribed. Be sure to keep it away from your eyes.

• For wounds, clean and dry the wound and surrounding skin carefully before applying ointment.

ELASE'S OTHER NAMES

Elase is a combination of two generic drugs: fibrinolysin and desoxyribonuclease.

SIDE EFFECTS

Call your doctor if you have any of these possible drug side effects.

Serious: none reported

Common: redness

Other: allergic reaction (redness with warmth, itching, or burning in treated area)

DRUG INTERACTIONS

Combining certain drugs may alter their action or produce unwanted side effects. Tell your doctor about other drugs you're taking.

• Apply a thin layer of ointment to the wound and cover with the prescribed dressing.

• Change the dressing at least once a day; wash away ointment and debris before reapplying ointment.

• For vaginal use, apply ointment with vaginal applicator as directed. Then insert a tampon. Remove the tampon before the next dose of ointment. Insert a new tampon after each dose.

• Store the ointment away from direct light and warmth.

If you miss a dose

Apply the missed dose as soon as possible. However, if it's almost time for your next dose, skip the missed dose and apply your next dose as scheduled. Don't apply a double dose.

If you suspect an overdose

Consult your doctor.

Warnings

• Make sure your doctor knows your medical history. Other medical conditions may affect your use of Elase.

• If you're nursing an infant, make sure you clean your breast thoroughly before beginning breastfeeding.

KEEP IN MIND...

* Keep ointment away from eyes.
* Clean and dry the wound before applying ointment.
* Change dressing at least once a day.
* Insert a fresh tampon after each vaginal application.
* Call your doctor if you notice such symptoms as redness, itching, warmth, or burning.

Elavil

E lavil is a tricyclic antidepressant that works primarily by maintaining levels of mood-altering chemicals in the brain.

Why it's prescribed

Doctors prescribe Elavil to relieve depression. It comes in tablets and syrup. Doctors usually prescribe the following amounts.

▶ **For depression,** in adults, 50 to 100 milligrams (mg) at bedtime, increased if needed. Maximum dosage is 300 mg a day. In older adults and adolescents, 10 mg three times a day and 20 mg at bedtime.

How to take Elavil

- Take Elavil exactly as directed.
- Take each dose with food.
- Don't stop taking Elavil abruptly. You may need to take it for several weeks before you begin to feel better.

If you miss a dose

Don't take a double dose. Adjust your schedule as follows:
- If you take one dose a day at bedtime and you miss a dose, don't take the missed dose in the morning. Call your doctor for directions.
- If you take more than one dose daily, take the missed dose as soon as possible. If it's almost time for your next dose, skip the missed dose and go back to your regular schedule.

ELAVIL'S OTHER NAMES

Elavil's generic name is amitriptyline. Other brand names include Emitrip, Endep, Enovil; and, in Canada, Apo-Amitriptyline, Levate, and Novotriptyn.

SIDE EFFECTS

Call your doctor if you have any of these possible drug side effects. Call *immediately* about any labeled "serious."

Serious: fast or irregular heartbeat, palpitations, heart attack (chest or arm pain, shortness of breath), congestive heart failure (shortness of breath, fatigue), seizures

Common: drowsiness, low blood pressure (dizziness, weakness), blurred vision, dry mouth, constipation, inability to urinate
Tips: Prevent dizziness by standing up slowly. Avoid activities that require alertness until you know how Elavil affects you. Relieve dry mouth with sugarless gum or hard candy, ice chips, or a saliva substitute. Avoid constipation by increasing fluids and fiber-rich foods in your diet.

Other: excitation, tremor, weakness, confusion, headache, nervousness, high blood pressure (headache, blurred vision), ringing in ears, nausea, vomiting, lack of appetite, rash, hives, skin sensitivity to sun, sweating
Tip: Wear protective clothing and use sunblock outdoors.

DRUG INTERACTIONS

Combining certain drugs may alter their action or produce unwanted side effects. Tell your doctor about other drugs you're taking, especially:
- Adrenalin
- alcohol
- antidepressants called MAO inhibitors, such as Marplan and Pamelor
- barbiturates such as Solfoton
- nonprescription drugs, especially for treating colds and allergies
- Ritalin
- Tagamet.

If you suspect an overdose

Contact your doctor *immediately.* Excessive Elavil can cause irregular heartbeats, inadequate breathing, and seizures.

Warnings

- Make sure your doctor knows your medical history. You may not be able to take this drug if you've had a recent heart attack or have seizures, inability to urinate, glaucoma, an overactive thyroid, heart or liver disease, or diabetes.

KEEP IN MIND...

* Stand up slowly to avoid dizziness.
* Protect skin from sun.
* Don't stop taking abruptly.

Eldepryl

Eldepryl is one of several drugs called monoamine oxidase (MAO) inhibitors. It acts on neurotransmitters — chemicals found mostly in the brain that affect movement.

Why it's prescribed

Doctors prescribe Eldepryl, usually along with a drug called Sinemet, to help manage the symptoms of Parkinson's disease. Eldepryl comes in tablets. Doctors usually prescribe the following amounts for adults.

▶ **To treat Parkinson's disease along with Sinemet,** 10 milligrams (mg) daily, divided into two equal doses. After 2 or 3 days of therapy, the doctor may gradually decrease the Sinemet dosage.

How to take Eldepryl

• Take the drug exactly as prescribed: 5 mg with breakfast and 5 mg with lunch.
• If you're also taking Sinemet, take both drugs at the same time.

If you miss a dose

Take the missed dose as soon as possible. However, if it's almost time for your next dose, skip the missed dose and take your next dose as scheduled. Don't take a double dose.

 If you suspect an overdose

Contact your doctor *immediately.* Excessive Eldepryl may cause low blood pressure (dizziness, weakness), agitation, and possibly sei-

ELDEPRYL'S OTHER NAME

Eldepryl's generic name is selegiline hydrochloride.

 SIDE EFFECTS

Call your doctor if you have any of these possible drug side effects. Call *immediately* about any labeled "serious."

Serious: fast or irregular heartbeat, palpitations, chest pain, severe headache

Common: dizziness, nausea
Tip: Stand up slowly to avoid dizziness, especially early in therapy.

Other: increased tremor and involuntary movements, loss of balance, restlessness, increased slowness, added difficulty with voluntary movements, facial grimacing, stiff neck, twitching, behavioral changes, fatigue, low blood pressure (dizziness, weakness), high blood pressure (headache, blurred vision), swelling of feet or hands, fainting, dry mouth, impaired sense of taste, vomiting, constipation, weight loss, poor appetite, difficulty swallowing, diarrhea, heartburn, enlarged prostate, sexual dysfunction, rash, hair loss, sweating, difficulty urinating, increased, decreased, or nighttime urination
Tip: For mouth dryness, use sugarless gum or hard candy or ice chips. If dryness continues more than 2 weeks, tell your doctor.

 DRUG AND FOOD INTERACTIONS

Combining certain drugs and certain foods may alter drug action or produce unwanted side effects. Tell your doctor about your diet and other drugs you're taking, especially:
• Demerol
• drugs that stimulate the nervous system, such as Bronkaid Mist, Catapres, and Neo-Synephrine
• foods high in the amino acid tyramine, including fermented foods, over-ripe fruit, and others (ask your doctor for a list).

zures, heart abnormalities, and coma.

 Warnings

• Make sure your doctor knows your medical history. Other medical conditions may affect your use of Eldepryl.
• Don't increase the amount you're taking. Taking more than 10 mg of Eldepryl a day will not improve its effect and may increase side effects.

• If any side effects become severe or last longer than 2 weeks, call your doctor.

 KEEP IN MIND...

∗ Don't take more than the prescribed amount.
∗ Avoid foods high in tyramine.
∗ Stand up slowly to avoid dizziness.

Elocon

Elocon is one of many drugs known as steroids or corticosteroids. Steroids are natural or man-made hormones that influence or control key processes throughout the body.

Why it's prescribed

Doctors prescribe Elocon to control the redness, itching, and inflammation associated with skin problems. Elocon is considered a medium-strength corticosteroid. It comes in a cream, a lotion, and an ointment. Doctors usually prescribe the following amounts for adults.

▶ **To relieve redness, itching, and swelling,** apply a thin film of cream or ointment to affected areas once a day. If you're using lotion, apply a few drops to affected areas and rub the lotion in until it disappears.

How to use Elocon

• Gently wash skin before applying Elocon.
• To prevent skin damage, rub it in gently.
• When treating hairy sites, part hair and apply directly to the skin.
• Avoid applying Elocon near your eyes or mucous membranes or in your ear canal.
• Leave the area unbandaged unless your doctor directs otherwise.
• If your doctor instructs you to use Elocon on a baby's diaper area, don't cover the medicated area with plastic pants or a tight diaper.

ELOCON'S OTHER NAME

Elocon's generic name is mometasone furoate.

 SIDE EFFECTS

Call your doctor if you have any of these possible drug side effects. Call *immediately* about any labeled "serious."

Serious: hormone suppression (decreased ability of body to cope with stress such as illness or surgery); painful, red skin; severe skin burning or blistering

Common: none reported

Other: burning, redness, itching, tissue shrinkage, skin irritation, acnelike eruptions, loss of pigmentation, allergic skin rash, high blood sugar (increased thirst, hunger, and urination; weight loss), high blood pressure (headache, blurred vision), weight gain, facial swelling

 DRUG INTERACTIONS

Combining certain drugs may alter their action or produce unwanted side effects. Tell your doctor about other drugs you're taking.

• Be sure to wash your hands after applying Elocon.

If you miss a dose

Apply the missed dose as soon as possible. However, if it's almost time for your next dose, skip the missed dose and apply your next dose as scheduled. Don't apply a double dose.

 If you suspect an overdose

Contact your doctor *immediately.* Excessive Elocon can cause high blood pressure (headache, blurred vision), weight gain, facial swelling, and high blood sugar (weight loss, increased hunger, thirst, and urination).

Warnings

• Make sure your doctor knows your medical history. Other medical conditions may affect your use of Elocon.
• If you need an antibiotic or antifungal drug to control an infection, stop using Elocon until the other infection is controlled, as directed by your doctor.
• Don't use leftover Elocon for other skin problems unless your doctor approves. And don't share leftover Elocon with friends or family.

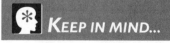 **KEEP IN MIND...**

∗ Use exactly the amount prescribed.

∗ Wash your hands after application.

∗ Leave the area unbandaged unless directed otherwise.

∗ Tell your doctor if you have skin ulcers or infection.

Emete-Con appears to affect the vomiting center of the brain, although the exact way it works is unknown.

Why it's prescribed

Doctors prescribe Emete-Con to control nausea and vomiting associated with anesthesia and surgery. It comes only in an injectable form for injection into a vein (intravenous injection) or a muscle (intramuscular injection).

▶ For nausea and vomiting after surgery, 50 milligrams by intramuscular injection; may be repeated in 1 hour, then every 3 to 4 hours as needed.

How to take Emete-Con

• A nurse or doctor will give you this drug.
• You'll probably receive the injection in a large muscle, such as the upper arm.
• The drug begins to take effect within 30 minutes. Effects last for 3 to 4 hours.
• Keep in mind the location of each injection, so that you can help in rotating injection sites to avoid pain and inflammation.

If you miss a dose

Not applicable because this drug is given only as needed.

EMETE-CON'S OTHER NAME

Emete-Con's generic name is benzquinamide hydrochloride.

SIDE EFFECTS

Call your doctor if you have any of these possible drug side effects. Call *immediately* about any labeled "serious."

Serious: irregular heartbeat (palpitations), high blood pressure (headache, blurred vision), low blood pressure (dizziness, weakness)

Common: drowsiness, fatigue, insomnia, restlessness, dizziness, dry mouth

Tips: To avoid dizziness, lie down after receiving Emete-Con. To relieve dry mouth, try ice chips or sugarless candy or gum.

Other: excitation, tremor, twitching, salivation, appetite loss, nausea, hives, rash, muscle weakness, flushing, hiccups, sweating, chills, fever, appetite and weight loss

DRUG INTERACTIONS

Combining certain drugs may alter their action or produce unwanted side effects. Tell your doctor about other drugs you're taking, especially:
• epinephrine (in nasal sprays).

If you suspect an overdose

Contact your doctor *immediately.* Excessive Emete-Con can cause drowsiness, restlessness, excitement, and nervousness.

Warnings

• Make sure your doctor knows your medical history. You may not be able to take Emete-Con if you have other medical problems, such as heart or blood vessel disease, irregular heartbeats, high blood pressure, a brain tumor, or intestinal obstruction.

• Use of Emete-Con during pregnancy and use in children are not recommended.
• Be aware that Emete-Con may mask symptoms of drug-induced hearing problems, brain tumor, or intestinal obstruction.

KEEP IN MIND...

* Don't use during pregnancy.
* Be aware of potential for dizziness.
* Lie down after receiving drug.
* May cause dry mouth.

Empirin with Codeine

Empirin with Codeine is a combination of aspirin and codeine. Researchers believe that the drug blocks pain impulses from reaching the brain.

Why it's prescribed

Doctors prescribe Empirin with Codeine to treat mild to moderately severe pain when nonprescription pain relievers are ineffective. It comes in tablets of varying strengths. Doctors usually prescribe the following amounts for adults.

▶ **For pain,** 1 or 2 tablets every 4 hours as needed.

How to take Empirin with Codeine

• Take Empirin with Codeine exactly as your doctor directs. This drug can become habit-forming, so don't take more than prescribed.
• To reduce stomach irritation, take this drug with food, milk, or water.
• Don't suddenly stop taking this drug after long-term use. Your doctor may reduce your dosage gradually to avoid withdrawal effects.

If you miss a dose

Not applicable because Empirin with Codeine is taken as needed.

If you suspect an overdose

Contact your doctor *immediately*. Excessive Empirin with Codeine can cause slow, shallow breathing;

EMPIRIN WITH CODEINE'S OTHER NAMES

Empirin with Codeine is a combination of two generic drugs: aspirin and codeine.

SIDE EFFECTS

Call your doctor if you have any of these possible drug side effects. Call *immediately* about any labeled "serious."

Serious: allergic reaction (trouble breathing, itching, rash), bone marrow suppression (fatigue, bleeding, bruising), fast pulse, hearing problems, ringing in ears, physical or psychological dependence on drug

Common: dizziness, shortness of breath, constipation, nausea, vomiting
Tips: To avoid dizziness, get up slowly from a sitting or lying position. To avoid constipation, drink more fluids and eat more high-fiber foods.

Other: headache, feeling of well-being, rash, itching, sweating, thirst, gout attack

DRUG INTERACTIONS

Combining certain drugs may alter their action or produce unwanted side effects. Tell your doctor about other drugs you're taking, especially:
• alcohol and drugs that slow down the central nervous system, such as muscle relaxants, narcotic pain relievers, cold and allergy drugs, seizure drugs, tranquilizers, and sleeping pills
• antacids
• anticoagulants (blood thinners) such as Coumadin
• diabetes drugs
• drugs that contain aspirin (such as Pepto-Bismol)
• Tylenol.

double vision, skin problems, garbled speech, hallucinations, and decreased consciousness (difficulty waking).

Warnings

• Make sure your doctor knows your medical history. You may not be able to take Empirin with Codeine if you've had an allergic reaction to aspirin or codeine or if you have gout or gallbladder disease.
• If you're pregnant or breast-feeding, tell the doctor before you take this drug.
• Be aware that older adults and children are especially sensitive to the effects of this drug. Never give this drug or any drug containing aspirin to a child or teenager who has a fever or other signs of a viral infection, such as chickenpox or flu, to reduce the risk of developing a potentially fatal disorder called Reye's syndrome.

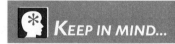 KEEP IN MIND...

* Take with food or fluids.

* Don't stop taking suddenly after long-term therapy.

* Don't take other products that contain aspirin.

E-Mycin

E-Mycin, an antibiotic, fights infection by preventing bacteria from reproducing.

Why it's prescribed

Doctors prescribe E-Mycin to treat a variety of infections. It comes in delayed-release tablets. Doctors usually prescribe the following amounts for adults; children's dosages are in parentheses.

▶ **For gonorrhea,** 250 milligrams (mg) every 6 hours for 7 days. Or 333 mg every 8 hours for 7 days.

▶ **To prevent endocarditis (heart valve infection) after dental procedures,** 1 gram (g) 1 hour before the procedure, then 500 mg 6 hours later. (Children: 20 mg for each 2.2 pounds [lb] of body weight 1 hour before the procedure, then 10 mg for each 2.2 lb 6 hours after.)

▶ **For intestinal amebiasis; respiratory, skin, and soft-tissue infections; syphilis; Legionnaire's disease; urinary tract, cervical, or rectal infection; and *Chlamydia* infection during pregnancy,** usually 250 mg every 6 hours, or 333 mg every 8 hours, or 500 mg every 12 hours. Dosage may be increased depending on nature and severity of infection. (Children: 30 to 50 mg for each 2.2 lb per day divided into equal doses. Dose may be doubled for severe infection.)

How to take E-Mycin

• Take all of the drug exactly as prescribed; no more, no less.

E-MYCIN'S OTHER NAMES

E-Mycin's generic name is oral erythromycin base. Other brand names include ERYC, PCE; and, in Canada, Apo-Erythro, Erybid, Erythromid, and Novo-rythro Encap.

 SIDE EFFECTS

Call your doctor if you have any of these possible drug side effects. Call *immediately* about any labeled "serious."

Serious: allergic reaction (severe facial and throat swelling, difficulty breathing, hives, rash)

Common: abdominal pain and cramping, nausea, vomiting, diarrhea
Tip: If the drug upsets your stomach, take it with food or milk, but not fruit juice.

Other: none reported

 DRUG INTERACTIONS

Combining certain drugs may alter their action or produce unwanted side effects. Tell your doctor about other drugs you're taking, especially:
• antibiotics, such as Cleocin and Lincocin
• anticoagulants (blood thinners) such as Coumadin
• Halcion, Versed
• Hismanal, Seldane, Theo-Dur
• Sandimmune
• Tegretol.

• Take E-Mycin with a full (8-ounce) glass of water 1 hour before meals or 2 hours after.
• Swallow the capsules whole.
• Finish all of the drug; don't stop early.

If you miss a dose

Take the missed dose as soon as possible. But don't take a double dose. If it's almost time for your next dose, adjust your schedule as follows, then resume your regular schedule.
• If you take two doses a day, space the missed dose and the next one 5 to 6 hours apart.
• If you take three or more doses a day, space the missed dose and the next one 2 to 4 hours apart.

If you suspect an overdose

Consult your doctor.

 Warnings

• Make sure your doctor knows your medical history. You may not be able to take E-Mycin if you have liver disease or a food or drug allergy.
• Tell the doctor that you're taking E-Mycin before any medical tests.

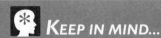 **KEEP IN MIND...**

* Take with water 1 hour before or 2 hours after meals.

* Reduce stomach upset by taking with food or milk, but not fruit juice.

* Report any trouble breathing.

Entex

Entex, a decongestant, narrows blood vessels in the nose, which thins secretions and clears nasal passages.

Why it's prescribed

Doctors prescribe Entex to relieve nasal congestion and clear thick mucus secretions that accompany sinus infection (sinusitis), lung infection (bronchitis), and throat infection (pharyngitis). It comes in capsules and liquid; Entex LA (long-acting) comes in tablets. Doctors usually prescribe the following amounts.

▶ **To relieve nasal congestion and thick mucus secretions,** in adults and children over age 12, 2 teaspoons (tsp) every 6 hours. For children ages 6 to 12, 1½ tsp; ages 4 to 6, 1 tsp; ages 2 to 4, ½ tsp. Not recommended for children under age 2. For Entex LA, in adults and children over age 12, 1 tablet every 12 hours; children ages 6 to 12, ½ tablet every 12 hours. Entex LA is not recommended for children under age 6.

How to take Entex

• Take Entex only as your doctor prescribes.
• Take each dose with fluid or food.

ENTEX'S OTHER NAMES

Entex is a combination of three generic drugs: phenylephrine hydrochloride, phenylpropanolamine hydrochloride, and guaifenesin. Other brand names include Banex Liquid, Despec, Dura-Gest, and Enomine.

 SIDE EFFECTS

Call your doctor if you have any of these possible drug side effects.

Serious: none reported

Common: nervousness, headache, nausea, insomnia, stomach irritation
Tips: Don't drive or perform other hazardous activities until you know how Entex affects you. Take it with food to avoid stomach irritation.

Other: inability to urinate (in men with an enlarged prostate)

 DRUG INTERACTIONS

Combining certain drugs may alter their action or produce unwanted side effects. Tell your doctor about other drugs you're taking, especially:
• antidepressants called MAO inhibitors, such as Nardil and Parnate.

• Don't crush or chew the capsules before swallowing them.
• Don't increase the amount or frequency of your dosage without consulting your doctor.

If you miss a dose

Take the missed dose as soon as possible. However, if it's almost time for your next dose, skip the missed dose and take your next dose as scheduled. Don't take a double dose.

 If you suspect an overdose

Contact your doctor *immediately*. Excessive Entex can cause high blood pressure (headache, blurred vision), fluttering feeling in the chest, vomiting, and numbness in the hands and feet.

 Warnings

• Make sure your doctor knows your medical history. You may not be able to take Entex if you have high blood pressure, diabetes, heart disease, an overactive thyroid, an enlarged prostate, or increased pressure in the eyes.
• If you're pregnant or breast-feeding, check with your doctor before taking this drug.
• Don't give Entex to children under age 2 or Entex LA to children under age 6.
• Be aware that older adults may be especially prone to Entex's side effects.

KEEP IN MIND...

* Don't crush or chew capsules.
* Take with food or fluid to avoid stomach irritation.
* Don't change dosage or frequency.
* Don't give to children under age 2.

Epifrin

Epifrin dilates the pupil of the eye by contracting its dilator muscle. The pupil dilates within a few minutes, which leads to a decrease in pressure within the eye.

Why it's prescribed

Doctors prescribe Epifrin to reduce pressure inside the eye (intraocular pressure) for people who have open-angle glaucoma. It comes as eyedrops. Doctors usually prescribe the following amounts for adults.

▶ **To reduce intraocular pressure in open-angle glaucoma,** 1 drop of 0.25%, 0.5%, 1%, or 2% solution once or twice a day.

How to use Epifrin

• Use the eyedrops exactly as your doctor directs.
• Wash your hands before and after using the eyedrops.
• Don't use Epifrin if the solution has darkened.
• Don't use Epifrin while wearing soft contact lenses; the lenses may discolor.
• To avoid contaminating the eyedrops, don't touch the dropper to your eye or the surrounding area.
• Press a finger against each tear duct for 1 minute after putting the drops in your eyes.

If you miss a dose

Apply the missed dose as soon as possible. However, if it's almost time for your next dose, skip the missed dose and apply your next dose as scheduled. Don't apply a double dose.

 SIDE EFFECTS

Call your doctor if you have any of these possible drug side effects. Call *immediately* about any labeled "serious."

Serious: blurred or decreased vision, sweating, trembling, paleness, feeling faint, fast, irregular, or pounding heartbeat

Common: headache, brow ache, sensitivity to light, stinging, burning, red, or watery eyes when inserting the drops
Tip: If you have any eye symptoms right after using the drops, dab your eyes with a tissue, but don't rub them.

Other: none reported

 DRUG INTERACTIONS

Combining certain drugs may alter their action or produce unwanted side effects. Tell your doctor about other drugs you're taking, especially:
• antidepressants, including MAO inhibitors, such as Marplan and Nardil
• certain decongestants and asthma drugs
• cold and allergy drugs
• drugs that affect the heart rate, such as Cardura, Lanoxin, Lopressor, and Minipress
• other drugs that dilate the pupil or lower pressure in eyes
• thyroid drugs.

 If you suspect an overdose

Contact your doctor *immediately.* Excessive Epifrin can cause increased blood pressure (headache, weakness in arms and legs), severe anxiety, nausea, vomiting, dilated pupils, and pale, cool skin.

Warnings

• Make sure your doctor knows your medical history. You may not be able to use Epifrin if you're allergic to it or if you have any type of glaucoma, brain damage, or heart disease.
• Your doctor may want to take special precautions if you are elderly or you have diabetes, high blood pressure, Parkinson's disease, an overactive thyroid, bronchial asthma, or no lenses in your eyes (as after cataract surgery).
• Expect your doctor to check the pressure in your eyes regularly.

 KEEP IN MIND...

∗ Press a finger against each tear duct after using drops.
∗ Don't use if the solution has darkened.
∗ Don't wear your soft contact lenses during therapy.
∗ Have pressure in eyes checked regularly.

EPIFRIN'S OTHER NAMES

Epifrin's generic name is epinephrine hydrochloride. Another brand name is Glaucon.

EpiPen contains a ready-to-inject dose of epinephrine. Used only in an emergency, this pen-shaped injector shrinks dilated blood vessels, increases the heart rate, strengthens the heartbeat, and opens the breathing passages.

Why it's prescribed

Doctors prescribe EpiPen for use at the start of a breathing emergency. The drug quickly treats the breathing difficulty, rashes, hives, swelling, and other serious symptoms that characterize severe allergic reactions. The EpiPen injects epinephrine just under the skin or into a muscle. Doctors usually prescribe the following amounts for adults and children.

▶ **For severe allergic reactions,** 1 EpiPen (delivers 0.30 milligrams [mg] of drug) or EpiPen Jr. (delivers 0.15 mg) injected under the skin or into a muscle, repeated as needed.

How to use the EpiPen

• Use EpiPen only in an emergency, as prescribed by your doctor.
• Select an injection site such as the thigh or upper arm below the shoulder. Don't use the buttocks.
• Aiming the EpiPen at the selected spot, push the plunger to allow the drug to enter your body. Then remove the EpiPen.
• Massage the site after injection to hasten response to the drug.

EPIPEN'S OTHER NAMES

EpiPen contains the generic drug epinephrine. Another brand name is Anakit.

SIDE EFFECTS

Call your doctor if you have any of these possible drug side effects. Call *immediately* about any labeled "serious."

Serious: high blood pressure (severe headache, nosebleed, blurred vision), fast or irregular pulse

Common: nervousness, headache, palpitations

Other: tremor, euphoria, anxiety, cold hands and feet, vertigo, sweating, disorientation, agitation, chest pain, shortness of breath, pallor, increased blood sugar (increased thirst, hunger, urination; weight loss)

DRUG INTERACTIONS

Combining certain drugs may alter their action or produce unwanted side effects. Tell your doctor about other drugs you're taking, especially:
• antidepressants, including MAO inhibitors, such as Elavil and Pamelor
• cold and allergy drugs
• Dopar
• Dopram
• heart drugs called beta blockers such as Lopressor
• Ritalin
• Sanorex
• thyroid hormones (Thyroid USP).

• EpiPen takes effect rapidly. The effect lasts a short time.

If you miss a dose

Use Epi-Pen in an emergency only.

If you suspect an overdose

Contact your doctor *immediately.* Excessive epinephrine can cause a fast rise in blood pressure, bleeding in the head, difficulty breathing, chest pain, cough, and anxiety.

Warnings

• Make sure your doctor knows your medical history. You may not be able to use the EpiPen if you have other medical problems, especially glaucoma, heart problems, an overactive thyroid, high blood pressure, diabetes, or an allergy to sulfites.
• If you're allergic to insect bites, always carry your EpiPen when outdoors.
• Carry medical identification that specifies your allergy.

KEEP IN MIND...

∗ Massage site after injection.

∗ Use only for emergencies.

∗ Carry identification that specifies your allergy.

Epitol

Epitol limits seizure activity. The drug probably curbs seizure-triggering impulses at sites in the brain where a seizure begins.

Why it's prescribed

Doctors prescribe Epitol to control some types of seizures. It's also used to treat pain from trigeminal neuralgia (sharp bursts of facial pain). Epitol comes in tablets. Doctors usually prescribe the following amounts for adults; children's dosages appear in parentheses.

▶ **For generalized tonic-clonic and complex partial seizures (mixed seizure patterns),** initially, 200 milligrams (mg) twice a day, increased at weekly intervals by 200 mg a day, as needed, divided into equal doses taken at 6- to 8-hour intervals. Dosage adjusted to minimum effective level when seizures are controlled. Maximum dosage: 1.2 grams (g) a day. (Children over age 15: same as adults. Children ages 12 to 15: same as adults, except for maximum dosage, which is 1 g. Children under age 12: initially, 100 mg twice a day, increased at weekly intervals by 100 mg a day. Maximum dosage is 1 g a day.)

▶ **For pain of trigeminal neuralgia,** initially, 100 mg twice a day, increased by 100 mg every 12 hours until pain subsides. Maximum dosage is 1.2 g a day. Maintenance dosage is 200 to 400 mg twice a day.

EPITOL'S OTHER NAMES

Epitol's generic name is carbamazepine. Other brand names include Tegretol; and, in Canada, Apo-Carbamazepine and Novo-carbamaz.

SIDE EFFECTS

Call your doctor if you have any of these possible drug side effects. Call *immediately* about any labeled "serious."

Serious: infection (fever, sore throat, chills, cough), blood problem (bleeding, bruising, fatigue, increased risk of infection), worsening of seizures (usually in people who have mixed seizure types), congestive heart failure (shortness of breath, anxiety, chest pain), hepatitis (yellow-tinged skin and eyes, itching), Stevens-Johnson syndrome (reddened, burnlike rash), altered blood pressure, irregular heartbeat, fainting, water intoxication (lethargy, vomiting, confusion, hostility)

Common: dizziness, drowsiness, clumsiness, nausea, vomiting, mouth sores, rash
Tips: Avoid activities that require full alertness or coordination until you know how Epitol affects you. Call the doctor right away if you develop mouth sores or a rash.

Other: drowsiness, fatigue, conjunctivitis, dry mouth and throat, blurred or double vision, uncontrollable eye movements, abdominal pain, diarrhea, appetite loss, inflamed mouth or tongue, increased urination, difficulty urinating, impotence, decreased amount of urine, dark urine, pale stools

DRUG INTERACTIONS

Combining certain drugs may alter their action or produce unwanted side effects. Tell your doctor about other drugs you're taking, especially:
• alcohol and other drugs that make you feel relaxed or sleepy, such as tranquilizers, sleeping pills, and cold and allergy medicines
• birth control pills
• Calan
• Cardizem
• Coumadin
• Danocrine
• Darvon
• E-Mycin, Vibramycin, and similar antibiotics
• Eskalith, Haldol
• Laniazid
• MAO inhibitors such as Marplan (don't take within 14 days of taking Epitol)
• other drugs for seizures (Solfoton, Dilantin, Depakene, Mysoline)
• Tagamet
• Theo-Dur.

How to take Epitol

- Take Epitol with meals, exactly as prescribed.
- If you're taking Epitol for seizures, don't stop using it without consulting your doctor, who may reduce the dosage gradually.
- Keep tablets in their original container, tightly closed and away from moisture.

If you miss a dose

Take the missed dose as soon as possible. However, if it's almost time for your next dose, skip the missed dose and take your next dose as scheduled. Don't take a double dose. If you miss more than one dose a day, check with your doctor.

If you suspect an overdose

Contact your doctor *immediately*. Excessive Epitol can cause a change in appetite, irregular breathing, rapid pulse, seizures, and coma.

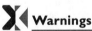 Warnings

- Make sure your doctor knows your medical history. You may not be able to take Epitol if you're allergic to it or to certain antidepressants, if you've taken an MAO inhibitor (a type of antidepressant) during the past 14 days, or if you have a history of bone marrow suppression.

- If you're pregnant or breast-feeding, consult your doctor before taking Epitol.
- If you're diabetic, monitor your blood sugar levels carefully. Epitol may alter them.
- Have regular checkups so the doctor can monitor your progress and make dosage changes. Also have regular eye exams during treatment.
- As a pain reliever, Epitol works only for certain kinds of pain. Don't take it for other types of discomfort.
- If you're taking Epitol for trigeminal neuralgia, your doctor will probably try to decrease your dosage or withdraw the drug every 3 months.
- Before medical tests, surgery, dental work, or emergency treatment, tell your doctor or dentist that you're taking Epitol.
- Carry or wear medical identification that says you're taking Epitol.

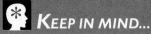

KEEP IN MIND...

* Take with meals.
* Store in tightly closed container away from moisture.
* Don't stop taking abruptly.
* Have regular eye and medical exams.

Epogen

E pogen is a man-made version of erythropoietin, a chemical that tells the body to make red blood cells. If there's not enough erythropoietin in the body, it won't make enough red blood cells, which can lead to severe anemia.

Why it's prescribed

Doctors prescribe Epogen to treat anemia caused by malfunctioning kidneys. It comes in an injectable form. Doctors usually prescribe the following amounts for adults.

▶ **For anemia associated with chronic kidney failure,** initially, 50 to 100 units for each 2.2 pounds (lb) of body weight three times a week. The dosage depends on the level of red blood cells.

▶ **For anemia in HIV-infected people treated with zidovudine,** 100 units for each 2.2 lb of body weight three times a week for 8 weeks or until the target level of red blood cells is reached.

▶ **For anemia related to cancer chemotherapy,** 150 units for each 2.2 lb of body weight three times a week for 8 weeks or until the target level of red blood cells is reached.

How to use Epogen

• When giving yourself injections, follow your doctor's instructions exactly. Epogen is injected just under the skin (subcutaneously).

EPOGEN'S OTHER NAMES

Epogen's generic name is epoetin alfa. Another brand name is Procrit.

 ## SIDE EFFECTS

Call your doctor if you have any of these possible drug side effects. Call *immediately* about any labeled "serious."

Serious: seizures, chest pain, shortness of breath, high blood pressure (headache, blurred vision)

Tip: To help control your blood pressure, follow your diet restrictions or drug therapy carefully.

Common: pain or discomfort in long limb bones and pelvis, sweating, chills (within 2 hours of an injection), iron deficiency (extreme fatigue), fast pulse, improved appetite

Tips: Most common side effects disappear after 12 hours. You may need supplemental iron therapy while taking Epogen.

Other: rash, hives, nausea, vomiting, diarrhea

 ## DRUG INTERACTIONS

Combining certain drugs may alter their action or produce unwanted side effects. Tell your doctor about other drugs you're taking.

If you miss a dose

Inject the missed dose as soon as possible. However, if it's almost time for the next dose, skip the missed dose and inject the next dose as scheduled. Don't inject a double dose.

 ## If you suspect an overdose

Contact your doctor *immediately.* Excessive Epogen can cause a blood disorder called polycythemia (headache, weakness, flushing, dizziness).

Warnings

• Make sure your doctor knows your medical history. You may not be able to use Epogen if you have a history of blood clots, heart disease, high blood pressure, bone problems, sickle-cell anemia, seizures, or an allergy to products derived from mammal cells.

• Your doctor will probably want to draw weekly blood specimens to monitor your red blood cell level.

 ## KEEP IN MIND...

∗ Give injections exactly as the doctor directs.

∗ Take an iron supplement if prescribed.

∗ Follow any special diet that the doctor prescribes.

Equanil relieves anxiety. The drug acts on parts of the nervous system.

Why it's prescribed

Doctors prescribe Equanil to help quell anxiety and nervous tension. It comes in tablets, capsules, and sustained-release capsules. Doctors usually prescribe the following amounts for adults and children over age 12; dosages for children ages 6 to 12 appear in parentheses.

▶ **For anxiety,** 1.2 to 1.6 grams (g) a day divided into three or four equal doses. Maximum dosage is 2.4 g a day. Or 400 to 800 milligrams (mg) of sustained-release capsules twice a day. (Children ages 6 to 12: 200 to 600 mg two or three times a day or 200 mg of sustained-release capsules twice a day.)

How to take Equanil

- Take exact amount prescribed.
- Take with food to reduce nausea.
- Don't stop taking Equanil abruptly after long-term therapy.

If you miss a dose

Take the missed dose as soon as possible. But if it's almost time for your next dose, skip the missed dose and take your next dose as scheduled. Don't take a double dose.

EQUANIL'S OTHER NAMES

Equanil's generic name is meprobamate. Other brand names include Meprospan, Miltown, Neuramate, Neurate, Probate, Sedabamate, SK-Bamate, Trancot, Tranmep; and, in Canada, Apo-Meprobamate, Meditran, Meprospan, and Novomepro.

SIDE EFFECTS

Call your doctor if you have any of these possible drug side effects. Call *immediately* about any labeled "serious."

Serious: severe anemia (fatigue), white-blood-cell deficiency (chills, fever, sore throat), low platelet count (bruising, bleeding), seizures (after stopping drug abruptly)

Common: drowsiness, dry mouth

Tips: Avoid activities that require full alertness or coordination until you know how Equanil affects you. For dry mouth, use sugarless gum or hard candy, ice chips, or a saliva substitute; if dryness continues more than 2 weeks, tell your doctor.

Other: slurred speech, headache, palpitations, rapid pulse, low blood pressure (dizziness, weakness), appetite loss, stomach upset, nausea, vomiting, diarrhea, inflammation of the mouth, itching, hives, rash

DRUG INTERACTIONS

Combining certain drugs may alter their action or produce unwanted side effects. Tell your doctor about other drugs you're taking, especially:

- alcohol and other drugs that depress the central nervous system, such as sedatives, tranquilizers, muscle relaxants, narcotic pain relievers, cold and allergy drugs, and seizure drugs
- antidepressants.

If you suspect an overdose

Contact your doctor *immediately.* Excessive Equanil can cause severe confusion, drowsiness, weakness, slurred speech, trouble breathing, staggering, slow heartbeat, unconsciousness, and death.

Warnings

- Make sure your doctor knows your medical history. You may not be able to take Equanil if you're allergic to similar drugs or if you have liver or kidney disease, seizures, suicidal tendencies, or an inherited disorder called porphyria.

- Don't take Equanil during pregnancy, especially the first trimester.
- Elderly or debilitated people usually receive a reduced dosage.
- Tell your doctor you're taking Equanil before having any lab tests.
- If you receive high doses of Equanil, your doctor will probably want to check your blood and your liver and kidney function periodically.

KEEP IN MIND...

- Take exact amount prescribed, preferably with food.
- Don't take if pregnant.
- Don't drink alcohol.

Ergamisol

Ergamisol is one of several drugs called immunomodulators. It helps restore a depressed immune system.

Why it's prescribed

Doctors prescribe Ergamisol in combination with a drug called Adrucil to treat people who have had surgery to remove certain colon cancers. Ergamisol comes in tablets. Doctors usually prescribe the following amounts for adults.

▶ **For treatment (along with Adrucil) of Dukes' stage C colon cancer after surgical removal,** 50 milligrams (mg) every 8 hours for 3 days, beginning 7 to 30 days after surgery, provided that the person is out of the hospital, moving about, and maintaining a normal diet; has well-healed wounds; and has recovered from any postoperative complications. Starting 21 to 34 days after surgery, Adrucil is given intravenously for 5 days along with the 3-day course of Ergamisol. Treatment then continues every 2 weeks for 1 year.

How to take Ergamisol

• Take Ergamisol exactly as prescribed.

If you miss a dose

Take the missed dose as soon as possible. However, if it's almost time for your next dose, skip the missed dose and take your next dose as scheduled. Don't take a double dose.

ERGAMISOL'S OTHER NAME

Ergamisol's generic name is levamisole hydrochloride.

 SIDE EFFECTS

Call your doctor if you have any of these possible drug side effects. Call *immediately* about any labeled "serious."

Serious: seizures, severe skin reaction, blood problems (chills, fever, signs of infection, easy bleeding or bruising)
Tip: Use a soft toothbrush and an electric razor to prevent excessive bleeding.

Common: dizziness, headache, pins-and-needles sensation, sleepiness, depression, nervousness, insomnia, anxiety, fatigue, altered taste or smell, nausea, vomiting, appetite loss, abdominal pain, diarrhea, mouth or lip sores, constipation, gas, stomach upset, dermatitis, itchiness, hives, hair loss, joint and muscle pain
Tips: If you develop diarrhea or swelling and inflammation in your mouth, notify your doctor, who will adjust your drug dosage. To prevent constipation, increase fluids and fiber in your diet.

Other: chest pain, swelling, blurred vision, conjunctivitis, shivering

 DRUG INTERACTIONS

Combining certain drugs may alter their action or produce unwanted side effects. Tell your doctor about other drugs you're taking, especially:
• alcohol
• anticoagulant drugs (blood thinners) such as Coumadin
• Dilantin.

If you suspect an overdose

Consult your doctor.

Warnings

• Make sure your doctor knows your medical history. You may not be able to take Ergamisol if you have liver or kidney disease.
• Your doctor will probably want to test your blood regularly during therapy. Be sure to keep all appointments.
• Try to avoid any contact with people who have infections.

• Tell your doctor if you develop unusual bruising or bleeding or persistent fever, sore throat, weakness, or other flulike symptoms.

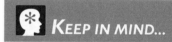 **KEEP IN MIND...**

* Take exactly as prescribed.
* Avoid people who have infections.
* Report flulike symptoms right away.

Ergostat

Ergostat relieves severe headache pain. It works by reducing the diameter of blood vessels and maintaining levels of certain chemicals in the brain.

Why it's prescribed

Doctors prescribe Ergostat to relieve migraine or cluster headaches. It comes in tablets to melt under your tongue, an inhaler, and suppositories. Doctors usually prescribe the following amounts for adults.

▶ **For cluster or migraine headache,** initially 2 milligrams (mg) orally or dissolved under the tongue, then 1 to 2 mg every hour orally (or every half-hour if dissolved under the tongue) to a maximum of 6 mg a day and 10 mg a week. If using an aerosol inhaler, 1 spray initially, repeated every 5 minutes as needed to a maximum of 6 sprays a day and 15 sprays a week. If using rectal suppositories, 1 suppository at start of the attack, repeated in 1 hour if needed. Maximum dosage is 2 suppositories per day, not more than 2 times a week.

How to take Ergostat

• Take Ergostat at the first sign of a headache. Then lie down in a quiet, dark room.
• While dissolving a tablet under your tongue, don't chew or swallow it, and don't eat, drink, or smoke.

ERGOSTAT'S OTHER NAMES

Ergostat's generic name is ergotamine tartrate. Other brand names include Ergomar, Medihaler-Ergotamine; and, in Canada, Gynergen.

 SIDE EFFECTS

Call your doctor if you have any of these possible drug side effects. Call *immediately* about any labeled "serious."

Serious: confusion, rapid or slow heartbeat, numbness or tingling in fingers or toes, shortness of breath, chest or stomach pain, bloating, weakness, leg swelling, increased headaches

Common: vomiting, abdominal cramps, itching, leg weakness, muscle pain

Other: diarrhea, dizziness, nausea, temporary changes in heart rhythm

 DRUG INTERACTIONS

Combining certain drugs may alter their action or produce unwanted side effects. Tell your doctor about other drugs you're taking, especially:
• alcohol
• antibiotics such as Ery-Tab
• any drug that causes excitement, difficulty sleeping, dry mouth, dizziness, or drowsiness
• epinephrine by injection (EpiPen)
• Inderal or other beta blockers (heart drugs).

• Don't take more than the prescribed amount of Ergostat without checking with your doctor.
• Don't stop taking this drug abruptly. Doing so could worsen your headaches.

If you miss a dose

Take the missed dose as soon as possible. However, if it's almost time for your next dose, skip the missed dose and take your next dose as scheduled. Don't take a double dose.

 If you suspect an overdose

Contact your doctor *immediately.* Excessive Ergostat can cause delirium, vomiting, severe shortness of breath, unconsciousness, and seizures.

Warnings

• Make sure your doctor knows your medical history. You may not be able to take Ergostat if you have high blood pressure or heart, blood vessel, kidney, liver, or thyroid disease.
• If you're pregnant or breast-feeding, check with your doctor before taking this drug.
• Avoid overexposure to cold weather because side effects may increase.

 KEEP IN MIND...

∗ Take at first sign of headache.
∗ Let tablets melt under tongue.
∗ Call doctor if fingers and toes tingle or become cold.

Ergotrate

Ergotrate belongs to a group of drugs called ergot alkaloids. It causes the muscles of the uterus to contract and shrinks associated blood vessels.

Why it's prescribed

Doctors prescribe Ergotrate after delivery, miscarriage, or abortion to prevent or treat excessive bleeding from the uterus. After an initial dose of Ergotrate by injection or intravenously, the doctor may prescribe tablets to take at home. Doctors usually prescribe the following amounts for adults.

▶ **For preventing or treating uterine bleeding,** 0.2 to 0.4 milligrams orally every 6 to 12 hours for 2 to 7 days.

How to take Ergotrate

• Don't take more of the drug or take it more often or for a longer time than prescribed.
• Store the drug in a light-resistant, airtight container. Don't take it if the tablets are discolored.

If you miss a dose

Skip the missed dose and take your next dose on schedule. Don't take a double dose.

If you suspect an overdose

Contact your doctor *immediately.* Excessive Ergotrate can cause vomiting, diarrhea, seizures, tingling and numbness in your hands and feet, and possibly gangrene.

ERGOTRATE'S OTHER NAME

Ergotrate's generic name is ergonovine.

 SIDE EFFECTS

Call your doctor if you have any of these possible drug side effects. Call *immediately* about any labeled "serious."

Serious: chest pain, blurred vision, seizures, wheezing or shortness of breath, irregular heartbeat, severe headache, rash

Common: uterine cramping, nausea, vomiting
Tip: Tell your doctor if you experience severe uterine cramps; your Ergotrate dose may need to be reduced.

Other: diarrhea, dizziness, mild headache, ringing in ears, stuffy nose, altered taste, sweating

 DRUG INTERACTIONS

Combining certain drugs may alter their action or produce unwanted side effects. Tell your doctor about other drugs you're taking, especially:
• certain anesthetics
• drugs for chest pain, such as Isordil and nitroglycerin
• other ergot alkaloids
• Parlodel
• tobacco.

Warnings

• Make sure your doctor knows your medical history. You may not be able to take Ergotrate if you have chest pain or other heart problems, blood vessel disease (such as Raynaud's disease), high blood pressure (now or in the past), toxemia, or kidney or liver disease; if you're overly sensitive to this drug; or if you have other drug or food allergies. Also report any new medical problems if they occur while taking this drug.
• If you're breast-feeding, check with your doctor before taking this drug.
• Make sure your doctor knows if you're on any special diet, such as a low-salt or low-sugar diet.

• If you have an infection, check with your doctor; Ergotrate's effect may be stronger.
• Don't smoke while taking Ergotrate; it may increase the risk of harmful side effects.
• If your bleeding doesn't slow down or if it becomes heavier, call your doctor as soon as possible.

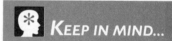 **KEEP IN MIND...**

* If the tablet is discolored, don't take it.
* Don't smoke while taking Ergotrate.
* Call doctor about severe cramps or continued bleeding.

Erycette

Erycette is a form of the antibiotic erythromycin that's applied to the skin. This drug kills certain types of bacteria.

Why it's prescribed

Doctors prescribe Erycette to control acne. It comes in an ointment, a gel, a swab, and a solution. Doctors usually prescribe the following amounts for adults and children.

▶ **For acne,** small amount applied to affected area twice a day.

How to use Erycette

• Before applying the ointment, wash the skin area gently with warm water and soap, rinse well, and pat dry.
• Apply drug to the whole area, not just to the lesions themselves.
• If you're using the ointment or gel, apply a thin film to cover the area lightly. If you're using the solution, dab Erycette on with an applicator tip or a moistened pad.
• After shaving, wait about 30 minutes before applying the swab, gel, or solution, because the alcohol in the drug may sting.
• Keep the drug away from your eyes, nose, and mouth. If you do get some in your eyes, immediately wash them out carefully with cool tap water.
• If you're using another drug on your skin along with Erycette, wait at

ERYCETTE'S OTHER NAMES

Erycette's generic name is topical erythromycin. Other brand names include Akne-Mycin, A/T/S, Del-Mycin, EryDerm, Erygel, Erymax, Ery-Sol, ETS, T-Stat; and, in Canada, Sans-Acne and Staticin.

SIDE EFFECTS

Call your doctor if you have any of these possible drug side effects. Call *immediately* about any labeled "serious."

Serious: severe allergic reaction (difficulty breathing, facial swelling)

Common: mild stinging
Tip: It's normal for your skin to sting somewhat after applying Erycette; if it continues to itch or burn, call your doctor.

Other: dry skin, itchiness, burning sensation, peeling, redness
Tip: Call the doctor if you develop a rash or dry or scaly skin.

DRUG INTERACTIONS

Combining certain drugs may alter their action or produce unwanted side effects. Tell your doctor about other drugs you're taking, especially:
• abrasive, astringent, or medicated soaps, cleansers, coverups, or cosmetics
• Accutane or other acne drugs that contain peeling agents
• alcohol.

least 1 hour before you apply the second drug to prevent skin irritation.
• It's important to use this drug exactly as prescribed; don't stop early and don't skip doses.

If you miss a dose

Apply the missed dose as soon as possible. However, if it's almost time for your next application, skip the missed dose and apply the next dose as scheduled. Don't apply a double dose.

If you suspect an overdose

Consult your doctor.

Warnings

• Make sure your doctor knows your medical history. You may not be able to use Erycette if you're allergic to any drug or food.

• Washing the affected area too often could dry your skin and make your acne worse. Wash with a mild, bland soap two or three times a day, unless you have oily skin. Check with your doctor for specific instructions.
• Wear only water-based cosmetics. Don't apply cosmetics heavily or frequently because your acne could worsen.
• Don't share your washcloths or towels with other people.

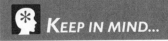

KEEP IN MIND...

* Apply drug to the whole area, not just to pimples.

* Avoid eyes, nose, and mouth.

* Call doctor if skin continues to burn and itch.

Ery-Tab

Ery-Tab, a form of the antibiotic erythromycin, fights infection by preventing bacteria from reproducing.

Why it's prescribed

Doctors prescribe Ery-Tab and other forms of erythromycin to treat a variety of infections. It comes in tablets, capsules, and an oral liquid. Doctors usually prescribe the following amounts for adults; children's dosages appear in parentheses.

▶ **For gonorrhea,** 250 milligrams (mg) every 6 hours for 7 days.

▶ To prevent endocarditis (heart valve infection) after dental procedures, 1 gram (g) 1 hour before the procedure, then 500 mg 6 hours later.

▶ **For intestinal amebiasis (parasitic infection); respiratory, skin, and soft-tissue infections; syphilis; Legionnaire's disease; urinary tract, cervical, or rectal infection; and *Chlamydia* infection,** usually 250 mg every 6 hours, or 333 mg every 8 hours, or 500 mg every 12 hours. Dosage may be increased, depending on nature and severity of infection. (Children: 30 to 50 mg for each 2.2 pounds [lb] of body weight per day in equally divided doses.)

▶ **For pneumonia in infants,** 50 mg for each 2.2 lb of body weight per day, divided into four equal doses, for at least 21 days.

ERY-TAB'S OTHER NAMES

Ery-Tab's generic name is oral erythromycin base. Other brand names include Eryc and PCE; and, in Canada, Apo-Erythro, Erybid, Eryc Sprinkle, Erythromid, and Novo-rythro.

SIDE EFFECTS

Call your doctor if you have any of these possible drug side effects. Call *immediately* about any labeled "serious."

Serious: severe allergic reaction (swelling in face and throat, difficulty breathing), rash or itchy skin

Common: abdominal pain and cramping, nausea, vomiting, diarrhea

Other: hives

DRUG INTERACTIONS

Combining certain drugs may alter their action or produce unwanted side effects. Tell your doctor about other drugs you're taking, especially:
- antibiotics, such as Cleocin and Lincocin
- anticoagulants (blood thinners) such as Coumadin
- Halcion, Tegretol, Theo-Dur
- Hismanal, Seldane
- Sandimmune.

How to take Ery-Tab

- Take all of the drug exactly as prescribed — no more, no less.
- Take it with a full (8-ounce) glass of water 1 hour before or 2 hours after meals.
- If the tablets are coated or the drug upsets your stomach, take the drug with food or milk. But don't take it with fruit juice.

If you miss a dose

Take the missed dose as soon as possible. If it's almost time for your next dose, and you take two doses a day, space the missed dose and the next one 5 to 6 hours apart. If you take three or more doses a day, space the missed dose and the next one 2 to 4 hours apart. Then resume your regular schedule.

 If you suspect an overdose

Consult your doctor.

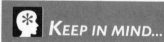

Warnings

- Make sure your doctor knows your medical history. You may not be able to take Ery-Tab if you have liver disease or if you're allergic to any antibiotic, another drug, or any food.
- Tell the doctor that you're taking Ery-Tab before you have medical tests because the drug may interfere with some test results.

KEEP IN MIND...

* Take entire prescription, even if you feel better.
* Take with water 1 hour before or 2 hours after meals.
* Tell your doctor if you have a rash or trouble breathing.

Eserine

Eserine contracts the muscles that control the iris, the colored portion of the eye. This dilates the pupils and reduces pressure in the eye.

Why it's prescribed

Doctors prescribe Eserine when pressure within the eye is abnormally high, as in glaucoma. Eserine comes in ointment (as sulfate) and eyedrops (as salicylate). Doctors usually prescribe the following amounts for adults and children.

▶ **For open-angle glaucoma,** 1 to 2 drops of solution in each eye two to four times a day, or a thin strip of ointment applied once or twice a day.

How to use Eserine

- Don't use the drug if the solution or ointment has darkened.
- Wash your hands before and after using Eserine.
- To avoid spreading infection, don't touch the applicator tip to your eye or to the surrounding skin.
- Don't exceed the prescribed dosage.
- Your doctor may have you use the ointment at night because of its longer period of action.
- Don't use any other eye preparation for at least 5 minutes after using eyedrops or 10 minutes after using ointment.

ESERINE'S OTHER NAMES

Eserine ointment's generic name is physostigmine sulfate. Another brand name is Isopto Eserine. Eserine solution's generic name is physostigmine salicylate.

 SIDE EFFECTS

Call your doctor if you have any of these possible drug side effects. Call *immediately* about any labeled "serious."

Serious: bronchial spasm (tightened airways, wheezing), pulmonary edema (shortness of breath, difficult breathing)

Common: blurred vision; pain in eyes, brows, and lids; sensitivity to light; cataracts (clouding of lens of the eye); reversible cysts (tiny fluid-filled sacs) in iris
Tip: Don't close your eye tightly or blink a lot just after using eyedrops.

Other: abdominal pain, diarrhea, excessive salivation
Tip: Avoid activities that require normal, sharp visual ability until you know how your body reacts to Eserine.

 DRUG INTERACTIONS

Combining certain drugs may alter their action or produce unwanted side effects. Tell your doctor about other drugs you're taking, especially:
- atropine sulfate
- drugs that slow heart rate, such as Duvoid and Pilocar
- Floropryl
- Inversine
- Phospholine Iodide.

If you miss a dose

Apply the missed dose as soon as possible. However, if it's almost time for your next dose, skip the missed dose and apply your next dose as scheduled. Don't use a double dose.

 If you suspect an overdose

Contact your doctor *immediately.* Excessive Eserine can cause headache, vomiting, diarrhea, asthmalike breathing attacks, restlessness, and confusion.

 Warnings

- Make sure your doctor knows your medical history. You may not be able to take Eserine if you're allergic to it or if you have an inflamed iris, a corneal injury, diabetes, intestinal or urinary tract obstruction, a slow heart rate, low blood pressure, or an allergy to sulfites.
- Keep all appointments so your doctor can check the pressure in your eyes.

 KEEP IN MIND...

* Don't use if solution or ointment darkens.
* Wash your hands before and after use.
* Avoid excessive blinking after using ointment.

Eskalith

Eskalith helps stabilize the condition of a person with manic-depressive illness (bipolar disorder) during the excited, or manic, state. It seems to work by reducing the amount of certain natural chemicals, which may be excessive during manic states.

Why it's prescribed

Doctors prescribe Eskalith to prevent or control mania, which typically causes an unusual sense of well-being or excessive anger or irritability in people with manic-depressive illness. Eskalith comes in capsules and controlled-release tablets (Eskalith CR). Doctors usually prescribe the following amounts for adults.

▶ **To prevent or control mania,** 300 milligrams (mg) three or four times a day, or 450 mg of Eskalith CR twice a day, increased as needed.

How to take Eskalith

• Take this drug exactly as your doctor directs.
• If you're taking controlled-release tablets, swallow them whole. Don't crush, break, or chew them.

If you miss a dose

Take the missed dose as soon as possible. However, if it's within 4 hours of the next dose (6 hours for controlled-release tablets), skip the

ESKALITH'S OTHER NAMES

Eskalith's generic name is lithium carbonate. Other brand names include Eskalith CR, Lithane, Lithobid, Lithonate; and, in Canada, Carbolith, Duralith, and Lithizine.

 SIDE EFFECTS

Call your doctor if you have any of these possible drug side effects. Call *immediately* about any labeled "serious."

Serious: coma, irregular heartbeats, dangerously low blood pressure leading to peripheral vascular collapse (dizziness; cold, discolored fingers or toes)

Common: frequent urination, headache, dizziness

Other: tremor, drowsiness, confusion, restlessness, extreme tiredness, muscle weakness, impaired speech, poor coordination, ringing in ears, blurred vision, dry mouth, metallic taste, sudden weight gain or swelling, nausea, vomiting, appetite loss, diarrhea, thirst, stomach upset, gas, rash, itching, diminished or absent sensation, hair loss, psoriasis, acne, increased blood sugar level (increased thirst, hunger, and urination), goiter, underactive thyroid (dry, rough skin; hair loss; feeling cold or sluggish), salt deficiency (abdominal cramps, extreme tiredness)
Tips: To help prevent upset stomach, take this drug with plenty of water and after meals. Weigh yourself regularly; call the doctor if you notice a sudden weight gain or swelling. Avoid driving and other activities that require alertness and good coordination until you know how you react to Eskalith.

 DRUG INTERACTIONS

Combining certain drugs may alter their action or produce unwanted side effects. Tell your doctor about other drugs you're taking, especially:
• Aldomet
• Amoline
• Benemid
• diuretics (water pills)
• nonsteroidal anti-inflammatory drugs, such as Advil
• sedatives, tranquilizers, and other drugs that cause sedation or reduce anxiety
• Tegretol
• thyroid hormones
• urine alkalinizers, such as sodium bicarbonate (baking soda) and sodium lactate.

missed dose and take the next dose as scheduled. Don't take a double dose.

 If you suspect an overdose

Contact your doctor *immediately*. Excessive Eskalith can cause vomiting, diarrhea, and death. A less severe overdose can cause extreme sleepiness, confusion, hand tremors, joint pain, poor coordination, stiff muscles, vision problems, seizures, extremely low blood pressure (severe dizziness and weakness;

cold, discolored fingers and toes), and coma.

✕ Warnings

• Make sure your doctor knows your medical history. You may not be able to take Eskalith if you have other problems, such as schizophrenia, diabetes, difficulty urinating, infection, kidney disease, heart disease, seizures, a thyroid disorder, Parkinson's disease, or psoriasis, or if you have a history of leukemia.
• Don't take this drug if you're pregnant.
• If you're breast-feeding, tell your doctor before you start taking Eskalith.
• Be aware that this drug may cause weak bones in children.
• Be aware that older adults may be especially prone to Eskalith's side effects.

• If you're diabetic, be aware that your insulin dosage may need to be changed after you start taking Eskalith.
• Call your doctor if you have an infection or illness that causes heavy sweating, vomiting, or diarrhea.
• Drink 2 to 3 quarts of fluid a day and use a normal amount of salt in your food, unless your doctor tells you otherwise.
• Don't go on a diet without first checking with your doctor.
• Keep medical appointments so your doctor can check drug effects and measure the amount of Eskalith in your blood.
• Carry medical identification stating that you're taking Eskalith.

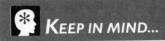

KEEP IN MIND...

∗ Take with plenty of water and after meals.

∗ Drink 2 to 3 quarts of fluid a day and use normal amount of salt in food.

∗ Avoid driving and other activities requiring alertness until your reaction to drug is known.

∗ Don't go on diet unless doctor approves.

∗ Call your doctor if you notice a sudden weight gain.

Estinyl

Estinyl mimics the action of natural estrogen, a female sex hormone.

Why it's prescribed

Doctors prescribe Estinyl to treat breast cancer (at least 5 years after menopause), deficient ovary function, menopausal symptoms, and some types of prostate cancer in men. Estinyl comes in tablets. Doctors usually prescribe the following amounts for adults.

▶ **For postmenopausal breast cancer,** 1 milligram (mg) three times a day for at least 3 months.

▶ **For deficient ovary function,** 0.05 mg once to three times a day for 2 weeks each month, followed by 2 weeks of progesterone therapy; continued for 3 to 6 months, followed by 2 months off.

▶ **For menopausal symptoms,** 0.02 to 0.05 mg a day for cycles of 3 weeks on, 1 week off.

▶ **For inoperable prostate cancer,** 0.15 to 2 mg a day.

How to take Estinyl

- Take Estinyl exactly as prescribed.
- Take it at the same time each day.
- To reduce nausea, take with food.

If you miss a dose

Take the missed dose as soon as possible. But if it's almost time for your next dose, skip the missed dose and take your next dose as scheduled. Don't take a double dose.

ESTINYL'S OTHER NAME

Estinyl's generic name is ethinyl estradiol.

SIDE EFFECTS

Call your doctor if you have any of these possible drug side effects. Call *immediately* about any labeled "serious."

Serious: sudden pain in chest or leg, shortness of breath, vision changes, or pain, numbness, or stiffness in legs or buttocks (typical of blood clots); abdominal pain; chest pain or pressure; swelling of hands or feet; yellow-tinged skin or eyes; dark urine; light-colored stools

Common: nausea, bloating or abdominal cramps, headache

Other: dizziness, involuntary movements, depression, lethargy, vomiting, diarrhea, constipation, appetite gain or loss, weight change, altered menstrual cycle, yeast infection, testicular atrophy or impotence, hives, acne, oily skin, hair growth or loss, breast changes (tenderness, enlargement, secretions), increased blood sugar (increased thirst, hunger, and urination), change in sex drive

DRUG INTERACTIONS

Combining certain drugs may alter their action or produce unwanted side effects. Tell your doctor about other drugs you're taking, especially:
- antibiotics
- anticoagulants (blood thinners) such as Coumadin
- Dantrium, Sandimmune, and other drugs that may damage the liver
- Nolvadex, Parlodel, Rifadin
- seizure drugs, such as Solfoton and Tegretol
- steroids.

If you suspect an overdose

Consult your doctor.

Warnings

- Make sure your doctor knows your medical history. You may not be able to take Estinyl if you're pregnant or if you've had blood clots, estrogen-related tumors, breast or reproductive organ cancer, menstrual abnormalities, asthma, depression, or heart, liver, kidney, or bone disease.
- Tell the doctor if you have a family history of breast or genital cancer, breast nodules, fibrocystic disease, or abnormal mammograms.
- If you're taking Estinyl for menopausal symptoms, you may bleed during the week you're off the drug.
- Examine your breasts regularly.

KEEP IN MIND...

* Take at same time each day.
* Take with food to reduce nausea.
* Examine breasts regularly.

Estrace

Estrace mimics the action of natural estrogen, a female sex hormone.

Why it's prescribed

Doctors prescribe Estrace to treat breast cancer in women and men, ovary disorders, menopausal symptoms, vaginal inflammation, and some types of prostate cancer in men. Estrace comes in tablets, skin patches, and a vaginal cream. Doctors usually prescribe the following amounts for adults.

▶ **For menopausal symptoms, deficient or malfunctioning ovaries, or hormone replacement for removed ovaries,** 1 to 2 milligrams (mg) orally each day, in cycles of 21 days on and 7 days off or 5 days on and 2 days off. Or 1 skin patch delivering 0.05 mg every 24 hours, applied twice a week in cycles of 3 weeks on and 1 week off.

▶ **For vaginal inflammation,** 2 to 4 grams (g) of vaginal cream daily for 1 to 2 weeks, then 1 g one to three times a week in a cyclic regimen. Use applicator provided.

▶ **For inoperable breast cancer in women and men,** 10 mg orally three times a day for 3 months.

▶ **For inoperable prostate cancer,** 1 to 2 mg orally three times a day.

How to use Estrace

• Take tablets at the same time each day.
• To reduce nausea, take Estrace with food or after meals.

ESTRACE'S OTHER NAMES

Estrace's generic name is estradiol. Another brand name is Estraderm.

SIDE EFFECTS

Call your doctor if you have any of these possible drug side effects. Call *immediately* about any labeled "serious."

Serious: sudden pain in chest or leg (typical of blood clots); abdominal pain; pain, numbness, or stiffness in legs or buttocks; chest pain or pressure; shortness of breath; severe headaches; visual disturbances, such as blind spots, flashing lights, or blurriness; breast lumps; swelling of hands or feet; yellow-tinged skin or eyes; dark urine; light-colored stools

Common: nausea, headache, dizziness, constipation

Other: involuntary movements, depression, lethargy, intolerance of contact lenses, vomiting, bloating, diarrhea, appetite or weight change, menstrual irregularities, altered cervical secretions, enlargement of uterine fibromas (noncancerous tumors), yeast infection, breast development, testicular atrophy or impotence in men, brown facial pigmentation, hives, acne, oily skin, hair growth or loss, breast changes (tenderness, enlargement, secretions), increased blood sugar (increased thirst, hunger, urination), excess calcium (constipation, fast heartbeats), folic acid deficiency (red or swollen mouth or tongue, diarrhea), change in sex drive

DRUG INTERACTIONS

Combining certain drugs may alter their action or produce unwanted side effects. Tell your doctor about other drugs you're taking, especially:

• antibiotics
• anticoagulants (blood thinners) such as Coumadin
• Dantrium, Rifadin, and other drugs toxic to the liver
• Nolvadex
• Parlodel
• Sandimmune
• seizure drugs, such as Solfoton and Tegretol
• steroids.

• Apply the skin patch to your abdomen or buttocks, not your breasts or waist.
• If you're switching from tablets to a skin patch, apply the first patch 1 week after you stop taking the tablets, sooner with your doctor's permission.
• If you're using vaginal cream, wash your genital area with soap and water before applying it. Use the cream at bedtime or lie flat for 30 minutes afterward.

If you miss a dose

Take the missed dose as soon as possible. However, if it's almost time for your next dose, skip the missed

Continued on next page ▶

dose and take your next dose as scheduled. Don't take a double dose.

 ### If you suspect an overdose

Consult your doctor.

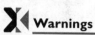 ### Warnings

• Make sure your doctor knows your medical history. You may not be able to take Estrace if you're pregnant or if you've had blood clots, estrogen-related tumors, breast or reproductive organ cancer, or abnormal menstrual bleeding or if you currently have heart disease, asthma, migraine headaches, depression, bone disease, or liver or kidney problems.

• Also tell the doctor if you have a family history (mother, grandmother, sister) of breast or genital cancer, breast nodules, fibrocystic disease, or abnormal mammogram results.

• You'll need a checkup before starting Estrace and during each year of therapy.

• You'll probably stop taking Estrace at least 1 month before having surgical procedures (such as knee or hip surgery) that cause you to be inactive for a long time and thus increase your risk of developing blood clots.

• If you're on cyclic therapy for menopausal symptoms, you may bleed during the week you're off the drug. You won't get pregnant, however, because you haven't ovulated.

• Examine your breasts regularly for lumps.

• If you're diabetic and your blood sugar rises, tell the doctor, who may adjust the amount of diabetes drug you're taking.

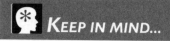 ## KEEP IN MIND...

* Report any family history of breast or genital cancer.

* Take tablets at same time each day.

* Don't place patch near breast or waist.

* Perform regular breast self-exams.

Estratab

Estratab mimics the action of natural estrogen, a female sex hormone.

Why it's prescribed

Doctors prescribe Estratab to treat breast cancer (at least 5 years after menopause), deficiency in ovary function, menopausal symptoms, and prostate cancer. It comes in tablets and coated tablets. Doctors usually prescribe the following amounts for adults.

▶ **For inoperable prostate cancer,** 1.25 to 2.5 milligrams (mg) three times a day.

▶ **For breast cancer in men and postmenapausal women,** 10 mg three times a day for 3 or more months.

▶ **For ovary deficiency,** 2.5 mg one to three times a day in cycles of 20 days on, 10 days off.

▶ **For vaginal inflammation, menopausal symptoms,** 0.3 to 1.25 mg or more daily in cycles of 3 weeks on, 1 week off.

How to take Estratab

• Take Estratab as prescribed at the same time each day.

If you miss a dose

Take the missed dose as soon as possible. But, if it's almost time for your next dose, skip the missed dose and take your next dose as scheduled. Don't take a double dose.

 If you suspect an overdose

Consult your doctor.

ESTRATAB'S OTHER NAMES

Estratab's generic name is esterified estrogens. Other brand names include Menest; and, in Canada, Neo-Estrone.

 SIDE EFFECTS

Call your doctor if you have any of these possible side effects. Call *immediately* about any effects labeled "serious."

Serious: blood clots (sudden pain in chest or leg), abdominal pain, shortness of breath, severe headache, visual disturbances (blind spots, flashing lights, blurriness), breast lumps, swelling of hands or feet, yellow-tinged skin or eyes, dark urine, light-colored stools
Tip: Regularly examine your breasts for lumps.

Common: nausea, headache, dizziness, weight changes
Tip: Take with food to reduce nausea.

Other: depression, lethargy, vomiting, bloating, constipation, increased or decreased appetite, altered menstrual flow, altered cervical secretions, yeast infection, impotence, brown facial pigmentation, hives, acne, oily skin, hair growth or loss, breast changes (tenderness, enlargement, secretion), increased blood sugar (increased thirst, hunger, and urination), change in sex drive
Tip: If you are diabetic and your blood sugar level rises, your doctor will adjust the amount of diabetes drug you take.

 DRUG INTERACTIONS

Combining certain drugs may alter their action or produce unwanted side effects. Tell your doctor about other drugs you're taking, especially:
• anticoagulants (blood thinners) such as Coumadin
• Dantrium and other drugs toxic to the liver
• Nolvadex, Parlodel, Rifadin, Sandimmune
• Solfoton, Tegretol
• steroids.

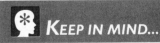 **Warnings**

• Make sure your doctor knows your medical history. You may not be able to take Estratab if you are pregnant, have a family history of breast or genital cancer, or have abnormal mammogram results, blood clots, estrogen-related tumors, breast or reproductive organ cancer, abnormal menstrual bleeding, heart or bone disease, asthma, depression, or liver or kidney problems.
• You'll probably stop taking Estratab at least 1 month before any surgery.

• If you're on cyclic therapy for menopausal symptoms, you may bleed during the week you're off the drug.

KEEP IN MIND...

* Report any family history of breast or genital cancer.
* Perform routine breast self-exams.
* Take at same time each day.

Eulexin

Eulexin is one of several anticancer drugs called antiandrogens, which block the action of the male sex hormone, testosterone.

Why it's prescribed

Doctors prescribe Eulexin to treat prostate cancer, usually in combination with another drug (such as Lupron). Eulexin blocks testosterone's action at the cell level, while the other drug reduces the body's ability to produce the hormone. Eulexin comes in capsules and, in Canada, tablets. Doctors usually prescribe the following amounts for adults.

▶ **For prostate cancer (stage D2),** 250 milligrams every 8 hours.

How to take Eulexin

• Take this drug and any drug prescribed with it exactly as your doctor has directed.
• Continue taking Eulexin for the full course of treatment, even after you begin to feel better. To prevent the cancer from recurring, don't stop taking the drug without first talking to your doctor.

If you miss a dose

Take the missed dose as soon as possible. However, if it's almost time for your next dose, skip the missed dose and take your next dose as scheduled. Don't take a double dose.

EULEXIN'S OTHER NAMES

Eulexin's generic name is flutamide. A brand name in Canada is Euflex.

 SIDE EFFECTS

Call your doctor if you have any of these possible drug side effects. Call *immediately* about any effects labeled "serious."

Serious: blue lips, dark urine, extreme dizziness, pain in right side, yellow-tinged eyes or skin, shortness of breath, weak and fast heartbeat

Common: drowsiness, confusion, numbness or tingling in hands or feet, diarrhea, nausea, vomiting, impotence, altered sex drive, hot flashes
Tips: Some side effects may worsen initially before they improve. Take the drug with food to reduce nausea. If you vomit shortly after taking a dose, check with your doctor to see whether you should take the dose again or wait until the next scheduled dose.

Other: swelling of hands or lower legs, high blood pressure (headache, blurred vision), liver changes (flulike symptoms, itching, abdominal tenderness), hepatitis (nausea, vomiting, yellow-tinged skin), rash, skin sensitivity to sun, breast enlargement

DRUG INTERACTIONS

Combining certain drugs may alter their action or produce unwanted side effects. Tell your doctor about other drugs you're taking, especially:
• Coumadin.

 If you suspect an overdose

Contact your doctor *immediately.* Excessive Eulexin can cause decreased activity, "goosebumps," vomiting, appetite loss, and crying.

Warnings

• Make sure your doctor knows your medical history. You may not be able to take Eulexin if you have certain liver problems.
• Schedule and keep regular medical checkups so your doctor can monitor your progress. Your doctor may want to test your liver function periodically.
• If you want to have children, talk to your doctor. Eulexin lowers your sperm count, and the drug used with it can cause possible permanent sterility.
• Keep in mind that you must take both of the drugs your doctor has prescribed for your therapy to be effective. Don't stop taking either of the drugs without first consulting your doctor.

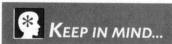 **KEEP IN MIND...**

* Take both drugs exactly as prescribed.

* Side effects may worsen before improving.

* If you vomit after taking a dose, call your doctor.

Eurax

Eurax is one of several drugs known as scabicides (which kill parasitic mites that live in human skin) and anti-pruritics (anti-itch compounds).

Why it's prescribed

Doctors prescribe Eurax to treat scabies (itch mite) infection and to reduce the itching associated with certain other skin conditions. Eurax comes in a cream and a lotion. Doctors usually prescribe the following amounts for adults and children.

▶ **For itch mite infection,** apply to your entire body, reapply after 24 hours, wait an additional 48 hours and then wash it off. Repeat treatment in 7 to 10 days if mites reappear or if new lesions develop.

▶ **For relief of itching,** apply to affected skin area as needed.

How to use Eurax

• For itch mite infection, scrub your entire body with soap and water. Remove any scales or crusts. Then apply a thin layer of cream over your entire body, from the chin down (pay special attention to folds, creases, and spaces between fingers and toes).

• Don't apply Eurax to your face, eyes, mucous membranes, or urinary opening. If you accidentally get Eurax in your eyes, flush them with water and notify the doctor.

EURAX'S OTHER NAME

Eurax's generic name is crotamiton.

SIDE EFFECTS

Call your doctor if you have any of these possible drug side effects.

Serious: none reported

Common: none reported

Other: skin irritation

Tip: Wash Eurax off your skin, stop using it, and tell your doctor right away if your skin becomes irritated or overly sensitive to the drug.

DRUG INTERACTIONS

Combining certain drugs may alter their action or produce unwanted side effects. Tell your doctor about other drugs you're taking.

If you miss a dose

Reapply Eurax if it's washed off during treatment time.

If you suspect an overdose

Consult your doctor, stop using Eurax, and wash the area well.

Warnings

• Make sure your doctor knows your medical history. You may not be able to use Eurax if your skin is broken or inflamed or if you're overly sensitive to the drug.

• Try not to use too much of the drug. For most adults, a single tube of cream contains enough for two full-body applications.

• After you wash Eurax off, change out of and sterilize all clothing and bed linen (by boiling, laundering, or dry-cleaning or by applying a very hot iron).

• Be sure to tell family members and sexual contacts about the possibility that they'll become infected.

• Use a condom during sexual intercourse to avoid scabies infection.

• If you develop dermatitis from scratching, your doctor may give you a steroid cream to help the area heal.

• You may continue to itch after the treatment ends. However, if it becomes intolerable, notify your doctor.

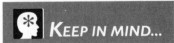

* Be sure to apply drug in skin folds and creases.

* Tell sexual contacts about your infection.

* Sterilize linens and clothes after treatment.

* Don't get Eurax in your eyes, mouth, or other mucous membranes.

Euthroid

 uthroid is a thyroid hormone replacement that's a combination of two drugs: levothyroxine and liothyronine. It stimulates the metabolism of all body tissues.

Why it's prescribed

Doctors prescribe Euthroid for hypothyroidism, when the thyroid gland doesn't produce enough thyroid hormone. It comes in tablets. Doctors usually prescribe the following amounts for adults and children, but dosages are individualized for each person.

▶ **For hypothyroidism,** initially, 12.5 micrograms (mcg) of levothyroxine and 3.1 mcg of liothyronine by mouth daily. Or, 25 mcg of levothyroxine and 6.25 mcg of liothyronine daily. Or, 30 mcg of levothyroxine and 7.5 mcg of liothyronine daily. Dosage is increased in increments at 2-week intervals.

How to take Euthroid

• Take Euthroid as prescribed. Establishing a successful dosing schedule may take some time.
• Take the drug at the same time each day, preferably before breakfast, to maintain constant hormone levels and avoid insomnia.
• Don't stop taking this drug without checking with your doctor.

If you miss a dose

Take the missed dose as soon as possible. However, if it's almost time

EUTHROID'S OTHER NAMES

Euthroid's generic name is liotrix. Another brand name is Thyrolar.

 SIDE EFFECTS

Call your doctor if you have any of these possible drug side effects. Call *immediately* about any labeled "serious."

Serious: chest pain, palpitations, irregular heartbeat, cardiac collapse (heart stoppage), shortness of breath

Common: sweating, nervousness, sleeplessness
Tip: Take the drug several hours before bedtime to improve sleep.

Other: twitching, tremors, increased blood pressure (headache, blurred vision), diarrhea, abdominal cramps, vomiting, weight loss, heat intolerance, menstrual changes

 DRUG INTERACTIONS

Combining certain drugs may alter their action or produce unwanted side effects. Tell your doctor about other drugs you're taking, especially:
• anticoagulants (blood thinners) such as Coumadin
• Colestid, Questran
• Dilantin (given intravenously)
• epinephrine and similar stimulants
• insulin and oral diabetes drugs.

for your next dose, skip the missed dose and take your next dose as scheduled. Don't take a double dose.

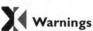 **If you suspect an overdose**

Contact your doctor *immediately.* Excessive Euthroid causes symptoms of hyperthyroidism, including weight loss, palpitations, nervousness, sweating, heat intolerance, headache, and insomnia.

 Warnings

• Make sure your doctor knows your medical history. You may not be able to take Euthroid if you are overly sensitive to the drug, have had a heart attack, or have Grave's disease (hyperactive thyroid), underactive adrenal glands, angina,

high blood pressure or other heart or circulatory problems, kidney problems, or diabetes.
• Once you've achieved a stable and successful dosing schedule, don't change to a different brand of thyroid hormone replacement.
• If you have no thyroid gland or if it produces no thyroid hormone, you may need to take Euthroid for the rest of your life.

KEEP IN MIND...

∗ Don't stop taking Euthroid without doctor's approval.

∗ Don't switch brand names without consultation.

∗ Be alert for symptoms of too much thyroid hormone.

Ex-Lax

Exlax is a stimulant laxative that makes the muscles of the intestine expel solid wastes more forcefully. The drug also brings extra fluids into the intestines.

Why it's taken

Ex-Lax is taken to help relieve occasional constipation. It comes in tablets, chewable tablets, and chewing gum. The following amounts are usually recommended for adults; children's dosages appear in parentheses.

▶ **For constipation,** 30 to 270 milligrams (mg), preferably at bedtime. (Children over age 12: same as adults. Children ages 6 to 12: 30 to 60 mg at bedtime. Children ages 2 to 6: 15 to 30 mg at bedtime.)

How to take Ex-Lax

• Arrange to take your Ex-Lax dose so its effect doesn't interfere with your sleep or scheduled activities.

If you miss a dose

Not applicable because Ex-Lax is used as needed.

EX-LAX'S OTHER NAMES

Ex-Lax's generic name is white phenolphthalein. Other brand names include Alophen Pills, Correctol, Modane, Phenolax, Evac-U-Lax, Ex-Lax Maximum Relief Formula, Ex-Lax Pills, Feen-A-Mint, Feen-A-Mint Gum, and Lax-Pills.

 SIDE EFFECTS

Call your doctor if you have any of these possible drug side effects. Call *immediately* about any labeled "serious."

Serious: weakness, low blood pressure (dizziness, weakness), severe abdominal pain, rash

Common: abdominal cramps

Other: diarrhea, nausea, vomiting, reduced bowel function with excessive use, discolored (pink or yellow-brown) urine, laxative dependence, changes in skin color, allergic reactions (difficulty breathing, hives, itching)

Tip: To avoid skin problems, avoid excessive sun exposure and don't take Ex-Lax with any other product containing phenolphthalein.

DRUG INTERACTIONS

Combining certain drugs may alter their action or produce unwanted side effects. Tell your doctor about other drugs you're taking.

 If you suspect an overdose

Consult your doctor. Excessive Ex-Lax can cause abdominal pain and diarrhea.

Warnings

• Make sure your doctor knows your medical history. You may not be able to take Ex-Lax if you have rectal bleeding, abdominal pain, nausea, vomiting, other symptoms of appendicitis, or a blocked or perforated intestine.
• Make sure your doctor knows if you're pregnant or breast-feeding before you begin taking Ex-Lax.
• Make sure your diet includes adequate fluids and such fiber-rich foods as bran and other cereals, fresh fruits, and vegetables.

• Review your diet for foods and medicines that could be causing constipation. Avoid these foods and talk with your doctor about the medicines.
• Keep this drug hidden from children; they could mistake it for candy.
• Ex-Lax's laxative action may linger for several days.

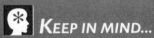 **KEEP IN MIND...**

∗ Plan doses so drug action doesn't interfere with activities.

∗ Increase fluids and fiber-rich foods.

∗ Remove constipation-causing foods from diet.

Famvir

Famvir is one of several drugs known as antivirals. It's especially effective against skin eruptions caused by the herpes zoster virus (also known as shingles).

Why it's prescribed

Doctors prescribe Famvir to help reduce the intensity and duration of herpes zoster infections. It comes in tablets. Doctors usually prescribe the following amounts for adults.

▶ **For acute herpes zoster infections,** 500 milligrams every 8 hours. For a person with kidney problems, the same amount every 12 or 24 hours.

How to take Famvir

• Take Famvir with or without food, whichever you prefer. However, if you experience nausea after taking the drug, take it with food.
• Store tablets at room temperature.

If you miss a dose

Take the missed dose as soon as possible. However, if it's almost time for your next dose, skip the missed dose and take your next dose as scheduled. Don't take a double dose.

FAMVIR'S OTHER NAME

Famvir's generic name is famciclovir.

 SIDE EFFECTS

Call your doctor if you have any of these possible drug side effects. Call *immediately* about any labeled "serious."

Serious: chills, extreme sleepiness

Common: headache, nausea
Tip: Take with meals to avoid nausea.

Other: fatigue, diarrhea, vomiting, sleepiness, itchiness, sore throat, sinus infection, back or joint pain, fever, pain, shivering

 DRUG INTERACTIONS

Combining certain drugs may alter their action or produce unwanted side effects. Tell your doctor about other drugs you're taking, especially:
• Benemid.

 If you suspect an overdose

Consult your doctor.

 Warnings

• Make sure your doctor knows your medical history. If you have kidney or liver problems, the doctor may adjust the amount of drug you take.
• Make sure your doctor knows if you're pregnant or breast-feeding before you begin taking Famvir.
• This drug is not recommended for children under age 18.
• Your doctor may want to test your blood frequently to check your kidney function. Therefore, keep all scheduled appointments.

• Because the herpes zoster virus may merely become inactive after treatment, it may recur later. Therefore, be aware of the early signs and symptoms of herpes zoster infection, which usually include tingling, itching, and pain. Treatment is most effective if you can start taking Famvir as early as possible in the course of the infection.

 KEEP IN MIND...

* Take with or without food.

* Learn to recognize the early symptoms of herpes zoster.

* Start Famvir as early as possible in the infection.

Fansidar

Fansidar is used in the treatment of infections, such as malaria, that are caused by one-celled animals called protozoa. It works by killing protozoa that invade the body.

Why it's prescribed

Doctors prescribe Fansidar to treat malaria in travelers and a disease called toxoplasmosis that's caused by protozoa found in raw meat and cat feces. It comes in tablets. Doctors usually prescribe the following amounts for adults; children's dosages appear in parentheses.

▶ **For malaria attack,** 2 to 3 tablets as a single dose. (Children ages 9 to 14: 2 tablets. Children ages 4 to 8: 1 tablet. Children under age 4: $\frac{1}{2}$ tablet.)

▶ **For preventing malaria,** 1 tablet once a week, or 2 tablets every 2 weeks. (Children ages 9 to 14: $\frac{3}{4}$ tablet once a week, or $1\frac{1}{2}$ tablets every 2 weeks. Children ages 4 to 8: $\frac{1}{2}$ tablet once a week, or 1 tablet every 2 weeks. Children under age 4: $\frac{1}{4}$ tablet once a week, or $\frac{1}{2}$ tablet every 2 weeks.)

How to take Fansidar

• Take Fansidar only as your doctor directs.
• Take with meals to minimize stomach distress.
• Take the first preventive dose of Fansidar 1 to 2 days before traveling to an infestation area. Continue doses while you're there and for 4 to 6 weeks after returning.

FANSIDAR'S OTHER NAME

Fansidar is a combination of the generic drugs pyrimethamine and sulfadoxine.

SIDE EFFECTS

Call your doctor if you have any of these possible drug side effects. Call *immediately* about any labeled "serious."

Serious: seizures, severe blood problems (fatigue, bleeding, bruising, dizziness, sore throat), severe skin problem such as Stevens-Johnson syndrome (reddened, burnlike rash), fever, yellow-tinged skin and eyes, burning and tingling of tongue

Common: skin sensitivity to sun, nausea, stomach pain, vomiting, diarrhea, allergic reaction (hives, itching), nervousness
Tips: Use sunscreen and wear protective clothing when outdoors. To reduce nausea and vomiting, take your doses with meals or a snack.

Other: weight loss

DRUG INTERACTIONS

Combining certain drugs may alter their action or produce unwanted side effects. Tell your doctor about other drugs you're taking, especially:
• birth control pills or estrogen supplements
• heart drugs, such as Pronestyl and Quinidex
• Mexate
• seizure drugs, such as Depakote and Dilantin
• sulfa drugs such as Bactrim
• sunscreens with PABA.

If you miss a dose

Take the missed dose as s1 oon as possible. However, if it's almost time for your next dose, skip the missed dose and go back to your regular schedule. Don't take a double dose.

If you suspect an overdose

Contact your doctor *immediately.* Excessive Fansidar can cause seizures and vomiting.

Warnings

• Make sure your doctor knows your medical history. You may not be able to take Fansidar if you're allergic to either of its components or to other drugs; if you have anemia or other blood disorders, kidney or liver problem, severe allergy or bronchial asthma, seizures, or G6PD deficiency (a chronic enzyme deficiency that causes anemia); or if you are in late pregnancy or are breast-feeding.

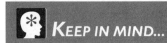

* Take with meals.

* Take drug 1 or 2 days before traveling.

* Report any rash, bleeding, skin problems, or infection.

Fastin

Fastin is an appetite suppressant that's chemically related to amphetamines; however, it has fewer side effects and less addictive potential than amphetamines.

Why it's prescribed

Doctors prescribe Fastin as a short-term aid in weight reduction for obese people. It comes in tablets, capsules, and slow-release capsules. Doctors usually prescribe the following amounts for adults.

▶ **For weight reduction,** 1 capsule a day.

How to take Fastin

• Take Fastin at least 6 hours before bedtime to avoid interfering with sleep. For best results, take it 2 hours after breakfast.
• Intermittent therapy (6 weeks on, 4 weeks off) works as well as continuous therapy.
• Don't take extra doses of Fastin.

If you miss a dose

Take the missed dose as soon as possible. However, if it's almost time for your next dose, skip the missed dose and take your next dose as scheduled. Don't take a double dose.

 If you suspect an overdose

Contact your doctor *immediately*. Excessive Fastin can cause restlessness, confusion, aggression, fatigue, depression, seizures, coma, and death.

FASTIN'S OTHER NAMES

Fastin's generic name is phentermine hydrochloride. Other brand names include Adipex-P, Obe-Nix, Obephen, Oby-Trim, Phentrol, Wilpowr, and Zantryl.

 SIDE EFFECTS

Call your doctor if you have any of these possible drug side effects.

Serious: none reported

Common: insomnia, palpitations, rapid heartbeat

Other: overstimulation, headache, euphoria, depression or anguish, dizziness, increased blood pressure (headache, blurred vision), dry mouth, altered taste, stomach upset, hives, impotence, altered sex drive

Tips: Avoid caffeine-containing beverages because they can increase Fastin's stimulant effect. Tell the doctor if the drug makes you feel overly stimulated.

 DRUG AND FOOD INTERACTIONS

Combining certain drugs and foods may alter drug action or produce unwanted side effects. Tell your doctor about your diet and other drugs you're taking, especially:
• ammonium chloride (diuretic or expectorant)
• antacids, baking soda
• antipsychotic drugs such as Haldol
• caffeine-containing beverages
• Diamox
• insulin and oral diabetes drugs
• MAO inhibitors and tricyclic antidepressants
• vitamin C.

Warnings

• Make sure your doctor knows your medical history. You may not be able to take Fastin if you have an overactive thyroid (hyperthyroidism), high blood pressure, advanced artery disease, heart disease, glaucoma, or very high sensitivity to stimulant drugs or if you are agitated or have taken certain antidepressants recently.
• Your doctor will probably require that you use Fastin in conjunction with a weight-reduction program.
• If you're diabetic, monitor your blood sugar level closely.

• After the first few weeks, you may develop a tolerance to Fastin and it won't work as well. Your doctor will probably stop your therapy for a while rather than increasing the dosage.
• When you stop taking Fastin, you may feel some fatigue and need more rest as the drug wears off.

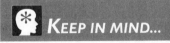 **KEEP IN MIND...**

∗ Don't take more than prescribed.

∗ Avoid caffeine-containing beverages.

∗ Follow a weight-loss plan.

Felbatol

Felbatol is an anticonvulsant, a drug that helps prevent seizures from starting or, if they've already begun, prevents them from continuing.

Why it's prescribed

Doctors prescribe Felbatol to control seizures in the treatment of epilepsy. It comes in tablets and a liquid. Doctors usually prescribe the following amounts.

▶ **For seizures in adults and children age 14 and older, when used as the only treatment,** initially 1,200 milligrams (mg) daily, divided into three or four equal doses, increased in 600-mg increments every 2 weeks to 2,400 mg a day and finally to 3,600 mg a day if needed and tolerated.

▶ **For seizures in adults and children age 14 and older, when used with other seizure drugs,** initially 1,200 mg daily, divided into three or four equal doses. Dosages for the other drugs are reduced by 20%. Felbatol dosage is increased by 1,200 mg a day in three to four equal doses at weekly intervals to a maximum of 3,600 mg a day; reductions in the dosage of other seizure drugs may be needed.

▶ **When switching to Felbatol from other seizure drugs in adults and children age 14 and over,** initially 1,200 mg a day, divided into three or four equal doses, while reducing the dosage of other drugs by one-third. The 2nd week, Felbatol increases to 2,400 mg a day while the other drugs are cut by another third. The 3rd week, Felbatol increases to 3,600 mg a day while the other drugs are reduced or removed as needed.

▶ **When switching to Felbatol from other seizure drugs in children ages 2 to 14,** 15 mg for each 2.2 pounds (lb) of body weight a day divided into three or four equal doses, while reducing other drug dosages by 20%. Each week, Felbatol is increased by 15 mg for each 2.2 lb a day to a maximum of 45 mg a day, while other drugs are reduced or removed.

How to take Felbatol

• Shake the liquid well before measuring dose.
• Don't stop taking Felbatol without checking with your doctor.

If you miss a dose

Take the missed dose as soon as possible. But, if it's almost time for your next dose, skip the missed dose and take your next dose as scheduled. Don't take a double dose.

FELBATOL'S OTHER NAME

Felbatol's generic name is felbamate.

 SIDE EFFECTS

Call your doctor if you have any of these possible drug side effects. Call *immediately* about any labeled "serious."

Serious: severe anemia (fatigue, dizziness), acute liver failure (yellow-tinged skin or eyes, seizures, confusion)

Common: insomnia, headache, fatigue, congestion, vomiting, constipation

Tip: Avoid activities that require full alertness or coordination until you know how Felbatol affects you.

Other: anxiety, blurred or double vision, rash, weight loss

 DRUG INTERACTIONS

Combining certain drugs may alter their action or produce unwanted side effects. Tell your doctor about other drugs you're taking, especially:
• Depakene, Dilantin, Tegretol.

If you suspect an overdose

Consult your doctor.

Warnings

• Make sure your doctor knows your medical history. You may not be able to take Felbatol if you're pregnant or breast-feeding.
• You'll need to have regular blood tests performed while taking Felbatol to check for possible liver damage or anemia.

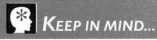 **KEEP IN MIND...**

∗ Shake liquid before taking.

∗ Don't stop taking this drug without doctor's permission.

∗ Routine blood testing is required while taking drug.

Feldene

Feldene reduces inflammation, pain, and fever. It belongs to a large group of drugs called nonsteroidal anti-inflammatory drugs (NSAIDs).

Why it's prescribed

Doctors prescribe Feldene to relieve the joint swelling, pain, and stiffness of arthritis. It comes in capsules. Doctors usually prescribe the following amounts for adults.
▶ **For arthritis,** 20 milligrams once or twice a day.

How to take Feldene

• Follow your doctor's instructions for taking this drug. It relieves pain in 15 to 30 minutes. But it may take several weeks before you start to feel the full effects of the drug.
• To reduce stomach upset, take Feldene with food, milk, or an antacid. Avoid lying down for 15 to 30 minutes after taking it to prevent the drug from irritating your esophagus.

If you miss a dose

Take the missed dose if you remember it within 2 hours. Otherwise, skip the missed dose and take your next dose as scheduled. Don't take a double dose.

 If you suspect an overdose

Contact your doctor *immediately*. Because Feldene persists in the body for a long time, the side ef-

FELDENE'S OTHER NAMES

Feldene's generic name is piroxicam. Brand names in Canada include Apo-Piroxicam and Novopirocam.

 SIDE EFFECTS

Call your doctor if you have any of these possible drug side effects. Call *immediately* about any labeled "serious."

Serious: stomach ulcers (severe abdominal or stomach pain; severe, continuing nausea or heartburn), bleeding in digestive tract (black, tarry stools; vomiting of blood or material that looks like coffee grounds), kidney damage (flank pain, blood in urine, decreased urine output), severe anemia (fatigue, weakness)

Common: stomach upset, nausea, sensitivity to sun
Tip: Use a sunscreen, wear protective clothing, and avoid prolonged exposure to sunlight. Feldene causes sensitivity to the sun more than other NSAIDs.

Other: headache, drowsiness, dizziness, tingling sensations, swelling of lower legs, anemia, slow blood clotting, itchiness, rash
Tip: Avoid activities that require full alertness or coordination until you know how Feldene affects you.

 DRUG INTERACTIONS

Combining certain drugs may alter their action or produce unwanted side effects. Tell your doctor about other drugs you're taking, especially:
• alcohol
• anticoagulants (blood thinners) such as Coumadin
• aspirin or other pain relievers
• Eskalith
• oral diabetes drugs
• steroids.

fects listed above may occur long after an overdose has occurred.

 Warnings

• Make sure your doctor knows your medical history. You may not be able to take Feldene if you are allergic to aspirin or related drugs or if you have kidney or liver problems, heart failure, ulcers, high blood pressure, or fluid retention.
• If you're pregnant or breast-feeding, check with your doctor before using this drug.

• Older adults may be especially prone to Feldene's side effects.
• If you have diabetes, Feldene may hide the signs of infection.

KEEP IN MIND...

* Take with food, milk, or antacids.
* Watch for signs of bleeding in digestive tract.
* May not feel better for a few weeks.

Feosol

Feosol is iron in a form known as ferrous sulfate. Iron is important in the formation of hemoglobin, a component of blood that enables it to carry oxygen through the body.

Why it's taken

Feosol is taken to help increase the body's iron stores, which in turn can increase the hemoglobin level. You can but Feosol without a prescription. It comes in tablets and capsules, slow-release tablets and capsules, elixir, syrup, solution, and drops. The following amounts are usually recommended for adults; children's dosages are in parentheses.

▶ **For iron deficiency,** 325 milligrams (mg) three or four times a day. Or, one extended-release capsule (160 to 525 mg) twice a day. (Children: 5 to 10 mg for each 2.2 pounds of body weight three times a day.)

How to take Feosol

• To promote iron absorption, take tablets with orange juice. Dilute liquid forms of Feosol in juice or water, but not in milk or antacids.
• Don't crush or chew slow-release tablets or capsules.
• It's best to take Feosol between meals. But if you experience stomach upset, take it with some food.

FEOSOL'S OTHER NAMES

Feosol's generic name is ferrous sulfate. Other brand names include Fer-In-Sol, Fer-In-Sol Drops, Fer-In-Sol Syrup, Fer-Iron Drops, Fero-Gradumet, Ferospace, Ferra-TD, and Ferralyn Lanacaps; and, in Canada, Apo-Ferrous Sulfate and Fero-Grad.

SIDE EFFECTS

Call your doctor if you have any of these possible drug side effects.

Serious: none reported

Common: nausea, constipation, black stools
Tips: Drink lots of fluids and eat plenty of fiber-rich foods to help avoid constipation. Black stools are usually a result of unabsorbed iron; however, you should call your doctor if you have black stools and continued abdominal pain.

Other: stomach pain, vomiting, diarrhea, stained teeth
Tip: To avoid staining your teeth, take liquid forms through a straw placed in the back of your mouth.

DRUG AND FOOD INTERACTIONS

Combining certain drugs and foods may alter their action or produce unwanted side effects. Tell your doctor about your diet and other drugs you're taking, especially:
• antacids
• antibiotics such as Achromycin
• Chloromycetin
• fluoroquinolones, such as Cipro and Floxin
• foods that can reduce oral iron absorption, including yogurt, cheese, eggs, milk, whole-grain breads and cereals, tea, and coffee
• Larodopa
• Questran
• vitamin E.

Coated tablets reduce stomach upset, but they also reduce the amount of iron absorbed.

If you miss a dose

Skip the missed dose and take your next dose as scheduled. Don't take a double dose.

 If you suspect an overdose

Contact your doctor *immediately.* Excessive Feosol can cause lethargy, nausea and vomiting, weak and rapid pulse, green and then tarry stools, dehydration, and coma. As few as 3 or 4 tablets can cause serious iron poisoning in children.

 Warnings

• Before taking Feosol, consult your doctor if you have stomach ulcers or ulcerative colitis or if you've received repeated blood transfusions.

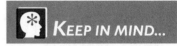

* Take with orange juice.
* Take with food if stomach upset occurs.
* Increase fluids and fiber in diet.

Fioricet

Fioricet is a combination of three drugs that relieve pain and aid relaxation.

Why it's prescribed

Doctors usually prescribe Fioricet to treat tension headaches when nonprescription pain relievers are ineffective. It comes in tablets. Doctors usually prescribe the following amount for adults.

▶ **For tension headaches,** 1 or 2 tablets every 4 hours as needed. Maximum daily dosage is 6 tablets.

How to take Fioricet

• Fioricet works best if you take it at the first sign of a headache.
• To minimize stomach upset, take Fioricet with milk or meals.
• Don't take more than 6 tablets a day.
• If you don't feel better in 45 to 60 minutes, call your doctor. Don't increase the dose on your own.
• Don't stop taking Fioricet suddenly; your doctor may reduce your dosage gradually before stopping.

If you miss a dose

Take the missed dose as soon as possible. However, if it's almost time for your next dose, skip the missed dose and take your next dose as scheduled. Don't take a double dose.

FIORICET'S OTHER NAMES

Fioricet is a combination of three generic drugs: acetaminophen, butalbital, and caffeine. Other brand names include Amaphen, Anolor-300, Anoquan, Butace, Dolmar, Esgic, Ezol, Femcet, Isocet, Isopap, Medigesic, Pacaps, Repan, and Two-Dyne.

SIDE EFFECTS

Call your doctor if you have any of these possible drug side effects. Call *immediately* about any labeled "serious."

Serious: reduced, shallow breathing; low blood pressure (dizziness, weakness); dependence; confusion; blood in urine or stools; bruising; hives; muscle cramps; white spots on the tongue; chest pain; allergic reaction (itchiness, rash, difficulty breathing or swallowing)

Common: dizziness, abdominal pain, nausea, vomiting
Tips: Get up slowly to avoid dizziness. Take the drug with food to avoid nausea. Avoid activities that require full alertness or coordination until you know how Fioricet affects you.

Other: none reported

DRUG INTERACTIONS

Combining certain drugs may alter their action or produce unwanted side effects. Tell your doctor about other drugs you're taking, especially:
• alcohol
• antihistamines or other drugs that make you feel relaxed or sleepy
• MAO inhibitors, such as Nardil and Parnate
• other drugs that contain acetaminophen (risk of liver damage)
• other narcotic pain relievers
• tranquilizers, such as Librium and Xanax.

 If you suspect an overdose

Contact your doctor *immediately.* Excessive Fioricet can lead to respiratory depression, low blood pressure, decreased level of consciousness, and death.

 Warnings

• Make sure your doctor knows your medical history, especially if you have a history of alcohol or drug abuse, asthma, depression, heart disease, an overactive thyroid, diabetes, or kidney, liver, or blood disorders.

• If you're pregnant or breast-feeding, check with your doctor before taking Fioricet.
• Because Fioricet is a narcotic, it can be habit-forming.
• Older adults may be especially prone to Fioricet's side effects.
• Call your doctor if your headaches worsen.

 KEEP IN MIND...

* Take as soon as headache begins.
* Take with milk or meals.
* Don't stop taking abruptly.

Fiorinal

Fiorinal is a combination of three drugs — butalbital, acetaminophen, and caffeine — that relieve pain and aid relaxation. Butalbital is a barbiturate (a form of narcotic), aspirin is a pain reliever, and caffeine reduces blood flow through blood vessels.

Why it's prescribed

Doctors prescribe Fiorinal to treat moderately severe tension headaches when over-the-counter pain relievers are ineffective. It comes in tablets. Doctors usually prescribe the following amount for adults.
▶ **For tension headaches,** 1 or 2 tablets every 4 hours as needed. Maximum dosage is 6 tablets a day.

How to take Fiorinal

• To reduce stomach irritation, take it with meals or a full glass (8 ounces) of milk or water.
• Don't take this drug if it has a strong, vinegar-like odor. The odor means that the aspirin part of the combination is breaking down and is no longer effective.
• Fiorinal works best if taken as soon as a headache begins.
• Don't take more than 6 tablets a day.
• If you don't feel better after several weeks, call your doctor. Don't in-

FIORINAL'S OTHER NAMES

Fiorinal is a combination of three generic drugs: aspirin, butalbital, and caffeine. Other brand names include Butalgen, Fiormor, Fortabs, Isobutal, Isolin, Isollyl, Isobutyl, Laniroif, Lanorinal, Marnal, Vibutal; and, in Canada, Tecnal.

 ## SIDE EFFECTS

Call your doctor if you have any of these possible drug side effects. Call *immediately* about any labeled "serious."

Serious: decreased and shallow breathing, low blood pressure (dizziness, weakness), confusion, dependence, ringing in ears, skin discoloration, chest tightness, hives, swelling, bruising, bleeding (bruising, black or bloody stools), white spots in mouth, allergic reaction (itchiness, rash, difficulty breathing or swallowing)

Common: bloated feeling, dizziness, abdominal pain, nausea, vomiting
Tips: When lying down or sitting, get up slowly to avoid dizziness. Increase amount of rest while taking the drug. Take the drug with food to reduce nausea. Avoid activities that require full alertness or coordination until you know how Fiorinal affects you.

Other: none reported

 ## DRUG INTERACTIONS

Combining certain drugs may alter their action or produce unwanted side effects. Tell your doctor about other drugs you're taking, especially:
• alcohol
• antacids
• anticoagulants (blood thinners) such as Coumadin
• antidepressants
• antihistamines or other drugs that make you feel relaxed or sleepy
• Anturane
• Benemid
• corticosteroids such as Prednisone
• Depakene, Depakote
• Dolobid
• Folex
• ibuprofen (NSAIDs), drugs that contain aspirin or salicylates
• insulin, oral diabetes drugs such as DiaBeta
• MAO inhibitors
• methotrexate
• oral contraceptives
• Tegretol
• Vancocin.

crease the dose on your own, and don't take it longer than the doctor ordered.
• If you're taking this drug regularly or in large amounts, don't stop taking it abruptly. Check with your doctor.

If you miss a dose

Take the missed dose as soon as possible. However, if it's almost time for your next dose, skip the missed

Continued on next page ▶

dose and take your next dose as scheduled. Don't take a double dose.

If you suspect an overdose

Contact your doctor *immediately*. Excessive Fiorinal can cause respiratory depression, low blood pressure, and confusion, ringing in the ears, fever, restlessness, decreased level of consciousness, and death.

Warnings

• Make sure your doctor knows your medical history. Tell your doctor if you have anemia, gout, peptic ulcer or other stomach problems, or heart, kidney, liver disease, because using this drug may make these conditions worse. Also tell your doctor if you have a vitamin K deficiency.

• If you're pregnant or breast-feeding, tell your doctor before you begin taking Fiorinal.

• Before surgery (including dental surgery) or emergency treatment, tell your doctor or dentist that you're taking this drug.

• If you have diabetes and take this drug regularly, it may cause false urine sugar test results. Check with your doctor if you notice any unusual changes.

• Because Fiorinal is a narcotic, it is potentially habit-forming. Take the drug only in the amount and frequency prescribed by your doctor.

• Because Fiorinal contains aspirin, never give it to a child or a teenager who has a fever or other signs of a viral infection, such as flu or chickenpox.

• Children and older adults may be especially prone to Fiorinal's side effects.

• Rebound headaches may occur after stopping the drug.

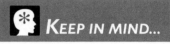 **KEEP IN MIND...**

* Take as soon as headache begins.

* Take with fluids or meals.

* Don't stop taking Fiorinal abruptly.

Flagyl

Flagyl kills certain microscopic parasites (amoebas, *Giardia*, *Trichomonas*) and other infection-causing organisms.

Why it's prescribed

Doctors prescribe Flagyl to treat infection of the sex organs (trichomoniasis), the intestine, or the liver. It comes in tablets and an oral suspension and may also be given intravenously. Doctors usually prescribe the following amounts for adults; children's dosages appear in parentheses.

▶ **For liver or intestinal parasitic infection,** 500 to 750 milligrams (mg) orally three times a day for 5 to 10 days. (Children: 35 to 50 mg for each 2.2 pounds [lb] of body weight divided into three equal doses a day for 10 days.)

▶ **For intestinal amebiasis,** 750 mg three times a day for 5 to 10 days. (Children: 35 to 50 mg for each 2.2 lb of body weight divided into three equal doses a day for 10 days.) Therapy with oral iodoquinol usually follows.

▶ **For parasitic infection of sex organs,** 250 mg three times a day for 7 to 10 days, or 2 grams (g) each day in a single dose or divided into two equal doses; leave 4 to 6 weeks between courses of therapy. (Children: 5 mg for each 2.2 lb three times a day for 7 days.)

▶ **For other intestinal parasitic infection,** 250 mg three times a day

FLAGYL'S OTHER NAMES

Flagyl's generic name is metronidazole. Other brand names include Metric 21, Protostat, and Trikacide. In Canada, Apo-Metronidazole, Novonidazol, and PMS Metronidazole.

SIDE EFFECTS

Call your doctor if you have any of these possible drug side effects. Call *immediately* about any labeled "serious."

Serious: seizures; pain, tingling, numbness, or weakness in your hands or feet

Common: headache, dizziness, light-headedness, diarrhea, nausea, vomiting, stomach pain, appetite loss, metallic taste, red-brown urine, alcohol-induced vomiting

Tip: Avoid activities that require full alertness or coordination until you know how Flagyl affects you.

Other: vertigo, lack of balance and coordination, confusion, irritability, depression, restlessness, fatigue, drowsiness, insomnia, swelling of lower legs, abdominal cramps, swollen tongue, constipation, dry mouth, frequent or difficult urination, decreased sex drive, dryness of vagina and vulva, painful sex, feeling of pelvic pressure, itchiness, rash, flushing, fever

DRUG INTERACTIONS

Combining certain drugs may alter their action or produce unwanted side effects. Tell your doctor about other drugs you're taking, especially:

• alcohol and products that contain alcohol such as cough syrup (avoid during therapy and for at least 48 hours after therapy is completed)
• Antabuse
• anticoagulants (blood thinners) such as Coumadin
• Dilantin
• drugs toxic to the liver
• Eskalith
• Tagamet.

for 5 to 7 days, or 2 g once a day for 3 days. (Children: 5 mg for each 2.2 lb three times a day for 5 to 7 days.)

▶ **For certain other bacterial infections:** therapy starts with an intravenous dose. Maintenance dose is 7.5 mg for each 2.2 lb orally or intravenously every 6 hours, with the first dose given 6 hours after the initial dose. Dosage should not exceed 4 g a day.

How to take Flagyl

• Don't take more Flagyl than your doctor prescribes.
• Crush the tablets before swallowing, if necessary.
• If this drug upsets your stomach, take it with meals.
• Space doses evenly to keep a steady level of Flagyl in your blood.

Continued on next page ▶

If you miss a dose

Take the missed dose as soon as possible. However, if it's almost time for your next dose, skip the missed dose and take your next dose as scheduled. Don't take a double dose.

If you suspect an overdose

Contact your doctor *immediately*. Excessive Flagyl can cause seizures.

Warnings

• Make sure your doctor knows your medical history. You may not be able to take Flagyl, especially if you have heart or liver disease, blood abnormalities, or central nervous system problems, such as seizures, retinal problems, or swelling (edema).

• If you're in the first 3 months of pregnancy or if you're breast-feeding, check with your doctor before taking this drug.

• If you're being treated for a sexually transmitted infection (trichomoniasis), your sexual partners should also seek treatment. Active sexual partners should be treated at the same time.

• To prevent reinfection, wash your hands after bowel movements and before handling and eating food. Avoid eating raw foods.

• If your're taking this drug to treat an intestinal infection, see your doctor for follow-up visits. You may need to provide stool specimens for 3 months after treatment ends to make sure your infection is gone.

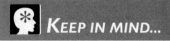

KEEP IN MIND...

* Crush before swallowing, if necessary.

* Avoid alcohol and products containing alcohol.

* Have sexual partners treated too.

F leet Phospho-Soda draws fluids into the small intestine, which softens stool and increases the volume of material inside the intestine. The added volume encourages bowel movements.

Why it's taken

Fleet Phospho-Soda (not to be confused with Fleet Enema) is taken to help relieve constipation. You can buy Fleet Phospho-Soda without a prescription. It comes in an oral solution. The following amounts are recommended for adults; children's dosages appear in parentheses.

▶ **For constipation,** 20 to 30 milliliters (ml) of solution mixed with 120 ml cold water taken once. (Children: 5 to 15 ml of solution mixed with 120 ml of cold water.)

How to take Fleet Phospho-Soda

• Take with a full (8-ounce) glass of cold water or fruit juice. Drink a second glass of water or fruit juice to provide more fluid for the laxative to work and to keep you from becoming dehydrated.

• This type of laxative — often called salts — produces rapid results and shouldn't be used for chronic constipation.

FLEET PHOSPHO-SODA'S OTHER NAME

Fleet Phospho-Soda is a combination of two generic drugs: sodium phosphate and sodium biphosphate.

SIDE EFFECTS

Call your doctor if you have any of these possible drug side effects. Call *immediately* about any labeled "serious."

Serious: continuous abdominal pain

Common: occasional abdominal cramping

Other: fluid and electrolyte disturbance (restlessness, shortness of breath, altered breathing, swelling), dehydration, laxative dependence with long-term use

Tip: Increase your fluid intake to avoid dehydration.

DRUG INTERACTIONS

Combining certain drugs may alter their action or produce unwanted side effects. Tell your doctor about other drugs you're taking.

Fleet Phospho-Soda usually starts working in 3 to 6 hours.

If you miss a dose

Not applicable.

If you suspect an overdose

Consult your doctor.

Warnings

• Make sure your doctor knows your medical history. You may not be able to use Fleet Phospho-Soda if you have abdominal pain, nausea, vomiting, a blocked or perforated intestine, lower-leg swelling, congestive heart failure, kidney problems, or an enlarged colon.

• Check with your doctor before using Fleet Phospho-Soda if you have large hemorrhoids or rectal irritation.

• Be careful if you're on a sodium-restricted diet; Fleet Phospho-Soda contains sodium compounds.

• Reduce your risk of future constipation by getting more exercise and adding water, fresh fruits and vegetables, and other fiber-rich foods to your diet.

• Frequent or prolonged use of laxatives can cause dependence on these products.

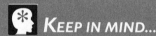
KEEP IN MIND...

* Take with two glasses of water or juice.

* Usually starts working 3 to 6 hours after taking.

* Don't use for chronic constipation.

* Anticipate absorption of salt from drug.

* Increase exercise, fluids, and fiber-rich foods.

Flexeril

Flexeril relaxes skeletal muscle spasms without affecting muscle function.

Why it's prescribed

Doctors prescribe Flexeril to relieve muscle pain, stiffness, and discomfort caused by strains, sprains, or injuries to your muscles. It comes in tablets. Doctors usually prescribe the following amounts for adults.

▶ **For short-term treatment of muscle spasm,** 20 to 40 milligrams (mg), divided into three or four equal doses a day for 7 days. Maximum dosage is 60 mg a day; maximum duration of treatment is 2 to 3 weeks.

How to take Flexeril

- Follow the label directions exactly.
- You may not notice Flexeril's effect until a day or two after you begin taking it.
- Don't stop taking Flexeril abruptly after long-term use without first asking your doctor. If you do, you could experience nausea, headache, and malaise.

If you miss a dose

If you remember within an hour or so of the missed dose, take it right away. Then go back to your regular schedule. If you don't remember until later, skip the missed dose and take your next dose on schedule. Don't take a double dose.

 If you suspect an overdose

Contact your doctor *immediately.* Excessive Flexeril can cause severe

FLEXERIL'S OTHER NAME

Flexeril's generic name is cyclobenzaprine hydrochloride.

 SIDE EFFECTS

Call your doctor if you have any of these possible drug side effects. Call *immediately* about any labeled "serious."

Serious: seizures

Common: drowsiness, constipation, heartburn or abdominal pain, dry mouth

Tips: Avoid activities that require full alertness or coordination until you know how Flexeril affects you. To relieve constipation, drink several extra glasses of water daily and eat more fiber-rich foods. If that doesn't help, check with your doctor about using a stool softener. If your mouth feels dry, try using sugarless hard candy or gum, ice chips, or a saliva substitute. If dry mouth lasts for more than 2 weeks, check with your doctor or dentist.

Other: euphoria, weakness, headache, insomnia, nightmares, tingling sensation, depression, visual disturbances, rapid heartbeat, abnormal taste, difficulty urinating, rash, hives, itchiness

 DRUG INTERACTIONS

Combining certain drugs may alter their action or produce unwanted side effects. Tell you doctor about other drugs you're taking, especially:
- alcohol and alcohol-containing products such as cough syrup
- antihistamines (used for treating colds, allergies, and hay fever)
- certain antidepressants (MAO inhibitors)
- muscle relaxants
- sedatives
- sleeping aids
- tranquilizers.

drowsiness, difficulty breathing, seizures, rapid or irregular heartbeat, and hallucinations.

✕ Warnings

- Make sure your doctor knows your medical history. You may not be able to take Flexeril if you have other medical problems, especially heart problems, an overactive thyroid, difficulty urinating, liver or kidney disease, or closed-angle glaucoma or if you've had a heart attack or taken certain antidepressant drugs (MAO inhibitors) recently.

❋ KEEP IN MIND...

* Increase fluids and fiber in diet.
* Call doctor about trouble urinating.
* Avoid alcohol.
* Don't stop drug suddenly.
* Check with doctor before taking any other drugs.

Florinef is a steroid that helps the body maintain a normal balance of certain important minerals.

Why it's prescribed

Doctors prescribe Florinef to supplement a low production of steroids in the body, which leads to conditions called adrenal insufficiency and adrenogenital syndrome. Florinef comes in tablets. Doctors usually prescribe the following amounts for adults.

▶ **For adrenal insufficiency (partial replacement) and adrenogenital syndrome,** 0.1 to 0.2 milligrams daily.

How to take Florinef

- Take the drug exactly as ordered.

If you miss a dose

Take the missed dose as soon as possible. But, if it's almost time for your next dose, skip the missed dose and take your next dose as scheduled. Don't take a double dose.

 If you suspect an overdose

Contact your doctor *immediately*. Excessive Florinef can disturb the levels of fluids and electrolytes in your body and can cause high blood pressure, swollen hands and feet, and heart problems.

 Warnings

- Make sure your doctor knows your medical history. You may not be able to take Florinef if you are overly sensitive to the drug or if

FLORINEF'S OTHER NAME

Florinef's generic name is fludrocortisone acetate.

 SIDE EFFECTS

Call your doctor if you have any of these possible drug side effects. Call *immediately* about any labeled "serious."

Serious: low potassium levels, cramps, heart palpitations, high blood pressure (headache, blurred vision)
Tip: Call your doctor if your symptoms worsen and you feel weak or dizzy when you stand up.

Common: sodium and water retention, sudden weight gain, mild swelling of hands and feet
Tip: Eat a low-sodium diet to minimize these problems.

Other: cough, difficulty swallowing, hives, itchiness, rash

DRUG INTERACTIONS

Combining certain drugs may alter their action or produce unwanted side effects. Tell your doctor about other drugs you're taking, especially:

- adrenocorticotropic hormone (ACTH)
- alcohol
- antibiotics, such as Mezlin, Pipracil, Ticar, and Timentin
- antifungal drugs, such as Fulvicin and Fungizone
- aspirin or other products containing salicylates
- baking soda
- barbiturates
- Butazolidin
- diuretics (water pills), such as Diamox and Lasix
- drugs that contain sodium, other steroids
- Geopen
- glaucoma drugs, such as Daranide and Neptazane
- heart drugs
- insulin
- laxatives (regularly)
- seizure drugs, such as Dilantin, Mysoline, and Tegretol
- tuberculosis drugs, such as Capastat and Rifampin
- vitamin B_{12} or D.

you have other medical problems, especially a fungal infection; an underactive thyroid; digestive problems; kidney, liver, or heart problems; high blood pressure; or bone disorders.

 KEEP IN MIND...

* Eat low-sodium diet, if prescribed.

* Report sudden weight gain or worsening of symptoms.

* Check with doctor before taking any other drugs.

Floropryl

Floropryl is one of several drugs called miotics, which cause the pupils of the eyes to contract.

Why it's prescribed

Doctors prescribe Floropryl to treat some forms of glaucoma and to diagnose and treat a few other eye diseases. It comes in an ointment. Doctors usually prescribe the following amounts for adults.

▶ **For glaucoma,** ¼-inch ribbon of ointment applied to each eye every 8 to 72 hours.

▶ **To diagnose convergent strabismus (crossed eyes),** ¼-inch ribbon of ointment applied to each eye each day at bedtime for 2 weeks.

▶ **To treat convergent strabismus (crossed eyes),** ¼-inch ribbon of ointment applied to each eye at bedtime for 2 weeks, then once every 2 to 7 days, depending on response, for 2 months.

▶ **For preoperative treatment of strabismus in children,** ¼-inch ribbon of ointment applied to each eye once each night.

How to use Floropryl

• Wash your hands before and after each application.

• To avoid contaminating the drug, don't touch the applicator tip to your eye or to any surface; wipe the tip with a clean tissue after use.

• Don't use more than your doctor ordered.

If you miss a dose

Take the missed dose as soon as possible if you remember on the same

FLOROPRYL'S OTHER NAME

Floropryl's generic name is isoflurophate.

SIDE EFFECTS

Call your doctor if you have any of these possible drug side effects.

Serious: none reported

Common: eye burning, blurred vision
Tip: Pat the eye gently after applying the drug; don't rub.

Other: headache, brow ache, unusual fatigue or weakness, slow or irregular heartbeat, retinal detachment (spots in field of vision, gradual painless vision loss leading to a veil-like obscuring of part of visual field), cysts in the iris (small, fluid-filled sacs in the colored part of the eye), changes in the eye's lens and conjunctiva (clouded vision, increased tearing), blocked tear ducts (swelling, redness), increased eye pressure (eye pain, vision loss), red eyes, eyelid twitching, nausea, vomiting, diarrhea, abdominal cramps or pain, loss of bladder control, sweating, flushing, vision changes

DRUG INTERACTIONS

Combining certain drugs may alter their action or produce unwanted side effects. Tell your doctor about other drugs you're taking, especially:

• antiarrhythmics, such as Norpace, Pronestyl and Quinidex
• antidepressants
• antihistamines
• antipsychotics
• Atrovent
• bladder-control drugs, such as Ditropan and Urispas
• Cyclogyl
• drugs for treating Parkinson's disease such as Symmetrol
• epinephrine
• insecticides or pesticides
• Isopto-Eserine
• local anesthetics such as cocaine
• muscle relaxants, such as Flexeril and Norflex
• muscle stimulants, such as Mestinon, Mytelase, and Prostigmin
• nausea drugs, such as Antivert, Bucladin, Marezine, and Phenergan
• Prioderm
• Ritalin
• steroids for eye conditions (Cyclogyl, Isopto Eserine)
• Tegretol
• Temaril.

day. However, if you're on an every-other-day dosing cycle and you remember on your off day, apply the drug on that day, skip a day, and then resume your every-other-day

schedule. If you remember when it's almost time for your next dose, skip the missed dose and apply your next dose as scheduled. Don't apply a double dose.

If you suspect an overdose

Consult your doctor.

Warnings

• Make sure your doctor knows your medical history. You may not be able to use Floropryl if you're overly sensitive to the drug, if you have acute closed-angle glaucoma, corneal abrasion, a history of retinal detachment, bronchial asthma, slow heartbeat, low blood pressure, seizures, spastic digestive disturbances, or Parkinson's disease or if you've had a heart attack.

• If you're pregnant or breast-feeding, tell your doctor before you start taking Floropryl.

• If your response to Floropryl decreases over time, the doctor may switch you to another similar drug for a short time.

• Be aware that long-term treatment with Floropryl raises the risk of cysts (small fluid-filled sacs) developing in the eyes. The risk is greatest for children.

• Your doctor will want to check the pressure in your eyes regularly.

• Avoid breathing the fumes from pesticides while using Floropryl. Certain pesticides add to Floropryl's effect on nerve impulse transmission.

• Wear or carry a medical identification that shows you're taking Floropryl.

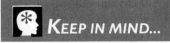

KEEP IN MIND...

* Keep applicator from touching eye.

* Avoid pesticides.

* Have eye pressure checked regularly.

* Don't use more than your doctor ordered.

Floxin

Floxin kills bacteria or prevents their growth in many areas of the body.

Why it's prescribed

Doctors prescribe Floxin to treat bacterial infections. It comes in tablets. Doctors usually prescribe the following amounts for adults.

▶ **For lower respiratory tract infections,** 400 milligrams (mg) every 12 hours for 10 days.

▶ **For cervicitis or urethritis caused by** *Chlamydia* **or gonorrhea,** 300 mg every 12 hours for 7 days.

▶ **For acute, uncomplicated gonorrhea,** 400 mg as a single dose.

▶ **For mild to moderate skin infections,** 400 mg every 12 hours for 10 days.

▶ **For cystitis,** 200 mg every 12 hours for 3 days.

▶ **For urinary tract infections,** 200 mg every 12 hours for 7 days. Complicated infections may require 10 days.

▶ **For prostatitis,** 300 mg every 12 hours for 6 weeks.

How to take Floxin

• Take Floxin exactly as ordered.
• For best results, take each dose with a full glass (8 ounces) of water. Drink several extra glasses of water every day unless your doctor tells you otherwise.
• Finish your prescription, even after you begin to feel better.

If you miss a dose

Take the missed dose as soon as possible. However, if it's almost time

FLOXIN'S OTHER NAME

Floxin's generic name is ofloxacin.

 ## SIDE EFFECTS

Call your doctor if you have any of these possible drug side effects. Call *immediately* about any labeled "serious."

Serious: seizures, severe allergic reaction (hives, difficulty breathing, facial swelling)

Common: headache, nausea
Tip: Take the drug with food to reduce nausea.

Other: dizziness, fatigue, lethargy, malaise, drowsiness, disturbed sleep, nervousness, light-headedness, chest pain, appetite loss, abdominal discomfort, diarrhea, vomiting, dry mouth, gas, altered taste, vaginal discharge, genital itching, joint and muscle pain, rash, skin sensitivity to sun, fever
Tips: Avoid activities that require full alertness or coordination until you know how Floxin affects you. For sun sensitivity, use a sunscreen and wear a hat and protective clothing when you go outdoors.

 ## DRUG INTERACTIONS

Combining certain drugs may alter their action or produce unwanted side effects. Tell your doctor about other drugs you're taking, especially:
• antacids with aluminum or magnesium, Carafate, iron supplements, and products containing zinc (take at least 2 hours before or after taking Floxin)
• anticoagulants (blood thinners) such as Coumadin
• cancer drugs
• Theo-Dur.

for your next dose, skip the missed dose and take your next dose as scheduled. Don't take a double dose.

 ### If you suspect an overdose

Consult your doctor.

 ### Warnings

• Make sure your doctor knows your medical history. You may not be able to take Floxin if you're overly sensitive to it or if you have seizures or kidney problems.
• Tell your doctor if you're pregnant or breast-feeding.

• If you're being treated for gonorrhea, your doctor may want you have a test for syphilis as well. Floxin will not cure syphilis, and it may hide the symptoms.

 ## KEEP IN MIND...

* Take with water and drink extra water each day.

* Finish entire amount prescribed.

* Protect skin from the sun.

Flumadine

Flumadine is an antiviral drug that works by interfering with the virus's ability to reproduce.

Why it's prescribed

Doctors prescribe Flumadine to prevent or treat Type A influenza, either alone or in combination with flu shots. It comes in tablets and syrup. Doctors usually prescribe the following amounts.

▶ **For influenza A in adults and children age 10 and above,** 100 milligrams (mg) twice a day.

▶ **For influenza A in children under age 10,** 5 mg for each 2.2 pounds of body weight once a day. Maximum dosage is 150 mg a day.

▶ **For influenza A in elderly people or those with severe liver or kidney problems,** 100 mg daily.

How to take Flumadine

• Start taking Flumadine within 48 hours of experiencing flu symptoms. Continue taking it for 7 days or as long as your doctor advises.

• Take Flumadine several hours before bedtime to avoid insomnia.

• Space your doses evenly and try not to miss any doses.

• Take the entire prescribed amount; don't stop when you begin to feel better.

If you miss a dose

Take the missed dose as soon as possible. However, if it's almost time for your next dose, skip the missed dose and take your next dose as

FLUMADINE'S OTHER NAME

Flumadine's generic name is rimantadine.

SIDE EFFECTS

Call your doctor if you have any of these possible drug side effects. Call *immediately* about any labeled "serious."

Serious: seizures, extremely low blood pressure (severe dizziness and weakness, fainting)
Tip: If you've had seizures in the past and you have one while taking Flumadine, stop taking it and call your doctor right away.

Common: none reported

Other: insomnia, headache, dizziness, nervousness, fatigue, weakness, eye pain, ringing in the ears, nausea, vomiting, loss of appetite, dry mouth, abdominal pain
Tips: To avoid nausea, take this drug with food. Avoid activities that require full alertness or coordination until you know how Flumadine affects you.

DRUG INTERACTIONS

Combining certain drugs may alter their action or produce unwanted side effects. Tell your doctor about other drugs you're taking.

---

scheduled. Don't take a double dose.

If you suspect an overdose

Consult your doctor. Excessive Flumadine may cause agitation, hallucinations, and irregular heartbeat.

Warnings

• Make sure your doctor knows your medical history. You may not be able to take Flumadine if you have a drug allergy, kidney or liver problems, or seizures.

• You may still be able to spread the flu, even when you're taking Flumadine. Minimize direct contact with others, especially people at great risk for infection, until your infection passes.

• Make sure your doctor knows if you're pregnant or breast-feeding before you begin taking Flumadine.

• Older adults may be especially prone to Flumadine's side effects.

• Don't give this drug to infants under age 1.

KEEP IN MIND...

∗ Start Flumadine as soon as possible after symptoms appear.

∗ Take entire amount prescribed, even if you feel better.

∗ Take several hours before bedtime.

∗ Minimize contact with others to avoid spreading flu.

Fluoritab

Fluoritab stabilizes the structure of bones and teeth. It promotes healthy tooth growth and prevents tooth decay.

Why it's taken

Fluoritab is taken to reduce or prevent tooth decay in adults and children. You can buy it without a prescription. Fluoritab comes in tablets, chewable tablets, lozenges, gel, drops, and an oral rinse. The following amounts are usually recommended.

▶ **To prevent tooth decay,** in adults and children over 6 years, 5 to 10 milliliters (ml) of oral rinse or a thin ribbon of gel applied to teeth with a toothbrush for at least 1 minute at bedtime. Children ages 4 to 6: 1-milligram (mg) tablet or lozenge daily. Children ages 2 to 3: 0.5-mg tablet or drops daily. Children under age 2: 0.25-mg tablet or drops daily.

How to use Fluoritab

• For best results, use Fluoritab just after brushing your teeth.

FLUORITAB'S OTHER NAMES

Fluoritab's generic name is sodium fluoride. Other brand names for tablets and lozenges include Fluorodex, Flura, Lozi-Tabs, Pediaflor, Pharmaflur, Phos-Flur; and, in Canada, Fluor-A-Day, Fluotic, Pedi-Dent, Solv-Flur. Brand names for topical sodium fluoride (gel, drops, or rinse) include ACT, Fluorigard, Fluorinse, Gel Kam, Gel-Tin, Karigel, Listermint with Fluoride, Minute Gel, Point Two, PreviDent, and Thera-Flur.

SIDE EFFECTS

Call your doctor if you have any of these possible drug side effects. Call *immediately* about any labeled "serious."

Serious: mottling of tooth enamel (fluorosis)
Tip: Tell your doctor if your teeth begin to look mottled; it could be a sign of too much Fluoritab.

Common: none reported

Other: headache, weakness, stomach upset, nausea, vomiting, bad taste (salty, soapy), allergic skin reactions (rash, itching), hives

DRUG AND FOOD INTERACTIONS

Combining certain drugs or foods may alter drug action or produce unwanted side effects. Tell your doctor about other drugs you're taking and your diet, especially:
• dairy products.

• Swish the rinse around and between your teeth for 1 minute; then spit it out.
• Take oral drops undiluted or mixed with nondairy food or fluids.
• Mix drops or rinses in plastic rather than glass containers.
• Don't swallow Fluoritab rinses or gels; especially don't allow children under age 3 to swallow them.
• Don't eat, drink, or rinse your mouth for 30 minutes after using Fluoritab.
• Don't take or use more than the prescribed amount.

If you miss a dose

Consult your doctor.

 ## If you suspect an overdose

Contact your doctor *immediately*. Especially in children, excessive Fluoritab can cause increased salivation, vomiting, diarrhea, seizures, and respiratory or heart failure.

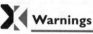 **Warnings**

• Make sure your doctor knows your medical history. You may not be able to use Fluoritab if you're overly sensitive to it, if you're on a low-sodium diet, or if you have joint pain, kidney problems, or a stomach ulcer.
• To be effective, fluoride supplements should last from infancy to age 14. Tell your doctor if you move to another area or your water supply changes.

 ## KEEP IN MIND...

∗ Don't take with dairy products.
∗ Use after brushing teeth.
∗ Don't eat or rinse mouth for 30 minutes after use.

Folvite

Folvite is a B vitamin (B_9) known as folic acid. It stimulates formation of normal blood cells.

Why it's prescribed

Doctors prescribe Folvite to help prevent or treat conditions resulting in anemia, such as alcoholism, chronic diarrhea, protracted fever, hemodialysis, intestinal problems, liver disease, or pregnancy. Folvite comes in tablets. Doctors usually prescribe the following amounts for adults; children's dosages appear in parentheses.

▶ **For vitamin B_9 anemia,** 0.4 to 1 milligram (mg) daily. (Children age 4 and over: same as adults. Children under age 4: up to 0.3 mg a day.)

▶ **In pregnant and lactating women,** 0.8 mg a day.

▶ **To prevent anemia with possible fetal damage during pregnancy,** up to 1 mg daily throughout pregnancy.

▶ **As a nutritional supplement,** 0.1 mg daily. (Children: 0.05 mg a day.)

▶ **To test folic acid deficiency in adults with megaloblastic anemia without masking pernicious anemia,** 0.1 to 0.2 mg for 10 days while maintaining a diet low in folic acid and vitamin B_{12}.

FOLVITE'S OTHER NAMES

Folvite's generic name is folic acid. A brand name in Canada is Novo-Folacid.

SIDE EFFECTS

Call your doctor if you have any of these possible drug side effects. Call *immediately* about any labeled "serious."

Serious: sudden asthmalike attack (wheezing, difficulty breathing)

Common: none reported

Other: allergic reaction (hives, itchiness, red skin), general malaise

DRUG INTERACTIONS

Combining certain drugs may alter their action or produce unwanted side effects. Tell your doctor about other drugs you're taking, especially:

- Azulfidine
- Chloromycetin
- Dilantin, Solfoton, and other seizure drugs
- Rheumatrex
- Trimpex.

How to take Folvite

- Follow your doctor's instructions exactly.
- Protect Folvite from heat and light; store it at room temperature.

If you miss a dose

Although you should try to remember to take Folvite every day, don't worry if you forget to take it, even for a few days. Don't make up missed doses, and don't take a double dose.

If you suspect an overdose

Consult your doctor.

Warnings

- Make sure your doctor knows your medical history. Be sure to tell your doctor if you have a condition called pernicious anemia, or if you have vitamin B_{12} deficiency.
- After your anemia is corrected, make sure you get adequate folic acid from your diet. Foods rich in folic acid include green vegetables, potatoes, fruits, grains, and organ meats.

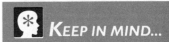

KEEP IN MIND...

* Take Folvite every day.
* Don't take if you have a vitamin B_{12} deficiency.
* Eat plenty of fresh foods containing folic acid.

Fosamax

Fosamax halts bone deterioration by stopping cells from reabsorbing minerals that build healthy bones.

Why it's prescribed

Doctors prescribe Fosamax to treat osteoporosis, or calcium and mineral loss that leaves bones porous and brittle, especially in women who are past menopause; and Paget's disease, which makes bones fragile, weak, and deformed. Fosamax comes in tablets. Doctors usually prescribe the following amounts for adults.

▶ **For osteoporosis in postmenopausal women,** 10 milligrams (mg) a day.

▶ **For Paget's disease,** 40 mg a day for 6 months.

How to take Fosamax

• Take Fosamax only as your doctor directs.

• Take Fosamax at least 30 minutes before your first food, beverage, or other medicines of the day. Waiting longer than 30 minutes improves absorption of the drug.

• Take Fosamax with a full glass of plain water only; food and other beverages can decrease the amount of medicine that your body absorbs.

• Don't lie down for at least 30 minutes after taking Fosamax. This helps the medicine stay in your stomach until it's absorbed and reduces the chance of stomach upset or heartburn.

If you miss a dose

Take the missed dose as soon as possible. However, if it's almost time

FOSAMAX'S OTHER NAME

Fosamax's generic name is alendronate sodium.

 SIDE EFFECTS

Call your doctor if you have any of these possible drug side effects.

Serious: none reported

Common: abdominal pain or bloating

Other: headache, nausea, indigestion, constipation, diarrhea, gas, acid regurgitation, ulcer, vomiting, difficulty swallowing, stomach upset, muscle or bone pain, taste change.

Tip: Take with food or use an antacid as directed by your doctor to prevent stomach upset.

 DRUG INTERACTIONS

Combining certain drugs may alter their action or produce unwanted side effects. Tell your doctor about other drugs you're taking, especially:

• antacids, calcium supplements (wait at least 30 minutes after taking Fosamax)

• aspirin, Tylenol, and other nonsteroidal anti-inflammatory drugs

• hormone replacement therapy.

for your next dose, skip the missed dose and go back to your regular dosing schedule. Don't take a double dose.

If you suspect an overdose

Contact your doctor *immediately*. Although no overdose of Fosamax has been reported, the most likely symptoms would be upset stomach, heartburn, ulcer, or other stomach-related problems and low calcium and phosphorus levels (difficulty swallowing, muscle spasms, and heart palpitations).

Warnings

• Make sure your doctor knows your medical history. You may not be able to take Fosamax if you have an allergy; a calcium deficiency, kidney disorder, ulcer, or other disorder of the stomach or digestive system; or trouble swallowing.

• Tell your doctor if you're pregnant or breast-feeding before you take Fosamax.

• Follow your doctor's instructions for correcting vitamin and mineral deficiencies before treatment begins. You may need to take calcium and vitamin D supplements if you don't get enough of these in your daily diet.

• Practice exercises that help increase bone mass, as your doctor directs. You may need to reduce cigarette smoking and alcohol use, as well, for the best results.

 KEEP IN MIND...

∗ Take calcium and vitamin supplements as directed.

∗ Take with plain water only.

∗ Stand or sit for 30 minutes after taking.

Foscavir

Foscavir inhibits cytomegalovirus (CMV) by preventing it from reproducing.

Why it's prescribed

Doctors prescribe Foscavir to treat an eye disorder called CMV retinitis in people with acquired immunodeficiency syndrome (AIDS). Foscavir is available only in an injectable form. Doctors usually prescribe the following amounts for adults.

▶ **For CMV retinitis in people with AIDS,** 60 milligrams (mg) for each 2.2 pounds (lb) of body weight injected into a vein every 8 hours for 2 to 3 weeks, then a maintenance dose of 90 mg for each 2.2 lb injected daily.

How to take Foscavir

• A nurse will administer this drug through an intravenous line, using an infusion pump.

If you miss a dose

Consult your doctor.

 ## If you suspect an overdose

Consult your doctor.

 ## Warnings

• Make sure your doctor knows your medical history. You may not be able to take Foscavir if you have other medical problems, especially

FOSCAVIR'S OTHER NAMES

Foscavir's generic name is foscarnet sodium (also known as phosphonoformic acid).

 ## SIDE EFFECTS

Call your doctor if you have any of these possible drug side effects. Call *immediately* about any labeled "serious."

Serious: seizures, meningitis (severe headache, neck stiffness, vomiting), encephalopathy (vomiting, seizures, lethargy), palpitations, high blood pressure (headache, blurred vision), low blood pressure (dizziness, weakness), bleeding from rectum, blood problems (bruising, bleeding, chills, fatigue, infection), coma

Common: headache, fatigue, violent shivering, dizziness, nausea, vomiting, diarrhea, cough, shortness of breath, rash, fever, pain at infusion site

Other: numbness, tingling, tremor, spasms, dementia, stupor, sensory disturbances, abnormal coordination, lip smacking, involuntary movements, change in speech, visual changes, abdominal pain, constipation, dry mouth, gas, increased urination, inability to urinate, urinary tract infections, increased sweating, leg cramps

DRUG INTERACTIONS

Combining certain drugs may alter their action or produce unwanted side effects. Tell your doctor about other drugs you're taking, especially:
• aminoglycosides, such as Amikin, Garamycin, and Nebcin
• amphotericin B such as Fungizone
• AZT
• pentamidin.

kidney problems, or if you have a sensitivity to this drug.
• Before you begin taking Foscavir and while you're taking it, your doctor may want you to have blood tests and 24-hour urine tests to monitor the condition of your kidneys. Be sure to keep all appointments for laboratory work.
• Your dosage will depend directly on the condition of your kidneys.
• Be aware that Foscavir may cause anemia, possibly severe enough to require blood transfusions.

• To minimize Foscavir's effect on your kidneys, you may need to drink more fluids while you're taking the drug.

 ## KEEP IN MIND...

* Report numbness or tingling in fingers or toes.

* Report any redness or pain at infusion site.

* Keep all appointments for lab tests.

Fragmin

Fragmin blocks steps in the blood clotting cycle, thereby preventing the formation of blood clots.

Why it's prescribed

Doctors prescribe Fragmin to prevent blood clots in people who are undergoing abdominal surgery. It's also used in people who are at risk for deep vein thrombosis (blood clots), including people who are over age 40, obese, undergoing surgery under general anesthesia lasting longer than 30 minutes, or have additional risk factors, such as cancer or a history of deep vein thrombosis or pulmonary embolism (blood clots in the lung). Fragmin comes only in an injectable form. Doctors usually prescribe the following amounts for adults.

▶ **To prevent clot formation after surgery,** 2,500 International Units injected under the skin daily, starting 1 to 2 hours before surgery and repeated once daily for 5 to 10 days after surgery.

How to take Fragmin

• A health care professional will administer injections of Fragmin.
• You'll receive the injections subcutaneously, probably in the skin around your navel or on your outer thigh. The site of the injection will vary from day to day.
• You'll be asked to sit or lie down to receive the injection. The person giving the injection will use thumb and forefinger to lift up a

FRAGMIN'S OTHER NAME

Fragmin's generic name is dalteparin sodium.

SIDE EFFECTS

Call your doctor if you have any of these possible drug side effects. Call *immediately* about any labeled "serious."

Serious: blood problems (fatigue, bruising, bleeding), pain at injection site, allergic reaction (difficulty breathing, facial or throat swelling)

Common: rash, itching

Other: fever, pinpoint red spots on skin

DRUG INTERACTIONS

Combining certain drugs may alter their action or produce unwanted side effects. Tell your doctor about other drugs you're taking, especially:
• anticoagulants (blood thinners) such as Coumadin
• antiplatelet agents, such as Persantine
• nonprescription drugs containing aspirin or other salicylates.

fold of skin, then insert the entire length of the needle at a 45- to 90-degree angle. The drug is never given directly into a muscle.

If you miss a dose

Consult your doctor.

If you suspect an overdose

Consult your doctor.

Warnings

• Make sure your doctor knows your medical history. You may not be able to take Fragmin if you're allergic to pork products or heparin; if you have a history of abnormal blood counts, stroke, or transient ischemic attacks; or if you have severe uncontrolled high blood pressure, a heart infection, a bleeding problem (particularly intestinal bleeding), ulcers or other intestinal disease, liver or kidney disease, or eye problems.

• Because you're taking Fragmin to prevent blood clots, your doctor will want to know if you develop any signs or symptoms of blood clots. Clots commonly form in the large veins of the legs, so notify your doctor about any redness, swelling, or pain in your legs or shortness of breath.
• Your doctor will probably want you to have periodic blood and stool tests during the course of treatment. Be sure to keep all appointments.

KEEP IN MIND...

∗ Report any bleeding or pain.
∗ Avoid aspirin.
∗ Keep appointments for lab tests.

Fulvicin

Fulvicin is an antifungal drug derived from penicillin. It kills fungal cells by preventing them from dividing.

Why it's prescribed

Doctors prescribe Fulvicin to treat fungal infections of the skin, scalp, fingernails, and toenails. In its microsize preparation (Fulvicin-U/F), it comes in tablets, capsules, and a liquid. In its ultramicrosize preparation (Fulvicin P/G), it comes in tablets. Doctors usually prescribe the following amounts for adults; children's dosages appear in parentheses.

▶ **For ringworm infections,** 500 milligrams (mg) of the microsize preparation daily in a single dose or divided into equal doses. Severe infections may require up to 1 gram (g) a day. Or, 330 to 375 mg of the ultramicrosize preparation daily in a single dose or divided into equal doses.

▶ **For athlete's foot, infections of the toenails and fingernails,** 0.75 to 1 g of the microsize preparation daily. Or, 660 to 750 mg of the ultramicrosize preparation daily, divided into equal doses. (Children over age 2: 11 mg of the microsize preparation for each 2.2 pounds [lb] of body weight daily. Or, 7.3 mg for each 2.2 lb a day of the ultramicrosize preparation.)

How to take Fulvicin

• Take Fulvicin with or after meals, preferably with fatty foods (for example, whole milk or ice cream) to reduce stomach upset.

FULVICIN'S OTHER NAMES

Fulvicin's generic name is griseofulvin. Other brand names Grifulvin and Grisactin.

 SIDE EFFECTS

Call your doctor if you have any of these possible drug side effects. Call *immediately* about any labeled "serious."

Serious: allergic reaction (rash, itching, wheezing), mouth sores, blood disorders (fever, chills, signs of infection)

Common: headache, skin sensitivity to sun
Tip: Use a sunscreen, wear protective clothing, and avoid intense sunlight.

Other: fatigue, confusion, dizziness, insomnia, vomiting, diarrhea, estrogen-like effects in children (enlarged breasts, appearance of pubic hair), white patches in mouth, lupuslike syndrome (aching joints)
Tip: Avoid activities that require full alertness or coordination until you know how Fulvicin affects you.

 DRUG INTERACTIONS

Combining certain drugs may alter their action or produce unwanted side effects. Tell your doctor about other drugs you're taking, especially:
• alcohol
• anticoagulants (blood thinners) such as Coumadin
• barbiturates such as Solfoton
• birth control pills (use additional birth control method).

• To help clear up your infection completely, take Fulvicin for the full time prescribed.

If you miss a dose

Take the missed dose as soon as possible. But if it's almost time for your next dose, skip the missed dose and take your next dose as scheduled. Don't take a double dose.

 If you suspect an overdose

Contact your doctor *immediately.* Excessive Fulvicin can cause confusion, blurred vision, nausea, vomiting, and diarrhea.

 Warnings

• Make sure your doctor knows your medical history. You may not be able to take Fulvicin if you're overly sensitive to the drug or allergic to penicillin or if you have lupus or blood, liver, or kidney disorders.
• Don't take during pregnancy.
• Keep your skin clean and dry during treatment.

 KEEP IN MIND...

* Keep skin clean and dry during therapy.
* Protect skin from sun.
* Use additional birth control if you take oral contraceptives.

Gammar is one of several drugs called immunizing agents. Made from blood plasma, it provides immunity to several diseases and increases the number of platelets, the blood cells required for blood to clot properly.

Why it's prescribed

Doctors prescribe Gammar to prevent or treat some illnesses caused by poor immunity. It comes in an injectable form. Doctors usually prescribe the following amounts for adults; children's dosages appear in parentheses.

▶ **For an immunune system deficiency (such as agammaglobulinemia or hypogammaglobulinemia),** 30 to 50 milliliters (ml) injected into a muscle once a month. (Children: 20 to 40 ml injected into a muscle once a month.)

▶ **To prevent hepatitis A in people who've been exposed to this virus,** 0.02 ml for each 2.2 pounds (lb) of body weight injected into a muscle as soon as possible after exposure. Up to 0.06 ml for each 2.2 lb may be given every 4 to 6 months if exposure will be 3 months of longer. (Children: same as adults.)

▶ **To prevent measles in people who've been exposed to this virus,** 0.25 ml for each 2.2 lb injected into a muscle within 6 days of exposure. (Children: same as adults.)

GAMMAR'S OTHER NAME

Gammar's generic name is immune globulin intramuscular (IGIM). Another brand name is Gamastan.

 SIDE EFFECTS

Call your doctor if you have any of these possible drug side effects. Call *immediately* about any labeled "serious."

Serious: severe allergic reaction (wheezing or closing up of throat, itching and reddened skin, and swelling of face, lips, throat, hands, and feet)

Common: none reported

Other: headache, hives, overall feeling of illness, fever, kidney dysfunction (swelling, weight gain, distended abdomen) and pain, redness, muscle stiffness at injection site
Tip: Use a different site for each injection.

 DRUG INTERACTIONS

Combining certain drugs may alter their action or produce unwanted effects. Tell your doctor about other drugs you're taking, especially:
• live-virus vaccines (consult your doctor before getting immunized during Gammar treatment).

How to take Gammar

• Take this drug exactly as your doctor directs.
• Be aware that this drug is usually injected by a health care professional into a large muscle, typically the buttock.

If you miss a dose

Consult your doctor.

 If you suspect an overdose

Consult your doctor.

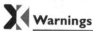 **Warnings**

• Make sure your doctor knows your medical history. You may not be able to take Gammar if you have other problems, such as an immune deficiency or a heart problem.

• If you were exposed to hepatitis A 6 weeks ago or earlier, you shouldn't receive this drug.
• If you're pregnant or breast-feeding, tell your doctor before you start taking Gammar.
• Be aware that, although Gammar is made from blood cells, it can't transmit hepatitis B or human immunodeficiency virus (HIV), the virus that causes AIDS.

KEEP IN MIND...

* Don't take this drug if exposure to hepatitis A occurred 6 weeks ago or longer.

* Don't get vaccines unless doctor approves.

* Use a different site for each injection.

Gantanol

antanol is one of several sulfa drugs that attack certain bacteria.

Why it's prescribed

Doctors prescribe Gantanol to treat bacterial infections. It comes in tablets and liquid. Doctors usually prescribe the following amounts for adults; children's dosages appear in parentheses.

▶ **For severe urinary tract and body-wide infections,** initially, 2 grams (g) for 1 day, then 1 g two or three times a day. (Children and infants over age 2 months: initially, 50 to 60 milligrams [mg] for each 2.2 pounds [lb] of body weight, then 25 to 30 mg for each 2.2 lb twice a day. Maximum dosage is 75 mg for each 2.2 lb a day.)

How to take Gantanol

• Take Gantanol at the same time every day to keep the amount of drug in your bloodstream constant.
• With each dose, drink a full glass (8 ounces) of water. Also drink several extra glasses of water throughout the day to help prevent kidney stones.
• Take all of the prescribed drug, even if you feel better after a few days.

If you miss a dose

Take the missed dose as soon as you can. But if it's almost time for your next dose and you take two doses a day, wait 5 to 6 hours after taking the missed dose and then take your next dose. If you take three or more doses a day, wait 2 to 4 hours after taking the missed dose and then take the next dose. After that, resume your regular schedule. Don't take a double dose.

GANTANOL'S OTHER NAMES

Gantanol's generic name is sulfamethoxazole. A brand name in Canada is Apo-Methoxazole.

 SIDE EFFECTS

Call your doctor if you have any of these possible drug side effects. Call *immediately* about any labeled "serious."

Serious: allergic reaction (rash, itchiness, wheezing), pallor, seizures, serious blood problems (sore throat, fever, unusual bruising, bleeding, or tiredness), serious skin reaction (redness, blistering, peeling, loosening of skin)

Common: diarrhea, headache, dizziness, loss of appetite, nausea, vomiting, yellow-tinged skin and eyes
Tip: Avoid activities that require full alertness or coordination until you know how Gantanol affects you.

Other: skin sensitivity to sunlight, depression, hallucinations, abdominal pain, tongue swelling, blood in urine, kidney stones
Tip: Avoid direct sunlight and ultraviolet light.

 DRUG INTERACTIONS

Combining certain drugs may alter their action or produce unwanted side effects. Tell your doctor about other drugs you're taking, especially:
• anticoagulants (blood thinners) such as Coumadin
• Dilantin
• diuretics (water pills) such as HydroDIURIL
• Mexate
• oral diabetes drugs
• para-aminobenzoic acid (PABA), found in some multivitamins and sunscreens.

more doses a day, wait 2 to 4 hours after taking the missed dose and then take the next dose. After that, resume your regular schedule. Don't take a double dose.

If you suspect an overdose

Contact your doctor *immediately.* Excessive Gantanol can cause unconsciousness, yellow-tinged skin and eyes, and death.

 Warnings

• Make sure your doctor knows your medical history. You may not be able to take Gantanol if you're allergic to this or other substances or if you have anemia, liver or kidney problems, asthma, urinary blockage, or a metabolism disorder.
• Make sure your doctor knows if you're pregnant or breast-feeding before you begin taking Gantanol.

 KEEP IN MIND...

* Take at same time every day.
* Drink extra water throughout the day.
* Avoid direct sunlight.

Gantrisin (for eyes)

Gantrisin (for eyes) is one of a group of antibiotics, called sulfa drugs, that attack bacteria.

Why it's prescribed

Doctors prescribe Gantrisin (for eyes) to treat eye infections. It comes in eyedrops and ointment. Doctors usually prescribe the following amounts for adults and children.
▶ **For conjunctivitis, corneal ulcers and other eye-surface infections,** 2 to 3 drops in each eye three or more times a day or a thin strip of ointment applied inside your lower eyelid one to three times a day and at bedtime.

How to use Gantrisin

• Wash your hands before and after using Gantrisin.
• To avoid contamination, don't touch the applicator to your eye or to the surrounding skin.
• After using eyedrops or ointment, keep your eyes closed and press a finger lightly against each tear duct for 1 to 2 minutes to allow the drug to cover your eye.
• Use the drug for the full time prescribed, even if your symptoms go away after a few days.

If you miss a dose

Apply the missed dose as soon as possible. However, if it's almost

GANTRISIN'S OTHER NAME

Gantrisin's generic name is sulfisoxazole diolamine.

 SIDE EFFECTS

Call your doctor if you have any of these possible drug side effects.

Serious: none reported

Common: temporary stinging, burning, or blurring
Tips: Your vision may be blurry just after using Gantrisin (for eyes) ointment. Keep your eyes closed for 1 or 2 minutes and your vision should clear. Don't blink excessively because the medicine won't stay in your eyes long enough to heal your infection.

Other: itchy, swollen, burning eyelids

 DRUG INTERACTIONS

Combining certain drugs may alter their action or produce unwanted side effects. Tell your doctor about other drugs you're taking, especially:
• Garamycin
• silver eye preparations (silver nitrate or mild silver protein).

time for your next dose, skip the missed dose and apply your next dose as scheduled. Don't apply a double dose.

 If you suspect an overdose

Consult your doctor.

Warnings

• Make sure your doctor knows your medical history. You may not be able to take Gantrisin if you've ever had an allergic reaction to any type of sulfa drug.
• Don't use leftover Gantrisin for a new eye infection. Throw away any leftover drug when your infection is cured.
• Don't share this drug with anyone. If someone in your family develops the same symptoms that you have, call your doctor.
• Tell the doctor that you're taking Gantrisin before you have any diagnostic tests.

KEEP IN MIND...

* Tell doctor if you're allergic to sulfa drugs.
* Wash hands before and after use.
* Don't touch applicator to your eye or skin.
* Finish entire amount prescribed, even if you feel better.
* Discard any leftover drug.

Gantrisin (oral)

Gantrisin is one of a group of antibiotics, called sulfa drugs, that attack bacteria.

Why it's prescribed

Doctors prescribe oral Gantrisin to treat infections. It comes in tablets and liquid. Doctors usually prescribe the following amounts for adults; children's dosages appear in parentheses.

▶ **For urinary tract and body-wide infections,** initially, 2 to 4 grams (g), then 4 to 8 g divided into four to six equal doses and given over 24 hours. (Children over age 2 months: initially, 75 milligrams [mg] per 2.2 pounds [lb] of body weight divided into four equal doses and spaced evenly over 24 hours. Then 150 mg per 2.2 lb divided into four equal doses.)

How to take Gantrisin

- Take on an empty stomach.
- Take at evenly spaced intervals day and night to keep a stable level of the drug in your system.
- Measure liquid Gantrisin in a special medicine spoon, not a household teaspoon.
- Drink a full glass (8 ounces) of water with every dose, and drink several extra glasses of water throughout the day.

If you miss a dose

Take the missed dose as soon as you can. But if it's almost time for your next dose and you take two doses a day, wait 5 to 6 hours after taking

GANTRISIN'S OTHER NAMES

Gantrisin's generic name is sulfisoxazole (also known as sulfafurazole). A Canadian brand name is Novosoxazole.

SIDE EFFECTS

Call your doctor if you have any of these possible drug side effects. Call *immediately* about any labeled "serious."

Serious: itching or rash, blistering or peeling skin, decreased urine output, difficulty swallowing, seizures, kidney problems (painful urination, blood in urine), blood problems (fever, chills, sore throat, bruising, bleeding, unusual weakness), severe allergic reaction (difficulty breathing, swelling of face and throat)

Common: diarrhea, headache, dizziness, appetite loss, nausea
Tip: Avoid activities that require full alertness or coordination until you know how Gantrisin affects you.

Other: depression, hallucinations, abdominal pain, swollen tongue, blood in urine, sensitivity to sun, hives
Tip: Wear a sunscreen (not containing PABA) and protective clothing outdoors; avoid intense sunlight.

DRUG INTERACTIONS

Combining certain drugs may alter their action or produce unwanted side effects. Tell your doctor about other drugs you're taking, especially:
- anticoagulants (blood thinners) such as Coumadin
- Mexate
- oral diabetes drugs
- PABA, found in some multivitamins and sunscreens.

the missed dose before taking the next dose. If you take three or more doses a day, wait 2 to 4 hours after taking the missed dose before taking the next dose. Then resume your regular schedule. Don't take a double dose.

If you suspect an overdose

Contact your doctor *immediately*. Excessive Gantrisin can cause dizziness, drowsiness, unconsciousness, blood problems, and yellow-tinged skin and eyes.

Warnings

- Make sure your doctor knows your medical history. You may not

be able to take Gantrisin if you're overly sensitive to it or if you have urinary blockage, liver or kidney disease, allergies, asthma, or a blood or metabolism problem.
- Tell your doctor if you're pregnant or breast-feeding before you begin taking Gantrisin.

KEEP IN MIND...

* Take on an empty stomach.
* Take day and night at evenly spaced intervals.
* Drink a full glass of water with each dose and several extra glasses during the day.

Garamycin (for eyes)

aramycin is an anti-bacterial drug that kills bacterial cells by interfering with their ability to reproduce.

Why it's prescribed

Doctors prescribe Garamycin to treat eye infections. It comes in eyedrops and ointment. Doctors usually prescribe the following amounts for adults and children.

▶ **For external eye infections,** 1 to 2 drops in each eye every 4 hours. Severe infections may require up to 2 drops every hour. If using ointment, apply small amounts two or three times a day.

How to use Garamycin

• Carefully follow your doctor's instructions.
• Wash your hands before and after using Garamycin.
• Wipe away any crusty drainage from your eyes before instilling drops.
• To avoid contamination, don't touch the applicator to your eye or to the surrounding skin.
• Keep your eyes closed, and press a finger lightly against each tear duct for 1 to 2 minutes after using drops or ointment to allow the medicine to cover your eye.

GARAMYCIN'S OTHER NAMES

Garamycin's generic name is gentamicin. Other brand names include Genoptic, Gentacidin; and, in Canada, Cidomycin.

• Finish taking your entire prescription, even after your eye infection seems to clear up. Stopping early invites a recurrent infection.
• Store this medicine away from heat.

If you miss a dose

Use the eyedrops or apply the ointment as soon as possible. But if it's almost time for the next dose, skip the missed dose and apply your next dose on schedule. Don't apply a double dose.

If you suspect an overdose

Consult your doctor.

Warnings

• Make sure your doctor knows your medical history. You may not be able to take Garamycin if you're allergic to this drug or to related an-

tibiotics, such as Amikin, Kantrex, neomycin, streptomycin, or Tobrex.
• Don't share your eyedrops with other family members.
• Don't share your towels or washcloths with others.
• Follow all of your doctor's recommendations exactly because complete vision loss can occur from certain bacteria.

SIDE EFFECTS

Call your doctor if you have any of these possible drug side effects.

Serious: none reported

Common: temporary eye irritation, blurred vision (if using ointment)
Tip: To avoid irritation, dab the eye with a tissue; don't rub.

Other: numbness of lower eyelid, dilated pupils

DRUG INTERACTIONS

Combining certain drugs may alter their action or produce unwanted side effects. Tell your doctor about other drugs you're taking.

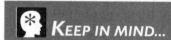
KEEP IN MIND...

* Wash your hands before and after use.

* Keep eyes closed for 1 to 2 minutes after use.

* Finish the entire amount prescribed.

* Don't share your eyedrops.

* Don't share towels or washcloths with others.

Glucophage

Glucophage decreases the amount of sugar (glucose) produced by the liver, reduces the amount of sugar absorbed by the intestine, and improves the body's sensitivity to insulin.

Why it's prescribed

Doctors prescribe Glucophage to help control blood sugar levels in non-insulin-dependent (type II) diabetes. It comes in tablets. Doctors usually prescribe the following amounts for adults.

▶ **To lower blood sugar levels in type II diabetes,** initially 500 milligrams (mg) twice a day with morning and evening meals, or 850 mg once a day with the morning meal. With 500-mg dose form, dosage may be increased by 500 mg a week to a maximum dosage of 2,500 mg a day if needed. With 850-mg dose form, dosage may be increased by 850 mg every other week to a maximum dosage of 2,550 mg a day if needed.

How to take Glucophage

• Never change the amount you take without your doctor's consent.

If you miss a dose

Consult your doctor.

If you suspect an overdose

Consult your doctor.

Warnings

• Make sure your doctor knows your medical history. You may not

GLUCOPHAGE'S OTHER NAME

Glucophage's generic name is metformin hydrochloride.

SIDE EFFECTS

Call your doctor if you have any of these possible drug side effects. Call *immediately* about any labeled "serious."

Serious: lactic acidosis (confusion, increased breathing rate, dizziness, tiredness, fainting, muscle pain)

Common: diarrhea, nausea, vomiting, abdominal bloating, gas, appetite loss

Tips: Take with food to reduce stomach upset. Stop taking Glucophage and call your doctor right away if you experience dehydration from diarrhea and vomiting (extreme dry mouth, decreased sweating and urination, thirst, weight loss).

Other: anemia, rash, dermatitis, unpleasant or metallic taste

DRUG INTERACTIONS

Combining certain drugs may alter their action or produce unwanted side effects. Tell your doctor about other drugs you're taking, especially:
• alcohol
• antiarrhythmics, such as Cardioquin, Lanoxin, and Procan SR
• antipsychotic drugs
• birth control pills, estrogens
• corticosteroids
• Dilantin
• diuretics (water pills), such as Dyrenium and Midamor
• heart drugs called calcium channel blockers, such as Adalat and Procardia
• iodine contrast agents used in diagnostic tests
• Laniazid
• morphine
• muscle relaxants such as quinine
• nicotinic acid
• thyroid replacement drugs
• ulcer drugs, such as Tagamet and Zantac
• Vancocin.

be able to take Glucophage if you're overly sensitive to it or if you have kidney problems, liver problems, metabolic acidosis, adrenal or pituitary insufficiency, or malnourishment.

• Your doctor will probably want to test your kidneys before starting you on Glucophage and at least once a year thereafter. If your kid-

neys begin to show problems, your doctor will probably switch you to a different drug.

• Monitor your blood sugar levels regularly and carefully. Tell your doctor if your blood sugar level stays too high. You may need insulin therapy during periods of stress,

Continued on next page ▶

such as when you have an infection, a fever, surgery, or some form of trauma.

• If your blood sugar level doesn't respond well enough to Glucophage alone, your doctor will probably add another drug to your therapy. If your blood sugar level doesn't respond to therapy at maximum dosages, you may need to switch to insulin.

• Follow your prescribed diet closely in addition to taking Glucophage.

• Stop taking Glucophage and call your doctor right away if you develop unexplained hyperventilation (rapid breathing, dizziness, tingling in fingers or feet), muscle pain, malaise, unusual sleepiness, or signs of lactic acidosis.

• Check with your doctor before taking any drug, including nonprescription drugs.

• Tell the doctor you're on Glucophage before having any diagnostic tests.

• Tell family members how to treat high and low blood sugar so they're prepared if you have a reaction and can't direct them.

• Wear or carry medical identification stating that you're a diabetic.

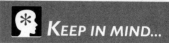

KEEP IN MIND...

* Take with food.
* Follow prescribed diet carefully.
* Check blood sugar level regularly.
* Teach family how to treat blood sugar reactions.

Glucotrol causes the pancreas to release insulin and reduce blood sugar levels.

Why it's prescribed

Doctors prescribe Glucotrol in combination with diet and exercise to control blood sugar levels in non-insulin-dependent (type II) diabetes. It comes in tablets and slow-release tablets. Doctors usually prescribe the following amounts.

▶ **To lower blood sugar levels or replace insulin therapy**, initially, 5 milligrams (mg) a day before breakfast. Usual maintenance dosage is 10 to 15 mg. Maximum recommended dosage is 40 mg a day. If insulin dosage is more than 20 units daily, therapy starts at usual dosage in addition to cutting the insulin dosage by 50%. If insulin dosage is less than 20 units, insulin may be discontinued.

How to take Glucotrol

• Take Glucotrol exactly as prescribed. Take it at the same time each day, about 30 minutes before a meal. If you take one dose a day, take it in the morning.

If you miss a dose

Take the missed dose as soon as possible. But if it's almost time for your next dose, skip the missed dose and take your next dose as scheduled. Don't take a double dose.

 If you suspect an overdose

Contact your doctor *immediately*. Excessive Glucotrol can cause leth-

GLUCOTROL'S OTHER NAME

Glucotrol's generic name is glipizide.

 ## SIDE EFFECTS

Call your doctor if you have any of these possible drug side effects. Call *immediately* about any labeled "serious."

Serious: low blood sugar (clammy skin, tremors, anxiety, fatigue)

Common: headache, nausea, vomiting, constipation

Other: nervousness, increased sweating, fast heartbeat, skin sensitivity to sun, dizziness, jaundice, rash, itchiness, facial flushing
Tip: To prevent skin reactions, wear a sunscreen and protective clothing outdoors and avoid intense sun.

 ## DRUG INTERACTIONS

Combining certain drugs may alter their action or produce unwanted side effects. Tell your doctor about other drugs you're taking, especially:
• alcohol
• antidepressants called MAO inhibitors
• anticoagulants (blood thinners), such as Coumadin and aspirin
• beta blockers such as Catapres, Inderal, Ismelin
• diuretics (water pills)
• seizure drugs such as Dilantin, Rifadin
• steroids
• sulfa antibiotics such as Bactrim.

---

argy, rapid heartbeat, seizures, and coma.

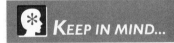 ## Warnings

• Make sure your doctor knows your medical history. You may not be able to take Glucotrol if you are overly sensitive to it; have had diabetic ketoacidosis; have other medical problems, especially liver or kidney problems or thyroid disease; or are elderly, pregnant, or breast-feeding.
• Monitor your blood sugar levels regularly. Tell your doctor if your blood sugar stays too high.
• Follow your prescribed diet and exercise plan carefully.
• If you develop new problems, especially infections, tell your doctor.

• Tell family members how to treat high and low blood sugar so they're prepared if you have a reaction and can't direct them.
• Carry medical identification that indicates diabetes.

KEEP IN MIND...

∗ Follow diet and exercise plan.

∗ Check blood sugar levels regularly.

∗ Teach family how to treat blood sugar reactions.

GoLYTELY

GoLYTELY is a laxative solution that can't be absorbed by the intestine, so it moves through the body quickly.

Why it's prescribed

Doctors prescribe GoLYTELY to clean out the intestines before examinations and tests. It comes in a powder for mixing into a solution. Doctors usually prescribe the following amounts for adults.

▶ **For bowel preparation before examination,** 8 ounces every 10 minutes until 48 ounces are consumed.

How to take GoLYTELY

- Use tap water to reconstitute the powder until you have 48 ounces of solution. Shake or stir it vigorously to ensure that all powder is dissolved.
- Don't add flavoring or other ingredients to the solution.
- Refrigerate reconstituted solution, but use within 48 hours.
- Fast for 3 or 4 hours before drinking the solution. Afterward, take only clear fluids until your examination is over.
- Allow yourself about 4 hours to drink the solution and empty your bowel. If your examination is early in the morning, drink the solution

 SIDE EFFECTS

Call your doctor if you have any of these possible drug side effects.

Serious: none reported

Common: nausea, bloating, abdominal cramps, vomiting

Other: hypothermia from chilled solution

Tip: It's okay to let the solution warm up while you drink it. Drinking a large amount of chilled solution could make you cold.

 DRUG INTERACTIONS

Combining certain drugs may alter their action or produce unwanted side effects. Tell your doctor about other drugs you're taking.

the evening before, as directed by your doctor.
- Drink a full glass of solution every 10 minutes. For best results, don't sip it; drink each glass quickly.
- Expect to have your first bowel movement within an hour of drinking your first glass of solution. Your intestines will be completely cleaned within about an hour after you finish drinking all the solution.

If you miss a dose

Not applicable.

 If you suspect an overdose

Consult your doctor.

 Warnings

- Make sure your doctor knows your medical history. You may not be able to take GoLYTELY if you have a blocked or perforated intestine, gastric retention (inability to empty the stomach properly), colitis, or an enlarged colon.

- Tell your doctor if you've ever had an allergic or unusual reaction to GoLYTELY or to any foods or dyes.
- Any drugs you take within an hour of starting your GoLYTELY solution could be washed out of your system. Ask your doctor what to do about conflicting medication schedules.

GoLYTELY's OTHER NAMES

GoLYTELY's generic name is polyethylene glycol (PEG) and electrolyte solution. Other brand names include Colovage, CoLyte, NuLYTELY, and OCL.

KEEP IN MIND...

* Mix powder and tap water to make 48 ounces.

* Fast for 3 to 4 hours before starting.

* Don't take any drugs within 1 hour of starting GoLYTELY.

* Drink a full glass of solution every 10 minutes.

* Drink the solution quickly; don't sip it.

Grisactin

Grisactin is an antifungal drug derived from penicillin. It kills fungal cells by preventing them from dividing.

Why it's prescribed

Doctors prescribe Grisactin to treat fungal infections of the skin, scalp, and nails. In its microsize form (Grisactin-U/F), it comes in tablets, capsules, and liquid. In its ultramicrosize form (Grisactin P/G), it comes in tablets. Doctors usually prescribe the following amounts for adults; children's dosages appear in parentheses.

▶ **For ringworm infections of the skin, scalp, or nails,** 500 milligrams (mg) of microsize form daily in a single dose or divided into equal doses. Severe infections may require up to 1 gram (g) a day. Or, 330 to 375 mg of ultramicrosize form daily in a single dose or divided into equal doses.

▶ **For athlete's foot, infections of the nails,** 0.75 to 1 g of microsize form daily. Or, 660 to 750 mg of ultramicrosize form daily, divided into equal doses. (Children over age 2: 11 mg of microsize form for each 2.2 pounds [lb] of body weight daily. Or, 7.3 mg for each 2.2 lb a day of ultramicrosize form.)

How to take Grisactin

• Take Grisactin with or after meals, preferably with fatty foods (for example, whole milk or ice cream) to reduce stomach upset.
• To help clear up your infection completely, take Grisactin for the full time prescribed.

GRISACTIN'S OTHER NAMES

Grisactin's generic name is griseofulvin. Other brand names include Fulvicin, Grifulvin V, and Grisactin Ultra.

SIDE EFFECTS

Call your doctor if you have any of these possible drug side effects. Call *immediately* about any labeled "serious."

Serious: allergic reaction (rash, itching, wheezing), fever, weakness, mouth sores, blood problems (fever, chills, signs of infection)

Common: headache, skin sensitivity to sun
Tip: Wear a sunscreen and wear protective clothing; avoid intense sunlight.

Other: hearing loss, fatigue, confusion, strange behavior, dizziness, insomnia, nausea, vomiting, excessive thirst, gas, diarrhea, estrogen-like effects in children (pubic hair, enlarged breasts), white patches in mouth, lupuslike syndrome (aching joints)
Tip: Avoid activities that require full alertness or coordination until you know how Grisactin affects you.

DRUG INTERACTIONS

Combining certain drugs may alter their action or produce unwanted side effects. Tell your doctor about other drugs you're taking, especially:
• alcohol
• anticoagulants (blood thinners) such as Coumadin
• barbiturates such as Solfoton
• birth control pills (use additional birth control method).

If you miss a dose

Take the missed dose as soon as possible. However, if it's almost time for your next dose, skip the missed dose and take your next dose as scheduled. Don't take a double dose.

If you suspect an overdose

Contact your doctor *immediately*. Excessive Grisactin can cause confusion, blurred vision, nausea, vomiting, and diarrhea.

Warnings

• Make sure your doctor knows your medical history. You may not be able to take Grisactin if you're allergic to the drug or to penicillin or if you have lupus or blood, liver, or kidney problems.
• Don't take Grisactin during pregnancy.
• Keep your skin clean and dry during treatment.

KEEP IN MIND...

∗ Keep skin clean and dry during therapy.

∗ Protect skin from sun.

∗ Use additional birth control if you take oral contraceptives.

Gyne-Lotrimin

Gyne-Lotrimin is a fungicide that kills fungi and prevents further spread in the body.

Why it's prescribed

Doctors prescribe Gyne-Lotrimin to treat fungal (yeast) infections of the vagina. It comes as a vaginal cream or vaginal tablet. The 100-milligram (mg) vaginal tablets and cream are available without a prescription, but the 500-mg tablets require a doctor's prescription. Doctors usually prescribe the following amounts for adults.

▶ **For vaginal yeast infection,** 100-mg tablet inserted in the vagina at bedtime for 7 consecutive days. Or, if you're not pregnant, you can insert two 100-mg tablets at bedtime for 3 consecutive days, or you can insert one 500-mg tablet one time at bedtime. If you use vaginal cream, insert one dose daily at bedtime for 7 to 14 days.

How to use Gyne-Lotrimin

• Unwrap a tablet, wet it with lukewarm water, and place it on the applicator. Or, fill the applicator with vaginal cream to the level indicated.
• Lie down with your knees apart, insert the applicator in your vagina, and deposit the tablet or cream.
• Apply a menstrual pad to keep the medication from leaking onto your clothes.

GYNE-LOTRIMIN'S OTHER NAMES

Gyne-Lotrimin's generic name is clotrimazole. Other brand names include Fem Care, Mycelex G, and Mycelex-7; and, in Canada, Canestin.

SIDE EFFECTS

Call your doctor if you have any of these possible drug side effects.

Serious: none reported

Common: mild vaginal burning or irritation
Tip: Check with your doctor if you feel burning or irritation in your vagina.

Other: none reported

DRUG INTERACTIONS

Combining certain drugs may alter their action or produce unwanted side effects. Tell your doctor about other drugs you're taking.

• Continue to use Gyne-Lotrimin for as long as prescribed, even if your symptoms soon clear up. Otherwise, your infection may return. Because fungal infections may be slow to clear up, you may need to use Gyne-Lotrimin every day for several weeks or more.

If you miss a dose

Insert the missed dose as soon as possible. However, if it's almost time for your next dose, skip the missed dose and insert your next dose as scheduled. Don't apply a double dose.

If you suspect an overdose

Consult your doctor.

Warnings

• Make sure your doctor knows your medical history, You may not be able to take Gyne-Lotrimin, especially if you have liver disease.
• If you're pregnant, don't use Gyne-Lotrimin without first checking with your doctor.

• If your symptoms don't improve in a few days, or if they get worse, call your doctor.
• You can help prevent reinfection by wearing cotton-crotch underwear and pantyhose.
• It's best to avoid having sex during your treatment. Ask your partner to wear a condom if you do have sex during treatment. Keep in mind that some vaginal preparations contain oil, which can weaken latex condoms. Also have your partner ask the doctor if he needs treatment as well.
• Most doctors advise against douching between doses. If you douche, use a vinegar-and-water douche.

KEEP IN MIND...

* Call doctor if vagina itches or burns.

* Wear cotton-crotch underwear and pantyhose.

* Use condoms and advise sex partner to be checked.

Halcion

Halcion is one of several drugs called sedative-hypnotics. It acts on the brain to produce calming effects.

Why it's prescribed

Doctors prescribe Halcion as a sleep aid. It comes in tablets. Doctors usually prescribe the following amounts.

▶ **For insomnia,** in adults under age 65, 0.125 to 0.5 milligrams (mg) at bedtime; in adults over age 65, 0.125 mg at bedtime, increased to 0.25 mg if needed.

How to take Halcion

- Follow your doctor's instructions exactly. Don't increase your dose, even if you think your current dose isn't working. Instead, call your doctor.
- Because Halcion begins to work right away, take it after you get in bed.
- Try additional ways to help yourself sleep, including warm milk, quiet music, avoiding alcohol near bedtime, regular exercise, and a consistent bedtime.
- Because Halcion can be habit-forming, don't take it for a longer time than your doctor prescribes.

If you miss a dose

Take the missed dose as soon as possible. However, if it's almost time for your next dose, skip the missed dose and take your next dose as scheduled. Don't take a double dose.

HALCION'S OTHER NAMES

Halcion's generic name is triazolam. A Canadian brand name is Apo-Triazo.

 SIDE EFFECTS

Call your doctor if you have any of these possible drug side effects. Call *immediately* about any labeled "serious."

Serious: slowed breathing

Common: drowsiness, dizziness, headache
Tips: Avoid activities that require full alertness or coordination until you know how Halcion affects you. If you feel overly tired in the morning, your dose may be too high; contact your doctor.

Other: rebound insomnia, amnesia, light-headedness, incoordination, confusion, depression, nausea, vomiting, dependence on drug
Tip: After you stop taking Halcion, you may have difficulty sleeping for the next few nights. This is not unusual and should stop on its own.

 DRUG INTERACTIONS

Combining certain drugs may alter their action or produce unwanted side effects. Tell your doctor about other drugs you're taking, especially:
- alcohol
- cigarettes (in high numbers)
- Dopar
- drugs that make you relax or feel sleepy, such as antihistamines, narcotic pain relievers, antidepressants, and barbiturates
- E-Mycin, Retrovir
- Haldol
- Tagamet.

 If you suspect an overdose

Contact your doctor *immediately.* Excessive Halcion can cause sleepiness, confusion, slurred speech, a slow heart rate, a staggering gait, and coma.

Warnings

- Make sure your doctor knows your medical history. You may not be able to take Halcion if you are overly sensitive to it or if you have sleep apnea, glaucoma, a muscle disorder, Parkinson's disease, depression, suicidal tendencies, a history of drug or alcohol abuse, or kidney, liver, or respiratory problems.
- Don't take this drug if you think you might be pregnant or if you're breast-feeding.
- Older adults may feel drowsy during the day after taking Halcion.

 KEEP IN MIND...

* Take Halcion after getting in bed.
* Expect brief insomnia when you stop taking Halcion.
* Morning "hangover" may mean your dosage is too high.

Haldol

Haldol is one of a group of drugs called neuroleptics that control hallucinations and agitation.

Why it's prescribed

Doctors prescribe Haldol to treat psychiatric conditions. It comes in tablets and liquid. Doctors usually prescribe the following amounts.

▶ **For strange (psychotic) behavior disorders,** in adults and children age 12 and over, dosage varies for each person; initial range is 0.5 to 5 milligrams (mg) two or three times a day; maximum dosage is 100 mg a day. Children ages 3 to 12: 0.05 to 0.15 mg for each 2.2 pounds (lb) of body weight a day. Severely disturbed children may require higher doses.

▶ **For nonpsychotic behavior disorders,** in children ages 3 to 12, 0.05 mg for each 2.2 lb a day. Maximum dosage is 6 mg a day.

▶ **For Tourette's syndrome,** in adults, 0.5 to 5 mg two or three times a day or as needed. In children ages 3 to 12, 0.075 mg for each 2.2 lb daily.

How to take Haldol

• Take this drug exactly as prescribed with food or milk.
• Take the liquid form by mouth only. If it doesn't come in a dropper bottle, use a specially marked measuring spoon, not a household teaspoon, to measure your dose.
• Don't stop taking it abruptly.

Side effects

Call your doctor if you have any of these possible drug side effects. Call *immediately* about any labeled "serious."

Serious: rapid heartbeat, difficulty breathing, profuse sweating, seizures

Common: nausea, temporary dry mouth and blurred vision, reduced perspiration, sensitivity to sun, involuntary movements, drowsiness
Tip: Avoid activities that require full alertness or coordination until you know how Haldol affects you.

Other: shaky tongue movement, inability to urinate menstrual irregularities, enlarged breasts in men, temporary blood problems (fever, chills, sore throat, unusual bruising or bleeding), heart problems (with high doses), rash

Drug interactions

Combining certain drugs may alter their action or produce unwanted side effects. Tell your doctor about other drugs you're taking, especially:
• alcohol and drugs that make you feel relaxed or sleepy
• Aldomet
• anticoagulants (blood thinners) such as Coumadin
• drugs used to treat Parkinson's disease and seizures
• Eskalith, Lithobid.

HALDOL'S OTHER NAMES

Haldol's generic name is haloperidol. Other brand names include Halperon; and, in Canada, Apo-Haloperidol and Novo-Peridol.

If you miss a dose

Take the missed dose as soon as possible, and space any doses remaining for that day at regular intervals. The next day, resume your regular schedule. Don't take a double dose.

If you suspect an overdose

Contact your doctor *immediately*. Excessive Haldol can cause unarousable sleep, agitation, seizures, and irregular heartbeats.

Warnings

• Make sure your doctor knows your medical history. You may not be able to take Haldol if you are overly sensitive to it, have Parkinson's disease, seizures, heart disease, glaucoma, inability to urinate, or may be pregnant or breast-feeding.
• If you experience trembling or uncontrolled movements, nausea, or vomiting after you stop taking Haldol, call your doctor right away.
• Children and older adults are especially sensitive to Haldol's side effects.

KEEP IN MIND...

* Take with food or milk.
* Tell doctor about any other drugs you're taking.
* Don't stop taking without consulting doctor.

Halog

Halog is one of a group of drugs called steroids. It stimulates the synthesis of the enzymes needed to decrease an inflammatory response.

Why it's prescribed

Doctors prescribe Halog to treat rashes and other skin conditions responsive to steroids. It comes in cream, ointment, and topical solution. Doctors usually prescribe the following amounts.

▶ **To relieve redness, swelling, itching, and discomfort from skin problems in adults and children,** apply two or three times a day.

How to use Halog

• Gently wash the affected area before applying Halog.
• Apply it sparingly and rub it in gently, leaving a thin coat.
• When treating hairy sites, part the hair and apply directly to skin.
• Don't get Halog in your eyes or ear canals or on mucous membranes or genitals.
• Don't cover or bandage the area being treated unless your doctor tells you to do so.
• To prevent your skin condition from recurring, continue using Halog for a few days after the problem clears up.

If you miss a dose

Apply the missed dose as soon as possible. But if it's almost time for your next dose, skip the missed

HALOG'S OTHER NAMES

Halog's generic name is halcinonide. Other brand names include Halog-E; and, in Canada, Halciderm.

dose and apply your next dose as scheduled. Don't apply a double dose.

 If you suspect an overdose

Contact your doctor *immediately*. Excessive Halog may cause signs of abnormally high blood sugar levels (excessive thirst, hunger, and urination; weight loss).

 Warnings

• Make sure your doctor knows your medical history. You may not be able to use Halog if you are overly sensitive to it or if you have cataracts, glaucoma, diabetes, tuberculosis, or infection or sores at the place you need to treat.
• If you need to take an antibiotic or antifungal drug, your doctor will ask you to stop using Halog until your other treatment has been completed.

• If you use Halog for a long time, over much of your body, or under a sealed dressing, you could absorb too much of the drug into your system. Call your doctor if you experience unusual symptoms.
• Don't use leftover Halog for a new skin condition without checking with your doctor first. Throw away leftover Halog when your condition clears up.

 SIDE EFFECTS

Call your doctor if you have any of these possible drug side effects. Call *immediately* about any labeled "serious."

Serious: bodywide effects such as hypothalamic-pituitary-adrenal suppression (weakness, dizziness, fever, vomiting, diarrhea, irregular heartbeat, low blood pressure), elevated blood sugar level (increased thirst, hunger, and urination), sugar in the urine

Common: skin softening and slight breakdown from moisture
Tip: Don't put plastic pants or tight diapers over areas being treated on children.

Other: burning, itching, redness, hair growth, pimplelike eruptions
Tip: Call your doctor if any skin problems develop.

DRUG INTERACTIONS

Combining certain drugs may alter their action or produce unwanted side effects. Tell your doctor about other drugs you're taking.

KEEP IN MIND...

* Apply sparingly.
* Avoid eyes, ears, mucous membranes, and genitals.
* Don't cover treated area.
* Call doctor if skin becomes more irritated.
* Continue Halog a few days after infection clears.

Halotestin

Halotestin is a synthetic androgen (male sex hormone) that has anticancer properties.

Why it's prescribed

Doctors prescribe Halotestin to treat hormone-related disorders. It comes in tablets. Doctors usually prescribe the following amounts.

▶ **For testicular deficiency,** 5 to 20 milligrams (mg) each day.

▶ **For reducing symptoms of breast cancer in women,** 10 to 40 mg daily, divided into equal doses spaced evenly throughout the day.

▶ **To reduce symptoms of menopause,** 1 to 2 mg twice a day for 21 days, then 7 days off. Cycle is repeated as necessary.

How to take Halotestin

• Take Halotestin with food or fluids to reduce nausea.

• Women with breast cancer may not feel Halotestin's effects for about 1 month after starting treatment.

If you miss a dose

Take the missed dose as soon as possible. However, if it's almost time for your next dose, skip the missed dose and take your next dose as scheduled. Don't take a double dose.

 If you suspect an overdose

Consult your doctor.

 Warnings

• Make sure your doctor knows your medical history. You may not be able to take Halotestin if you

HALOTESTIN'S OTHER NAMES

Halotestin's generic name is fluoxymesterone. Another brand name is Android-F.

 SIDE EFFECTS

Call your doctor if you have any of these possible drug side effects. Call *immediately* about any labeled "serious."

Serious: liver cell tumors

Common: decreased breast size

Other: change in appetite, bladder irritability, blood problems (fever, chills, sore throat, unusual tiredness, bruising, bleeding), yellow-tinged skin and eyes, increased calcium level (confusion, vomiting, constipation), androgenic effects in women (acne, swelling, weight gain, hair growth, hoarseness, clitoral enlargement, changes in sex drive, male-pattern baldness), low-estrogen effects in women (flushing; vaginitis, including itching, dryness, and burning; vaginal bleeding; mood swings; menstrual irregularities), excessive hormonal effects in men (stunted growth in boys, acne, painful erection, growth of body and facial hair, enlargement of penis, reduced testicle size in adults, impotence, breast growth)

Tips: For swelling in your lower legs or hands, your doctor may put you on a sodium-restricted diet and may give you a diuretic (water pill). If you're a man and experience painful erections or excessive sexual stimulation, call your doctor so your dosage can be decreased. If you're a woman, tell your doctor if you experience hair growth or other male-type changes. These changes will stop when therapy ends but will probably not reverse.

 DRUG INTERACTIONS

Combining certain drugs may alter their action or produce unwanted side effects. Tell your doctor about other drugs you're taking, especially:

• anticoagulants (blood thinners) such as Coumadin
• birth control pills
• drugs toxic to the liver
• insulin and oral diabetes drugs.

are overly sensitive to it or to aspirin; if you have heart, liver, or kidney problems; or if you're a man with an enlarged prostate or prostate or breast cancer.

• Make sure your doctor knows if you're pregnant or breast-feeding before you begin taking Halotestin.

• If you're diabetic, check your blood sugar level regularly and watch for low blood sugar.

• Use a nonhormonal birth control method.

 KEEP IN MIND...

* If diabetic, be alert for episodes of low blood sugar.

* Use nonhormonal birth control during therapy.

* Watch for possibly irreversible sexual changes.

Halotex

Halotex is one of a group of drugs known as antifungals that kill fungi (such as yeasts) by destroying their cell walls.

Why it's prescribed

Doctors prescribe Halotex for fungal infections that can occur in many different areas of the body. It comes in a cream and a topical solution. Doctors usually prescribe the following amounts for adults.

▶ **For superficial fungal infections of the feet, scalp, skin, fingernails, or toenails,** apply liberally twice a day for 2 to 3 weeks. Lesions between fingers and toes or other enclosed areas that are subject to friction may require 4 weeks of treatment.

How to use Halotex

- Use Halotex exactly as your doctor directs.
- Wash your hands well before and after applying Halotex.
- Apply liberally to the affected area.
- Avoid getting the drug in your eyes.
- Use Halotex for the full time prescribed by your doctor, even if your infection clears up before the prescription ends.

HALOTEX'S OTHER NAME

Halotex's generic name is haloprogin.

SIDE EFFECTS

Call your doctor if you have any of these possible drug side effects.

Serious: none reported

Common: stinging after applying solution
Tip: Stinging usually subsides in a short time.

Other: burning sensation, skin irritation, water-filled blisters, minor skin softening and breakdown from moisture, itching, worsening of pre-existing lesions

DRUG INTERACTIONS

Combining certain drugs may alter their action or produce unwanted side effects. Tell your doctor about other drugs you're taking.

If you miss a dose

Apply the missed dose as soon as possible. However, if it's almost time for your next dose, skip the missed dose and apply your next dose as scheduled. Don't apply a double dose.

If you suspect an overdose

Consult your doctor.

Warnings

- Make sure your doctor knows your medical history. You may not be able to use Halotex if you are overly sensitive to it.
- Tell your doctor if your skin becomes more irritated after you start using Halotex or if the condition hasn't improved after 4 weeks of treatment.
- Make sure your doctor knows if you're pregnant or breast-feeding before you begin taking Halotex.
- If an allergic reaction occurs, such as redness and itching, wash the medicine off your skin and call your doctor.

KEEP IN MIND...

* Keep drug out of eyes.
* Take entire amount prescribed, even if condition improves.
* Call doctor if skin problem worsens.

Herplex Liquifilm

Herplex Liquifilm is an antiviral drug. It kills viruses by interfering with their ability to reproduce.

Why it's prescribed

Doctors prescribe Herplex Liquifilm to treat certain viral eye infections. It comes in eyedrops and ointment. Doctors usually prescribe the following amounts for adults and children.

▶ **For herpes simplex infection of the cornea,** 1 drop of solution in the eye every hour during the day and every 2 hours at night. Or a ⅜-inch strip of ointment every 4 hours or five times a day, with the last dose at bedtime.

How to use Herplex Liquifilm

- Use the drug exactly as prescribed.
- Wash your hands before and after using Herplex Liquifilm.
- Clean around your eyes before applying the drug.
- Close your eyes gently after applying the drug. Don't blink. Keep your eyes closed for 1 to 2 minutes so the drug can reach the infection. If using eyedrops, hold a finger lightly on the inner corner of the treated eye for 1 minute to keep the solution from being absorbed by your tear duct.
- To avoid contamination, don't touch the applicator tip to your eye, surrounding skin, or any other surface.

HERPLEX LIQUIFILM'S OTHER NAMES

Herplex's generic name is idoxuridine. Another brand name is Stoxil.

 SIDE EFFECTS

Call your doctor if you have any of these possible drug side effects.

Serious: none reported

Common: sensitivity to sunlight
Tip: If Herplex Liquifilm makes your eyes more sensitive to light, wear sunglasses and avoid bright lights.

Other: allergic reaction (itching, swelling, redness, pain, constant burning), blurred or dimmed vision, corneal ulcer, slower corneal wound healing

 DRUG INTERACTIONS

Combining certain drugs may alter their action or produce unwanted side effects. Tell your doctor about other drugs you're taking, especially:
- other eye drugs, especially those that contain boric acid.

- Store eyedrops in the refrigerator in a tightly closed, light-resistant container.
- Use Herplex Liquifilm for the entire time prescribed, even if your symptoms improve.
- Don't use this drug for more than 21 consecutive days.

If you miss a dose

Apply the missed dose as soon as possible. However, if it's almost time for your next dose, skip the missed dose and apply your next dose as scheduled. Don't apply a double dose.

 If you suspect an overdose

Consult your doctor.

Warnings

- Make sure your doctor knows your medical history. You may not be able to use Herplex Liquifilm if you've ever had an unusual reaction to this drug or iodine.

- If you're pregnant or think you may be, check with your doctor before using Herplex Liquifilm.
- Don't share this drug with family members. Use separate washcloths and towels to help prevent the spread of infection.
- Throw away any leftover Herplex Liquifilm after treatment ends.
- If your symptoms don't get better within 1 week, tell your doctor.

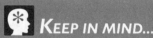 **KEEP IN MIND...**

∗ Don't touch applicator tip to any surface.

∗ Tell doctor if you have constant itching, swelling, or burning.

∗ Don't use for more than 21 days.

Hexalen

Hexalen is an anticancer drug. It interferes with the metabolism and growth of cancer cells.

Why it's prescribed

Doctors prescribe Hexalen to treat ovarian cancer. It comes in capsules. Doctors usually prescribe the following amounts for adults.
▶ **For ovarian cancer,** 260 milligrams per square meter of body size, divided into four equal doses and taken with meals and at bedtime for 14 or 21 consecutive days in a 28-day cycle.

How to take Hexalen

• Take Hexalen with meals to help minimize stomach upset.

If you miss a dose

Take the missed dose as soon as possible. But if it's almost time for your next dose, skip the missed dose and take your next dose as scheduled. Don't take a double dose.

 If you suspect an overdose

Consult your doctor.

 Warnings

• Make sure your doctor knows your medical history. You may not be able to take Hexalen if you're overly sensitive to it or if you have kidney or liver disease, an infection, bone marrow suppression, neurologic problems, or recent exposure to chickenpox or shingles.

 SIDE EFFECTS

Call your doctor if you have any of these possible drug side effects. Call *immediately* about any labeled "serious."

Serious: seizures, blood problems (fatigue, bruising, bleeding, fever, chills, signs of infection)

Common: nausea, vomiting, mood changes, dizziness, drowsiness
Tip: Your doctor can usually treat nausea and vomiting; however, you may have to stop taking Hexalen if you develop severe stomach distress.

Other: appetite loss, loss of balance, tingling sensation, slow reflexes, fatigue, rash, hair loss, changes in kidney function (decreased amount of urine)

DRUG INTERACTIONS

Combining certain drugs may alter their action or produce unwanted side effects. Tell your doctor about other drugs you're taking, especially:
• antidepressants called MAO inhibitors such as Elavil
• antifungal drugs, such as Ancobon and Fungizone
• antiviral drugs, such as Cytovene and Retrovir
• Chloromycetin
• colchicine
• Imuran
• radiation treatments or cancer drugs, such as Intron A and Mithracin
• Tagamet
• thyroid drugs
• vaccinations.

• Don't become pregnant while taking Hexalen because the drug will harm a developing fetus.
• Don't receive any vaccinations while taking Hexalen or afterward without checking with your doctor. Avoid people who have infections or who have recently taken an oral polio vaccine. If that's not possible, wear a protective mask over your nose and mouth.
• Ask your doctor what you should use to brush your teeth, and talk to your doctor before having any dental work.
• Call your doctor right away if you think you're getting an infection or

if you have fever, chills, cough or hoarseness, back or side pain, or difficult urination.

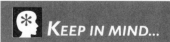 **KEEP IN MIND...**

＊ Take Hexalen with meals.

＊ Avoid people with infections or those who have recently received oral polio vaccination.

＊ Don't get pregnant while taking the drug.

Hismanal

Hismanal is an antihistamine. It interferes with the development of allergy-related inflammation but isn't as sleep-inducing as some other antihistamines.

Why it's prescribed

Doctors prescribe Hismanal to relieve or prevent the symptoms of hay fever and other allergies. It comes in tablets by prescription only; in Canada, it's a liquid that's available without a prescription. Doctors usually prescribe the following amounts for adults and children over 12.

▶ **To relieve symptoms of chronic hives and seasonal allergies,** one 10-milligram tablet daily.

How to take Hismanal

- Take Hismanal on an empty stomach 1 hour before or 2 hours after a meal.
- Take Hismanal only once a day.
- Don't increase the dosage, even if your symptoms persist or worsen.

If you miss a dose

Take the missed dose as soon as possible. But if it's almost time for your next dose, skip the missed dose and take your next dose as scheduled. Don't take a double dose.

If you suspect an overdose

Call your doctor *immediately*. Excessive Hismanal can cause serious irregularities in your heartbeat.

HISMANAL'S OTHER NAME

Hismanal's generic name is astemizole.

SIDE EFFECTS

Call your doctor if you have any of these possible drug side effects.

Serious: none reported

Common: none reported

Other: headache, nervousness, dizziness, drowsiness, irregular heartbeat with high doses, dry mouth, sore throat, conjunctivitis, nausea, diarrhea, abdominal pain, increased appetite, joint pain, yellow-tinged skin and eyes

Tip: Avoid activities that require full alertness or coordination until you know how Hismanal affects you.

DRUG INTERACTIONS

Combining certain drugs may alter their action or produce unwanted side effects. Tell your doctor about other drugs you're taking, especially:

- alcohol
- antifungal drugs, such as Nizoral and Sporanox
- aspirin
- certain antibiotics such as E-Mycin.

Warnings

- Make sure your doctor knows your medical history. You may not be able to take Hismanal if you're overly sensitive to it or to certain antifungal drugs or antibiotics or if you have other medical problems, especially asthma, other lower respiratory disorders, enlarged prostate, low potassium level, urinary tract blockage or difficulty urinating, glaucoma, or kidney or liver problems.
- Tell your doctor if you're breastfeeding or if you become pregnant while taking this drug.
- Check with your doctor first before starting any other drugs, either prescription or nonprescription.
- Be aware that children and older adults are especially sensitive to Hismanal's side effects.

- Tell the doctor you're taking this drug before you have skin tests for allergies because it may affect the test results. If you're scheduled for allergy tests, stop taking Hismanal 4 days ahead of time, or as directed by your doctor.

KEEP IN MIND...

- Take once a day on an empty stomach.
- Don't increase dosage without doctor's permission.
- Don't take large amounts of aspirin without doctor's approval.
- Stop Hismanal 4 days before allergy tests.

HIVID

HIVID retards the spread of human immunodeficiency virus (HIV), which causes acquired immunodeficiency syndrome (AIDS).

Why it's prescribed

Doctors prescribe HIVID to help slow the advancement of HIV infections and to help slow destruction of the immune system. It comes in film-coated tablets. Doctors usually prescribe the following amounts for adults and children age 13 or over who weigh at least 65 pounds.

▶ **For advanced HIV infection,** 0.75 milligrams every 8 hours, taken with another HIV drug.

How to take HIVID

• For best results, don't take HIVID with food.
• Take HIVID at regular intervals throughout the day and night to keep a steady level of the drug in your body.
• Store HIVID in a dry spot, not in the bathroom or near a sink; moisture can make this drug break down.
• Finish the entire prescription, even if you begin to feel better before finishing.

If you miss a dose

Take the missed dose as soon as possible. However, if it's almost time for your next dose, skip the missed dose and take your next dose as scheduled. Don't take a double dose.

HIVID's OTHER NAME

HIVID's generic name is zalcitabine.

 SIDE EFFECTS

Call your doctor if you have any of these possible drug side effects. Call *immediately* about any labeled "serious."

Serious: congestive heart failure (shortness of breath, fatigue), pancreatitis (abdominal pain, unrelieved vomiting)

Common: peripheral neuropathy (numbness and pain in hands and feet)
Tip: Your doctor may adjust your dosage if this side effect is persistent.

Other: headache, fatigue, depression, abnormally increased muscle tone, weakness, anxiety, sore throat, cough, nausea, vomiting, diarrhea, abdominal pain, appetite loss, anemia, blood problems, itchiness, night sweats, rash, fever, shivering, weight loss, altered liver function
Tips: Keep yourself dry and warm. Practice good mouth care; treat sore throat with frequent gargling.

 DRUG INTERACTIONS

Combining certain drugs may alter their action or produce unwanted side effects. Tell your doctor about other drugs you're taking, especially:
• drugs that cause peripheral neuropathy, such as Adalat, Antabuse, Apresoline, Chloromycetin, Dapsone, Dilantin, Diodoquint, Doriden, Flagyl, gold salts, Laniazid, Oncovin, Platinol, Trecator, and Virazole
• drugs that may impair kidney function, such as Foscavir, Fungizone, Mycifradin Sulfate, and Nebcin
• NebuPent.

 If you suspect an overdose

Consult your doctor.

 Warnings

• Make sure your doctor knows your medical history. You may not be able to take HIVID if you are overly sensitive to it or if you have a nerve disorder, kidney or liver problems, pancreatitis, or congestive heart failure.

• Make sure your doctor knows if you're pregnant or breast-feeding before you begin taking HIVID.

KEEP IN MIND...

* Take on an empty stomach.

* Space doses at regular intervals through day and night.

* Report numbness or burning in hands or feet.

Humorsol

Humorsol is applied directly to the eye, where it frees a chemical that causes the pupils to become smaller.

Why it's prescribed

Doctors prescribe these eyedrops to treat glaucoma, crossed eyes (strabismus), and other eye conditions and to diagnose certain eye problems. Doctors usually prescribe the following amounts for adults.

▶ **For primary open-angle glaucoma, or acute angle-closure glaucoma after iris surgery,** 1 drop in eye once or twice a day.

▶ **For strabismus,** 1 drop in eye once a day for 2 to 3 weeks, reduced to 1 drop every 2 days for 3 to 4 weeks. After reevaluation, 1 drop once or twice a week to once every 2 days. Dosage then reevaluated every 4 to 12 weeks.

How to use Humorsol

• Wash your hands before and after applying the drops.
• Don't touch the applicator tip to your eye or any other surface.
• After applying the drops, press your finger against the inner corner of your eye for 1 minute to help your eye absorb the drug.

If you miss a dose

Don't apply a double dose. Adjust your schedule as follows:
• If you apply one dose every other day, apply the missed dose as soon as possible. If you don't remember that day, don't apply a dose until

HUMORSOL'S OTHER NAME

Humorsol's generic name is demecarium bromide.

SIDE EFFECTS

Call your doctor if you have any of these possible drug side effects. Call *immediately* about any labeled "serious."

Serious: retinal detachment

Common: increased tear production, blurred vision

Other: brow pain, unusual fatigue or weakness, headache, slow pulse, palpitations, cysts on the iris, clouding of the lens of the eye, increased pressure in the eye, eye pain or irritation, blocked tear ducts, twitching eyelids, vision disturbances, nausea, vomiting, diarrhea, loss of bladder control

DRUG INTERACTIONS

Combining certain drugs may alter their action or produce unwanted side effects. Tell your doctor about other drugs you're taking, especially:
• drugs that reduce bronchial secretions
• drugs used to treat myasthenia gravis or spastic disorders of the digestive tract
• insecticides
• Pro-Banthine.

the next day. Then skip a day and apply the next dose as scheduled.
• If you apply one dose a day, apply the missed dose as soon as possible. However, if you don't remember until the next day, skip the missed dose and apply the next dose as scheduled.
• If you apply several doses a day, apply the missed dose as soon as possible. But if it's almost time for the next dose, skip the missed dose and apply the next dose as scheduled.

If you suspect an overdose

Consult your doctor.

Warnings

• Make sure your doctor knows your medical history. You may not

be able to use Humorsol if you have other medical problems.
• Don't use Humorsol if you're pregnant or breast-feeding.
• Be aware that children are more prone to some side effects, such as eye cysts.
• Don't breathe in even small amounts of insecticides because they may increase your risk of side effects.

KEEP IN MIND...

∗ Wash hands before and after applying.
∗ Don't touch applicator tip to eye or any other surface.
∗ Don't breathe in insecticides.

Hydrea

Hydrea interferes with the growth of cancer cells, eventually leading to their destruction.

Why it's prescribed

Doctors prescribe Hydrea to treat some cancers. It comes in capsules. Doctors usually prescribe the following amounts for adults.

▶ **For melanoma, resistant chronic myelocytic leukemia, head and neck cancers, and ovarian cancer,** 80 milligrams (mg) for each 2.2 pounds (lb) of body weight as a single dose every 3 days or 20 to 30 mg for each 2.2 lb as a single daily dose.

How to take Hydrea

• If you can't swallow the capsules, you may empty the contents into water and then drink the fluid immediately.

• Don't stop taking this drug, even if it causes nausea, vomiting, or diarrhea. Instead, call your doctor. If you vomit shortly after you take a dose, call your doctor for instructions on whether to take the dose again or wait until the next scheduled dose.

If you miss a dose

Don't take the missed dose or double the next dose. Resume your regular schedule and call your doctor.

HYDREA'S OTHER NAME

Hydrea's generic name is hydroxyurea.

SIDE EFFECTS

Call your doctor if you have any of these possible drug side effects. Call *immediately* about any labeled "serious."

Serious: blood problems (infection, easy bruising or bleeding, fatigue)
Tips: Watch for symptoms of infection, such as fever and sore throat, and call your doctor if you have any. Take your temperature daily. Avoid people with infections. Stay alert for symptoms of bleeding, such as easy bruising, nosebleeds, bleeding gums, and black, tarry stools. Avoid injury and be careful when using a toothbrush or razor.

Common: appetite loss, nausea, vomiting, diarrhea
Other: drowsiness, hallucinations, mouth sores, rash, itching, joint pain

DRUG INTERACTIONS

Combining certain drugs may alter their action or produce unwanted side effects. Tell your doctor about other drugs you're taking, especially:
• other cancer drugs.

If you suspect an overdose

Contact your doctor *immediately*. Excessive Hydrea can affect the immune system and cause mouth and digestive tract ulcers, facial redness, rash, disorientation, hallucinations, and kidney problems.

Warnings

• Make sure your doctor knows your medical history. You may not be able to take Hydrea if you have other problems, especially anemia, gout, or a kidney disorder.
• Don't take Hydrea if you're pregnant or breast-feeding. Avoid getting pregnant while taking this drug.

• Be aware that older adults are especially prone to Hydrea's side effects.
• Be aware that radiation therapy may increase side effects.
• Drink extra fluids if your doctor instructs you to do so.

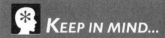

KEEP IN MIND...

* Drink extra fluids if instructed.
* Don't stop taking if nausea, vomiting, or diarrhea occurs.
* Watch for symptoms of infection.
* Avoid injury and bruising.

HydroDIURIL

HydroDIURIL is a diuretic (water pill). It rids the body of excess water by increasing urination. This, in turn, helps lower blood pressure.

Why it's prescribed

Doctors prescribe HydroDIURIL to treat high blood pressure and swelling (edema). It comes in tablets and a liquid. Doctors usually prescribe the following amounts for adults; children's dosages appear in parentheses.

▶ **For high blood pressure,** 25 to 50 milligrams (mg) every day as a single dose or divided into two equal doses, increased or decreased according to blood pressure.

▶ **For swelling,** 25 to 100 mg a day or intermittently. (Children ages 2 to 12: 37.5 to 100 mg a day divided into two equal doses. Children under age 2: 12.5 to 37.5 mg a day divided into two equal doses.)

How to take HydroDIURIL

• To avoid waking up to urinate, take in the morning. If you're taking more than one daily dose, take the last dose before 6 p.m.

• Measure the liquid form with a specially marked dropper or medicine spoon.

• If you take HydroDIURIL for high blood pressure, don't stop taking it suddenly, even if you feel well.

HYDRODIURIL'S OTHER NAMES

HydroDIURIL's generic name is hydrochlorothiazide. Other brand names include Esidrix, Hydro-Chlor, Hydro-D, Oretic; and, in Canada, Apo-Hydro, Diuchlor H, Neo-Codema, Novo-Hydrazide, and Urozide.

 ## SIDE EFFECTS

Call your doctor if you have any of these possible drug side effects. Call *immediately* about any labeled "serious."

Serious: blood problems (fatigue, infection, abnormal bleeding), hepatic encephalopathy (confusion, tremor, slurred speech)

Common: dizziness when standing up, appetite loss, nausea

Other: dehydration, stomach pain, excessive or frequent urination, sensitivity to sunlight, shortness of breath, cough, fever, rash, overall feeling of illness, difficulty waking, muscle weakness and cramps, increased thirst and hunger, gout

Tip: Call your doctor if you have muscle weakness or cramps.

 ## DRUG INTERACTIONS

Combining certain drugs may alter their action or produce unwanted side effects. Tell your doctor about other drugs you're taking, especially:

• alcohol
• barbiturates
• blood pressure drugs
• Colestid, Questran (take at least 1 hour before HydroDIURIL)
• Crystodigin, Lanoxin
• diabetes drugs
• Lithobid
• narcotic pain relievers
• nonsteroidal anti-inflammatory drugs, such as Advil.

If you miss a dose

Take the missed dose as soon as possible. But if it's almost time for the next dose, skip the missed dose and take your next dose as scheduled. Don't take a double dose.

 ## If you suspect an overdose

Contact your doctor *immediately.* Excessive HydroDIURIL can cause diarrhea, vomiting, increased urination, sluggishness, and coma.

 ## Warnings

• Make sure your doctor knows your medical history. You may not be able to take HydroDIURIL if you have other medical problems or if you're pregnant or breast-feeding.

• If you're diabetic, be aware that HydroDIURIL may interfere with the results of sugar tests.

• Eat potassium-rich foods, take a potassium supplement, and decrease your salt intake, as directed.

 ## KEEP IN MIND...

* Take last dose before 6 p.m.
* Don't stop taking suddenly.
* Eat foods high in potassium.

Hygroton

Hygroton is a diuretic (water pill). It rids the body of excess water by increasing urination. This, in turn, helps lower blood pressure.

Why it's prescribed

Doctors prescribe Hygroton to treat high blood pressure and swelling (edema). It comes in tablets. Doctors usually prescribe the following amounts for adults; children's dosage appears in parentheses.

▶ **For high blood pressure or swelling,** 25 to 100 milligrams (mg) a day or up to 200 mg on alternate days. (Children: 2 mg for each 2.2 pounds of body weight three times a week.)

How to take Hygroton

• Take this drug exactly as your doctor directs.
• To avoid waking up to urinate, take in the morning. If you're taking more than one daily dose, take the last dose before 6 p.m.
• If you're taking Hygroton for high blood pressure, don't stop taking it suddenly even if you feel well.

If you miss a dose

Take the missed dose as soon as possible. But if it's almost time for the next dose, skip the missed dose and take the next dose as scheduled. Don't take a double dose.

HYGROTON'S OTHER NAMES

Hygroton's generic name is chlorthalidone. Other brand names include Thalitone; and, in Canada, Apo-Chlorthalidone, Novo-Thalidone, and Uridon.

 SIDE EFFECTS

Call your doctor if you have any of these possible drug side effects. Call *immediately* about any labeled "serious."

Serious: blood problems (fatigue, infection, abnormal bleeding), hepatic encephalopathy (confusion, tremor, slurred speech)

Common: none reported

Other: dizziness when standing up, appetite loss, nausea, stomach pain, impotence, excessive or frequent urination, sensitivity to sunlight, shortness of breath, cough, fever, rash, overall feeling of illness, difficulty waking, muscle weakness and cramps, increased thirst and hunger, gout
Tip: Call your doctor if you have muscle weakness or cramps.

 DRUG INTERACTIONS

Combining certain drugs may alter their action or produce unwanted side effects. Tell your doctor about other drugs you're taking, especially:
• alcohol
• barbiturates
• Colestid, Questran (take at least 1 hour before Hygroton)
• Crystodigin, Lanoxin
• Lithobid
• narcotic pain relievers
• nonsteroidal anti-inflammatory drugs, such as Advil.

 If you suspect an overdose

Contact your doctor *immediately*. Excessive Hygroton can cause diarrhea, vomiting, increased urination, sluggishness, and possibly coma.

Warnings

• Make sure your doctor knows your medical history. You may not be able to take Hygroton if you have other medical problems.
• If you're pregnant or breast-feeding, check with your doctor before you start taking Hygroton.
• Be aware that older adults are especially prone to side effects.

• If you're diabetic, be aware that Hygroton may increase your blood sugar level.
• Eat potassium-rich foods, take a potassium supplement, and decrease your salt intake, as directed by your doctor.

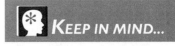 **KEEP IN MIND...**

* Take last dose before 6 p.m.
* Don't stop taking suddenly.
* Eat potassium-rich foods.

Hylorel

Hylorel lowers high blood pressure by causing blood vessels to relax, which allows more blood to pass through them, and by slowing the heart rate.

Why it's prescribed

Doctors prescribe Hylorel to control high blood pressure. It comes in tablets. Doctors usually prescribe the following amounts for adults.
▶ **For high blood pressure,** at first, 5 milligrams (mg) twice a day, adjusted until blood pressure is controlled. Usual dosage is 20 to 75 mg a day, divided into two equal doses. Maximum dosage is 400 mg a day, divided into three or four equal doses.

How to take Hylorel

• Take this drug exactly as your doctor directs.
• Continue to take it even if you feel well. You may have to take Hylorel for the rest of your life.

If you miss a dose

Take the missed dose as soon as possible. However, if it's almost time for the next dose, skip the missed dose and take the next dose as scheduled. Don't take a double dose.

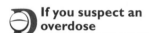 **If you suspect an overdose**

Contact your doctor *immediately*. Excessive Hylorel can cause dizziness, weakness, fainting, and blurred vision.

HYLOREL'S OTHER NAME

Hylorel's generic name is guanadrel sulfate.

 SIDE EFFECTS

Call your doctor if you have any of these possible drug side effects.
Serious: none reported
Common: fatigue, low blood pressure (dizziness, weakness)
Tips: Avoid strenuous exercise, hot showers, and hot weather. These conditions may cause your blood pressure to drop too low. To help prevent dizziness, rise slowly and avoid sudden position changes.

Other: drowsiness, faintness, swelling, diarrhea, dry mouth, impotence, difficulty ejaculating
Tip: To relieve dry mouth, use ice chips or sugarless candy or gum.

 DRUG INTERACTIONS

Combining certain drugs may alter their action or produce unwanted side effects. Tell your doctor about other drugs you're taking, especially:
• amphetamines, such as Dexedrine and Pondimin
• diuretics (water pills), such as Lasix
• MAO inhibitors, such as Nardil and Parnate, and tricyclic antidepressants, such as Elavil (don't take within 1 week of taking Hylorel)
• other blood pressure drugs
• phenothiazines (used for anxiety, nausea, vomiting, or psychosis), such as Haldol
• Ritalin.

 Warnings

• Make sure your doctor knows your medical history. You may not be able to take Hylorel if you have other medical problems.
• If you're pregnant, check with your doctor before taking Hylorel.
• Be aware that older adults may be especially prone to Hylorel's side effects, especially dizziness.
• Schedule checkups regularly so your doctor can monitor your progress and check for any side effects.
• Call your doctor if you have a fever because your dosage may need to be changed.

• Before you undergo any surgical procedures (including dental surgery), tell your doctor or dentist that you're taking Hylorel.

KEEP IN MIND...

* Stand up slowly to avoid dizziness.

* Use ice chips or sugarless chewing gum or hard candy to relieve dry mouth.

* Keep taking even if you feel well.

Hypotears

Hypotears is an artificial tear preparation that supplements the tears produced by the eye.

Why it's used

Hypotears is used to relieve dryness or irritation of the eye caused by reduced tear flow. You can buy Hypotears without a prescription. It comes in eyedrops. The following amounts are usually recommended for adults and children.

▶ **For insufficient tear production,** 1 or 2 drops in the eye three or four times a day or as needed.

How to use Hypotears

• If you're treating yourself, read the package instructions carefully to find out how much to use and how to apply it.
• Don't use this preparation with a contact lens in place.
• Wash your hands before and after using the preparation.
• To use the drops, gently pull your lower eyelid away from the eye to form a pouch. Don't blink as you drop the dose into your eye.
• To prevent contamination, don't touch the tip of the dropper or container to your eye, the surrounding area, or any other surface.

 SIDE EFFECTS

Call your doctor if you have any of these possible drug side effects.

Serious: none reported

Common: none reported

Other: eye burning or pain (when first used), blurred vision, crust formation on eyelids and eyelashes

Tip: Dab your eyes with a tissue after applying Hypotears. Don't rub them.

 DRUG INTERACTIONS

Combining certain products may alter drug action or produce unwanted side effects. Tell your doctor about other products you're using, especially:
• other eye irrigating solutions, such as Liquifilm Forte or Tears Naturale.

• Keep your eyes closed for a minute to allow your eye to absorb the drug.
• Store Hypotears with the bottle tightly closed.

If you miss a dose

Apply the missed dose as soon as possible. However, if it's almost time for the next dose, skip the missed dose and apply the next dose as scheduled. Don't apply a double dose.

 If you suspect an overdose

Contact your doctor *immediately.* Excessive Hypotears can cause eye redness and burning. If swallowed, this drug can cause seizures, low blood pressure (dizziness, weakness), vomiting, and rash.

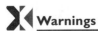 **Warnings**

• Before you start using Hypotears, consult your doctor if you have any allergies to the ingredients in this drug (including the preservatives), to contact lens solutions, or to any other substance. You may not be able to use Hypotears.
• Don't share this drug because doing so could spread infection.
• Stop using this drug and contact your doctor if your eye condition persists or gets worse.

 KEEP IN MIND...

∗ Wash hands before and after using drug.

∗ Don't touch dropper or container to eye or other surface.

∗ Don't use these eyedrops while wearing contact lenses.

∗ Don't share these eyedrops with other people.

Hytrin

Hytrin relaxes the blood vessels so that blood passes through them more easily, helping to lower blood pressure. In men with an enlarged prostate gland, it also increases the flow of urine and relieves pressure in the urethra.

Why it's prescribed

Doctors prescribe Hytrin to reduce high blood pressure or to treat symptoms of an enlarged prostate. Hytrin comes in tablets. Doctors usually prescribe the following amounts for adults.

▶ **For high blood pressure,** 1 milligram (mg), increased gradually according to person's response. Usual dosage is 1 to 5 mg a day. Maximum dosage is 20 mg a day.

▶ **For symptoms of enlarged prostate,** 1 mg, increased in steps to 2 mg, 5 mg, or 10 mg once a day to achieve best response.

How to take Hytrin

• Take this drug exactly as your doctor directs.

• Because your first dose may make you drowsy or dizzy, take it at bedtime, and be careful if you need to get up during the night.

• Don't stop taking Hytrin suddenly, even if you feel well.

If you miss a dose

Take the missed dose as soon as possible if you remember it the same day. If you don't remember until

the next day, skip the missed dose and take the next dose as scheduled. If you miss several doses, call your doctor before resuming the drug. Don't take a double dose.

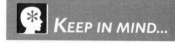

If you suspect an overdose

Contact your doctor *immediately.* Excessive Hytrin can cause low blood pressure (dizziness, weakness) and shock (clammy skin, difficulty waking).

Warnings

• Make sure your doctor knows your medical history. You may not be able to take Hytrin if you have other problems, such as chest pain, heart disease, or kidney disease.

• If you're pregnant or breast-feeding, tell your doctor before you start taking Hytrin.

• Be aware that older adults are especially prone to Hytrin's side effects.

• Check your blood pressure frequently, if instructed by your doctor.

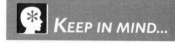

KEEP IN MIND...

* Take this drug at bedtime.
* Don't stop taking suddenly.
* Don't drive until you know how drug affects you.

SIDE EFFECTS

Call your doctor if you have any of these possible drug side effects. Call *immediately* about any labeled "serious."

Serious: palpitations, difficulty breathing or shortness of breath

Common: dizziness, swelling of lower legs or feet, stuffy nose

Tips: To reduce dizziness when standing up, rise slowly to your feet. If you start to feel light-headed when standing, lie down so you won't faint; then sit up for a few moments before standing. Hytrin is more likely to cause dizziness when you drink alcohol, stand for a long time, or exercise (especially in hot weather).

Other: lack of energy, drowsiness, headache, nervousness, numbness or tingling sensations, fast pulse, sinus pain, blurred vision, nausea, impotence, decreased sex drive, weight gain, back or muscle pain

Tip: Until you know how this drug affects you, don't drive or do anything else that requires you to be fully alert.

DRUG INTERACTIONS

Combining certain drugs may alter their action or produce unwanted side effects. Tell your doctor about other drugs you're taking, especially:
• other blood pressure drugs.

Ilotycin eye ointment

Ilotycin eye ointment is an antibiotic applied directly to the eye. It eliminates infection by stopping the bacteria from producing proteins, which eventually kills the bacteria or prevents their growth.

Why it's prescribed

Doctors prescribe Ilotycin eye ointment to treat various eye infections. Doctors usually prescribe the following amounts for adults and children.

► **For acute and chronic pinkeye (conjunctivitis), trachoma (chlamydial eye infection), and other eye infections, ribbon of ointment ⅓ inch long applied directly to the affected eye up to six times a day, depending on the severity of the infection.**

How to use Ilotycin eye ointment

• Use this drug exactly as your doctor directs.
• Wash your hands before and after applying this drug.
• To prevent contamination, don't touch the applicator tip to your eye, the surrounding area, or any other surface.
• After applying the ointment, close your eye and keep it closed for 1 or 2 minutes.
• Close the container tightly and store it fully closed at room temperature.

ILOTYCIN'S OTHER NAME

Ilotycin's generic name is erythromycin.

SIDE EFFECTS

Call your doctor if you have any of these possible drug side effects.

Serious: none reported

Common: none reported

Other: slow healing of corneal wounds, blurred vision, infection (with long-term use), allergic reactions (itching and burning eyes, hives, skin irritation)

Tip: If you develop symptoms of an allergic reaction, stop using this drug and call your doctor immediately.

DRUG INTERACTIONS

Combining certain drugs may alter their action or produce unwanted side effects. Tell your doctor about other drugs you're taking.

• To help clear up your infection, keep taking this drug for the full treatment time.
• Don't flush your eye with water or apply any nonprescription eyedrops to it after you've applied Ilotycin eye ointment; doing so could reduce the amount of the drug in your eye.

If you miss a dose

Apply the missed dose as soon as possible. However, if it's almost time for the next dose, skip the missed dose and apply the next dose as scheduled. Don't apply a double dose.

If you suspect an overdose

Consult your doctor.

Warnings

• Make sure your doctor knows your medical history. You should not use Ilotycin eye ointment if you're allergic to it.
• If you're pregnant or breast-feeding, tell your doctor before you begin using this drug.
• If your symptoms don't improve within a few days or if they get worse, call your doctor.
• Don't share this eye ointment, washcloths, or towels with family members. If anyone in your household develops the same symptoms, call the doctor.

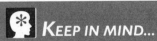

* Don't touch applicator tip to eye or other surface.

* Keep eye closed for 1 or 2 minutes after applying.

* Don't share this drug with family members.

* Keep using for full treatment time.

Imitrex

Imitrex is used to treat severe migraine headaches. It's thought to work by slowing the activity of nerves in the brain.

Why it's prescribed

Doctors prescribe Imitrex to relieve attacks of migraine. It comes in tablets. It's also available in an injectable form. Doctors usually prescribe the following amounts for adults.

▶ **For acute migraine attacks,** 25 to 100 milligrams (mg) orally with fluid, repeated once if no relief is obtained after 2 hours. Or 6 mg injected under the skin. Maximum recommended dosage is 300 mg orally or two 6-mg injections a day.

How to take Imitrex

• Take this drug exactly as your doctor directs. For best results, take it as soon as symptoms appear.
• If you're taking the tablets, swallow them whole. Don't break, crush, or chew them.
• If you're self-administering the injection, follow the doctor's or nurse's instructions closely. Make sure you understand how to load the injector, administer the injection, and dispose of used syringes.
• After the injection, expect to feel relief from migraine in 1 to 2 hours.

If you miss a dose

Not applicable because drug is taken only as needed.

IMITREX'S OTHER NAME

Imitrex's generic name is sumatriptan succinate.

 ## SIDE EFFECTS

Call your doctor if you have any of these possible drug side effects. Call *immediately* about any labeled "serious."

Serious: potentially fatal irregular heartbeat; persistent or severe chest pain, heaviness, pressure, or tightness
Common: dizziness, vertigo, tingling; warm, hot, or burning sensation
Other: drowsiness; headache; anxiety; overall feeling of illness; fatigue; weakness; difficulty swallowing; discomfort in throat, nose, sinus, mouth, jaw, or tongue; altered vision; abdominal discomfort; skin inflammation (especially at injection site); light-headedness; cold sensation; neck pain; muscle ache or cramps
Tip: If redness or pain at the injection site doesn't subside within 1 hour, call your doctor.

 ## DRUG INTERACTIONS

Combining certain drugs may alter their action or produce unwanted side effects. Tell your doctor about other drugs you're taking, especially:
• ergot and ergot derivatives, such as Ergostat (don't take within 24 hours of taking Imitrex)
• drugs for depression called MAO inhibitors, such as Marplan and Nardil (don't take within 14 days of taking Imitrex).

 ### If you suspect an overdose

Contact your doctor *immediately.* Excessive Imitrex can cause seizures, tremor, redness of the arms and legs, slow breathing, bluish skin, poor coordination, enlarged pupils, and paralysis.

Warnings

• Make sure your doctor knows your medical history. You may not be able to take Imitrex if you have other problems, such as chest pain, fast or irregular heartbeat, heart or blood vessel disease, high blood pressure, or kidney or liver disease, or if you have ever had a heart attack or stroke.

• If you're pregnant or breast-feeding or if you intend to become pregnant, tell your doctor before you start taking Imitrex.
• Don't take Imitrex to try to prevent migraine attacks or reduce their frequency.

 ## KEEP IN MIND...

* Don't break, crush, or chew tablets.
* Take as soon as migraine symptoms occur.
* Use only to relieve migraines, not to prevent them.

Imagedium

Imodium

Imodium relieves diarrhea. It slows movements of the intestines and helps the intestinal contents stay in the digestive tract longer.

Why it's prescribed

Doctors prescribe Imodium for acute, nonspecific diarrhea and for chronic diarrhea. You can also buy Imodium without a prescription. It comes in tablets, capsules, and an oral liquid. Doctors usually prescribe the following amounts for adults; children's dosages appear in parentheses.

▶ **For acute, nonspecific diarrhea,** at first, 4 milligrams (mg), then 2 mg after each unformed stool. Maximum dosage is 16 mg a day. (Children ages 8 to 12: 10 milliliters [ml] or 2 mg three times on first day. Subsequent doses of 5 ml [1 mg] for each 2.2 pounds of body weight may be given after each unformed stool. Maximum dosage is 6 mg a day. Children ages 6 to 8: 10 ml [2 mg] twice on first day. If diarrhea persists, contact doctor. Children ages 2 to 6: 5 ml three times on first day. If diarrhea persists, call doctor.)

▶ **For chronic diarrhea,** at first, 4 mg, then 2 mg after each unformed stool until diarrhea subsides. Dosage adjusted to person's response.

How to take Imodium

• If you're treating yourself, follow the instructions on the package carefully. Don't take more than the recommended amount.

IMODIUM'S OTHER NAMES

Imodium's generic name is loperamide. Imodium A-D is the nonprescription form.

SIDE EFFECTS

Call your doctor if you have any of these possible drug side effects.

Serious: none reported

Common: constipation

Other: drowsiness, fatigue, dizziness, dry mouth, nausea, vomiting, rash; abdominal pain, swelling, or discomfort

DRUG INTERACTIONS

Combining certain drugs may alter their action or produce unwanted side effects. Tell your doctor about other drugs you're taking.

• If you're taking Imodium by prescription, follow your doctor's instructions carefully.

• After the first dose, take Imodium after each passage of unformed stool until your diarrhea stops (unless the doctor tells you otherwise).

If you miss a dose

If you're taking Imodium on a regular schedule, skip the missed dose and take the next dose as scheduled. Don't take a double dose.

If you suspect an overdose

Contact your doctor *immediately*. Excessive Imodium can cause constipation, abdominal pain and bloating, drowsiness, and fatigue.

Warnings

• Make sure your doctor knows your medical history. You may not be able to take Imodium if you have other medical problems.

• If you're pregnant or breast-feeding, check with your doctor before you start taking Imodium.

• Don't give this drug to children under age 2.

• Be aware that losing fluid from diarrhea can be dangerous, especially for children and older adults. Call your doctor right away if you have signs of dehydration (dry mouth, increased thirst, decreased urination, dizziness, light-headedness, wrinkled skin).

• Until your stools become solid, replace the fluid your body has lost from diarrhea. Drink plenty of clear liquids that don't contain caffeine.

• If your diarrhea doesn't stop after 2 days or if you develop a fever, stop taking Imodium and call your doctor.

KEEP IN MIND...

* Call doctor immediately about symptoms of dehydration.

* Take after each unformed stool until diarrhea stops.

* Drink plenty of clear liquids.

* Call doctor if diarrhea doesn't stop after 2 days or if fever develops.

Imuran

Imuran suppresses the immune system. By stopping the body's natural defenses from working normally, it helps prevent rejection of transplanted organs and relieves symptoms of immune system diseases such as rheumatoid arthritis.

Why it's prescribed

Doctors prescribe Imuran to prevent organ rejection in people who've receive kidney transplants or to treat severe rheumatoid arthritis. Imuran comes in tablets. It's also available in an injectable form. Doctors usually prescribe the following amounts.

▶ **To suppress the immune system in people who've received a kidney transplant,** at first, 3 to 5 milligrams (mg) for each 2.2 pounds (lb) of body weight orally every day, usually starting on day of transplantation. The usual daily dosage is 1 to 3 mg for each 2.2 lb.

▶ **For severe, refractory rheumatoid arthritis in adults,** initially, 1 mg for each 2.2 lb of body weight orally as a single dose or divided into two equal doses each day, increased after 6 to 8 weeks, as needed, by 0.5 mg for each 2.2 lb a day (to maximum of 2.5 mg for each 2.2 lb a day) every 4 weeks.

How to take Imuran

• Take this drug exactly as your doctor directs.
• If you vomit after taking a dose, notify your doctor before taking another dose.

IMURAN'S OTHER NAME

Imuran's generic name is azathioprine.

SIDE EFFECTS

Call your doctor if you have any of these possible drug side effects. Call *immediately* about any labeled "serious."

Serious: stomach pain, liver problems (clay-colored stools, dark urine, itching, yellow-tinged skin and eyes), fatigue, weakness, infection (fever, chills, wet cough), unusual bruising or bleeding (tarry stools, bloody urine)

Common: none reported

Other: mouth sores, nausea, vomiting, diarrhea, appetite loss, foul-smelling stools that float, inflammation of esophagus (difficulty swallowing, fever, sore throat), rash, itching, joint pain, muscle wasting, hair loss
Tips: To minimize nausea and vomiting, take this drug with or just after meals. If gastrointestinal symptoms become bothersome, call your doctor; you may need a dosage adjustment.

DRUG INTERACTIONS

Combining certain drugs may alter their action or produce unwanted side effects. Tell your doctor about other drugs you're taking, especially:
• blood pressure drugs, such as Capoten, Lotensin, and Vasotec
• Cytoxan
• Leukeran
• Sandimmune
• steroids, such as Decadron and Prednisone
• vaccines
• Zyloprim.

• Store Imuran away from heat and direct light. Don't store it in a damp place, such as the bathroom or near the kitchen sink; moisture can cause the drug to deteriorate.
• Don't stop taking Imuran without first consulting your doctor.

If you miss a dose

Adjust your schedule as follows:
• If you take one dose a day, don't take the missed dose or double the next dose. Instead, take your next dose as scheduled and consult your doctor.
• If you take more than one dose a day, take the missed dose as soon as possible. However, if it's almost time for the next dose, take both doses together; then resume your usual schedule. If you miss more than one dose, notify your doctor.

 ## If you suspect an overdose

Contact your doctor *immediately.* Excessive Imuran can cause nausea, vomiting, diarrhea, and decreased blood cell counts (fatigue, infection, bleeding, bruising).

Warnings

• Make sure your doctor knows your medical history. You may not be able to take Imuran if you have other medical problems, such as liver or kidney disease, gout, herpes zoster (shingles), infection, pancreatitis, or recent exposure to chickenpox.

• Avoid getting pregnant or breast-feeding during Imuran therapy and for 4 months afterward. If you do become pregnant, stop taking Imuran and notify your doctor.

• Schedule regular medical check-ups so your doctor can monitor Imuran's effectiveness and check for side effects.

• Because Imuran increases your risk of infection, avoid people with known infections. Remember to wash your hands frequently.

• Avoid contact with people who have just received the oral polio vaccine. Don't have any immunizations or vaccinations without checking with your doctor first.

• Because Imuran puts you at risk for unusual bleeding, be careful not to cut yourself using a toothbrush, dental floss, or a razor. Also, avoid contact sports and other activities in which bruises, cuts, and other injuries are likely to occur. Be sure to wear your seatbelt every time you're in a vehicle.

• If you need dental work done, try to schedule it before starting treatment with Imuran. If you need dental work done after you've started taking Imuran, make sure your dentist knows you're using this drug.

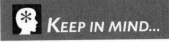

KEEP IN MIND...

* Take drug with or after meals to minimize stomach upset.

* Don't stop taking drug unless doctor approves.

* Avoid people with infections and activities that increase your risk of injury.

* Call doctor about symptoms of infection or unusual bleeding.

Inderal

Inderal is one of a group of drugs called beta blockers. It regulates the heartbeat, reduces high blood pressure, and decreases the heart's oxygen needs. It also helps prevent migraine headaches by preventing the arteries from narrowing.

Why it's prescribed

Doctors prescribe Inderal to relieve angina (chest pain) and to treat certain heart conditions. It may also be used to prevent severe migraine or vascular headaches, to calm tremors, and to treat some other conditions. Inderal comes in tablets, extended-release capsules, and a liquid. It's also available in an injectable form. Doctors usually prescribe the following amounts for adults.

▶ **For chest pain,** 10 to 20 milligrams (mg) orally three or four times a day, or one 80-mg extended-release capsule a day. Dosage is then increased at 7- to 10-day intervals.

▶ **To help prevent death after heart attack,** 180 to 240 mg orally a day divided into three or four equal doses starting 5 to 21 days after heart attack.

▶ **For certain types of irregular heartbeats,** usually 10 to 30 mg orally three or four times a day (after starting drug intravenously).

▶ **For high blood pressure,** at first, 80 mg orally a day divided into two

SIDE EFFECTS

Call your doctor if you have any of these possible drug side effects. Call *immediately* about any labeled "serious."

Serious: heart failure (shortness of breath, fatigue)

Common: fatigue, lethargy, slow pulse, dizziness, weakness, increased airway resistance (wheezing), rash

Tips: Call your doctor if you feel dizzy, start wheezing, develop a rash, or have a very slow pulse (especially if it's less than 50 beats per minute). To minimize dizziness, rise slowly from a sitting or lying position and avoid sudden changes in position. Make sure you know how you react to the drug before you drive or perform other activities that might be dangerous if you're not fully alert.

Other: vivid dreams, hallucinations, depression, leg pain and weakness when walking, nausea, vomiting, diarrhea, fever, joint pain

DRUG INTERACTIONS

Combining certain drugs may alter their action or produce unwanted side effects. Tell your doctor about other drugs you're taking, especially:
• diabetes drugs
• Dilantin
• drugs for heart conditions, especially Calan, Cardizem, Crystodigin, Isuprel, and Lanoxin
• epinephrine preparations, such as Bronkaid, Medihaler, and Primatene Mist
• Haldol
• Rifadin
• Serpalan
• Tagamet
• Thorazine.

---

to four equal doses, or 1 extended-release capsule once a day, increased every 3 to 7 days to maximum of 640 mg a day. Usual dosage is 160 to 480 mg a day.

▶ **To prevent severe migraine or vascular headache,** at first, 80 mg orally a day divided into equal doses, or 1 extended-release capsule a day. Usual dosage is 160 to 240 mg a day divided into three or four equal doses.

▶ **For essential tremor,** at first, 40 mg orally three times a day. Usual

dosage is 120 to 320 mg a day divided into three equal doses.

▶ **For hypertrophic subaortic stenosis,** 20 to 40 mg orally three or four times a day, or 80 to 160 mg extended-release capsules once a day.

▶ **For additional therapy in pheochromocytoma,** 60 mg orally a day divided into equal doses for 3 days before surgery.

How to take Inderal

• Take this drug exactly as your doctor directs. Take it with meals, preferably at the same time each day.

• Take your pulse once a day, preferably before the first dose. If your pulse rate is less than 50 beats per minute, don't take the dose; call your doctor as soon as possible.

• Don't stop taking Inderal suddenly; doing so could worsen your chest pain.

If you miss a dose

Take the missed dose right away if you remember within 1 hour or so. However, if it's within 8 hours of the next regular dose, skip the missed dose and take the next dose as scheduled. Don't take a double dose.

If you suspect an overdose

Contact your doctor *immediately*. Excessive Inderal can cause severe high blood pressure (dizziness, weakness), a fast pulse, heart failure (shortness of breath, fatigue), and closing up of the throat.

Warnings

• Make sure your doctor knows your medical history. You may not be able to take Inderal if you have other problems, such as a heart problem, asthma, lung disease, diabetes, low blood sugar, an overactive thyroid, or liver disease.

• If you're pregnant or breast-feeding, check with your doctor before you start taking Inderal.

• Be aware that older adults may be especially prone to Inderal's side effects.

• If you're diabetic, be aware that this drug may hide some symptoms of low blood sugar.

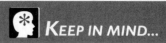

KEEP IN MIND...

* Take with meals.

* If pulse is below 50, call doctor and don't take dose.

* Don't stop taking suddenly.

* Don't drive until you know how you react to drug.

Indocin

Indocin is one of a group of drugs called nonsteroidal anti-inflammatory drugs (NSAIDs). It's thought to reduce pain, inflammation, and fever by inhibiting the production of hormones called prostaglandins and by impeding the action of certain other body substances.

Why it's prescribed

Doctors prescribe Indocin to treat various inflammatory conditions, such as arthritis. It comes in capsules, sustained-release capsules, a liquid, and suppositories. It's also available in an injectable form. Doctors usually prescribe the following amounts for adults.

▶ **For moderate to severe rheumatoid arthritis or osteoarthritis, or ankylosing spondylitis (chronic inflammatory disease of the spine),** 25 milligrams (mg) orally or rectally two or three times a day, increased by 25 or 50 mg a day every 7 days up to 200 mg a day. Or 75 mg in sustained-release capsules orally once a day in morning or at bedtime, increased, if needed, to 75 mg twice a day.

▶ **For acute gouty arthritis,** 50 mg orally three times a day, reduced as soon as possible, then discontinued.

▶ **For acute painful shoulder (bursitis or tendinitis),** 75 to 150 mg orally three or four times a day for 7 to 14 days.

INDOCIN'S OTHER NAMES

Indocin's generic name is indomethacin. Other brand names include Indameth, Indocin SR; and, in Canada, Apo-Indomethacin, Indocid, Indocid SR, and Novomethacin.

SIDE EFFECTS

Call your doctor if you have any of these possible drug side effects. Call *immediately* about any labeled "serious."

Serious: seizures; heart failure (shortness of breath, fatigue, wheezing, restlessness); blood in urine, stools, or vomit; acute kidney failure (reduced urination); blood problems (bleeding, bruising, fatigue, fever, infection); Stevens-Johnson syndrome (burnlike rash); severe allergic reaction (hivelike rash, itching); swelling of face, lips, hands, and feet; low blood sugar (difficulty concentrating, shakiness, headache, cold sweats, anxiety, cool and pale skin); salt deficiency (abdominal cramps, extreme tiredness), potassium deficiency (diarrhea, irritability, numbness)

Common: headache, dizziness, vomiting, peptic ulcers

Other: depression, drowsiness, confusion, numbness or tingling in arms or legs, high blood pressure (severe headache, nosebleeds, blurred vision), damage to eyes, hearing loss, ringing in ears, appetite loss, stomach pain

Tip: Don't drive or perform other activities requiring alertness until you know how you react to this drug.

DRUG INTERACTIONS

Combining certain drugs may alter their action or produce unwanted side effects. Tell your doctor about other drugs you're taking, especially:
- alcohol
- antibiotics, such as Amikin, Garamycin, Myciguent, Netromycin, and streptomycin
- aspirin
- Benemid
- blood pressure drugs
- corticosteroids
- diuretics (water pills)
- Dolobid
- Dyrenium
- Lanoxin
- Lithobid
- Mexate
- other NSAIDs, such as Advil and Motrin
- Sandimmune.

How to take Indocin

• Take this drug exactly as your doctor directs. Take the capsules or liquid on a full stomach or with an antacid, unless your doctor instructs otherwise. Don't mix the liquid with the antacid or any other liquid before taking it; take the antacid first. Take capsules with a full glass (8 ounces) of water, and don't lie down for 15 to 30 minutes afterward.

• If you're taking the sustained-release capsules, swallow them whole. Don't crush, break, or chew them.

• If you're using a suppository, be sure to keep it in place for at least 1 hour.

If you miss a dose

Don't take a double dose. Adjust your schedule as follows:

• If you're using the capsules, liquid, or suppositories, take the missed dose as soon as possible. However, if it's almost time for the next dose, skip the missed dose and take the next dose as scheduled.

• If you're taking sustained-release capsules once or twice a day, take the missed dose if it's no more than 2 hours after the scheduled time. However, if it's later, skip the missed dose and take the next dose as scheduled.

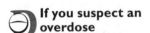

If you suspect an overdose

Contact your doctor *immediately*. Excessive Indocin can cause dizziness, nausea, vomiting, intense headache, confusion, drowsiness, ringing in the ears, sweating, blurred vision, numbness, tingling sensations, and seizures.

Warnings

• Make sure your doctor knows your medical history. You may not be able to take Indocin if you have other problems, such as seizures, Parkinson's disease, a digestive disorder, mental illness or depression, or kidney, liver, or heart disease.

• Don't take Indocin if you've had a bad reaction or an asthma attack after taking aspirin or other NSAIDs, such as Advil.

• Don't use the suppositories if you've had rectal bleeding recently or if you've ever had rectal inflammation.

• If you're pregnant or think you may be, check with your doctor before you start taking Indocin.

• Don't breast-feed while taking Indocin.

• Be aware that older adults may be especially prone to Indocin's side effects.

• Don't use Indocin regularly to relieve pain or reduce fever.

• If you have high blood pressure, you may need to take your blood pressure regularly. Report any increased readings to your doctor immediately.

• If you're on long-term oral therapy, be aware that you'll need to schedule regular eye exams, hearing tests, and blood and kidney tests so that your doctor can monitor for harmful levels of the drug in your blood.

• Be aware that this drug may mask signs and symptoms of infection.

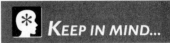

KEEP IN MIND...

* Take capsules with full glass of water; then stay upright for 15 to 30 minutes.

* Don't crush, break, or chew sustained-release capsules.

* Don't use Indocin regularly to relieve pain or reduce fever.

* Don't take this drug if you're allergic to aspirin or other NSAIDs, such as Advil or Motrin.

Inflamase

Inflamase is a corticosteroid (a cortisone-like drug) that's applied directly to the eye. It relieves eye inflammation and discomfort, probably by reducing the number of blood cells in the inflamed area.

Why it's prescribed

Doctors prescribe Inflamase to reduce inflammation of the eye. It comes in eyedrops. Doctors usually prescribe the following amounts for adults and children.

▶ **For inflammation of the eye,** 1 to 2 drops in eye. In severe conditions, drops may be used hourly, then gradually tapered as inflammation subsides. In mild conditions, drops may be used up to six times a day.

How to use Inflamase

• Use this drug exactly as your doctor directs. Shake the container well just before applying the drops.
• Be sure to wash your hands before and after applying Inflamase.
• To prevent contamination, don't touch the tip of the dropper to your eye, the surrounding area, or any other surface.
• After applying the drops, press your finger against the inner corner of your eye to help your eye absorb

INFLAMASE'S OTHER NAMES

Inflamase's generic name is prednisolone acetate. Other brand names include AK-Pred, Hydeltrasol Ophthalmic, Inflamase Forte, and Ocu-Pred.

SIDE EFFECTS

Call your doctor if you have any of these possible drug side effects.

Serious: none reported

Common: none reported

Other: glaucoma (increased pressure within the eye), various corneal problems; with excessive or long-term use, worsening of glaucoma, cataracts, vision problems, damage to optic nerve

DRUG INTERACTIONS

Combining certain drugs may alter their action or produce unwanted side effects. Tell your doctor about other drugs you're taking.

---

the drug. Keep your eye closed for 1 or 2 minutes.
• Close the container tightly and store it fully closed.

If you miss a dose

Apply the missed dose as soon as possible. However, if it's almost time for the next dose, skip the missed dose and apply the next dose as scheduled. Don't apply a double dose.

If you suspect an overdose

Consult your doctor.

Warnings

• Make sure your doctor knows your medical history. You may not be able to use Inflamase if you have other problems, such as a scratched cornea, an eye infection or disease (including cataracts or glaucoma), or diabetes.
• If you're pregnant, tell your doctor before you start using Inflamase.

• Don't wear contact lenses while using this drug because doing so may lead to infection. Ask your eye doctor how long you should wait before wearing contact lenses.
• Don't use leftover Inflamase for a new eye inflammation.
• Don't share this drug with family members. If anyone in your household develops similar symptoms, call the doctor.

 KEEP IN MIND...

* Wash hands before and after using.
* Don't touch tip of dropper to eye or other surface.
* Don't share drug with family members.
* Don't wear contact lenses while using.
* Don't use leftover drug for new eye inflammation.

Insulin

Insulin is a hormone normally produced by the pancreas that helps the body turn food into energy. Diabetes occurs when the body doesn't use insulin properly or doesn't make enough of it. When this happens, the person may need insulin injections to control the blood sugar (glucose) level. Insulin helps transport glucose to muscle and fat cells, which use it for energy. It also has other important functions in the body. Most insulin used today is synthetic human insulin. However, some is derived from beef or pork.

INSULIN'S OTHER NAMES

Brand names for regular (rapid-acting) insulin include Humulin R, Novolin R, Novolin R PenFill, Regular (Concentrated) Iletin II, and Regular Iletin I.

Brand names for isophane insulin suspension (neutral protamine Hagedorn insulin, or NPH) include Humulin N, Novolin N, Novolin N PenFill, and NPH Insulin.

Brand names for isophane insulin suspension with insulin injection include Humulin 50/50, Humulin 70/30, Novolin 70/30, and Novolin 70/30 PenFill.

Brand names for insulin zinc suspension (lente) include Humulin L, Lente Iletin II, Lente Insulin, and Novolin L.

Brand names for insulin zinc suspension (extended, or ultralente) include Humulin U and Ultralente Insulin.

 SIDE EFFECTS

Call your doctor if you have any of these possible drug side effects. Call *immediately* about any labeled "serious."

Serious: low blood sugar (difficulty concentrating, shakiness, headache, cold sweats, anxiety, cool and pale skin), severe allergic reaction (itching, hives, rash, difficulty breathing, or wheezing)

Tips: Watch for symptoms of low blood sugar, especially if you delay or miss a meal or snack, exercise more than usual, or drink alcoholic beverages. Frequent or severe low blood sugar may require your insulin dosage or type to be changed. If you have symptoms of low blood sugar, eat or drink something that contains sugar, such as glucose tablets or fruit juice. If possible, check your blood sugar level to confirm that it's low. If symptoms don't go away in 15 minutes, again eat or drink something sugary and wait another 15 minutes. If symptoms still don't go away, seek emergency medical care immediately. If you develop symptoms of an allergic reaction, immediately contact your doctor, who may change your type of insulin.

Common: skin changes at injection sites

Tip: Call your doctor if you see pitting, thickening, or other skin changes at injection sites.

Other: swelling, redness, high blood sugar level (excessive thirst, hunger, and urination)

 DRUG INTERACTIONS

Combining certain drugs may alter their action or produce unwanted side effects. Tell your doctor about other drugs you're taking, especially:
- Achromycin
- alcohol
- aspirin
- Atromid-S
- beta blockers, such as Lopressor and Tenormin
- birth control pills
- Choloxin
- Dilantin (high doses)
- diuretics (water pills) such as Lasix
- epinephrine preparations, such as Bronkaid and Primatene Mist
- Ismelin
- MAO inhibitors, such as Nardil and Parnate
- Pondimin
- Proglycem
- steroids, such as Anadrol and Orasone.

Continued on next page ▶

Why it's prescribed

Doctors prescribe insulin to treat type I (insulin-dependent) diabetes or to treat type II (non-insulin-dependent) diabetes that's not controlled by diet and oral diabetes drugs. Insulin comes in an injectable form.

▶ **For type I diabetes or for type II diabetes not controlled by diet and oral diabetic drugs,** dosage for an adult or child is set and adjusted by doctor according to person's blood sugar levels.

How to take insulin

• Keep unopened bottles of insulin refrigerated until needed. Never freeze insulin or expose it to hot temperatures or sunlight.

• Follow your doctor's instructions exactly on the kind of insulin to use, the correct dose, the number of injections to take each day, when to take them, and how to prepare and administer the injection.

• Remove insulin from the refrigerator and allow it to reach room temperature before injecting it.

• Don't use insulin that looks lumpy or grainy, seems unusually thick, sticks to the bottle, or appears even a little discolored or if the bottle looks frosty. Use regular insulin (short-acting) only if it's clear and colorless.

• Don't use insulin after the expiration date shown on the package.

• If you're mixing more than one type of insulin in the same syringe, first draw into the syringe the same amount of air as the amount of insulin you'll be withdrawing from each bottle. If you're mixing regular insulin with another insulin, always draw up the regular insulin first. When mixing two types of insulin other than regular insulin, you can draw them in any order, but use the same order each time.

• Inject insulin into fatty tissue on your thigh, abdomen, upper arm, or buttocks. The abdomen is preferred because insulin is absorbed into the bloodstream most evenly from here. Rotate among sites within the same anatomic area, such as moving from left to right in rows, from the top to the bottom of the area. Inject each new dose at least 1 inch from the previous site.

• Rapid-acting insulin takes effect within ½ to 1½ hours; intermediate-acting insulin, within 1 to 2½ hours; and long-acting insulin, within 4 to 8 hours. Drug effects last 5 to 7 hours with rapid-acting regular insulin, 12 to 16 hours with rapid-acting semilente insulin, 18 to 24 hours with intermediate-acting insulin, and 36 hours with long-acting insulin.

If you miss a dose

Follow your doctor's instructions. What you must do depends on the type and amount of insulin you're taking and how much time has elapsed since your last insulin injection.

If you suspect an overdose

Contact your doctor *immediately*. Excessive insulin can cause a fast pulse, palpitations, anxiety, hunger, nausea, sweating, tremor, pallor, restlessness, headache, and difficulty speaking and moving.

Warnings

• Make sure your doctor knows your medical history. Other problems may affect your insulin use.

• If you become pregnant, your doctor will adjust your insulin therapy.

• Schedule appointments regularly so your doctor can check your condition and adjust your insulin therapy as needed.

• Follow your prescribed diet and exercise plan strictly.

• Learn how to check your own blood sugar level and your urine for ketones.

• If you become sick with a cold, fever, or the flu, ask your doctor about changing the dose. Take your insulin even if you feel too sick to eat, especially if you have nausea, vomiting, or diarrhea.

• Be alert for symptoms of high blood sugar, which can appear if you're not getting enough insulin. Contact your doctor if you experience excessive thirst, hunger, and urination or if your blood sugar levels are high even without symptoms. If left untreated, high blood sugar can cause diabetic coma, an emergency condition.

• Keep a glucagon kit and a syringe and needle available, and teach your family how to prepare and use it if you develop severe low blood sugar. Keep a quick-acting, sugary food handy to treat low blood sugar symptoms.

• Carry medical identification stating that you have diabetes and listing your insulin type and dosage.

KEEP IN MIND...

* Don't use lumpy, grainy, unusually thick, or discolored insulin.

* Inject insulin into thigh, abdomen, upper arm, or buttocks.

* Rotate injection sites.

* Ask doctor what dose to take when ill.

* Check blood sugar level and urine for ketones.

* Learn how to handle symptoms of high and low blood sugar.

Intal

Intal is an asthma drug. It stops inflammatory cells in the lungs from releasing substances that lead to asthma symptoms or bronchospasm (closing up of the throat).

Why it's prescribed

Doctors prescribe Intal to treat asthma, to prevent asthma attacks brought on by exercise, and to treat and prevent some allergies. It comes in an inhaler, capsules (for oral solution), a nasal solution, a nebulizer solution, and eyedrops. Doctors usually prescribe the following amounts.

▶ **As part of a drug regimen in severe asthma,** adults and children age 5 and older: 2 sprays by inhaler four times a day at regular intervals. Or 20 milligrams (mg) by nebulizer four times a day at regular intervals.

▶ **To prevent and treat nasal inflammation due to allergy,** adults and children age 5 and older: 1 spray by inhaler in each nostril three to six times a day, at regular intervals.

▶ **To prevent asthma attacks caused by exercise,** adults and children age 5 and older: 2 sprays by inhaler no more than 1 hour before exercise.

▶ **For allergic eye disorders,** adults and children age 4 and older: 1 to 2 drops in each eye four to six times a day at regular intervals.

INTAL'S OTHER NAMES

Intal's generic name is cromolyn sodium. Other brand names include Gastrocrom, Intal Aerosol Spray, Intal Nebulizer Solution, Nalcrom, Nasalcrom, Opticrom; and, in Canada, Rynacrom.

SIDE EFFECTS

Call your doctor if you have any of these possible drug side effects. Call *immediately* about any labeled "serious."

Serious: closing up of throat (after inhaling dry powder), pneumonia (fever, cough)

Common: irritation of throat and trachea, dizziness, headache

Other: stuffy nose, nausea, inflammation of esophagus (difficulty swallowing), painful or frequent urination, cough, wheezing, rash, hives, joint swelling and pain, increased tearing; swelling of face, lips, hands, and feet

DRUG INTERACTIONS

Combining certain drugs may alter their action or produce unwanted side effects. Tell your doctor about other drugs you're taking.

How to use Intal

• Use this drug exactly as your doctor directs. Use it only after the acute asthma attack is under control, your airway is clear, and you can inhale on your own.
• If you're using the aerosol, your doctor may recommend a spacer device. If so, closely follow the doctor's instructions and manufacturer's directions.
• If you're using the eyedrops, be sure to wash your hands before and after applying them. Don't touch the applicator tip to your eye or any other surface.

If you miss a dose

If you take Intal regularly, take the missed dose as soon as possible. Then take any remaining doses for that day at regularly spaced intervals. Don't take a double dose.

 If you suspect an overdose

Consult your doctor.

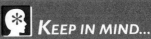Warnings

• Make sure your doctor knows your medical history before you use Intal.
• If you're pregnant or breast-feeding, tell your doctor before you start taking Intal.
• If you're also taking a steroid or bronchodilator, keep taking it even if your asthma seems better, unless your doctor tells you not to.
• If your symptoms don't improve within 4 weeks or if they get worse, call your doctor.

KEEP IN MIND...

∗ Use only after acute asthma attack is under control.

∗ If using a spacer device, follow doctor's and manufacturer's instructions.

∗ Call doctor if symptoms get worse or if they don't improve within 4 weeks.

Intron A

Intron A is a manmade version of an interferon — a substance naturally produced by the body to help fight infections and tumors. Researchers suspect that Intron A fights infection by stopping viral cells from multiplying. It seems to fight cancer by preventing tumor cells from increasing in number and by altering the body's immune response.

Why it's prescribed

Doctors prescribe Intron A to treat certain cancers and some types of hepatitis. It's available in an injectable form. Doctors usually prescribe the following amounts for adults.

▶ **For hairy-cell leukemia,** 2 million units per square meter of body surface area injected into a muscle or under the skin three times a week.

▶ **For AIDS-related Kaposi's sarcoma,** 30 million units per square meter of body surface area injected into a muscle or under the skin three times a week.

▶ **For chronic hepatitis B,** 30 to 35 million units a week injected into a muscle or under the skin, given as 5 million units a day or 10 million units three times a week, for 16 weeks.

▶ **For chronic hepatitis non-A, non-B/C,** 3 million units injected into a muscle or under the skin three times a week.

How to take Intron A

• If you'll be self-administering this drug, take it exactly as your doctor

INTRON A'S OTHER NAME

Intron A's generic name is recombinant interferon alfa-2b.

 SIDE EFFECTS

Call your doctor if you have any of these possible drug side effects. Call *immediately* about any labeled "serious."

Serious: too few white blood cells (infection)
Tips: Try to avoid people with infections. Call your doctor right away if you develop symptoms of infection, such as a fever, sore throat, or chills.

Common: fatigue, appetite loss, nausea, flulike symptoms (fever, chills, muscle ache, headache), joint pain
Tips: To ease flulike symptoms, take Tylenol. Also, check your temperature, if directed by your doctor.

Other: dizziness, confusion, numbness or tingling, mood changes, difficulty thinking or concentrating, difficulty sleeping, sedation, reduced sensations, memory loss, agitation, weakness, lack of energy, chest pain, vision or hearing problems, stye, stuffy or runny nose, sinus inflammation, sore throat, diarrhea, vomiting, stomach upset, constipation, belching, dry mouth, bad taste in mouth, mouth sores, difficulty breathing, cough, rash, dry skin, itching, slight hair loss or thinning, hives, skin inflammation, rigid muscles, leg cramps, bone disorders, back pain, increased sweating, decreased sex drive, migraine; joint pain, redness, or swelling
Tips: Any hair that falls out while you're taking this drug should grow back after you complete the treatment. If drowsiness occurs, take Intron A at bedtime. To relieve dry mouth, use sugarless gum or hard candy or ice chips.

 DRUG INTERACTIONS

Combining certain drugs may alter their action or produce unwanted side effects. Tell your doctor about other drugs you're taking, especially:
• drugs that relax you or make you sleepy, such as cold and allergy drugs, sedatives, tranquilizers, narcotic pain relievers, barbiturates, seizure drugs, and muscle relaxants
• Retrovir (AZT)
• Theo-Dur
• vaccines that contain live viruses (postpone immunizations).

directs. Also, closely follow the patient instructions that come with each package of Intron A. Make sure you understand how to prepare and give the injection and how to dispose of used syringes.

If you miss a dose

Don't take the missed dose or double the next dose. Call your doctor for instructions.

If you suspect an overdose

Consult your doctor.

Warnings

• Make sure your doctor knows your medical history. You may not be able to take Intron A if you have other problems, such as seizures, diabetes, a blood clotting disorder, heart or blood vessel disorders, or lung, kidney, or liver disease.

• If you're pregnant or breast-feeding, tell your doctor before you start taking Intron A.

• Be aware that older adults may be especially prone to side effects of Intron A.

• Schedule regular medical check-ups so your doctor can check your progress and evaluate the drug's effectiveness. The doctor may also order routine blood tests and X-rays while you're taking this drug.

• Drink plenty of fluids to help prevent low blood pressure — especially when you first start taking Intron A.

• Call your doctor immediately if you notice unusual bleeding or bruising or other symptoms of bleeding, such as pinpoint red spots on your skin, blood in your stools or urine, or black, tarry stools. Take care when using a toothbrush, dental floss, and a razor. Avoid contact sports and other activities in which injury and bruising are likely to occur.

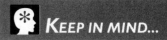

* Take drug at bedtime if drowsiness occurs.

* Drink plenty of fluids.

* Avoid people with infections and activities that increase risk of injury.

* Call doctor about symptoms of infection or bleeding.

Ipecac syrup

Ipecac syrup causes vomiting. Used in the emergency treatment of some types of poisoning, it works by stimulating the stomach lining and the part of the brain that controls vomiting.

Why it's prescribed

Doctors prescribe ipecac syrup to cause vomiting in people who've ingested certain toxic substances. You can also buy ipecac syrup without a prescription. Doctors usually prescribe the following amounts for adults; children's dosages appear in parentheses.

▶ **To induce vomiting in poisoning,** 30 milliliters (ml), followed by 8 to 12 ounces of water. (Children age 12 and older: same as adults. Children ages 1 to 12: 15 ml, followed by 8 ounces of water or milk. Children ages 6 months to 1 year: 5 ml, followed by 4 to 8 ounces of water or milk, repeated once, if needed, after 20 minutes.)

How to take ipecac syrup

• Take this drug only as directed by your doctor or poison control center. Don't take more of it than prescribed because this can damage your heart or even cause death.
• Drink water after taking ipecac syrup to help it cause vomiting. Don't take ipecac syrup with a carbonated beverage.
• This drug should cause vomiting within 20 to 30 minutes of the first dose. If it doesn't, take a second

IPECAC SYRUP'S OTHER NAME

Ipecac syrup is the generic name of this drug. It has no brand names.

SIDE EFFECTS

Call your doctor if you have any of these possible drug side effects.
Serious: none reported
Common: none reported
Other: slow pulse, dizziness, weakness, diarrhea

◆ DRUG INTERACTIONS

Combining certain drugs may alter their action or produce unwanted side effects. Tell your doctor about other drugs you're taking, especially:
• activated charcoal (take after ipecac-induced vomiting has stopped, usually around 30 minutes).

dose. If you still don't vomit, contact your doctor immediately or seek emergency care.

If you miss a dose

Not applicable because this drug is taken only as needed.

 ## If you suspect an overdose

Contact your doctor *immediately.* Excessive ipecac syrup can cause diarrhea, persistent nausea or vomiting, stomach pain or cramps, irregular heartbeats, low blood pressure (dizziness, weakness), inflammation of the heart muscle (chest pain, shortness of breath, fatigue, restlessness), difficulty breathing, and unusual fatigue or weakness.

◆ Warnings

• Before taking ipecac syrup, be sure to tell the health care professional treating or advising you if you've ever had a heart problem.
• Don't take ipecac syrup if you've ingested kerosene, gasoline, paint thinner, or a caustic substance, such as lye. If you do, a serious injury may occur.

• Don't give ipecac syrup to someone who's unconscious or very drowsy because the vomited substance may enter the lungs.
• Before giving ipecac syrup, call your doctor, a poison control center, or an emergency department for instructions.
• If you have a child over age 1 in your household, keep 1 ounce (30 ml) of ipecac syrup available for emergencies.

 ## KEEP IN MIND...

* Drink water after taking.

* Don't take with carbonated beverage.

* If vomiting doesn't occur after second dose, seek emergency treatment.

* Don't take after ingesting kerosene, gasoline, paint thinner, or caustic substances.

Ismelin

Ismelin lowers blood pressure. It works by regulating nerve impulses, which widens the blood vessels and helps blood pass through them more easily.

Why it's prescribed

Doctors prescribe Ismelin to reduce high blood pressure. It comes in tablets. Doctors usually prescribe the following amounts for adults.
▶ **For moderate to severe high blood pressure or for high blood pressure caused by a kidney disorder,** 10 milligrams (mg) a day, increased by 10 mg every week or month, as needed. Usual dosage is 25 to 50 mg a day. Maximum dosage is 300 mg a day.

How to take Ismelin

• Take this drug exactly as your doctor directs.
• Keep taking Ismelin even if you feel well. You may have to take it for the rest of your life.

If you miss a dose

Take the missed dose as soon as possible. However, if it's almost time for the next dose, skip the missed dose and take the next dose as scheduled. Don't take a double dose.

If you suspect an overdose

Contact your doctor *immediately.* Excessive Ismelin can cause low

ISMELIN'S OTHER NAMES

Ismelin's generic name is guanethidine monosulfate. A Canadian brand name is Apo-Guanethidine.

 SIDE EFFECTS

Call your doctor if you have any of these possible drug side effects. Call *immediately* about any labeled "serious."

Serious: heart failure (shortness of breath, fatigue, restlessness), irregular heartbeat (dizziness, fluttering in chest)

Common: dizziness (especially when standing up), weakness, fainting, slow pulse, stuffy nose, diarrhea, generalized swelling, weight gain, inability to ejaculate

Other: dry mouth

 DRUG INTERACTIONS

Combining certain drugs may alter their action or produce unwanted side effects. Tell your doctor about other drugs you're taking, especially:
• alcohol
• amphetamines, such as Didrex, Pondimin, and Tenuate
• Larodopa
• Levophed
• MAO inhibitors, such as Nardil and Parnate, and tricyclic antidepressants, such as Elavil
• phenothiazines (used for anxiety, nausea, vomiting, or psychosis)
• Ritalin.

blood pressure (dizziness, weakness), blurred vision, fainting, a slow pulse, and severe diarrhea.

 Warnings

• Make sure your doctor knows your medical history. You may not be able to take Ismelin if you have other problems, such as heart or blood vessel disease, a peptic ulcer, kidney disease, or bronchial asthma.
• Be aware that older adults may be especially prone to Ismelin's side effects.
• Schedule appointments regularly so your doctor can check your progress.
• Follow any special diet, such as a low-salt diet, the doctor prescribes.

• Learn how to take your blood pressure, and take it regularly.
• Consult your doctor before taking any other drugs, including nonprescription drugs.
• Before having surgery (including dental surgery), tell the doctor or dentist that you're taking Ismelin.

 KEEP IN MIND...

∗ Keep taking even if you feel well.
∗ Take blood pressure regularly.
∗ Follow any prescribed diets.

ISMO

ISMO is one of several heart drugs called nitrates. It works by relaxing the blood vessels, which boosts the supply of blood and oxygen to the heart and eases the heart's workload.

Why it's prescribed

Doctors prescribe ISMO to help prevent chest pain (angina). It comes in tablets and extended-release tablets. Doctors usually prescribe the following amounts for adults.

▶ **To treat acute attacks of chest pain or to prevent chest pain in situations in which it's likely to occur,** 30 to 60 milligrams (mg) once a day on arising, increased to 120 mg once a day after several days, if needed.

How to take ISMO

• Take this drug exactly as your doctor directs. ISMO takes effect in about 1 hour.
• Don't suddenly stop taking ISMO if you've been taking it regularly. Doing so could trigger an angina attack.

If you miss a dose

Take the missed dose as soon as possible. However, if it's within 2 hours of the next dose (or within 6 hours if you're taking the extended-release tablets), skip the missed dose

ISMO'S OTHER NAMES

ISMO's generic name is isosorbide mononitrate. Other brand names include IMDUR and Monoket.

 SIDE EFFECTS

Call your doctor if you have any of these possible drug side effects. Call *immediately* about any labeled "serious."

Serious: palpitations

Common: headache, dizziness (especially when standing up), fast pulse, swollen ankles, flushing

Tips: After taking a dose, you may get a headache that lasts a short time. Try taking aspirin or Tylenol for relief. If your headaches are severe or persistent, or if you suddenly *stop* getting headaches, check with your doctor — the drug may not be working as well anymore. To minimize dizziness, rise to your feet slowly. Go up and down stairs carefully, and lie down at the first sign of dizziness.

Other: weakness, fainting, nausea, vomiting, allergic reaction (rash, hives)

 DRUG INTERACTIONS

Combining certain drugs may alter their action or produce unwanted side effects. Tell your doctor about other drugs you're taking, especially:
• alcohol
• blood pressure drugs.

and take the next dose as scheduled. Don't take a double dose.

 If you suspect an overdose

Contact your doctor *immediately*. Excessive ISMO can cause increased pressure within the skull (persistent throbbing headache, confusion, fever, vertigo, palpitations, vision disturbances, nausea, vomiting, fainting, difficulty breathing, sweating) and heart block (slow pulse, paralysis, coma, seizures, death).

 Warnings

• Make sure your doctor knows your medical history. You may not be able to take ISMO if you have other medical problems.
• If you're pregnant or breast-feeding, tell your doctor before you start taking ISMO.
• Keep ISMO within easy reach at all times.
• Call your doctor if you find any partially dissolved tablets in your stools.

 KEEP IN MIND...

* Don't stop taking suddenly.
* Keep within reach at all times.
* Call doctor about severe or persistent headache.

Isoptin

Isoptin blocks calcium from entering the heart muscle, thereby slowing heart contractions. It also widens blood vessels, allowing more oxygen-carrying blood to reach and nourish the heart.

Why it's prescribed

Doctors prescribe Isoptin for chest pain, fast or irregular heartbeats, or high blood pressure. It comes in tablets and in sustained-release tablets (Isoptin SR). It's also available in an injectable form. Doctors usually prescribe the following amounts for adults.

▶ **For chest pain, high blood pressure, or irregular heartbeat,** 80 to 120 milligrams (mg) three times a day, increased weekly as necessary; some people may require up to 480 mg a day. Or for high blood pressure, 180 mg of sustained-release tablets once a day in the morning, increased as needed.

How to take Isoptin

• Take Isoptin only as your doctor directs. If you're taking the sustained-release tablet, swallow it whole; don't crush or chew it.
• Keep taking Isoptin even if you feel well. Stopping suddenly could worsen your condition.

ISOPTIN'S OTHER NAMES

Isoptin's generic name is verapamil. The generic name of Isoptin SR (sustained-release form) is verapamil hydrochloride. Other brand names include Calan, Verelan; and, in Canada, Apo-Verap, Novo-Veramil, and Nu-Verap.

 SIDE EFFECTS

Call your doctor if you have any of these possible drug side effects. Call *immediately* about any labeled "serious."

Serious: shortness of breath, difficulty breathing except when upright, wheezing, palpitations, irregular heartbeat, swollen legs, pale or bluish skin

Common: constipation, dizziness
Tips: Avoid constipation by increasing fluids and high-fiber foods in your diet. Prevent dizziness by standing up slowly and taking care when walking.

Other: nausea, headache, slow pulse, fatigue
Tips: Take your doses with food to avoid nausea, although food may decrease your body's ability to absorb the sustained-release form, requiring a change in dosage. Try to get extra rest while taking this drug.

 DRUG INTERACTIONS

Combining certain drugs may alter their action or produce unwanted side effects. Tell your doctor about other drugs you're taking, especially:
• drugs for high blood pressure, seizures, tuberculosis, or glaucoma
• Eskalith
• heart drugs (except nitroglycerin as needed for chest pain).

If you miss a dose

Take the missed dose as soon as possible. However, if it's almost time for your next dose, skip the missed dose and take your next dose as scheduled. Don't take a double dose.

 If you suspect an overdose

Contact your doctor *immediately*. Excessive Isoptin can cause extreme low blood pressure (dizziness, weakness), heart attack (chest pain, shortness of breath), and sudden death.

 Warnings

• Make sure your doctor knows your medical history. You may not be able to take Isoptin if you have other problems, especially another heart or blood vessel disorder or kidney or liver disease.
• If you're pregnant or breast-feeding, tell your doctor before you begin taking Isoptin.

 KEEP IN MIND...

* Take this drug with food.
* Don't crush or chew sustained-release tablets.
* Increase fluids and fiber in diet.
* Don't stop taking this drug suddenly.

Isopto Atropine

Isopto Atropine enlarges the pupil of the eye. It works by relaxing the sphincter muscle of the iris. This prevents the pupil from reacting to light.

Why it's prescribed

Doctors prescribe Isopto Atropine before eye examinations, before and after eye surgery, and to treat some eye conditions. This drug comes in an eye ointment and eyedrops. Doctors usually prescribe the following amounts for adults; children's dosage appears in parentheses.

▶ **For acute inflammation of the iris or for uveitis (inflammation of the uveal tract of the eye),** 1 to 2 drops in eye up to four times a day, or small strip of ointment applied to space inside lower eyelid up to three times a day. (Children: 1 to 2 drops of 0.5% solution in eye up to three times a day, or small strip of ointment applied to space inside lower eyelid up to three times a day.)

How to use Isopto Atropine

• Use this drug exactly as your doctor directs.
• Wash your hands before and after applying this drug.
• To prevent contamination, don't touch the applicator tip to your eye or any other surface.

ISOPTO ATROPINE'S OTHER NAMES

Isopto Atropine's generic name is atropine sulfate. Another brand name is Atropisol.

 ## SIDE EFFECTS

Call your doctor if you have any of these possible drug side effects.
Serious: none reported
Common: blurred vision, unusual sensitivity of the eyes to light
Other: irritability, confusion, sleepiness, poor coordination, eye crusting or drainage (with prolonged use), pinkeye, allergic reaction of eye (itching, redness), swelling within eye, dry eye, eye pain, dry mouth, swollen stomach (in infants), dry skin, flushing, fever

 ## DRUG INTERACTIONS

Combining certain drugs may alter their action or produce unwanted side effects. Tell your doctor about other drugs you're taking.

If you miss a dose

Don't apply a double dose. Adjust your schedule as follows:
• If you apply one dose a day, apply the missed dose as soon as possible. However, if you don't remember until the next day, skip the missed dose and apply the next dose as scheduled.
• If you apply more than one dose a day, apply the missed dose as soon as possible. However, if it's almost time for the next dose, skip the missed dose and apply the next dose as scheduled.

 ## If you suspect an overdose

Consult your doctor.

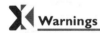 ## Warnings

• Make sure your doctor knows your medical history. You may not be able to use Isopto Atropine if you have other medical problems.
• If you're pregnant or breast-feeding, tell your doctor before you start using Isopto Atropine.
• Be aware that children with blond hair and blue eyes as well as older adults may be especially prone to this drug's side effects.
• Don't ingest this drug because it can cause poisoning (symptoms include disorientation and confusion).

 ## KEEP IN MIND...

* Wash hands before and after using.
* Don't touch applicator tip to eye or other surface.
* Older adults and blond, blue-eyed children are more prone to side effects.

Isopto Eserine

Isopto Eserine makes the pupil of the eye smaller and causes the ciliary muscle of the eye to contract. As a result, the flow of fluid from the eye chamber increases, reducing the pressure within the eye.

Why it's prescribed

Doctors prescribe Isopto Eserine to treat some types of glaucoma. It comes in eyedrops and an ointment. Doctors usually prescribe the following amounts for adults and children.

▶ For open-angle glaucoma, 1 to 2 drops in the eye two to four times a day, or thin strip of ointment applied to eye one to three times a day.

How to use Isopto Eserine

• Use this drug exactly as your doctor directs.
• Wash your hands before and after applying this drug.
• To prevent contamination, don't touch the applicator tip to your eye or any other surface.

If you miss a dose

Don't apply a double dose. Adjust your schedule as follows:
• If you apply one dose a day, apply the missed dose as soon as possible. However, if you don't remember

ISOPTO ESERINE'S OTHER NAMES

Isopto Eserine's generic name is physostigmine salicylate. The brand name of a similar drug, physostigmine sulfate, is Eserine Sulfate.

 SIDE EFFECTS

Call your doctor if you have any of these possible drug side effects. Call *immediately* about any labeled "serious."

Serious: slow or irregular pulse

Common: blurred vision, change in near or distance vision
Tip: Don't drive or perform other hazardous activities until your vision clears.

Other: headache, weakness, twitching eyelids, watery eyes, nausea, vomiting, diarrhea, loss of bladder control, sweating, shortness of breath; eye pain, burning, redness, stinging, or irritation

 DRUG INTERACTIONS

Combining certain drugs may alter their action or produce unwanted side effects. Tell your doctor about other drugs you're taking, especially:
• belladonna alkaloids used in the eye, such as AK-Homatropine and atropine
• other glaucoma drugs, such as Floropryl and Phospholine Iodide.

until the next day, skip the missed dose and apply the next dose as scheduled.
• If you apply more than one dose a day, apply the missed dose as soon as possible. However, if it's almost time for the next dose, skip the missed dose and apply the next dose as scheduled.

If you suspect an overdose

Contact your doctor *immediately.* Excessive Isopto Eserine can cause headache, nausea, vomiting, diarrhea, blurred vision, nearsightedness, excessive tearing, closing up of the throat, low blood pressure (dizziness, weakness), poor coordination, excessive sweating, slow pulse, excessive salivation, restlessness or agitation, and confusion.

Warnings

• Make sure your doctor knows your medical history. You may not be able to use Isopto Eserine if you have another eye problem.

KEEP IN MIND...

* Wash hands before and after using.

* Don't touch applicator tip to eye or other surface.

* Avoid driving until vision clears.

Isopto Hyoscine

Isopto Hyoscine enlarges the pupil of the eye. It works by relaxing the sphincter muscle of the iris. This prevents the pupil from reacting to light.

Why it's prescribed

Doctors prescribe Isopto Hyoscine before eye examinations, before and after eye surgery, and to treat some eye conditions. Isopto Hyoscine comes in eyedrops. Doctors usually prescribe the following amounts for adults; children's dosage appears in parentheses.

▶ For acute inflammation of the iris or for uveitis (inflammation of the uveal tract of the eye), 1 to 2 drops in the eye one to three times a day. (Children: 1 drop in the eye one to three times a day.)

How to use Isopto Hyoscine

- Use this drug exactly as your doctor directs.
- Wash your hands before and after using this drug.
- To prevent contamination, don't touch the applicator tip to your eye or any other surface.

If you miss a dose

Don't apply a double dose. Adjust your schedule as follows:
- If you apply one dose a day, apply the missed dose as soon as possible. However, if you don't remember until the next day, skip the missed dose and apply the next dose as scheduled.
- If you apply more than one dose a day, apply the missed dose as soon

SIDE EFFECTS

Call your doctor if you have any of these possible drug side effects. Call *immediately* about any labeled "serious."

Serious: fast or irregular pulse, hallucinations

Common: blurred vision, unusual sensitivity of eyes to light
Tips: Don't drive or perform other hazardous activities until your vision clears. Wear dark glasses if your eyes become sensitive to light.

Other: poor coordination, irritability, confusion, deliriousness, sleepiness, eye crusting or drainage (with prolonged use), pinkeye, dry eyes, increased pressure within eye (headache, eye pain), dry mouth, dry skin, skin inflammation, flushing, fever
Tip: To relieve dry mouth, use ice chips or sugarless hard candy or gum.

DRUG INTERACTIONS

Combining certain drugs may alter their action or produce unwanted side effects. Tell your doctor about other drugs you're taking.

as possible. However, if it's almost time for the next dose, skip the missed dose and apply the next dose as scheduled.

If you suspect an overdose

Contact your doctor *immediately.* Excessive Isopto Hyoscine can cause excitability and seizures followed by depression, disorientation, confusion, hallucinations, delusions, anxiety, agitation, restlessness, dry mucous membranes, difficulty swallowing, urine retention, fast pulse, fast breathing, fever, high blood pressure (severe headache, dizziness, numbness in the arms and legs), and flushed, hot, dry skin.

Warnings

- Make sure your doctor knows your medical history. You may not

be able to use Isopto Hyoscine if you have other problems, such as heart disease, glaucoma, or other eye problems.
- If you're pregnant or breast-feeding, tell your doctor before you start using Isopto Hyoscine.
- Be aware that older adults, children with blond hair and blue eyes, and infants may be especially prone to this drug's side effects.

KEEP IN MIND...

- ✳ Wash hands before and after using.
- ✳ Don't touch applicator tip to eye or other surface.
- ✳ Avoid driving until vision clears.

ISOPTO HYOSCINE'S OTHER NAME

Isopto Hyoscine's generic name is scopolamine hydrobromide.

Isordil

sordil relaxes the blood vessels, boosting the supply of blood and oxygen to the heart and easing the heart's workload.

Why it's prescribed

Doctors prescribe Isordil to treat attacks of angina (chest pain). It comes in tablets, extended-release tablets, chewable tablets, sublingual (under-the-tongue) tablets, capsules, sustained-release capsules, and a topical spray. Doctors usually prescribe the following amounts for adults.

▶ **For acute chest pain,** 2.5 to 5 milligrams (mg) sublingual tablets every 5 to 10 minutes, as needed, to a maximum of three doses in 30 minutes. Or 5 to 10 mg chewable tablets, as needed.

▶ **To prevent chest pain in situations in which it's likely to occur,** 5 to 30 mg orally three or four times a day, using smallest effective dose. Or 40 mg sustained-release capsules or extended-release tablets every 6 to 12 hours. Or 2.5 to 10 mg sublingual tablets every 2 to 3 hours. Or 5 to 10 mg chewable tablets every 2 to 3 hours.

How to take Isordil

• Take this drug exactly as directed.
• At the first sign of chest pain, place a sublingual tablet under your tongue and let it dissolve. Don't chew or swallow it.

ISORDIL'S OTHER NAMES

Isordil's generic name is isosorbide dinitrate. Other brand names include Dilatrate-SR, Iso-Bid, Isonate, Isorbid, Isotrate, Sorbitrate, Sorbitrate SA; and, in Canada, Apo-ISDN, Cedocard-SR, Coradur, Coronex, and Novosorbide.

 SIDE EFFECTS

Call your doctor if you have any of these possible side effects.

Serious: palpitations, fainting

Common: headache, dizziness (especially when standing up), fast pulse, swollen ankles, flushing, weakness

Other: fainting, nausea, vomiting, allergic reaction (rash, hives)

 DRUG INTERACTIONS

Combining certain drugs may alter their action or produce unwanted side effects. Tell your doctor about other drugs you're taking, especially:
• alcohol
• blood pressure drugs.

• Chew the chewable tablets well, and hold them in your mouth for about 2 minutes before swallowing.
• If you still have chest pain after taking three sublingual or chewable tablets in 15 minutes, seek emergency care.
• Take oral forms of the drug with 8 ounces of water on an empty stomach (30 minutes before or 1 to 2 hours after a meal). Swallow extended-release tablets or sustained-release capsules whole. Don't crush, break, or chew them.
• Don't suddenly stop using this drug after long-term use.

If you miss a dose

Take the missed dose as soon as possible. However, if it's within 2 hours of the next dose (or within 6 hours if you're taking extended-release tablets or sustained-release capsules), skip the missed dose and take the next dose as scheduled. Don't take a double dose.

If you suspect an overdose

Contact your doctor *immediately.* Excessive Isordil can cause headache, confusion, fever, vertigo, palpitations, vision disturbances, nausea, vomiting, fainting, difficulty breathing, sweating, and slow pulse.

Warnings

• Make sure your doctor knows your medical history before you start taking Isordil.
• If you're pregnant or think you may be, check with your doctor before taking this drug.

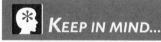 **KEEP IN MIND...**

* Place sublingual tablet under tongue at first sign of chest pain.

* Seek emergency care if chest pain persists after 3 tablets in 15 minutes.

* Don't stop taking suddenly.

Kaopectate

Kaopectate helps to halt diarrhea by decreasing the fluid content of the stool, making it more solid.

Why it's taken

Kaopectate is taken to treat diarrhea. You can buy it without a prescription. Kaopectate comes in liquids of varying strengths. The following amounts are recommended for adults; children's dosages appear in parentheses.
▶ **For mild diarrhea,** 60 to 120 milliliters (ml) of regular-strength liquid or 45 to 90 ml of concentrated liquid after each bowel movement.
• Children over age 12: 60 ml of regular-strength or 45 ml of concentrated liquid after each bowel movement.
• Children ages 6 to 12: 30 to 60 ml of regular-strength or 30 ml of concentrated liquid after each bowel movement.
• Children ages 3 to 5: 15 to 30 ml of regular-strength or 15 ml of concentrated liquid after each bowel movement.)

How to take Kaopectate

• If you're treating yourself, carefully follow the instructions on the bottle. If your doctor has prescribed this drug, follow any special directions.
• Shake the bottle vigorously before pouring your dose.

KAOPECTATE'S OTHER NAMES

Kaopectate is a combination of the generic drugs kaolin and pectin. Other brand names include Kapectolin, K-P, K-Pek; and, in Canada, Donnagel-MB and Kao-Con.

SIDE EFFECTS

Call your doctor if you have any of these possible drug side effects.
Serious: none reported

Common: none reported

Other: constipation, nutritional deficiencies (with chronic use because this drug absorbs nutrients); fecal impaction or ulcers in infants, older adults, and people weakened by illness (with chronic use)

DRUG INTERACTIONS

Combining certain drugs may alter their action or produce unwanted side effects. Tell your doctor about other drugs you're taking, especially:
• Achromycin, Lincocin
• Aralen
• Bentyl
• caffeine, Theo-Dur
• Lanoxin
• other oral drugs (take 2 to 3 hours before or after Kaopectate).

If you miss a dose

Not applicable because this drug is taken only as needed.

If you suspect an overdose

Consult your doctor.

Warnings

• Don't take Kaopectate if you must avoid constipation.
• If you're pregnant or breast-feeding, check with your doctor before you use Kaopectate.
• Don't give Kaopectate to children under age 3 because they may develop severe health problems from the fluid loss caused by diarrhea. Call the doctor instead.
• Be aware that older adults may also experience serious health problems due to fluid loss.
• During the first 24 hours, drink plenty of clear liquids, such as apple juice, broth, plain gelatin, and decaffeinated tea. (Call your doctor for specific guidelines on fluid replacement for a child.) Eat bland foods, such as applesauce, bread, cooked cereals, and crackers.
• Call your doctor if you have severe dehydration (dizziness, dry mouth, increased thirst, decreased urination, wrinkled skin).
• If you still have diarrhea after taking Kaopectate for more than 48 hours, don't take any more; call your doctor promptly.

KEEP IN MIND...

* Shake bottle vigorously before using.
* Drink plenty of clear fluids.
* Eat bland foods.
* Call doctor right away if diarrhea persists after 48 hours.

Kayexalate

Kayexalate is used to treat hyperkalemia — excessive potassium in the blood. It works by exchanging sodium ions for potassium ions in the digestive tract. The resin attaches to the potassium ions and is then eliminated from the body.

Why it's prescribed

Doctors prescribe Kayexalate to reduce the amount of potassium in the blood. It comes in a powder and a liquid. Doctors usually prescribe the following amounts for adults; children's dosages appear in parentheses.

▶ **For excessive potassium in the blood,** 15 grams (g) one to four times a day in water or sorbitol (3 to 4 milliliters per gram of resin). (Children: 1 g of resin for each milliequivalent of potassium to be removed.)

How to take Kayexalate

• Take this drug exactly as directed.
• Mix Kayexalate only with water or sorbitol for oral use. Never mix it with orange juice to disguise its taste because orange juice is rich in potassium. To make Kayexalate taste better, chill it.

If you miss a dose

If you're taking the drug once a day, take the missed dose as soon as

KAYEXALATE'S OTHER NAMES

Kayexalate's generic name is sodium polystyrene sulfonate. Other brand names include Kionex, SPS Suspension, and, in Canada, K-Exit.

 SIDE EFFECTS

Call your doctor if you have any of these possible drug side effects. Call *immediately* about any labeled "serious."

Serious: potassium deficiency (irritability, confusion, irregular heartbeat, severe muscle weakness, paralysis)

Common: constipation, diarrhea

Other: appetite loss, stomach upset, nausea, vomiting, calcium or magnesium deficiency (muscle spasms, seizures, irregular heartbeat), sodium retention (swelling, weight gain)

 DRUG INTERACTIONS

Combining certain drugs may alter their action or produce unwanted side effects. Tell your doctor about other drugs you're taking, especially:
• antacids
• laxatives.

possible. If you're taking it four times a day, take the missed dose as soon as you remember if it's within 2 hours of the next dose. Don't take a double dose.

 If you suspect an overdose

Contact your doctor *immediately.* Excessive Kayexalate can cause a potassium deficiency, which leads to irritability, confusion, irregular heartbeat, severe muscle weakness, and possibly paralysis.

Warnings

• Make sure your doctor knows your medical history. You may not be able to take Kayexalate if you have other problems, such as a heart condition, high blood pressure, or swelling anywhere in your body.

• If you are pregnant or breast-feeding, consult your doctor before taking Kayexalate.
• Keep all medical appointments so your doctor can check your progress and monitor your blood's potassium level.
• If you want to try the powder form of the drug, ask your pharmacist or a dietitian to supply recipes for Kayexalate cookies and candy.

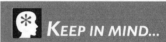 **KEEP IN MIND...**

* Mix only with water or sorbitol for oral use.

* Never mix with orange juice.

* Call doctor about irritability, confusion, irregular heartbeat, severe muscle weakness, or paralysis.

K-Dur

K-Dur is a potassium supplement. It replaces the body's potassium and maintains a normal level of potassium in the blood.

Why it's prescribed

Doctors prescribe K-Dur to increase the potassium level in people who don't get enough potassium in their regular diet or have lost much potassium due to illness or certain drugs. K-Dur comes in tablets, controlled-release tablets and capsules, enteric-coated tablets, an oral liquid, a powder for oral use, and an injectable form. Doctors usually prescribe the following amounts for adults; children's dosage appears in parentheses.

▶ **For potassium deficiency,** 40 to 100 milliequivalents (mEq) orally a day divided into three or four equal doses for treatment, or 20 mEq for prevention. Further dosages depend on blood potassium level. (Children: 3 mEq for each 2.2 pounds of body weight a day.)

How to take K-Dur

• Take this drug exactly as your doctor directs.
• Don't crush the controlled-release tablets or capsules or enteric-coated tablets; swallow them whole.

K-DUR'S OTHER NAMES

K-Dur's generic name is potassium chloride. Other brand names include Cena-K, K+10, Kaochlor 10%, Kaochlor S-F 10%, Kaon-Cl 20%, Kato, Klor-Con, Klorvess, Klotrix, K-Lyte/Cl, K-Norm, K-Tab, Micro-K, Rum-K, Slow-K, and Ten-K.

SIDE EFFECTS

Call your doctor if you have any of these possible drug side effects. Call *immediately* about any labeled "serious."

Serious: life-threatening low blood pressure and heart block (extreme dizziness, irregular or slow heartbeat), fluttering in chest, reduced urination, cold or graying skin

Common: nausea, vomiting, stomach pain, diarrhea, stomach ulcers
Tip: To prevent stomach upset, take the drug with meals or liquids.

Other: numbness, prickling, or tingling sensations in arms and legs; listlessness; confusion; weakness or heaviness of limbs; muscle paralysis

DRUG AND FOOD INTERACTIONS

Combining certain drugs and foods may alter drug action or produce unwanted side effects. Tell your doctor about your diet and other drugs you're taking, especially:
• diuretics (water pills), such as Aldactone, Dyrenium, and Midamor
• drugs used to treat high blood pressure or heart failure, particularly Accupril, Altace, Capoten, Lotensin, Monopril, Prinivil, and Vasotec
• salt substitutes containing potassium, low-sodium foods, and milk containing potassium.

• Dilute the oral liquid or powder in at least half a glass (4 ounces) of cold water or juice.

If you miss a dose

Take the missed dose as soon as possible if you remember within 2 hours. If you don't remember until later, skip the missed dose and take the next dose as scheduled. Don't take a double dose.

 If you suspect an overdose

Contact your doctor *immediately.* Excessive K-Dur can cause life-threatening heart problems (slow or irregular heartbeat), weakness, muscle paralysis, and difficulty breathing and swallowing.

 Warnings

• Make sure your doctor knows your medical history before you take K-Dur.
• Older adults may be more prone to excess potassium when taking K-Dur.

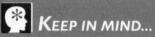 KEEP IN MIND...

* Don't crush tablets or capsules.

* Dilute oral liquid or powder in 4 ounces of cold water or juice.

* Don't use salt substitutes or eat low-sodium foods.

Keflex

Keflex is an antibiotic. It works by damaging the cell walls of bacteria, which eventually kills the bacteria.

Why it's prescribed

Doctors prescribe Keflex to treat infections in various parts of the body. It comes in tablets, capsules, and a liquid. Doctors usually prescribe the following amounts for adults; children's dosage appears in parentheses.

▶ **For infections of the respiratory tract, digestive tract, skin, soft tissues, bones, joints, or middle ear,** 250 milligrams (mg) to 1 gram every 6 hours. (Children: 6 to 12 mg for each 2.2 pounds [lb] of body weight every 6 hours. Maximum dosage is 25 mg for each 2.2 lb of body weight every 6 hours.)

How to take Keflex

• Take this drug exactly as your doctor directs.
• If your doctor has prescribed Benemid to help Keflex work better, take this drug exactly as directed also.
• If you're taking Keflex liquid, shake the bottle well before using and store it in the refrigerator.
• Discard any unused liquid after 14 days.
• To make sure your infection clears up completely, take Keflex for the entire time prescribed, even if you feel better.

KEFLEX'S OTHER NAMES

Keflex's generic name is cephalexin monohydrate. Other brand names include Cefanex, C-Lexin; and, in Canada, Apo-Cephalex and Novolexin.

 SIDE EFFECTS

Call your doctor if you have any of these possible drug side effects. Call *immediately* about any labeled "serious."

Serious: severe allergic reaction (rash, itching, restlessness, difficulty breathing), blood problems (fatigue, dizziness, infection)

Common: nausea, appetite loss, diarrhea, hives; red, raised blotchy rash

Other: dizziness, headache, numbness or tingling sensations, severe inflammation of colon (abdominal pain, diarrhea), vomiting, tongue inflammation, stomach upset or cramps, anal or genital itching, bladder or rectal spasms, yeast infection of mouth or genitals (sore mouth or tongue, vaginal itching or discharge)

DRUG INTERACTIONS

Combining certain drugs may alter their action or produce unwanted side effects. Tell your doctor about other drugs you're taking, especially:
• diarrhea drugs (may prolong diarrhea).

If you miss a dose

Take the missed dose as soon as possible. But, if it's almost time for the next dose and you take three or more doses a day, space the missed dose and the next dose 2 to 4 hours apart. Then resume your normal schedule. Don't take a double dose.

 If you suspect an overdose

Contact your doctor *immediately.* Excessive Keflex can cause seizures, numbness and tingling sensations, muscle spasms, and pain in the fingertips and toes.

 Warnings

• Make sure your doctor knows your medical history. You may not be able to take Keflex if you have other medical problems.

• If you're pregnant or breast-feeding, check with your doctor before you start taking Keflex.
• If you're diabetic, be aware that Keflex may cause false-positive results for urine sugar on the copper sulfate test (Clinitest). But glucose enzymatic tests (Clinistix, Tes-Tape) aren't affected.
• Check with your doctor before taking new drugs (prescription or nonprescription) or if new medical problems develop.
• If your symptoms persist or worsen after a few days, call your doctor.

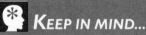 **KEEP IN MIND...**

* Shake liquid well before use.

* Take entire amount prescribed.

* Call doctor if symptoms don't subside in several days or if they get worse.

Kemadrin

Kemadrin helps treat the loss of muscle control caused by some diseases and drugs. Researchers suspect that it works by inhibiting the parts of the brain that control movement.

Why it's prescribed

Doctors prescribe Kemadrin to treat Parkinson's disease and to control severe side effects of certain drugs. It comes in tablets. Doctors usually prescribe the following amounts for adults.

▶ **For Parkinson's disease or severe side effects of drugs,** at first, 2.5 milligrams (mg) three times a day after meals, increased as needed to 5 mg three times a day after meals and, occasionally, 5 mg at bedtime.

How to take Kemadrin

• Take this drug exactly as your doctor directs.
• Don't stop taking Kemadrin without first checking with your doctor, who may want you to reduce the amount you're taking gradually before you stop taking it completely.

If you miss a dose

Take the missed dose as soon as possible. However, if it's within 2 hours of the next dose, skip the missed dose and take the next dose

SIDE EFFECTS

Call your doctor if you have any of these possible drug side effects.

Serious: none reported

Common: dry mouth, constipation
Tip: To relieve dry mouth, try ice chips, cool drinks, or sugarless gum or hard candy.

Other: light-headedness, giddiness, blurred vision, enlarged pupils, nausea, vomiting, stomach upset, rash, muscle weakness
Tips: Don't drive or perform other dangerous activities until you know how you react to this drug. To decrease stomach upset, take Kemadrin after meals.

DRUG INTERACTIONS

Combining certain drugs may alter their action or produce unwanted side effects. Tell your doctor about other drugs you're taking.

as scheduled. Don't take a double dose.

If you suspect an overdose

Contact your doctor *immediately.* Excessive Kemadrin can cause agitation and restlessness followed by depression, disorientation, confusion, hallucinations, delusions, anxiety, blurred vision, dry mucous membranes, difficulty swallowing, inability to urinate, fever, high blood pressure (headache, blurred vision), fast pulse, fast breathing, and flushed, hot, dry skin.

Warnings

• Make sure your doctor knows your medical history. You may not be able to take Kemadrin if you have other problems, such as glaucoma, high blood pressure, an enlarged prostate, heart or blood vessel disease, kidney

or liver disease, myasthenia gravis, blockage of the bowel, or uncontrollable movements of the hands, mouth, or tongue.
• If you're pregnant or breast-feeding, tell your doctor before you start taking Kemadrin.
• Be aware that older adults may be especially prone to Kemadrin's side effects.
• Keep all medical appointments so your doctor can check your progress and monitor drug effects.

KEEP IN MIND...

* Take after meals to decrease stomach upset.

* Don't stop taking unless doctor approves.

* Don't drive until your reaction to drug is known.

KEMADRIN'S OTHER NAMES

Kemadrin's generic name is procyclidine hydrochloride. Canadian brand names include PMS Procyclidine and Procyclid.

Kenacort

Kenacort is a cortisone-like drug used to relieve inflammation, swelling, redness, itching, and allergic reactions.

Why it's prescribed

Doctors prescribe Kenacort to treat Addison's disease (nonfunctioning adrenal glands), to reduce inflammation, or to suppress the body's immune system. It comes in tablets. Doctors usually prescribe the following amounts for adults; children's dosages appear in parentheses.

▶ **For severe inflammation or immune system suppression,** 4 to 60 milligrams (mg) a day in a single dose or divided into equal doses. (Children: 416 micrograms [mcg] to 1.7 mg for each 2.2 pounds [lb] of body weight per day in a single dose or divided into equal doses.)

▶ **For Addison's disease or adrenal insufficiency,** 4 to 12 mg a day in a single dose or divided into equal doses. (Children: 117 mcg for each 2.2 lb a day in a single dose or divided into equal doses.)

How to take Kenacort

- Take this drug exactly as directed.
- If you're taking one dose a day, take it in the morning.
- Don't stop taking this drug abruptly or without your doctor's approval.

If you miss a dose

Adjust your schedule as follows:
- If you take one dose a day, take the missed dose as soon as possible; then take your next scheduled dose.
- If you take several doses a day, take the missed dose as soon as possible;

 KENACORT'S OTHER NAMES

Kenacort's generic name is triamcinolone. Another brand name is Aristocort.

 SIDE EFFECTS

Call your doctor if you have any of these possible drug side effects. Call *immediately* about any labeled "serious."

Serious: congestive heart failure (shortness of breath, swelling), high blood pressure (headache, blurred vision)

Common: feeling of unusual well-being, trouble sleeping, fatigue, muscle weakness, joint pain, fever, nausea, ulcers, dizziness, fainting
Tips: To improve your sleep, take your last dose several hours before bedtime. To reduce stomach irritation, take your doses with food.

Other: uncharacteristic behavior, cataracts, glaucoma, increased appetite, delayed wound healing, skin eruptions, osteoporosis, abnormal hair growth, infections, high blood sugar level (increased urination, thirst, and hunger), growth retardation in children

 DRUG INTERACTIONS

Combining certain drugs may alter their action or produce unwanted side effects. Tell your doctor about other drugs you're taking, especially:
- anticoagulants (blood thinners) such as Coumadin
- aspirin, Advil, and other nonsteroidal anti-inflammatory drugs
- barbiturates, Dilantin, Rifadin
- Diuril, HydroDIURIL
- skin-test antigens (delay testing until end of Kenacort therapy)
- vaccines and toxoids (get doctor's approval before immunizations).

then resume your regular schedule. If you don't remember until the next dose is due, take a double dose.

 If you suspect an overdose

Contact your doctor *immediately.* Excessive Kenacort can cause muscle weakness, swelling, rounding of the face, and fat deposits on the torso.

Warnings

- Before taking Kenacort, inform your doctor if you've ever had stomach ulcers, kidney disease, high blood pressure, osteoporosis, diabetes, underactive thyroid, cirrhosis, colitis, blood clot, seizures, myasthenia gravis, heart failure, tuberculosis, herpes of the eye, or emotional instability, or if you're pregnant or breast-feeding.
- This drug may make older adults more prone to osteoporosis.
- If you're diabetic, this drug may increase your insulin requirements.
- Carry medical identification stating that you use Kenacort.

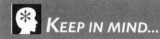 **KEEP IN MIND...**

- * Don't stop taking abruptly.
- * Carry medical identification.
- * Call doctor about headache or vision or breathing problems.

Kerlone

Kerlone is a beta blocker — a drug that interferes with the action of a specific part of the nervous system. It lowers blood pressure, possibly by slowing the pulse and decreasing the amount of blood expelled by the heart.

Why it's prescribed

Doctors prescribe Kerlone to reduce high blood pressure. It comes in tablets. Doctors usually prescribe the following amounts for adults.

▶ **For high blood pressure (used alone or with other drugs),** 10 milligrams (mg) once a day, increased to 20 mg once a day if desired response doesn't occur in 7 to 14 days.

How to take Kerlone

- Take this drug exactly as your doctor directs.
- Keep taking Kerlone even if you feel well. You may have to take it for the rest of your life.
- Don't stop taking this drug suddenly because doing so could cause serious medical problems.

If you miss a dose

Take the missed dose as soon as possible. However, if it's within 8 hours of the next dose, skip it and take the next dose as scheduled. Don't take a double dose.

 If you suspect an overdose

Contact your doctor *immediately.* Excessive Kerlone can cause dou-

KERLONE'S OTHER NAME

Kerlone's generic name is betaxolol hydrochloride.

 SIDE EFFECTS

Call your doctor if you have any of these possible drug side effects. Call *immediately* about any labeled "serious."

Serious: closing up of the throat, heart failure (shortness of breath, difficulty breathing, unusually fast pulse, cough, fatigue with exertion), slow pulse, chest pain, low blood pressure (dizziness, weakness), poor circulation (coolness, pain, bluish gray skin in arms and legs)

Common: none reported

Other: swelling, fainting, dizziness (especially when standing up), fatigue, headache, sluggishness, anxiety, gas, constipation, nausea, diarrhea, vomiting, appetite loss, dry mouth

 DRUG INTERACTIONS

Combining certain drugs may alter their action or produce unwanted side effects. Tell your doctor about other drugs you're taking, especially:
- calcium channel blockers, such as Calan and Cardizem
- Serpasil
- Xylocaine.

ble vision, slow pulse, low blood pressure (dizziness, weakness), heart block (dizziness), shock (extremely low blood pressure, severe dizziness), wheezing or difficulty breathing, bluish skin, fatigue, sleepiness, headache, sedation, coma, slowed breathing, seizures, nausea, vomiting, diarrhea, low blood sugar level (anxiety, clammy skin, tremor), hallucinations, and nightmares.

 Warnings

- Make sure your doctor knows your medical history. You may not be able to take Kerlone if you have other medical problems, such as heart disease, asthma, or emphysema.
- If you're pregnant or breast-feeding, tell your doctor before you start taking Kerlone.

- Be aware that older adults may be especially prone to Kerlone's side effects.
- Keep all medical appointments so your doctor can monitor your progress and check for any side effects.
- Follow any special prescribed diet, such as a low-salt diet.
- Ask your doctor for instructions on taking your blood pressure, and take it regularly.

KEEP IN MIND...

* Keep taking this drug even if you feel well.

* Follow any special diet that the doctor recommends.

* Take your blood pressure regularly.

Klonopin

Klonopin is one of a group of drugs called benzodiazepines, which slow down the central nervous system. Researchers suspect that it acts by making a brain chemical called GABA more available to nerve cells.

Why it's prescribed

Doctors prescribe Klonopin to control some types of seizures. It comes in tablets and drops for oral use. It's also available in an injectable form. Doctors usually prescribe the following amounts for adults; children's dosages appear in parentheses.

▶ **For various types of seizures,** no more than 1.5 milligrams (mg) orally a day divided into three equal doses, increased by 0.5 to 1 mg, if needed, every 3 days until seizures are controlled. If taken in unequal doses, largest dose is taken at bedtime. Maximum dosage is 20 mg a day. (Children up to age 10 or weighing up to 66 pounds [lb]: 0.01 to 0.03 mg for each 2.2 lb of body weight orally a day [but not more than 0.05 mg for each 2.2 lb a day] divided into two or three equal doses. Increased by 0.25 to 0.5 mg every third day to a maximum of 0.1 to 0.2 mg for each 2.2 lb every day, as needed.)

How to take Klonopin

• Take this drug in regularly spaced doses exactly as your doctor directs.

KLONOPIN'S OTHER NAME

Klonopin's generic name is clonazepam. Another brand name is Rivotril.

 SIDE EFFECTS

Call your doctor if you have any of these possible drug side effects. Call *immediately* about any labeled "serious."

Serious: slowed or difficult breathing, blood problems (fatigue, bleeding, bruising, increased risk of infection, fever, chills)

Common: drowsiness, incoordination, increased salivation, unusual behavior

Tip: Check with your doctor if you become drowsy, your mouth starts to water, or you notice changes in your behavior.

Other: slurred speech, tremor, confusion, mental disturbances, agitation, double vision, abnormal eye movements, sore gums, constipation, stomach pain, nausea, vomiting, change in appetite, abnormal thirst, painful urination, bedwetting, excessive nighttime urination, inability to urinate, rash

 DRUG INTERACTIONS

Combining certain drugs may alter their action or produce unwanted side effects. Tell your doctor about other drugs you're taking, especially:
• alcohol and other drugs that make you relaxed or sleepy.

• Don't stop taking this drug suddenly because this could cause your seizures to get worse.

If you miss a dose

Take the missed dose as soon as possible. However, if it's almost time for the next dose, skip the missed dose and take the next dose as scheduled. Don't take a double dose.

 If you suspect an overdose

Contact your doctor *immediately.* Excessive Klonopin can cause incoordination, confusion, coma, decreased reflexes, and low blood pressure (dizziness, weakness).

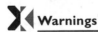 **Warnings**

• Make sure your doctor knows your medical history. You may not be able to take Klonopin if you have other problems, such as liver disease or acute angle-closure glaucoma, or if you're sensitive to other benzodiazepines.
• If you're pregnant or breast-feeding, check with your doctor before you start taking Klonopin.
• Carry medical identification stating that you're taking Klonopin.

 KEEP IN MIND...

∗ Don't stop taking suddenly.
∗ Avoid driving until you know how you react to drug.
∗ Call doctor if breathing becomes slow or difficult.
∗ Carry medical identification.

Kwell

Kwell is believed to interfere with certain cells in scabies and lice, causing seizures and death in the insects.

Why it's prescribed

Doctors prescribe Kwell to treat scabies and lice infestations. It comes in a cream, lotion, and shampoo. The cream and lotion are used to treat scabies; the shampoo is used to treat lice. Doctors usually prescribe the following amounts for adults and children.

▶ **For scabies or lice,** thin layer of cream or lotion applied over entire skin surface (scabies) or hairy areas (lice) and left on for 8 to 12 hours, repeated in 1 week if needed. Or shampoo applied to hair and lathered for 4 to 5 minutes.

How to use Kwell

• Use this drug exactly as your doctor directs. Don't use more than your doctor has ordered, and don't use it more often or for a longer time than ordered because this could cause poisoning.
• To use the cream or lotion, apply a thin layer to freshly washed and dried skin. Use enough to cover the entire skin surface from your neck down. Rub in the cream or lotion well; then leave it on. After the prescribed number of hours, wash thoroughly.
• To use the shampoo, apply it undiluted to freshly washed and dried hair. Apply enough to thoroughly

KWELL'S OTHER NAMES

Kwell's generic name is lindane. Other brand names include Bio-Well, Kildane, Scabene; and, in Canada, GBH and Kwellada.

SIDE EFFECTS

Call your doctor if you have any of these possible drug side effects. Call *immediately* about any labeled "serious."

Serious: seizures

Common: dizziness, irritation (with repeated use)

Other: none reported

DRUG INTERACTIONS

Combining certain drugs may alter their action or produce unwanted side effects. Tell your doctor about other drugs you're taking.

wet the affected areas and the surrounding hair-covered areas. Rub the shampoo into your hair and scalp. If you're taking a bath, make sure the shampoo doesn't drip onto your body or into the bath water. Leave it on for 4 to 5 minutes; then add enough water to create a lather. Rinse your hair thoroughly; then dry it with a clean towel. Use a fine-toothed comb dipped in white vinegar to remove any remaining lice eggs from your dried hair.
• Keep Kwell away from your eyes, nose, mouth, and lips. If it gets in your eyes, *immediately* flush your eyes with water and call your doctor.
• Don't inhale Kwell's vapors.
• Don't use Kwell on open cuts, sores, or inflamed areas of your skin.

If you miss a dose

Not applicable because this drug is used only as needed.

If you suspect an overdose

Contact your doctor *immediately* if you accidentally swallow Kwell. Ingestion can cause stimulation of

the central nervous system (anxiety, restlessness), dizziness, seizures, and death.

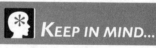
Warnings

• Make sure your doctor knows your medical history. You may not be able to use Kwell if you have other medical problems, especially a history of seizures.
• If you're pregnant or breast-feeding, tell your doctor before using Kwell.

KEEP IN MIND...

* Don't use more often or for longer than ordered.
* Don't swallow or inhale this drug.
* Keep Kwell away from eyes, nose, mouth, and lips.
* Don't use on open cuts, sores, or inflamed areas.

Kytril

Kytril helps prevent nausea and vomiting by attaching to receptors in the brain region that controls vomiting. It may also block chemicals in other parts of the nervous system.

Why it's prescribed

Doctors prescribe Kytril to prevent nausea and vomiting caused by some drugs used to treat cancer. Kytril comes in tablets. It's also available in an injectable form. Doctors usually prescribe the following amounts for adults.

▶ **To prevent nausea and vomiting associated with drug treatment for cancer,** 1 milligram orally up to 1 hour before cancer drug and repeated 12 hours later.

How to take Kytril

- Take this drug exactly as your doctor directs.

If you miss a dose

Consult your doctor.

If you suspect an overdose

Consult your doctor. Excessive Kytril can cause a slight headache.

Warnings

- Make sure your doctor knows your medical history. You may not be able to use Kytril if you have

---

KYTRIL'S OTHER NAME

Kytril's generic name is granisetron hydrochloride.

SIDE EFFECTS

Call your doctor if you have any of these possible drug side effects. Call *immediately* about any labeled "serious."

Serious: irregular heartbeat, severe allergic reaction (hives, chest pain, difficulty breathing)

Common: headache, weakness, drowsiness
Tip: Rest frequently to relieve weakness. Don't drive or perform other tasks that require full alertness until you know how Kytril affects you.

Other: high blood pressure (headache, blurred vision), diarrhea, constipation, fever, unusual taste in mouth
Tip: To prevent constipation, drink plenty of fluids and eat high-fiber foods, such as fruits, vegetables, and whole-grain products.

DRUG INTERACTIONS

Combining certain drugs may alter their action or produce unwanted side effects. Tell your doctor about other drugs you're taking, especially:
- antibiotics such as erythromycin
- birth control pills that contain estrogen
- MAO inhibitors, such as Nardil and Parnate
- seizure drugs such as Dilantin
- tuberculosis drugs, such as Laniazid and Rifadin.

---

other medical problems, such as kidney failure, liver disease, a drug allergy, or an allergy to other substances, such as preservatives and dyes.
- If you're pregnant or breast-feeding, tell your doctor before you begin taking Kytril.
- Kytril is used for nausea and vomiting caused by drug treatment for cancer. Do not take it for nausea and vomiting from any other cause.
- Some people who are undergoing cancer treatment find that eating smaller meals more frequently also helps ease nausea and vomiting.

- If nutrition becomes a problem, ask your doctor if you should add supplements to your diet, such as Ensure.

KEEP IN MIND...

* Take only for nausea and vomiting caused by use of cancer drugs.

* Take exactly as directed.

* Call doctor right away if you experience symptoms of severe allergic reaction.

Lamictal

Lamictal is used in the treatment of epilepsy to help control seizures. It reduces seizures by stopping the release of certain chemicals in the brain that affect the nervous system.

Why it's prescribed

Doctors prescribe Lamictal to help control seizures. It comes in tablets. Doctors usually prescribe the following amounts for adults.

▶ **For seizures in epilepsy,** 50 milligrams (mg) once a day for 2 weeks, followed by 100 mg a day divided into two equal doses for 2 weeks. Usual dosage is 300 to 500 mg a day divided into two equal doses. For people also taking valproic acid, 25 mg every other day for 2 weeks, followed by 25 mg a day for 2 weeks. Thereafter, no more than 150 mg a day divided into two equal doses.

How to take Lamictal

• Take Lamictal only as your doctor directs.
• Don't suddenly stop taking Lamictal; seizures may occur more frequently. Check with your doctor about gradually stopping treatment over at least 2 weeks.

If you miss a dose

Take the missed dose as soon as you remember. However, if it's almost time for your next dose, skip the missed dose and go back to your regular schedule. Don't take a double dose.

LAMICTAL'S OTHER NAME

Lamictal's generic name is lamotrigine.

 SIDE EFFECTS

Call your doctor if you have any of these possible drug side effects. Call *immediately* about any labeled "serious."

Serious: rash

Tip: A rash may or may not be a serious side effect. If you develop one, report it to your doctor immediately to see whether or not you should continue taking Lamictal.

Common: dizziness, headache, incoordination, sleepiness, blurred or double vision, nausea, vomiting, weight gain

Other: insomnia, tremor, depression, anxiety, seizures, irritability, decreased memory, restlessness, mood swings, vertigo, mind racing, palpitations, uncontrollable rapid eye movements, diarrhea, abdominal pain, constipation, weight loss, dry mouth, cough, difficulty breathing, itching, hot flashes, hair loss, acne, slurred speech, muscle spasm, fever, infection, neck pain, overall feeling of illness, chills, menstrual changes

 DRUG INTERACTIONS

Combining certain drugs may alter their action or produce unwanted side effects. Tell your doctor about other drugs you're taking, especially:
• folate inhibitors, such as Bactrim and Rheumatrex
• seizure drugs, such as Dilantin, Mysoline, Solfoton, and Tegretol
• valproic acid.

 If you suspect an overdose

Contact your doctor *immediately*. Excessive Lamictal can cause dizziness, headache, drowsiness, and coma.

 Warnings

• Make sure your doctor knows your medical history. You may not be able to take Lamictal if you have other medical problems, such as kidney, liver, or heart disease, or if you're allergic to this or other drugs.

• Make sure your doctor knows if you're pregnant or breast-feeding before you begin taking Lamictal.
• Schedule regular follow-up visits so that your doctor can check your progress.

KEEP IN MIND...

∗ Take only as directed.

∗ Dosage reduced when combined with other drugs.

∗ To avoid seizures, don't stop taking suddenly.

Lamisil

Lamisil is a fungus-fighting drug. It works by destroying the fungus's cell walls, which kills the fungus or prevents its growth.

Why it's prescribed

Doctors prescribe Lamisil to treat ringworm of the body and fungal infections of the foot (athlete's foot) or groin (jock itch). It comes in a cream. Doctors usually prescribe the following amounts for adults.

▶ **For ringworm of the body and fungal infection of the groin,** small amount applied to affected and immediate surrounding areas once or twice a day for at least 1 week.

▶ **For athelete's foot,** small amount applied to affected and immediate surrounding areas twice a day for at least 1 week.

How to use Lamisil

• Use this drug exactly as your doctor directs.
• Use Lamisil for the full time prescribed, even if your symptoms start to clear up after several days. If you stop using it too soon, your symptoms may return.
• Keep Lamisil away from your eyes, mouth, and mucous membranes. This drug is for external use only.
• Don't cover the medicated areas with an airtight dressing unless the

LAMISIL'S OTHER NAME

Lamisil's generic name is terbinafine hydrochloride.

 SIDE EFFECTS

Call your doctor if you have any of these possible drug side effects.

Serious: none reported

Common: none reported

Other: skin irritation, burning, itching, or dryness

Tip: Stop using the drug and call your doctor if you experience skin irritation or other skin problems.

 DRUG INTERACTIONS

Combining certain drugs may alter their action or produce unwanted side effects. Tell your doctor about other drugs you're taking.

doctor tells you to; doing so could result in skin irritation.

If you miss a dose

Apply the missed dose as soon as possible. However, if it's almost time for the next dose, skip the missed dose and apply the next dose as scheduled.

If you suspect an overdose

Contact your doctor *immediately.* Excessive Lamisil can cause irregular pulse, seizures, nausea, and vomiting.

 Warnings

• Make sure your doctor knows your medical history. You may not be able to use Lamisil if you have other medical problems.
• If you're pregnant or breast-feeding, tell your doctor before you start using Lamisil.

• Be aware that Lamisil is not recommended for use in children under age 12.
• Don't use Lamisil for more than 4 weeks.
• Call your doctor if the infection doesn't clear up. But keep in mind that you may continue to see improvement for up to 4 weeks after completing the treatment.

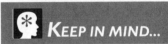 **KEEP IN MIND...**

* Keep away from eyes, mouth, and mucous membranes.

* Don't cover medicated areas with dressing.

* Keep using for full time prescribed.

* Stop using and call doctor if skin becomes irritated.

* Drug isn't recommended for children under age 12.

Laniazid

Laniazid is a drug for tuberculosis. It works by inhibiting the growth of the bacteria that cause tuberculosis.

Why it's prescribed

Doctors prescribe Laniazid to treat tuberculosis. It comes in tablets and a liquid. It's also available in an injectable form. Doctors usually prescribe the following amounts for adults; children's dosages appear in parentheses.

▶ **To treat active tuberculosis,** 5 milligrams (mg) for each 2.2 pounds (lb) of body weight orally every day in a single dose, up to 300 mg per day, continued for 6 months to 2 years. (Infants and children: 10 to 20 mg for each 2.2 lb orally every day in a single dose, up to 300 to 500 mg per day.)

▶ **To prevent tuberculosis in people who've been exposed to tuberculosis or those with positive skin tests whose diagnostic findings suggest nonprogressive tuberculosis,** 300 mg orally a day in a single dose, continued for 6 months to 1 year. (Infants and children: 10 mg for each 2.2 lb orally every day in a single dose, up to 300 mg per day, continued for 1 year.)

How to take Laniazid

• Take this drug exactly as directed, at the same time each day.
• Keep taking Laniazid for the full time prescribed, even if you feel

LANIAZID'S OTHER NAMES

Laniazid's generic name is isoniazid (also called INH). Other brand names include Nydrazid and, in Canada, Isotamine and PMS-Isoniazid.

 SIDE EFFECTS

Call your doctor if you have any of these possible drug side effects. Call *immediately* about any labeled "serious."

Serious: blood problems (bruising, fatigue, dizziness, increased risk of infection), allergic reaction (fever, rash, swollen lymph glands)

Common: peripheral neuropathy (numbness, tingling, and coolness in arms and legs), nausea, vomiting, stomach upset

Other: constipation, dry mouth, yellow-tinged skin and eyes, stiff joints, increased thirst and urination, strange behavior

 DRUG AND FOOD INTERACTIONS

Combining certain drugs and foods may alter drug action or produce unwanted side effects. Tell your doctor about your diet and other drugs you're taking, especially:
• alcohol
• Antabuse
• antacids that contain aluminum, such as Basaljel and AlternaGEL
• corticosteroids such as Orasone
• Dilantin, Tegretol
• laxatives (take at least 1 hour after Laniazid)
• tuna.

better. You may need to take this drug for 1 year or even longer.

If you miss a dose

Take the missed dose as soon as possible. But, if it's almost time for the next dose, skip the missed dose and take the next dose as scheduled. Don't take a double dose.

 If you suspect an overdose

Contact your doctor *immediately.* Excessive Laniazid can cause nausea, vomiting, slurred speech, dizziness, blurred vision, and visual hallucinations. Severe overdose can cause stupor or coma, difficulty breathing, seizures, and death.

 Warnings

• Make sure your doctor knows your medical history. You may not be able to take Laniazid if you have other medical problems.
• If you're pregnant or breast-feeding, tell your doctor before taking Laniazid.

KEEP IN MIND...

* Take with food or non-aluminum antacid if drug upsets stomach.
* Take drug for full time prescribed.
* Avoid eating tuna.

Lanoxin

Lanoxin is a type of heart drug. It provides more calcium to the heart and slows electrical impulses through crucial parts of the heart, making the heart stronger and more efficient.

Why it's prescribed

Doctors prescribe Lanoxin to treat some heart conditions. It comes in tablets, capsules, and an elixir. It's also available in an injectable form. Doctors usually prescribe the following amounts for adults; children's dosages vary with age and height.

▶ **For congestive heart failure and certain irregular heartbeats,** initially, 0.5 to 1 milligram (mg) orally divided into equal doses over 24 hours; maintenance dosage is 0.125 to 0.5 mg a day. Depending on response, larger doses may be needed to treat irregular heartbeats. Frail and underweight older adults may require a lower maintenance dose.

How to take Lanoxin

• Take this drug exactly as your doctor directs.
• As directed, check your pulse rate before each dose. If it's much slower or faster than usual (or less than 50 beats per minute), call your doctor.
• Don't stop taking Lanoxin without first checking with your doctor.

SIDE EFFECTS

Call your doctor if you have any of these possible drug side effects. Call *immediately* about any labeled "serious."

Serious: irregular heartbeat (palpitations, shortness of breath, dizziness, sweating), hallucinations, yellow-green halos around visual images, double vision, light flashes

Common: fatigue, weakness, agitation, blurred vision, nausea

Other: headache, overall feeling of illness, vertigo, numbness or tingling sensations, unusual sensitivity of eyes to light, vomiting, diarrhea

DRUG INTERACTIONS

Combining certain drugs may alter their action or produce unwanted side effects. Tell your doctor about other drugs you're taking, especially:
• antacids, Reglan
• antibiotics, such as erythromycin
• anticholinergics, such as atropine and Pro-Banthine
• cholesterol-lowering drugs, such as Colestid and Questran
• diuretics (water pills) such as Lasix
• other heart drugs, especially Calan, Cardioquin, and Cardizem.

Stopping suddenly may cause a serious heart problem.

If you miss a dose

Take the missed dose as soon as possible if you remember within 12 hours. But if you don't remember until later, skip the missed dose and take the next dose as scheduled. Don't take a double dose.

If you suspect an overdose

Contact your doctor *immediately*. Excessive Lanoxin can cause potassium excess (palpitations, nausea, vomiting, and fast, irregular pulse).

Warnings

• Make sure your doctor knows your medical history. You may not be able to take Lanoxin if you have other medical problems.
• If you're pregnant or breast-feeding, tell your doctor before taking Lanoxin.

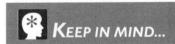

KEEP IN MIND...

∗ Check pulse before each dose, if instructed; call doctor if pulse is less than 50.

∗ Don't stop taking without first checking with doctor.

∗ Call doctor right away about irregular heartbeat, hallucinations, or visual disturbances.

Lariam

Lariam is an antimalaria drug. It seems to work by killing the parasites that cause malaria or by preventing their growth.

Why it's prescribed

Doctors prescribe Lariam to treat malaria or to prevent it in people who live in or plan to travel to an area where there's a good chance of getting malaria. Lariam comes in tablets. Doctors usually prescribe the following amounts for adults; children's dosages appear in parentheses.

▶ **To treat acute malaria,** 1,250 milligrams (mg) as a single dose, followed by treatment with another drug, such as primaquine, to avoid relapse. (Children over age 2: 16.5 mg for each 2.2 pounds of body weight as a single dose.)

▶ **To prevent malaria,** 250 mg once a week, starting 1 week before the person enters malaria-prone area and continuing for 4 weeks after leaving area. In a person who returns from such an area without malaria after prolonged stay, treatment ends after three doses. (Children over age 2: 62.5 to 250 mg once a week, based on age and body weight.)

How to take Lariam

• Take this drug exactly as your doctor directs. Take it with a full glass (at least 8 ounces) of water. Don't take it on an empty stomach.
• If you're taking Lariam to prevent malaria, try to take it on the same day every week.

LARIAM'S OTHER NAME

Lariam's generic name is mefloquine hydrochloride.

 SIDE EFFECTS

Call your doctor if you have any of these possible drug side effects. Call *immediately* about any labeled "serious."

Serious: slow pulse, seizures, emotional disturbances

Common: nausea

Other: dizziness, fainting, headache, palpitations, ringing in ears, appetite loss, vomiting, diarrhea, stomach upset, rash, fatigue, fever, chills

Tip: Avoid driving and other dangerous activities until you know how you react to the drug.

 DRUG INTERACTIONS

Combining certain drugs may alter their action or produce unwanted side effects. Tell your doctor about other drugs you're taking, especially:
• beta blockers, such as Tenormin
• Depakene
• other drugs to treat malaria.

If you miss a dose

Take the missed dose as soon as possible. However, if it's almost time for the next dose, skip the missed dose and take the next dose as scheduled. Don't take a double dose.

 If you suspect an overdose

Contact your doctor *immediately.* Excessive Lariam can cause slow pulse, depression, seizures, and hallucinations.

 Warnings

• Make sure your doctor knows your medical history. You may not be able to take Lariam if you have other problems, such as heart disease, or a history of seizures or mental illness.

• If you're pregnant or breast-feeding, tell your doctor before you start taking Lariam.
• Be aware that Lariam is not recommended for children who are younger than age 2 or who weigh less than 33 pounds.
• If you're taking Lariam to treat malaria, call your doctor if your symptoms don't improve within a few days or if they get worse.
• If you'll be taking Lariam for a long time, get your eyes examined periodically.

 KEEP IN MIND...

* Take with full glass of water.
* Call doctor if symptoms don't improve within several days or if they get worse.
* Avoid driving until you know how you react to drug.

Larodopa

Larodopa improves muscle control in conditions caused by a decrease in dopamine, which transmits nerve impulses.

Why it's prescribed

Doctors prescribe Larodopa to treat Parkinson's disease or parkinson-like symptoms caused by injury. It comes in tablets. Doctors usually prescribe the following amounts for adults and children over age 12.

▶ **For Parkinson's disease or parkinson-like symptoms,** initially, 0.5 to 1 gram (g) daily, divided into two or more equal doses. Dosage should be increased by no more than 0.75 g per day, every 3 to 7 days.

How to take Larodopa

• Take no more than your doctor prescribes.
• If you have trouble swallowing the tablets, crush them and mix them with applesauce.
• Protect this drug from heat, light, and moisture. If the tablets darken, don't take them.
• Larodopa may not take effect for several weeks. If you don't think the drug is working, don't stop taking it; call your doctor.

If you miss a dose

Take the missed dose as soon as possible. However, if your next scheduled dose is within 2 hours, skip the missed dose and resume your regular schedule. Don't take a double dose.

LARODOPA'S OTHER NAMES

Larodopa's generic name is levodopa. Another brand name is Dopar.

 SIDE EFFECTS

Call your doctor if you have any of these possible drug side effects. Call *immediately* about any labeled "serious."

Serious: depression or mood changes, unusual or uncontrollable movements, difficulty urinating, light-headedness or dizziness, irregular heartbeat, severe nausea or vomiting, eyelid spasms, shortness of breath

Common: dark sweat and urine

Other: fatigue, anxiety, confusion, constipation, insomnia, aggressive behavior, disturbing dreams, euphoria, flushing, blurred vision, increased salivation, dry mouth, bitter taste, gas, stomach upset, increased sex drive, painful erections, liver problems (yellow-tinged skin and eyes)

Tip: To avoid constipation, increase fluids and fiber in your diet.

 DRUG AND FOOD INTERACTIONS

Combining certain drugs and foods may alter drug action or produce unwanted side effects. Tell your doctor about your diet and other drugs you're taking, especially:
• antacids, Reglan
• antidepressants called MAO inhibitors
• antipsychotic drugs
• decongestants, asthma drugs, and other stimulants
• Dilantin
• foods high in protein or vitamin B_6 (such as avocados, bacon, liver, peas, pork, and tuna)
• Matulane.

 If you suspect an overdose

Contact your doctor *immediately.* Excessive Larodopa can cause muscle and eyelid twitching, palpitations, or an irregular heartbeat.

 Warnings

• Make sure your doctor knows your medical history. You may not be able to take Larodopa if you have severe heart, kidney, liver, or lung problems; peptic ulcer; psychiatric illness; irregular heartbeat; or endocrine disease or if you're pregnant or breast-feeding.
• If you have diabetes, the doctor may need to adjust your diabetes drug and change urine sugar tests.

 KEEP IN MIND...

* Avoid foods high in protein and vitamin B_6.

* Urine and sweat may darken.

* Don't take darkened tablets.

Lasix

Lasix is one of several potent diuretics (water pills). It prevents sodium and chloride from being reabsorbed in the kidneys, which increases the flow of urine, helping to rid the body of excess water.

Why it's prescribed

Doctors prescribe Lasix to stimulate urination and reduce the amount of water in the body. This may help to improve the condition of people with swelling (edema), high blood pressure, or heart failure. Lasix comes in tablets and a liquid. It's also available in an injectable form. Doctors usually prescribe the following amounts for adults; children's dosages appear in parentheses.

▶ **For swelling,** 20 to 80 milligrams (mg) orally a day in morning, second dose in 6 to 8 hours; increased gradually up to 600 mg a day, if needed. (Infants and children: 2 mg for each 2.2 pounds [lb] of body weight orally a day, increased by 1 to 2 mg for each 2.2 lb in 6 to 8 hours, if needed.)

▶ **For high blood pressure,** 40 mg orally twice a day, adjusted according to person's response.

How to take Lasix

• Take this drug exactly as your doctor directs, preferably with food or milk to reduce stomach upset.
• Take a single dose in the morning after breakfast or, if you're tak-

LASIX'S OTHER NAMES

Lasix's generic name is furosemide. Other brand names include Myrosemide and, in Canada, Apo-Furosemide, Furoside, Lasix Special, Novosemide, and Uritol.

 ## SIDE EFFECTS

Call your doctor if you have any of these possible drug side effects. Call *immediately* about any labeled "serious."

Serious: bleeding, bruising, fatigue, muscle weakness and cramps

Common: none reported

Other: dehydration (dry mouth, increased thirst, decreased urination, dizziness, light-headedness, wrinkled skin), stomach upset, diarrhea, increased blood sugar level (increased thirst, hunger, and urination)

 ## DRUG INTERACTIONS

Combining certain drugs may alter their action or produce unwanted side effects. Tell your doctor about other drugs you're taking, especially:
• blood pressure drugs such as Capoten
• heart drugs, such as Cordarone and Lanoxin
• nonsteroidal anti-inflammatory drugs such as Advil
• oral diabetes drugs.

ing more than one dose a day, take the last dose no later than 6 p.m., unless your doctor tells you otherwise. This should prevent you from being awakened at night by the need to urinate, which is caused by Lasix.
• Use a special measuring spoon, not a household teaspoon, to measure each liquid dose accurately.

If you miss a dose

Take the missed dose as soon as possible. However, if it's almost time for the next dose, skip the missed dose and take the next dose as scheduled. Don't take a double dose.

 ## If you suspect an overdose

Contact your doctor *immediately.* Excessive Lasix can cause your body to lose potassium and fluid, which may trigger reduced urination, irregular pulse, confusion, lethargy, and muscle cramps.

Warnings

• Make sure your doctor knows your medical history. You may not be able to take Lasix if you have other medical problems.
• If you're pregnant or breast-feeding, tell your doctor before you start taking Lasix.
• If you're diabetic, be aware that Lasix may affect your blood sugar level.

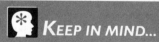 ## KEEP IN MIND...

* Take single dose in morning, or take last dose of day by 6 p.m.
* Take with food or milk to reduce stomach upset.
* Call doctor about muscle weakness and cramps.

Lescol

Lescol reduces the amount of cholesterol (a type of fat) in the blood by interfering with the body's cholesterol production.

Why it's prescribed

Doctors prescribe Lescol to help lower cholesterol levels in the blood and thus reduce the risk of some heart and blood vessel diseases. Lescol comes in capsules. Doctors usually prescribe the following amounts for adults.

▶ **To reduce levels of low-density lipoprotein (the "bad" cholesterol) and total cholesterol in people with high cholesterol levels,** initially 20 milligrams (mg) at bedtime, increased as needed to maximum of 40 mg a day.

How to take Lescol

- Take this drug exactly as your doctor directs.
- For best results, take Lescol at bedtime. However, you may take it with or between meals.
- Don't suddenly stop taking this drug until your doctor tells you to. Doing so could affect your blood cholesterol level.

If you miss a dose

Adjust your schedule as follows:
- Take the missed dose as soon as possible. However, if it's almost time for the next dose, skip the missed dose and take the next dose as scheduled. Don't take a double dose.

LESCOL'S OTHER NAME

Lescol's generic name is fluvastatin sodium.

SIDE EFFECTS

Call your doctor if you have any of these possible drug side effects. Call *immediately* about any labeled "serious."

Serious: hemolytic anemia (bleeding, fatigue), allergic reaction (closing up of throat; swelling of face, lips, hands, and feet)

Common: muscle pain, tenderness, fever, constipation

Other: stomach upset, impotence, nausea, too few white blood cells (increased risk of infection), too few blood-clotting cells (abnormal bleeding), sinus inflammation, insomnia

DRUG INTERACTIONS

Combining certain drugs may alter their action or produce unwanted side effects. Tell your doctor about other drugs you're taking, especially:
- alcohol
- anticoagulants (blood thinners) such as Coumadin
- drugs that suppress the immune system, such as Sandimmune
- Lanoxin
- other cholesterol-lowering drugs, such as Lopid and Questran (take at least 4 hours before or after Lescol)
- Rifadin
- Tagamet and other ulcer drugs.

- If you normally take your dose at bedtime but don't remember it until morning, don't take the missed dose in the morning. Skip the missed dose and take the next dose as scheduled.

 ## If you suspect an overdose

Consult your doctor.

Warnings

- Make sure your doctor knows your medical history. You may not be able to take Lescol if you have other problems, such as liver or kidney disease, or a history of alcohol abuse.
- Don't take Lescol if you're pregnant or breast-feeding. Consult your doctor if you're planning to become pregnant or if you think you may be pregnant.
- Stay on a standard low-cholesterol diet while taking Lescol. Exercise and weight control are essential in controlling your condition.

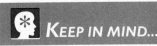

- Take at bedtime for best results.
- Follow low-cholesterol diet.
- Don't stop taking unless directed by doctor.

Leukeran

Leukeran interferes with the growth of cancer cells, leading to their destruction.

Why it's prescribed

Doctors prescribe Leukeran to treat some types of cancer, especially leukemia and lymphoma. It comes in tablets. Doctors usually prescribe the following amounts for adults; children's dosages appear in parentheses.

▶ **For chronic lymphocytic leukemia or malignant lymphoma (such as Hodgkin's disease),** 0.1 to 0.2 milligrams (mg) for each 2.2 pounds (lb) of body weight daily for 3 to 6 weeks; afterward usual dosage is 4 to 10 mg a day. (Children: 0.1 to 0.2 mg for each 2.2 lb a day as a single dose or divided into equal doses.)

How to take Leukeran

• Take this drug exactly as your doctor directs.
• Don't stop taking Leukeran even if it causes nausea or vomiting; your doctor can suggest ways to lessen these effects.
• If you vomit shortly after taking a dose, ask your doctor whether to take the dose again or wait until the next scheduled dose.

If you miss a dose

Don't take a double dose. Adjust your schedule as follows:
• If you take one dose a day, take the missed dose as soon as possible, then go back to your regular schedule. However, if you don't remember until the next day, skip the

LEUKERAN'S OTHER NAME

Leukeran's generic name is chlorambucil.

SIDE EFFECTS

Call your doctor if you have any of these possible drug side effects. Call *immediately* about any labeled "serious."

Serious: blood problems (unusual bleeding, bruising, fatigue, increased risk of infection), pulmonary fibrosis (shortness of breath, cough), allergic reaction (rash), seizures, liver problems (yellow-tinged skin and eyes), skin inflammation and peeling
Tips: Use caution when brushing or flossing your teeth or using a razor. Avoid situations in which injury or bruising could occur, and try to avoid people with known infections.

Common: nausea, vomiting, mouth sores, infertility

Other: bone marrow suppression (fever, chills, cough), gout and kidney problems (joint pain, swelling in feet or legs, low back or side pain)
Tip: Drink extra fluids to help avoid kidney problems.

DRUG INTERACTIONS

Combining certain drugs may alter their actions or produce unwanted side effects. Tell your doctor about other drugs you're taking, especially:
• anticoagulants (blood thinners)
• aspirin.

missed dose and take the next dose as scheduled.
• If you take more than one dose a day, take the missed dose as soon as possible. However, if it's almost time for the next dose, skip the missed dose and take the next dose as scheduled.

If you suspect an overdose

Contact your doctor *immediately.* In adults, excessive Leukeran can cause fever, chills, unusual bleeding, seizures, and agitation; in children, vomiting, poor coordination, abdominal pain, muscle twitching, and seizures.

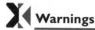

Warnings

• Make sure your doctor knows your medical history. You may not be able to take Leukeran if you have other medical problems.
• If you're of child-bearing age, be sure to use an effective birth control method during Leukeran treatment. Call your doctor right away if you think you've become pregnant.

KEEP IN MIND...

* Drink extra fluids.
* Keep taking even if nausea or vomiting occurs.
* Use effective birth control while taking Leukeran.

Levatol

Levatol is one of a group of drugs called beta blockers, which interfere with the action of the nervous system by slowing down the heart, decreasing the amount of blood it pumps, and lowering blood pressure.

Why it's prescribed

Doctors prescribe Levatol to treat high blood pressure. It comes in tablets. Doctors usually prescribe the following amounts for adults.
▶ **For mild to moderately high blood pressure,** 20 milligrams once a day. Usually given with other drugs that lower blood pressure, such as diuretics (water pills).

How to take Levatol

• Take this drug exactly as your doctor directs. Try not to miss any doses; your condition may worsen if you don't take Levatol regularly.
• If the doctor wants you to, count your pulse before each dose. If it's much slower or faster than usual, postpone the dose and call the doctor immediately.
• Don't stop taking Levatol before consulting your doctor.

If you miss a dose

Take the missed dose as soon as possible. However, if it's within 8 hours of the next dose, skip the missed dose and take the next dose as scheduled. Don't take a double dose.

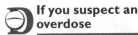 **If you suspect an overdose**

Contact your doctor immediately. Excessive Levatol can cause a slow

LEVATOL'S OTHER NAME

Levatol's generic name is penbutolol sulfate.

 SIDE EFFECTS

Call your doctor if you have any of these possible drug side effects. Call *immediately* about any labeled "serious."

Serious: shortness of breath, closing up of throat, difficulty breathing, wheezing, hallucinations, lethargy, confusion, chest pain, rash, swelling of ankles and feet

Common: dizziness, slow pulse

Other: headache, fatigue, numbness or tingling sensations, sleep disturbances, light-headedness, cold hands and feet, sore throat, stomach pain, gas, nausea, constipation, vomiting, decreased sex drive, frequent urination, sweating
Tip: Make sure you know how this drug affects you before you drive or perform other hazardous activities.

DRUG INTERACTIONS

Combining certain drugs may alter their action or produce unwanted side effects. Tell your doctor about other drugs you're taking, especially:
• asthma drugs such as Theo-Dur
• diabetes drugs, including insulin
• Hytrin
• Klonopin
• nonsteroidal anti-inflammatory drugs such as Advil
• other drugs used to lower blood pressure, relieve chest pain, or treat heart conditions

pulse, closing up of the throat, heart failure (difficulty breathing, swelling in the arms and legs), and severe low blood pressure (extreme dizziness, weakness).

 Warnings

• Make sure your doctor knows your medical history. You may not be able to take Levatol if you have other medical problems.
• If you're pregnant or breast-feeding, check with your doctor before you start taking Levatol.
• If you have diabetes, be aware that this drug may cause your blood

sugar level to fall or may mask signs of low blood sugar.
• Before you have surgery (including dental surgery), tell your doctor or dentist that you're taking this drug.

 KEEP IN MIND...

* Avoid driving until you know how you react to this drug.
* Don't stop taking this drug suddenly.
* You may have to take your pulse before each dose.

Levo-Dromoran

Levo-Dromoran is a narcotic pain reliever. It activates the body's internal pain-relief system, changing the body's perception of pain.

Why it's prescribed

Doctors prescribe Levo-Dromoran to treat moderate to severe pain. It comes in tablets and is also available in an injectable form. Doctors usually prescribe the following amounts for adults.

▶ **For moderate to severe pain,** 2 to 3 mg orally every 6 to 8 hours as needed.

How to take Levo-Dromoran

• Take this drug exactly as your doctor directs. Take only the amount prescribed.

• If you're giving yourself the injection at home, make sure you understand your doctor's instructions and follow them carefully.

• Don't stop taking this drug suddenly without first checking with your doctor. Levo-Dromoran is a narcotic. If you use it for a long time, you may become dependent on it and have withdrawal symptoms when you stop taking it.

If you miss a dose

Take the missed dose as soon as possible. However, if it's almost time for the next dose, skip the missed dose and take the next dose as scheduled. Don't take a double dose.

LEVO-DROMORAN'S OTHER NAME

Levo-Dromoran's generic name is levorphanol tartrate.

 SIDE EFFECTS

Call your doctor if you have any of these possible drug side effects. Call *immediately* about any labeled "serious."

Serious: seizures, low blood pressure (dizziness, weakness), slow or difficult breathing, difficulty urinating

Common: drowsiness, nausea, vomiting
Tips: Take with food to help prevent nausea. Avoid driving or operating machinery until you know how you react to this drug.

Other: sweating, allergic reaction (itching, hives)

 DRUG INTERACTIONS

Combining certain drugs may alter their action or produce unwanted side effects. Tell your doctor about other drugs you're taking, especially:
• alcohol and other drugs that relax you or make you sleepy, such as sleeping pills, antidepressants, drugs for anxiety, narcotic pain relievers, and cold and allergy medicines
• Dilantin
• Lanoxin
• Rifadin
• Tagamet

 If you suspect an overdose

Contact your doctor *immediately.* Excessive Levo-Dromoran can cause slow or difficult breathing, seizures, weakness, dizziness, restlessness, nervousness, confusion, and severe drowsiness.

 Warnings

• Make sure your doctor knows your medical history. You may not be able to take Levo-Dromoran if you have other problems, such as irregular heartbeats, a liver or kidney problem, seizures, or a respiratory disorder, or if you've recently had a head injury. Also tell your doctor if you've ever been addicted to any drug.

• Don't take Levo-Dromoran if you're allergic to it or to similar drugs, such as codeine and morphine.

• If you're pregnant or breast-feeding, tell your doctor before you start taking Levo-Dromoran.

• Be aware that older adults may be especially prone to Levo-Dromoran's side effects.

KEEP IN MIND...

* Avoid driving while taking drug.

* Don't stop taking suddenly.

* Take with food to help prevent nausea.

Levoxyl

Levoxyl is a thyroid hormone that stimulates the body's metabolism.

Why it's prescribed

Doctors prescribe Levoxyl to supplement the amount of hormone produced by the thyroid gland. It comes in tablets. Doctors usually prescribe the following amounts for adults; older adults' and children's dosages follow.

▶ **For thyroid hormone replacement,** 0.025 to 0.05 milligrams (mg) a day, increased by 0.025 mg every 2 to 4 weeks until desired response occurs. Maintenance dosage: 0.1 to 0.2 mg a day.
• Adults over age 65: 0.0125 to 0.025 mg a day, increased by 0.025 mg every 3 to 4 weeks, as needed.
• Children over age 10: 2 to 3 micrograms (mcg) for each 2.2 pounds (lb) of body weight daily.
• Children ages 6 to 10: 4 to 5 mcg for each 2.2 lb daily.
• Children ages 1 to 5: 3 to 5 mcg for each 2.2 lb.
• Children under age 1: 5 to 6 mcg for each 2.2 lb.)

How to take Levoxyl

• Take Levoxyl exactly as your doctor directs. Don't take more or less of it than prescribed, and don't take it more often than prescribed. Your doctor may have to adjust the dosage repeatedly.
• Take this drug at the same time each morning, preferably before

LEVOXYL'S OTHER NAMES

Levoxyl's generic name is levothyroxine sodium. Other brand names include Levothroid, Synthroid; and, in Canada, Eltroxin.

SIDE EFFECTS

Call your doctor if you have any of these possible drug side effects. Call *immediately* about any labeled "serious."

Serious: chest pain or fast pulse (palpitations, dizziness)
Tip: If you have heart disease, Levoxyl may cause you to develop chest pain or shortness of breath when you exert yourself. If this occurs, reduce your physical exercise.

Common: nervousness, insomnia, tremors

Other: increased blood pressure (headache, blurred vision), appetite change, nausea, diarrhea, headache, leg cramps, weight loss, sweating, heat intolerance, fever, menstrual irregularities, partial hair loss in children
Tip: In a child who's taking Levoxyl, partial hair loss may occur during the first 4 months of treatment. However, hair growth usually returns to normal, even when the child continues to take the drug.

DRUG INTERACTIONS

Combining certain drugs may alter their action or produce unwanted side effects. Tell your doctor about other drugs you're taking, especially:
• allergy and cold medicines
• amphetamines
• anticoagulants (blood thinners) such as Coumadin
• asthma drugs and drugs used to treat other lung conditions
• blood pressure drugs
• certain antidepressants, such as Elavil, Pamelor, and Sinequan
• Colestid
• diet pills
• epinephrine and similar drugs
• estrogens
• insulin and oral diabetes drugs
• Questran.

breakfast, to maintain constant hormone levels and avoid insomnia.
• Once you've achieved the correct dosage, don't change brand names.
• If you're taking Levoxyl for an underactive thyroid gland, realize that it may take several weeks before you notice any change in your condition.
• Don't stop taking this drug without first talking with your doctor,

who may want to decrease the dosage gradually.

If you miss a dose

Take the missed dose as soon as possible. However, if it's almost time for your next dose, skip the missed dose and take your next dose as scheduled. Don't take a double dose. If you miss two or more doses in a row, call your doctor.

Continued on next page ▶

If you suspect an overdose

Contact your doctor *immediately*. Excessive Levoxyl can cause chest pain, nervousness, insomnia, hand tremor, a rapid pulse or palpitations, nausea, headache, fever, sweating, and shortness of breath.

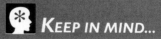

Warnings

• Make sure your doctor knows your medical history. You may not be able to take Levoxyl if you're allergic to it or if you have other medical problems, such as diabetes, coronary artery disease, angina, high blood pressure, oxygen deficiency, untreated Graves' disease, an underactive adrenal or pituitary gland, myxedema (severe hypothyroidism), or kidney problems, or if you've recently had a heart attack or stroke.

• Call your doctor if you become pregnant or start breast-feeding while taking Levoxyl.

• Be aware that older adults may be more sensitive to Levoxyl's effects.

• Your doctor may want to check your blood periodically while you're taking Levoxyl to make sure that you're taking the right amount of the drug.

KEEP IN MIND...

* Take at same time each morning, before breakfast.

* Don't change dosage or stop taking without doctor's approval.

* Don't change brand names.

* Don't expect full effect for several weeks.

Levsin

Levsin blocks certain types of nervous stimulation, slowing down the movements of the digestive tract and decreasing the amount of acid formed in the stomach.

Why it's prescribed

Doctors prescribe Levsin to relieve spasms and cramps of the bowels and stomach. Levsin comes in tablets, an elixir, and an oral solution. It's also available in sublingual tablets, extended-release capsules (Levbid), and an injectable form. Doctors usually prescribe the following amounts for adults; children's dosages are in parentheses.

▶ **For digestive disorders caused by spasms or as part of a drug regimen for stomach ulcers,** 0.125 to 0.25 milligrams (mg) orally or under the tongue three or four times a day before meals and at bedtime; or 0.375 mg of extended-release capsules every 8 to 12 hours. Maximum dosage is 1.5 mg a day. (Children age 12 and older: same as adults. Children ages 2 to 11: one-half of adult dose orally, but not more than 0.75 mg a day. Children under age 2: one-fourth of adult dose orally, but not more than 0.075 mg a day.)

How to take Levsin

• Take this drug exactly as your doctor directs, 30 minutes to 1 hour before meals and at bedtime.

LEVSIN'S OTHER NAMES

Levsin's generic name is hyoscyamine sulfate. Other brand names include Anaspaz, Cystospaz-M, Gastrosed, and Levsinex Timecaps.

 SIDE EFFECTS

Call your doctor if you have any of these possible drug side effects.

Serious: none reported

Common: confusion or excitement (in older adults), palpitations, blurred vision, dry mouth, difficulty urinating, inability to urinate
Tip: Drink plenty of fluids to help prevent constipation.

Other: headache, difficulty sleeping, drowsiness, nervousness, weakness, fast pulse, enlarged pupils, paralysis of certain eye muscles, unusual sensitivity to light, difficulty swallowing, heartburn, loss of taste, nausea, vomiting, impotence, hives, decreased sweating, fever, allergic reaction (itching, rash, shortness of breath)

 DRUG INTERACTIONS

Combining certain drugs may alter their action or produce unwanted side effects. Tell your doctor about other drugs you're taking, especially:
• antacids (take at least 2 hours before or after taking Levsin)
• antihistamines (used to treat colds and allergies)
• Demerol
• drugs for Parkinson's disease or for irregular heartbeat
• phenothiazines (used for anxiety, nausea, vomiting, or strange behavior)
• tricyclic antidepressants.

Take the bedtime dose at least 2 hours after your last meal of the day.

If you miss a dose

Take the missed dose as soon as possible. But if it's almost time for the next dose, skip the missed dose and take the next dose as scheduled. Don't take a double dose.

 If you suspect an overdose

Contact your doctor *immediately.* Excessive Levsin can cause inability to breathe, depression, confusion, hallucinations, delusions, anxiety, agitation, dry mucous membranes, difficulty swallowing, inability to urinate, fever, fast pulse and breathing, headache, blurred vision, and flushed, hot, dry skin.

Warnings

• Make sure your doctor knows your medical history. You may not be able to take Levsin if you have other medical problems or are pregnant or breast-feeding.
• Children and older adults may be more prone to side effects.

 KEEP IN MIND...

* Take 30 minutes to 1 hour before meals and at bedtime.
* Take bedtime dose at least 2 hours after last meal.
* Increase fluid intake.

Librium

Librium slows down the nervous system by inhibiting activity in several parts of the brain. This has a calming effect.

Why it's prescribed

Doctors prescribe Librium to relieve mild to moderate anxiety and tension or to treat alcohol withdrawal symptoms. It comes in tablets, capsules, and an injectable form. Doctors usually prescribe the following amounts.

▶ **For mild to moderate anxiety,** 5 to 10 milligrams (mg) orally three or four times a day. (Children over age 6: 5 mg orally three or four times a day. Maximum dosage is 10 mg three or four times a day.)

▶ **For severe anxiety,** 20 to 25 mg orally three or four times a day.

▶ **For withdrawal symptoms of acute alcoholism,** 50 to 100 mg orally, repeated in 2 to 4 hours as needed. Maximum dosage is 300 mg a day.

How to take Librium

• Take this drug exactly as your doctor directs. Don't take more than the prescribed amount to avoid drug dependence.

• If you've been taking Librium for a long time, don't suddenly stop taking it. Unpleasant withdrawal symptoms may occur. Call your doctor, who will advise you on how to reduce your dosage before completely stopping this drug.

LIBRIUM'S OTHER NAMES

Librium's generic name is chlordiazepoxide hydrochloride. Other brand names include Libritabs, Poxi; and, in Canada, Apo-Chlordiazepoxide, Novopoxide, and Solium.

 ## SIDE EFFECTS

Call your doctor if you have any of these possible drug side effects. Call *immediately* about any labeled "serious."

Serious: suicidal tendencies

Common: drowsiness, hangover, inflammation of veins, swelling
Tip: Avoid driving or performing other activities requiring alertness until you know how you react to this drug.

Other: fainting, restlessness, strange behavior, dizziness, weakness, vision disturbances, nausea, vomiting, stomach upset, loss of bladder control, inability to urinate, menstrual irregularities

 ## DRUG INTERACTIONS

Combining certain drugs may alter their action or produce unwanted side effects. Tell your doctor about other drugs you're taking, especially:
• alcohol and other drugs that make you relaxed or sleepy, such as cold and allergy medicines, sedatives, tranquilizers, narcotic pain relievers, barbiturates, drugs to control seizures, and muscle relaxants
• Lanoxin
• nicotine
• Tagamet and other ulcer drugs.

If you miss a dose

Take the missed dose as soon as possible. But if it's almost time for the next dose, skip the missed dose and take the next dose as scheduled. Don't take a double dose.

 ### If you suspect an overdose

Contact your doctor *immediately.* Excessive Librium can cause sleepiness, confusion, coma, decreased reflexes, difficulty breathing, dizziness, weakness, slow pulse, slurred speech, unsteady gait, and poor coordination.

 ## Warnings

• Make sure your doctor knows your medical history. You may not be able to take Librium if you have other medical problems, especially depression, porphyria, liver or kidney disease, or a drug allergy.

• If you're pregnant or breast-feeding, tell your doctor before you start taking Librium.

 ## KEEP IN MIND...

* Don't take more than prescribed to avoid drug dependence.

* Don't suddenly stop taking the drug.

* Avoid driving until you know your reaction to drug.

Lidex

Lidex is a steroid that's applied to the skin to relieve skin inflammation, swelling, itching, and redness.

Why it's prescribed

Doctors prescribe Lidex to help relieve redness, swelling, itching, and other discomfort caused by skin problems. It comes in a cream, an ointment, a gel, and a topical solution. Doctors usually prescribe the following amounts for adults and children.

▶ **For skin inflammation,** small amount applied to affected area three or four times a day.

How to use Lidex

• Apply the drug exactly as your doctor directs. First, gently wash the affected skin area. Then rub Lidex in gently, leaving a thin coat. If the area is hairy, part the hair and apply Lidex directly on the skin.

• Don't get Lidex in your eyes. If you do, flush your eyes with water. Also, don't get it in your ear canal or near your mucous membranes, such as your mouth or nostrils.

• If you're applying Lidex to a child's diaper area, avoid using tight-fitting diapers or plastic pants. They may cause unwanted side effects.

• Don't bandage or wrap the skin being treated unless your doctor tells you to. If the doctor instructs you to use an airtight covering

LIDEX'S OTHER NAMES

Lidex's generic name is fluocinonide. Other brand names include Lidex-E, Topsyn; and, in Canada, Lidemol.

 SIDE EFFECTS

Call your doctor if you have any of these possible drug side effects. Call *immediately* about any labeled "serious."

Serious: growth retardation and delayed weight gain in children
Tip: Children and teenagers who use Lidex should have frequent checkups so the doctor can monitor their growth and weight.

Common: tearing or softening of skin; secondary infection; skin color changes; reddish purple lines on arms, face, legs, trunk, or groin; heat rash (with use of airtight dressing)

Other: burning, inflammation, rash, itching, irritation, dryness, or redness of skin; pinpoint red blisters; inflammation of hair follicles; acne or oily skin; irritation of skin around mouth; filling out of face; rapid weight gain or loss; increased hair growth (especially on face); unusual hair loss; unusual weakness (especially of arms, legs, and trunk); fever (in worsening infection)

DRUG INTERACTIONS

Combining certain drugs may alter their action or produce unwanted side effects. Tell your doctor about other drugs you're taking.

---

such as plastic wrap or a special patch over Lidex, make sure you understand how to apply it.

• Wash your hands after applying.

If you miss a dose

Apply the missed dose as soon as possible. However, if it's almost time for the next dose, skip the missed dose and apply the next dose as scheduled. Don't apply a double dose.

 If you suspect an overdose

Consult your doctor.

 Warnings

• Make sure your doctor knows your medical history. You may not be able to use Lidex if you have

other medical problems, such as diabetes, cataracts, glaucoma, or tuberculosis.

• Before you start using Lidex, tell your doctor if you're pregnant. Call your doctor if you become pregnant while using Lidex.

• Don't apply Lidex to your breasts before breast-feeding.

 KEEP IN MIND...

∗ Wash hands after applying.

∗ Don't cover treated area unless doctor directs.

∗ Don't get drug in eyes.

Lincocin

Lincocin is an antibiotic that destroys bacteria by preventing them from producing needed proteins.

Why it's prescribed

Doctors prescribe Lincocin to treat infections in various parts of the body. It comes in regular capsules and capsules for children. It's also available in an injectable form. Doctors usually prescribe the following amounts for adults; children's dosages appear in parentheses.

▶ **For infection of the respiratory tract, skin, soft tissues, urinary tract, bone (osteomyelitis), or bloodstream,** 500 milligrams (mg) orally every 6 to 8 hours, but not more than 8 grams a day. (Children over age 1 month: 30 to 60 mg for each 2.2 pounds of body weight orally every day divided into equal doses given every 6 to 8 hours.)

How to take Lincocin

• Take this drug exactly as your doctor directs. Unless the doctor tells you otherwise, take it with a full glass (8 ounces) of water on an empty stomach 1 hour before or 2 hours after meals.
• To help clear up your infection, keep taking Lincocin for the full treatment time, even if you start to feel better after a few days.
• If your symptoms don't get better within a few days or if they get worse, call your doctor.

LINCOCIN'S OTHER NAME

Lincocin's generic name is lincomycin hydrochloride.

 SIDE EFFECTS

Call your doctor if you have any of these possible drug side effects. Call *immediately* about any labeled "serious."

Serious: allergic reaction (swelling of face, hives, difficulty breathing, tightness in chest), severe colitis (severe cramps or pain in abdomen, blood and mucus in stool)

Common: tender abdomen, persistent or severe watery diarrhea, fever, infection
Tips: If Lincocin causes diarrhea, don't take a drug for diarrhea without first checking with your doctor. Such a drug may make your diarrhea worse. Avoid contact with people who are sick.

Other: dizziness, headache, tongue inflammation, ringing in ears, nausea, vomiting, mouth sores, anal itching, vaginal inflammation, unexplained bruising, tiny red or purple spots on skin, abnormal bleeding, rash, hives, yellow-tinged skin and eyes, swelling of face, neck, lips, hands, and feet

 DRUG INTERACTIONS

Combining certain drugs may alter their action or produce unwanted side effects. Tell your doctor about other drugs you're taking, especially:
• drugs for diarrhea such as Kaopectate (take these only if the doctor approves and always at least 2 hours before Lincocin).

If you miss a dose

Take the missed dose as soon as possible. However, if it's almost time for the next dose, skip the missed dose and take the next dose as scheduled. Don't take a double dose.

 If you suspect an overdose

Consult your doctor.

 Warnings

• Make sure your doctor knows your medical history. You may not be able to take Lincocin if you have other problems, such as liver, kidney, stomach, or bowel disease.

• Before having surgery (including dental surgery), tell your doctor or dentist that you're taking Lincocin.

 KEEP IN MIND...

* Take with full glass of water.

* Keep taking for full treatment time.

* Call doctor if symptoms don't get better in few days.

* Don't take a drug for diarrhea unless doctor approves.

Lioresal

Lioresal relaxes the muscles. It seems to work by reducing the transmission of nerve impulses from the spinal cord to muscles.

Why it's prescribed

Doctors prescribe Lioresal to relax the muscles and relieve spasms, cramping, and tightness caused by such disorders as multiple sclerosis and spinal injuries. It comes in tablets. It's also available in an injectable form. Doctors usually prescribe the following amounts for adults.

▶ **For relief of spastic muscles in multiple sclerosis or spinal cord injury,** at first, 5 milligrams (mg) orally three times a day for 3 days, then 10 mg three times a day for 3 days, 15 mg three times a day for 3 days, and 20 mg three times a day for 3 days. Dosage increased according to person's response to maximum of 80 mg a day.

How to take Lioresal

• Take this drug exactly as your doctor directs.
• Don't stop taking Lioresal suddenly because this may cause unwanted effects. Instead, call your doctor, who will tell you how to reduce your dosage gradually before stopping completely.

If you miss a dose

Take the missed dose as soon as possible if you remember within about an hour. However, if you don't remember until later, skip the missed

LIORESAL'S OTHER NAME

Lioresal's generic name is baclofen.

 SIDE EFFECTS

Call your doctor if you have any of these possible drug side effects. Call *immediately* about any labeled "serious."

Serious: seizures

Common: nausea, dizziness, drowsiness, weakness, fatigue
Tips: To prevent nausea, take Lioresal with milk or meals. Don't drive, operate machinery, or do anything else that could be hazardous if you aren't alert, well coordinated, and able to see well.

Other: headache, confusion, difficulty speaking, stuffy nose, difficulty sleeping, blurred vision, constipation, frequent urination, rash, itching, swollen ankles, excessive sweating, increased blood sugar level (increased thirst and urination), weight gain

 DRUG INTERACTIONS

Combining certain drugs may alter their action or produce unwanted side effects. Tell your doctor about other drugs you're taking, especially:
• alcohol and other drugs that make you relaxed or sleepy, such as cold and allergy medicines, sedatives, tranquilizers, narcotic pain relievers, barbiturates, drugs to control seizures, and muscle relaxants.

dose and take the next dose as scheduled. Don't take a double dose.

 If you suspect an overdose

Contact your doctor *immediately*. Excessive Lioresal can cause vomiting, poor muscle tone, absence of reflexes, increased saliva production, drowsiness, vision disturbances, seizures, slow breathing, and coma.

Warnings

• Make sure your doctor knows your medical history. You may not be able to take Lioresal if you have other medical problems.
• If you're breast-feeding or become pregnant while taking Lioresal, contact your doctor.

• Be aware that older adults may be especially prone to Lioresal's side effects.
• If you're diabetic, be aware that Lioresal may raise your blood sugar level. Call your doctor if you notice a change.

 KEEP IN MIND...

* Take with milk or meals.
* Don't stop taking suddenly.
* Avoid driving and other activities requiring alertness until you know how you react to drug.

Lithobid

Lithobid helps stabilize the condition of a person with manic-depressive illness (bipolar disorder) during the excited, or manic, state. It seems to work by reducing the amount of certain natural chemicals, which may be excessive during manic states.

Why it's prescribed

Doctors prescribe Lithobid to prevent or control mania, which typically causes an unusual sense of well-being or excessive anger or irritability in people with manic-depressive illness. It comes in tablets and controlled-release tablets. It's also available in capsules (Eskalith) and a sugarless syrup (Lithium Citrate Syrup). Doctors usually prescribe the following amounts for adults.

▶ **To prevent or control mania,** 300 to 600 milligrams up to four times a day, increased as needed.

How to take Lithobid

• Take this drug exactly as your doctor directs.
• If you're taking controlled-release tablets, swallow them whole. Don't crush, break, or chew them.
• If you're taking the syrup, first shake the bottle well. Dilute the syrup in fruit juice or another flavored beverage before taking it.

LITHOBID'S OTHER NAMES

Lithobid's generic name is lithium carbonate. Other brand names include Eskalith, Eskalith CR, Lithane, Lithonate; and, in Canada, Carbolith, Duralith, and Lithizine.

 ## SIDE EFFECTS

Call your doctor if you have any of these possible drug side effects. Call *immediately* about any labeled "serious."

Serious: coma, irregular heartbeat, dangerously low blood pressure leading to peripheral vascular collapse (dizziness, cold, discolored fingers or toes)

Common: frequent urination, headache, dizziness

Other: tremor, drowsiness, confusion, restlessness, lethargy, muscle weakness, impaired speech, poor coordination, ringing in ears, blurred vision, dry mouth, metallic taste, nausea, vomiting, appetite loss, diarrhea, thirst, stomach upset, gas, rash, itching, diminished or absent sensation, hair loss, psoriasis, acne, increased blood sugar level (increased thirst and urination), goiter (swelling of neck), underactive thyroid (hair loss, slow pulse, sensitivity to cold, weight gain, constipation, absent menstrual cycle, incoordination), salt deficiency, swollen ankles and wrists

Tips: To help prevent upset stomach, take this drug with plenty of water and after meals. Weigh yourself regularly. Call the doctor if you notice a sudden weight gain or swelling. Avoid driving and other activities that require alertness and good coordination until you know how you react to Lithobid.

 ## DRUG INTERACTIONS

Combining certain drugs may alter their action or produce unwanted side effects. Tell your doctor about other drugs you're taking, especially:
• Aldomet
• Amoline
• Benemid
• diuretics (water pills)
• nonsteroidal anti-inflammatory drugs such as Advil
• sedatives, tranquilizers, and other drugs that cause sedation or reduce anxiety
• Tegretol
• thyroid hormones
• urine alkalinizers, such as sodium bicarbonate (baking soda) and sodium lactate.

If you miss a dose

Take the missed dose as soon as possible. However, if it's within 4 hours of the next dose (6 hours for controlled-release tablets), skip the missed dose and take the next dose as scheduled. Don't take a double dose.

If you suspect an overdose

Contact your doctor *immediately*. Excessive Lithobid can cause vomiting, diarrhea, and death. A less severe overdose can cause sedation, confusion, hand tremor, joint pain, poor coordination, stiff muscles, vision problems, seizures, extremely low blood pressure (extreme dizziness and weakness, fainting), cold discolored fingers and toes, and coma.

Warnings

• Make sure your doctor knows your medical history. You may not be able to take Lithobid if you have other problems, such as schizophrenia, brain disease, diabetes, difficulty urinating, infection, kidney disease, heart disease, seizures, thyroid disease, Parkinson's disease, psoriasis, or a history of leukemia, or if you're an asthmatic with an allergy to aspirin.
• Don't take this drug if you're pregnant.
• If you're breast-feeding, tell your doctor before you start taking Lithobid.
• Be aware that older adults may be especially prone to Lithobid's side effects.
• Be aware that this drug may cause weak bones in children.

• If you're diabetic, be aware that your insulin dosage may need to be changed after you start taking Lithobid.
• Call your doctor if you have an infection or illness that causes heavy sweating, vomiting, or diarrhea.
• Drink 2 to 3 quarts of fluid a day and use a normal amount of salt in your food, unless the doctor tells you otherwise.
• Keep in mind that it may be take 1 to 3 weeks before you notice Lithobid's effects. Your doctor may prescribe another drug until Lithobid takes effect.
• Avoid large amounts of caffeine (found in coffee, tea, cola, chocolate, and some diet pills), which can interfere with Lithobid's effectiveness.
• Don't change to another brand of lithium before checking with your doctor.
• Teach family members the signs and symptoms of Lithobid overdose, which can be very serious.
• Don't go on a diet without first checking with your doctor.
• Keep medical appointments so the doctor can check drug effects and measure the amount of Lithobid in your blood.
• Carry medical identification stating that you're taking Lithobid.

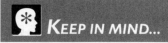

* Take with plenty of water and after meals.
* Drink 2 to 3 quarts of fluid a day, and use normal amount of salt in food.
* Avoid driving and other activities requiring alertness until you know how you react to drug.
* Don't go on diet unless doctor approves.
* Call your doctor if you notice a sudden weight gain.

Lodine

Lodine is a nonsteroidal anti-inflammatory drug (NSAID) that seems to work by inhibiting production of a hormone called prostaglandin and by impeding the action of other body substances.

Why it's prescribed

Doctors prescribe Lodine to reduce pain or relieve inflammation and other symptoms of arthritis. It comes in tablets and capsules. Doctors usually prescribe the following amounts for adults.

▶ **To relieve pain and symptoms of arthritis,** 200 to 400 milligrams (mg) every 6 to 8 hours as needed, up to 1,200 mg a day. For people who weigh 132 pounds (lb) or less, total daily dose shouldn't exceed 20 mg for each 2.2 lb of body weight.

How to take Lodine

• Take this drug exactly as your doctor directs.

If you miss a dose

If you're taking Lodine on a regular schedule, take the missed dose as soon as possible. However, if it's almost time for the next dose, skip the missed dose and take the next dose as scheduled. Don't take a double dose.

 If you suspect an overdose

Consult your doctor.

LODINE'S OTHER NAME

Lodine's generic name is etodolac.

 SIDE EFFECTS

Call your doctor if you have any of these possible drug side effects. Call *immediately* about any labeled "serious."

Serious: heart failure (shortness of breath, fatigue, anxiety), kidney failure (decreased urination), Stevens-Johnson syndrome (reddened skin, burnlike rash)

Common: weakness, dizziness, overall feeling of illness, stomach upset, gas, diarrhea
Tip: To help prevent stomach upset, take Lodine with milk or meals.

Other: depression, drowsiness, light-headedness, confusion, nervousness, difficulty sleeping, anemia, high blood pressure (headache, blurred vision), flushing, palpitations, swelling, ringing in ears, sensitivity of skin or eyes to sunlight, dry mouth, nausea, constipation, black and tarry stools, vomiting, appetite loss, mouth sores, thirst, painful or frequent urination, infection, abnormal bleeding, yellow-tinged skin or eyes, asthma, rash, itching, chills, fever, weight gain
Tip: Avoid driving and other activities requiring alertness until you know how you react to this drug.

 DRUG INTERACTIONS

Combining certain drugs may alter their action or produce unwanted side effects. Tell your doctor about other drugs you're taking, especially:
• alcohol
• antacids
• anticoagulants (blood thinners) such as Coumadin
• aspirin
• Lanoxin
• Lithobid
• Mexate
• Sandimmune.

✕ Warnings

• Make sure your doctor knows your medical history. You may not be able to take Lodine if you have other problems, such as bleeding in the digestive tract or kidney or liver disease, or if you've ever had an allergic reaction to aspirin.
• If you're pregnant or breast-feeding, tell your doctor before you start taking Lodine.

• Before you have surgery or dental work, tell the doctor or dentist that you're taking Lodine.

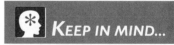 **KEEP IN MIND...**

* Take with milk or meals.
* Don't drive until you know how you react to drug.
* Tell doctor if you're pregnant.

Loestrin Fe

L oestrin Fe is an oral contraceptive, or birth control pill. When taken on a regular schedule, this drug stops ovulation (release of eggs from the ovaries), preventing pregnancy.

Why it's prescribed

Doctors prescribe Loestrin Fe to prevent pregnancy. It comes in tablets. Doctors usually prescribe the following amounts for adults.

▶ **For contraception,** 1 tablet a day, starting on day 5 of menstrual cycle (first day of menstrual period is day 1). With 20- and 21-tablet packages, new dosing cycle begins 7 days after last tablet is taken. With 28-tablet packages, dosage is 1 tablet a day without interruption (extra tablets are placebos or contain iron).

How to take Loestrin Fe

• Take this drug exactly as your doctor directs to prevent pregnancy. Be sure to take the tablets in the order in which they come in the container.
• Try to take doses at the same time each day, no more than 24 hours apart.

If you miss a dose

Adjust your schedule as follows:
• If you miss one tablet, take it as soon as possible, or take two tablets the next day and return to your regular schedule.
• If you miss tablets 2 days in a row, take two tablets on the day you re-

LOESTRIN FE'S OTHER NAMES

Loestrin Fe is a combination of the generic drugs ethinyl estradiol, norethindrone acetate, and ferrous fumarate.

 SIDE EFFECTS

Call your doctor if you have any of these possible drug side effects. Call *immediately* about any labeled "serious."

Serious: blood clots (chest pain or pressure; shortness of breath; abdominal pain; numbness, stiffness, or pain in the legs or buttocks; severe headache; visual disturbances; swelling of the hands or feet), eruptions of skin or mucous membranes

Common: headache, dizziness, nausea, abdominal pain and bloating, vomiting, blood in stool or vomit, spotting or other changes in vaginal bleeding
Tip: Call your doctor if headache, dizziness, spotting, and other bleeding changes last longer than 6 months.

Other: depression, lethargy, high blood pressure (prolonged headache, blurred vision, nosebleeds), swelling, worsening of near-sightedness or astigmatism, inability to wear contact lenses, vomiting, diarrhea, constipation, changes in appetite, weight gain, inflammation of pancreas (pain in abdomen, back, or chest; clay-colored stools; nausea; vomiting; yellow-tinged skin and eyes), inflammatory bowel disease (stool incontinence, abdominal pain, weight loss), menstrual irregularities, abnormal vaginal discharge, vaginal yeast infection, gallbladder disease (severe, persistent abdominal pain), liver tumors (yellow-tinged skin and eyes), rash, acne, oily skin, changes in skin color, breast changes (tenderness, enlargement, or secretions); increased blood sugar level (increased thirst, hunger, and urination; weight loss), too much calcium in blood (increased thirst and urination, constipation), folic acid deficiency (fatigue, weakness, palpitations, nausea, weight loss), change in sex drive

 DRUG INTERACTIONS

Combining certain drugs may alter their action or produce unwanted side effects. Tell your doctor about other drugs you're taking, especially:
• anticoagulants (blood thinners) such as Coumadin
• Barbita
• drugs that can damage the liver such as Dantrium
• Parlodel
• Rifadin
• Sandimmune
• steroids
• Tamofen
• Tegretol.

member and two tablets the next day; then resume your normal schedule. After missing two doses, use a second birth control method for 7 days.

• If you miss three or more tablets, discard the remaining tablets in

Continued on next page ▶

your monthly package and use a different birth control method. If your next menstrual period doesn't start on schedule, have a pregnancy test before you start a new dosing cycle. If your menstrual period begins, start a new dosing cycle 7 days after you took the last tablet.

If you suspect an overdose

Contact your doctor *immediately*. Excessive Loestrin Fe can cause nausea and vomiting.

Warnings

• Make sure your doctor knows your medical history. You may not be able to take Loestrin Fe if you are over age 40 (35 if you smoke) or have other problems, such as stroke, heart attack, blood clots, coronary artery disease, breast or liver cancer, high blood pressure, lupus, migraine headaches, epilepsy, asthma, diabetes, irregular periods, kidney or gallbladder disease, double vision, eye lesions or tumors, liver disease, or high cholesterol.
• Don't take Loestrin Fe if you're pregnant.
• If you're breast-feeding, tell your doctor before you start taking Loestrin Fe.

• If you're diabetic, be aware that the dosage of your diabetes drug may need to be changed after you start taking Loestrin Fe.
• Use an extra birth control method, such as condoms, for the first week after you start taking this drug.
• Keep an extra month's supply of Loestrin Fe on hand so you won't run out.
• If you miss two menstrual periods in a row, stop taking Loestrin Fe and call your doctor.
• Have regular gynecologic checkups and Pap tests. Never go more than 12 months without seeing your doctor.
• Before surgery (including dental surgery), tell your doctor or dentist that you're taking a birth control pill.
• If you decide you want to get pregnant, consult with your doctor, who may advise you to wait 2 months after stopping Loestrin Fe before trying to get pregnant.
• Schedule regular checkups with your doctor to have blood tests (to check for side effects) and to measure your blood pressure. You can also check your own blood pressure regularly.
• Record your baseline weight before you start taking this drug, and then weigh yourself monthly. Notify your doctor if you gain more than 5 pounds a month without an increase in your food intake.

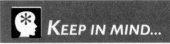

* Take tablets in proper order.
* Take doses at same time each day.
* Use extra birth control method for first week.

Lomotil

Lomotil helps stop diarrhea. It slows down intestinal activity by decreasing the activity of certain muscles in the large and small intestines.

Why it's prescribed

Doctors prescribe Lomotil to treat diarrhea. It comes in tablets and a liquid. Doctors usually prescribe the following amounts for adults; children's dosages are in parentheses.

▶ **For diarrhea,** 5 milligrams (mg) four times a day, adjusted as needed. (Children over age 12: same as adults. Children ages 2 to 12: 0.3 to 0.4 mg for each 2.2 pounds of body weight of the liquid daily divided into four equal doses. Maintenance dosage is reduced, as needed, up to 75%.)

How to take Lomotil

• Take this drug exactly as your doctor directs.
• If you're taking the liquid, measure the correct amount with a special measuring spoon or dropper, not a regular household teaspoon.

If you miss a dose

If you're taking Lomotil on a regular schedule, take the missed dose as soon as possible. However, if it's almost time for the next dose, skip the missed dose and take the next dose as scheduled. Don't take a double dose.

LOMOTIL'S OTHER NAMES

Lomotil is a combination of the generic drugs diphenoxylate hydrochloride and atropine sulfate. Other brand names include Lofene, Logen, Lomanate, and Lonox.

SIDE EFFECTS

Call your doctor if you have any of these possible drug side effects. Call *immediately* about any labeled "serious."

Serious: swelling of face, lips, throat, hands, or feet

Common: sedation, dizziness, dry mouth

Other: headache, drowsiness, lethargy, restlessness, depression, unusual feeling of well-being, fast pulse, enlarged pupils, nausea, vomiting, abdominal discomfort or bloating, appetite loss, inability to urinate, slowed breathing, rash, itching

DRUG INTERACTIONS

Combining certain drugs may alter their action or produce unwanted side effects. Tell your doctor about other drugs you're taking, especially:
• alcohol and other drugs that make you relaxed or sleepy, including sedatives, tranquilizers, narcotic pain relievers, barbiturates, drugs to control seizures, and muscle relaxants
• MAO inhibitors such as Marplan.

If you suspect an overdose

Contact your doctor *immediately.* Excessive Lomotil can cause drowsiness, low blood pressure (dizziness, weakness), seizures, slower or arrested breathing, blurred vision, flushing, dryness of the mouth and mucous membranes, and strange behavior.

Warnings

• Make sure your doctor knows your medical history. You may not be able to take Lomotil if you have other medical problems.
• If you're pregnant or breast-feeding, check with your doctor before you start taking Lomotil.
• Don't give this drug to a child under age 2 because of the high risk of side effects.

• Don't take this drug for any bout of diarrhea other than the prescribed condition. It can make certain forms of diarrhea worse.
• Call your doctor if diarrhea continues after 2 days or if you develop a fever.
• To help replace fluid lost in your stools, drink clear liquids, such as apple juice, broth, ginger ale, or tea. Eat bland foods, such as plain bread or crackers, cooked cereals, and applesauce.

KEEP IN MIND...

* Drink clear liquids and eat bland foods.

* Call doctor if diarrhea continues after 2 days.

* Don't give to children under age 2.

Loniten

Loniten widens the blood vessels so that blood can pass through them more easily, which helps to reduce blood pressure.

Why it's prescribed

Doctors prescribe Loniten to treat very high blood pressure. It comes in tablets. Doctors usually prescribe the following amounts for adults; children's dosages appear in parentheses.

▶ **For very high blood pressure,** initially 5 milligrams (mg) as a single dose. Effective dosage usually ranges from 10 to 40 mg a day. Maximum dosage is 100 mg a day. (Children age 12 and older: same as adults. Children under age 12: 0.2 mg for each 2.2 pounds [lb] of body weight [maximum 5 mg] as a single daily dose. Effective dosage usually ranges from 0.25 to 1 mg for each 2.2 lb a day. Maximum dosage is 50 mg a day.)

How to take Loniten

• Take this drug exactly as your doctor directs. To control your blood pressure, you must keep taking it regularly. You may have to take it for the rest of your life.
• Don't stop taking this drug suddenly because doing so could worsen your condition. Instead, call your doctor, who may recommend ways to ease unpleasant side effects.

LONITEN'S OTHER NAME

Loniten's generic name is minoxidil.

 SIDE EFFECTS

Call your doctor if you have any of these possible drug side effects. Call *immediately* about any labeled "serious."

Serious: heart failure (shortness of breath, anxiety, fatigue), Stevens-Johnson syndrome (reddened skin, burnlike rash)

Common: swelling, fast pulse, heart problems (overall swelling, dry cough, fast pulse, dizziness and weakness from low blood pressure), increased hair growth

Other: rash, breast tenderness, weight gain
Tips: Weigh yourself every week. Call the doctor if you suddenly gain 5 pounds or more or if your feet or lower legs start to swell.

 DRUG INTERACTIONS

Combining certain drugs may alter their action or produce unwanted side effects. Tell your doctor about other drugs you're taking, especially:
• Ismelin.

If you miss a dose

Take the missed dose as soon as possible if you remember it within a few hours. However, if you don't remember until the next day, skip the missed dose and take the next dose as scheduled. Don't take a double dose.

 If you suspect an overdose

Contact your doctor *immediately.* Excessive Loniten can cause low blood pressure (dizziness, weakness), a fast pulse, headache, and flushing.

Warnings

• Make sure your doctor knows your medical history. You may not be able to take Loniten if you have other problems, such as heart or blood vessel disease, chest pain, or blood vessel disease, chest pain, kidney disease, or pheochromocytoma, or if you've recently had a heart attack or stroke.
• If you're pregnant or breast-feeding, tell your doctor before you start taking Loniten.
• Be aware that older adults may be especially prone to Loniten's side effects.
• Keep all medical appointments so the doctor can check your progress and monitor drug effects.
• Follow any special diet the doctor prescribes, such as a low-salt diet.

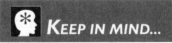 **KEEP IN MIND...**

* Don't suddenly stop taking.
* Follow prescribed diet.
* Call doctor about sudden gain of 5 pounds or more or foot or lower leg swelling.

Lo/Ovral

Lo/Ovral is an oral contraceptive, or birth control pill. When taken on a regular schedule, this drug stops ovulation (the release of eggs from the ovaries) and changes the body's hormone balance, preventing pregnancy.

Why it's prescribed

Doctors prescribe Lo/Ovral to prevent pregnancy. It comes in tablets. Doctors usually prescribe the following amounts for adults.

▶ **For contraception,** 1 tablet a day, starting on day 5 of menstrual cycle (first day of menstrual period is day 1). With 20- and 21-tablet packages, new dosing cycle begins 7 days after last tablet is taken. With 28-tablet packages, dosage is 1 tablet a day without interruption (extra tablets are placebos or contain iron).

How to take Lo/Ovral

• Take this drug exactly as your doctor directs to prevent pregnancy. Be sure to take the tablets in the order in which they come in the container.
• Try to take doses at the same time each day, no more than 24 hours apart.

If you miss a dose

Adjust your schedule as follows:
• If you miss one tablet, take it as soon as possible, or take two tablets the next day and return to your regular schedule.

LO/OVRAL'S OTHER NAMES

Lo/Ovral is a combination of the generic drugs ethinyl estradiol and norgestrel. Another brand name is Ovral.

 SIDE EFFECTS

Call your doctor if you have any of these possible drug side effects. Call *immediately* about any labeled "serious."

Serious: blood clots (chest pain or pressure; shortness of breath; abdominal pain; numbness, stiffness, or pain in the legs or buttocks; severe headache; vision disturbances; swelling of the hands or feet), eruptions of skin or mucous membranes

Common: headache, dizziness, nausea, decreased blood flow to bowel (abdominal pain and bloating, nausea, vomiting, blood in stool or vomit), spotting or other changes in vaginal bleeding, breast tenderness
Tips: If nausea persists or becomes bothersome, take Lo/Ovral with food or immediately after eating. Call your doctor if headache, dizziness, breast tenderness, spotting, and other bleeding changes last longer than 6 months.

Other: depression, lethargy, migraine, high blood pressure (headache, blurred vision, nosebleeds), swelling, worsening of near-sightedness or astigmatism, inability to wear contact lenses, vomiting, diarrhea, constipation, changes in appetite, weight gain, inflammation of pancreas (pain in abdomen, back, or chest; clay-colored stools; nausea; vomiting; yellow-tinged skin and eyes), inflammatory bowel disease (stool incontinence, abdominal pain, weight loss), menstrual irregularities, abnormal vaginal discharge, vaginal yeast infection, gallbladder disease (severe abdominal pain, bloating, gas), liver tumors (yellow-tinged skin and eyes), rash, acne, oily skin, changes in skin color, breast changes (such as enlargement or secretions), increased blood sugar level (increased thirst, hunger, and urination; weight loss), too much calcium in blood (increased thirst and urination, constipation), folic acid deficiency (fatigue, weakness, palpitations, nausea, weight loss), change in sex drive

 DRUG INTERACTIONS

Combining certain drugs may alter their action or produce unwanted side effects. Tell your doctor about other drugs you're taking, especially:
• anticoagulants (blood thinners)
• Barbita
• drugs that can damage the liver such as Dantrium
• Parlodel
• Rifadin
• Sandimmune
• steroids
• Tamofen
• Tegretol.

Continued on next page ▶

• If you miss tablets 2 days in a row, take two tablets on the day you remember and two tablets the next day; then resume your normal schedule. After missing two doses, use a second birth control method for 7 days.

• If you miss three or more tablets, discard the remaining tablets in your monthly package and use a different birth control method. If your next menstrual period doesn't start on schedule, have a pregnancy test before you start a new dosing cycle. If your menstrual period begins, start a new dosing cycle 7 days after you took the last tablet.

 ## If you suspect an overdose

Contact your doctor. Excessive Lo/Ovral can cause nausea and vomiting.

Warnings

• Make sure your doctor knows your medical history. You may not be able to take Lo/Ovral if you are over age 40 (35 if you smoke) or have medical problems, such as stroke, heart attack, blood clots, coronary artery disease, breast or liver cancer, high blood pressure, lupus, migraine headaches, epilepsy, asthma, diabetes, irregular periods, kidney or gallbladder disease, double vision, or eye tumors.

• Don't take Lo/Ovral if you're pregnant.

• If you're breast-feeding, tell your doctor before you start taking Lo/Ovral.

• If you're diabetic, be aware that the dosage of your diabetes drug may need to be changed after you start taking Lo/Ovral.

• Use an extra birth control method, such as condoms, for the first week that you take Lo/Ovral.

• Keep an extra month's supply of Lo/Ovral on hand so you won't run out.

• If you miss two menstrual periods in a row, stop taking Lo/Ovral and call your doctor.

• Have regular gynecologic checkups and Pap tests. Never go more than 12 months without seeing your doctor.

• Schedule regular checkups to have blood tests performed to monitor for possible side effects.

• Take your blood pressure regularly, or have your doctor check it.

• Record your weight before you start taking Lo/Ovral. Tell your doctor if you gain more than 5 pounds a month, especially if you haven't increased your food intake.

• Before surgery (including dental surgery), tell your doctor or dentist that you're taking a birth control pill.

• If you decide you want to get pregnant, consult your doctor, who may advise you to wait 2 months after stopping Lo/Ovral before trying to get pregnant.

 ## KEEP IN MIND...

* Take tablets in correct order.

* Take doses at same time each day.

* Use extra birth control method for first week.

* If you miss two periods in a row, stop taking the pills and call doctor.

Lopid

Lopid reduces the levels of fatty substances (cholesterol and triglycerides) in the blood. It seems to work by reducing cholesterol formation, helping to move cholesterol out of body tissues, and decreasing the body's fat production. It also raises levels of the "good" cholesterol (high-density-lipoprotein cholesterol, or HDL).

Why it's prescribed

Doctors prescribe Lopid to reduce cholesterol and triglyceride (fat) levels in the blood. It comes in tablets and capsules. Doctors usually prescribe the following amounts for adults.

▶ To reduce high blood fat levels in people who don't respond to dietary changes or who can't tolerate or don't respond to other drugs (such as niacin), 1,200 milligrams a day divided into two equal doses.

How to take Lopid

• Take this drug exactly as your doctor directs. If your doctor tells you to take two doses a day, take one dose 30 minutes before breakfast and the second dose 30 minutes before your evening meal.
• Don't stop taking Lopid without first consulting your doctor. If you stop taking it, your cholesterol and triglyceride levels could rise again.

LOPID'S OTHER NAME

Lopid's generic name is gemfibrozil.

 ## SIDE EFFECTS

Call your doctor if you have any of these possible drug side effects.

Serious: none reported

Common: abdominal or stomach pain, diarrhea, nausea
Tip: If these symptoms persist or become severe, call your doctor.

Other: blurred vision, headache, dizziness, vomiting, gas, anemia (fatigue, pale skin), too few white blood cells (persistent infection), bile duct obstruction (clay-colored stools, abdominal pain, weight loss), rash or inflammation, itching pain in arms or legs
Tip: Don't drive or perform other activities requiring alertness and clear vision until you know how you react to Lopid.

 ## DRUG INTERACTIONS

Combining certain drugs may alter their action or produce unwanted side effects. Tell your doctor about other drugs you're taking, especially:
• anticoagulants (blood thinners) such as Coumadin
• Mevacor.

If you miss a dose

Take the missed dose as soon as possible. But if it's almost time for the next dose, skip the missed dose and take the next dose as scheduled. Don't take a double dose.

 ## If you suspect an overdose

Consult your doctor.

Warnings

• Make sure your doctor knows your medical history. You may not be able to take Lopid if you have other problems, such as kidney or liver disease, gallstones, or gallbladder disease.
• If you're pregnant or breast-feeding, check with your doctor before you start taking Lopid.
• Carefully follow the special diet your doctor has ordered for you so that Lopid can work properly.

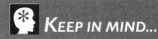 ## KEEP IN MIND...

∗ Follow special prescribed diet.

∗ Don't stop taking unless doctor approves.

∗ Call doctor about persistent or severe abdominal or stomach pain, diarrhea, or nausea.

∗ Don't drive until you know how you react to drug.

Lopressor

Lopressor reduces the strength of heart contractions, slows the pulse rate, reduces the heart's workload, and lowers the heart's oxygen needs.

Why it's prescribed

Doctors prescribe Lopressor to treat high blood pressure or to relieve chest pain. It comes in tablets and in an injectable form. A similar form of the drug also is available in extended-release tablets. Doctors usually prescribe the following amounts for adults.

▶ **For high blood pressure,** initially 50 milligrams (mg) orally twice a day or 100 mg once a day, then 100 to 450 mg a day divided into two or three equal doses. Or 50 to 100 mg of extended-release tablets once a day. Dosage is adjusted as needed and tolerated at intervals of at least 1 week to maximum of 400 mg a day.

▶ **For chest pain,** initially 100 mg orally a day as a single dose or divided into two equal doses, increased every week until adequate response or marked decrease in pulse rate occurs. Or 100 mg of extended-release tablets once a day. Dosage adjusted as needed and tolerated at intervals of at least 1 week to maximum of 400 mg a day.

LOPRESSOR'S OTHER NAMES

Lopressor's generic name is metoprolol tartrate. Canadian brand names include Apo-Metoprolol, Betaloc, Betaloc Durules, Lopresor, Novometoprol, and Nu-Metop. A similar generic drug, metoprolol succinate, has the brand name Toprol-XL.

SIDE EFFECTS

Call your doctor if you have any of these possible drug side effects. Call *immediately* about any labeled "serious."

Serious: heart failure (shortness of breath, fatigue), severe allergic reaction (swelling of face or throat, difficulty breathing)

Common: dizziness, weakness, slow pulse

Tips: Avoid hazardous activities such as driving until you know how you react to this drug. Ask your doctor if you should take your pulse regularly while taking Lopressor. If so, take it as instructed; if it's below 50 beats per minute, don't take your next dose and call your doctor.

Other: fatigue, peripheral vascular disease (coldness, numbness, or tingling in hands or feet), nausea, vomiting, diarrhea, rash, fever, joint pain

DRUG INTERACTIONS

Combining certain drugs may alter their action or produce unwanted side effects. Tell your doctor about other drugs you're taking, especially:
• barbiturates (used for sedation or seizures), such as Barbita and Seconal
• Indocin
• insulin and oral diabetes drugs
• other drugs for high blood pressure or heart disease, such as Cardizem, digoxin, and verapamil
• Rifadin
• Tagamet
• Thorazine.

How to take Lopressor

• Take this drug exactly as your doctor directs. To help the drug work better, take it with meals.
• Don't stop taking Lopressor, even if you're feeling well or side effects occur. Instead, check with your doctor.
• Store this drug at room temperature and away from light.

If you miss a dose

Take the missed dose as soon as possible. However, if it's within 4 hours of the next regular dose, skip the missed dose and take the next dose as scheduled. Don't take a double dose.

If you suspect an overdose

Contact your doctor *immediately.* Excessive Lopressor can cause severe low blood pressure (dizziness, weakness), slow pulse, heart failure (shortness of breath, fatigue, anxiety), and closing up of the throat.

Warnings

• Make sure your doctor knows your medical history. You may not be able to take Lopressor if you have other problems, such as heart or blood vessel disease, diabetes, kidney or liver disease, depression, hay fever, hives, bronchitis, emphysema, an unusually slow pulse, or an overactive thyroid.

• Don't take Lopressor if you have a history of asthma. Notify your doctor if you experience shortness of breath.

• If you're pregnant or breast-feeding, check with your doctor before you start taking Lopressor.

• Be aware that older adults may be especially prone to Lopressor's side effects.

• If you're diabetic, Lopressor may lower your blood sugar level and mask signs of low blood sugar (such as a change in your pulse rate). Also, the dosage of your diabetes drug may need to be changed.

• Follow any special diet that your doctor prescribes.

• Don't stop taking Lopressor abruptly; doing so could lead to a heart attack (chest pain, shortness of breath, anxiety).

• Be aware that Lopressor can mask the signs of shock (very low blood pressure and cold, clammy skin).

• Before any surgical procedure (including dental work), notify your doctor or dentist that you're taking Lopressor.

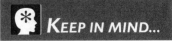 **KEEP IN MIND...**

* Take with meals.
* Don't stop taking unless doctor approves.
* Drug may lower blood sugar level of diabetics.
* Don't drive until you know how you react to this drug.

Lorabid

Lorabid is an antibiotic that eliminates infection by damaging the bacterial cell wall, which eventually destroys the bacteria.

Why it's prescribed

Doctors prescribe Lorabid to treat bacterial infections in various parts of the body. It comes in pulvules (which look like capsules) and a powder for an oral suspension. Doctors usually prescribe the following amounts for adults; children's dosages appear in parentheses (except for acute middle ear infection and impetigo).

▶ **For acute bronchitis, pneumonia, or skin, bladder, or kidney infection,** 200 to 400 milligrams (mg) every 12 hours for 7 to 14 days.

▶ **For sore throat, sinus inflammation, or tonsillitis,** 200 to 400 mg every 12 hours for 10 days. (Children: 15 mg for each 2.2 pounds [lb] of body weight daily divided into equal doses given every 12 hours for 10 days.)

▶ **For acute middle ear infection in children,** 30 mg for each 2.2 lb (oral suspension) each day divided into equal doses given every 12 hours for 10 days.

▶ **For impetigo in children,** 15 mg for each 2.2 lb each day divided into equal doses given every 12 hours for 7 days.

How to take Lorabid

• Take this drug exactly as your doctor directs. Take it on an empty

LORABID'S OTHER NAME

Lorabid's generic name is loracarbef.

SIDE EFFECTS

Call your doctor if you have any of these possible drug side effects. Call *immediately* about any labeled "serious."

Serious: eruptions on skin and mucous membranes, severe allergic reaction (difficulty breathing, swelling of the face and throat, hives)

Common: nausea, diarrhea, appetite loss, blotchy rash with red raised areas

Other: headache, sleepiness, nervousness, insomnia, dizziness, vomiting, abdominal pain, intestinal inflammation, vaginal yeast infection, too few white blood cells (persistent infection), too few blood-clotting cells (abnormal bleeding), itching

DRUG INTERACTIONS

Combining certain drugs may alter their action or produce unwanted side effects. Tell your doctor about other drugs you're taking, especially:
• Benemid.

stomach, at least 1 hour before or 2 hours after meals.

• To help clear up your infection, keep taking Lorabid for the full time prescribed, even if you feel better.

If you miss a dose

Take the missed dose as soon as possible. However, if it's almost time for the next dose, skip the missed dose and take the next dose as scheduled. Don't take a double dose.

If you suspect an overdose

Contact your doctor *immediately.* Excessive Lorabid can cause nausea, vomiting, stomach pain, and diarrhea.

Warnings

• Make sure your doctor knows your medical history. You may not be able to take Lorabid if you have other problems, such as kidney disease, or if you are allergic to any antibiotics.

• If you're pregnant or breast-feeding, tell your doctor before you start taking Lorabid.

• If your symptoms don't improve within a few days or if they get worse, call your doctor.

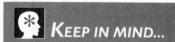
KEEP IN MIND...

* Take on empty stomach.
* Keep taking for full time prescribed.
* Call doctor if symptoms don't improve or if they get worse within several days.

Lortab 5/500

L ortab 5/500 is a combination of a narcotic pain reliever and acetaminophen (Tylenol). It reduces pain and fever and alters the brain's perception of pain.

Why it's prescribed

Doctors prescribe Lortab 5/500 to relieve pain. It comes in tablets, capsules, and a liquid. Doctors usually prescribe the following amounts for adults.

▶ **For moderate to moderately severe pain,** 1 or 2 tablets every 4 to 6 hours, up to 8 tablets a day. Or 1 capsule or 1 to 3 teaspoons every 4 to 6 hours, as needed.

How to take Lortab 5/500

• Take this drug exactly as your doctor orders. Don't take more than prescribed. If you don't think it's working, call your doctor.
• If you take Lortab 5/500 regularly, don't stop taking it abruptly.

If you miss a dose

Take the missed dose as soon as possible. But if it's almost time for your next dose, skip the missed dose and take your next dose as scheduled. Don't take a double dose.

 If you suspect an overdose

Contact your doctor *immediately.* Excessive Lortab 5/500 can cause low blood sugar (dizziness, tiredness), decreased urine output, inter-

nal bleeding, nausea, vomiting, slow and shallow breathing, cold and clammy skin, extremely low blood pressure (extreme dizziness and weakness), and unconsciousness.

 Warnings

• Make sure your doctor knows your medical history. You may not be able to take Lortab 5/500 if you're allergic to it or if you have a brain disease or head injury, a digestive disorder, seizures, asthma or another chronic lung disease, liver or kidney problems, an underactive

 SIDE EFFECTS

Call your doctor if you have any of these possible drug side effects. Call *immediately* about any labeled "serious."

Serious: seizures

Common: dizziness, light-headedness, fainting, drowsiness, nausea, vomiting, tiredness, weakness
Tips: If you feel dizzy, light-headed, or nauseous, lie down for awhile after taking each dose. If you're not fully alert, don't drive or perform other activities that could be dangerous. To minimize dizziness and light-headedness, get up slowly after sitting or lying down.

Other: vision changes, constipation, dry mouth, headache, appetite loss, nervousness, sleeplessness or disturbing dreams
Tips: To reduce constipation, drink plenty of water and eat fiber-rich foods, such as whole grains, vegetables, and fruits.

 DRUG INTERACTIONS

Combining certain drugs may alter their action or produce unwanted side effects. Tell your doctor about other drugs you're taking, especially:
• alcohol and other drugs that make you feel relaxed or sleepy, such as tranquilizers, sleeping pills, and cold and allergy drugs
• antidepressants, such as MAO inhibitors (Nardil, Parnate) and tricyclic antidepressants (Elavil)
• AZT
• other drugs that contain acetaminophen
• Tegretol
• Trexan.

thyroid, an enlarged prostate, gallbladder disease, heart disease, alcohol or drug problems, or mental illness.
• Before surgery, dental procedures, or emergency treatment, tell your doctor or dentist that you're taking Lortab 5/500.

LORTAB 5/500's OTHER NAMES

Lortab 5/500 is a combination of two generic drugs: acetaminophen and hydrocodone bitartrate. Another brand name is Vicodin.

KEEP IN MIND...

* Take only as directed.
* Don't stop taking abruptly.
* Increase fluids and fiber in diet.

Lotensin

Lotensin causes blood vessels to relax and lowers blood pressure. It also helps prevent further weakening of the heart after a heart attack.

Why it's prescribed

Doctors prescribe Lotensin to treat high blood pressure. It comes in tablets. Doctors usually prescribe the following amounts for adults.

▶ **For high blood pressure in people who aren't taking a diuretic (water pill),** initially 10 milligrams (mg) a day, gradually increased as needed and tolerated. Most people take 20 to 40 mg a day in one dose or divided into two equal doses.

▶ **For people who are taking a diuretic,** 5 mg a day.

How to take Lotensin

• Take this drug exactly as your doctor directs. Take it on an empty stomach 1 hour before meals, unless the doctor tells you otherwise.

• Keep taking Lotensin even if you feel well. You may have to take it for the rest of your life.

If you miss a dose

Take the missed dose as soon as possible. However, if it's almost time for the next dose, skip the missed dose and take the next dose as scheduled. Don't take a double dose.

If you suspect an overdose

Contact your doctor *immediately.* Excessive Lotensin can cause low

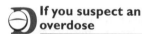

LOTENSIN'S OTHER NAME

Lotensin's generic name is benazepril hydrochloride.

SIDE EFFECTS

Call your doctor if you have any of these possible drug side effects. Call *immediately* about any labeled "serious."

Serious: throat swelling, difficulty breathing

Common: headache, cough

Other: low blood pressure (dizziness, weakness), anxiety, memory loss, depression, difficulty sleeping, nervousness, numbness or tingling, fainting, chest pain, swelling, palpitations, nausea, vomiting, abdominal pain, constipation, allergic reaction (rash, skin inflammation), itching, skin sensitivity to sunlight, unusual bruising, pinpoint red or purple spots on skin, swelling of hands or feet, arthritis, impotence, heavy sweating, muscle pain, weight gain

Tips: Until you know how Lotensin affects you, don't drive or do anything else that requires you to be fully alert. Call your doctor right away if you experience severe nausea, vomiting, or diarrhea.

DRUG INTERACTIONS

Combining certain drugs may alter their action or produce unwanted side effects. Tell your doctor about other drugs you're taking, especially:

• alcohol
• diuretics (water pills), such as HydroDIURIL and Vaseretic
• Lithobid
• other blood pressure drugs
• salt substitutes containing potassium.

blood pressure (dizziness, weakness).

Warnings

• Make sure your doctor knows your medical history. You may not be able to take Lotensin if you have other medical problems.

• If you're pregnant or breast-feeding, tell your doctor before you start taking Lotensin. If you become pregnant during treatment, stop taking the drug and call your doctor.

• Keep all medical appointments so your doctor can check your progress.

• Before any surgery (including dental surgery), tell your doctor or dentist that you're taking Lotensin.

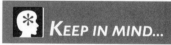

KEEP IN MIND...

* Take on empty stomach.

* Check with doctor before taking other drugs.

* Avoid driving until you know your reaction to the drug.

* Call doctor about severe vomiting or diarrhea.

Lotrimin

Lotrimin is applied to the skin to treat fungal infections. It works by altering the cell walls of the fungus, which prevents the fungus from growing.

Why it's prescribed

Doctors prescribe Lotrimin to treat fungal infections of the skin. It comes in a cream, a lotion, and a topical solution. Doctors usually prescribe the following amounts for adults and children.

▶ **For fungal infections of the skin (such as athlete's foot and jock itch),** a thin strip applied and massaged into affected and surrounding area morning and evening for 2 to 8 weeks.

How to use Lotrimin

• Apply this drug exactly as your doctor directs.
• Clean the affected area before applying Lotrimin. Apply enough Lotrimin to cover the affected skin area, and rub it in gently. Don't put a bandage over the treated area unless your doctor tells you to do so.
• Continue to use Lotrimin, even if your symptoms clear up in a few days. If you stop using it too soon, your infection may return. Because fungal infections may be slow to

LOTRIMIN'S OTHER NAMES

Lotrimin's generic name is clotrimazole. Other brand names include Lotrimin AF, Mycelex; and, in Canada, Canesten Cream, Clotrimaderm Cream, Myclo Cream, and Neo-Zol Cream.

clear up, you may need to use Lotrimin every day for several weeks or more.

If you miss a dose

Apply the missed dose as soon as possible. However, if it's almost time for the next dose, skip the missed dose and apply the next dose as scheduled.

If you suspect an overdose

Wash off the cream and consult your doctor.

Warnings

• Make sure your doctor knows your medical history. You may not be able to use Lotrimin if you have other medical problems, such as liver disease.
• If you're pregnant or breast-feeding, tell your doctor before you start using Lotrimin.

• Don't use Lotrimin on children under age 3.
• If your skin problem doesn't improve within 4 weeks or if it gets worse, call your doctor.
• Avoid getting Lotrimin in your eyes.
• Be aware that Lotrimin may stain your clothing.

SIDE EFFECTS

Call your doctor if you have any of these possible drug side effects.

Serious: none reported

Common: redness of skin

Other: blistering, swelling, cracking, itching, burning, stinging, or peeling of skin; hives

Tip: Call your doctor if you develop skin redness, blistering, swelling, burning, or stinging.

DRUG INTERACTIONS

Combining certain drugs may alter their action or produce unwanted side effects. Tell your doctor about other drugs you're taking.

KEEP IN MIND...

* Don't bandage treated area unless doctor tells you to do so.

* Keep using, even if symptoms clear up in a few days.

* Call doctor if skin problem doesn't improve within 4 weeks or if you notice signs of irritation.

Lotrisone

Lotrisone helps kill or prevent the growth of fungi. It also relieves the itching, burning, swelling, and redness that often occur with fungal infections.

Why it's prescribed

Doctors prescribe Lotrisone to treat fungal infections, such as athlete's foot, jock itch, and ringworm. It comes in a cream. Doctors usually prescribe the following amounts for adults and children over age 12.

▶ **For athlete's foot, jock itch, and ringworm,** a small amount applied to affected skin twice a day.

How to use Lotrisone cream

- Apply this drug exactly as your doctor directs. Don't apply it more frequently without your doctor's approval.
- Make sure the affected skin is clean and dry before applying the cream.
- Apply Lotrisone to the affected area with clean fingers.
- If desired, apply a dry gauze dressing over the area to protect clothing.

LOTRISONE'S OTHER NAMES

Lotrisone is a combination of the generic drugs clotrimazole and betamethasone dipropionate. A Canadian brand name is Lotriderm.

SIDE EFFECTS

Call your doctor if you have any of these possible drug side effects.

Serious: none reported

Common: none reported

Other: blistering, burning, peeling, itching, and redness
Tip: Call your doctor if you develop redness, blistering, burning, or peeling after first applying the cream or after continued use.

INTERACTIONS

Combining certain drugs may alter their action or produce unwanted side effects. Tell your doctor about other drugs you're taking.

- Continue using Lotrisone for the full length of treatment, even if your symptoms seem to be getting better.

If you miss a dose

Apply the missed dose as soon as possible. However, if it's almost time for the next dose, skip the missed dose and apply the next dose as scheduled.

If you suspect an overdose

Consult your doctor.

Warnings

- Make sure your doctor knows your medical history. You may not be able to use Lotrisone if you're allergic to it.
- If you're pregnant or breast-feeding, check with your doctor before using Lotrisone.

- Lotrisone can raise blood sugar levels, so use it with caution if you have severe diabetes. Consult your doctor if you notice a change.
- Wear light, loose clothing during treatment to prevent the clothing from sticking to the cream, which could increase your risk of developing irritation.
- Store Lotrisone away from light and heat.

KEEP IN MIND...

* Apply to clean, dry skin.
* Wear loose clothing during treatment.
* Continue treatment even if condition improves.
* Be alert for elevated blood sugar levels if diabetic.

Lovenox

Lovenox is a blood thinner, or anticoagulant. It interferes with blood clotting by speeding the formation of a natural substance that limits clotting and by altering the activities of several substances that can cause clotting.

Why it's prescribed

Doctors prescribe Lovenox for several days after hip or knee replacement surgery to prevent blood clots from forming in the legs. (Clots are most likely to form when a person is confined to bed and can't walk.) A blood clot in the leg may travel to the pulmonary artery, causing a life-threatening condition called pulmonary embolism. Lovenox is available in an injectable form. Doctors usually prescribe the following amounts for adults.

▶ **To prevent pulmonary embolism and blood clots in leg after hip or knee replacement surgery,** 30 milligrams injected under the skin twice a day for 7 to 10 days. Initial dose given as soon as possible after surgery, but no later than 24 hours afterward.

How to take Lovenox

• If you're administering this drug to yourself at home, follow your doctor's instructions on how to inject yourself.
• After injection, don't massage the area where you injected the drug. Watch for symptoms of bleeding at this area, such as bruising.

LOVENOX'S OTHER NAME

Lovenox's generic name is enoxaparin sodium.

 SIDE EFFECTS

Call your doctor if you have any of these possible drug side effects. Call *immediately* about any labeled "serious."

Serious: abnormal bleeding (bleeding gums, bruises on your arms or legs, tiny purple or red spots on skin, nosebleeds, black tarry stools, blood in urine, vomiting of bright red blood), extreme fatigue

Common: none reported

Other: confusion, swelling, nausea, fever, pain; irritation, pain, redness, or other problems at injection site
Tip: Use a different site (on abdomen, thighs, or upper arms) for each injection.

 DRUG INTERACTIONS

Combining certain drugs may alter their action or produce unwanted side effects. Tell your doctor about other drugs you're taking, especially:
• aspirin or other salicylates (including nonprescription drugs)
• drugs that lower platelet count such as Pepcid
• other anticoagulants (blood thinners).

• Place used syringes in a disposable, puncture-resistant container, or discard them as instructed by your doctor.

If you miss a dose

Take the missed dose as soon as possible. But if it's almost time for the next dose, skip the missed dose and take the next dose as scheduled. Don't take a double dose.

 If you suspect an overdose

Contact your doctor *immediately.* Excessive Lovenox can cause bleeding complications.

 Warnings

• Make sure your doctor knows your medical history. You may not be able to take Lovenox if you have other problems, such as bleeding or blood vessel problems, blood disease, high blood pressure, heart infection, kidney or liver disease, or an ulcer; are allergic to pork, heparin, or insulin; have recently given birth, injured your head or body, or had any surgery (including dental surgery); or are pregnant or breast-feeding.
• Keep all follow-up appointments. Your doctor will want to check your platelet count often.
• Tell all your doctors and your dentist that you're using Lovenox.

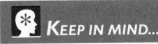 **KEEP IN MIND...**

∗ Rotate injection sites.
∗ Don't massage injection site.
∗ Call doctor about symptoms of abnormal bleeding.

Loxitane

Loxitane helps control symptoms of psychosis, a type of mental illness. It seems to work by affecting certain chemicals in the brain.

Why it's prescribed

Doctors prescribe Loxitane to treat mental illnesses, such as schizophrenia and bipolar disorder (manic-depression). It comes in tablets, capsules, and an oral liquid. It's also available in an injectable form. Doctors usually prescribe the following amounts for adults.

▶ **For psychotic disorders,** 10 milligrams (mg) orally two to four times a day, rapidly increasing to 60 to 100 mg orally a day for most people. Dosage varies among individuals.

How to take Loxitane

- Take this drug exactly as your doctor directs.
- If you're taking the liquid, measure the correct amount with a specially marked measuring spoon or dropper, not a regular household teaspoon. Dilute it with orange or grapefruit juice just before taking it.
- Don't stop taking this drug without consulting your doctor, who may want to reduce your dosage gradually.

If you miss a dose

Take the missed dose as soon as possible. But if it's within 1 hour of the next dose, skip the missed dose and take the next dose as scheduled. Don't take a double dose.

LOXITANE'S OTHER NAMES

Loxitane's generic name is loxapine succinate. A Canadian brand name is Loxapac.

 ## SIDE EFFECTS

Call your doctor if you have any of these possible drug side effects. Call *immediately* about any labeled "serious."

Serious: fever, rigid muscles, coma

Common: lip smacking; puffing of cheeks; uncontrollable tongue, mouth, arm, or leg movements; sedation; restlessness; blurred vision; dry mouth; constipation, inability to urinate; skin sensitivity to sunlight
Tip: To relieve dry mouth, use sugarless gum or hard candy.

Other: dizziness, difficulty speaking or swallowing, masklike facial expression, shuffling walk, slow or stiff movements, shaking of hands, fast pulse, dark urine, menstrual irregularities, enlarged breasts, allergic reactions (rash, fever, swelling), weight gain, increased appetite, stomach upset
Tips: Avoid driving or doing anything else that could be dangerous until you know how Loxitane affects you. Rise to your feet slowly to avoid dizziness. To help prevent stomach upset, take Loxitane with food or a full glass (8 ounces) of water or milk.

DRUG INTERACTIONS

Combining certain drugs may alter their action or produce unwanted side effects. Tell your doctor about other drugs you're taking, especially:
- alcohol and other drugs that relax or make you sleepy, including cold and allergy medicines, sedatives, tranquilizers, narcotic pain relievers, barbiturates, drugs to control seizures, and muscle relaxants.

 ## If you suspect an overdose

Contact your doctor *immediately.* Excessive Loxitane can cause extremely deep sleep and possibly a coma, lip smacking, chewing motions, uncontrollable arm and leg movements, abnormal muscle movements, agitation, seizures, irregular heartbeats, fever or low body temperature, and dramatic changes in blood pressure and heart rate, which can cause dizziness and fainting.

Warnings

- Make sure your doctor knows your medical history. You may not be able to take Loxitane if you have other medical problems.

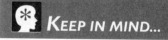 ## KEEP IN MIND...

- Take with food or full glass of water or milk.
- Dilute liquid form with orange or grapefruit juice.
- Avoid driving until you know how you react to this drug.
- Stand slowly to avoid dizziness.

Lozol

Lozol, a diuretic (water pill), makes the body excrete more sodium, which reduces the amount of water in the body. This, in turn, lowers blood pressure. Lozol also relaxes blood vessels so blood can pass through them more easily.

Why it's prescribed

Doctors prescribe Lozol to treat high blood pressure and swelling (edema). It comes in tablets. Doctors usually prescribe the following amounts for adults.

▶ **For high blood pressure,** initially 1.25 milligrams (mg) a day in the morning, increased to 2.5 mg a day after 4 weeks, if needed, then to 5 mg a day after 4 more weeks, if needed.

▶ **For swelling,** initially 2.5 mg a day in the morning, increased to 5 mg a day after 1 week, if needed.

How to take Lozol

• Take this drug exactly as your doctor directs.

• Because Lozol will make you urinate more, take it in the morning to avoid nighttime urination.

• If you're taking Lozol for high blood pressure, be sure to keep taking it even if you feel well.

If you miss a dose

Take the missed dose as soon as possible. However, if it's almost time for the next dose, skip the missed dose and take the next dose as scheduled. Don't take a double dose.

LOZOL'S OTHER NAMES

Lozol's generic name is indapamide. A Canadian brand name is Lozide.

 SIDE EFFECTS

Call your doctor if you have any of these possible drug side effects.

Serious: none reported

Common: none reported

Other: headache, irritability, nervousness, dizziness (especially when standing up), light-headedness, weakness, dehydration, appetite loss, nausea, inflammation of pancreas (nausea, vomiting, abdominal pain, clay-colored stools, indigestion), frequent or nighttime urination, skin inflammation, skin sensitivity to sunlight, rash, muscle cramps or spasms, too little potassium in blood (muscle cramps or weakness), imbalances of body's fluid and salt levels (dry mouth, thirst, unusual tiredness), gout

Tips: To offset potassium loss, ask your doctor about eating potassium-rich foods, such as citrus fruits, tomatoes, bananas, dates, and apricots, or taking a potassium supplement. Call your doctor if you have muscle cramps or weakness.

 DRUG INTERACTIONS

Combining certain drugs may alter their action or produce unwanted side effects. Tell your doctor about other drugs you're taking, especially:

• Crystodigin, Lanoxin
• nonsteroidal anti-inflammatory drugs such as Advil
• Proglycem.

 If you suspect an overdose

Contact your doctor *immediately.* Excessive Lozol can cause stomach irritation, increased urination, lethargy, and coma.

Warnings

• Make sure your doctor knows your medical history. You may not be able to take Lozol if you have other medical problems.

• Schedule medical appointments regularly so your doctor can check your progress.

• Follow any special diet your doctor prescribes.

• Call your doctor if you develop severe vomiting or diarrhea. These conditions may lead to a dangerous loss of water and potassium, which can worsen some side effects.

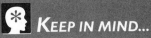 **KEEP IN MIND...**

∗ Take in morning.

∗ Follow prescribed diet.

∗ Eat potassium-rich foods if directed.

∗ Call doctor about muscle weakness or cramps or severe vomiting or diarrhea.

Ludiomil

Ludiomil is a tricyclic anti-depressant. It seems to help lift depression by increasing the amounts of certain crucial chemicals in the brain.

Why it's prescribed

Doctors prescribe Ludiomil to relieve depression. It comes in tablets. Doctors usually prescribe the following amounts for adults.

▶ **For depression,** initially 75 milligrams (mg) a day for people with mild to moderate depression, increased to 150 mg a day, if needed. Maximum dosage is 225 mg a day.

How to take Ludiomil

• Take this drug exactly as your doctor directs.
• Don't stop taking it without consulting your doctor first.

If you miss a dose

Don't take a double dose. Adjust your schedule as follows:
• If you take one dose a day, don't take the missed dose at bedtime because this may cause unpleasant effects during the day. Call your doctor for instructions.
• If you take more than one dose a day, take the missed dose as soon as possible. But if it's almost time for your next dose, skip the missed dose and take your next dose as scheduled.

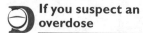 **If you suspect an overdose**

Contact your doctor *immediately*. Excessive Ludiomil can cause agita-tion, irritation, confusion, hallucinations, fever, tremor, seizures, inability to urinate, dry mucous membranes, enlarged pupils, constipation, low body temperature, decreased reflexes, sedation, low blood pressure (dizziness, weakness, fainting), bluish skin, and heart abnormalities (such as a fast pulse).

LUDIOMIL'S OTHER NAME

Ludiomil's generic name is maprotiline hydrochloride.

 SIDE EFFECTS

Call your doctor if you have any of these possible drug side effects. Call *immediately* about any labeled "serious."

Serious: seizures

Common: drowsiness, dizziness (especially when standing up), blurred vision, inability to urinate, fast pulse, sweating

Other: excitation, tremor, weakness, confusion, headache, nervousness, restlessness, ringing in ears, enlarged pupils, dry mouth, constipation, nausea, vomiting, appetite loss, skin sensitivity to sunlight, allergic reaction (rash, fever, hives, swelling)

Tip: To help prevent constipation, drink plenty of fluids and eat high-fiber foods.

 DRUG INTERACTIONS

Combining certain drugs may alter their action or produce unwanted side effects. Tell your doctor about other drugs you're taking, especially:
• alcohol and other drugs that make you relaxed or sleepy, such as cold and allergy medicines, sedatives, tranquilizers, narcotic pain relievers, barbiturates, drugs to control seizures, and muscle relaxants
• epinephrine
• Klonopin
• Levophed
• MAO inhibitors, such as Marplan and Nardil
• Ritalin
• Tagamet.

• Be aware that you may need to take Ludiomil for several weeks before you notice its effects.

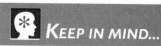 **KEEP IN MIND...**

* Drug may not take effect for several weeks.
* Don't stop taking suddenly.
* Drink plenty of fluids and eat high-fiber foods.

Warnings

• Make sure your doctor knows your medical history. You may not be able to take Ludiomil if you have other medical problems.

Lugol's solution

Lugol's solution is a treatment for overactive thyroid. It works by acting directly on the thyroid gland to block the production and release of thyroid hormone.

Why it's prescribed

Doctors prescribe Lugol's solution to prepare the thyroid gland for surgery, to treat acute episodes of overactive thyroid (thyroid crisis), and to treat hyperthyroidism. It comes in a liquid. Doctors usually prescribe the following amounts for adults; children's dosages appear in parentheses.

▶ **To prepare a person for thyroid surgery,** 0.1 to 0.3 milliliters (ml) three times a day for 10 to 14 days before surgery. (Children: same as adults.)

▶ **For thyroid crisis,** 1.8 ml (30 drops) a day. (Children: same as adults.)

▶ **For hyperthyroidism,** 0.1 to 0.3 ml three times a day. (Children over age 10: 100 mg three times a day, followed by maintenance dosage of 25 mg three times a day up to a maximum of 100 mg twice a day. Children ages 6 to 10: 50 to 150 mg divided into equal doses taken every 8 hours.)

How to take Lugol's solution

• Take this drug exactly as your doctor directs. Don't stop taking it suddenly because doing so could cause a serious medical problem.

• Take the liquid by mouth even if it comes in a dropper bottle. Take it in a full glass (8 ounces) of water

LUGOL'S SOLUTION'S OTHER NAME

Lugol's solution's generic name is strong iodine solution.

SIDE EFFECTS

Call your doctor if you have any of these possible drug side effects. Call *immediately* about any labeled "serious."

Serious: allergic reaction (fever, swollen glands, rash, joint pain)

Common: nausea, metallic taste

Other: fever, headache, runny nose, inflammation of salivary glands, tooth stains, swelling around eyes, pinkeye, warm and reddened skin, stomach upset, nausea, vomiting, diarrhea (sometimes bloody), acnelike rash, sores on mucous membranes

Tips: To avoid tooth stains, drink the liquid through a straw. If the drug upsets your stomach, take it after meals or with food or milk.

DRUG INTERACTIONS

Combining certain drugs may alter their action or produce unwanted side effects. Tell your doctor about other drugs you're taking, especially:

• drugs for high blood pressure or heart conditions, including Aldactone, Catapres, Midamor, and Vasotec

• Lithobid

• other antithyroid drugs.

or in fruit juice, milk, or broth to improve its taste and reduce stomach upset. Drink all the liquid. Don't use it if it's brownish yellow.

If you miss a dose

Take the missed dose as soon as possible. But if it's almost time for the next dose, skip the missed dose and take the next dose as scheduled. Don't take a double dose.

If you suspect an overdose

Contact your doctor *immediately.* Excessive Lugol's solution can cause skin hemorrhages and swelling of the face, lips, tongue, throat, hands, and feet.

Warnings

• Make sure your doctor knows your medical history. You may not be able to take Lugol's solution if you have other problems, such as kidney disease, tuberculosis, or too much potassium in the blood, or if you're allergic to sulfites.

• If you're pregnant or breast-feeding, tell your doctor before you start taking Lugol's solution.

• Follow any special diet that the doctor has prescribed.

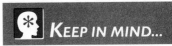

KEEP IN MIND...

∗ Don't stop taking suddenly.

∗ Drink liquid through straw.

∗ Take after meals or with food or milk to reduce stomach upset.

Lupron

Lupron is a cancer-fighting drug. It works by first stimulating and then inhibiting the release of certain hormones. This action suppresses the body's production of testosterone, a male hormone.

Why it's prescribed

Doctors prescribe Lupron to treat prostate cancer and endometriosis (in which tissue normally found only in the lining of the uterus is found outside this area). It comes in an injectable form. Doctors usually prescribe the following amounts for adults.

▶ **For advanced prostate cancer,** 1 milligram (mg) injected under the skin daily or 7.5 mg injected into a muscle monthly.

▶ **For endometriosis,** 3.75 mg injected into a muscle once a month for up to 6 months.

How to use Lupron

• Use this drug exactly as your doctor directs. If you'll be injecting Lupron under the skin, make sure you understand the doctor's instructions on how to do so. Also, be sure to read the manufacturer's directions in the package.

• Use only the disposable syringes provided by the manufacturer.

• Don't stop using Lupron without first consulting your doctor, even if the drug causes side effects or makes your symptoms worsen temporarily.

LUPRON'S OTHER NAMES

Lupron's generic name is leuprolide acetate. Another brand name is Lupron Depot.

 SIDE EFFECTS

Call your doctor if you have any of these possible drug side effects. Call *immediately* about any labeled "serious."

Serious: heart attack (chest or arm pain, shortness of breath, anxiety, indigestion), pulmonary embolism (extreme shortness of breath, anxiety, pale skin)

Common: hot flashes, temporary worsening of cancer symptoms

Other: dizziness, depression, headache, irregular pulse, swelling of lower legs or feet, nausea, vomiting, bone pain (during first week of treatment), decreased sex drive, skin reactions at injection site, enlarged breasts, impotence, miscarriage, birth defects, sterility in men (likely to be temporary)

 DRUG INTERACTIONS

Combining certain drugs may alter their action or produce unwanted side effects. Tell your doctor about other drugs you're taking.

If you miss a dose

If you use Lupron every day, inject the missed dose as soon as possible. But if you don't remember until the next day, skip the missed dose and inject the next dose as scheduled. Don't inject a double dose.

 If you suspect an overdose

Consult your doctor.

Warnings

• Make sure your doctor knows your medical history. You may not be able to use Lupron if you have other medical problems.

• Don't use this drug if you're pregnant or breast-feeding or if you intend to have children in the future. Be sure to use an effective nonhormonal birth control method during Lupron treatment. If you think you've become pregnant while using Lupron, stop taking it and call your doctor immediately.

• Be aware that Lupron may cause sterility in men, though it may be temporary. Discuss this with your doctor before taking this drug.

• If you're taking Lupron for endometriosis, be aware that you may have irregular menstrual periods or none at all during treatment. If your periods don't become regular within 2 to 3 months after stopping Lupron, call your doctor.

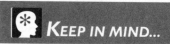 **KEEP IN MIND...**

* Use only syringes provided by manufacturer.

* Before starting therapy, tell doctor if you want to have children.

* Don't stop taking drug unless doctor approves.

Luvox

Luvox is a drug that acts on the nervous system. It seems to relieve obsessive-compulsive disorder by increasing levels of a brain chemical called serotonin.

Why it's prescribed

Doctors prescribe Luvox for obsessive-compulsive disorder. It comes in tablets. Doctors usually prescribe the following amounts for adults.

▶ **For obsessive-compulsive disorder,** initially 50 milligrams (mg) a day at bedtime, increased by 50 mg every 4 to 7 days until maximum benefit achieved. Maximum dosage is 300 mg a day. Total daily doses of more than 100 mg should be divided into two equal doses.

How to take Luvox

• Take this drug exactly as your doctor directs.
• Don't stop taking Luvox without first checking with your doctor even if it doesn't seem to be working. You may need to take it for a few weeks before your condition improves.

If you miss a dose

Consult your doctor.

 If you suspect an overdose

Consult your doctor.

 Warnings

• Make sure your doctor knows your medical history. You may not be able to take Luvox if you have other medical problems, such as seizures, mania, or liver disease.
• If you become pregnant or intend to get pregnant during Luvox therapy, tell your doctor.
• Be aware that this drug may be less effective if you smoke during treatment.

LUVOX'S OTHER NAME

Luvox's generic name is fluvoxamine maleate.

 SIDE EFFECTS

Call your doctor if you have any of these possible drug side effects.

Serious: none reported

Common: headache, weakness, sleepiness or difficulty sleeping, agitation, nausea, vomiting

Other: nervousness, dizziness, tremor, anxiety, depression, restlessness, strange taste in mouth, palpitations, decreased vision in one eye, diarrhea, constipation, stomach upset, appetite loss, gas, tooth disorder, difficulty swallowing, dry mouth, decreased sex drive, abnormal ejaculation, frequent urination, inability to urinate, impotence, difficulty having an orgasm, upper respiratory tract infection, difficulty breathing, yawning, sweating, flulike symptoms, chills

Tip: Avoid driving or doing anything else that could be dangerous until you know how Luvox affects you.

 DRUG INTERACTIONS

Combining certain drugs may alter their action or produce unwanted side effects. Tell your doctor about other drugs you're taking, especially:
• alcohol
• allergy drugs, such as Hismanal and Seldane
• anticoagulants (blood thinners) such as Coumadin
• benzodiazepines (drugs used to treat anxiety)
• beta blockers such as Inderal
• Cardizem
• Clozaril
• Lithobid
• MAO inhibitors such as Marplan (stop taking for at least 14 days before you start taking Luvox)
• methadone
• Tegretol
• Theo-Dur
• tricyclic antidepressants, such as Elavil and Tofranil
• tryptophan.

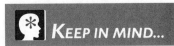 **KEEP IN MIND...**

* Avoid driving until you know how you react to drug.

* Don't take within 14 days of taking MAO inhibitor.

* Don't stop taking unless doctor approves.

Lysodren

Lysodren acts on the adrenal glands, which sit on top of the kidneys. It works by decreasing the amount of cortisone-like hormones (called adrenocorticoids) produced by the adrenal glands.

Why it's prescribed

Doctors prescribe Lysodren to treat some cancers that affect the adrenal cortex (the larger portion of the adrenal glands). It comes in tablets. Doctors usually prescribe the following amounts for adults.

▶ **For inoperable cancer of the adrenal cortex,** initially 2 to 6 grams (g) a day divided into three or four equal doses, increased to 9 to 10 g a day divided into three or four equal doses. Dosage is adjusted until maximum tolerated dosage is achieved.

How to take Lysodren

• Take this drug exactly as your doctor directs.
• Don't stop taking Lysodren suddenly because this may cause unpleasant side effects.

If you miss a dose

Take the missed dose as soon as possible. However, if it's almost time for the next dose, skip the missed dose, and take the next dose as scheduled. Don't take a double dose. Also check with your doctor.

LYSODREN'S OTHER NAME

Lysodren's generic name is mitotane.

 ## SIDE EFFECTS

Call your doctor if you have any of these possible drug side effects.

Serious: none reported

Common: depression, sleepiness, lethargy, vertigo, severe nausea
Tip: Until you know how this drug affects you, avoid driving or doing anything else that could be dangerous if you're not fully alert.

Other: brain damage (with long-term, high-dose therapy), vomiting, diarrhea, appetite loss, skin inflammation, rash, increased cholesterol level, adrenal gland dysfunction (weight loss, nausea, vomiting, salt craving, dizziness), vision disturbances, bladder infection (frequent or painful urination), high blood pressure (headache, blurred vision, nosebleeds)

DRUG INTERACTIONS

Combining certain drugs may alter their action or produce unwanted side effects. Tell your doctor about other drugs you're taking, especially:
• alcohol and other drugs that make you relaxed or sleepy, such as cold and allergy medicines, sedatives, barbiturates, tranquilizers, narcotic pain relievers, muscle relaxants, antidepressants, and drugs to control seizures.

 ### If you suspect an overdose

Contact your doctor *immediately.* Excessive Lysodren can cause vomiting, weakness, numbness of the arms and legs, diarrhea, fearfulness, and excitement.

Warnings

• Make sure your doctor knows your medical history. You may not be able to take Lysodren if you have other medical problems.
• Before taking this drug, tell your doctor if you're pregnant or breast-feeding.
• Schedule medical appointments regularly so your doctor can check your progress and monitor drug effects.

• Be aware that Lysodren may make you more vulnerable to infection. Call your doctor right away if you develop symptoms of infection (such as a fever, chills, or a sore throat), if you become ill, or if you suffer an injury.

 ### KEEP IN MIND...

* Don't stop taking drug abruptly.

* Avoid driving until you know how you react to drug.

* Call doctor right away if you have an infection, illness, or injury.

Maalox

Maalox is an antacid that relieves symptoms of heartburn and acid indigestion. It works by causing a chemical reaction that neutralizes acids found in the stomach.

Why it's taken

Maalox is a nonprescription drug taken for upset stomach. It comes in a liquid suspension and chewable tablets. The following amounts are usually recommended for adults.

▶ **For upset stomach,** 2 tablespoons or 1 or 2 tablets after meals and at bedtime.

How to take Maalox

• If you're treating yourself, follow the directions on the label or package exactly.
• If your doctor has given you special instructions on how to use Maalox and how much to take, follow the doctor's instructions.
• Don't take more than the recommended dose.
• Shake the liquid suspension well before measuring.
• If you're taking the chewable tablets, chew them well to allow for better absorption. Then drink milk or water.
• Don't take Maalox within 2 to 3 hours of other drugs.

MAALOX'S OTHER NAMES

Maalox is a combination of the generic compounds aluminum hydroxide and magnesium hydroxide. Brand names of drugs with similar generic compounds include Almag, Gelusil, Mintox, Rulox, and Unival. Canadian brand names include Almagel 200, Amphojel 500, and Diovol.

 SIDE EFFECTS

Call your doctor if you have any of these possible drug side effects. Call *immediately* about any labeled "serious."

Serious: bone pain, constipation, appetite loss, mood changes, tiredness, slowed breathing

Common: none reported

Other: mild constipation, diarrhea, cramps, whitish stools
Tip: Avoid constipation by increasing fluids and high-fiber foods in your diet.

 DRUG INTERACTIONS

Combining certain drugs may alter their action or produce unwanted side effects. Tell your doctor about other drugs you're taking, especially:
• Achromycin, Cipro, Hiprex, Nizoral (take 2 to 3 hours before or after Maalox)
• other oral drugs (take 2 hours before or after Maalox).

• If you're using Maalox to relieve heartburn or acid indigestion, don't take it for more than 2 weeks unless your doctor tells you to.
• If you're using Maalox to relieve ulcer symptoms, take it exactly as directed and for the full time prescribed by the doctor. For best results, take it 1 to 3 hours after meals and at bedtime (unless the doctor puts you on a different schedule).

If you miss a dose

Not applicable because this drug is taken only as needed.

 If you suspect an overdose

Consult your doctor.

Warnings

• Make sure your doctor knows your medical history. You may not be able to take Maalox if you have other problems, such as Alzheimer's disease, constipation, inflamed bowel, diarrhea, or liver or kidney disease, or if you're an older adult with bone problems.
• If your stomach condition doesn't improve or if it recurs, consult your doctor.
• Have regular checkups, especially if you're taking Maalox for a long time.

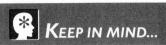 **KEEP IN MIND...**

∗ Don't take within 2 to 3 hours of other drugs.

∗ Take only recommended dose.

∗ Call doctor if stomach condition doesn't improve.

∗ Increase fluids and high-fiber foods.

Macrodantin

Macrodantin is an infection-fighting drug that eliminates bacterial infections, possibly by interfering with bacterial enzymes or by altering bacterial cell walls.

Why it's prescribed

Doctors prescribe Macrodantin to treat urinary tract infections. It comes in tablets, capsules, and an oral suspension. Doctors usually prescribe the following amounts for adults; children's dosages are in parentheses.

▶ **For urinary tract infection,** 50 to 100 milligrams (mg) four times a day with milk or meals. (Children over age 12: same as adults. Children ages 1 month to 12 years: 5 to 7 mg for each 2.2 pounds [lb] of body weight daily divided into four equal doses.)

▶ **For long-term suppression of urinary tract infection, 50 to 100 mg a day at bedtime. (Children: 1 to 2 mg for each 2.2 lb a day at bedtime.)**

How to take Macrodantin

• Take this drug exactly as your doctor directs. To decrease stomach upset, take it with food or milk.
• Shake the oral suspension well before each dose, and use a specially marked measuring spoon to measure doses accurately.
• Take Macrodantin for the full time prescribed, even if you feel better after a few days.

MACRODANTIN'S OTHER NAMES

Macrodantin's generic name is nitrofurantoin. Other brand names include Furadantin, Furalan, Furatoin, Nitrofuracort; and, in Canada, Apo-Nitrofurantoin.

SIDE EFFECTS

Call your doctor if you have any of these possible drug side effects. Call *immediately* about any labeled "serious."

Serious: serious blood problems in people with G6PD deficiency (chills, fever, abdominal pain), Stevens-Johnson syndrome (reddened skin, burnlike rash), asthma attack in people with history of asthma, allergic reaction (closing up of throat, hives, or swelling of face, lips, hands, or feet), hepatitis (yellow-tinged skin or eyes, clay-colored stools)

Common: appetite loss, nausea, vomiting, diarrhea, pain and tingling in fingers and toes (with high doses)

Other: headache; dizziness; drowsiness; stomach pain; too few blood-clotting cells (abnormal bruising and bleeding); bleeding ulcers of mouth, rectum, and vagina; rash or skin inflammation; itching; temporary hair loss or thinning; fever after taking the drug; cough; chest pain

DRUG INTERACTIONS

Combining certain drugs may alter their action or produce unwanted side effects. Tell your doctor about other drugs you're taking, especially:
• antacids that contain magnesium such as Maalox (take at least 1 hour before or after Macrodantin)
• drugs used to treat gout such as Benemid
• other drugs for urinary tract infections, such as NegGram and Noroxin.

If you miss a dose

Take the missed dose as soon as possible. If it's almost time for the next dose and you're taking three or more doses a day, space the missed dose and the next dose 2 to 4 hours apart. Don't take a double dose.

If you suspect an overdose

Contact your doctor. Excessive Macrodantin can cause nausea and vomiting.

Warnings

• Make sure your doctor knows your medical history. You may not

be able to take Macrodantin if you have other medical problems.
• If you're pregnant or breast-feeding, check with your doctor before taking Macrodantin.
• If you're diabetic, don't use the copper sulfate test (Clinitest) to test your urine sugar; Macrodantin may cause a false-positive result.

 KEEP IN MIND...

∗ Take with food or milk.
∗ Shake oral suspension vigorously.
∗ Keep taking for full time prescribed.

Mag-Ox 400

Mag-Ox 400 is an antacid. It decreases the amount of acid in the digestive tract and reduces the activity of pepsin, a stomach enzyme. It also strengthens the stomach lining.

Why it's taken

Mag-Ox 400 is taken to relieve heartburn, sour stomach, or acid indigestion; to produce a laxative effect (when taken in higher doses); or to increase the magnesium level in people with too little magnesium in the blood. You can buy Mag-Ox 400 without a prescription. It comes in tablets, capsules, and a liquid. The following amounts are usually recommended for adults.

▶ **As an antacid,** 140 milligrams (mg) with water or milk after meals and at bedtime.

▶ **As a laxative,** 4 grams with water or milk, usually at bedtime.

▶ **To increase magnesium levels,** 400 to 840 mg a day.

How to take Mag-Ox 400

• If you're treating yourself, closely follow the instructions on the label.
• If your doctor has given you special instructions on how to use Mag-Ox 400 and how much to take, follow the doctor's instructions.

If you miss a dose

If you're taking Mag-Ox 400 on a regular schedule, take the missed dose as soon as possible. However,

SIDE EFFECTS

Call your doctor if you have any of these possible drug side effects.

Serious: none reported

Common: diarrhea

Other: nausea, stomach pain, too much magnesium in the blood (dizziness, weakness, nausea, vomiting, decreased reflexes, slow breathing)

Tip: Call your doctor if you develop symptoms of excessive magnesium.

DRUG INTERACTIONS

Combining certain drugs may alter their action or produce unwanted side effects. Tell your doctor about other drugs you're taking, especially:
• antibiotics, Cardioquin, Dolobid, iron, Laniazid, Lanoxin
• enteric-coated drugs (take at least 1 hour before or after Mag-Ox 400)
• other oral drugs (take 1 to 2 hours before or after taking Mag-Ox 400)
• phenothiazines (used for anxiety, nausea or vomiting, or psychosis)
• Zyloprim (take at least 1 to 2 hours before or after Mag-Ox 400).

if it's almost time for the next dose, skip the missed dose and take the next dose as scheduled. Don't take a double dose.

If you suspect an overdose

Consult your doctor.

Warnings

• Make sure your doctor knows your medical history. You may not be able to take Mag-Ox 400 if you have other medical problems, such as kidney disease, colitis, severe constipation, hemorrhoids, an inflamed or blocked bowel, intestinal or rectal bleeding, prolonged diarrhea, swelling, or heart or liver disease, or if you have a colostomy or an ileostomy.

• If you're pregnant, tell your doctor before you start taking this drug.
• If you're taking Mag-Ox 400 to relieve heartburn and your condition doesn't improve after 2 weeks, call your doctor.

KEEP IN MIND...

* Don't take within 1 to 2 hours of other oral drugs.

* Call doctor if you have dizziness, weakness, nausea, vomiting, decreased reflexes, or slow breathing.

* Call doctor if heartburn doesn't improve within 2 weeks.

Mandelamine

Mandelamine is an infection-fighting drug that also helps to keep the urine acidic. It works by changing to formaldehyde, which has an antibacterial action.

Why it's prescribed

Doctors prescribe Mandelamine to help prevent or treat chronic infections of the urinary tract. It comes in tablets, enteric-coated tablets, film-coated tablets, and an oral suspension. Doctors usually prescribe the following amounts for adults; children's dosages appear in parentheses.

▶ **For long-term prevention or treatment of chronic urinary tract infections,** 1 gram (g) every 12 hours. (Children over age 12: same as adults. Children ages 6 to 12: 500 milligrams to 1 g every 12 hours.)

How to take Mandelamine

• Take this drug exactly as your doctor directs. For Mandelamine to work, your urine must be acidic (pH of 5.5 or below). Before you start taking this drug, test your urine acidity with nitrazine (pH) paper, as instructed by the doctor.
• If you're taking the enteric-coated tablets, swallow them whole. Don't break or crush them.
• If you're taking the oral suspension, use a specially marked measur-

SIDE EFFECTS

Call your doctor if you have any of these possible drug side effects.

Serious: none reported

Common: none reported

Other: nausea, vomiting, diarrhea, stomach cramps, appetite loss, rash; with high doses, painful, bloody, or frequent urination

Tip: Call your doctor if you experience burning or see blood when you urinate.

DRUG INTERACTIONS

Combining certain drugs may alter their action or produce unwanted side effects. Tell your doctor about other drugs you're taking, especially:
• Diamox (a diuretic, or water pill)
• urine alkalinizing agents, such as sodium bicarbonate (baking soda) and sodium lactate.

ing spoon, not a household teaspoon, to measure doses accurately.
• Keep taking Mandelamine for the full time prescribed, even if you feel better in a few days.

If you miss a dose

Take the missed dose as soon as possible. However, if it's almost time for the next dose, skip the missed dose and take the next dose as scheduled. Don't take a double dose.

If you suspect an overdose

Consult your doctor.

Warnings

• Make sure your doctor knows your medical history. You may not be able to take Mandelamine if you have other problems, such as kidney or liver disease.
• If instructed by the doctor, drink cranberry and prune juices. Avoid

foods that make the urine less acidic, such as citrus fruits and juices and milk and other dairy products. Also avoid antacids.
• Drink eight 8-ounce glasses of fluids daily.
• Call your doctor if your symptoms don't improve within a few days or if they get worse.

KEEP IN MIND...

* Don't break or crush enteric-coated tablets.
* Test urine acidity before taking.
* Drink cranberry and prune juice.
* Drink eight full glasses of fluids a day.
* Take drug for full time prescribed.

MANDELAMINE'S OTHER NAMES

Mandelamine's generic name is methenamine mandelate. Brand names of a similar generic drug, methenamine hippurate, include Hiprex, Urex; and, in Canada, Hip-Rex.

Marezine

Marezine is an antihistamine that helps to halt nausea and vomiting. It seems to work by affecting nerve pathways that originate in the inner ear.

Why it's prescribed

Doctors prescribe Marezine to prevent and treat nausea, vomiting, and dizziness caused by motion sickness. Marezine comes in tablets. It's also available in an injectable form. Doctors usually prescribe the following amounts for adults; children's dosages appear in parentheses.

▶ **To prevent or treat motion sickness,** 50 milligrams (mg) orally $\frac{1}{2}$ hour before travel, then every 4 to 6 hours, as needed, to maximum of 200 mg a day. (Children over age 12: same as adults. Children ages 6 to 12: 25 mg orally every 4 to 6 hours, as needed, to maximum of 75 mg a day.)

How to take Marezine

• Take this drug exactly as your doctor directs.
• To reduce stomach upset, take Marezine with food, water, or milk.

If you miss a dose

If you're taking Marezine on a regular schedule, take the missed dose as soon as possible. However, if it's

SIDE EFFECTS

Call your doctor if you have any of these possible drug side effects.

Serious: none reported

Common: drowsiness
Tip: Until you know how Marezine affects you, avoid driving or doing anything else that could be dangerous if you're not fully alert.

Other: dizziness, hallucinations, weakness, blurred vision, constipation, dry mouth, inability to urinate
Tips: To relieve dry mouth, use ice chips or sugarless candy or gum. Call your doctor if this problem lasts more than 2 weeks.

DRUG INTERACTIONS

Combining certain drugs may alter their action or produce unwanted side effects. Tell your doctor about other drugs you're taking, especially:
• alcohol and other drugs that make you relaxed or sleepy, such as cold and allergy medicines, sedatives, tranquilizers, narcotic pain relievers, barbiturates, drugs to control seizures, and muscle relaxants.

almost time for the next dose, skip the missed dose and take the next dose as scheduled. Don't take a double dose.

If you suspect an overdose

Contact your doctor *immediately*. Excessive Marezine can cause sedation, reduced alertness, arrested breathing, and heart and blood vessel dysfunction. In some people, it may cause difficulty sleeping, hallucinations, tremor, or seizures.

Warnings

• Make sure your doctor knows your medical history. You may not be able to take Marezine if you have other problems, such as glaucoma, heart problems, an enlarged

prostate, or a blockage in the bowel or urinary tract.
• If you're pregnant or breast-feeding, tell your doctor before you start taking Marezine.
• Be aware that children and older adults may be especially prone to Marezine's side effects.

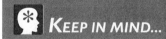

* Take with food, water, or milk.

* Avoid driving and other activities requiring alertness until you know how you react to drug.

* Use ice chips or sugarless candy or gum to relieve dry mouth.

MAREZINE'S OTHER NAMES

Marezine's generic name is cyclizine hydrochloride. In Canada, a similar generic drug, cyclizine lactate, is sold under the brand name Marzine.

Marinol

Marinol, derived from a component of marijuana, helps to prevent and treat nausea and vomiting that haven't responded to other drugs. It works by inhibiting the part of the brain that controls vomiting.

Why it's prescribed

Doctors prescribe Marinol to prevent nausea and vomiting caused by treatment with cancer-fighting drugs or to stimulate the appetite of people with AIDS. It comes in capsules. Doctors usually prescribe the following amounts.

▶ **For nausea and vomiting associated with cancer chemotherapy,** 5 milligrams (mg) per square meter of body surface area (m^2) 1 to 3 hours before chemotherapy is administered. Then, same dose every 2 to 4 hours after chemotherapy for total of four to six doses a day. If needed, dosage increased in increments of 2.5 mg per m^2 to maximum of 15 mg per m^2 per dose. (Children: same as adults.)

▶ **To stimulate appetites of people with AIDS,** 2.5 mg twice a day before lunch and dinner.

How to take Marinol

• Take this drug exactly as your doctor directs.
• Don't take more Marinol than prescribed, and don't take it longer than prescribed. Overuse of this drug can cause physical and psychological dependence.

MARINOL'S OTHER NAME

Marinol's generic name is dronabinol.

SIDE EFFECTS

Call your doctor if you have any of these possible drug side effects.

Serious: none reported

Common: dizziness, drowsiness, unusual sense of well-being, poor coordination, dry mouth

Tips: If you feel dizzy or faint when you stand, rise to your feet slowly. Avoid driving or doing anything else that requires alertness and good coordination until you know how Marinol affects you.

Other: sense of unreality, disorientation, hallucinations, headache, irritability, weakness, memory lapse, muddled thinking, paranoia, disturbances in sensations or perceptions, numbness or tingling sensations, fast pulse, vision disturbances

DRUG INTERACTIONS

Combining certain drugs may alter their action or produce unwanted side effects. Tell your doctor about other drugs you're taking, especially:
• alcohol and other drugs that make you relaxed or sleepy, such as cold and allergy medicines, sedatives, tranquilizers, narcotic pain relievers, barbiturates, drugs to control seizures, and muscle relaxants.

If you miss a dose

Take the missed dose as soon as possible. But if it's almost time for the next dose, skip the missed dose and take the next dose as scheduled. Don't take a double dose.

If you suspect an overdose

Consult your doctor.

Warnings

• Make sure your doctor knows your medical history. You may not be able to take Marinol if you have heart disease, high blood pressure, a mental disorder, or a history of drug or alcohol abuse.
• Don't use Marinol if you've ever had a bad reaction to sesame oil or marijuana.
• If you're pregnant or breast-feeding, tell your doctor before you start taking Marinol.
• Be aware that children and older adults may be especially prone to Marinol's side effects.
• Be aware that Marinol's effects may last for days after you take a dose.

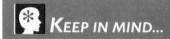

KEEP IN MIND...

* Avoid driving until you know how you react to drug.
* Stand up slowly to avoid dizziness.
* Don't overuse to avoid drug dependence.
* Drug's effects may last for days after taking a dose.

Marplan

Marplan is one of a group of antidepressants called MAO inhibitors. It works by blocking the action of monoamine oxidase, an enzyme in the brain.

Why it's prescribed

Doctors prescribe Marplan to treat depression. It comes in tablets. Doctors usually prescribe the following amounts for adults.

▶ **For depression,** 30 milligrams (mg) a day as a single dose or divided into equal doses, reduced to 10 to 20 mg a day when condition improves.

How to take Marplan

• Take this drug exactly as your doctor directs. You may take it with or without food.
• Don't stop taking Marplan suddenly because this can cause restlessness, anxiety, hallucinations, headache, and weakness. Instead, call your doctor, who will tell you how to reduce your dosage gradually before stopping completely.

If you miss a dose

Take the missed dose as soon as possible. However, if it's within 2 hours of the next dose, skip the missed dose and take the next dose as scheduled. Don't take a double dose.

 If you suspect an overdose

Contact your doctor *immediately.* Excessive Marplan can cause palpi-

MARPLAN'S OTHER NAME

Marplan's generic name is isocarboxazid.

 SIDE EFFECTS

Call your doctor if you have any of these possible drug side effects. Call *immediately* about any labeled "serious."

Serious: irregular heartbeats

Common: dizziness when standing up
Tip: To prevent dizziness when standing up, rise to your feet slowly.

Other: vertigo, weakness, hyperactivity, increased reflexes, tremor, muscle twitching, mania, difficulty sleeping, confusion, poor memory, fatigue, increased blood pressure (headache, blurred vision, nosebleeds), dry mouth, appetite loss, nausea, diarrhea, constipation, rash, swelling of lower legs, sweating, weight changes, changes in sex drive
Tip: Avoid driving and other dangerous activities that require clear vision until you know how Marplan affects you.

 DRUG AND FOOD INTERACTIONS

Combining certain drugs and foods may alter drug action or produce unwanted side effects. Tell your doctor about your diet and other drugs you're taking, especially:
• alcohol and other drugs that make you relaxed or sleepy, such as sedatives, barbiturates, tranquilizers, narcotic pain relievers, muscle relaxants, and cold and allergy medicines
• amphetamines
• blood pressure drugs
• diabetes drugs, including insulin
• foods and beverages that contain caffeine (such as chocolate, coffee, cola, and tea)
• foods high in tyramine or tryptophan, such as fava or broad beans, aged cheese, Chianti wine, beer, avocados, chicken livers, chocolate, bananas, soy sauce, smoked or pickled meat, meat tenderizers, salami, and bologna
• Larodopa
• other drugs for depression
• Ritalin.

tations, rapid and irregular heartbeat, frequent severe headaches, severe low blood pressure (extreme dizziness and weakness), insomnia, restlessness, anxiety, irritability, confusion, and seizures.

Warnings

• Make sure your doctor knows your medical history. You may not be able to take Marplan if you have other problems, such as heart or

Continued on next page ▶

blood vessel disease, chest pain, high blood pressure, Parkinson's disease, kidney or liver disease, an overactive thyroid, pheochromocytoma, diabetes, seizures, mental illness, asthma, bronchitis, or frequent or severe headaches; if you abuse alcohol; or if you've recently had a heart attack or stroke.

• If you're pregnant or breast-feeding, tell your doctor before you start taking Marplan.

• Be aware that older adults may be especially prone to Marplan's side effects.

• If you're diabetic, be aware that Marplan may change the amount of insulin or other diabetes drugs that you need.

• Don't take any other drugs, especially nonprescription drugs, without first consulting your doctor. Combining other drugs with Marplan can be dangerous.

• To avoid a severe rise in blood pressure and other serious problems, you must avoid certain foods, beverages, and drugs while taking Marplan and for 14 days afterward. Ask your doctor for a complete list of foods, beverages, and drugs to avoid.

• Before undergoing surgery (including dental surgery), tell your doctor or dentist that you're taking Marplan.

KEEP IN MIND...

* Don't stop taking drug abruptly.

* Can be taken with or without food.

* Don't take other drugs without doctor's approval.

* Don't eat foods high in tyramine or tryptophan.

Matulane

Matulane is a cancer-fighting drug that stops the growth of cancer cells by damaging their chromosomes and preventing them from producing protein and basic genetic material.

Why it's prescribed

Doctors prescribe Matulane to treat several types of cancer. It comes in capsules. Doctors usually prescribe the following amounts for adults; children's dosage appears in parentheses. (Dosages differ with the individual, depending on body weight and on other drugs that are prescribed with Matulane. For example, the MOPP regimen includes Mustargen, Oncovin, Matulane, and prednisone.)

▶ **For Hodgkin's disease and other cancers treated with MOPP regimen,** 2 to 4 milligrams (mg) for each 2.2 pounds (lb) of body weight daily in a single dose or divided into equal doses for first week. Then 4 to 6 mg for each 2.2 lb daily until white blood cell count or platelet count falls below a certain level. After these blood counts improve, maintenance dosage of 1 to 2 mg for each 2.2 lb a day is resumed. (Children: 50 mg for each square meter [m^2] of body surface a day for first week; then 100 mg per m^2 until response or toxicity occurs. Maintenance dosage is 50 mg per m^2 a day.)

MATULANE'S OTHER NAMES

Matulane's generic name is procarbazine hydrochloride. Another brand name is Natulan.

SIDE EFFECTS

Call your doctor if you have any of these possible drug side effects. Call *immediately* about any labeled "serious."

Serious: abnormal bleeding (easy bruising, nosebleeds, bleeding gums, or black, tarry stools), infection, fever, sore throat, fatigue, difficulty breathing, chest pain, dry cough, rapid or irregular heartbeat, severe headache, stiff neck

Common: hallucinations, nausea, vomiting
Tips: To reduce nausea and vomiting, take Matulane at bedtime or divided into equal doses. Ask your doctor or pharmacist about other ways to ease nausea and vomiting.

Other: nervousness, depression, difficulty sleeping, nightmares, numbness or tingling sensations, confusion, seizures, blurred vision, abnormal sensitivity to light, appetite loss, mouth sores, dry mouth, difficulty swallowing, diarrhea, constipation, skin inflammation, hair loss or thinning
Tips: Use sugarless gum, or hard candy or ice chips to relieve dry mouth. If diarrhea or constipation becomes bothersome, call your doctor.

DRUG AND FOOD INTERACTIONS

Combining certain drugs and foods may alter drug action or produce unwanted side effects. Tell your doctor about your diet and other drugs you're taking, especially:
• alcohol and other drugs that make you relaxed or sleepy, such as cold and allergy medicines, sedatives, tranquilizers, narcotic pain relievers, barbiturates, drugs to control seizures, and muscle relaxants
• decongestants
• drugs and foods high in tyramine, such as Chianti wine and aged cheese
• Lanoxin
• local anesthetics such as lidocaine
• tricyclic antidepressants such as Elavil.

How to take Matulane

• Take this drug exactly as your doctor directs. Don't take more or less than indicated, and don't take it more often than indicated.
• Don't stop taking Matulane, even if it makes you feel ill, without consulting your doctor.

If you miss a dose

If you remember within a few hours, take the missed dose immediately. However, if you don't remember for several hours or until it's almost time for the next dose,

Continued on next page ▶

skip the missed dose and take the next dose as scheduled. Don't take a double dose.

If you suspect an overdose

Contact your doctor *immediately*. Excessive Matulane can cause nausea, vomiting, muscle and joint pain, fever, weakness, skin inflammation, hair loss, numbness or tingling sensations, hallucinations, tremor, seizures, coma, and bone marrow suppression (fatigue, dizziness, bleeding, bruising, fever, susceptibility to infection).

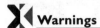 Warnings

• Make sure your doctor knows your medical history. You may not be able to take Matulane if you have other problems, such as heart or blood vessel disease, chest pain, diabetes, seizures, an infection, or liver or kidney disease.

• Tell your doctor if you're pregnant or breast-feeding or if you intend to have children in the future.

• Be aware that older adults may be especially prone to Matulane's side effects.

• If you're diabetic, be aware that Matulane can change the amount of diabetes drugs you need.

• If you vomit soon after taking a dose, check with your doctor to find out whether you should take another dose right away or wait until it's time for the next scheduled dose.

• Check with your doctor before you receive vaccinations or take new drugs, even aspirin.

• Ask your doctor to give you a complete list of foods to avoid.

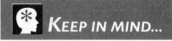 KEEP IN MIND...

* Take at bedtime or divided into equal doses to reduce nausea and vomiting.

* Avoid foods high in tyramine.

* Call doctor if you have symptoms of infection or bleeding.

* Don't stop taking without consulting your doctor.

Maxair

Maxair is a bronchodilator, a drug that widens the air passages and makes breathing easier. It works by stimulating special cell structures called beta receptors, which cause smooth muscles in the lungs to relax.

Why it's prescribed

Doctors prescribe Maxair to treat symptoms of asthma, chronic bronchitis, emphysema, and other lung diseases. It comes in an aerosol inhaler. Doctors usually prescribe the following amounts for adults and children age 12 and older.

▶ **To prevent or reverse asthma or bronchospasm (wheezing),** 1 or 2 inhalations (0.2 to 0.4 milligrams), repeated every 4 to 6 hours. Don't exceed 12 inhalations a day.

How to use Maxair

• Follow your doctor's instructions for using Maxair. Don't use more of it or use it more often than prescribed.
• Shake the aerosol canister well before each use. Keep the spray away from your eyes because it may cause irritation.
• Don't take more than two inhalations at one time unless your doctor instructs otherwise. Wait 1 to 2 minutes after the first inhalation to make sure a second inhalation is necessary.
• If you're also using a steroid inhaler, use Maxair first; then wait

MAXAIR'S OTHER NAME

Maxair's generic name is pirbuterol.

 SIDE EFFECTS

Call your doctor if you have any of these possible drug side effects.

Serious: none reported

Common: none reported

Other: tremor, nervousness, dizziness, difficulty sleeping, headache, fast pulse, palpitations, increased blood pressure (headache, blurred vision, nosebleeds), throat dryness or irritation

Tip: If Maxair makes your throat and mouth feel dry, try rinsing your mouth with water after each dose.

 DRUG INTERACTIONS

Combining certain drugs may alter their action or produce unwanted side effects. Tell your doctor about other drugs you're taking, especially:
• blood pressure drugs such as Inderal
• drugs for depression, such as MAO inhibitors and tricyclic antidepressants.

about 5 minutes before using the steroid.

If you miss a dose

If you're using the inhaler on a regular schedule, take the missed dose as soon as possible. Then take any remaining doses for that day at regularly spaced intervals. Don't take a double dose.

 If you suspect an overdose

Contact your doctor *immediately*. Excessive Maxair can cause chest pain, high blood pressure (headache, blurred vision, nosebleeds), and a fast pulse.

Warnings

• Make sure your doctor knows your medical history. You may not be able to take Maxair if you have

other problems, such as heart disease or seizures.
• If you're pregnant or breast-feeding, check with your doctor before you start taking Maxair.
• If the dosage you've been using no longer seems to work, check with your doctor. This may mean your condition is getting worse.

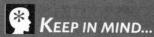 **KEEP IN MIND...**

* Keep spray out of eyes.

* Rinse mouth with water after each dose if throat and mouth feel dry.

* Call doctor if you develop nervousness, dizziness, headaches, trouble sleeping, palpitations, or a fast pulse.

Maxaquin

Maxaquin is an infection-fighting drug. It kills bacteria by preventing them from reproducing.

Why it's prescribed

Doctors prescribe Maxaquin to treat bacterial infections of various parts of the body. It comes in film-coated tablets. Doctors usually prescribe the following amounts for adults.

▶ **For acute bacterial flare-ups of chronic bronchitis or for uncomplicated urinary tract infections,** 400 milligrams (mg) a day for 10 days.

▶ **For complicated urinary tract infections,** 400 mg a day for 14 days.

How to take Maxaquin

• Take this drug exactly as your doctor directs.

• For best results, take Maxaquin on an empty stomach 1 hour before or 2 hours after a meal.

If you miss a dose

Take the missed dose as soon as possible. But if it's almost time for the next dose, skip the missed dose and take the next dose as scheduled. Don't take a double dose.

If you suspect an overdose

Consult your doctor.

Warnings

• Make sure your doctor knows your medical history. You may not

---

MAXAQUIN'S OTHER NAME

Maxaquin's generic name is lomefloxacin hydrochloride.

SIDE EFFECTS

Call your doctor if you have any of these possible drug side effects. Call *immediately* about any labeled "serious."

Serious: seizures, coma, allergic reaction (hives, wheezing, and swelling of face, lips, hands, and feet), heart attack (chest or arm pain, anxiety, shortness of breath), heart failure (shortness of breath, chest pain, anxiety), pulmonary embolism (shortness of breath, anxiety), high blood pressure (headache, blurred vision, nosebleeds), irregular pulse, fast or slow pulse, bleeding in digestive tract, painful or bloody urination, inability to urinate, rash or peeling of skin

Common: dizziness, headache, diarrhea, nausea, sensitivity to sunlight
Tips: Avoid sun exposure during treatment and for several days afterward. Wear a sunblock and protective clothing when going outside.

Other: abnormal dreams, fatigue, overall feeling of illness, weakness, agitation, anxiety, confusion, feeling of unreality, depression, increased or decreased appetite, difficulty sleeping or excessive sleepiness, tremor, numbness or tingling sensations, muscle or joint pain, flushing, fainting, blue-tinged skin, pinkeye, eye pain, earache, ringing in ears, tongue discoloration, dry mouth, abdominal pain, vomiting, gas, constipation, testicular pain, swollen lymph glands, cough, increased sputum, itching, eczema, hives, increased sweating, taste distortion, thirst, back pain, flulike symptoms, decreased heat tolerance, low blood sugar level (tremor, fast pulse, sweating), gout, vaginal bleeding, discharge, or inflammation

DRUG INTERACTIONS

Combining certain drugs may alter their action or produce unwanted side effects. Tell your doctor about other drugs you're taking, especially:
• antacids, Carafate (take at least 4 hours before or 2 hours after taking Maxaquin)
• anticoagulants (blood thinners) such as Coumadin
• Benemid
• Sandimmune
• Tagamet.

---

be able to take Maxaquin if you have other problems, such as seizures, brain or spinal cord disease, or kidney or liver disease.

• If you're pregnant or breast-feeding, tell your doctor before you start taking Maxaquin.

• If your symptoms don't improve within a few days or if they get worse, call your doctor.

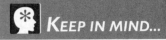

* Take 1 hour before or 2 hours after meals.

* Avoid sun exposure.

* Call doctor if symptoms get worse or don't improve within a few days.

Maxidex

Maxidex is a steroid applied directly to the eye to treat certain eye disorders. It seems to work by reducing the number of white blood cells at the inflamed area.

Why it's prescribed

Doctors prescribe Maxidex to prevent permanent damage to the eye resulting from some eye problems or to relieve eye irritation or redness. Maxidex comes in eyedrops. Doctors usually prescribe the following amounts for adults and children.

▶ **For eye inflammation, for corneal injury due to burns or foreign bodies, or for allergic pinkeye,** 1 to 2 drops into space behind lower eyelid. In severe conditions, drops may be used hourly. In mild conditions, drops may be used four to six times a day. As condition improves, reduce dosage to twice, then once a day. Treatment may range from a few days to several weeks.

How to use Maxidex

• Use this drug exactly as your doctor directs.
• Shake the container well before using the eyedrops.
• Wash your hands before and after using Maxidex.
• To prevent contamination, don't touch the applicator tip to any surface, including your eye. Close the bottle tightly after use and keep it closed.

MAXIDEX'S OTHER NAME

Maxidex's generic name is dexamethasone.

SIDE EFFECTS

Call your doctor if you have any of these possible drug side effects. Call *immediately* about any labeled "serious."

Serious: increased pressure within eye (headache, eye pain); thinning of cornea; poor corneal wound healing; increased susceptibility to corneal infection; corneal ulcers; mild blurred vision; burning, stinging, or redness of eyes; watery eyes; glaucoma flare-up; cataracts; decreased vision; optic nerve damage (night blindness, decreased vision)
Tip: Stop using Maxidex and call your doctor *right away* if you notice any changes in your vision or other problems with your eyes, such as burning, stinging, redness, or wateriness.

Common: none reported

Other: weight loss, nausea, vomiting, dizziness, salt craving

DRUG INTERACTIONS

Combining certain drugs may alter their action or produce unwanted side effects. Tell your doctor about other drugs you're taking.

If you miss a dose

Apply the missed dose as soon as possible. However, if it's almost time for the next dose, skip the missed dose and apply the next dose as scheduled. Don't apply a double dose.

If you suspect an overdose

Consult your doctor.

 ## Warnings

• Make sure your doctor knows your medical history. You may not be able to use Maxidex if you have other problems, such as cataracts, diabetes, glaucoma, a scratched cornea, or herpes or tuberculosis of the eye.
• If you're pregnant, tell your doctor before you start taking Maxidex.
• Be aware that children younger than age 2 may be especially prone to Maxidex's side effects.

• Don't rub or scratch around your eye while using Maxidex.
• If your eye condition doesn't improve within 7 days or if it gets worse, call your doctor.
• Don't share this drug with family members. If a family member has similar symptoms, call the doctor.
• Once your eye infection is cured, don't save any leftover drug or use it for a new eye infection.

KEEP IN MIND...

∗ Shake container well before using.

∗ Wash hands before and after using.

∗ Don't touch applicator tip to any surface.

∗ Call doctor if eye condition doesn't improve within 7 days or gets worse.

Mebaral

Mebaral, a barbiturate, slows down the nervous system, causing drowsiness. It also halts seizures, probably by making the brain less vulnerable to stimulation.

Why it's prescribed

Doctors prescribe Mebaral to control some types of seizures and to treat anxiety. It comes in tablets. Doctors usually prescribe the following amounts for adults; children's dosages appear in parentheses.

▶ **For seizures,** 400 to 600 milligrams (mg) once a day or divided into equal doses. (Children age 5 and over: 32 to 64 mg three or four times a day. Children under age 5: 16 to 32 mg three or four times a day.)

▶ **To relieve anxiety, tension, and apprehension,** 32 to 100 mg three or four times a day. (Children: 1.6 to 3 mg three or four times a day.)

How to take Mebaral

• Take this drug exactly as your doctor directs. Mebaral can become habit-forming, so don't use more of it than prescribed.

• If you're taking Mebaral to control seizures, you must take it daily in regularly spaced doses for it to work properly. Don't miss any doses.

• Don't stop taking this drug suddenly because this could make your seizures worse. Call your doctor, who will instruct you on how to reduce your dosage gradually.

MEBARAL'S OTHER NAME

Mebaral's generic name is mephobarbital.

 SIDE EFFECTS

Call your doctor if you have any of these possible drug side effects. Call *immediately* about any labeled "serious."

Serious: blood problems (fever, weakness, and bleeding ulcers of mouth, rectum, or vagina), slow breathing, skin and mucous membrane eruptions, abdominal pain, weight loss, diarrhea, constipation

Common: dizziness, "hangover" feeling
Tip: Until you know how this drug affects you, don't drive or perform other activities that could be dangerous if you're not fully alert.

Other: headache, confusion, excitation, worsening pain, drowsiness, weakness, slow pulse, nausea, vomiting, stomach pain, worsening porphyria (sensitivity to light, abdominal pain, numbness and tingling), hives, rash, blisters, tiny red or purplish spots on skin, bruising, allergic reactions (facial swelling)
Tip: Consult your doctor if nausea and vomiting become bothersome.

 DRUG INTERACTIONS

Combining certain drugs may alter their action or produce unwanted side effects. Tell your doctor about other drugs you're taking, especially:
• alcohol and other drugs that make you relaxed or sleepy, such as cold and allergy medicines, sedatives, tranquilizers, narcotic pain relievers, other barbiturates, and muscle relaxants
• anticoagulants (blood thinners)
• Chloromycetin
• corticosteroids
• Crystodigin
• Depakene
• drugs used to treat depression
• estrogens and birth control pills
• Fulvicin
• Rifadin
• Vibramycin.

If you miss a dose

If you take Mebaral every day, take the missed dose as soon as possible. However, if it's almost time for the next dose, skip the missed dose and take the next dose as scheduled. Don't take a double dose.

If you suspect an overdose

Contact your doctor *immediately.* Excessive Mebaral can cause slowing of the nervous system, slowed breathing, absence of reflexes, small pupils, decreased urination, fast pulse, low blood pressure (dizziness and weakness), low body temperature, coma, and shock.

⊁ Warnings

• Make sure your doctor knows your medical history. You may not be able to take Mebaral if you have other problems, such as asthma, heart disease, diabetes, depression, suicidal tendencies, an overactive thyroid, porphyria, kidney or liver disease, an underactive adrenal gland, or a history of alcohol or drug abuse.

• If you're pregnant or breast-feeding, tell your doctor before you start taking Mebaral.

• Be aware that children and older adults may be more prone to Mebaral's side effects.

• If you have seizures at night, ask your doctor if you can take the total or largest dose at night.

• If your condition doesn't improve in a few weeks, consult your doctor; don't increase your dosage on your own.

• Call your doctor if you notice symptoms of drug dependence, such as a need to increase your dosage to get the same effects as before or a strong desire to keep taking Mebaral.

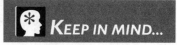 KEEP IN MIND...

∗ For seizures, take daily in regularly spaced doses.

∗ Don't stop taking suddenly.

∗ Don't take more than prescribed.

Meclomen

Meclomen is a nonsteroidal anti-inflammatory drug (NSAID). It seems to reduce pain, inflammation, and fever by interfering with the production and action of certain body substances.

Why it's prescribed

Doctors prescribe Meclomen to relieve pain, treat menstrual discomfort, and relieve symptoms of arthritis. It comes in capsules. Doctors usually prescribe the following amounts for adults.

▶ **For rheumatoid arthritis and osteoarthritis,** 200 to 400 milligrams (mg) a day divided into three or four equal doses.

▶ **For mild to moderate pain,** 50 to 100 mg every 4 to 6 hours. Maximum dosage is 400 mg a day.

▶ **For menstrual discomfort,** 100 mg three times a day.

How to take Meclomen

• Take this drug exactly as your doctor directs.

• Take the capsules with 8 ounces of water; then stay upright for 15 to 30 minutes.

• If you're taking Meclomen for arthritis, be sure to take it regularly for best results. It may take several weeks before you start to feel better.

If you miss a dose

If you take Meclomen regularly, take the missed dose as soon as possible. But if it's almost time for the next dose, skip the missed dose and

MECLOMEN'S OTHER NAME

Meclomen's generic name is meclofenamate.

SIDE EFFECTS

Call your doctor if you have any of these possible drug side effects. Call *immediately* about any labeled "serious."

Serious: stomach ulcer (abdominal pain, bloody vomit), liver damage (abdominal pain, nausea, vomiting, yellow-tinged skin and eyes), blood problems (fever, weakness, bleeding ulcers of mouth, rectum, or vagina), aplastic anemia (bleeding, bruising, signs of infection)

Common: dizziness, headache, stomach pain, gas, diarrhea
Tip: To reduce stomach upset, take this drug with food or an antacid.

Other: fatigue, overall feeling of illness, difficulty sleeping, nervousness, swelling, blurred vision, eye irritation, nausea, vomiting, hemorrhage (feeling faint, cool or clammy, fast heartbeat, bleeding), painful or bloody urination, pain in side, infection, abnormal bleeding, rash, hives

DRUG INTERACTIONS

Combining certain drugs may alter their action or produce unwanted side effects. Tell your doctor about other drugs you're taking, especially:

• alcohol
• anticoagulants (blood thinners) such as Coumadin
• aspirin
• corticosteroids
• diuretics (water pills)
• drugs for high blood pressure
• other NSAIDs such as Advil.

take the next dose as scheduled. Don't take a double dose.

If you suspect an overdose

Contact your doctor *immediately*. Excessive Meclomen can cause restlessness, agitation, irrational behavior, and seizures.

 ## Warnings

• Make sure your doctor knows your medical history. You may not be able to take Meclomen if you have other medical problems or if you've ever had a bad reaction to aspirin or another pain reliever.

• If you're pregnant or breast-feeding, tell your doctor before you start taking Meclomen.

• Be aware that older adults may be especially prone to Meclomen's side effects.

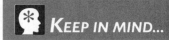

KEEP IN MIND...

* Take with full glass of water.

* Stay upright for 15 to 30 minutes after taking drug.

* To reduce stomach upset, take with food or antacid.

Medihaler-Iso

Medihaler-Iso is a broncho-dilator — a drug that opens the air passages in the lungs and makes breathing easier. It works by relaxing the smooth muscles in the lungs.

Why it's prescribed

Doctors prescribe Medihaler-Iso to relieve wheezing and closing up of the throat (bronchospasm), shortness of breath caused by asthma, bronchitis, or emphysema. It comes in an aerosol inhaler. Doctors usually prescribe the following amounts for adults and children.

▶ **For bronchospasm or acute episodes of shortness of breath,** 1 inhalation initially, repeated if needed after 2 to 5 minutes. May take third inhalation 10 minutes after second one. Don't take more than 3 inhalations for each attack. Maintenance dosage is 1 to 2 inhalations four to six times a day.

How to use Medihaler-Iso

• Use this drug exactly as your doctor directs.
• If you think you need more than one inhalation, wait at least 2 minutes before the second inhalation.
• Don't use this drug if the solution is discolored or cloudy.
• If you're also using a steroid inhaler, use Medihaler-Iso first; then wait about 5 minutes before using the steroid.
• Medihaler-Iso starts to work 2 to 5 minutes after inhalation. Its effect lasts 30 minutes to 2 hours.

MEDIHALER-ISO'S OTHER NAME

Medihaler-Iso's generic name is isoproterenol sulfate.

 SIDE EFFECTS

Call your doctor if you have any of these possible drug side effects. Call *immediately* about any labeled "serious."

Serious: swelling and inflammation of air passages (wheezing, difficulty breathing)

Common: headache, palpitations, fast pulse, chest pain, high blood pressure (headache, blurred vision, nosebleeds) followed by low blood pressure (dizziness, weakness, fainting)

Other: mild tremor, weakness, dizziness, nervousness, difficulty sleeping, dry mouth and throat, nausea, vomiting, sweating, flushing, high blood sugar level (weight loss, increased thirst, hunger, and urination)

Tips: To avoid possible difficulty sleeping, don't take this drug at bedtime. If your mouth and throat become dry after using Medihaler-Iso, rinse your mouth with water after each dose.

 DRUG INTERACTIONS

Combining certain drugs may alter their action or produce unwanted side effects. Tell your doctor about other drugs you're taking, especially:
• Adrenalin, Bronkaid, Primatene Mist
• blood pressure drugs such as Inderal
• decongestants.

If you miss a dose

Not applicable because this drug is taken only as needed.

 If you suspect an overdose

Contact your doctor *immediately*. Excessive use of Medihaler-Iso can cause very low blood pressure (extreme dizziness and weakness), irregular pulse, severe tremor, nausea, and vomiting.

 Warnings

• Make sure your doctor knows your medical history. You may not be able to use Medihaler-Iso if you have other problems, such as irregular heartbeats, chest pain, heart or blood vessel disease, seizures, diabetes, high blood pressure, brain damage, or an overactive thyroid.
• If you're pregnant or breast-feeding, tell your doctor before you start taking Medihaler-Iso.

 KEEP IN MIND...

* Wait at least 2 minutes before taking second inhalation.

* Rinse mouth with water after each dose if drug makes mouth and throat dry.

* Avoid taking at bedtime.

Medrol

Medrol is one of several drugs called corticosteroids. It decreases inflammation by stabilizing certain cell membranes. It also suppresses the body's immune response, stimulates the bone marrow, and influences the body's use of proteins, fats, and carbohydrates.

Why it's prescribed

Doctors prescribe Medrol to treat severe inflammation caused by allergies, asthma, skin problems, or arthritis and sometimes to suppress the immune response. Medrol comes in tablets. Doctors usually prescribe the following amounts for adults and children.

▶ **For severe inflammation or immunosuppression,** 2 to 60 milligrams a day divided into four equal doses.

How to take Medrol

• Take this drug exactly as your doctor directs. Read the prescription label carefully, and take only the amount prescribed.
• Take the tablets in the morning unless the doctor tells you otherwise. Taking them with food helps prevent stomach upset.
• Don't stop taking Medrol suddenly after long-term use; this action could be fatal. Check with your doctor for instructions on reducing the dosage gradually.

MEDROL'S OTHER NAMES

Medrol's generic name is methylprednisolone. Another brand name is Meprolone.

SIDE EFFECTS

Call your doctor if you have any of these possible drug side effects. Call *immediately* about any labeled "serious."

Serious: congestive heart failure (shortness of breath, anxiety, fatigue), adrenal insufficiency (fatigue, muscle weakness, joint pain, fever, appetite loss, nausea, dizziness, fainting)

Common: unusual feeling of well-being, difficulty sleeping, stomach ulcer

Other: strange behavior, high blood pressure (headache, blurred vision, nosebleeds), swelling, cataracts, glaucoma, increased appetite, inflammation of pancreas (nausea, vomiting, abdominal pain, clay-colored stools), delayed wound healing, acne, skin eruptions, muscle weakness, osteoporosis, unusual hair growth, susceptibility to infection, too little potassium (increased thirst and urination, decreased alertness), high blood sugar level (weight loss, increased thirst, hunger, and urination), growth suppression in children

DRUG INTERACTIONS

Combining certain drugs may alter their action or produce unwanted side effects. Tell your doctor about other drugs you're taking, especially:
• anticoagulants (blood thinners) such as Coumadin
• aspirin and nonsteroidal anti-inflammatory drugs, such as Advil and Indocin
• barbiturates
• Dilantin
• Rifadin
• some diuretics (water pills)
• vaccines.

If you miss a dose

Adjust your schedule as follows:
• If you take one dose every other day and you remember the missed dose on the same morning you're scheduled to take it, take the missed dose immediately; then resume your regular schedule. If you don't remember the missed dose until later in the day, take it the next morning; then skip a day and start your regular schedule again. Don't take a double dose.
• If you take one dose a day, take the missed dose as soon as possible; then resume your regular schedule. If you don't remember it until the next day, skip the missed dose. Don't take a double dose.
• If you take several doses a day, take the missed dose as soon as possible; then take the next dose as scheduled. If you don't remember

until it's time for the next regular dose, take the two doses together.

If you suspect an overdose

Consult your doctor.

Warnings

• Make sure your doctor knows your medical history. You may not be able to take Medrol if you have other problems, such as a stomach or intestinal disorder, diabetes, infection, glaucoma, high blood pressure, kidney stones, a high cholesterol level, an overactive or underactive thyroid, myasthenia gravis, lupus, or bone, heart, liver, or kidney disease; if you have a history of tuberculosis; or if you've recently had surgery or a serious injury.

• If you're pregnant or breast-feeding, tell your doctor before you start taking Medrol.

• Be aware that older adults are especially prone to Medrol's side effects.

• If you have diabetes, you may need to change the dosage of your diabetes drugs. Call your doctor for instructions.

• Be aware that stopping this drug suddenly can cause difficulty breathing, dizziness, fainting, fatigue, weakness, joint pain, and fever.

• Follow any special diet your doctor has prescribed (for example, low-salt, high-potassium). The doctor may also want you to add protein to your diet and take potassium supplements.

• Have regular medical exams so the doctor can check your progress.

• Call the doctor if you experience swelling or a sudden weight gain of 5 to 10 pounds with no corresponding increase in food intake.

• Carry medical identification stating that you're taking Medrol.

• Before surgery (including dental surgery), tell your doctor or dentist that you're taking Medrol.

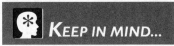

KEEP IN MIND...

* Take tablets in morning with food.

* Don't stop taking suddenly after long-term use.

* Follow special diet if prescribed.

Megace

Megace is a progestin, or female hormone, used to treat certain cancers of the breast and uterus. It works by changing the tumor's hormonal environment and altering tumor growth. It also stimulates the appetite.

Why it's prescribed

Doctors prescribe Megace to treat some breast and uterine tumors and to stimulate the appetite in people with certain conditions. Megace comes in tablets and a liquid. Doctors usually prescribe the following amounts for adults.

▶ **For breast cancer,** 40 milligrams (mg) four times a day.

▶ **For endometrial cancer,** 40 to 320 mg a day divided into equal doses.

▶ **To treat prolonged appetite loss (anorexia), malnutrition, weakness, and wasting caused by serious illness or unexplained significant weight loss in people with AIDS,** 800 mg (liquid form) a day divided into equal doses.

How to take Megace

• Take this drug, as directed, at the same time each day.

If you miss a dose

Take the missed dose as soon as possible. However, if it's almost time

MEGACE'S OTHER NAME

Megace's generic name is megestrol acetate.

 SIDE EFFECTS

Call your doctor if you have any of these possible drug side effects.

Serious: none reported

Common: none reported

Other: high blood pressure (headache, blurred vision, nosebleeds), swelling, blood clots, nausea, vomiting, breakthrough menstrual bleeding, weight gain, increased appetite, carpal tunnel syndrome (pain in wrist and hand), hair loss, unusual hair growth (especially on face), breast tenderness

Tips: To help prevent nausea, take Megace with food. If you experience breast tenderness, avoid beverages and foods containing caffeine, such as coffee, tea, and chocolate.

 DRUG INTERACTIONS

Combining certain drugs may alter their action or produce unwanted side effects. Tell your doctor about other drugs you're taking.

for the next dose, skip the missed dose and take the next dose as scheduled. Don't take a double dose.

 If you suspect an overdose

Consult your doctor.

Warnings

• Make sure your doctor knows your medical history. You may not be able to take Megace if you have other problems, such as asthma, diabetes, seizures, heart or blood vessel disease, a high cholesterol level, kidney or liver disease, gallbladder disease, migraine headaches, depression, or stroke, or if you have a history of blood clots.

• Don't take this drug if you know that you're allergic to it.

• Don't take Megace if you're pregnant or breast-feeding.

• Schedule regular medical appointments so your doctor can check your progress.

• Be aware that your response to this drug will not be immediate.

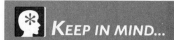 **KEEP IN MIND...**

* Take at same time each day.

* Take with food to prevent nausea.

* Don't take if pregnant or breast-feeding.

* See doctor regularly.

Mellaril

Mellaril is one of a group of drugs called phenothiazines — drugs used to treat such disorders as psychosis, anxiety, nausea, and vomiting. Researchers suspect it works by blocking the brain's receptors for a substance called dopamine.

Why it's prescribed

Doctors prescribe Mellaril for psychotic disorders (mental illness), depression, and agitation. Mellaril comes in tablets, an oral concentrate, and an oral suspension. Doctors usually prescribe the following amounts for adults; children's dosages appear in parentheses.

▶ **For psychosis,** initially 50 to 100 milligrams (mg) three times a day, gradually increased to 800 mg a day, if needed, divided into equal doses. (Children: 25 mg two or three times a day at first, increased gradually until desired response is achieved. Maximum dosage is 3 mg for each 2.2 pounds [lb] of body weight daily.)

▶ **For short-term treatment of depression with anxiety or treatment of multiple symptoms (such as agitation, anxiety, depressed mood, tension, sleep disturbances, and fears),** initially 25 mg a day. Maximum daily dosage is 200 mg. (Children ages 2 to 12: 0.5 to 3 mg for each 2.2 lb of body weight daily divided into equal doses.)

MELLARIL'S OTHER NAMES

Mellaril's generic name is thioridazine hydrochloride. Other brand names include Mellaril Concentrate; and, in Canada, Apo-Thioridazine, Novo-Ridazine, and PMS Thioridazine.

 ## SIDE EFFECTS

Call your doctor if you have any of these possible drug side effects. Call *immediately* about any labeled "serious."

Serious: rigid muscles, fever, decreased alertness, blood pressure changes (dizziness and weakness or headache and blurred vision), blood problems (fever, weakness, bleeding ulcers of mouth, rectum, or vagina), stomach upset
Tip: To prevent stomach upset, take this drug with food or a glass of water.

Common: rapid, wormlike movements of tongue and uncontrollable movements of mouth, jaw, arms, or legs; sedation, dizziness when standing up, eye changes (difficulty seeing colors or at night), blurred vision, dry mouth, constipation, inability to urinate, skin sensitivity to sunlight
Tips: Call your doctor *right away* if you have any uncontrollable movements. If you experience dry mouth, use sugarless gum or hard candy or ice chips. Avoid sun exposure. Use a sunblock and wear protective clothing when going outdoors.

Other: unusual restlessness, fast pulse, dark urine, menstrual irregularities, enlarged breasts, reduced ability to ejaculate, allergic reaction (rash, fever, hives, yellow-tinged skin and eyes), weight gain, increased appetite

 ## DRUG INTERACTIONS

Combining certain drugs may alter their action or produce unwanted side effects. Tell your doctor about other drugs you're taking, especially:
• alcohol and other drugs that make you relaxed or sleepy, such as cold and allergy medicines, sedatives, tranquilizers, narcotic pain relievers, barbiturates, drugs to control seizures, and muscle relaxants
• antacids (take at least 2 hours before or after taking Mellaril)
• blood pressure drugs such as Aldomet and Catapres
• Lithobid.

How to take Mellaril

• Take this drug exactly as your doctor directs.
• If Mellaril comes in a bottle with a dropper, use the dropper to measure each dose. Dilute the dose in half a glass (4 ounces) of fruit juice, soda, milk, water, or semisolid food.
• If you're using the liquid form, shake the bottle well before using.

• Don't let the drug touch your skin or clothes; it could cause a rash.
• Don't stop taking Mellaril unless your doctor tells you to; sudden withdrawal may cause a severe reaction.

Continued on next page ▶

If you miss a dose

Don't take a double dose. Adjust your schedule as follows:
• If you take one dose a day and you remember the missed dose on the day it's scheduled to be taken, take it as soon as possible. Otherwise, skip the missed dose and take the next dose as scheduled.
• If you take more than one dose a day and you remember the missed dose within 1 hour, take it right away. Otherwise, skip the missed dose and take the next dose as scheduled.

If you suspect an overdose

Contact your doctor *immediately*. Excessive Mellaril can cause very deep sleep, coma, unusual restlessness, abnormal involuntary muscle movements, agitation, seizures, irregular heartbeats, fever or low body temperature, and high or low pulse rate, high blood pressure (headache, blurred vision), low blood pressure (dizziness, weakness, fainting, especially when changing positions).

Warnings

• Make sure your doctor knows your medical history. You may not be able to take Mellaril if you have other problems, such as a blood disorder, breast cancer, difficulty urinating, kidney disease, an enlarged prostate, glaucoma, heart or blood vessel disease, lung disease, Parkinson's disease, seizures, stomach ulcers, or a history of alcohol abuse.
• If you're pregnant or breast-feeding, tell your doctor before you start taking Mellaril.
• Be aware that children and older adults may be especially prone to Mellaril's side effects.

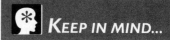

KEEP IN MIND...

* Take with food or water.
* Don't let drug touch skin or clothes.
* Don't stop taking suddenly.
* Call doctor if you have uncontrollable movements of mouth, tongue, cheeks, jaw, arms, or legs.

Mepron

Mepron helps to treat a certain type of pneumonia in people whose immune systems can't protect them from disease. Mepron attacks and destroys the organism that causes this type of pneumonia.

Why it's prescribed

Doctors prescribe Mepron to fight pneumonia in some people with cancer or AIDS. They also give it to recipients of transplanted organs. Mepron is especially useful for people who can't tolerate the drugs usually prescribed for this type of infection. The drug comes in tablets. Doctors usually prescribe the following amounts for adults.

▶ **For mild to moderate pneumonia,** 750 milligrams three times a day for 21 days.

How to take Mepron

• Take Mepron with meals to help the body absorb the drug.
• Take the drug exactly as your doctor directs, for the full time prescribed, to prevent the infection from returning.

If you miss a dose

Take the missed dose as soon as possible to keep a constant amount of the drug in your body. However, if

MEPRON'S OTHER NAME

Mepron's generic name is atovaquone.

it's almost time for your next dose, skip the missed dose and go back to your regular schedule. Don't take a double dose.

If you suspect an overdose

Consult your doctor.

Warnings

• Make sure your doctor knows your medical history. You may not be able to take Mepron if you're allergic to it.

• Make sure your doctor knows if you're pregnant or breast-feeding before you begin taking Mepron.
• Be aware that older adults may be more prone to Mepron's side effects.

SIDE EFFECTS

Call your doctor if you have any of these possible drug side effects.

Serious: none reported

Common: headache, sleeplessness, cough, nausea, diarrhea, rash, fever
Tips: These common side effects may go away as your body adjusts to this drug. However, you should check with your doctor if they persist or get worse. If you experience nausea, try taking Mepron with food.

Other: weakness, dizziness, vomiting, constipation, stomach pain, itching, infection in the mouth
Tip: Drink more fluids and eat more high-fiber foods to avoid constipation.

DRUG INTERACTIONS

Combining certain drugs may alter their action or produce unwanted side effects. Tell your doctor about other drugs you're taking, especially:
• Coumadin
• Rifadin.

KEEP IN MIND...

* Take the full amount prescribed.
* Take the drug with food to improve absorption.
* Don't take a double dose.
* Consult your doctor if side effects persist or get worse.

Mesantoin

Mesantoin helps to control epileptic seizures. It works by regulating nerve impulses in the brain.

Why it's prescribed

Doctors prescribe Mesantoin to control seizures. It's especially useful for people who aren't helped by less powerful drugs. Mesantoin comes in tablets. Doctors usually prescribe the following amounts for adults; children's dosages appear in parentheses.

▶ **For seizures,** 50 to 100 milligrams (mg) once a day, increased by 50 to 100 mg at weekly intervals. The usual dosage is 200 to 800 mg a day divided into three equal doses. (Children: at first, 50 to 100 mg per day, increased by 50 to 100 mg at weekly intervals. The usual dosage is 100 to 400 mg or 100 to 450 mg for each square meter of body surface area a day divided into three equal doses.)

How to take Mesantoin

- Take Mesantoin exactly as your doctor directs.
- Don't stop taking Mesantoin suddenly. Check with your doctor if you develop problems while taking your normal dosage.

If you miss a dose

Don't take a double dose. Adjust your schedule as follows:
- If you take one dose a day, take the missed dose as soon as possible. However, if you remember a day late, skip the missed dose and go back to your regular schedule.

SIDE EFFECTS

Call your doctor if you have any of these possible drug side effects. Call *immediately* about any labeled "serious."

Serious: severe blood disorders (marked by fatigue, bleeding, bruising, fever, chills, increased risk of infection), severe skin inflammation and peeling, difficulty breathing, chest tightness

Common: drowsiness, rash

Other: incoordination, fatigue, irritability, rapid jerky movements, depression, tremor, insomnia, dizziness, inflamed eye area, double vision, rapid eye movements, swollen gums, nausea and vomiting (with prolonged use), hairiness, skin sensitivity to sunlight, water retention (swelling, weight gain), slurred speech, lymph node or joint disorders

DRUG INTERACTIONS

Combining certain drugs may alter their action or produce unwanted side effects. Tell your doctor if you regularly drink alcohol or if you're taking:
- Antabuse, Bactrim, Butazol, Chloromycetin, Folvite, or Laniazid
- aspirin and aspirin-containing products
- cold and allergy drugs, such as Actifed and Benadryl
- Depakene or Dilantin
- Tagamet
- Valium.

- If you take more than one dose a day, take the missed dose as soon as possible. However, if it's within 4 hours of your next dose, skip the missed dose and go back to your regular schedule. If you miss doses for two or more days in a row, check with your doctor.

If you suspect an overdose

Contact your doctor *immediately.* An overdose of Mesantoin can cause restlessness, dizziness, drowsiness, nausea, vomiting, rapid eye movements, poor coordination, and slurred speech.

Warnings

- Make sure your doctor knows your medical history. You may not be able to take Mesantoin if you're allergic to it.
- Tell your doctor if you're pregnant or breast-feeding before taking Mesantoin.

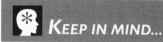 KEEP IN MIND...

* Don't stop taking suddenly.
* Report fever, bleeding, or rash.
* Don't drink alcohol while taking this drug.

Mestinon

Mestinon helps to control — but not cure — myasthenia gravis, a muscle disorder that weakens muscles of the face, lips, tongue, neck, and throat. This drug relieves flare-ups of muscle weakness and fatigue. At times, doctors use Mestinon as an antidote; the drug can counteract the effects of muscle relaxants that are used during surgery.

Why it's prescribed

Doctors prescribe Mestinon to relieve the muscle weakness and fatigue of myasthenia gravis. It's also used to treat infants born to mothers with myasthenia gravis. Mestinon comes in tablets, syrup, and timed-release tablets. It's also available in an injectable form. Doctors usually prescribe the following amounts for adults; children's dosages appear in parentheses.

▶ **For myasthenia gravis,** 60 to 120 milligrams (mg) orally every 3 or 4 hours. Usual dosage is 600 mg a day; maximum dosage is 1,500 mg a day. Or 180 to 540 mg timed-release tablets (1 to 3 tablets) twice a day, with at least 6 hours between doses. Dosage is adjusted according to the person's response and tolerance of the drug's side effects.(Children: 7 mg for each 2.2 pounds of body weight divided into five or six equal doses.)

MESTINON'S OTHER NAMES

Mestinon's generic name is pyridostigmine bromide. Other brand names include Mestinon Timespans and Regonol.

SIDE EFFECTS

Call your doctor if you have any of these possible drug side effects. Call *immediately* about any labeled "serious."

Serious: seizures, tightening of throat, difficulty breathing, slow pulse, low blood pressure (dizziness, fainting), blood clots

Common: none reported

Other: headache (with high doses), weakness, sweating, tiny pupils, abdominal cramps, nausea, vomiting, diarrhea, heavy salivation, increased bronchial secretions, muscle cramps or spasms
Tip: Take with food or milk to avoid nausea.

DRUG INTERACTIONS

Combining certain drugs may alter their action or produce unwanted side effects. Tell your doctor about other drugs you're taking, especially:
- aminoglycosides, such as Mycifradin, Nebcin, and Tobrex
- atropine sulfate, Darbid
- corticosteroids, such as Decadron, Kenalog, and Topicort
- Phillips' Milk of Magnesia, Riopan
- Procan SR, Quinaglute Dura-tabs.

How to take Mestinon

- Take Mestinon exactly as your doctor directs. This drug takes effect 20 to 45 minutes after taking tablets or syrup, 30 to 60 minutes after taking timed-release tablets. Effects last for 3 to 6 hours after regular tablets or syrup, 6 to 12 hours after timed-release tablets.
- Take Mestinon on time, in evenly spaced doses. If you're taking timed-release tablets, take them at the same time each day, at least 6 hours apart. Don't stop taking the drug abruptly.
- For best results, take this drug with food or milk.
- Don't crush or chew timed-release tablets before taking; swallow them whole so the drug is absorbed slowly.

- If you have difficulty swallowing the sweet syrup or can't tolerate the flavor, pour the measured dose over ice chips.

If you miss a dose

Take the missed dose as soon as possible. However, if it's almost time for your next dose, skip the missed dose and go back to your regular schedule. Don't take a double dose.

If you suspect an overdose

Contact your doctor *immediately.* An overdose of Mestinon can cause nausea, vomiting, diarrhea, blurred vision, pinpoint pupils, tearing eyes, wheezing and cough-

Continued on next page ▶

ing, low blood pressure (dizziness, fainting), poor coordination, heavy sweating, paralysis, fast or slow pulse, heavy salivation, restlessness or agitation, and muscle weakness, cramps, or spasms.

Warnings

• Make sure your doctor knows your medical history. You may not be able to take Mestinon if you're allergic to it or to similar drugs or if you have other problems, such as an intestinal or urinary tract blockage, bronchial asthma, or a slow or irregular heartbeat.

• Make sure your doctor knows if you're pregnant or breast-feeding before you begin taking Mestinon.
• Mestinon tablets may become discolored, but this will not affect how well they work.
• Be aware that you may need to take Mestinon throughout your life to control weakness and fatigue. Carry medical identification that lets others know you have myasthenia gravis.
• If weakness and fatigue return, notify your doctor. You may have developed a tolerance to Mestinon.

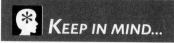

KEEP IN MIND...

* Take drug on time, in evenly spaced doses.
* Don't crush timed-release tablets.
* Don't stop taking abruptly.
* Don't take double doses.

Metamucil

Metamucil is a laxative that absorbs water and expands to increase the bulk and moisture content of the stool. This encourages a bowel movement. This type of laxative is especially helpful for people who are weakened by illness and for those with constipation resulting from childbirth, irritable bowel syndrome, and other intestinal disorders. Metamucil is also used to treat chronic laxative abuse and to empty the colon before barium enema examinations.

Why it's taken

Doctors prescribe Metamucil to encourage bowel movements and relieve constipation. Most people, though, buy Metamucil themselves since it's available without a prescription. The drug comes in chewable pieces, powder, effervescent powder, granules, and wafers. The following amounts are usually recommended for adults; children's dosages appear in parentheses.

▶ **For constipation and bowel management,** 1 to 2 rounded teaspoons (tsp) of sugar-free form or 1 tablespoon of regular form in full glass (8 ounces) of liquid once,

SIDE EFFECTS

Call your doctor if you have any of these possible drug side effects. Call *immediately* about any labeled "serious."

Serious: severe constipation, difficulty swallowing, rash, abdominal obstruction (severe abdominal pain)

Common: none reported

Other: nausea, vomiting, diarrhea (with excessive use); intestinal blockage (if drug is taken in dry form); abdominal cramps, especially in severe constipation

DRUG INTERACTIONS

Combining certain drugs may alter their action or produce unwanted side effects. Tell your doctor about other drugs you're taking, especially the following (all of these should be taken 2 hours before or after Metamucil):

• aspiring and aspirin-containing products
• Lanoxin
• oral anticoagulants (blood thinners) such as Coumadin.

METAMUCIL'S OTHER NAMES

Metamucil's generic name is psyllium hydrophilic mucilloid. Other brand names include Cilium, Fiberall, Hydrocil Instant, Konsyl, Modane Bulk, Naturacil, Prodiem, Pro-Lax, Reguloid, Serutan, Siblin, Syllact, Versabran, V-Lax; and, in Canada, Fibrepur, Karacil, and Prodiem Plain.

twice, or three times a day, followed by second glass of liquid. Or 1 packet dissolved in water once, twice, or three times a day. (Children over age 6: 1 level tsp in half a glass [4 ounces] of liquid at bedtime, or 2 wafers one to three times a day.)

How to take Metamucil

• Take Metamucil exactly as your doctor directs. This drug begins to take effect in 12 to 72 hours, but peak effects may not occur for 3 days.
• If you're treating yourself, read the package instructions carefully before taking Metamucil.
• If you're using the dry powder or granule form, always mix your dose with liquid. Never swallow the dry powder or granules without liquid, and avoid inhaling the powder, which may cause allergic reactions.

• After mixing, drink the liquid mixture immediately or it may congeal.
• Drink lots of fluids while taking Metamucil to enhance its effects and to prevent intestinal blockage. Take a full glass of cold water, milk, or fruit juice with each dose. Then drink a second glass. Throughout the day, drink 6 to 8 full glasses of liquid.
• When using the powder, take care not to generate "dust;" this could cause an allergic reaction.

If you miss a dose

Not a problem. Take the drug only as needed.

If you suspect an overdose

No cases of Metamucil overdose have been reported. However, the

Continued on next page ▶

overuse of laxatives can lead to dependence on them. In severe cases, this overuse can damage the nerves, muscles, and other tissues of the digestive tract.

Warnings

• Make sure your doctor knows your medical history. You may not be able to take Metamucil if you're allergic to it or to similar drugs; if you're on a low-salt diet (Metamucil is high in sodium); if you must limit foods such as bread, cheese, and eggs; or if you have other medical problems, such as difficulty swallowing, ulcers or another digestive disorder, or abdominal pain, nausea, vomiting, or other symptoms of appendicitis.

• Make sure your doctor knows if you're pregnant or breast-feeding before you begin taking Metamucil.
• Before giving Metamucil to children under age 6, check with the doctor.
• If you're a diabetic, check the label and use a brand of bulk-forming laxative that doesn't contain sugar.
• If you're allergic to the contents of NutraSweet, don't use Metamucil.
• Don't take Metamucil before meals; it tends to make you feel full and may reduce your appetite.
• It's important to take Metamucil with at least 8 ounces of a liquid because of the risk of choking.
• Follow your doctor's additional recommendations for exercise and diet. Add bran and other cereals as well as fresh fruits and vegetables to your daily diet.

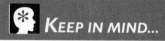

KEEP IN MIND...

* Report abdominal pain, nausea, vomiting, or difficulty swallowing to your doctor.
* Drink plenty of fluids.
* Don't take Metamucil without fluid.
* Don't take Metamucil before meals.

Mevacor

Mevacor lowers the levels of cholesterol and other fats in the blood by blocking a substance the body needs to make cholesterol.

Why it's prescribed

Doctors prescribe Mevacor to reduce cholesterol levels and to prevent problems caused by cholesterol buildup in the heart's blood vessels. It comes in tablets. Doctors usually prescribe the following amounts for adults.

▶ **To reduce cholesterol,** at first, 20 milligrams (mg) once a day with the evening meal. For very high cholesterol, initial dose is 40 mg. Recommended daily dosage is 20 to 80 mg in one or two doses.

How to take Mevacor

• Take Mevacor exactly as your doctor directs. Drug effects last for 4 to 6 weeks after stopping continuous treatment.
• Take Mevacor with food for the best results. If you're taking one dose a day, take it with your evening meal. If you're taking two doses a day, take them with meals or snacks.
• Don't stop taking Mevacor without your doctor's approval. When you stop treatment, your blood cholesterol level may increase again.
• Store tablets at room temperature in a light-resistant container.

If you miss a dose

Take the missed dose as soon as possible. However, if it's almost time

MEVACOR'S OTHER NAME

Mevacor's generic name is lovastatin.

SIDE EFFECTS

Call your doctor if you have any of these possible side effects. Call *immediately* about any labeled "serious."

Serious: blurred vision, fever, unusual weakness or fatigue, muscle aches or cramps, severe muscle breakdown

Common: headache, dizziness

Other: numbness or tingling in hands and feet, blurred vision, constipation, diarrhea, stomach upset, gas, abdominal pain or cramps, heartburn, unusual taste, nausea, rash, itching

DRUG INTERACTIONS

Combining certain drugs may alter their action or produce unwanted side effects. Tell your doctor about other drugs you're taking, especially:
• alcohol
• oral anticoagulants (blood thinners) such as Coumadin
• Sandimmune and other drugs that affect the immune system, such as E-Mycin, Lopid, and Niacor.

for your next dose, skip the missed dose and resume your regular schedule. Don't take a double dose.

If you suspect an overdose

Consult your doctor.

Warnings

• Make sure your doctor knows your medical history. You may not be able to take Mevacor if you're allergic to it or to other drugs; if you have low blood pressure, uncontrolled seizures, liver disease, or a severe metabolic or hormone disorder; if you've had an organ transplant or are about to have major surgery (including dental surgery); or if you're a heavy drinker.
• Before taking this drug, tell your doctor if you're pregnant or breastfeeding, or if you plan to become pregnant or breast-feed soon.

Mevacor can cause serious problems in a fetus or breast-feeding baby.
• While taking this drug, follow your doctor's recommendations for special diet (low-fat, low-cholesterol diet, for example).
• Have regular medical checkups so the doctor can make sure the drug is working properly and detect any side effects.
• Have periodic eye exams to check for cataracts.

KEEP IN MIND...

* Take with food.
* Follow doctor's advice about diet.
* Don't take if you have liver disease.

Mexitil

Mexitil is a drug that's used to regulate heartbeats. It affects nerve impulses in the heart so that the heart beats in a normal and steady rhythm.

Why it's prescribed

Doctors prescribe Mexitil to control life-threatening irregular heartbeats. Mexitil comes in capsules. It's also available in an injectable form. Doctors usually prescribe the following amounts for adults.

▶ **For irregular heartbeats,** 200 to 400 milligrams (mg) orally followed by 200 mg every 8 hours. The dosage may be increased every 2 to 3 days to 400 mg every 8 hours. People who respond well to a 12-hour schedule may be given up to 450 mg every 12 hours.

How to take Mexitil

• Take Mexitil exactly as your doctor directs.
• Take it with meals or antacids to avoid stomach upset.
• Take doses at evenly spaced intervals to keep a constant amount of drug in the blood.

If you miss a dose

Take the missed dose as soon as possible. However, if it's almost time for your next dose, skip the missed dose and resume your regular schedule. Don't take a double dose.

MEXITIL'S OTHER NAME

Mexitil's generic name is mexiletine hydrochloride.

 SIDE EFFECTS

Call your doctor if you have any of these possible drug side effects. Call *immediately* about any labeled "serious."

Serious: new or worsened irregular heartbeat

Common: tremor, dizziness
Tips: Mild shaking and dizziness may go away as your body adjusts to the drug; don't drive or perform activities that require mental alertness until you know how this drug affects you.

Other: blurred or double vision, rapid eye movements, incoordination, confusion, nervousness, headache, low blood pressure (dizziness, weakness), slow or irregular heartbeat, palpitations, chest pain, nausea, vomiting, rash

 DRUG AND FOOD INTERACTIONS

Combining certain drugs and foods may alter their action or produce unwanted side effects. Tell your doctor about your diet and other drugs you're taking, especially:
• antacids, atropine sulfate, narcotics
• Dilantin, Rifadin, Solfoton
• methylxanthines, such as caffeine and Theo-Dur
• Reglan
• Tagamet
• urine acidifiers, such as baking soda and cranberry juice
• urine alkalinizers.

 If you suspect an overdose

Contact your doctor *immediately.* An early sign of overdose is usually a fine tremor of the hands. This progresses to dizziness and later to poor muscle coordination and rapid eye movements as the amount of drug in the body increases.

 Warnings

• Make sure your doctor knows your medical history. You may not be able to take Mexitil if you have other problems, such as congestive heart failure or other heart problems or a pacemaker, low blood pressure (dizziness and fainting), or a seizure disorder.
• Make sure your doctor knows if you're pregnant or breast-feeding before you begin taking Mexitil.

 KEEP IN MIND...

* Take at regular intervals.
* Take with meals or antacids.
* Don't drive until you know how drug affects you.

Miacalcin

Miacalcin helps to treat conditions that lead to bone loss or excess calcium in the blood. It works by halting the mineral loss and physical breakdown of bone.

Why it's prescribed

Doctors prescribe Miacalcin to treat bone loss due to Paget's disease, osteoporosis in older women, and other conditions such as excess calcium in the blood. It's available only in an injectable form. Doctors usually prescribe the following amounts for adults.

▶ **For Paget's disease,** 0.5 milliliters (ml) injected just under the skin (subcutaneously) daily or 0.25 ml every other day.

▶ **For excess blood calcium,** 4 international units (IU) for each 2.2 pounds of body weight injected just under the skin every 12 hours. Dosage is increased as needed.

▶ **For osteoporosis in postmenopausal women,** 100 IU injected just under the skin every other day.

How to take Miacalcin

• Take Miacalcin exactly as your doctor directs.
• Take it at bedtime, if possible, to minimize nausea and vomiting.

SIDE EFFECTS

Call your doctor if you have any of these possible drug side effects. Call *immediately* about any labeled "serious."

Serious: severe allergic reaction (swelling, difficulty breathing)

Common: headache, nausea, inflammation at injection site

Other: unusual taste, diarrhea, drastic appetite and weight loss, increased urination, rash, face flushing; hand swelling, tingling, and tenderness; hypercalcemia relapse (bone pain, kidney stones, increased urination, loss of appetite, nausea, vomiting, thirst, constipation, sluggishness, slow pulse, muscle weakness, pathologic fracture, psychosis, and coma), calcium deficiency (lockjaw), high blood sugar (increased thirst and urination, weight loss)

DRUG INTERACTIONS

Combining certain drugs may alter their action or produce unwanted side effects. Tell your doctor about other drugs you're taking.

• Your face may flush and feel warm soon after your injection; this effect usually lasts about 1 hour.

If you miss a dose

Take the missed dose as soon as possible. However, if it's almost time for your next dose, skip the missed dose and go back to your regular schedule. Don't take a double dose.

If you suspect an overdose

Contact your doctor *immediately*. Excessive Miacalcin can cause nausea and vomiting.

Warnings

• Make sure your doctor knows your medical history. You may not be able to take Miacalcin if you're allergic to this or other drugs.

• Tell your doctor if you're pregnant or breast-feeding before you begin taking Miacalcin.
• If your symptoms subside after 6 months, treatment may be stopped until they return.
• If you're taking Miacalcin for osteoporosis, your doctor may recommend calcium and vitamin D supplements.
• If the drug loses its effectiveness, increased dosages are of no value.

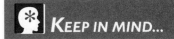

KEEP IN MIND...

* Take this drug at bedtime, if possible.
* Face flushing may occur.
* Take calcium and vitamin D supplements, if directed.

Micro-K Extencaps

Micro-K Extencaps are a type of potassium supplement. This drug replaces the body's potassium and maintains a normal level of potassium in the blood.

Why it's prescribed

Doctors prescribe Micro-K Extencaps to increase the potassium level in people who don't get enough potassium in their regular diet or who have lost much potassium because of illness or certain drugs. It comes in extended-release capsules containing different amounts of potassium. Doctors usually prescribe the following amounts for adults.

▶ **To prevent potassium deficiency,** 2 or 3 capsules a day, or 2 Micro-K 10 Extencaps a day divided into equal doses.

▶ **For potassium deficiency,** 5 to 12 capsules a day, or 4 to 10 Micro-K 10 Extencaps a day divided into equal doses.

How to take Micro-K Extencaps

• Take this drug exactly as your doctor directs.
• Swallow the capsules whole. Don't crush or chew them.

If you miss a dose

Take the missed dose as soon as possible if you remember within 2

 ## SIDE EFFECTS

Call your doctor if you have any of these possible drug side effects. Call *immediately* about any labeled "serious."

Serious: life-threatening low blood pressure and heart block (extreme dizziness), fluttering in chest, reduced urination, cold or graying skin

Common: nausea, vomiting, stomach pain
Tip: To reduce possible stomach upset, take the drug with or after meals with a full glass (8 ounces) of water or fruit juice.

Other: numbness, prickling, or tingling sensations in arms and legs; listlessness; confusion; weakness or heaviness of limbs; muscle paralysis; diarrhea; stomach ulcers

DRUG AND FOOD INTERACTIONS

Combining certain drugs and foods may alter drug action or produce unwanted side effects. Tell your doctor about your diet and other drugs you're taking, especially:
• diuretics (water pills) that decrease potassium excretion, such as Aldactone, Dyrenium, and Midamor
• drugs used to treat high blood pressure or heart failure, particularly Accupril, Altace, Capoten, Lotensin, Monopril, Prinivil, Vasotec, and Zestril
• salt substitutes containing potassium, low-sodium foods, and milk containing potassium.

hours. However, if you don't remember until later, skip the missed dose and take the next dose as scheduled. Don't take a double dose.

 ## If you suspect an overdose

Contact your doctor *immediately.* Excessive Micro-K Extencaps can cause life-threatening heart problems, weakness, muscle paralysis, respiratory distress, and difficulty swallowing.

Warnings

• Make sure your doctor knows your medical history. You may not

be able to take Micro-K Extencaps if you have other medical problems.
• Be aware that older adults may be more prone to high blood levels of potassium when taking this drug.

KEEP IN MIND...

∗ Take with or after meals with full glass of liquid.

∗ Don't crush or chew capsules.

∗ Don't use salt substitutes or eat low-sodium foods.

MICRO-K EXTENCAPS' OTHER NAMES

Micro-K Extencaps' and Micro-K 10 Extencaps' generic name is potassium chloride. Other brand names include K-Lease and K-Norm.

Micronase

Micronase helps to treat diabetes that begins in adulthood (type II or non-insulin-dependent diabetes). Micronase reduces the amount of sugar in the blood by increasing the amount of insulin the body produces. It's used in conjunction with a special diet to lower blood sugar levels.

Why it's prescribed

Doctors prescribe Micronase to treat type II diabetes. It comes in tablets. Doctors usually prescribe the following amounts for adults.
▶ **For type II diabetes,** at first, 2.5 to 5 milligrams (mg) once a day with breakfast; 1.25 mg a day for people more sensitive to the drug. Later, the customary dosage is 1.25 to 20 mg a day in one dose or divided into two equal doses.
▶ **To replace insulin therapy,** if the insulin dosage is more than 40 units a day, starting with 5 mg once a day in addition to half of the insulin dosage.

How to take Micronase

• Take Micronase only as your doctor directs. This drug takes effect in 1 hour, and effects last for 24 hours.
• Although most people take this drug once a day, people taking more than 10 mg a day may have better results with twice-a-day dosage. Check with your doctor.
• Store Micronase at room temperature in a tightly closed container.

MICRONASE'S OTHER NAMES

Micronase's generic name is glyburide. Other brand names include DiaBeta, Glynase Pres Tab, and, in Canada, Euglucon.

 SIDE EFFECTS

Call your doctor if you have any of these possible drug side effects. Call *immediately* about any labeled "serious."
Serious: low blood sugar (shakiness, weakness)
Tip: Carry a piece of candy or sugar, in case you start to feel as though your blood sugar is low.
Common: none reported
Other: nausea, stomach fullness, heartburn, liver disorder, rash, itching, facial flushing

 DRUG INTERACTIONS

Combining certain drugs may alter their action or produce unwanted effects. Tell your doctor about other drugs you're taking, especially:
• alcohol
• anabolic steroids such as nandrolone
• aspirin and aspirin-containing products
• Atromid-S
• blood pressure drugs, such as Catapres and Ismelin
• Butazolidin
• corticosteroids, such as Cortone, Decadron, and Topicort
• Dilantin
• diuretics (water pills), such as HydroDIURIL and Vaseretic
• heart drugs called beta blockers, such as Inderal and Lopressor
• MAO inhibitors, such as Eldepryl and Nardil
• oral anticoagulants (blood thinners) such as Coumadin
• Reglan
• Rifadin
• sulfonamides such as Bactrim.

If you miss a dose

Take the missed dose as soon as possible. However, if it's almost time for your next dose, skip the missed dose and go back to your regular schedule. Don't take a double dose.

If you suspect an overdose

Contact your doctor *immediately*. An overdose of Micronase can cause mild stomach pain, an anxious feeling, chills, cold sweats, confusion, seizures, difficulty concentrating, drowsiness, excessive hunger, fast pulse, headache, nausea or vomiting, shakiness, unsteady walk, unusual tiredness or weakness, vision changes, and cool, pale skin. It can lead to unconsciousness.

Warnings

• Make sure your doctor knows your medical history. You may not be able to take Micronase if you are

Continued on next page ▶

allergic to it or have complications due to diabetes or liver or kidney problems.

• Make sure your doctor knows if you're pregnant or breast-feeding before you begin taking Micronase.

• Micronase is not recommended for children.

• Be aware that older adults and people who are weakened by illness or malnourished may be more sensitive to Micronase's side effects.

• If you're under stress due to infection, fever, surgery, or an injury, you may also need insulin therapy. When switching from insulin to Micronase, you may need to be hospitalized so doctors can monitor the effects of the transition.

• While taking this drug, follow your doctor's recommendations about the treatment regimen, avoiding infection, and adhering to diet, weight reduction, exercise, and personal hygiene programs.

• Follow your doctor's instructions for checking your blood sugar levels and correcting high or low levels. Don't change your dosage without the doctor's consent; report abnormal blood or urine sugar test results.

• Carry candy or another source of sugar to treat mild episodes of low blood sugar. Severe episodes may require hospital treatment.

• Carry medical identification that lets others know you have diabetes.

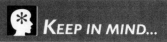

KEEP IN MIND...

∗ Check your blood sugar levels regularly.

∗ Don't change your dosage without your doctor's approval.

∗ Carry candy or sugar for mild low blood sugar.

∗ Carry medical identification stating that you have diabetes.

Midamor

Midamor is a type of diuretic (water pill). This drug helps control high blood pressure by reducing the amount of water in the body. It causes water loss without removing potassium from the body.

Why it's prescribed

Doctors prescribe Midamor to treat high blood pressure and to control water retention in people with congestive heart failure. Midamor comes in tablets. Doctors usually prescribe the following amounts for adults.

▶ **For high blood pressure and water retention**, usually 5 milligrams (mg) a day, increased to 10 mg a day if necessary. Maximum dosage is 20 mg a day.

How to take Midamor

• Take Midamor exactly as your doctor directs. This drug begins to take effect within 2 hours; effects last for 24 hours.
• Take Midamor in the morning to avoid nighttime urination. If you take more than one dose a day, take the last dose before 6:00 p.m.
• Take Midamor with meals or milk to avoid upset stomach.

If you miss a dose

Take the missed dose as soon as possible. But if it's almost time for your next dose, skip the missed dose and go back to your regular schedule. Don't take a double dose.

MIDAMOR'S OTHER NAME

Midamor's generic name is amiloride hydrochloride.

 SIDE EFFECTS

Call your doctor if you have any of these possible drug side effects.
Serious: none reported
Common: headache, nausea, drastic appetite and weight loss, diarrhea, vomiting
Other: weakness, dizziness, abdominal pain, constipation, impotence, too much potassium in the blood (nervousness, irregular heartbeat, shortness of breath, and numbness or tingling in hands, feet, or lips), increased skin sensitivity to sunlight
Tips: Stand up slowly to avoid dizziness. Avoid direct sunlight when possible, wear protective clothing, and use a sunblock with a skin protection factor (SPF) of 15 or higher.

 DRUG INTERACTIONS

Combining certain drugs may alter their action or produce unwanted side effects. Tell your doctor about other drugs you're taking, especially:
• Eskalith, Lithobid
• heart drugs called ACE inhibitors, such as Vasotec
• nonsteroidal anti-inflammatory drugs, such as Advil and Motrin
• potassium-sparing diuretics, such as Aldactone
• potassium supplements.

 If you suspect an overdose

Contact your doctor *immediately*. Excessive Midamor can cause dehydration and electrolyte disturbance (fluttering in chest, nausea, vomiting, feeling of ill-being).

 Warnings

• Make sure your doctor knows your medical history. You may not be able to take Midamor if you're allergic to it or if you have other problems, especially kidney or liver disorders, diabetes, or too much potassium in your blood.

• Make sure your doctor knows if you're pregnant before you start taking Midamor or if you become pregnant while taking it.
• Older adults may be more prone to Midamor's side effects.
• Before undergoing surgery (including dental surgery), tell the doctor or dentist that you're taking Midamor.

 KEEP IN MIND...

∗ Take in the morning or before 6:00 p.m.
∗ Take with meals or milk.
∗ Don't take extra potassium.

Minipress helps to lower blood pressure. It works by relaxing the blood vessels so that blood can pass through them more easily, which reduces pressure.

Why it's prescribed

Doctors prescribe Minipress to treat high blood pressure. It may be prescribed alone or with another drug. Minipress comes in capsules. Doctors usually prescribe the following amounts for adults.

▶ **For mild to moderate high blood pressure,** at first, test dose of 1 milligram (mg) at bedtime to prevent a condition called "first-dose syncope" (dizziness and an irregular heartbeat). Then 1 mg three times a day, increased slowly to a maximum of 20 mg a day. After this adjustment, the customary dosage is 6 to 15 mg a day divided into three equal doses. If other blood pressure drugs are added, the Minipress dosage is decreased to 1 to 2 mg three times a day.

How to take Minipress

• Take Minipress exactly as your doctor directs. This drug takes effect in 30 to 90 minutes but may not achieve its full effect until 3 to 4 weeks after treatment begins. Effects last about 7 to 10 hours.
• Take your first dose at bedtime. If the first dose of Minipress causes dizziness and an irregular heartbeat, take care not to fall if you get out of bed during the night.
• Take your doses at the same times every day.

MINIPRESS'S OTHER NAME

Minipress's generic name is prazosin hydrochloride.

SIDE EFFECTS

Call your doctor if you have any of these possible drug side effects.
Serious: none reported
Common: dizziness, palpitations, nausea, dry mouth
Tips: Prevent dizziness by rising slowly and avoiding sudden position changes. Relieve dry mouth with sugarless gum, hard candy, or ice chips.
Other: dizziness after first dose, headache, drowsiness, weakness, depression, blurred vision, vomiting, diarrhea, abdominal cramps, constipation, persistent painful erection, impotence

DRUG INTERACTIONS

Combining certain drugs may alter their action or produce unwanted side effects. Tell your doctor about other drugs you're taking, especially:
• heart drugs called beta blockers, such as Inderal and Tenormin.

• Don't stop taking Minipress suddenly; if mildly unpleasant side effects occur, check with your doctor.

If you miss a dose

Take the missed dose as soon as possible. However, if it's almost time for your next dose, skip the missed dose and take your next dose on schedule. Don't take a double dose.

If you suspect an overdose

Contact your doctor *immediately.* Excessive Minipress can cause low blood pressure (dizziness, fainting) and drowsiness.

Warnings

• Make sure your doctor knows your medical history. You may not be able to take Minipress if you have chest pain, kidney disease, or a heart condition.

• Make sure your doctor knows if you're pregnant or breast-feeding before you begin taking Minipress.
• Be aware that older adults may be especially vulnerable to side effects from Minipress, particularly dizziness and light-headedness.
• While taking this drug, follow your doctor's recommendations for a special low-salt diet, which helps keep blood pressure down.
• While taking Minipress, see your doctor for regular checkups, even if you feel well, to check your progress and change the drug dosage if necessary.

KEEP IN MIND...

* Take first dose at bedtime.
* Take at the same times every day.
* Avoid salty foods.
* Don't stop taking suddenly.

Minocin

Minocin is an antibiotic used to treat infections caused by certain bacteria. It's especially useful in treating gonorrhea, syphilis, and other infections in people who can't tolerate penicillin. Minocin works by inhibiting and killing infection-causing bacteria.

Why it's prescribed

Doctors prescribe Minocin to treat gonorrhea and other infections. Minocin comes in tablets, capsules, and an oral liquid. It's also available in an injectable form. Doctors usually prescribe the following amounts for adults; children's dosages appear in parentheses.

▶ **For infections (trachoma, amebiasis),** 200 mg orally at first, then 100 mg every 12 hours or 50 mg four times a day. (Children over age 8: at first, 4 mg for each 2.2 pounds [lb] of body weight orally, followed by 2 mg for each 2.2 lb every 12 hours.)

▶ **For gonorrhea,** at first, 200 mg orally, then 100 mg every 12 hours for at least 4 days.

▶ **For syphilis,** at first, 200 mg orally, then 100 mg every 12 hours for 10 to 15 days.

▶ **For person who carries but hasn't been infected by certain bacteria,** 100 mg orally every 12 hours for 5 days.

▶ **For uncomplicated infection of the urethra, cervical area (in women), or rectal area,** 100 mg orally twice a day for at least 5 days.

MINOCIN'S OTHER NAMES

Minocin's generic name is minocycline hydrochloride. Another brand name is Dynacin.

SIDE EFFECTS

Call your doctor if you have any of these possible drug side effects. Call *immediately* about any labeled "serious."

Serious: increased pressure on the brain (headache, sleepiness), severe allergic reaction (difficulty breathing, sweating, chest pain, reddened, burnlike rash), blood problems (bleeding, bruising, fatigue, fever, chills, increased risk of infection), liver problems (nausea, vomiting, yellow-tinged skin and eyes)
Tips: Avoid contact with people who are ill or infected. To minimize fatigue, try to avoid strenuous physical activity.

Common: light-headedness, dizziness, drastic appetite and weight loss, nausea, diarrhea, rash, skin sensitivity to sunlight, darkened skin, hives, blood clots
Tips: Avoid driving and other activities that require mental alertness until you know how Minocin affects you. Avoid direct sunlight and ultraviolet light; use a sunscreen.

Other: difficulty swallowing, inflamed tongue, yeast infection of the mouth and throat (white patches in mouth, pain with swallowing), stomach upset, enterocolitis (profuse watery diarrhea, vomiting, abdominal pain and bloating), anal or genital sores, other infections; permanent tooth discoloration, enamel defects, and poor bone growth in children under age 8
Tips: Check your tongue for signs of a yeast infection. Follow your doctor's recommendations for good mouth care.

DRUG INTERACTIONS

Combining certain drugs may alter their action or produce unwanted side effects. Tell your doctor about other drugs you're taking, especially:

• antacids (including sodium bicarbonate)
• birth control pills
• iron products (take 3 hours before or 2 hours after taking Minocin)
• laxatives containing aluminum, magnesium, or calcium (take 2 hours before or 1 hour after Minocin)
• oral anticoagulants (blood thinners) such as Coumadin
• penicillin, Bicillin-LA, Pen-Vee K
• zinc.

How to take Minocin

• Take Minocin exactly as your doctor directs.
• Take Minocin with food and a full glass (8 ounces) of water. Don't take within 1 hour of bedtime to avoid heartburn or stomach upset.

• Store tablets and capsules at room temperature, away from heat and moisture, in a tightly closed container.
• Store the liquid form at room temperature. Do not freeze it.

Continued on next page ▶

If you miss a dose

Take the missed dose as soon as possible to keep a constant level of the drug in your body. However, if it's almost time for your next dose, skip the missed dose and go back to your regular schedule. Don't take a double dose.

 ## If you suspect an overdose

Contact your doctor *immediately*. An overdose of Minocin can cause nausea, vomiting, and diarrhea.

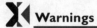 ## Warnings

• Make sure your doctor knows your medical history. You may not be able to take Minocin if you're allergic to it or to other tetracycline antibiotics or if you have other medical problems, such as kidney or liver disorders.

• Make sure your doctor knows if you're pregnant or breast-feeding before you begin taking Minocin. Using this drug during the last half of pregnancy can cause permanent tooth discoloration, enamel defects, and poor bone growth in the fetus. For the same reason, this drug is not recommended for children under age 8.

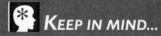 ## KEEP IN MIND...

* Keep this drug away from light, heat, and moisture.

* Take with food and a full glass of water.

* Check your tongue for signs of a yeast infection.

* Avoid contact with people who are ill or have infections.

Miostat

Miostat is a solution that's used in the eye to contract the muscles of the iris. It's used to prepare the eye during surgery and to treat some types of glaucoma.

Why it's prescribed

Doctors prescribe Miostat to cause a certain response of the eye muscles during surgery and for long-term use by people with glaucoma. It's especially useful for people resistant or allergic to other eyedrops. Miostat comes in eyedrops. It's also available in an injectable form. Doctors usually prescribe the following amounts for adults.

▶ **For glaucoma**, 1 to 2 drops in the eye every 4 to 8 hours.

How to use Miostat

• Use Miostat exactly as your doctor directs in the amount prescribed. Miostat drops take effect in 10 to 20 minutes; the effects last for about 8 hours after it's used.

• Wash your hands before and after using Miostat.

• Tilt your head back, gently pull the lower eyelid away from the eye, and drop Miostat into this space.

• To avoid contaminating the drug, don't touch the tip of the dropper to your eye or any other surface.

• Press your fingers lightly on the inside corners of your closed eyelids for 1 minute after drops are instilled.

MIOSTAT'S OTHER NAMES

Miostat's generic name is carbachol. Another brand name is Isopto Carbachol.

SIDE EFFECTS

Call your doctor if you have any of these possible drug side effects.

Serious: none reported

Common: temporarily blurred or poor vision at night or in dim light
Tip: Avoid using machines or driving until blurring subsides; blurred vision usually diminishes with regular use of Miostat.

Other: headache, eye spasm, bloodshot eyes, eye and brow pain, abdominal cramps, diarrhea, asthma, sweating, flushing

DRUG INTERACTIONS

Combining certain drugs may alter their action or produce unwanted side effects. Tell your doctor about other drugs you're taking, especially:
• pilocarpine (another glaucoma drug).

If you miss a dose

Apply the missed dose as soon as possible. However, if it's almost time for your next dose, skip the missed dose and go back to your regular schedule. Don't apply a double dose.

If you suspect an overdose

Contact your doctor *immediately*. Excessive Miostat can cause pinpoint pupils, flushing, vomiting, slow pulse, wheezing and congestion, sweating, tearing, involuntary urination, low blood pressure (dizziness, weakness), and seizures. If a person accidentally swallows Miostat, vomiting is usually spontaneous.

Warnings

• Make sure your doctor knows your medical history. You may not be able to use Miostat if you're allergic to it or to similar drugs or if you have certain forms of glaucoma, eye inflammation, a heart problem, asthma, an ulcer, an overactive thyroid, intestinal spasm, Parkinson's disease, or a urinary tract obstruction.

• Make sure your doctor knows if you're pregnant or breast-feeding before you begin using Miostat.

• If you're using Miostat for glaucoma, arrange for regular checkups by an eye doctor.

• If you have hazel or brown eyes, you may need a stronger solution or more frequent use because the eye pigment may absorb the drug.

• If your eyes stop responding to this drug, your doctor may have you switch to another drug for a short time.

KEEP IN MIND...

* Takes effect in 10 to 20 minutes.

* Don't allow dropper to touch any surface.

* Long-term use may be needed for glaucoma.

Moban

Moban helps to treat severe mental and emotional illnesses. This drug probably works by affecting certain activities in the brain.

Why it's prescribed

Doctors prescribe Moban to treat psychotic conditions. It comes in tablets and an oral liquid. Doctors usually prescribe the following amounts for adults.

▶ **For psychotic conditions,** at first, 50 to 75 milligrams (mg) a day, increased to 100 to 225 mg a day in 3 or 4 days. The usual long-term dosage for mild cases is 5 to 15 mg three or four times a day; for moderately severe cases, 10 to 25 mg three or four times a day; and for severe cases, 225 mg a day. Older adults and people who are ill may be started on a lower dose.

How to take Moban

• Take Moban exactly as your doctor directs in the amount prescribed. This drug is thought to take full effect after several weeks of treatment; effects last for 24 to 36 hours.
• You can take the oral liquid undiluted or mix it with water, milk, fruit juice, or a carbonated beverage.
• Take Moban with food or a full glass (8 ounces) of water or milk to reduce stomach irritation.
• Some people can take Moban in a single daily dose. Check with your doctor.
• Talk to your doctor before you stop taking this drug. Your dosage may need to be reduced gradually.

SIDE EFFECTS

Call your doctor if you have any of these possible drug side effects. Call *immediately* about any labeled "serious."

Serious: sleepiness, difficulty talking or swallowing, loss of balance, muscle spasms, restlessness, trembling hands, liver problems (nausea, vomiting, yellow-tinged skin or eyes), blood problems (bleeding, bruising, fatigue, fever, chills, increased risk of infection), neuroleptic malignant syndrome (rare; high fever, muscle spasms, slowed breathing)
Tips: Avoid contact with people who are ill or infected. To minimize fatigue, avoid strenuous physical activity.

Common: tardive dyskinesia (a movement disorder that causes lip smacking or puckering, cheek puffing, rapid or wormlike tongue movements, and other uncontrollable movements of the mouth, tongue, cheeks, jaw, arms, and legs), drowsiness, dizziness, blurred vision, inability to urinate, dry mouth, constipation, skin sensitivity to sunlight
Tips: Tardive dyskinesia may occur after long-term use and may disappear after stopping treatment or last for life. To avoid dizziness, stand up or change positions slowly. Don't drive or perform other activities that require mental alertness until you know how this drug affects you; drowsiness and dizziness usually subside after the first few weeks. To relieve dry mouth, try sugarless gum, hard candy, or ice chips. Wear sunscreen and protective clothing to avoid reactions to sunlight.

Other: fast pulse, dark urine, menstrual irregularities, allergic reactions (rash, hives, swelling); in men, breast enlargement and inhibited ejaculation

DRUG INTERACTIONS

Combining certain drugs may alter their action or produce unwanted side effects. Tell your doctor about other drugs you're taking, especially:
• alcohol and other drugs that relax you and make you feel sleepy, such as barbiturates (Solfoton), sedatives (Valium), and cold and allergy drugs (Benadryl)
• antacids and diarrhea drugs (don't take within 2 hours of taking Moban).

• Store this drug at room temperature and away from light.

If you miss a dose

Take the missed dose as soon as possible. However, if it's within 2 hours of your next regular dose, skip the missed dose and resume your regular schedule. Never take a double dose.

If you suspect an overdose

Contact your doctor *immediately.* An overdose can cause deep, unarousable sleep, low blood pressure (dizziness, weakness) or high blood pressure (headache, blurred vision), involuntary movements, agitation, seizures, irregular heartbeat or other heart problems, and high or low body temperature.

✕ Warnings

• Make sure your doctor knows your medical history. You may not be able to use Moban if you have other problems, such as heart, lung, or liver disease; a blocked intestine; difficulty urinating; an enlarged prostate; glaucoma; seizures; or Parkinson's disease. You also may not be able to use it if you're allergic to it or similar drugs or if you've ever had brain damage or a head injury.

• Make sure your doctor knows if you're pregnant or breast-feeding before you begin taking Moban.

• Don't give Moban to children under age 12 unless directed by your doctor.

• Be aware that older adults may be especially prone to Moban's side effects.

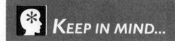

KEEP IN MIND...

* Take liquid undiluted or mixed with a beverage.

* Take tablets with food, water, or milk to reduce stomach upset.

* Don't stop taking Moban suddenly.

* Don't give to children under age 12 unless directed.

Monistat

Monistat is an antibiotic. It's used to treat fungal infections, such as athlete's foot and vaginal yeast infections.

Why it's prescribed

Doctors prescribe Monistat to treat fungal infections, such as athlete's foot, jock itch, and vaginal yeast infections. You can also buy Monistat without a prescription. It comes in cream, powder, spray, vaginal cream, and vaginal suppositories. Doctors usually prescribe the following amounts for adults and children (except when used for vaginal infection).

▶ **For athlete's foot or jock itch,** a small amount applied twice a day for 2 to 4 weeks.

▶ **For a fungal skin infection called tinea versicolor,** a small amount applied once a day for 2 weeks.

▶ **For vaginal yeast infection in women,** 1 applicatorful or 100 milligrams (mg) by suppository (Monistat 7) in vagina at bedtime for 7 days.

How to use Monistat

• Use Monistat only as your doctor directs. If you're treating yourself, follow the package instructions.
• Shake the spray well before applying. Spray it on the affected area from 4 to 6 inches away.
• When using the spray on your feet, spray it between your toes, on your feet, and in your socks and shoes. Don't inhale the spray.

MONISTAT'S OTHER NAMES

Monistat's generic name is miconazole nitrate. Another brand name is Micatin.

SIDE EFFECTS

Call your doctor if you have any of these possible drug side effects. Call *immediately* about any labeled "serious."

Serious: rash, burning, redness, blistering, or other skin irritation

Common: none reported

Other: abdominal pain or cramps

DRUG INTERACTIONS

Combining certain drugs may alter their action or produce unwanted side effects. Tell your doctor about other drugs you're taking.

• When using the powder on your feet, sprinkle it between your toes, on your feet, and in your socks and shoes.
• When using the vaginal cream or suppositories, insert the applicator or suppository high into your vagina at bedtime.
• Use Monistat for the full treatment time, even if your condition improves. If it doesn't improve within 4 weeks or if it gets worse, call your doctor.

If you miss a dose

Apply the missed dose as soon as possible. But if it's almost time for your next dose, skip the missed dose and resume your regular schedule. Don't apply a double dose.

If you suspect an overdose

Consult your doctor.

Warnings

• Make sure your doctor knows your medical history. You may not be able to use Monistat if you're allergic to it or if you have liver disease.

• Make sure your doctor knows if you're pregnant or breast-feeding before you begin using Monistat.
• When using the cream, don't apply an airtight dressing (such as plastic wrap) over the treated area unless the doctor tells you to.
• If you're already using another vaginal drug, consult your doctor or pharmacist before using a vaginal form of Monistat.
• When using the vaginal form, wear a sanitary pad to prevent clothing stains, don't use tampons, and don't use a latex diaphragm or condoms.
• Don't stop using Monistat if you have sexual intercourse during treatment (though it's best to abstain). Your sexual partner may also need to be treated.

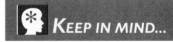

KEEP IN MIND...

* Use only as directed.
* If using spray form, don't inhale.
* If using cream, don't apply airtight dressing.

Photoguide to tablets and capsules

The following photoguide provides full–color photographs of some of the most commonly prescribed tablets and capsules in the United States. Shown here in actual size, the tablets and capsules are organized alphabetically for quick reference.

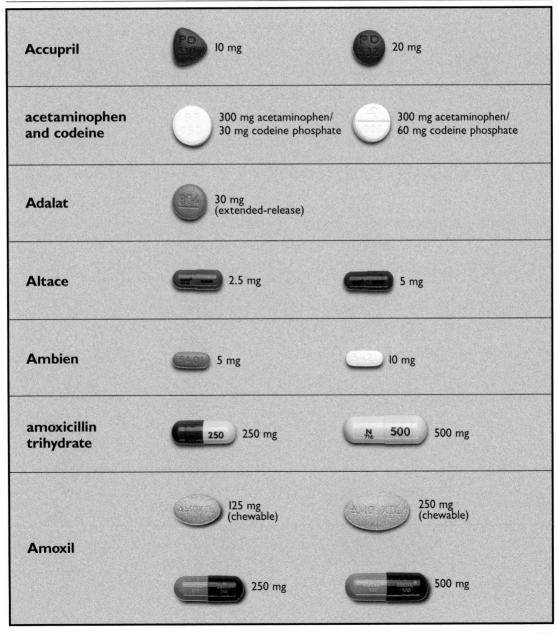

Accupril 10 mg 20 mg

acetaminophen and codeine 300 mg acetaminophen/ 30 mg codeine phosphate 300 mg acetaminophen/ 60 mg codeine phosphate

Adalat 30 mg (extended-release)

Altace 2.5 mg 5 mg

Ambien 5 mg 10 mg

amoxicillin trihydrate 250 mg 500 mg

Amoxil 125 mg (chewable) 250 mg (chewable) 250 mg 500 mg

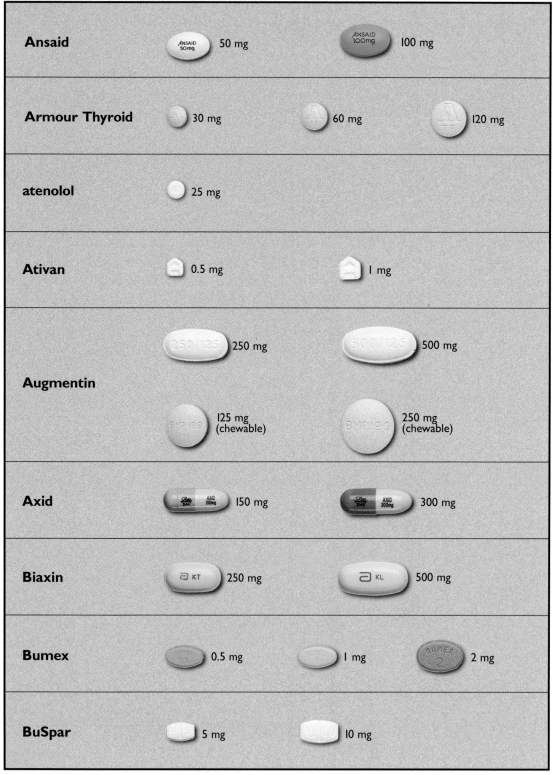

Ansaid	50 mg	100 mg
Armour Thyroid	30 mg / 60 mg	120 mg
atenolol	25 mg	
Ativan	0.5 mg	1 mg
Augmentin	250 mg / 500 mg / 125 mg (chewable)	250 mg (chewable)
Axid	150 mg	300 mg
Biaxin	250 mg	500 mg
Bumex	0.5 mg / 1 mg	2 mg
BuSpar	5 mg	10 mg

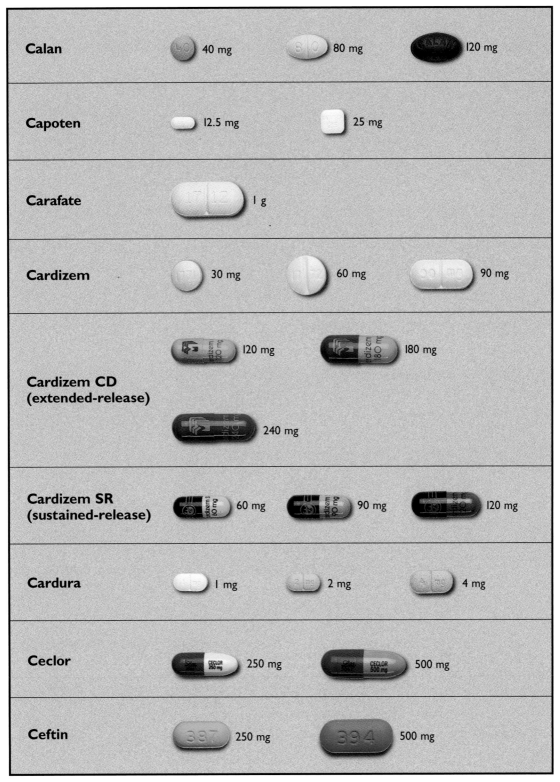

Calan	40 mg	80 mg	120 mg
Capoten	12.5 mg	25 mg	
Carafate	I g		
Cardizem	30 mg	60 mg	90 mg
Cardizem CD (extended-release)	120 mg	180 mg	
	240 mg		
Cardizem SR (sustained-release)	60 mg	90 mg	120 mg
Cardura	I mg	2 mg	4 mg
Ceclor	250 mg	500 mg	
Ceftin	250 mg	500 mg	

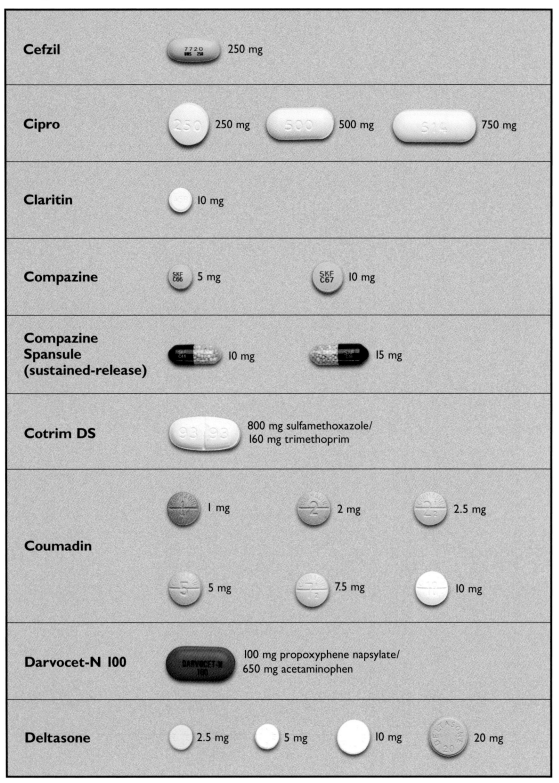

Cefzil — 250 mg

Cipro — 250 mg — 500 mg — 750 mg

Claritin — 10 mg

Compazine — 5 mg — 10 mg

Compazine Spansule (sustained-release) — 10 mg — 15 mg

Cotrim DS — 800 mg sulfamethoxazole/ 160 mg trimethoprim

Coumadin — 1 mg — 2 mg — 2.5 mg — 5 mg — 7.5 mg — 10 mg

Darvocet-N 100 — 100 mg propoxyphene napsylate/ 650 mg acetaminophen

Deltasone — 2.5 mg — 5 mg — 10 mg — 20 mg

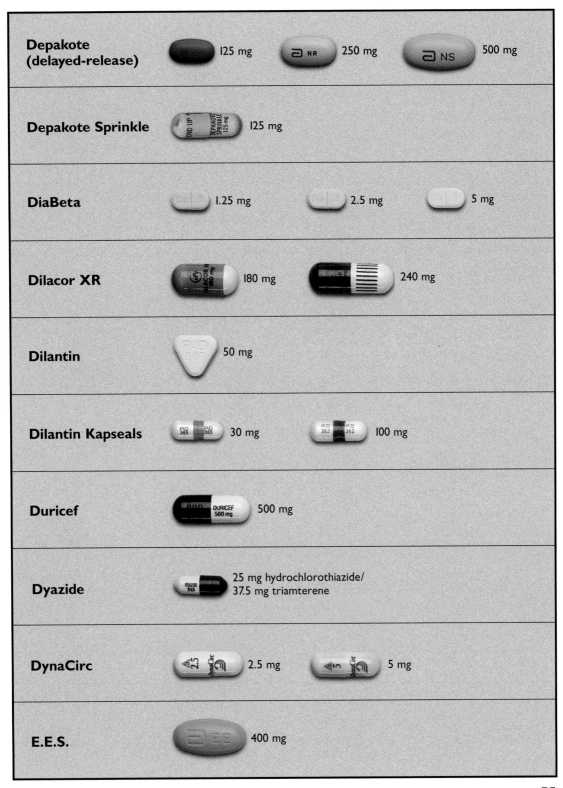

Depakote (delayed-release)	125 mg	250 mg	500 mg
Depakote Sprinkle	125 mg		
DiaBeta	1.25 mg	2.5 mg	5 mg
Dilacor XR	180 mg	240 mg	
Dilantin	50 mg		
Dilantin Kapseals	30 mg	100 mg	
Duricef	500 mg		
Dyazide	25 mg hydrochlorothiazide/ 37.5 mg triamterene		
DynaCirc	2.5 mg	5 mg	
E.E.S.	400 mg		

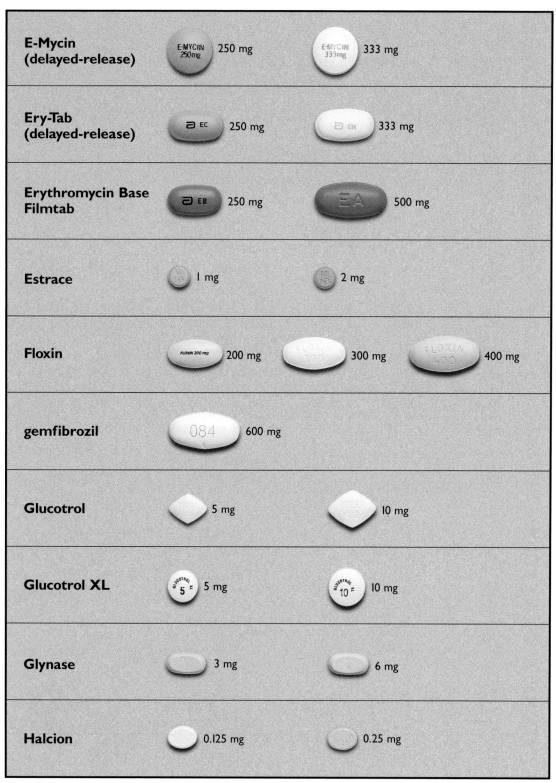

E-Mycin (delayed-release)	E-MYCIN 250mg — 250 mg	E-MYCIN 333mg — 333 mg
Ery-Tab (delayed-release)	EC — 250 mg	ER — 333 mg
Erythromycin Base Filmtab	EB — 250 mg	EA — 500 mg
Estrace	1 mg	2 mg
Floxin	FLOXIN 200 mg — 200 mg / FLOXIN 300 — 300 mg / FLOXIN 400 — 400 mg	
gemfibrozil	084 — 600 mg	
Glucotrol	5 mg	10 mg
Glucotrol XL	GLUCOTROL 5 XL — 5 mg	GLUCOTROL 10 XL — 10 mg
Glynase	3 mg	6 mg
Halcion	0.125 mg	0.25 mg

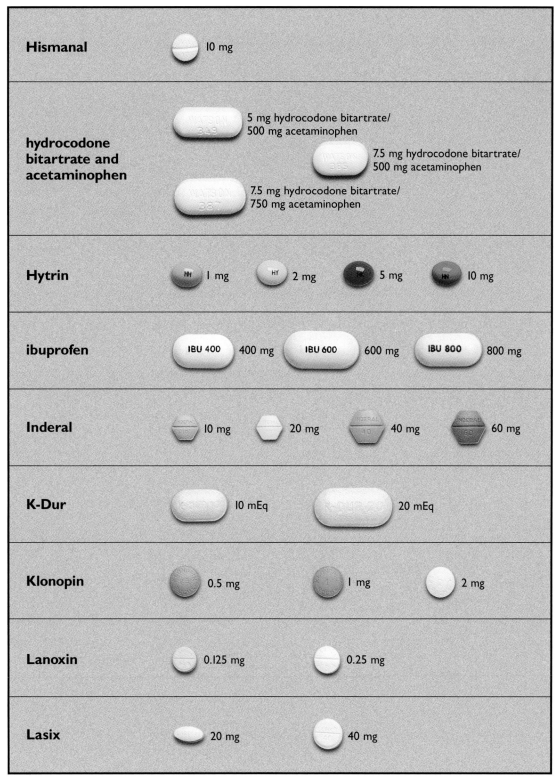

Hismanal 10 mg

hydrocodone bitartrate and acetaminophen
- 5 mg hydrocodone bitartrate/ 500 mg acetaminophen
- 7.5 mg hydrocodone bitartrate/ 500 mg acetaminophen
- 7.5 mg hydrocodone bitartrate/ 750 mg acetaminophen

Hytrin 1 mg 2 mg 5 mg 10 mg

ibuprofen 400 mg 600 mg 800 mg

Inderal 10 mg 20 mg 40 mg 60 mg

K-Dur 10 mEq 20 mEq

Klonopin 0.5 mg 1 mg 2 mg

Lanoxin 0.125 mg 0.25 mg

Lasix 20 mg 40 mg

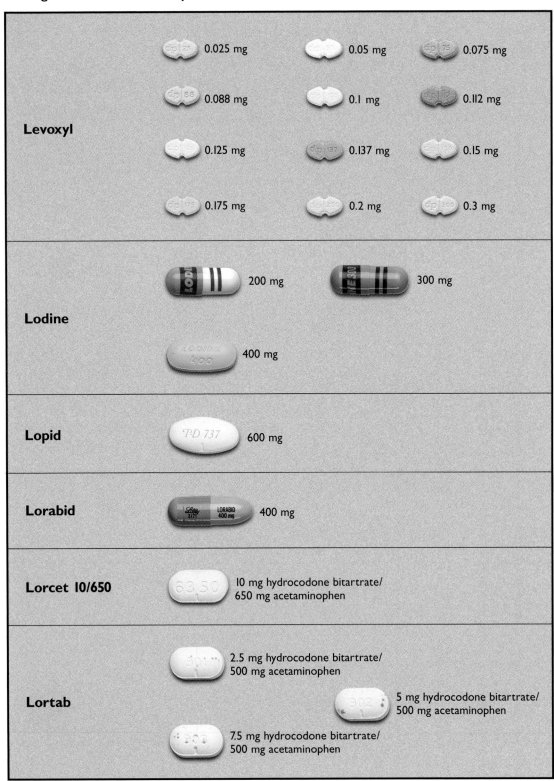

Levoxyl

0.025 mg · 0.05 mg · 0.075 mg

0.088 mg · 0.1 mg · 0.112 mg

0.125 mg · 0.137 mg · 0.15 mg

0.175 mg · 0.2 mg · 0.3 mg

Lodine

200 mg · 300 mg

400 mg

Lopid

600 mg

Lorabid

400 mg

Lorcet 10/650

10 mg hydrocodone bitartrate/
650 mg acetaminophen

Lortab

2.5 mg hydrocodone bitartrate/
500 mg acetaminophen

5 mg hydrocodone bitartrate/
500 mg acetaminophen

7.5 mg hydrocodone bitartrate/
500 mg acetaminophen

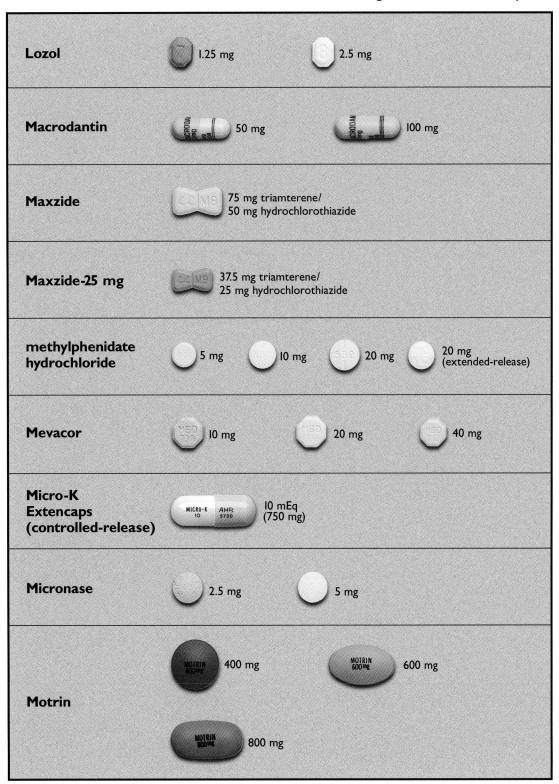

Lozol   1.25 mg   2.5 mg

Macrodantin   50 mg   100 mg

Maxzide   75 mg triamterene/ 50 mg hydrochlorothiazide

Maxzide-25 mg   37.5 mg triamterene/ 25 mg hydrochlorothiazide

methylphenidate hydrochloride   5 mg   10 mg   20 mg   20 mg (extended-release)

Mevacor   10 mg   20 mg   40 mg

Micro-K Extencaps (controlled-release)   10 mEq (750 mg)

Micronase   2.5 mg   5 mg

Motrin   400 mg   600 mg   800 mg

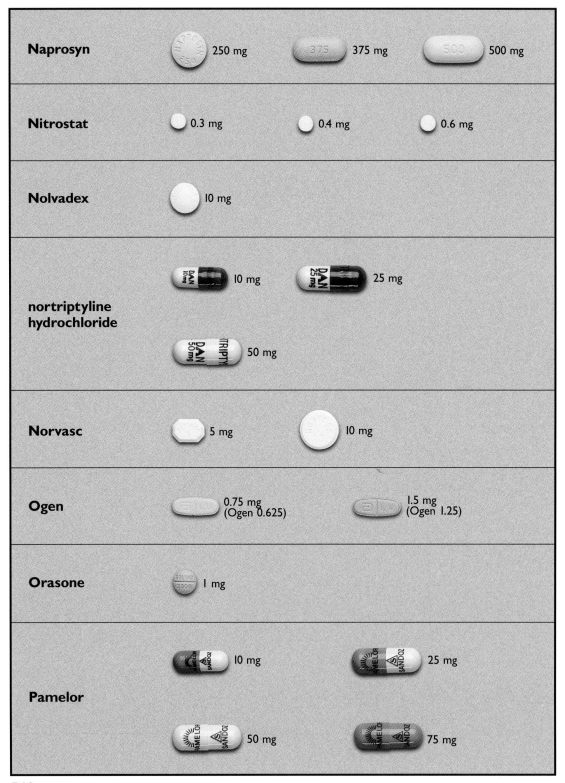

Naprosyn	250 mg	375 mg	500 mg
Nitrostat	0.3 mg	0.4 mg	0.6 mg
Nolvadex	10 mg		
nortriptyline hydrochloride	10 mg	25 mg	
	50 mg		
Norvasc	5 mg	10 mg	
Ogen	0.75 mg (Ogen 0.625)	1.5 mg (Ogen 1.25)	
Orasone	1 mg		
Pamelor	10 mg	25 mg	
	50 mg	75 mg	

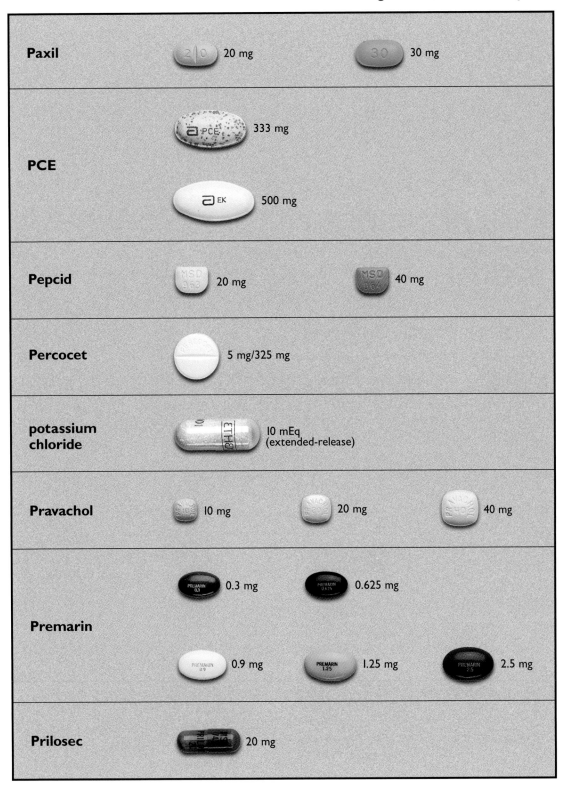

Paxil   20 mg   30 mg

PCE   333 mg   500 mg

Pepcid   20 mg   40 mg

Percocet   5 mg/325 mg

potassium chloride   10 mEq (extended-release)

Pravachol   10 mg   20 mg   40 mg

Premarin   0.3 mg   0.625 mg   0.9 mg   1.25 mg   2.5 mg

Prilosec   20 mg

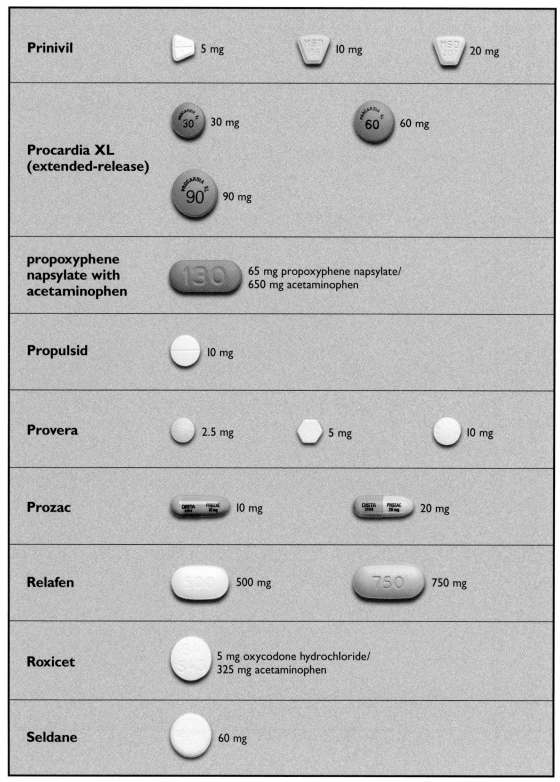

Prinivil 5 mg 10 mg 20 mg

Procardia XL (extended-release) 30 mg 60 mg 90 mg

propoxyphene napsylate with acetaminophen 65 mg propoxyphene napsylate/ 650 mg acetaminophen

Propulsid 10 mg

Provera 2.5 mg 5 mg 10 mg

Prozac 10 mg 20 mg

Relafen 500 mg 750 mg

Roxicet 5 mg oxycodone hydrochloride/ 325 mg acetaminophen

Seldane 60 mg

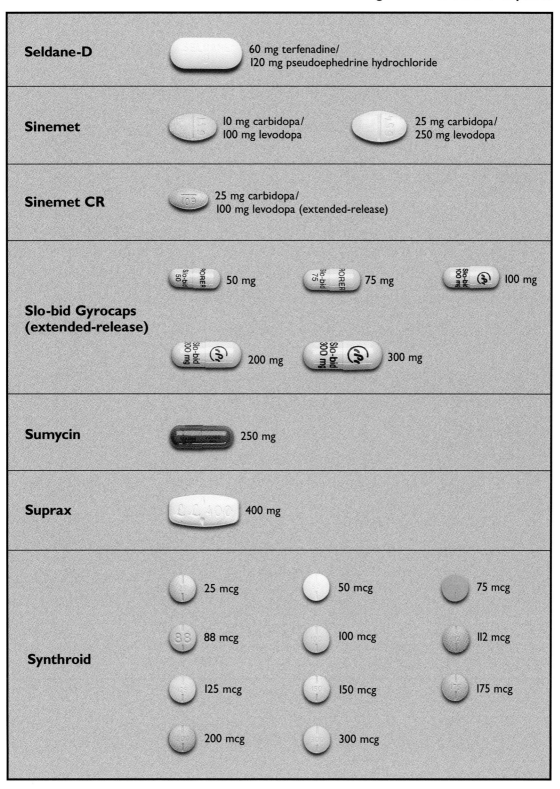

Seldane-D — 60 mg terfenadine/ 120 mg pseudoephedrine hydrochloride

Sinemet — 10 mg carbidopa/ 100 mg levodopa — 25 mg carbidopa/ 250 mg levodopa

Sinemet CR — 25 mg carbidopa/ 100 mg levodopa (extended-release)

Slo-bid Gyrocaps (extended-release) — 50 mg — 75 mg — 100 mg — 200 mg — 300 mg

Sumycin — 250 mg

Suprax — 400 mg

Synthroid — 25 mcg — 50 mcg — 75 mcg — 88 mcg — 100 mcg — 112 mcg — 125 mcg — 150 mcg — 175 mcg — 200 mcg — 300 mcg

Photoguide to Tablets and Capsules

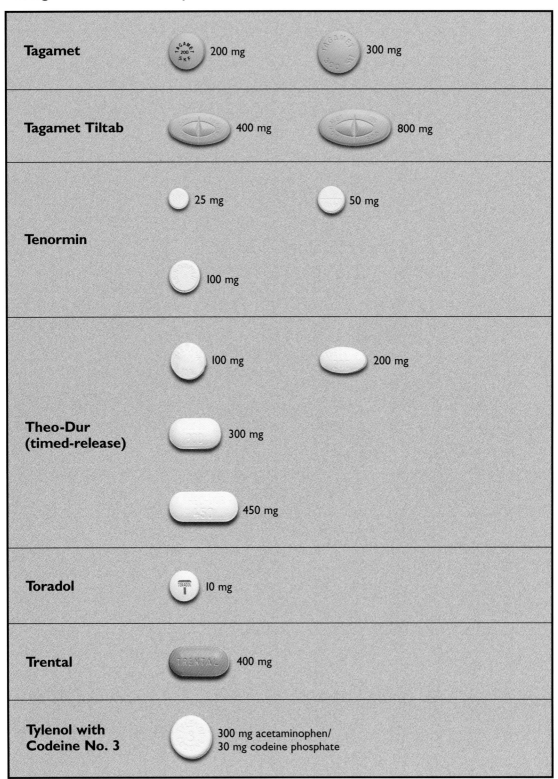

Tagamet	200 mg	300 mg
Tagamet Tiltab	400 mg	800 mg
Tenormin	25 mg	50 mg
	100 mg	
Theo-Dur (timed-release)	100 mg	200 mg
	300 mg	
	450 mg	
Toradol	10 mg	
Trental	400 mg	
Tylenol with Codeine No. 3	300 mg acetaminophen/ 30 mg codeine phosphate	

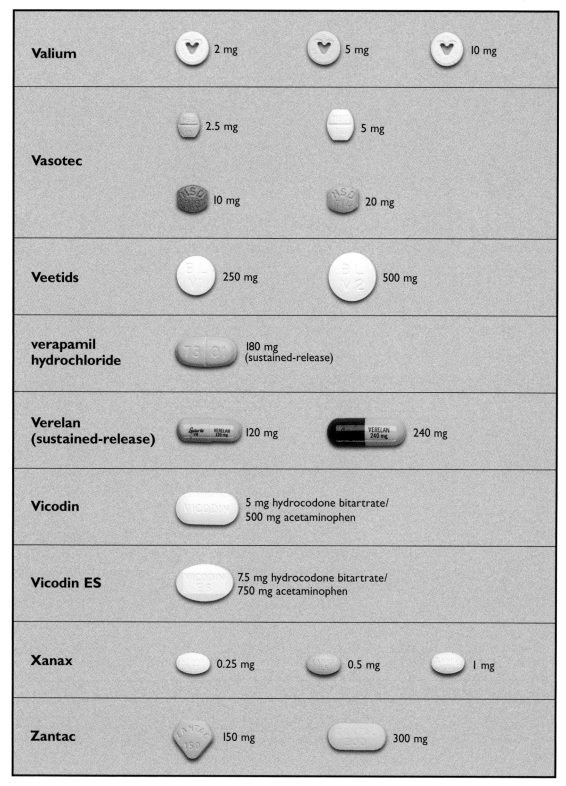

Valium	2 mg		5 mg		10 mg
Vasotec	2.5 mg		5 mg		
	10 mg		20 mg		
Veetids	250 mg		500 mg		
verapamil hydrochloride	180 mg (sustained-release)				
Verelan (sustained-release)	120 mg		240 mg		
Vicodin	5 mg hydrocodone bitartrate/ 500 mg acetaminophen				
Vicodin ES	7.5 mg hydrocodone bitartrate/ 750 mg acetaminophen				
Xanax	0.25 mg		0.5 mg		1 mg
Zantac	150 mg		300 mg		

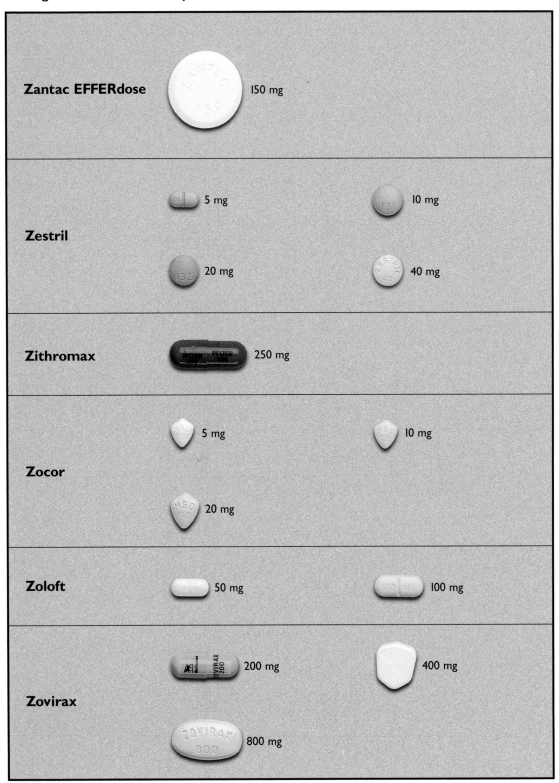

Zantac EFFERdose   150 mg

Zestril
5 mg   10 mg
20 mg   40 mg

Zithromax   250 mg

Zocor
5 mg   10 mg
20 mg

Zoloft   50 mg   100 mg

Zovirax   200 mg   400 mg
800 mg

Monopril

Monopril is a blood pressure drug known as an ACE inhibitor. It works by relaxing blood vessels, which lowers blood pressure and increases the supply of blood and oxygen to the heart.

Why it's prescribed

Doctors prescribe Monopril to treat high blood pressure. It comes in tablets. Doctors usually prescribe the following amounts for adults.

▶ **For high blood pressure,** at first, 10 milligrams (mg) once a day. Usual dosage is 20 to 40 mg a day. Maximum dosage is 80 mg a day. Total dosage is divided into several smaller doses if needed.

How to take Monopril

• Take Monopril exactly as your doctor directs. This drug begins to take effect within 1 hour; effects last about 24 hours.

If you miss a dose

Take the missed dose as soon as possible. However, if it's almost time for your next dose, skip the missed dose and go back to your regular schedule. Don't take a double dose.

 If you suspect an overdose

No cases of Monopril overdose have been reported.

MONOPRIL'S OTHER NAME

Monopril's generic name is fosinopril sodium.

 SIDE EFFECTS

Call your doctor if you have any of these possible drug side effects. Call *immediately* about any labeled "serious."

Serious: stroke, liver problems (yellow-tinged skin or eyes), blood problems (bleeding, bruising, fatigue, fever, chills, increased risk of infection), low blood pressure (dizziness, weakness), fluttering in chest, heart attack (chest pain), palpitations, high blood pressure (headache, blurred vision), bronchospasm (difficulty breathing, facial swelling), raised red wheals

Common: dry, persistent, tickling, nonproductive cough

Other: headache, dizziness, fatigue, sleep disturbance, drowsiness, fainting, memory disturbances, mood changes, flushing, limping, nausea, vomiting, diarrhea, heartburn, appetite change, weight change, sexual dysfunction, frequent urination, hoarseness, hives, rash, skin sensitivity to sunlight, itching, fever, joint or muscle pain, gout

DRUG INTERACTIONS

Combining certain drugs may alter their action or produce unwanted side effects. Tell your doctor about other drugs you're taking, especially:
• antacids (take at least 2 hours before or after Monopril)
• diuretics (water pills) or other blood pressure drugs
• Eskalith, Lithobid
• potassium supplements, sodium substitutes containing potassium.

Warnings

• Make sure your doctor knows your medical history. You may not be able to take Monopril if you're allergic to it or to other ACE inhibitors or if you have diabetes or kidney or liver disorders.
• Make sure your doctor knows if you're pregnant or breast-feeding before you begin taking Monopril. If you get pregnant while taking this drug, notify your doctor.
• If your doctor prescribes a low-potassium diet while you're taking Monopril, don't use salt substitutes that contain potassium. Call the doctor if you develop signs of too much potassium, such as confusion, irregular heartbeat, nervousness, shortness of breath or difficulty breathing, a weak or heavy feeling in the legs, or numbness or tingling in the hands, feet, or lips.

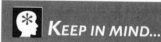 **KEEP IN MIND...**

∗ Daily dosage may be divided with doctor's consent.

∗ Don't take during pregnancy.

∗ Don't use salt substitutes containing potassium.

Motrin

Motrin is a one of a large group of drugs called nonsteroidal anti-inflammatory drugs (NSAIDs). This popular drug relieves symptoms of arthritis and other problems, such as inflammation, swelling, stiffness, and joint pain. It seems to work by stopping the body from producing substances called prostaglandins.

Why it's prescribed

Doctors prescribe Motrin to relieve joint pain, swelling, and other symptoms of arthritis. Motrin doesn't cure the condition. The drug is also used to reduce fever and some types of pain with inflammation, such as menstrual pain. You can buy Motrin without a prescription. It comes in tablets, extended-release tablets, caplets, an oral liquid, and a cream. Doctors usually prescribe the following amounts for adults; children's dosages appear in parentheses.

▶ **For arthritis**, 300 to 800 milligrams (mg) orally three or four times a day, but no more than 3.2 grams (g) per day.

▶ **For mild to moderate pain and menstrual pain**, 400 mg orally every 4 to 6 hours as needed.

▶ **For fever**, 200 to 400 mg orally every 4 to 6 hours, but no more

MOTRIN'S OTHER NAMES

Motrin's generic name is ibuprofen. Other brand names include Advil, Excedrin-IB, Genpril, Haltran, Ibuprin, Ibuprohm, Ibu-Tab, Medipren, Midol-200, Nuprin, Pamprin-IB, Rafen, Trendar; and, in Canada, Apo-Ibuprofen and Novo-Profen.

SIDE EFFECTS

Call your doctor if you have any of these possible drug side effects. Call *immediately* about any labeled "serious."

Serious: intestinal bleeding (dark or bloody stools or vomit), prolonged bleeding from a cut or sore, wheezing, difficulty breathing, Stevens-Johnson syndrome (reddened, burnlike rash), high blood pressure (headache, blurred vision), reversible kidney failure (decreased urination), liver problems (yellow-tinged skin or eyes), congestive heart failure (chest pain, difficulty breathing)

Common: headache, drowsiness, dizziness, puffy arms and legs, ringing in ears, nausea, undetected internal blood loss (pale skin, weakness), stomach ulcer, rash
Tip: Take Motrin with food or milk to prevent nausea.

Other: inability to think clearly, vision disturbances, itching, hives, skin sensitivity to sunlight, water retention (swelling, weight gain)

DRUG INTERACTIONS

Combining certain drugs may alter their action or produce unwanted effects. Tell your doctor about other drugs you're taking, especially:
- alcohol
- anticoagulants (blood thinners) such as Coumadin
- aspirin
- blood pressure drugs such as thiazide diuretics (water pills)
- corticosteroids, such as Decadron and Kenalog
- Eskalith, Lithobid.

than 1.2 g a day for no longer than 3 days. (Children age 6 months to 12 years: if fever is below 102.5°F [39.2°C], 5 mg for each 2.2 pounds [lb] of body weight orally every 6 to 8 hours; if fever is higher, 10 mg for each 2.2 lb every 6 to 8 hours, but no more than 40 mg for each 2.2 lb a day.)

▶ **For joint pain and swelling**, 4- to 10-cm strip of cream applied to the skin and massaged briskly three times a day.

How to take Motrin

- Take Motrin exactly as your doctor directs. Motrin begins to take effect against pain and fever within

30 minutes; against arthritis, within 7 days. Effects last 4 hours or more. Although Motrin reduces pain at low dosages, it doesn't relieve inflammation at dosages below 400 mg four times a day.

- If you buy Motrin without a prescription, don't take more than 1.2 g a day.

If you miss a dose

Adjust your schedule as follows:
- If you're taking this drug on a regular schedule, take the missed dose as soon as possible. However, if it's almost time for your next dose, skip the missed dose and go back to

your regular schedule. Don't take a double dose.

• If you're taking the extended-release form, take the missed dose if you remember within an hour or two. If more time has elapsed, skip the missed dose and go back to your regular schedule. Don't take a double dose.

 ## If you suspect an overdose

Contact your doctor *immediately*. Excessive Motrin may cause dizziness, drowsiness, burning sensations, vomiting, nausea, abdominal pain, headache, sweating, flickering movement of the eyeball, difficult or absent breathing, and blue-colored lips, nailbeds, or skin.

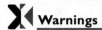 ## Warnings

• Make sure your doctor knows your medical history. You may not be able to take Motrin if you're allergic to it or to similar drugs, including aspirin; if you have other problems, such as nasal polyps, severe hives, stomach or intestinal disorders, an ulcer, high blood pressure, or a blood coagulation defect; or if you have a history of heart, liver, or kidney disease.

• Don't use Motrin during pregnancy or while breast-feeding.

• Watch for the signs and symptoms of digestive tract bleeding — such as bloody or dark stools or vomit — and contact the doctor *immediately* if any of these occur.

• If you're treating yourself, don't take the drug for longer than 3 days.

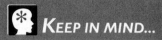 ## KEEP IN MIND...

* Take with food or milk.

* Don't use Motrin when pregnant or breast-feeding.

* Call doctor if you have symptoms of intestinal bleeding.

* Drug won't relieve inflammation at dosages below 400 mg four times a day.

MS Contin

MS Contin, a form of morphine, relieves severe pain. It acts on the brain and nervous system to change how a person perceives and responds to pain.

Why it's prescribed

Doctors prescribe MS Contin to relieve severe pain, such as that caused by a heart attack. It comes in tablets, sustained-release tablets, immediate-release tablets, an oral liquid, syrup, and suppositories. It's also available in an injectable form. Doctors usually prescribe the following amounts for adults.

▶ **For severe pain,** 10 to 30 milligrams (mg) orally or 10 to 20 mg rectally every 4 hours, as needed. Or 15 to 30 mg sustained-release tablets every 12 hours.

How to take MS Contin

• Take MS Contin exactly as your doctor directs in the amount prescribed. This drug begins to take effect within 1 hour after an oral dose and 20 to 60 minutes after a rectal dose. Effects last 4 to 5 hours with oral use, 8 to 12 hours with sustained-release tablets, and 4 to 5 hours with suppositories.
• Take MS Contin on a regular schedule; don't wait until your pain is severe. An around-the-

SIDE EFFECTS

Call your doctor if you have any of these possible drug side effects. Call *immediately* about any labeled "serious."

Serious: seizures (with large doses); slow breathing; fast, slow, or pounding heartbeat; wheezing or difficulty breathing; swollen hands and face; heavy sweating; hallucinations; confusion; dizziness; weakness or tiredness

Common: sedation, sleepiness, feeling of well being, low blood pressure (dizziness, weakness), nausea, vomiting, constipation, inability to urinate, physical dependence

Tips: For severe constipation with long-term use, take a laxative as your doctor directs and eat a well-balanced, high-fiber diet, including bran, fruit, and raw, leafy vegetables. Your doctor may recommend another drug for nausea or vomiting; wait until the nausea subsides before eating your meals. Be careful getting out of bed or walking, and don't drive or perform other hazardous activities that require mental alertness until you know how this drug affects you.

Other: nightmares (with long-acting oral forms), intestinal disorder (vomiting, constipation, abdominal pain), blood problems (unusual bleeding or bruising, red pinpoint rash), itching

DRUG INTERACTIONS

Combining certain drugs may alter their action or produce unwanted side effects. Tell your doctor about other drugs you're taking, especially:
• alcohol and other drugs that relax you or make you sleepy, such as MAO inhibitors (Nardil), other narcotic pain relievers, sedatives (Valium), tranquilizers (Xanax), tricyclic antidepressants (Elavil), sleeping pills (Halcion), and cold and allergy drugs (Benadryl).

MS Contin's OTHER NAMES

MS Contin's generic name is morphine sulfate. Other brand names include Astramorph PF, Duramorph, Infumorph 500, MSIR, Oramorph SR, RMS Uniserts, Roxanol; and, in Canada, Epimorph, Morphine H.P., and Statex.

clock dosage schedule is best for managing severe, chronic pain.
• Don't break, crush, or chew sustained-release tablets before swallowing them.
• Use a measuring spoon (not a household teaspoon) to measure the liquid form of the drug. Mix the drug with juice to improve its taste.
• Your doctor may instruct you to take the liquid by drops under your tongue to improve absorption of the drug.

• To use the suppositories, remove the foil wrapper and moisten the suppository with cold water. Lie on your side. Using your finger, push the suppository well up into your rectum. You don't have to refrigerate the suppositories.
• Don't stop taking MS Contin suddenly if you've been using it regularly; ask the doctor how to stop taking it gradually to avoid unpleasant withdrawal symptoms.

If you miss a dose

If you're taking this drug on a regular schedule, take the missed dose as soon as possible. But if it's almost time for your next dose, skip the missed dose and resume your regular schedule. Never take a double dose.

 If you suspect an overdose

Contact your doctor *immediately*. Excessive MS Contin can cause slow breathing and pinpoint pupils. Other signs are low blood pressure (dizziness, weakness), slow pulse, low body temperature, shock, breathing interruption, fluid in the lungs, seizures, and heart, lung, and blood circulation failure.

 Warnings

• Make sure your doctor knows your medical history. You may not be able to take MS Contin if you're allergic to it or similar drugs or if you have other problems, such as asthma or upper airway obstruction, a head injury, seizures, lung disease, a prostate problem, gallbladder problems, severe liver or kidney disease, acute abdominal conditions, an underactive thyroid, Addison's disease, or a constricted urethra.

• If you're pregnant or breast-feeding, check with your doctor before taking this drug.

• Be aware that children and older adults are especially prone to this drug's side effects.

• When taking MS Contin after surgery, follow your doctor's instructions for turning, coughing, and breathing deeply to prevent the lungs from collapsing.

• Long-term use of this drug can lead to physical or psychological dependence on it.

KEEP IN MIND...

* Take on a regular schedule to manage pain.

* Don't break, crush, or chew sustained-release tablets.

* Mix liquid drug with juice.

* Wait for nausea to pass before eating.

* Long-term use can lead to dependence.

* Don't stop taking suddenly.

Mucomyst

Mucomyst is used to relieve the congestion that makes breathing difficult in bronchitis and other lung diseases. Mucomyst liquefies or dissolves mucus so that it can be coughed up.

Why it's prescribed

Doctors prescribe Mucomyst to relieve congestion due to pneumonia, bronchitis, tuberculosis, cystic fibrosis, emphysema, or collapsed lung; to treat complications after some surgery; and to treat overdose of acetaminophen (Tylenol). Mucomyst comes in a liquid that can be inhaled or, for acetaminophen overdose, taken orally. It's also available in an injectable form. Doctors usually prescribe the following amounts for adults and children.

▶ **For lung disorders and surgery complications,** 1 to 2 milliliters (ml) 10% or 20% solution by inhalation as often as every hour; or 3 to 5 ml 20% solution or 6 to 10 ml 10% solution by inhalation every 2 to 6 hours as needed.

▶ **For acetaminophen overdose,** at first, 140 milligram (mg) for each 2.2 pounds (lb) of body weight orally, followed by 70 mg for each 2.2 lb orally every 4 hours for 17 doses.

How to use Mucomyst

• Use Mucomyst only as directed.
• Clear your airway by coughing before and after inhaling the drug.

MUCOMYST'S OTHER NAMES

Mucomyst's generic name is acetylcysteine. Another brand name is Mucosil.

 SIDE EFFECTS

Call your doctor if you have any of these possible drug side effects. Call *immediately* about any labeled "serious."

Serious: wheezing, difficulty breathing (especially in patients with asthma)

Common: runny nose, bloody sputum, inflamed mouth lining, nausea, vomiting
Tip: Perform mouth care frequently to prevent mouth irritation.

Other: drowsiness

 DRUG INTERACTIONS

Combining certain drugs may alter their action or produce unwanted side effects. Tell your doctor about other drugs you're taking, especially:
• activated charcoal (for treating acetaminophen overdose)
• antibiotics, such as tetracyclines, E-Mycin, amphotericin B, and ampicillin.

• Use a plastic, glass, stainless steel, or other noncorroding metal nebulizer (device that turns liquid to mist) as your doctor directs.
• When used for acetaminophen overdose, the oral dose is diluted with cola, fruit juice, or water before taking. Tell your doctor if you vomit within 1 hour of receiving Mucomyst so that the dose can be repeated.

If you miss a dose

Take the missed dose as soon as possible and the rest of that day's doses at evenly spaced intervals.

 If you suspect an overdose

Consult your doctor.

 Warnings

• Make sure your doctor knows your medical history. You may not be able to use Mucomyst if you have other problems, such as a severe breathing disorder, or if you're allergic to it or to other drugs, foods, or substances.
• Make sure your doctor knows if you're pregnant or breast-feeding before you begin using Mucomyst.
• Be aware that Mucomyst may have a foul taste or smell that goes away soon after using it.

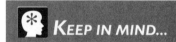 **KEEP IN MIND...**

* Clear airway by coughing before and after using.
* Use recommended nebulizer.
* May be used for acetaminophen overdose.
* Foul taste or smell is temporary.

Myambutol

Myambutol is used to treat the lung disease tuberculosis. It prevents reproduction of the bacteria that cause this disease.

Why it's prescribed

Doctors prescribe Myambutol to treat tuberculosis. It comes in tablets. Doctors usually prescribe the following amounts for adults and children over age 13.

▶ **For tuberculosis in people who haven't received treatment before,** 15 milligrams (mg) for each 2.2 pounds (lb) of body weight once a day in a single dose.

▶ **For re-treatment of tuberculosis,** 25 mg for each 2.2 lb once a day for 60 days with at least one other tuberculosis drug, then decreased to 15 mg for each 2.2 lb as a single dose each day.

How to take Myambutol

• Take Myambutol exactly as your doctor directs, preferably at the same time each day. You may need to take it for a year or more.
• Take Myambutol with food if it upsets your stomach.
• Take Myambutol with other drugs your doctor prescribes, to prevent the development of drug-resistant organisms.
• Keep taking Myambutol as directed, even after you feel better, to make sure the tuberculosis clears up completely.

If you miss a dose

Take the missed dose as soon as possible. However, if it's almost time

MYAMBUTOL'S OTHER NAMES

Myambutol's generic name is ethambutol hydrochloride. A Canadian brand name is Etibi.

 SIDE EFFECTS

Call your doctor if you have any of these possible drug side effects. Call *immediately* about any labeled "serious."

Serious: severe allergic reactions (facial and throat swelling, difficulty breathing, chest pain), blurred vision, blindness, eye pain, trouble differentiating between red and green, chills or fever, pain or swelling in the joints (especially in the feet); burning, numbness, tingling, or weakness in hands or feet; coughing up mucus tinged with blood

Common: gout, kidney stones (back pain, pain with urination, bloody urine)
Tip: Increase your intake of fluids to prevent kidney stones.

Other: headache, dizziness, confusion, hallucinations, appetite and weight loss, nausea, vomiting, abdominal pain, fever, general feeling of illness, itching, rash
Tips: Many side effects subside after extended use of Myambutol. Because this drug can affect alertness and vision, don't drive or perform dangerous activities until you know how it affects you.

 DRUG INTERACTIONS

Combining certain drugs may alter their action or produce unwanted side effects. Tell your doctor about other drugs you're taking, especially:
• aluminum salts, such as AlternaGEL, Basaljel, and Phosphaljel (take several hours before or after Myambutol).

for your next dose, skip the missed dose and go back to your regular schedule. Don't take a double dose.

 If you suspect an overdose

Consult your doctor.

 Warnings

• Make sure your doctor knows your medical history. You may not be able to take Myambutol if you have eye nerve damage, cataracts, recurrent eye infections, or vision problems related to diabetes, gout, or kidney disease.
• Make sure your doctor knows if you're pregnant or breast-feeding before you begin taking this drug.

• Be aware that Myambutol is not given to children under age 13.
• Check with the doctor if your symptoms don't disappear or you feel worse after 2 to 3 weeks of Myambutol treatment.

KEEP IN MIND...

* May be prescribed for a year or more.

* Take with food to avoid stomach upset.

* Have eye exams and blood tests regularly.

Mycelex

Mycelex is an antibiotic used to treat fungal infections. It works by destroying the infection-causing fungus.

Why it's prescribed

Doctors prescribe Mycelex to treat athlete's foot and other fungal infections that affect the skin and mucous membranes. You can also buy Mycelex without a prescription. It comes in throat lozenges, cream, lotion, liquid, and vaginal cream and tablets. Doctors usually prescribe the following amounts for adults and children.

▶ **For external fungal infections,** a small amount applied to affected and surrounding area morning and evening for 2 to 8 weeks.

▶ **For infection of the vulva and vagina,** two 100-milligram (mg) vaginal tablets inserted once a day at bedtime for 3 days, or one 500-mg vaginal tablet daily at bedtime for 3 days, or 1 applicatorful vaginal cream once a day at bedtime for 7 to 14 days.

▶ **For infection of the mouth and throat,** lozenge dissolved in mouth over 15 to 30 minutes five times a day for 14 days.

How to use Mycelex

• Use Mycelex only as your doctor directs. If you're treating yourself, follow the package instructions. You may need to use Mycelex every day for several weeks or more.

MYCELEX'S OTHER NAMES

Mycelex's generic name is clotrimazole. Other brand names include Gyne-Lotrimin and, in Canada, Canesten.

 SIDE EFFECTS

Call your doctor if you have any of these possible drug side effects. Call *immediately* about any labeled "serious."

Serious: severe irritation

Common: with vaginal use, mild burning or irritation and skin redness

Other: with lozenges, nausea and vomiting and liver problems (yellow-tinged skin and eyes); blistering, water retention (swelling, weight gain), itching, burning, stinging, peeling, hives, skin fissures, general irritation

 DRUG INTERACTIONS

Combining certain drugs may alter their action or produce unwanted side effects. Tell your doctor about other drugs you're taking.

• Wash your hands before and after applying Mycelex. Also, clean the affected area before applying.

• When using throat lozenges, hold the lozenge in your mouth and let it dissolve slowly and completely. Try not to swallow your saliva during this time. Don't chew the lozenges or swallow them whole.

• If your symptoms don't improve within a week or if they become worse, check with your doctor.

If you miss a dose

Apply the missed dose as soon as possible. However, if it's almost time for your next dose, skip the missed dose and apply your next dose on schedule.

 If you suspect an overdose

Consult your doctor.

 Warnings

• Make sure your doctor knows your medical history. You may not be able to use Mycelex if you are allergic to it or if you have liver disease.

• Tell your doctor if you're pregnant or breast-feeding before using Mycelex.

• Don't use Mycelex cream in or around the eyes.

• Be aware that Mycelex may stain clothing.

• Don't use airtight wrappings or dressings over the treated area without your doctor's consent.

• Frequent or persistent yeast infections may be a symptom of a more serious medical problem. Check with your doctor.

 KEEP IN MIND...

* Don't use airtight dressings over treated area.

* Let lozenges dissolve slowly.

* Keep using as prescribed even after symptoms clear up.

Myciguent

Myciguent is an antibiotic that's used to treat minor skin infections, burns, or wounds. Myciguent kills bacteria that may occur with these conditions.

Why it's taken

Doctors prescribe Myciguent to prevent or treat skin infections and to prevent bacterial infection with minor burns and wounds. You can buy Myciguent without a prescription. It comes in cream and ointment forms. Doctors usually prescribe the following amounts for adults and children.

▶ **To prevent or treat bacterial infections,** small amount of cream or ointment rubbed into the affected area one to three times a day.

How to use Myciguent

• Use Myciguent exactly as your doctor directs. If you buy Myciguent without a prescription, follow the package instructions carefully.
• Before applying Myciguent, wash the affected area with soap and water; then dry it thoroughly. Apply a generous amount to the affected area and rub it in gently. If you're using the cream form, rub it in until it disappears.
• Keep using Myciguent for the full term of treatment, even if your symptoms go away, to keep the infection from coming back.

MYCIGUENT'S OTHER NAMES

Myciguent's generic name is neomycin sulfate. Other brand names include Neo-Rx and, in Canada, Mycifradin.

SIDE EFFECTS

Call your doctor if you have any of these possible drug side effects. Call *immediately* about any labeled "serious."

Serious: fever, rash, itching, redness, increasing skin irritation

Common: none reported

Other: hives

DRUG INTERACTIONS

Combining certain drugs may alter their action or produce unwanted side effects. Tell your doctor about other drugs you're taking, especially:
• any other drug that's applied to the same skin area as Myciguent.

If you miss a dose

Apply the missed dose as soon as possible. However, if it's almost time for your next regular treatment, skip the one you missed and resume your regular schedule.

If you suspect an overdose

Wash off the cream and consult your doctor.

Warnings

• Make sure your doctor knows your medical history. You may not be able to use Myciguent if you have other problems, such as a kidney problem or an extensive skin condition, or if you're allergic to it or other drugs, especially antibiotics.
• Make sure your doctor knows if you're pregnant or breast-feeding before you begin using Myciguent.
• Don't use Myciguent in or around the eyes.

• Cover the treated area with a gauze dressing if you like. Don't use an airtight dressing without your doctor's consent.
• Don't apply this drug to a puncture wound, deep wound, serious burn, or raw area unless your doctor approves.
• Don't use Myciguent for a long time without your doctor's approval; prolonged use may allow other harmful organisms to flourish.
• If your skin condition doesn't improve within 1 week or if it gets worse, call your doctor or pharmacist.

KEEP IN MIND...

* Don't apply in or near eyes.
* Gently rub in cream or ointment.
* Use entire amount prescribed even after symptoms subside.
* For short-term use only.
* Not for serious burns or wounds.

Mycobutin

Mycobutin helps to treat AIDS and other conditions that weaken the body's response to disease. This drug prevents the spread of *Mycobacterium avium* complex (MAC), an illness that's caused by bacteria.

Why it's prescribed

Doctors prescribe Mycobutin to prevent the spread of MAC in people with AIDS and other immunity-suppressing conditions. The drug comes in capsules. Doctors usually prescribe the following amounts for adults.

▶ **To prevent MAC from spreading,** 300 milligrams (mg) as a single dose or split into two equal doses a day.

How to take Mycobutin

- Take Mycobutin only as your doctor directs.
- If you have difficulty swallowing the capsules, mix them with soft foods, such as applesauce or pudding.
- Take the drug with high-fat meals, for slower absorption into the body.

If you miss a dose

Take the missed dose as soon as possible. However, if it's almost time for your next dose, skip the missed

MYCOBUTIN'S OTHER NAME

Mycobutin's generic name is rifabutin.

 ## SIDE EFFECTS

Call your doctor if you have any of these possible drug side effects. Call *immediately* about any labeled "serious."

Serious: extreme sensitivity to light, excessive tearing, eye pain, blood problems (bleeding, bruising, fatigue, chills, fever, increased risk of infection) *Tips:* Avoid people who may be ill or have an infection. Avoid strenuous physical activity.

Common: rash; discolored urine, feces, sputum, saliva, tears, and skin *Tips:* Mycobutin may discolor urine, feces, sputum, saliva, tears, and skin brownish orange; avoid wearing soft contact lenses because they may be permanently stained.

Other: eye inflammation, stomach upset, belching, gas, nausea, vomiting, abdominal pain, fever, muscle pain or inflammation, peculiar taste

 ## DRUG INTERACTIONS

Combining certain drugs may alter their action or produce unwanted side effects. Tell your doctor about other drugs you're taking, especially:
- birth control pills
- drugs metabolized by the liver, such as Rifampin and Verapamil
- Retrovir (AZT).

dose and go back to your regular schedule. Don't take a double dose.

 ### If you suspect an overdose

Consult your doctor.

Warnings

- Make sure your doctor knows your medical history. You may not be able to take Mycobutin if you're allergic to it or other drugs or if you have active tuberculosis or a blood disorder.
- While you're taking Mycobutin, check with your doctor before you take any other drugs.

- Take Mycobutin with other drugs only as your doctor prescribes.

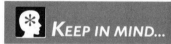 ## KEEP IN MIND...

- Mix with soft foods to ease swallowing.
- Take with high-fat foods for slower absorption.
- Take with other drugs only as directed.
- May stain soft contact lenses.

Mycolog II

ycolog II is a combination of two drugs used to treat fungal infections, such as *Candida* (*Monilia*). The antifungal portion kills or prevents the growth of infection-causing fungus. The other portion—an anti-inflammatory drug—relieves redness, swelling, itching, and other symptoms.

Why it's prescribed

Doctors prescribe Mycolog II to treat fungal skin infections and conditions such as diaper rash, and to relieve the discomfort they cause. It comes in cream and an ointment. Doctors usually prescribe the following amounts.

▶ **For fungal skin infection, diaper rash,** a thin layer applied to the affected area twice a day.

How to use Mycolog II

• Use Mycolog II only as your doctor directs; don't use it more often than prescribed or for a longer time than recommended.
• To apply, rub a small amount into the affected area gently and thoroughly. Keep Mycolog II away from your eyes.
• Use Mycolog II for the full treatment period, even if symptoms go away, to stop the infection from coming back.

MYCOLOG II'S OTHER NAME

Mycolog II is a combination of the generic drugs nystatin and triamcinolone.

 SIDE EFFECTS

Call your doctor if you have any of these possible drug side effects. Call *immediately* about any labeled "serious."

Serious: blistering, burning, dryness, itching, peeling

Common: dry skin

Other: with long-term use: acne or oily skin; increased growth or loss of hair; reddish purple lines on arms, face, legs, trunk, or groin; thin skin that bruises easily

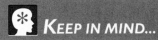 **DRUG INTERACTIONS**

Combining certain drugs may alter their action or produce unwanted side effects. Tell your doctor about other drugs you're taking.

If you miss a dose

Apply the missed dose as soon as possible. But if it's almost time for your next dose, skip the missed dose and apply your next dose on schedule.

If you suspect an overdose

Consult your doctor.

 Warnings

• Make sure your doctor knows your medical history. You may not be able to use Mycolog II if you have diabetes; if you're allergic to this or other antifungals; or if you have had herpes, chickenpox, tuberculosis, or viral skin infections.
• Make sure your doctor knows if you're pregnant or breast-feeding before you begin using Mycolog II.
• Don't put a bandage, wrap, or other tight dressing over the treated area without your doctor's consent. Wear loose-fitting clothing when using Mycolog II on your groin area.
• If you're using Mycolog II to treat a child's diaper rash, don't use tight-fitting diapers and plastic pants.
• Don't use Mycolog II for other skin problems without first checking with your doctor.
• If your skin problem doesn't clear up after 2 to 3 weeks of treatment, call your doctor.

 KEEP IN MIND...

∗ Don't use more than recommended.

∗ Keep away from eyes.

∗ Don't use airtight dressing over treated area.

∗ Don't use tight-fitting diapers or plastic pants over area treated for diaper rash.

∗ Use for full treatment period, even if you feel better.

Mydriacyl

Mydriacyl causes the pupils of the eye to dilate (become larger) and prevents the eye from adjusting to see near and far objects. It's used to make eye examinations easier to perform.

Why it's prescribed

Doctors prescribe Mydriacyl to dilate the pupils so that they can see the inner workings of the eye more clearly. It comes in eyedrops. Doctors prescribe the following amounts for adults and children.
▶ **For eye exams,** 1 or 2 drops of 0.5% or 1% solution in each eye 15 to 20 minutes before exam, repeated every 30 minutes if needed.

How to use Mydriacyl

• Your eye doctor will administer Mydriacyl eyedrops in the office before your eye exam.
• Mydriacyl takes effect within 15 minutes; effects may last up to 7 hours.

If you miss a dose

Not applicable because this drug is given in doctor's office.

 If you suspect an overdose

Tell your doctor *immediately*. Excessive Mydriacyl can cause dry, flushed skin; dry mouth; delirium; hallucinations; and fast pulse.

MYDRIACYL'S OTHER NAMES

Mydriacyl's generic name is tropicamide. Another brand name is Tropicacyl.

 SIDE EFFECTS

Call your doctor if you have any of these possible drug side effects. Call *immediately* about any labeled "serious."
Serious: behavioral disturbances in children
Tip: The doctor will probably stop using Mydriacyl on your child if behavioral changes occur.
Common: temporary stinging when applied, blurred vision, eye sensitivity to light, dry throat
Tips: Avoid hazardous activities, such as operating machinery or driving, until temporary blurring subsides. Ease light sensitivity by wearing sunglasses.
Other: incoordination, irritability, confusion, sleepiness, hallucinations, increased pressure in eye (headache, eye pain), dry mouth, dry skin, flushing, fever

 DRUG INTERACTIONS

Combining certain drugs may alter their action or produce unwanted side effects. Tell your doctor about other drugs you're taking.

Warnings

• Make sure your doctor knows your medical history. You may not be able to use these drops if you have other problems, especially narrow-angle glaucoma, increased pressure in the eye, brain damage (in children), Down's syndrome, or any drug allergies.
• Inform your doctor if you're pregnant or breast-feeding before the doctor administers the drops.
• Be aware that older adults and children (especially those with blond hair or blue eyes) may be more prone to this drug's side effects.
• Take sunglasses with you to the doctor's office. Your eyes will probably be very sensitive to light after the exam. Check with your doctor if these effects last more than 24 hours after the medication is stopped.
• Keep in mind that you may not be able to drive for a while after the exam because you'll have trouble focusing. Arrange for transportation home that doesn't involve your driving.

 KEEP IN MIND...

∗ Inform the doctor if you have narrow-angle glaucoma.

∗ Wear sunglasses after the exam.

∗ Avoid driving until blurred vision subsides.

Myidil

Myidil is an antihistamine. It blocks the effects of substances in the body called histamines, which cause itching, sneezing, runny nose, and watery eyes.

Why it's prescribed

Doctors prescribe Myidil to treat or prevent colds and allergy symptoms. It comes in tablets and syrup. Doctors usually prescribe the following amounts for adults; children's dosage appears in parentheses.

▶ **For colds and allergies,** 2.5 milligrams (mg) every 4 to 6 hours. Maximum dosage is 10 mg a day. (Children age 6 to 12 years: 1.25 mg every 4 to 6 hours. Maximum dosage is 5 mg a day. Children age 4 to 5 years: 0.9 mg every 4 to 8 hours. Maximum dosage is 3.75 mg a day. Children age 2 to 3 years: 0.6 mg every 6 to 8 hours. Maximum dosage is 2.5 mg a day. Children age 4 months to 1 year: 0.3 mg every 6 to 8 hours. Maximum dosage is 1.25 mg a day.)

How to take Myidil

• Take Myidil only as your doctor directs. This drug begins to take effect in 15 to 60 minutes; its effects last 4 to 8 hours.
• Take Myidil with food or milk to reduce stomach upset.

If you miss a dose

If you're taking Myidil on a regular schedule, take the missed dose as

MYIDIL'S OTHER NAMES

Myidil's generic name is triprolidine hydrochloride. Another brand name is Alleract.

 SIDE EFFECTS

Call your doctor if you have any of these possible drug side effects.

Serious: none reported

Common: drowsiness, stimulation, dry mouth

Tips: Don't drink alcohol and avoid driving or other activities that require alertness until you know how this drug affects you. Sugarless gum, hard candy, or ice chips may relieve dry mouth.

Other: dizziness, confusion, restlessness, sleeplessness, drastic appetite and weight loss, diarrhea or constipation, nausea, vomiting, frequent urination or inability to urinate, hives, rash

 DRUG INTERACTIONS

Combining certain drugs may alter their action or produce unwanted side effects. Tell your doctor about other drugs you're taking, especially:
• allergy skin tests (stop taking Myidil 4 days before)
• drugs for depression called MAO inhibitors such as Eldepryl
• drugs that relax you or make you sleepy, such as sleeping pills and sedatives.

soon as possible. However, if it's almost time for your next dose, skip the missed dose and go back to your regular schedule. Don't take a double dose.

 If you suspect an overdose

Contact your doctor immediately. Excessive Myidil can cause very opposite effects: slowing of the nervous system (sedation, reduced alertness, interrupted breathing, severe heart problems) or stimulation of the nervous system (sleeplessness, hallucinations, tremor, or seizures).

Warnings

• Make sure your doctor knows your medical history. You may not be able to take Myidil if you have asthma, glaucoma, overactive thyroid, heart disease, high blood pressure, prostate problem, bladder blockage, and stomach ulcers, or if you're allergic to antihistamines.
• Make sure your doctor knows if you're pregnant or breast-feeding before you begin taking Myidil.
• Children under age 12 should receive Myidil only if prescribed by a doctor.

 KEEP IN MIND...

＊ Take with food or milk.
＊ Stop taking 4 days before allergy tests.
＊ Don't give to children under age 12 without doctor's consent.

Mylanta

Mylanta, an antacid, causes a chemical reaction that neutralizes acids found in the stomach.

Why it's taken

Mylanta is taken to relieve symptoms of acid indigestion or ulcers. You can buy Mylanta without a prescription. It comes in a liquid suspension and chewable tablets. The following amounts are usually recommended for adults.

▶ **For upset stomach,** 2 tablespoons or 1 tablet after meals and at bedtime.

How to take Mylanta

• If you're treating yourself, follow the directions on the label or package exactly. Don't take more than the recommended dose.
• If your doctor has given you special instructions on how to use Mylanta and how much to take, follow the doctor's instructions.
• Shake the liquid suspension well before measuring. Then take it with milk or water.
• If you're taking the chewable tablets, chew well to improve absorption.

MYLANTA'S OTHER NAMES

Mylanta is a combination of the generic drugs aluminum hydroxide, magnesium hydroxide, and simethicone. Mylanta Double Strength is available with twice the amount of the ingredients listed above. Other brand names include Almacone, Alamag Plus, Aludrox, Extra Strength Mintox, Gelusil, Maalox Plus Extra Strength, Mi-Acid, Mygel, Simaal Gel; and, in Canada, Amphojel Plus and Diovol Plus.

 SIDE EFFECTS

Call your doctor if you have any of these possible drug side effects. Call *immediately* about any labeled "serious."

Serious: bone pain, constipation, appetite loss, mood changes, tiredness, slowed breathing

Common: none reported

Other: mild constipation, diarrhea, cramps, whitish stools
Tip: Avoid constipation by increasing fluids and high-fiber foods in your diet.

 DRUG INTERACTIONS

Combining certain drugs may alter their action or produce unwanted side effects. Tell your doctor about other drugs you're taking, especially:
• prescription and nonprescription drugs (take 2 hours before or after Mylanta).

• For best results, drink a glass of milk or water after taking Mylanta.
• If you're taking Mylanta to relieve heartburn or acid indigestion, don't take it for more than 2 weeks unless your doctor tells you to.
• If you're taking Mylanta to relieve symptoms of an ulcer, take it exactly as directed and for the full time prescribed by the doctor. For best results, take it 1 to 3 hours after meals and at bedtime (unless the doctor puts you on a different schedule).

If you miss a dose

Not applicable because Mylanta is taken only as needed.

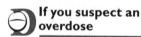 **If you suspect an overdose**

Consult your doctor.

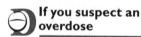 **Warnings**

• Make sure your doctor knows your medical history. You may not be able to take Mylanta if you have

other medical problems, such as Alzheimer's disease, constipation, inflamed bowel, diarrhea, or liver or kidney disease.
• If you're an older adult and have bone problems, check with your doctor before taking this drug.
• If your stomach condition doesn't improve or if it recurs, consult your doctor.
• Have regular checkups, especially if you're taking Mylanta for a long time.

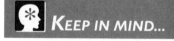 **KEEP IN MIND...**

∗ Don't take longer than 2 weeks.

∗ Don't take if you have kidney disease.

∗ Increase fluid intake.

Myleran

Myleran interferes with the growth of cancer cells by preventing them from reproducing.

Why it's prescribed

Doctors prescribe Myleran to treat leukemia and other types of cancer. It comes in tablets. Doctors usually prescribe the following amounts for adults; children's dosages appear in parentheses.

▶ **For leukemia,** 4 to 8 milligrams (mg) a day until the desired response occurs. The drug may be tried again if it doesn't stop the growth of cancer cells. (Children: 0.06 to 0.12 mg for each 2.2 pounds of body weight per day.)

How to take Myleran

• Take Myleran only as your doctor directs. This drug begins to take effect in 1 to 2 weeks.
• Take Myleran at the same time each day for the best effect.
• Drink extra fluids when taking Myleran, to prevent kidney problems.
• If you vomit shortly after taking a dose, check with your doctor to find out whether to repeat the dose or not.

If you miss a dose

Skip the missed dose and go back to your regular schedule. Don't take a double dose.

If you suspect an overdose

Contact your doctor *immediately.* Excessive Myleran can cause fever,

---

MYLERAN'S OTHER NAME

Myleran's generic name is busulfan.

SIDE EFFECTS

Call your doctor if you have any of these possible drug side effects. Call *immediately* about any labeled "serious."

Serious: seizures, blood problems (fever, chills, increased risk of infection, fatigue, bleeding, bruising), irreversible lung tissue disorder ("busulfan lung," in which the lung tissue becomes hard, breathing difficult)

Common: none reported

Other: unusual tiredness or weakness, nausea, vomiting, diarrhea, cracked and peeling lips, inflamed tongue, menstrual disorder, testicular wasting, impotence, persistent cough, difficulty breathing, temporary skin darkening, rash, hives, inability to sweat, breast enlargement in men, hair loss, wasting syndrome (fatigue, weight loss, weakness, low blood pressure)

DRUG INTERACTIONS

Combining certain drugs may alter their action or produce unwanted side effects. Tell your doctor about other drugs you're taking, especially:
• anticoagulants (blood thinners), such as Coumadin and aspirin
• radiation treatment or cancer drugs such as thioguanine.

---

chills, an increased risk of infection, bleeding gums, nosebleeds, blood in stool, and easy bruising.

Warnings

• Make sure your doctor knows your medical history. You may not be able to take Myleran if you're allergic to it or if you have other medical problems, such as seizures, a history of head trauma, or a form of leukemia that's resistant to this drug (chronic myelogenous leukemia in the "blastic" phase and children with chronic myelogenous leukemia).
• Women should prevent pregnancy during their treatment. If you're breast-feeding, stop while taking Myleran.
• Watch for and report signs of infection (fever, sore throat, fatigue)

and bleeding (easy bruising, nosebleeds, bleeding gums, bloody stool). Check your temperature daily.
• Call your doctor if you have a persistent cough and difficulty breathing.

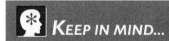 KEEP IN MIND...

∗ Take at same time each day.
∗ Drink extra fluids to prevent kidney problems.
∗ Check body temperature daily; report fever and signs of bleeding or infection.
∗ Prevent pregnancy during treatment.

Mylicon

Mylicon relieves pain and other symptoms of too much gas in the stomach and digestive system. The drug destroys mucus-surrounded gas bubbles in the stomach and intestines.

Why it's taken

Doctors prescribe Mylicon to treat bloating, pain, and flatulence caused by gas bubbles in the digestive system. You can buy Mylicon without a prescription. It comes in tablets, chewable tablets, capsules, and oral drops. Doctors usually recommend the following amounts for adults and children over age 12.

▶ **For gas and bloating,** 40 to 125 milligrams after each meal and at bedtime.

How to take Mylicon

• Take Mylicon only as directed. Although this drug doesn't prevent gas, it begins to take effect immediately to break up existing gas bubbles.
• If you're using the chewable tablets, be sure to chew them thoroughly before swallowing. That way, you'll get the best results.
• If you're taking the oral drops, carefully measure each dose. Use

---

MYLICON'S OTHER NAMES

Mylicon's generic name is simethicone. Other brand names include Extra Strength Gas-X, Mylanta Gas; and, in Canada, Ovol, Ovol-40, and Ovol-80.

 SIDE EFFECTS

Call your doctor if you have any of these possible drug side effects.
Serious: none reported
Common: none reported
Other: excessive belching, gas

 DRUG INTERACTIONS

Combining certain drugs may alter their action or produce unwanted side effects. Tell your doctor about other drugs you're taking.

---

the specially marked dropper that comes with the drug.

If you miss a dose

If you take Mylicon on a regular schedule, take the missed dose as soon as you can. However, if it's almost time for your next dose, skip the missed dose and go back to your regular schedule. Don't take a double dose.

 If you suspect an overdose

Consult your doctor.

 Warnings

• Make sure your doctor knows your medical history. You may not be able to take Mylicon if you're allergic to it or other drugs, foods, or other substances.
• Check with your doctor if you're pregnant or breast-feeding. Be assured, though, that Mylicon isn't absorbed into the body and isn't likely to cause problems during pregnancy or breast-feeding.

• Follow your doctor's recommendations for changing positions frequently and walking to aid in passing gas.
• Follow your doctor's advice for developing regular bowel habits. To help prevent gas, avoid foods that seem to cause gas. Also, chew food thoroughly and slowly and avoid fizzy drinks. If you smoke, avoid lighting up before meals.

✱ KEEP IN MIND...

✱ Usually not for children under age 12.

✱ Take after each meal and at bedtime.

✱ If taking tablets, chew thoroughly before swallowing.

✱ If taking oral drops, measure carefully.

✱ Takes effect immediately.

Mysoline

Mysoline is a seizure-fighting drug. It works by controlling nerve impulses in the brain.

Why it's prescribed

Doctors prescribe Mysoline to treat epilepsy and other seizure disorders. It comes in tablets and an oral liquid. Doctors usually prescribe the following amounts for adults; children's dosages appear in parentheses.

▶ **For seizures,** at first, 100 to 125 milligrams (mg) at bedtime on days 1 to 3; then 100 to 125 mg twice a day on days 4 to 6; then 100 to 125 mg on days 7 to 9. After that, the usual amount increases to 250 mg three times a day or even four times a day, if needed. (Children age 8 and over: same as adult dosages. Children under age 8: at first, 50 mg at bedtime, then 50 mg twice a day, then 100 mg twice a day followed by maintenance dosage of 125 to 250 mg three times a day.)

How to take Mysoline

• Take Mysoline only as your doctor directs. It may take 2 or more weeks for this drug's full effect.
• Take Mysoline in regularly spaced doses to make sure there's enough drug in your body to prevent seizures.
• Don't suddenly stop taking Mysoline, because seizures may worsen.

MYSOLINE'S OTHER NAMES

Mysoline's generic name is primidone. Canadian brand names include Apo-Primidone, PMS-Primidone, and Sertan.

SIDE EFFECTS

Call your doctor if you have any of these possible drug side effects. Call *immediately* about any labeled "serious."

Serious: slowed breathing, double vision, nausea, vomiting, blood problems (bruising, bleeding, fatigue, fever, chills)

Common: drowsiness, dizziness, fatigue, incoordination
Tips: Avoid driving or other hazardous activities that require mental alertness until you're familiar with how this drug affects you.

Other: emotional disturbances, irritability, rapid uncontrollable eye movements, swollen eyelids, drastic appetite and weight loss, thirst, impotence, rash, hair loss, water retention (swelling, weight gain)

DRUG INTERACTIONS

Combining certain drugs may alter their action or produce unwanted side effects. Tell your doctor about other drugs you're taking, especially:
• alcohol and drugs that make you relaxed or sleepy (muscle relaxants, anesthetics, sleeping pills, cold and flu remedies)
• Dilantin
• Tegretol.

Check with your doctor about reducing your dosage gradually.

If you miss a dose

Take the missed dose as soon as possible. But if it's within 1 hour of your next dose, skip the missed dose and take your next dose on schedule. Don't take a double dose.

If you suspect an overdose

Contact your doctor *immediately.* Excessive Mysoline can cause confusion, uncontrolled rolling or rapid movement of the eyeballs, double vision, and shortness of breath.

Warnings

• Make sure your doctor knows your medical history. You may not be able to take Mysoline if you have other problems, such as asthma or another lung disease, blood disorder, or liver disease, or if you're allergic to it or other anti-seizure drugs.
• If you're pregnant or breast-feeding, don't use Mysoline without your doctor's consent.
• Older adults may be especially prone to Mysoline's side effects.

KEEP IN MIND...

∗ Takes effect in 2 weeks or more.
∗ Take in regularly spaced doses.
∗ Don't stop taking suddenly.

Naftin

Naftin is an antibiotic that's used to treat athlete's foot and other common skin infections that are caused by certain types of fungus. Naftin kills the infection-causing fungus.

Why it's prescribed

Doctors prescribe Naftin to treat fungal infections of the skin, such as athlete's foot, jock itch, and ringworm. Naftin comes in a cream and a gel. Doctors usually prescribe the following amounts for adults.

▶ **For fungal infections,** a small amount of cream applied to the affected area once a day. Or a small amount of gel applied twice a day in the morning and evening.

How to use Naftin

- Use Naftin only as your doctor directs.
- Wash your hands before and after using Naftin.
- Apply enough cream to cover the affected skin and surrounding areas. Rub it in gently.
- When using Naftin to treat athlete's foot, dry your feet carefully. Wear cotton socks and change them at least daily. After the Naftin has been absorbed, apply an antifungal, talcum, or another bland, absorbent powder to the affected area. Sprinkle powder on your feet, between your toes, and in your socks and shoes once or twice a day.
- If you're using Naftin to treat jock itch, dry your groin area carefully after bathing. Wear loose-fitting, cotton underwear. After the

Naftin has been absorbed, apply an antifungal, talcum, or another bland, absorbent powder to your groin area. Use the powder once or twice a day.
- If you're using Naftin to treat ringworm, dry yourself carefully after bathing. Try to prevent moisture buildup on the affected skin areas. Avoid high heat and humidity. Don't wear tight-fitting, poorly ventilated clothing. After the Naftin cream has been absorbed into your skin, sprinkle an antifungal, talcum, or another bland, absorbent powder on the affected areas.
- Use Naftin for the full treatment time prescribed, to keep the infection from coming back.

If you miss a dose

Apply the missed dose as soon as you remember. However, if it's almost time for your next application, skip the one you missed and resume your regular schedule.

If you suspect an overdose

Consult your doctor.

 ## SIDE EFFECTS

Call your doctor if you have any of these possible drug side effects.

Serious: none reported

Common: burning, stinging

Tip: Burning or stinging usually go away over time as your body adjusts to this drug.

Other: dryness, itching, irritation

 ## DRUG INTERACTIONS

Combining certain drugs may alter their action or produce unwanted side effects. Tell your doctor about other drugs you're taking.

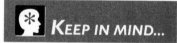 Warnings

- You may not be able to use Naftin if you're allergic to it.
- Make sure your doctor knows if you're pregnant or breast-feeding before you use Naftin.
- Keep Naftin away from your eyes, nose, and mouth.
- Don't use an airtight dressing over the treated area unless directed by your doctor.
- Call your doctor if your skin condition doesn't improve after 1 month of treatment or if it gets worse.
- Stop using this drug and check with your doctor if irritation or sensitivity develops during treatment.

KEEP IN MIND...

* If treating athlete's foot, wear cotton socks and change them daily.
* Don't use airtight dressings over treated area.
* Use for entire treatment time even if symptoms subside.

NAFTIN'S OTHER NAME

Naftin's generic name is naftifine.

Nalfon

Nalfon is a nonsteroidal anti-inflammatory drug (NSAID). It relieves inflammation, swelling, stiffness, and joint pain by blocking the body's production of substances called prostaglandins.

Why it's prescribed

Doctors prescribe Nalfon to relieve symptoms of some types of arthritis and other mild to moderate pain. Nalfon comes in tablets and capsules. Doctors usually prescribe the following amounts for adults.

▶ **For arthritis,** 300 to 600 milligrams (mg) three or four times a day. The maximum dosage is 3.2 grams a day.

▶ **For mild to moderate pain,** 200 mg every 4 to 6 hours, as needed.

How to take Nalfon

• Take Nalfon as your doctor directs.
• Take Nalfon 30 minutes before or 2 hours after meals. If the drug upsets your stomach, take it with food.
• Nalfon takes effect in 15 to 30 minutes, and pain relief lasts for 4 to 6 hours. For arthritis, the full effects may take 2 to 4 weeks to begin.

If you miss a dose

Take the missed dose as soon as you remember. However, if it's almost time for your next dose, skip the missed dose and go back to your regular schedule. Don't take a double dose.

NALFON'S OTHER NAMES

Nalfon's generic name is fenoprofen calcium.

 ## SIDE EFFECTS

Call your doctor if you have any of these possible drug side effects. Call *immediately* about any labeled "serious."

Serious: heart failure (difficulty breathing, cough); kidney problems (decreased urine output); ulcers; severe cramps; pain or burning in stomach; severe, continuing nausea; heartburn; stomach bleeding (vomit tinged with blood or that looks like coffee grounds, bloody or tarry stools); severe skin peeling; blood problems (fatigue, prolonged bleeding of a cut or sore)

Common: headache, sleepiness, heartburn, nausea, itching, skin sensitivity to sunlight
Tips: Don't drive or perform other activities that require alertness until you know how this drug affects you. Wear sunscreen and protective clothing.

Other: drowsiness, dizziness, swollen arms and legs, hearing problem, vomiting, constipation, drastic appetite and weight loss, rash, hives

 ## DRUG INTERACTIONS

Combining certain drugs may alter their action or produce unwanted side effects. Tell your doctor about other drugs you're taking, especially:
• alcohol
• aspirin, Tylenol
• corticosteroids, such as Decadron and Kenacort
• oral anticoagulants (blood thinners) such as Coumadin
• oral diabetes drugs such as Micronase
• diuretics (water pills) such as Lasix.

 ## If you suspect an overdose

Contact your doctor *immediately.* Excessive Nalfon can cause severe kidney problems (reduced urine), fast pulse, dizziness, drowsiness, confusion, nausea, vomiting, headache, ringing in the ears, and blurred vision.

Warnings

• Make sure your doctor knows your medical history. You may not be able to take Nalfon if you're allergic to it or other drugs or if you

have poor kidney or liver function, heart disease or high blood pressure, ulcers, asthma, or if you're pregnant or breast-feeding.
• Older adults may be especially prone to Nalfon's side effects.

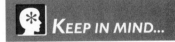 ## KEEP IN MIND...

* Take 30 minutes before or 2 hours after meals.
* Watch for bloody stools.
* Avoid alcohol, aspirin, and Tylenol.

Naphcon

Naphcon relieves inflammation and itching in and around the eye. It's thought to relieve these symptoms by narrowing the blood vessels in the membranes around the eye.

Why it's prescribed

Doctors prescribe Naphcon to treat minor eye irritations caused by colds, pollution, pollen, dust, swimming, or wearing contact lenses. You can also buy Naphcon without a prescription. It comes in eyedrops. Doctors usually prescribe the following amounts for adults.

▶ **For inflammation and itching,** 1 to 3 drops of 0.1% solution (prescription strength) in the eye every 3 to 4 hours or 1 to 2 drops of 0.012% to 0.03% solution (nonprescription strength) up to four times a day.

How to use Naphcon

• Use Naphcon only as directed. Redness usually goes away within 10 minutes. Effects last for 2 to 6 hours.
• Wash your hands before and after using Naphcon.
• Pull lower lid away from the eye and put drops in the space that's created. Close the eye gently and press lightly on the inside corners of the closed eyelids for 1 minute after drops are instilled.
• Don't touch the dropper to your eye any other surface, to avoid contamination.

NAPHCON'S OTHER NAMES

Naphcon's generic name is naphazoline hydrochloride. Other brand names include Ak-Con, Albalon Liquifilm, Allerest, Clear Eyes, Degest 2, Estivin II, Naphcon Forte, VasoClear, and Vasocon Regular.

 SIDE EFFECTS

Call your doctor if you have any of these possible drug side effects. Call *immediately* about any labeled "serious."

Serious: extreme sensitivity to light, blurred vision, pain, eyelid swelling

Common: stinging eyes
Tip: Dab eyes with a tissue; do not rub.

Other: headache, dizziness, nervousness, weakness, temporary stinging, dilated pupils, eye irritation, pain, increased pressure in the eye (headache, blurred vision), nausea, heavy sweating

 DRUG INTERACTIONS

Combining certain drugs may alter their action or produce unwanted side effects. Tell your doctor about other drugs you're taking, especially:
• drugs for depression, such as tricyclic antidepressants (such as Elavil) or MAO inhibitors (such as Eldepryl).

• Don't use more than the recommended dosage. Symptoms may get worse with overuse.

If you miss a dose

Take the missed dose as soon as possible. However, if it's almost time for your next dose, skip the missed dose and go back to your regular schedule. Don't take a double dose.

 If you suspect an overdose

Contact your doctor *immediately.* Excessive Naphcon can cause low body temperature, drowsiness, slow pulse, or severe weakness.

 Warnings

• Make sure your doctor knows your medical history. You may not be able to use Naphcon if you have other problems, such as glaucoma, overactive thyroid, heart disease, high blood pressure, or diabetes, or

if you're allergic to Naphcon or any of its ingredients.
• Make sure your doctor knows if you're pregnant or breast-feeding before you begin taking Naphcon.
• Don't use 0.1% eyedrop solution in children; this concentration of the drug can cause severe sedation and coma in children, especially infants.
• Keep container tightly closed when not in use.
• Stop using this drug and check with your doctor if pain or vision change occurs, or if irritation gets worse or lasts for more than 3 days.

KEEP IN MIND...

* Wash your hands before and after using.
* Don't touch dropper to eye or any surface.
* Don't use more than recommended dosage.
* Report pain or vision change.

Naprosyn

Naprosyn is a nonsteroidal anti-inflammatory drug (NSAID). Doctors suspect that the drug relieves pain by blocking the body's production of a hormone called prostaglandin.

Why it's prescribed

Doctors prescribe Naprosyn to treat mild to moderate pain associated with menstruation, gout attacks, or symptoms of arthritis. A nonprescription brand of this drug is available: Aleve. Naprosyn comes in film-coated tablets. Doctors usually prescribe the following amounts for adults.

▶ **For rheumatoid arthritis or osteoarthritis,** 250 to 500 milligrams (mg) twice a day. Maximum dose is 1,500 mg a day.

▶ **For juvenile arthritis** (children's dosage only), 10 mg for each 2.2 pounds of body weight twice a day.

▶ **For acute gout attack,** initially, 750 mg, followed by 250 mg every 8 hours until attack subsides.

▶ **For mild to moderate pain, pain associated with menstruation, or severe tendinitis or bursitis,** 500 mg, followed by 250 mg every 6 to 8 hours as needed.

How to take Naprosyn

• If you're treating yourself, check the label carefully and take only the prescribed amount.

NAPROSYN'S OTHER NAMES

Naprosyn's generic name is naproxen sodium. Other brand names include Aleve, Anaprox; and, in Canada, Apo-Naproxen, Novonaprox, and Nu-Naprox.

SIDE EFFECTS

Call your doctor if you have any of these possible drug side effects. Call *immediately* about any labeled "serious."

Serious: peptic ulcer (nausea, vomiting, heartburn, dark or bloody vomit or stools), blood problems (bleeding of gums, fatigue, fever, chills), kidney problems (decreased urination), liver problems (nausea, vomiting, yellow-tinged skin and eyes), shortness of breath, hives

Common: headache, drowsiness, dizziness, swelling of the feet or lower legs, ringing in the ears, nausea, itching, confusion

Tips: Avoid potentially hazardous activities, such as driving a car, until you know how Naprosyn affects you. Take doses with food to avoid stomach upset.

Other: mood changes, palpitations, vision disturbances, painful urination

DRUG INTERACTIONS

Combining certain drugs may alter their action or produce unwanted side effects. Tell your doctor about other drugs you're taking, especially:

• alcohol
• aspirin and other anticoagulants (blood thinners), such as Coumadin
• Benemid
• diuretics (water pills) and other blood pressure drugs
• protein-bound drugs, such as Coumadin and Dilantin
• Mexate
• oral diabetes drugs
• steroids

• Take each dose with a full glass (8 ounces) of water. Stay upright for about 30 minutes afterward.

• This drug starts to relieve pain within 1 hour and starts to relieve arthritis symptoms within 14 days. Pain relief lasts about 7 hours.

• If you're an arthritis-sufferer, be aware that the drug may take a month to achieve its full effect.

If you miss a dose

Take the missed dose as soon as possible. However, if it's almost time for your next dose, skip the missed dose and take your next dose as scheduled. Don't take a double dose.

If you suspect an overdose

Contact your doctor *immediately.* Excessive Naprosyn can cause drowsiness, nausea, and vomiting.

Continued on next page ▶

Warnings

• Before taking Naprosyn, consult your doctor if you have a stomach or intestinal disorder, ulcers, kidney disease, or heart or blood vessel disease.

• Don't take this drug if you're allergic to aspirin.

• If you're pregnant, check with your doctor before taking this drug.

• Older adults may be especially prone to stomach upset from Naprosyn.

• If you're taking Naprosyn (prescription), don't take Aleve (nonprescription) at the same time.

• Before giving a urine specimen, tell the lab staff that you're taking Naprosyn.

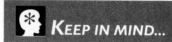

KEEP IN MIND...

* Take with full glass of water.

* Stay upright for 30 minutes.

* Don't take Naprosyn and Aleve at the same time.

Nardil

Nardil blocks the effects of a substance called monoamine oxidase (MAO) on the nervous system.

Why it's prescribed

Doctors prescribe Nardil to treat depression. It comes in tablets. Doctors usually prescribe the following amounts for adults.

▶ **For depression,** 15 milligrams (mg) three times a day, increased rapidly to 60 mg a day. Maximum dosage is 90 mg a day.

How to take Nardil

• Take Nardil only as your doctor directs.
• Nardil begins to take effect in 7 to 10 days; full effects may take 4 to 8 weeks.

If you miss a dose

Take the missed dose as soon as possible. However, if it's within 2 hours of your next dose, skip the missed dose and go back to your regular schedule. Don't take a double dose.

If you suspect an overdose

Contact your doctor *immediately.* Signs of overdose may develop slowly (within 24 to 48 hours) and may last for up to 2 weeks. These may include frequent headaches, agitation, flushing, rapid pulse, high blood pressure (headache, blurred vision), low blood pressure (dizziness, weakness), palpitations, restlessness, seizures, heart and lung failure, and coma.

NARDIL'S OTHER NAME

Nardil's generic name is phenelzine sulfate.

SIDE EFFECTS

Call your doctor if you have any of these possible drug side effects. Call *immediately* about any labeled "serious."

Serious: irregular heartbeats, high blood pressure (headache, blurred vision), palpitations

Common: dizziness, drowsiness, sleeplessness, drastic appetite and weight loss, weakness, fatigue
Tip: To avoid dizziness, get out of bed and stand up slowly.

Other: headache, hyperactivity, tremor, muscle twitching, mania, confusion, impaired memory, dry mouth, nausea, constipation, swollen arms and legs, heavy sweating, weight changes

DRUG AND FOOD INTERACTIONS

Combining certain drugs and certain foods may alter drug action or produce unwanted side effects. Tell your doctor about your diet and other drugs you're taking, especially:
• alcohol, caffeine, foods high in tryptophan (broad beans) or tyramine (aged cheese, Chianti wine, beer, avocados, chicken livers, chocolate, bananas, meat tenderizers)
• Aramine, Ritalin
• barbiturates (such as Solfoton), dextromethorphan (as in Benylin), Levoprome, narcotics, other sedatives, tricyclic antidepressants (such as Elavil)
• blood pressure drugs such as HydroDIURIL
• cold, hay fever, or diet medicines
• insulin, oral diabetes drugs (such as Micronase)
• other MAO inhibitors, such as Parnate and Eldepryl.

X Warnings

• Make sure your doctor knows your medical history. You may not be able to take Nardil if you have other medical problems, especially an adrenal tumor, high blood pressure, or heart, liver, or lung disease; or if you're allergic to other antidepressants.
• Make sure your doctor knows if you're pregnant or breast-feeding before you begin taking Nardil.
• Nardil may hide the warning signs of an angina attack.

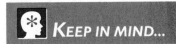 KEEP IN MIND...

∗ Take as directed.
∗ May take several weeks to reach full effect.
∗ Schedule regular follow-up visits to check progress.

Nasacort

Nasacort is a steroid that's used to treat stuffy nose, irritation, and other symptoms of hay fever and other allergic reactions. Nasacort reduces symptoms by reducing inflammation in the nasal passages.

Why it's prescribed

Doctors prescribe Nasacort to treat nasal problems caused by hay fever and other allergic reactions. It comes in a nasal aerosol. Doctors usually prescribe the following amounts for adults and children age 12 and over.

▶ **For hay fever and allergies,** at first, 2 sprays (110 micrograms [mcg]) in each nostril once a day, increased as needed up to 440 mcg a day either in a single dose or divided into up to four doses a day. After desired effect is obtained, dosage may be decreased to as little as 1 spray (55 mcg) in each nostril daily.

How to use Nasacort

• Use Nasacort only as your doctor directs. Symptoms may decrease within 12 hours; effects may last for several days after treatment is stopped.
• Use Nasacort on a regular schedule for greatest effectiveness, but don't use more than the prescribed dosage.
• Shake the container before using; blow your nose to clear your nasal passages; tilt your head slightly forward and insert nozzle into

NASACORT'S OTHER NAME

Nasacort's generic name is triamcinolone acetonide.

 SIDE EFFECTS

Call your doctor if you have any of these possible drug side effects.
Serious: none reported
Common: nose irritation, headache
Other: dry mucous membranes, nasal and sinus congestion, sore throat, sneezing, nosebleed

 DRUG INTERACTIONS

Combining certain drugs may alter their action or produce unwanted side effects. Tell your doctor about other drugs you're taking, especially:
• other steroids.

nostril, pointing away from the septum (center of your nose). Hold the other nostril closed and then inhale gently and spray. Shake the container again and repeat in the other nostril.

If you miss a dose

Take the missed dose if you remember within an hour. However, if it's almost time for your next dose, skip the missed dose and go back to your regular schedule. Don't take a double dose.

 If you suspect an overdose

Consult your doctor.

 Warnings

• Make sure your doctor knows your medical history. You may not be able to use Nasacort if you have other problems, such as tuberculosis; a fungal, bacterial, or viral infection or herpes; if you're allergic to it, its ingredients, or other drugs; or if you've had nasal ulcers, recent nasal surgery, or trauma. (Nasacort slows wound healing).

• Make sure your doctor knows if you're pregnant or breast-feeding before you begin taking Nasacort.
• Avoid people with chickenpox or measles; if you're exposed to either, let your doctor know.
• Watch for signs of nasal infection (redness, discolored nasal discharge). If these occur, check with your doctor.
• Discard the canister after 100 dosages. Don't break the canister, incinerate it, or store it in extreme heat; the contents are under pressure and may explode.
• If you don't feel better after 2 to 3 weeks of treatment, or if your condition worsens, call your doctor.

KEEP IN MIND...

* Take on schedule for best results.
* Don't use more than prescribed.
* Shake container before each use.

Nasalide

 Nasalide is used to treat stuffy nose, irritation, and other symptoms of hay fever and other allergies. Nasalide works by decreasing nasal inflammation.

Why it's prescribed

Doctors prescribe Nasalide to treat nasal stuffiness and inflammation caused by hay fever and other allergies. It comes in a nasal inhalant and a liquid solution in a spray pump bottle. Doctors usually prescribe the following amounts for adults; children's dosages appear in parentheses.

▶ **For hay fever and allergies,** starting dose is 2 sprays, or 50 micrograms [mcg], in each nostril twice a day. Total daily dosage is 200 mcg. If necessary, dosage may be increased to 2 sprays in each nostril three times a day. Maximum dosage is 8 sprays a day in each nostril or 400 mcg a day. (Children age 6 to 14: starting dose is 1 spray [25 mcg] in each nostril three times a day or 2 sprays [50 mcg] in each nostril twice a day. Total daily dosage is 150 to 200 mcg. Maximum dosage is 4 sprays a day in each nostril [200 mcg a day].)

How to use Nasalide

• Use Nasalide only as your doctor directs. This drug should begin to take effect within a few days, but in some cases beneficial effects may not be seen until after 2 to 3 weeks of treatment.

NASALIDE'S OTHER NAME

Nasalide's generic name is flunisolide.

 SIDE EFFECTS

Call your doctor if you have any of these possible drug side effects.

Serious: none reported

Common: temporary mild nasal burning and stinging

Other: headache, nasal congestion, fungal infection, sneezing, nosebleed, watery eyes, nausea, vomiting

DRUG INTERACTIONS

Combining certain drugs may alter their action or produce unwanted side effects. Tell your doctor about other drugs you're taking.

• Use Nasalide on a regular schedule for greatest effectiveness, but don't use more than the prescribed dosage.

• Shake the container before using; blow your nose to clear your nasal passages; tilt your head slightly forward and insert nozzle into nostril, pointing away from the septum (center of your nose). Hold the other nostril closed and then inhale gently and spray. Shake the container again and repeat in the other nostril.

• Clean the nosepiece with warm water if it becomes clogged.

If you miss a dose

Take the missed dose if you remember within an hour or so. However, if it's almost time for your next dose, skip the missed dose and go back to your regular schedule. Do not take a double dose.

 If you suspect an overdose

Consult your doctor.

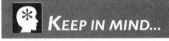 **Warnings**

• Make sure your doctor knows your medical history. You may not be able to use Nasalide if you have other problems, such as an infection of the nose or sinuses, tuberculosis, or a fungal, bacterial, or viral infection or herpes; if you're allergic to it or any of its ingredients, or to other drugs; or if you've had nasal ulcers, surgery, or trauma.

• Make sure your doctor knows if you're pregnant or breast-feeding before you begin taking Nasalide.

• Stop taking Nasalide and check with your doctor if you don't feel better within 3 weeks.

KEEP IN MIND...

∗ Take on schedule for greatest effectiveness.

∗ Usually takes effect within a few days.

∗ Clean nosepiece with warm water after use.

Navane is used to treat nervous, mental, and emotional illnesses. It works by blocking dopamine receptors in the brain. Blocking dopamine decreases hallucinations and agitation.

Why it's prescribed

Doctors prescribe Navane to treat mild to severe psychoses (nervous, mental, and emotional illnesses). Navane comes in capsules and an oral liquid. It's also available in an injectable form. Doctors usually prescribe the following amounts for adults.

▶ **For mild to moderate psychosis,** at first, 2 milligrams (mg) orally three times a day, increased gradually to 15 mg a day as needed.

▶ **For severe psychosis,** at first, 5 mg orally twice a day, increased gradually to 15 to 30 mg a day as needed. Maximum recommended dosage is 60 mg a day.

How to take Navane

• Take Navane only as your doctor directs. Dosages of Navane vary from person to person; occasionally, a single daily dose may be sufficient.

• When taking the oral liquid, use the bottle dropper to measure the exact dose. Then dilute the dose in half a glass (4 ounces) of water, milk, soda, or tomato or fruit juice.

• You may not notice Navane's effects for several weeks.

NAVANE'S OTHER NAME

Navane's generic name is thiothixene (capsules) or thiothixene hydrochloride (liquid).

SIDE EFFECTS

Call your doctor if you have any of these possible drug side effects. Call *immediately* about any labeled "serious."

Serious: liver disorder (nausea, vomiting, yellow-tinged skin and eyes), blood disorder (fatigue, bleeding, bruising, chills, fever, increased risk for infection), uncontrollable movements of mouth, tongue, cheeks, jaw, or arms and legs; fever; sore throat; fast pulse; rapid breathing; profuse sweating; fainting or dizziness; difficulty urinating; blurred vision

Common: "prickly" feeling, decreased muscle tone, dizziness, blurred vision, dry mouth, constipation, sensitivity to sunlight, reduced sweating
Tips: To relieve dry mouth, try sugarless gum or hard candy. Use sunblock and wear protective clothing to avoid reactions to sunlight. For dizziness, stand and change positions slowly. Avoid activities that require alertness or coordination until you know how this drug affects you; dizziness usually subside after a few weeks. Avoid getting overheated.

Other: sedation, fast or changed heartbeat, menstrual irregularities, breast development in men, inhibited ejaculation, allergic reactions (itching, hives, difficulty breathing), weight gain, increased appetite, neuroleptic malignant syndrome (fever, muscle rigidity, confusion)

DRUG INTERACTIONS

Combining certain drugs may alter their action or produce unwanted side effects. Tell your doctor about other drugs you're taking, especially:
• alcohol and other drugs that make you relaxed or sleepy (sedatives, sleeping pills, allergy medicines, pain relievers, and muscle relaxants).

• Don't suddenly stop taking Navane unless your doctor tells you to.

If you miss a dose

Take the missed dose as soon as possible. But if it's within 2 hours of your next dose, skip the missed dose and take your next dose as scheduled. Don't take a double dose.

If you suspect an overdose

Contact your doctor *immediately*. Excessive Navane can cause high blood pressure (headache, blurred vision), low blood pressure (dizziness, weakness), uncontrollable movements, agitation, seizures, palpitations, high or low body temperature, tremor, and deep, unarousable sleep.

✕ Warnings

• Make sure your doctor knows your medical history. You may not be able to take Navane if you have other problems, such as a blood or bone marrow disorder, heart or lung problems, seizures, glaucoma, enlarged prostate, Parkinson's disease, urine retention, tumors, low calcium level, or kidney or liver disease; if you're allergic to it or other drugs; or if you have a history of circulation problems, a head injury, or coma.

• Make sure your doctor knows if you're pregnant or breast-feeding before you begin taking Navane.

• Navane is not recommended for children under age 12.

• With long-term use, schedule appointments for regular blood tests and eye exams.

• Be aware that tardive dyskinesia—a condition that causes uncontrollable movements of the tongue, lips, or other body parts—may occur after prolonged use; it may not appear until months or years later, and may disappear or last for life, even after you stop taking this drug.

• Be aware that after abrupt withdrawal of long-term treatment, you may experience stomach upset, nausea, vomiting, dizziness, tremor, feeling of warmth or cold, sweating, fast pulse, headache, or sleeplessness.

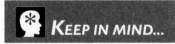

KEEP IN MIND...

* Takes effect in several weeks.
* Dilute liquid concentrate in a beverage.
* Don't suddenly stop taking Navane.

NebuPent

NebuPent is used to prevent or treat a type of pneumonia in people whose immune systems can no longer fight disease, such as people with AIDS. NebuPent destroys the tiny organisms (*Pneumocystis carinii*) that cause this pneumonia.

Why it's prescribed

Doctors prescribe NebuPent to prevent or treat some pneumonia in people with AIDS and others whose immune systems are depressed. NebuPent comes in an aerosol form that's inhaled. It's also available in an injectable form. Doctors usually prescribe the following amounts for adults; children's dosage appears in parentheses.

▶ **To treat pneumonia,** by injection once a day for 14 days. (Children: same as adult dosage.)

▶ **To prevent pneumonia,** 300 milligrams inhaled through aerosol device (nebulizer) once every 4 weeks.

How to use NebuPent

• Use NebuPent only as your doctor directs. Use aerosol form only with Respirgard II nebulizer made by Marquest.

• Use the aerosol device as directed until the chamber is empty. This may take as long as 45 minutes.

NEBUPENT'S OTHER NAMES

NebuPent's generic name is pentamidine isethionate. Other brand names include Pentacarinat, Pentam 300, and Pneumopent.

 ## SIDE EFFECTS

Call your doctor if you have any of these possible drug side effects. Call *immediately* about any labeled "serious."

Serious: decreased urination, sore throat and fever, easy bleeding or bruising; diarrhea, vomiting, bronchospasm, low blood sugar (anxiety, chills, cold sweats, cool and pale skin, headache, increased hunger, nervousness), low blood pressure (dizziness, fainting), kidney problems (decreased urine output), liver problems (yellow-tinged skin and eyes)

Common: cough
Tip: Don't smoke during treatment; smoking can cause coughing and difficulty breathing.

Other: confusion, hallucinations, fast pulse, nausea, drastic appetite and weight loss, metallic taste, facial flushing, itching, fever

 ## DRUG INTERACTIONS

Combining certain drugs may alter their action or produce unwanted side effects. Tell your doctor about other drugs you're taking, especially:

• Aerosporin, Coly-Mycin, Fungizone, Platinol, Vancocin
• aminoglycosides such as Nebcin, Garamycin
• other drugs to treat breathing problems
• Retrovir (AZT).

• Keep taking this drug as prescribed, even after you begin to feel better, to prevent pneumonia from coming back.

If you miss a dose

Take the missed dose as soon as possible.

 ## If you suspect an overdose

Consult your doctor.

 ## Warnings

• Make sure your doctor knows your medical history. You may not be able to take NebuPent if you have other problems, such as anemia or other blood disorders, asthma, diabetes, high or low blood pressure, or kidney, heart, or liver disease, or if you're allergic to it or other drugs.

• If you're pregnant or breast-feeding, check with your doctor before using NebuPent.

 ## KEEP IN MIND...

* Use recommended nebulizer only.

* Takes up to 45 minutes to inhale dosage.

* Take entire prescription even if symptoms subside.

* Don't smoke, to avoid coughing and difficulty breathing.

NegGram

NegGram, an antibiotic, kills the organisms that flourish in urinary infections.

Why it's prescribed

Doctors prescribe NegGram to treat urinary tract infections. It comes in tablets and an oral liquid. Doctors usually prescribe the following amounts for adults; children's dosages appear in parentheses.

▶ **For urinary tract infections**, 1 gram (g) four times a day for 7 to 14 days; 2 g a day for long-term use. (Children over age 3 months: 55 milligrams [mg] for each 2.2 pounds [lb] of body weight each day, divided into four equal doses a day for 7 to 14 days; 33 mg for each 2.2 lb a day for long-term use.)

How to take NegGram

• Take NegGram only as your doctor directs.
• When taking the oral liquid, use a specially marked measuring spoon, not a household teaspoon.
• For best results, take NegGram with a full glass (8 ounces) of water on an empty stomach (1 hour before or 2 hours after meals). If NegGram upsets your stomach, take with food or milk.
• Take NegGram for the full prescribed time and don't skip doses, even if you feel better after a few days. Call your doctor if your symptoms don't improve within 2 days or if they get worse.

If you miss a dose

Take the missed dose as soon as you remember. However, if it's almost time for your next dose and the doctor has prescribed three or more doses a day, space the missed dose and the next dose 2 to 4 hours apart, or double your next dose. Then go back to your regular schedule.

If you suspect an overdose

Contact your doctor *immediately*. Excessive NegGram can cause seizures, lethargy, nausea, vomiting, mental problems (excitement, depression, paranoia), increased pressure inside the skull (sleepiness), and metabolic acidosis (vomiting, nausea, fast breathing).

Warnings

• Make sure your doctor knows your medical history. You may not be able to take NegGram if you have other medical problems, especially seizures, liver or kidney problems, brain or spinal cord damage, a blood or blood vessel disorder, lung disease, or diabetes, or if you're allergic to this or other drugs.
• If you're pregnant or breast-feeding, check with your doctor before taking this drug.
• If you're diabetic, be aware that NegGram will affect results of urine sugar tests. Consult your doctor before adjusting your diabetes drug dosage.

SIDE EFFECTS

Call your doctor if you have any of these possible drug side effects. Call *immediately* about any labeled "serious."

Serious: seizures, blood problems (bleeding, bruising, fatigue, fever, chills, increased risk for infection), increased pressure inside the skull that causes bulging of the soft spot on top of head in infants and children, vision changes, hallucinations, mood changes, pale skin, pale stools, severe stomach pain, yellow-tinged skin or eyes

Common: abdominal pain, nausea, vomiting, diarrhea
Tip: Abdominal pain, nausea, and vomiting usually subside as your body adjusts to the drug.

Other: drowsiness, weakness, headache, dizziness, vertigo, confusion, hallucinations, sensitivity to light, itching, hives, rash

DRUG INTERACTIONS

Combining certain drugs may alter their action or produce unwanted side effects. Tell your doctor about other drugs you're taking, especially:
• anticoagulants (blood thinners), such as Coumadin and dicumarol.

NEGGRAM'S OTHER NAME

NegGram's generic name is nalidixic acid.

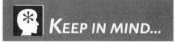

* Call your doctor if you see no improvement in 2 days.
* Take on an empty stomach.
* Take only as directed.
* Take for full prescribed time, even after you feel better.

Nembutal

Nembutal belongs to a group of drugs called barbiturates, which act by slowing down the central nervous system.

Why it's prescribed

Doctors prescribe Nembutal to relax a person before surgery and to treat insomnia and other conditions. Nembutal comes in capsules, an elixir, and suppositories. It's also available in an injectable form. Doctors usually prescribe the following amounts for adults; children's dosages appear in parentheses.

▶ **For sedation,** 20 to 40 milligrams (mg) orally two to four times a day. (Children: 2 to 6 mg for each 2.2 pounds [lb] orally a day divided into three equal doses. Maximum dosage is 100 mg a day.)

▶ **For insomnia,** 100 mg orally at bedtime or 120 or 200 mg rectally. (Children age 2 months to 1 year: 30 mg rectally. Children age 1 to 4 years: 30 or 60 mg rectally. Children age 5 to 11 years: 60 mg rectally. Children age 12 to 14 years: 60 or 120 mg rectally.)

How to take Nembutal

• Take Nembutal only as your doctor directs. This drug begins to take effect within 15 minutes after oral or rectal use; effects last 1 to 4 hours.

• To use a suppository, wash your hands and remove the foil wrapper;

NEMBUTAL'S OTHER NAMES

Nembutal's generic name is pentobarbital sodium. Other brand names include Nembutal Sodium and, in Canada, Nova Rectal and Novopentobarb.

SIDE EFFECTS

Call your doctor if you have any of these possible drug side effects. Call *immediately* about any labeled "serious."

Serious: skin eruptions (may follow high fever, inflamed mouth or nose, or headache), Stevens-Johnson syndrome (reddened, burn-like rash), liver problems (nausea, yellow-tinged skin and eyes), blood problems (bruising, bleeding, fever, chills, increased risk for infection)

Common: drowsiness, lethargy, "hangover" feeling

Tips: Morning "hangover" is common after dose that suppresses dreaming; dreaming may increase after drug is stopped. Don't drive or perform activities that require you to be fully alert if you become drowsy or lethargic.

Other: unusual excitement in older people, nausea, vomiting, rash, hives

DRUG INTERACTIONS

Combining certain drugs may alter their action or produce unwanted side effects. Tell your doctor about other drugs you're taking, especially:

• corticosteroids, anticoagulants (blood thinners) such as Coumadin
• alcohol or other drugs that make you relaxed or sleepy, including many allergy and cold medicines, narcotic pain relievers, and sleeping pills
• drugs for depression called MAO inhibitors such as Eldepryl
• estrogens (hormones) and birth control pills
• Fulvicin
• other antifungal drugs
• Rifadin
• Vibramycin.

---

then moisten the suppository with cold water. Next, lie down on your side and use your finger to push the suppository well up into your rectum. Wash your hands afterward.

• To ensure accurate dosage, don't divide suppositories.

• Store Nembutal in its original container at room temperature.

• Don't suddenly stop taking Nembutal, to avoid withdrawal symptoms. Check with your doctor about gradually stopping your use of this drug.

If you miss a dose

If you're taking Nembutal regularly, take the missed dose as soon as possible. However, if it's almost time for your next dose, skip the missed dose and go back to your regular schedule. Don't take a double dose.

 If you suspect an overdose

Contact your doctor *immediately.* Excessive Nembutal can cause severe drowsiness, confusion, or weakness; shortness of breath; slow pulse; slow or troubled breathing; slurred speech; staggering; coma; pinpoint pupils; bluish or clammy skin; and low blood pressure (dizziness, weakness, fainting). Overdose can be fatal.

✗◀ Warnings

• Make sure your doctor knows your medical history. You may not be able to take Nembutal if you have other medical problems, such as a blood or liver disorder, pain, depression, suicidal tendencies, or a history of drug abuse, or if you're allergic to this or other drugs.

• If you're pregnant or breast-feeding, check with your doctor before using this drug.
• Be aware that older adults and people who are ill may be especially prone to Nembutal's side effects.
• Nembutal can become habit-forming; don't take it longer than your doctor recommends, to avoid drug dependence. Also, this drug no longer promotes sleep after 14 days of continued use.

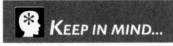

KEEP IN MIND...

* Take only as directed.
* Can become habit-forming.
* Don't suddenly stop taking.
* Don't divide suppositories.

Neo-Synephrine (eyedrops)

Neo-Synephrine eyedrops act on muscles in the eye to dilate the pupil and stop the lens from flattening and rounding.

Why it's prescribed

Doctors prescribe Neo-Synephrine eyedrops to relieve eye redness and discomfort, dilate the pupils, and treat certain eye problems (adhesion of iris). This drug comes in eyedrops, available in three different strengths — 0.12%, 2.5%, 10%. You can buy the 0.12% strength without a prescription. Doctors usually prescribe the following amounts for adults; children's dosages appear in parentheses.

▶ **For chronic dilated pupil,** 1 drop of 2.5% or 10% solution in the eyes two or three times a day. (Adolescents: same as adults. Children: 1 drop of 2.5% solution in the eyes two or three times a day.)

▶ **For iris that's attached to lens,** 1 drop of 10% solution.

How to use Neo-Synephrine eyedrops

• Use Neo-Synephrine eyedrops only as your doctor directs. If you bought this drug without a prescription, carefully follow the package directions.

• Wash your hands before and after using.

NEO-SYNEPHRINE'S OTHER NAMES

Neo-Synephrine (eyedrops)'s generic name is phenylephrine hydrochloride. Other brand names include AK-Dilate, I-Phrine 2.5%, Isopto Frin, Mydfrin, and Prefrin Liquifilm.

 SIDE EFFECTS

Call your doctor if you have any of these possible drug side effects. Call *immediately* about any labeled "serious."

Serious: high blood pressure (headache, blurred vision), fast or abnormal heartbeat, palpitations, glaucoma, allergic inflammation

Common: headache, burning or stinging (after using drops), blurred vision, bloodshot eyes

Other: brow pain, iris floaters, pallor, trembling, sweating, rash

DRUG INTERACTIONS

Combining certain drugs may alter their action or produce unwanted side effects. Tell your doctor about other drugs you're taking, especially:
• atropine for external use
• beta blockers, such as Inderal and Lopressor
• Ismelin, Lanoxin
• Parkinson's disease drugs such as Sinemet
• tricyclic antidepressants (such as Elavil) and MAO inhibitors (such as Eldepryl).

• Don't touch the tip of the dropper to your eye or any other surface, to avoid contamination.

• This drug takes effect rapidly. Effects last for about 3 to 7 hours.

If you miss a dose

Use the missed dose as soon as possible. However, if it's almost time for your next dose, skip the missed dose and use your next dose on schedule. Don't use a double dose.

 If you suspect an overdose

Contact your doctor *immediately.* Excessive Neo-Synephrine eyedrops can cause palpitations, vomiting, and high blood pressure (headache, blurred vision).

Warnings

• Make sure your doctor knows your medical history. You may not be able to use Neo-Synephrine eyedrops if you have glaucoma, high blood pressure, heart problems, diabetes, an overactive thyroid, or drug allergies; or if you wear soft contact lenses.

• Make sure your doctor knows if you're pregnant or breast-feeding before you begin using Neo-Synephrine (eyedrops).

• Don't use this drug if it turns brown or cloudy.

• If your eyes don't return to normal after 12 hours, call your doctor.

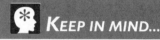 **KEEP IN MIND...**

* Don't touch dropper to eye or any surface.

* Don't use cloudy solution.

* Check with doctor if effects last more than 12 hours.

Neo-Synephrine Nasal Spray

Neo-Synephrine Nasal Spray narrows dilated blood vessels in the nose and nasal passages, reducing nasal congestion.

Why it's prescribed

Doctors prescribe Neo-Synephrine Nasal Spray to relieve stuffy nose. You can buy Neo-Synephrine Nasal Spray without a prescription. It comes in nose spray; other brands come in nose drops and a nose jelly. Doctors usually prescribe the following amounts for adults; children's dosages appear in parentheses.

▶ **For nasal congestion,** 2 to 3 drops or 1 to 2 sprays in each nostril or small amount of jelly inside nose every 4 hours, as needed. (Children age 12 and older: same as adults. Children age 6 to 12: 2 to 3 drops or 1 to 2 sprays of 0.25% solution in each nostril. Children under age 6: 2 to 3 drops of 0.125% solution in each nostril every 4 hours, as needed.)

How to use Neo-Synephrine Nasal Spray

• Use this drug as your doctor directs. It takes effect rapidly; effects last for up to 4 hours.
• If you're treating yourself, follow the package directions carefully.

NEO-SYNEPHRINE NASAL SPRAY'S OTHER NAMES

Neo-Synephrine Nasal Spray's generic name is phenylephrine hydrochloride. Other brand names include Alconefrin Nasal Spray 25, Duration, Nostril Spray Pump Mild, Rhinall, and Vicks Sinex.

 SIDE EFFECTS

Call your doctor if you have any of these possible drug side effects. Call *immediately* about any labeled "serious."

Serious: high blood pressure (headache, blurred vision)

Common: fast pulse, palpitations

Other: headache, tremor, dizziness, nervousness, pallor, temporary burning or stinging, dry nose, rebound nasal congestion, nausea

 DRUG INTERACTIONS

Combining certain drugs may alter their action or produce unwanted side effects. Tell your doctor about other drugs you're taking.

• Before using, blow your nose.
• To use the spray, sniff briskly while squeezing the bottle into your nostril. Spray once or twice; then wait a few minutes for the drug to work. Blow your nose and repeat until the complete dose is taken.
• Don't use Neo-Synephrine Nasal Spray longer than necessary; overuse can make your condition worse.

If you miss a dose

Take the missed dose right away if it's within 1 hour. If you don't remember until later, skip the missed dose and take your next dose on schedule. Don't take a double dose.

 If you suspect an overdose

Contact your doctor *immediately.* Excessive Neo-Synephrine Nasal Spray can cause palpitations, irregular heartbeat, tingling or other strange sensation, vomiting, and high blood pressure (headache, blurred vision).

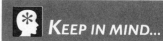 **Warnings**

• Make sure your doctor knows your medical history. You may not be able to use Neo-Synephrine if you have heart or blood vessel disease, high blood pressure, glaucoma, diabetes, an overactive thyroid, liver or pancreas problems, or drug allergies.
• Tell your doctor if you're pregnant or breast-feeding.
• Before having a hearing test, tell the doctor that you're using Neo-Synephrine.
• If your symptoms don't improve after 3 days of treatment, check with your doctor.

KEEP IN MIND...

∗ Gently blow nose before using.
∗ Don't share this drug.
∗ Don't use more than 3 days without doctor's consent.

Neurontin

Neurontin is used to help control seizures in epilepsy. How Neurontin reduces seizures is not fully understood.

Why it's prescribed

Doctors prescribe Neurontin to reduce seizures. It comes in capsules. Doctors usually prescribe the following amounts for adults.

▶ **For seizures in epilepsy,** 300 milligrams (mg) at bedtime on day 1; 300 mg twice a day on day 2; then 300 mg three times a day on day 3. Dosage increased as needed and tolerated to 1,800 mg a day divided into equal doses. Dosages up to 3,600 mg a day have been well tolerated.

How to take Neurontin

• Take Neurontin only as your doctor directs. This drug may be taken with or without meals.
• Take your first dose at bedtime to avoid drowsiness, dizziness, fatigue, and incoordination.
• Don't suddenly stop taking Neurontin. Your doctor will stop treatment gradually over at least 1 week, or will substitute a different drug for that time, to avoid bringing on seizures.

If you miss a dose

Take the missed dose as soon as possible. However, if it's almost time for your next dose, skip the missed

NEURONTIN'S OTHER NAME

Neurontin's generic name is gabapentin.

 SIDE EFFECTS

Call your doctor if you have any of these possible drug side effects.

Serious: none reported

Common: sleepiness, dizziness, incoordination, fatigue, rapid eye movements, tremor, double vision or other vision problem, stuffy or runny nose

Tip: Avoid driving or operating heavy machinery until you know how this drug affects you.

Other: nervousness, slurred speech, memory loss, depression, abnormal thinking, twitching, poor muscle coordination, swollen arms and legs, irritated or dry throat, coughing, nausea, vomiting, stomach upset, dry mouth, constipation, impotence, blood problems (fever, chills, cough, hoarseness, lower back or side pain, painful or difficult urination), itching, abrasion, dental problems, increased appetite, weight gain, back pain, muscle pain, fractures

 DRUG INTERACTIONS

Combining certain drugs may alter their action or produce unwanted side effects. Tell your doctor about other drugs you're taking, especially:
• antacids (take at least 2 hours before or after Neurontin).

dose and go back to your regular schedule. Don't take a double dose.

 If you suspect an overdose

Contact your doctor *immediately.* Excessive Neurontin can cause double vision, slurred speech, drowsiness, lethargy, and diarrhea.

Warnings

• Make sure your doctor knows your medical history. You may not be able to take Neurontin if you have other problems, especially kidney disease, or if you're allergic to the drug.

• Tell your doctor if you're pregnant or breast-feeding before you begin taking Neurontin.
• Check with your doctor about gradually switching from other seizure drugs to Neurontin.

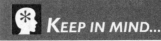 **KEEP IN MIND...**

∗ Take with or without meals.

∗ Take first dose at bedtime to avoid side effects.

∗ Don't suddenly stop taking; seizures may occur.

Niacor

Niacor replaces niacin—a necessary B vitamin—in the body and helps the body process fats and prevent cholesterol buildup.

Why it's prescribed

Doctors prescribe Niacor to treat niacin deficiency and related diseases, such as pellagra and Hartnup disease, or to help reduce elevated cholesterol levels. You can also buy Niacor without a prescription. It comes in tablets, timed-release tablets, timed-release capsules, and an oral liquid. It's also available in an injectable form. Doctors usually prescribe the following amounts for adults; children's dosages appear in parentheses.

▶ **For daily use, recommended daily allowances (RDA) are:**
• Neonates and infants to age 6 months: 5 milligrams (mg).
• Infants age 6 months to 1 year: 6 mg.
• Children age 1 to 3 years: 9 mg.
• Children age 4 to 6 years: 12 mg.
• Children age 7 to 10 years: 13 mg.
• Boys age 11 to 14 years: 17 mg.
• Boys age 15 to 18 years: 20 mg.
• Men age 19 to 50 years: 19 mg.
• Men age 51 years and over: 15 mg.
• Women age 11 to 50 years: 15 mg.
• Women age 51 years and over: 13 mg.
• Pregnant women: 17 mg.
• Breast-feeding women: 20 mg.

NIACOR'S OTHER NAMES

Niacor's generic name is niacin (also known as vitamin B_3 or nicotinic acid). Other brand names include Niac, Nico-400, Nicobid, Nicolar, Nicotinex, and Slo-Niacin.

▶ **For pellagra (severe niacin deficiency)**, 300 to 500 mg orally. (Children: up to 300 mg a day orally.) After symptoms subside, good nutrition and supplements prevent recurrence.
▶ **For Hartnup disease,** 50 to 200 mg orally once a day.
▶ **For niacin deficiency,** up to 100 mg orally once a day.
▶ **For high cholesterol levels,** 1 to 2 grams (g) orally three times a day with or after meals, increased gradually to 6 g a day.

How to take Niacor

• Take Niacor only as your doctor directs, in the amount prescribed. Don't take large doses of Niacor without your doctor's consent.
• When taking timed-release tablets, swallow them whole. If the tablets are scored, you may break them before swallowing, but don't crush or chew them.
• When taking timed-release capsules, swallow them without chewing or crushing. If too large to swallow, open the capsules and mix the contents with jelly or jam and swallow without chewing.

If you miss a dose

Adjust your schedule as follows:
• When taking Niacor without a prescription, missing 1 or 2 days won't drastically affect you.
• When taking Niacor to reduce cholesterol, take the missed dose as soon as possible. However, if it's almost time for your next dose, skip the missed dose and go back to your regular schedule. Don't take a double dose.

 If you suspect an overdose

Consult your doctor. However, because niacin dissolves in water and is flushed through the body, overdose is rare in people whose kidneys are working properly.

Continued on next page ▶

 SIDE EFFECTS

Call your doctor if you have any of these possible drug side effects. Call *immediately* about any labeled "serious."

Serious: with timed-release forms: darkened urine, light gray stools, appetite loss, liver problems (severe stomach pain, yellow skin or eyes)

Common: flushing or warmth, nausea, vomiting, diarrhea
Tip: Take with milk or meals to avoid nausea and diarrhea.

Other: dizziness, temporary headache, ulcer aggravation, itching, dry skin, tingling, high blood sugar (increased thirst, hunger, and urination)

 DRUG INTERACTIONS

Combining certain drugs may alter their action or produce unwanted side effects. Tell your doctor about other drugs you're taking, especially:
• blood pressure drugs (Cardura, Catapres, Inderal, Lopressor, Minipress).

✕ Warnings

• Make sure your doctor knows your medical history. You may not be able to take Niacor if you have other problems, such as diabetes, bleeding problems, glaucoma, gout, low blood pressure, ulcers, or gall-bladder, heart, or liver disease, or if you're allergic to this or other drugs.

• If you're pregnant or breast-feeding, check with your doctor before taking Niacor.

• Check with your doctor before you stop taking Niacor if you're being treated for high cholesterol.

• Follow your doctor's recommendations to lower your cholesterol level; follow any special diet your doctor recommends (such as a low-fat, low-cholesterol diet) while taking Niacor.

• Be aware that Niacor is a vitamin supplement only; follow your doctor's recommendations for eating a varied, well-balanced diet that includes niacin-rich meat, eggs, and dairy foods.

• If your doctor directs, take aspirin (325 mg orally 30 minutes before niacin dose) to possibly reduce the flushing response to niacin. Timed-release Niacor may prevent the excessive flushing that occurs with large doses. However, check with your doctor before changing the form of Niacor that you take.

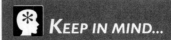

KEEP IN MIND...

* Take with milk or meals to avoid diarrhea or upset stomach.

* Don't crush or chew timed-release tablets or capsules.

* Check with doctor before you stop taking.

* Follow your doctor's diet recommendations.

* Take aspirin or a timed-release form to reduce flushing.

Niclocide

Niclocide is used to treat parasitic worm infestations. Tapeworms from fish, beef, and pork are killed on contact with this drug, and are eliminated in the stool.

Why it's prescribed

Doctors prescribe Niclocide to treat tapeworm infestations. It's ineffective against other worms (for example, pinworms or roundworms). Niclocide comes in chewable tablets. Doctors usually prescribe the following amounts for adults; children's dosages appear in parentheses.

▶ **For tapeworms (from fish, beef, or pork),** 4 tablets, or 2 grams (g), chewed thoroughly as a single dose. (Children over age 2 and weighing more than 75 pounds [lb]: 3 tablets [1.5 g] chewed thoroughly as a single dose. Children over age 2 and weighing 24 to 74 lb: 2 tablets [1 g] chewed thoroughly as a single dose.)

▶ **For dwarf tapeworm,** 4 tablets chewed thoroughly once a day for 7 days. (Children over age 2 and weighing more than 75 lb: 3 tablets [1.5 g] chewed thoroughly on the first day, then 2 tablets [1 g] daily for the next 6 days. Children over age 2 and weighing 24 to 74 kg: 2 tablets [1 g] chewed thoroughly on the first day, then 1 tablet [0.5 g] a day for the next 6 days.)

How to take Niclocide

• Take Niclocide only as your doctor directs. Take a drug to prevent

NICLOCIDE'S OTHER NAME

Niclocide's generic name is niclosamide.

SIDE EFFECTS

Call your doctor if you have any of these possible drug side effects.

Serious: none reported

Common: nausea, vomiting, drastic appetite and weight loss

Other: drowsiness, dizziness, headache, mouth irritation, bad taste in mouth, diarrhea, rash, itching in anal area

DRUG INTERACTIONS

Combining certain drugs may alter their action or produce unwanted side effects. Tell your doctor about other drugs you're taking.

vomiting before you take Niclocide. You may also be directed to take a laxative 2 hours after you take Niclocide to eliminate the killed worms and to prevent worm eggs from moving into the stomach.

• Take tablets as a single dose after breakfast.

• Chew tablets thoroughly and wash them down with water; for children, crush and mix the tablets with water or applesauce.

• When taking for dwarf tapeworms, drink fruit juices to help eliminate intestinal mucus that protects the tapeworms.

If you miss a dose

Take the missed dose as soon as possible. However, if it's almost time for your next dose, skip the missed dose and go back to your regular schedule. Don't take a double dose.

 If you suspect an overdose

Contact your doctor *immediately.* Overdose is treated by a fast-acting laxative and an enema.

Warnings

• Make sure your doctor knows your medical history. You may not be able to take Niclocide if you're allergic to this or other drugs.

• Tell your doctor if you're pregnant or breast-feeding before you take Niclocide.

• Schedule a follow-up visit so your doctor can make sure the tapeworms are gone.

• Practice good hand-washing techniques as instructed by your doctor. Also, don't prepare food for others during infestation.

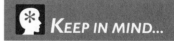 KEEP IN MIND...

* Take as a single dose after breakfast.

* Chew tablets thoroughly before swallowing with water.

* For dwarf tapeworms, drink fruit juices during treatment.

* Wash hands thoroughly; don't prepare food while infected.

Nicoderm

Nicoderm provides a controlled dosage of nicotine through the skin to relieve the anxiety, tremors, and palpitations that characterize withdrawal from smoking.

Why it's prescribed

Doctors prescribe Nicoderm to help people quit smoking. It's prescribed as part of a supervised program of education, counseling, and psychological support. Nicoderm comes in a series of adhesive skin patches that deliver different amounts of nicotine into the body. Doctors usually prescribe the following amounts for adults.

▶ **For smoking withdrawal**, at first, 1 patch, delivering the largest dosage of nicotine, applied once a day in the morning to a nonhairy part of body and removed before bedtime. After 4 to 12 weeks (depending on brand used), dosage tapered to next largest patch, followed in 2 to 4 weeks by patch with lowest nicotine dosage. Treatment is then stopped in 2 to 4 weeks.

How to take Nicoderm

• Take Nicoderm only as your doctor directs. To prevent nicotine overdose, don't smoke during treatment with Nicoderm.
• Follow package instructions carefully regarding when and how often to apply a new patch and how long to leave it on. A new patch is

NICODERM'S OTHER NAMES

Nicoderm's generic name is nicotine transdermal system. Other brand names include Habitrol, Nicotrol, and ProStep.

 SIDE EFFECTS

Call your doctor if you have any of these possible drug side effects.

Serious: none reported

Common: headache, sleeplessness, overall rash; itching, burning, or rash where patch was applied

Tips: The first patch may cause mild itching, tingling, and burning; these symptoms should go away within 1 hour. If skin under the patch becomes red or swollen or if a rash appears, remove the patch and call your doctor to check for allergy.

Other: sleepiness, dizziness, irritated nose or throat, abdominal pain, constipation, stomach upset, nausea, menstrual irregularity or absence, back pain, muscle pain, sweating

 DRUG INTERACTIONS

Combining certain drugs may alter their action or produce unwanted side effects. Tell your doctor about other drugs you're taking, especially:
• caffeine, Inderal, Serax, Talwin, Theo-Dur, Tofranil, Tylenol
• Cardura, Minipress
• insulin
• nonprescription decongestants.

usually applied every day, preferably at the same time each day.
• Apply the patch to a hairless part of your body, such as the outer part of your upper arm, or your stomach or back above the waist. Choose an area that's free from cuts and irritation.
• Nicotine evaporates from the patch after it's opened, so apply the patch promptly. Don't fold or cut the patch before applying it. Don't store at temperatures above 86° F.
• Press the patch firmly to your skin. Then wash your hands with water only; soap can cause unwanted nicotine absorption.
• To avoid skin irritation, apply each new patch to a different site. Wait at least 1 week before reusing a site.

• After removal, fold the patch in half, bringing the adhesive sides together. If the patch comes in a protective pouch, place the used patch in the pouch and discard it where children and animals can't reach it. Used patches contain enough nicotine to poison children and pets.
• Use Nicoderm for the full time prescribed; don't stop using it suddenly.

If you miss a dose

Apply a new patch as soon as you remember. Then change the patch at the regular time. If the patch falls off, apply a new one, then change it at your usual time.

If you suspect an overdose

Contact your doctor *immediately*. Symptoms of nicotine overdose may include severe headache, vomiting, diarrhea, dizziness, weakness, or confusion.

Warnings

• Make sure your doctor knows your medical history. You may not be able to use Nicoderm if you have other problems, such as an overactive thyroid, high blood pressure, hyperthyroidism, adrenal tumor, diabetes, ulcers, kidney or liver disease, heart rhythm problems, or angina (chest pain); if you're allergic to the drug or any ingredient of the patch; or if you've recently had a heart attack.

• If you're pregnant, don't use Nicoderm. If you become pregnant while using it, stop using the patch until you've checked with your doctor.

• If you're breast-feeding, check with your doctor before using Nicoderm.

• Use Nicoderm patches as you follow the other parts of your smoke-ending program.

• Don't use nicotine patches for more than 3 months. Ongoing use can be dangerous and habit-forming.

• If you can't stop cigarette smoking during the first 4 weeks of therapy, you may need counseling to find out why the treatment isn't working. You may want to try this treatment again after a short time.

KEEP IN MIND...

* Don't smoke during treatment.

* Place on skin that's free from cuts and irritation.

* Wash hands with water (no soap) after applying patch.

* Remove patch before bedtime.

* Discard where children and animals can't reach.

* Place each new patch on different skin area.

* Don't stop using suddenly or continue use for more than 3 months.

Nicorette

Nicorette provides a controlled dosage of nicotine to relieve the anxiety, tremors, and palpitations that characterize withdrawal from smoking.

Why it's prescribed

Doctors prescribe Nicorette to help people quit smoking. It's prescribed as part of a supervised program. Nicorette is especially useful for people with high "physical" nicotine dependence; that is, people who smoke more than 15 cigarettes a day. Nicorette comes in chewing gum squares. Doctors usually prescribe the following amounts for adults.

▶ **For nicotine withdrawal,** at first, one 2-milligram (mg) square; highly dependent people start treatment with 4-mg squares. One piece of gum chewed slowly and intermittently for 30 minutes whenever the urge to smoke occurs; usually 9 to 12 pieces of gum a day for the first month. For people using 4-mg squares, maximum dosage is 20 pieces a day. For people using 2-mg squares, maximum dosage is 30 pieces a day.

How to take Nicorette

• Take Nicorette only as your doctor directs; also, read the instruction sheet that comes in the package.
• Chew gum slowly and intermittently (chew several times, then place between cheek and gums) for about 30 minutes, so the nicotine is absorbed slowly and evenly and to avoid side effects.

NICORETTE'S OTHER NAME

Nicorette's generic name is nicotine polacrilex.

 SIDE EFFECTS

Call your doctor if you have any of these possible drug side effects.

Serious: none reported

Common: none reported

Other: dizziness, light-headedness, fast or irregular heartbeat, sore throat, jaw muscle ache (from chewing), nausea, vomiting, indigestion, hiccups

 DRUG INTERACTIONS

Combining certain drugs may alter their action or produce unwanted side effects. Tell your doctor about other drugs you're taking, especially:
• beta blockers, such as Inderal
• Darvon.

• Gradually stop using the gum after 3 months; don't use Nicorette for longer than 6 months. For gradual withdrawal, cut gum in halves or quarters and mix with other sugarless gum.

If you miss a dose

While using this treatment, carry nicotine gum with you at all times, to avoid reverting to cigarettes when the gum is not readily available. Don't chew double your normal amount.

If you suspect an overdose

Contact your doctor *immediately.* Excessive Nicorette can cause, in the following order: nausea or vomiting; heavy salivation; severe abdominal or stomach pain; severe diarrhea; cold sweat; severe headache; drooling; hearing and vision disturbance; confusion; low blood pressure (severe dizziness and weakness, fainting); severe difficulty breathing; fast, weak, or irregular heartbeat; and seizures.

✕ Warnings

• Make sure your doctor knows your medical history. You may not be able to take Nicorette if you have other problems, such as severe irregular heartbeats, severe chest pain (angina), overactive thyroid, adrenal tumor, diabetes, ulcer, mouth or throat inflammation, or a jaw or dental problem that might be worsened by chewing gum; if you're allergic to this or other drugs; or if you've recently had a heart attack.
• If you're pregnant, don't use Nicorette. If you're breast-feeding, make sure your doctor knows before you begin using Nicorette.

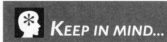 **KEEP IN MIND...**

* Chew gum slowly and intermittently for about 30 minutes.
* Don't use longer than 6 months.
* Carry at all times, to avoid cigarette use.

Nilstat (oral)

Nilstat, an antibiotic, fights fungal infections by destroying the membrane around fungal cells, thereby killing the fungus.

Why it's prescribed

Doctors prescribe oral Nilstat to treat fungal infections that affect the mouth and throat, intestines, or vagina. It comes in tablets and an oral liquid. Doctors usually prescribe the following amounts for adults; children's dosages appear in parentheses.

▶ **For intestinal infections,** 500,000 to 1 million units three times a day.

▶ **For infections of the mouth or intestine,** 400,000 to 600,000 units four times a day. (Children over age 3 months: 250,000 to 500,000 units four times a day. Newborns and premature infants: 100,000 units four times a day.)

▶ **For vaginal infections,** 1 vaginal tablet once or twice a day for 14 days.

How to take Nilstat

• Take Nilstat only as your doctor directs.

NILSTAT'S OTHER NAMES

Nilstat's generic name is nystatin. Other brand names include Mycostatin, Nystex, and, in Canada, Nadostine.

 SIDE EFFECTS

Call your doctor if you have any of these possible drug side effects.

Serious: none reported

Common: none reported

Other: transient nausea, vomiting, or diarrhea

 DRUG INTERACTIONS

Combining certain drugs may alter their action or produce unwanted side effects. Tell your doctor about other drugs you're taking.

• When taking the oral liquid, swish the dose in your mouth, gargle, and swallow.

• Take your entire prescription as your doctor directs, even if your symptoms disappear. If you stop too soon your infection may return.

If you miss a dose

Take the missed dose as soon as possible. However, if it's almost time for your next dose, skip the missed dose and go back to your regular schedule. Don't take a double dose.

 If you suspect an overdose

Contact your doctor. Excessive Nilstat can cause nausea, vomiting, and diarrhea.

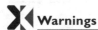 **Warnings**

• Make sure your doctor knows your medical history. You may not be able to take Nilstat if you have

diabetes or if you're allergic to this or other drugs.

• Tell your doctor if you're pregnant or breast-feeding before you begin taking Nilstat.

• With oral or intestinal infection, follow your doctor's recommendations for good oral hygiene during treatment. Overuse of mouthwash or poorly fitting dentures, especially in older people, may promote infection.

• Check with your doctor or pharmacist about how to store this drug. Don't allow the oral liquid to freeze.

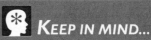 **KEEP IN MIND...**

* Swish oral liquid in mouth before swallowing.

* For infants, swab inside of mouth with the drug.

* Follow doctor's recommendations for oral hygiene.

Nilstat (for skin)

Nilstat fights fungal infections by destroying the membrane around fungal cells, thereby killing the fungus.

Why it's prescribed

Doctors prescribe Nilstat for the skin to treat certain fungal infections, called *Candida*, that affect the skin or vagina and vulva. It comes in cream, ointment, powder, and vaginal tablets. Doctors usually prescribe the following amounts for adults; children's dosages appear in parentheses.

▶ **For skin infections,** small amount of cream, ointment, or powder applied to affected area up to several times a day. (Children: same as adult dosage.)

▶ **For vulvovaginal infection,** 1 vaginal tablet inserted into vagina once or twice a day for 14 days.

How to use Nilstat

• Use Nilstat only as your doctor directs.

• For a skin infection, apply just enough cream or ointment to cover the affected area. When using the powder on your feet, sprinkle it between your toes, on your feet, and in socks and shoes.

• When using cream or ointment, don't cover treated skin with a bandage, wrap, or other airtight dressing without your doctor's consent.

• Refrigerate vaginal tablets.

 SIDE EFFECTS

Call your doctor if you have any of these possible drug side effects.

Serious: none reported

Common: none reported

Other: skin reaction, from preservatives in some brands (redness; itching; irritation, including vaginal irritation)

 DRUG INTERACTIONS

Combining certain drugs may alter their action or produce unwanted side effects. Tell your doctor about other drugs you're taking.

• For a vaginal infection, insert the tablets with an applicator, which your doctor will tell you how to use. Keep using this drug during menstruation.

• Use Nilstat for as long as your doctor prescribes, even if your symptoms disappear. If you stop using it too soon your infection may return.

If you miss a dose

Apply the missed dose as soon as possible. However, if it's almost time for your next dose, skip the missed dose and go back to your regular schedule. Don't apply a double dose.

 If you suspect an overdose

Consult your doctor.

 Warnings

• Make sure your doctor knows your medical history. You may not be able to use Nilstat if you're allergic to this or other drugs, foods, or preservatives.

• Tell your doctor if you're pregnant or breast-feeding before you begin taking Nilstat. Check with your doctor before using the applicator to insert vaginal tablets during pregnancy.

• When using vaginal tablets, expect some vaginal drainage. Wear a sanitary napkin to protect your clothing.

• If you have a vaginal infection, wear only freshly washed cotton underwear or pantyhose with cotton crotches instead of synthetics, to prevent reinfecting yourself.

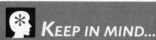 **KEEP IN MIND...**

* Don't cover treated skin with airtight dressing.
* Refrigerate vaginal tablets.
* Keep using vaginal tablets during menstruation.
* Wear sanitary napkin to protect clothing from vaginal drainage.
* Keep using as prescribed even if symptoms disappear.

NILSTAT'S OTHER NAMES

Nilstat's generic name is topical nystatin. Other brand names include Mycostatin and, in Canada, Nadostine.

Nitro-Dur

Nitro-Dur releases a steady, controlled amount of nitroglycerin into the body through the skin. It regulates the flow of oxygen-rich blood to the heart and reduces the heart's workload.

Why it's prescribed

Doctors prescribe Nitro-Dur to prevent chest pain (angina) attacks. It comes in adhesive skin patches that supply various amounts of the drug. Doctors usually prescribe the following amounts for adults.

▶ **To prevent chest pain,** 1 skin patch applied once a day.

How to use Nitro-Dur

• Use Nitro-Dur only as your doctor directs.
• Nitro-Dur begins to take effect within 30 minutes. Effects last up to 24 hours with patch on, but only for several minutes after removing the patch.
• Apply the patch to a clean, dry skin area with little or no hair and no cuts, scars, or irritation. Don't place the patch on the lower part of your arm or leg because the drug won't work as well at these sites.
• To keep your body from building up resistance to this drug, remove the patch in the early evening and apply a new patch the next morning. Always remove the previous patch before applying a new one.
• To prevent skin irritation or other problems, apply each new patch to a different skin area.

NITRO-DUR'S OTHER NAMES

Nitro-Dur's generic name is topical nitroglycerin. Other brand names include Transderm-Nitro.

 SIDE EFFECTS

Call your doctor if you have any of these possible drug side effects. Call *immediately* about any labeled "serious."

Serious: severe or prolonged headache, dry mouth, blurred vision

Common: fast pulse, skin flushing, headache, nausea, vomiting, restlessness, dizziness

Tip: These side effects usually go away as your body adjusts to the drug. If they persist or worsen, call your doctor.

Other: weakness, fainting, rash

 DRUG INTERACTIONS

Combining certain drugs may alter their action or produce unwanted side effects. Tell your doctor about other drugs you're taking, especially:
• alcohol
• other heart or blood pressure drugs.

• Don't suddenly stop using Nitro-Dur; this may bring on angina attacks. Your doctor may want to reduce your dosage gradually.

If you miss a dose

Apply a new patch as soon as possible. Then resume your regular schedule.

 If you suspect an overdose

Contact your doctor *immediately.* Excessive Nitro-Dur can cause persistent throbbing headache, palpitations, vision disturbances, flushing, sweating, nausea, vomiting, abdominal pain and cramps, bloody diarrhea, low blood pressure (dizziness, weakness), deep or difficult breathing, slow breathing, slow pulse, confusion, fever, or seizures.

 Warnings

• Make sure your doctor knows your medical history. You may not be able to use Nitro-Dur if you have glaucoma, kidney or liver disease, an overactive thyroid, severe anemia, or a drug allergy; if you've recently had a heart attack, stroke, or head injury; or if you're pregnant or breast-feeding.
• Older adults may be especially sensitive to Nitro-Dur's side effects.
• Don't remain close to a microwave oven when wearing a patch. Leaking radiation can heat the patch's metallic backing and cause burns.
• Don't trim or cut the patch to adjust the dosage. If you think this drug isn't working properly, check with your doctor.

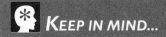 **KEEP IN MIND...**

∗ Place patch on clean, dry hairless skin, free of cuts or scars.

∗ Place each new patch on a different skin area.

∗ Don't suddenly stop using.

Nitrol

Nitrol increases the flow of oxygen-rich blood to the heart and reduces the heart's workload.

Why it's prescribed

Doctors prescribe Nitrol ointment to relieve chest pain (angina). It comes in an ointment. Doctors usually prescribe the following amounts for adults.

▶ **To prevent chest pain,** start with ½ inch of ointment, increasing by ½-inch increments until headache occurs, then decreasing to previous dose. Dosage range is ½ to 5 inches. Usual dose is 1 to 2 inches.

How to use Nitrol

• Use Nitrol only as your doctor directs.
• Nitrol begins to take effect in 30 minutes; effects last 4 to 8 hours.
• Remove all excess ointment from previous site before applying the next dose.
• Measure the prescribed amount on the application paper, then place the paper on any nonhairy area.
• Avoid getting ointment on fingers.
• If using Tape-Surrounded Appli-Ruler (TSAR) system, keep the TSAR on your skin to protect your clothing and to make sure the ointment stays in place.
• Apply each dose to a different area of skin, to prevent skin irritation and other problems.
• Don't suddenly stop using Nitrol; this may bring on angina attacks.

NITROL'S OTHER NAME

Nitrol's generic name is nitroglycerin ointment.

 SIDE EFFECTS

Call your doctor if you have any of these possible drug side effects. Call *immediately* about any labeled "serious."

Serious: severe or prolonged headache, dry mouth, blurred vision

Common: headache (sometimes throbbing), dizziness, fast pulse, flushing, palpitations, weakness
Tips: Sit up and stand slowly to avoid dizziness; use stairs carefully; lie down at the first sign of dizziness.

Other: fainting, nausea, vomiting, rash, allergic reaction (rash)

 DRUG INTERACTIONS

Combining certain drugs may alter their action or produce unwanted side effects. Tell your doctor about other drugs you're taking, especially:
• alcohol
• other heart or blood pressure drugs.

Your doctor may want to reduce your dosage gradually.

If you miss a dose

Apply the missed dose as soon as possible. If your next scheduled application is within 2 hours, skip the missed dose and resume your regular schedule. Don't apply a double dose.

 If you suspect an overdose

Contact your doctor *immediately.* Excessive Nitrol can cause bluish lips, fingernails, or palms of the hands; extreme dizziness or fainting; feeling of extreme pressure in the head; shortness of breath; unusual tiredness or weakness; weak and fast pulse; fever; and seizures.

 Warnings

• Make sure your doctor knows your medical history. You may not be able to use Nitrol if you have other medical problems, especially glaucoma, kidney or liver disease, an overactive thyroid, or severe anemia; if you're allergic to this or other drugs; or if you've recently had a heart attack, stroke, or head injury.
• Tell your doctor if you're pregnant or breast-feeding before you begin taking Nitrol.
• Be aware that older adults may be especially sensitive to Nitrol's side effects.

KEEP IN MIND...

∗ Don't rub ointment into skin.
∗ Cover treated area, as instructed.
∗ Don't get ointment on fingers.
∗ Don't suddenly stop using Nitrol ointment.

Nitrostat

Nitrostat relaxes the arteries of the heart, allowing more oxygen-rich blood to reach and nourish the heart.

Why it's prescribed

Doctors prescribe Nitrostat to relieve angina attacks. Nitrostat comes in sublingual (under-the-tongue) tablets. Doctors usually prescribe the following amounts for adults.

▶ **To prevent angina,** 1 sublingual tablet dissolved under the tongue as soon as angina begins, repeated in 5 minutes if needed.

▶ **To prevent angina before physical activity,** 1 sublingual tablet 5 or 10 minutes before activity.

How to take Nitrostat

- Take Nitrostat only as your doctor directs.
- Place the sublingual tablet under your tongue and allow it to dissolve. Don't swallow, crush, or chew the tablet.
- Don't eat, drink, smoke, or use chewing tobacco while the tablet is dissolving in your mouth.
- Don't take more than three sublingual tablets. Call your doctor if these don't relieve your chest pain.
- Store Nitrostat in a cool, dark place. Remove the cotton from the top of the container, because it can absorb the drug.
- To ensure freshness, discard any leftover Nitrostat every 3 months and replace it.

NITROSTAT'S OTHER NAMES

Nitrostat's generic name is nitroglycerin (also called glyceryl trinitrate). Another brand name is Nitrolingual.

 SIDE EFFECTS

Call your doctor if you have any of these possible drug side effects. Call *immediately* about any labeled "serious."

Serious: severe or prolonged headache, dry mouth, blurred vision

Common: fast pulse, flushing, headache, nausea, vomiting, dizziness
Tip: These side effects usually go away as your body adjusts to the drug. If they persist or worsen, call your doctor.

Other: weakness, fainting, rash, restlessness

 DRUG INTERACTIONS

Combining certain drugs may alter their action or produce unwanted side effects. Tell your doctor about other drugs you're taking, especially:
- alcohol
- other heart or blood pressure drugs.

If you miss a dose

Not applicable because Nitrostat is taken only as needed.

 ## If you suspect an overdose

Contact your doctor *immediately.* Excessive Nitrostat can cause persistent throbbing headache, palpitations, vision disturbances, flushing, sweating (with skin later becoming cold and bluish), nausea, vomiting, abdominal pain and cramps, bloody diarrhea, dizziness, deep or difficult breathing, slow breathing, slow pulse, confusion, fever, paralysis, coma, seizures, blood circulation collapse, and death.

Warnings

- Make sure your doctor knows your medical history. You may not be able to take Nitrostat if you've had a head injury, heart attack, or stroke, or if you have anemia, glaucoma, or kidney, liver, or thyroid disease.
- Tell your doctor if you're pregnant or breast-feeding before you begin taking Nitrostat.
- Older adults may be prone to Nitrostat's side effects.
- Carry Nitrostat with you at all times in case of an angina attack. Carry the drug in its original container in a jacket pocket or purse, not in a pocket close to the body.

 KEEP IN MIND...

- Don't take more than three tablets.
- Don't carry in pocket close to body.
- Replace sublingual tablets every 3 months.

Nizoral (oral)

Nizoral, an antibiotic, fights fungal infections by destroying fungal cell walls, thereby killing the fungus.

Why it's prescribed

Doctors prescribe oral Nizoral to treat serious fungal infections of the mouth and throat (thrush), skin, or throughout the body. It's *not* used for minor infections of the skin or nails. Nizoral comes in tablets and an oral liquid. Doctors usually prescribe the following amounts for adults; children's dosages appear in parentheses.

▶ **For fungal infections,** at first, 200 milligrams (mg) a day in a single dose, increased to 400 mg once a day as needed. (Children age 2 and over weighing more than 88 pounds [lb]: same as adult dosage. Children age 2 and over weighing less than 88 lb: 3.3 to 6.6 mg for each 2.2 lb of body weight daily as one dose.)

How to take Nizoral

• Take Nizoral only as your doctor directs, for the time prescribed, even if your symptoms disappear. Minimum treatment time is 7 to 14 days, but may last up to 6 months.
• For conditions that cause you to have no stomach acid, your doctor may prescribe a special solution. A pharmacist will prepare the solution for you. Add it to 1 to 2 teaspoons of water in a glass. Drink it through a straw placed far back in

NIZORAL'S OTHER NAME

Nizoral's generic name is ketoconazole.

 ## SIDE EFFECTS

Call your doctor if you have any of these possible drug side effects. Call *immediately* about any labeled "serious."

Serious: liver problems (unusual fatigue, yellow-tinged skin and eyes, dark urine, pale stools), persistent nausea, appetite loss

Common: nausea, vomiting, headache
Tip: To reduce nausea, divide your daily dose into two and take with meals.

Other: nervousness, dizziness, abdominal pain, diarrhea, constipation, itching, breast enlargement and tenderness in men

 ## DRUG INTERACTIONS

Combining certain drugs may alter their action or produce unwanted side effects. Tell your doctor about other drugs you're taking, especially:
• alcohol
• antacids, anticholinergics, histamine blockers such as Axid and Pepcid (wait at least 2 hours after taking Nizoral before taking these drugs)
• Hismanal, Seldane
• Laniazid, Rifadin
• Propulsid.

your mouth and away from your teeth. Then swish half a glass (4 ounces) of water around in your mouth and swallow it.

If you miss a dose

Take the missed dose as soon as possible. If it's almost time for your next dose, space the missed dose and the next dose 10 to 12 hours apart. Then go back to your normal schedule. Don't take a double dose.

 ### If you suspect an overdose

Contact your doctor *immediately*. Excessive Nizoral can cause dizziness, ringing in the ears, headache, nausea, vomiting, diarrhea, or signs of adrenal crisis (abdominal pain, decreased level of wakefulness).

 ### Warnings

• Make sure your doctor knows your medical history. You may not be able to take Nizoral if you have liver disease or a drug allergy.
• If you're pregnant, check with your doctor before taking Nizoral.
• Don't breast-feed while you're taking Nizoral and for 48 hours after you stop taking it.

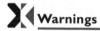 ## KEEP IN MIND...

* Treatment lasts 1 week to 6 months.
* Take with food.
* Not for minor infections.

Nizoral (for skin)

Nizoral, an antibiotic, fights fungal (yeast) infections by destroying fungal cell walls, thereby killing the fungus.

Why it's prescribed

Doctors prescribe Nizoral for the skin to treat minor fungus infections of the skin and scalp, such as jock itch, seborrhea, and minor infections of the fingers and nails. It comes in cream and shampoo. Doctors usually prescribe the following amounts for adults.

▶ **For minor fungal infections,** a small amount applied to the affected and surrounding areas once a day for at least 2 weeks; for seborrhea, apply twice a day for 4 weeks. When using shampoo, wet hair, lather, and massage for 1 minute. Then, rinse, lather, and leave on scalp for 3 minutes before rinsing. Shampoo twice weekly for 4 weeks, with at least 3 days between shampoos.

How to use Nizoral

• Use Nizoral only as your doctor directs, for the full time prescribed, even if your symptoms disappear. If you stop using this drug too soon, your symptoms may return.
• Wash your hands before and after applying the cream. Apply enough cream to cover the affected area and surrounding skin. Rub it in gently. Keep Nizoral away from your eyes.

NIZORAL'S OTHER NAME

Nizoral's generic name is ketoconazole.

 SIDE EFFECTS

Call your doctor if you have any of these possible drug side effects. Call *immediately* about any labeled "serious."

Serious: persistent skin irritation, itching, or stinging

Common: none reported

Other: swelling, inflammation

 DRUG INTERACTIONS

Combining certain drugs may alter their action or produce unwanted side effects. Tell your doctor about other drugs you're taking, including:
• alcohol.

If you miss a dose

Skip the missed dose and apply the next dose at the regularly scheduled time. Don't apply a double dose.

 If you suspect an overdose

Consult your doctor.

Warnings

• Make sure your doctor knows your medical history. You may not be able to use Nizoral if you're allergic to any drugs, foods, dyes, or preservatives.
• Tell your doctor if you're pregnant or breast-feeding before you begin using Nizoral.
• When using Nizoral to treat a skin infection, keep your skin clean and dry.
• When using Nizoral to treat jock itch, wear loose-fitting cotton underwear and use talcum or other bland, absorbent powder on your skin between Nizoral applications.
• When using Nizoral to treat athlete's foot, wear clean cotton socks and change them often to keep your feet dry. Wear sandals or shoes with lots of air holes. Apply talcum or another absorbent powder between your toes, on your feet, and in your socks and shoes once or twice a day, between applications of Nizoral.
• Check with the doctor if your condition worsens with treatment.

 KEEP IN MIND...

∗ For minor infections.
∗ Use for full time prescribed, even if symptoms subside.
∗ Wash hands before and after applying cream.
∗ Keep skin clean and dry; use talcum powder as directed.

Noctec

Noctec is one of several drugs called sedatives and hypnotics. It depresses the central nervous system.

Why it's prescribed

Doctors prescribe Noctec to treat insomnia or to relax people who are nervous or anxious, are about to have surgery or a brain scan, or are experiencing alcohol withdrawal. Noctec comes in capsules, syrup, and rectal suppositories. Doctors usually prescribe the following amounts for adults; children's dosages appear in parentheses, except for use in brain scans.

▶ **As sedative,** 250 milligrams (mg) orally or rectally three times a day after meals. (Children: 8.3 mg for each 2.2 pounds [lb] of body weight or 250 mg for each square meter of body surface area orally or rectally three times a day. Maximum dosage is 500 mg three times a day.)

▶ **For insomnia,** 500 mg to 1 gram (g) orally or rectally 15 to 30 minutes before bedtime. (Children: 50 mg for each 2.2 lb or 1.5 g for each square meter orally or rectally 15 to 30 minutes before bedtime. Maximum single dose is 1 g.)

▶ **Before surgery,** 500 mg to 1 g orally or rectally 30 minutes before surgery.

▶ **Before brain scan in children,** 20 to 25 mg for each 2.2 lb orally or rectally.

NOCTEC'S OTHER NAMES

Noctec's generic name is chloral hydrate. Other brand names include Aquachloral Supprettes and, in Canada, Novo-Chlorhydrate.

 SIDE EFFECTS

Call your doctor if you have any of these possible drug side effects. Call *immediately* about any labeled "serious."

Serious: extreme drowsiness, swallowing or breathing difficulties, blood problems (fatigue, chills, fever, increased risk of infection), seizures, allergic reaction (rash, hives)

Common: nausea, vomiting, diarrhea, drowsiness, dizziness, hangover
Tip: Don't drive or participate in activities that take alertness or coordination if you feel drowsy or dizzy.

Other: nightmares, incoordination, unusual excitement, gas

 DRUG INTERACTIONS

Combining certain drugs may alter their action or produce unwanted side effects. Tell your doctor about other drugs you're taking, especially:
• alcohol and other drugs that make you relaxed or sleepy, such as allergy and cold medicines, narcotic pain relievers, muscle relaxants, and anesthetics
• alkaline solutions such as sodium bicarbonate
• anticoagulants (blood thinners) such as Coumadin
• Dilantin.

▶ **For alcohol withdrawal symptoms,** 500 mg to 1 g orally or rectally every 6 hours as needed, up to 2 g a day.

How to take Noctec

• Take Noctec only as your doctor directs. This drug begins to take effect within 30 minutes. Effects last 4 to 8 hours.
• Double-check dose, especially when giving Noctec to children. Fatal overdoses have occurred.
• When taking Noctec to help you sleep, take it 15 to 30 minutes before bedtime.
• Take capsules after meals. Swallow the capsule whole, and drink a full glass (8 ounces) of liquid to avoid stomach upset.
• Mix each syrup dose in half a glass (4 ounces) of juice or other liquid before taking it to disguise the flavor of the drug and prevent stomach upset.
• If you're using a suppository and it's too soft to insert, chill it briefly or run cold water over it before removing the foil wrapper. Wash your hands before and after inserting suppository. To use, remove the wrapper and moisten the suppository with cold water. Lie on your side and use your finger to push the suppository gently into your rectum. Store suppositories in refrigerator.
• Don't stop taking Noctec without consulting your doctor; your dosage will be gradually reduced to prevent withdrawal effects.

If you miss a dose

Skip the missed dose. Take your next dose on schedule. Don't take a double dose.

If you suspect an overdose

Contact your doctor *immediately*. Excessive Noctec can cause stupor, coma, shallow or absent breathing, pinpoint pupils, low blood pressure (dizziness, weakness, fainting), low body temperature, closing up of the throat, internal bleeding (bruising, pain), and liver damage (nausea, vomiting, yellow-tinged skin and eyes).

Warnings

• Make sure your doctor knows your medical history. You may not be able to take Noctec if you have other problems, such as heart, liver, stomach, intestinal, kidney, blood, or emotional disorders; if you're allergic to this or other drugs; or if you have a history of drug dependence or abuse.

• If you're pregnant or breast-feeding, check with your doctor before taking Noctec.

• Don't use Noctec for extended lengths of time. This drug is ineffective after 14 days of continued use. Long-term use may cause drug dependence, and you may experience withdrawal symptoms if you stop taking the drug suddenly.

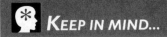

KEEP IN MIND...

* Overuse may lead to dependence.

* Double-check dose; fatal overdoses have occurred.

* To promote sleep, take before bedtime.

* Take capsules after meals.

* Mix syrup with juice to mask flavor.

* Store suppositories in refrigerator.

* Don't suddenly stop taking.

Nolvadex

Nolvadex blocks the effects of the hormone estrogen in the body, but the exact way it works isn't fully understood.

Why it's prescribed

Doctors prescribe Nolvadex to treat breast cancer in both women and men. It comes in tablets and in enteric-coated tablets that dissolve only after reaching the intestine. Doctors usually prescribe the following amounts for adults.

▶ **For breast cancer**, 10 milligrams two to three times a day.

How to take Nolvadex

• Take Nolvadex only as your doctor directs. This drug begins to take effect in 4 to 10 weeks, but may take several months; effects may last for several weeks after drug is stopped.

• Keep taking this drug even if it makes you feel nauseated.

• When taking enteric-coated tablets, swallow them whole; don't crush or break them before swallowing.

If you miss a dose

Skip the dose entirely, and take your next regular dose as scheduled. Call your doctor for further advice. If you vomit shortly after taking a dose of Nolvadex, call your doctor to find out whether or

NOLVADEX'S OTHER NAMES

Nolvadex's generic name is tamoxifen citrate. Canadian brand names include Alpha-Tamoxifen, Nolvadex-D, Novo-Tamoxifen, Tamofen, Tamone, and Tamoplex.

 SIDE EFFECTS

Call your doctor if you have any of these possible drug side effects.

Serious: none reported

Common: nausea
Tip: Sip fluids throughout the day to reduce nausea.

Other: vomiting, drastic appetite and weight loss, vaginal discharge and bleeding, blood problems (easy bruising and bleeding, black or tarry stools, dizziness), rash, temporary bone or tumor pain, hot flashes
Tip: Bone pain during treatment usually means this drug is working. Use aspirin or Tylenol to relieve pain.

 DRUG INTERACTIONS

Combining certain drugs may alter their action or produce unwanted side effects. Tell your doctor about other drugs you're taking, especially:

• antacids (don't take within 2 hours of Nolvadex)
• birth control pills.

not to take the dose again. Don't take a double dose.

 If you suspect an overdose

Consult your doctor.

 Warnings

• Make sure your doctor knows your medical history. You may not be able to take Nolvadex if you have other problems, such as a blood disorder; if you're allergic to this or other drugs; or if you've ever had cataracts or other eye problems.

• Tell your doctor if you're pregnant or breast-feeding before you begin taking Nolvadex. Short-term treatment induces ovulation. Use a barrier method of birth control (such as a condom or diaphragm) and tell your doctor immediately if you think you've become pregnant while taking this drug.

• Follow your doctor's recommendations for eating a high-calorie diet while taking Nolvadex.

• Have regular gynecologic exams because this drug may increase the risk of uterine cancer.

 KEEP IN MIND...

* Treatment may take several months.

* Eat a high-calorie diet while taking this drug.

* Swallow coated tablets whole; don't crush or break.

* Avoid pregnancy during treatment.

* Have regular gynecologic exams to check for uterine cancer.

Nordryl

Nordryl inhibits histamine, a body substance that causes itching, sneezing, runny nose, and watery eyes.

Why it's taken

Nordryl is taken to relieve stuffy nose, hay fever symptoms, nonproductive cough, difficulty sleeping, and motion sickness. It's also used to reduce tremor and stiffness in Parkinson's disease. You can buy Nordryl without a prescription. It comes in capsules, an elixir, a syrup, and an injectable form. The following amounts are usually recommended for adults; children's dosages appear in parentheses.

▶ **For runny nose, allergy symptoms, motion sickness, and Parkinson's disease,** 25 to 50 milligrams (mg) orally three or four times a day. (Children age 12 and over: same as adults. Children younger than age 12: 5 mg for each 2.2 pounds of body weight orally each day; maximum dosage is 300 mg a day.)

▶ **For sedation,** 25 to 50 mg orally as needed.

▶ **As a nighttime sleep aid,** 50 mg orally at bedtime.

▶ **For a nonproductive cough,** 25 mg orally every 4 to 6 hours, but no more than 150 mg a day. (Children ages 6 to 12: 12.5 mg orally every 4 to 6 hours, but no more than 75 mg a day. Children ages 2 to 6: 6.25

NORDRYL'S OTHER NAMES

Nordryl's generic name is diphenhydramine hydrochloride. Other brand names include AllerMax, Banophen, Beldin, Belix, Bena-D, Benadryl, Benahist, Benylin Cough, Hydramine, and Phendry.

SIDE EFFECTS

Call your doctor if you have any of these possible drug side effects.

Serious: none reported

Common: drowsiness, nausea, dry mouth

Tips: Make sure you know how you react to this drug before you drive or perform other tasks that require you to be fully alert. To reduce nausea, take doses with food, milk, or water. To relieve dry mouth, use sugarless hard candy or gum, ice chips, or a saliva substitute.

Other: confusion, headache, palpitations, stuffy nose, hives

DRUG INTERACTIONS

Combining certain drugs may alter their action or produce unwanted side effects. Tell your doctor about other drugs you're taking, especially:
• alcohol and other drugs that make you relaxed or sleepy, such as narcotic painkillers and tranquilizers
• MAO inhibitors, such as Nardil.

mg orally every 4 to 6 hours, but no more than 25 mg a day.)

How to take Nordryl

• If you're treating yourself, follow the directions on the label. If the doctor prescribed this drug, follow any special directions.
• If you're taking Nordryl to prevent motion sickness, take it at least 1 to 2 hours before traveling.

If you miss a dose

If you're taking this drug regularly and you miss a dose, take the missed dose as soon as possible. But if it's almost time for your next dose, skip the missed dose and take your next dose as scheduled. Don't take a double dose.

If you suspect an overdose

Contact your doctor *immediately*. Excessive Nordryl can cause drowsiness, seizures, coma, and stoppage of breathing.

Warnings

• Make sure your doctor knows your medical history. You may not be able to take Nordryl if you have asthma, glaucoma, a bladder disorder, heart disease, or if you're pregnant or breast-feeding.
• Children and older adults are especially prone to side effects.
• Nordryl can hide signs of aspirin overdose, such as ringing in ears.

KEEP IN MIND...

* Take at least 1 to 2 hours before traveling.
* Don't drive until you know how drug affects you.
* Take with food, milk, or water.

Norflex

Norflex relaxes muscles and relieves muscle pain, most likely by changing how a person perceives pain.

Why it's prescribed

Doctors prescribe Norflex to treat strains, sprains, or other muscle injuries. Norflex comes in tablets and extended-release tablets. It's also available in an injectable form. Doctors usually prescribe the following amounts for adults.

▶ **For muscle pain,** 100 milligrams orally twice a day, or by injection. Oral therapy is begun 12 hours after last injection.

How to take Norflex

• Take Norflex only as your doctor directs. This drug begins to take effect within 1 hour.
• Check all dosages carefully before swallowing, to avoid a dangerous overdose.

If you miss a dose

Take the missed dose if you remember within an hour or so. However, if more time has lapsed, skip the missed dose and go back to your regular schedule. Don't take a double dose.

 If you suspect an overdose

Contact your doctor *immediately*. Excessive Norflex may cause dry

NORFLEX'S OTHER NAMES

Norflex's generic name is orphenadrine citrate. Other brand names include Banflex, Flexoject, Myolin, and Orphenate.

 SIDE EFFECTS

Call your doctor if you have any of these possible drug side effects. Call *immediately* about any labeled "serious."

Serious: severe allergic reaction (facial and throat swelling, difficulty breathing, chest pain), anemia (fatigue)

Common: drowsiness, dry mouth
Tips: Relieve dry mouth with cool drinks, sugarless gum, or hard candy. Avoid tasks that require alertness if you're drowsy.

Other: disorientation, restlessness, irritability, weakness, headache, dizziness, hallucinations, sleeplessness, palpitations, fast pulse, dilated pupils, blurred vision, difficulty swallowing, increased pressure in the eyes (headache, eye pain), constipation, nausea, vomiting, intestinal disorder, difficulty urinating, inability to urinate

 DRUG INTERACTIONS

Combining certain drugs may alter their action or produce unwanted side effects. Tell your doctor about other drugs you're taking, especially:
• alcohol or other drugs that make you relaxed or sleepy (sedatives, sleeping pills), propoxyphene.

mouth, enlarged pupils, blurred vision, flushing, fever, slowed breathing, low blood pressure (dizziness, weakness), confusion, and decreased urine output.

 Warnings

• Make sure your doctor knows your medical history. You may not be able to take Norflex if you have another problem, such as glaucoma, a prostate problem, intestine or bladder obstruction, muscle weakness and fatigue, ulcers, fast or irregular heartbeats, or heart disease, or if you're allergic to this or other products.
• Tell your doctor if you're pregnant or breast-feeding before you begin taking Norflex.

• Schedule regular follow-up visits during long-term treatment so that your doctor can check your progress.

KEEP IN MIND...

* Begins to take effect within 1 hour.

* Check dosages carefully, to avoid overdose.

* Go for regular checkups during long-term treatment.

* Never take a double dose if you miss a dose.

Norlutin

Norlutin is an artificial form of the female hormones called progestins, which regulate the menstrual cycle. It also suppresses ovulation.

Why it's prescribed

Doctors prescribe Norlutin to treat abnormal or absent menstruation and a condition called endometriosis, in which tissue like that found in the uterine lining grows in the pelvis or abdominal wall. It's also prescribed to prevent pregnancy. Norlutin comes in tablets. Doctors usually prescribe the following amounts for adults.

▶ **For absent menstruation or abnormal bleeding from the uterus,** 5 to 20 milligrams (mg) once a day on days 5 to 25 of menstrual cycle.
▶ **For endometriosis,** 10 mg once a day for 14 days, increased by 5 mg a day every 2 weeks, up to 30 mg a day.
▶ **For birth control,** at first, 0.35 mg on the first day of menstruation, and one pill every day thereafter.

How to take Norlutin

• Take Norlutin only as your doctor directs.
• Take at the same time each day for best results and to reduce side effects.
• If any unusual symptoms occur, stop taking Norlutin immediately and call the doctor.

If you miss a dose

Adjust your schedule as follows:

NORLUTIN'S OTHER NAMES

Norlutin's generic name is norethindrone. Other brand names include Micronor and Nor-Q.D.

 SIDE EFFECTS

Call your doctor if you have any of these possible drug side effects. Call *immediately* about any labeled "serious."

Serious: vision disturbances, migraine, high blood pressure (headache, blurred vision), blood clots (shortness of breath; pain in chest, legs, or buttocks), high blood sugar (increased hunger, thirst, and urination)

Common: water retention (decreased urination, swelling, weight gain), nausea, vomiting, breakthrough bleeding; breast tenderness, enlargement, or secretion
Tip: Reducing high-salt foods helps lessen water retention.

Other: dizziness, lethargy, depression, abdominal cramps, abnormal or absent menstruation, vaginal yeast infection, abnormal secretions, yellow-tinged skin and eyes, skin pigment blotches, rash, decreased sex drive

 DRUG INTERACTIONS

Combining certain drugs may alter their action or produce unwanted side effects. Tell your doctor about other drugs you're taking, especially:
• Parlodel
• Rifadin, Solfoton, Tegretol.

• If you're not taking Norlutin for birth control, take the missed dose as soon as possible. If it's almost time for your next dose, skip the missed dose and return to your regular schedule. Don't take a double dose.
• When taking Norlutin for birth control, stop taking immediately and use another method of birth control until your period begins.

 If you suspect an overdose

Consult your doctor.

 Warnings

• Make sure your doctor knows your medical history. You may not be able to use Norlutin if you have diabetes, seizures, migraines, heart or kidney disease, asthma, depression, or a drug allergy; or if you've had a blood clotting disorder or stroke, breast cancer, vaginal bleeding, liver disease, or abortion.
• If you're pregnant, don't use Norlutin. This drug may cause birth defects and masculine traits in a female fetus.
• Perform routine monthly breast self-examination.

 KEEP IN MIND...

∗ Take at same time each day.
∗ Perform routine monthly breast self-exam.
∗ If you miss a dose, use other birth control method until your period begins.

Normodyne

Normodyne is one of a group of drugs called beta blockers. It affects nerve impulses in the body to decrease the heart's need for blood and oxygen; this reduces the heart's workload and helps the heart beat more regularly.

Why it's prescribed

Doctors prescribe Normodyne to treat high blood pressure. It comes in tablets and in an injectable form. Doctors usually prescribe the following amounts for adults.

▶ **For high blood pressure,** 100 milligrams (mg) orally twice a day with or without a diuretic (water pill). If needed, dosage is increased to 200 mg twice a day after 2 days, with further increases every 2 to 3 days until best response is reached. Usual maintenance dosage is 200 to 400 mg twice a day.

How to take Normodyne

• Take Normodyne only as your doctor directs. This drug begins to take effect within 20 minutes after oral dose. Effects last 12 to 24 hours.
• Don't suddenly stop taking Normodyne; angina (chest pain) and heart attack may occur.

If you miss a dose

Take the missed dose as soon as possible. However, if it's within 8

 ## SIDE EFFECTS

Call your doctor if you have any of these possible drug side effects.
Serious: none reported
Common: low blood pressure (dizziness, weakness), blood circulation problem (cold hands or feet)
Tips: Dizziness tends to occur early in treatment, in people also taking diuretics (water pills), and with higher dosages. To avoid dizziness, sit or stand slowly and avoid sudden position changes. Follow your doctor's suggestion to take a dose at bedtime or to take smaller doses three times a day.

Other: vivid dreams, fatigue, headache, scalp tingling, slow pulse, stuffy nose, nausea, vomiting, diarrhea, sexual dysfunction, inability to urinate, difficulty breathing, rash

 ## DRUG INTERACTIONS

Combining certain drugs may alter their action or produce unwanted side effects. Tell your doctor about other drugs you're taking, especially:
• halothane
• insulin and oral diabetes drugs
• Tagamet.

hours of your next dose, skip the missed dose and go back to your regular schedule. Don't take a double dose.

 ## If you suspect an overdose

Contact your doctor *immediately*. Signs of overdose may occur in the following order: slow pulse, severe dizziness or fainting, fast or irregular heartbeat, difficulty breathing, bluish fingernails or palms of hands, seizures.

Warnings

• Make sure your doctor knows your medical history. You may not be able to take Normodyne if you have other problems, such as asthma, a heart or lung disorder, severe slow pulse, severe low blood pressure, liver failure, bronchitis, emphysema, vascular disease, or adrenal tumor, or if you're allergic to this or other drugs.
• Tell your doctor if you're pregnant or breast-feeding before you begin taking Normodyne.

 ## KEEP IN MIND...

* To reduce dizziness, take a dose at bedtime or three smaller doses a day.
* Don't suddenly stop taking.
* Slow pulse may be first sign of overdose.

Noroxin

Noroxin, an antibiotic, prevents the spread of and kills infection-causing bacteria.

Why it's prescribed

Doctors prescribe Noroxin to treat bacterial infections of the urinary tract and gonorrhea. It comes in tablets. Doctors usually prescribe the following amounts for adults.

▶ **For uncomplicated urinary tract infections,** 400 milligrams (mg) twice a day for 7 to 10 days.

▶ **For complicated urinary tract infections,** 400 mg twice a day for 10 to 21 days.

▶ **For cystitis (a urinary infection),** 400 mg twice a day for 3 days.

▶ **For gonorrhea,** 800 mg as a single dose, followed by treatment with another drug for other infections.

How to take Noroxin

• Take Noroxin only as your doctor directs. For best results, take the drug at evenly spaced times during the day and night. For example, if you take two doses a day, you might take one dose at 8 a.m. and the other at 8 p.m.

• Take 1 hour before or 2 hours after meals because food may hinder absorption of the drug.

• Take your tablet with a full glass (8 ounces) of water and drink several more glasses of water throughout the day while taking Noroxin.

• Keep taking Noroxin, even after you begin to feel better, to stop your infection from coming back.

NOROXIN'S OTHER NAME

Noroxin's generic name is norfloxacin.

 SIDE EFFECTS

Call your doctor if you have any of these possible drug side effects. Call *immediately* about any labeled "serious."

Serious: severe allergic reactions (wheezing, difficulty breathing, hives or rash), seizures

Common: none reported

Other: fatigue, sleepiness, headache, dizziness, nausea, constipation, gas, heartburn, dry mouth, blood problems (cough, chest soreness, skin inflammation or infection), rash, sensitivity to light, arthritis, muscle pain, joint pain or swelling, fever

 DRUG INTERACTIONS

Combining certain drugs may alter their action or produce unwanted side effects. Tell your doctor about other drugs you're taking, especially:

• antacids, iron supplements, Carafate (take these 2 hours before or after Noroxin)
• Benemid
• cyclosporine
• Macrodantin
• oral anticoagulants (blood thinners) such as Coumadin
• other drugs for urinary tract infections
• Theo-Dur.

If you miss a dose

Take the missed dose as soon as possible. But if it's almost time for your next dose, skip the missed dose and go back to your regular schedule. Don't take a double dose.

 If you suspect an overdose

Consult your doctor.

Warnings

• Make sure your doctor knows your medical history. You may not be able to take Noroxin if you have a seizure disorder or kidney disease or if you're allergic to this or other drugs.

• If you're pregnant or breast-feeding, don't use Noroxin unless your doctor tells you to.

• Don't give Noroxin to infants, children, or adolescents because it may cause bone problems.

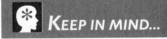 **KEEP IN MIND...**

* Take at evenly spaced times, day and night.

* Take on empty stomach with water.

* Drink extra water throughout the day.

* Don't give to infants, children, or adolescents.

Norpace

Norpace is used to correct an irregular heartbeat or to slow an overactive heart. Norpace regulates the heart's muscle contractions so that the heart pumps blood regularly and efficiently.

Why it's prescribed

Doctors prescribe Norpace to correct an irregular or fast heartbeat. Norpace comes in capsules and extended-release capsules. It's also available in an injectable form. Doctors usually prescribe the following amounts for adults; children's dosages appear in parentheses.

▶ **For irregular or fast heartbeat,** for adults weighing more than 110 pounds (lb): 150 milligrams (mg) capsules every 6 hours or 300 mg extended-release capsules every 12 hours. For adults weighing 110 lb or less, dosage is individualized. (Children under age 1: 10 to 30 mg for each 2.2 lb of body weight orally a day. Children age 1 to 4: 10 to 20 mg for each 2.2 lb orally a day. Children age 4 to 12: 10 to 15 mg for each 2.2 lb a day. Children age 12 to 18: 6 to 15 mg for each 2.2 lb a day. Children's dosages are divided into equal amounts and given every 6 hours.)

▶ **For irregular or fast heartbeats and advanced kidney disease,** de-

NORPACE'S OTHER NAMES

Norpace's generic name is disopyramide. A Canadian brand name is Rythmodan. Other brand names of disopyramide phosphate include Norpace CR and, in Canada, Rythmodan LA.

 SIDE EFFECTS

Call your doctor if you have any of these possible drug side effects. Call *immediately* about any labeled "serious."

Serious: severe heart disorder (chest pain, shortness of breath, anxiety), irregular heartbeats, sudden weight gain, swelling of ankles or fingers

Common: low blood pressure (dizziness, weakness, fainting), blurred vision, dry eyes, dry nose, constipation, dry mouth
Tip: To relieve dry mouth, try chewing gum, hard candy, or ice chips. Use a cool mist humidifier to help with mouth, nose, and eye dryness.

Other: dizziness, agitation, depression, fatigue, muscle weakness, fainting, water retention (decreased urination, swelling, weight gain), nausea, vomiting, drastic appetite and weight loss, abdominal pain, difficulty urinating or inability to urinate, yellow-tinged skin and eyes, rash, low blood sugar (drowsiness, headache, nervousness, cold sweats, confusion), aches, pain

 DRUG INTERACTIONS

Combining certain drugs may alter their action or produce unwanted side effects. Tell your doctor about other drugs you're taking, especially:
• alcohol
• Calan
• Colace
• Dilantin
• drugs for irregular heart rhythms, such as Inderal, Procan SR, Quinaglute Dura-Tabs
• Rifadin.

pending on test results, 100 mg every 8 hours, every 12 hours, or every 24 hours.

How to take Norpace

• Take Norpace only as your doctor directs. This drug begins to take effect within to 3 hours. Effects last for 1½ to 8½ hours after last dose.
• Take Norpace on time and exactly as prescribed. You may need to use an alarm clock to awaken you for night doses.
• When switching from regular to extended-release capsules, take an

extended-release capsule 6 hours after the last regular capsule was taken.
• Don't break, crush, or chew the extended-release capsules before swallowing.
• When giving to young children, the pharmacist may prepare oral liquid from 100-mg capsules and cherry syrup.
• Store at room temperature in a tightly closed container.
• Check with your doctor before you stop taking Norpace. Stopping suddenly can cause a serious change in heart function.

If you miss a dose

Take the missed dose as soon as possible unless it's within 4 hours of the next scheduled dose. In that case, skip the missed dose and take your next dose on schedule. Don't take a double dose.

If you suspect an overdose

Contact your doctor *immediately*. Excessive Norpace can cause severe low blood pressure (severe dizziness and weakness, fainting), irregular or slow heartbeat, labored breathing due to congestive heart failure, loss of consciousness, or seizures.

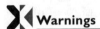

Warnings

• Make sure your doctor knows your medical history. You may not be able to take Norpace if you have other problems, such as severe muscle weakness and fatigue, glaucoma, difficulty urinating, other heart conditions, or liver or kidney disease, or if you're allergic to this or other drugs.

• If you're pregnant or breast-feeding, check with your doctor before taking Norpace.

• If you have diabetes or congestive heart failure, watch for symptoms of low blood sugar (headache, shakiness, cold sweats, excessive hunger, weakness). If these occur, eat or drink a sugary food and call your doctor *right away*.

• Follow your doctor's recommendation for managing constipation with proper diet or bulk laxatives.

• Keep all doctor's appointments. Your doctor may want to follow blood levels closely.

• Older adults may be more prone to Norpace's side effects.

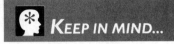

KEEP IN MIND...

* Take Norpace on time, day and night.

* Don't break, crush, or chew extended-release capsules.

* Don't suddenly stop taking.

Norplant

Norplant slowly releases hormones into the bloodstream, which prevents an egg from becoming attached to the uterus. It also can prevent ovulation.

Why it's prescribed

Doctors prescribe Norplant as a contraceptive. It comes in capsules that are implanted under a woman's skin. Doctors usually prescribe the following amounts.

▶ **To preventing pregnancy,** six capsules implanted under the skin of the upper arm during the first 7 days after the onset of menstruation.

How to use Norplant

• Use Norplant only as your doctor directs.
• Your doctor will make a small cut in your upper arm, implant six capsules, and close the skin over them. Norplant works as a contraceptive for about 5 years.

If you miss a dose

Call the doctor right away if one of the capsules falls out before your skin heals; this could reduce the contraceptive effect.

 If you suspect an overdose

Contact your doctor *immediately*. If more than six capsules are implanted, fluid retention and associated problems as well as irregular uterine bleeding may occur. Your doctor must make sure old capsules are

NORPLANT'S OTHER NAME

Norplant's generic name is levonorgestrel.

 SIDE EFFECTS

Call your doctor if you have any of these possible drug side effects. Call *immediately* about any labeled "serious."

Serious: vision change or contact lens intolerance, pain in stomach or muscles, discharge from breasts or vagina, blood clot in lungs

Common: menstrual changes (spotting and irregular, prolonged, or absent bleeding), nausea, inflammation of cervix or vagina, muscle or bone pain, difficulty removing implants
Tip: Menstrual changes usually subside over time.

Other: headache, nervousness, dizziness, appetite change, rash, acne, hairiness or hair loss, breast pain, organ enlargement, weight gain; infection, pain, or itching at implant site

 DRUG INTERACTIONS

Combining certain drugs may alter their action or produce unwanted side effects. Tell your doctor about other drugs you're taking, especially:
• Dilantin, Rifadin, Tegretol.

removed before a new set is implanted.

X **Warnings**

• Make sure your doctor knows your medical history. You may not be able to use Norplant if you have breast cancer, unusual genital bleeding, diabetes, depression or an emotional disorder, or liver, kidney, or heart disease; if you're allergic to any drugs; or if you must stay in bed for a long time.
• Norplant must be removed if you become pregnant. Don't assume you're pregnant if you miss a menstrual period. However, if your period still doesn't come after 6 or more weeks (after a pattern of regular periods), you may be pregnant.
• If you're breast-feeding, check with your doctor before the implants are inserted.

• Follow any special diet that's recommended. Norplant can cause you to retain water, so your doctor may want you to limit salt in your diet if you have heart or kidney disease.
• Have a physical exam at least every year so the doctor can check for any problems caused by Norplant.

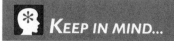 **KEEP IN MIND...**

* Works for about 5 years.
* Capsules must be removed if pregnancy occurs.
* Follow recommended diet.

Norpramin

Norpramin is one of a group of drugs called tricyclic antidepressants, which increase the body's level of natural substances that alleviate depression.

Why it's prescribed

Doctors prescribe Norpramin to relieve depression. It comes in capsules and tablets. Doctors usually prescribe the following amounts for adults; older adults' and adolescents' dosages appear in parentheses.

▶ **For depression,** 100 to 200 milligrams (mg) each day divided into equal doses, increased to maximum of 300 mg a day. Or entire dosage at bedtime. (Older adults and adolescents: 25 to 100 mg a day divided into equal doses, increased gradually to maximum of 150 mg a day if needed.)

How to take Norpramin

• Take Norpramin only as your doctor directs. This drug is thought to take effect in 2 to 4 weeks or longer.
• Take with food (including bedtime dose) unless your doctor tells you to take it on an empty stomach.
• Don't suddenly stop taking this drug; check with your doctor about gradually reducing your dosage.

If you miss a dose

Adjust your schedule as follows:
• If you normally take one dose a day at bedtime and you miss a dose,

NORPRAMIN'S OTHER NAMES

Norpramin's generic name is desipramine hydrochloride. Another brand name is Pertofrane.

 SIDE EFFECTS

Call your doctor if you have any of these possible drug side effects. Call *immediately* about any labeled "serious."

Serious: seizures, high blood pressure (headache, blurred vision)

Common: drowsiness, dizziness, fast pulse or other heart changes, blurred vision, dry mouth, constipation, inability to urinate, sweating
Tips: Avoid driving and hazardous activities that require alertness and coordination until you know how this drug affects you; dizziness usually subsides after a few weeks. Relieve dry mouth with sugarless hard candy, gum, or saliva substitutes. Increase the amount of fluids you drink to avoid urine retention. Take a stool softener or eat a high-fiber diet to reduce constipation.

Other: excitation, tremor, weakness, confusion, headache, nervousness, extrapyramidal reactions (spastic muscles, poor coordination, tremor), dizziness on standing, ringing in the ears, enlarged pupils, nausea, vomiting, drastic appetite and weight loss, intestinal disorder, rash, hives, sensitivity to light, allergic reaction (rash, itching)

DRUG INTERACTIONS

Combining certain drugs may alter their action or produce unwanted side effects. Tell your doctor about other drugs you're taking, especially:
• alcohol and other drugs that make you relaxed or sleepy, such as sedatives
• Catapres
• epinephrine (Adrenalin)
• other drugs for depression and other psychiatric disorders, such as MAO inhibitors
• Ritalin
• Tagamet.

call your doctor about what to do. Don't take the missed dose in the morning. It may cause disturbing side effects during waking hours.
• If you take more than one dose a day, take the missed dose as soon as possible. However, if it's almost time for your next dose, skip the missed dose and take your next dose on schedule. Don't take a double dose.
• Store tablets away from heat at room temperature.

 If you suspect an overdose

Contact your doctor *immediately*. Signs of overdose in the first 12 hours may include agitation, irritation, confusion, hallucinations, incoordination or muscle spasms, fever, seizures, urine retention, dry nose and mucous membranes, enlarged pupils, constipation, and in-

Continued on next page ▶

testinal disorder. This is followed by low body temperature, decreased or absent reflexes, sedation, low blood pressure (dizziness, weakness), bluish lips and nails, and heart irregularities.

✕ Warnings

• Make sure your doctor knows your medical history. You may not be able to take Norpramin if you have other problems, such as breathing problems, overactive thyroid, diabetes, seizures, urine retention, glaucoma, enlarged prostate, or heart, liver, or kidney disease; or if you're allergic to this or other drugs.
• If you're pregnant or breast-feeding, check with your doctor before taking Norpramin.

• If you have diabetes and the results of your blood or urine sugar tests change, check with your doctor.
• Before you have any medical tests, tell the doctor you're taking Norpramin because this drug can affect some test results.
• Record mood changes during treatment and check with your doctor to find out if your dosage is correct.
• If you will be undergoing surgery, tell your doctor that you are taking Norpramin. The dosage will have to be reduced gradually before surgery.
• Norpramin is not usually recommended for children.

 KEEP IN MIND...

* Takes effect in 2 to 4 weeks or longer.
* Take with food.
* Don't suddenly stop taking.
* Schedule regular checkups to monitor progress.
* Drug may change results of blood or urine sugar tests in diabetics.

Norvasc

Norvasc inhibits the flow of calcium into the heart and blood vessels. This relaxes the blood vessels and increases blood flow to the heart, thus reducing the heart's workload.

Why it's prescribed

Doctors prescribe Norvasc to relieve angina (chest pain) and to treat high blood pressure. It comes in tablets. Doctors usually prescribe the following amounts for adults.

▶ **For angina,** at first, 10 milligrams (mg) per day. Small, frail, or older adults or those with liver insufficiency should begin with 5 mg a day. Most people require 10 mg a day for good results.

▶ **For high blood pressure,** at first, 5 mg per day. Small, frail, or older adults; those currently taking other blood pressure drugs; or those with liver insufficiency should begin with 2.5 mg a day, adjusted according to the person's response and tolerance. Maximum daily dosage is 10 mg.

How to take Norvasc

• Take Norvasc only as your doctor directs. This drug's effects peak in 6 to 9 hours; the effects last for 24 hours.
• Keep taking Norvasc as directed, even when you're feeling better.
• Take additional drugs (such as nitroglycerin tablets), as directed, for sudden angina attacks during treatment.

NORVASC'S OTHER NAME

Norvasc's generic name is amlodipine besylate.

 SIDE EFFECTS

Call your doctor if you have any of these possible drug side effects. Call *immediately* about any labeled "serious."

Serious: signs of congestive heart failure (swelling of hands and feet, shortness of breath), increased angina, low blood pressure (dizziness, weakness), especially in the elderly.

Common: headache, water retention (decreased urination, swelling, weight gain)
Tip: Reduce the salt in your diet to avoid water retention.

Other: fatigue, sleepiness, dizziness, flushing, palpitations, nausea, abdominal pain

 DRUG INTERACTIONS

Combining certain drugs may alter their action or produce unwanted side effects. Tell your doctor about other drugs you're taking, especially:
• other drugs for high blood pressure or angina.

If you miss a dose

Take the missed dose as soon as possible. But if you miss a daily dose completely, skip the missed dose and go back to your regular schedule. Don't take a double dose.

 If you suspect an overdose

Contact your doctor *immediately.* Excessive Norvasc can cause nausea, weakness, dizziness, drowsiness, confusion, slurred speech, low blood pressure (dizziness, weakness), and slow pulse.

Warnings

• Make sure your doctor knows your medical history. You may not be able to take Norvasc if you have other problems, such as liver disease or heart or artery problems such as congestive heart failure or coronary artery disease, or if you're allergic to this or other drugs.
• Tell your doctor if you're pregnant or breast-feeding before you begin taking Norvasc.
• Be aware that older adults may be more sensitive to Norvasc's side effects.

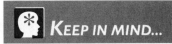 **KEEP IN MIND...**

* Take as directed, even when feeling better.
* Take additional drugs for sudden angina attacks.
* Older adults may be more sensitive to effects.

Nuprin is a nonsteroidal anti-inflammatory drug (NSAID). It reduces inflammation, pain, and fever, probably by stopping the body from producing substances called prostaglandins.

Why it's taken

Nuprin is taken to reduce fever and some types of pain with inflammation, such as menstrual pain. You can buy Nuprin without a prescription. It comes in tablets. The following amounts are usually recommended for adults; children's dosages appear in parentheses.

▶ **For mild to moderate pain and menstrual pain,** 200 to 400 mg every 4 to 6 hours as needed.

▶ **For fever,** 200 to 400 mg every 4 to 6 hours, but no more than 1.2 grams (g) a day and not for longer than 3 days. (Children age 6 months to 12 years: if fever is below 102.5° F, 5 mg for each 2.2 pounds [lb] of body weight every 6 to 8 hours; if fever is higher, 10 mg for each 2.2 lb every 6 to 8 hours, but not more than 40 mg for each 2.2 lb a day.)

How to take Nuprin

• Follow the manufacturer's or your doctor's directions exactly. Nuprin

NUPRIN'S OTHER NAMES

Nuprin's generic name is ibuprofen. Other brand names include Advil, Excedrin IB, Genpril, Haltran, Ibuprin, Ibuprohm, Ibu-Tab, Medipren, Midol-200, Motrin, Pamprin-IB, Rufen, Trendar; and, in Canada, Apo-Ibuprofen and Novo-Profen.

 ## SIDE EFFECTS

Call your doctor if you have any of these possible drug side effects. Call *immediately* about any labeled "serious."

Serious: gastrointestinal bleeding (vomiting dark material or blood, dark or bloody stools), prolonged bleeding from a cut or sore, bronchial spasm (wheezing, difficulty breathing), Stevens-Johnson syndrome (reddened, burnlike rash), high blood pressure (headache, blurred vision), fast or irregular pulse, decreased urine output, liver problems (yellow-tinged skin or eyes)

Common: headache, drowsiness, dizziness, puffy arms and legs, ringing in ears, indigestion, nausea, stomach ulcer, rash
Tip: Take with food to avoid indigestion.

Other: confusion, mood changes, vision disturbances, itching, hives, sensitivity to sunlight, swelling

 ## DRUG INTERACTIONS

Combining certain drugs may alter their action or produce unwanted side effects. Tell your doctor about other drugs you're taking, especially:
• alcohol
• anticoagulants (blood thinners) such as Coumadin
• aspirin; corticosteroids, such as Decadron and Kenacort
• blood pressure drugs and thiazide diuretics (water pills) such as HydroDIURIL and Vaseretic
• lithium.

begins to take effect against pain and fever within 30 minutes; against arthritis symptoms, within 7 days. Effects last 4 hours or more. Although Nuprin reduces pain at low dosages, anti-inflammatory effects don't occur at dosages below 400 mg four times a day.

If you miss a dose

• If you're taking this drug on a regular schedule, take the missed dose as soon as possible. But if it's almost time for your next dose, skip the missed dose and go back to your regular schedule. Don't take a double dose.

 ## If you suspect an overdose

Contact your doctor *immediately.* Excessive Nuprin may cause dizziness, drowsiness, burning or other strange feelings, vomiting, nausea, abdominal pain, headache, sweating, flickering movement of the eyeball, difficult or absent breathing, and bluish coloration of lips, nailbeds, or skin.

✕ Warnings

• Before taking Nuprin, consult your doctor if you have nasal polyps, severe hives, stomach or intestinal disorders, ulcer, high blood pressure, a blood coagulation defect, an allergy to aspirin, or heart, liver, or kidney disease.

• Don't use Nuprin during pregnancy or while breast-feeding.
• Don't take Nuprin for longer than 3 days.

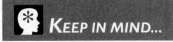

KEEP IN MIND...

* Take with food.
* Won't reduce inflammation at dosages below 400 mg four times a day.
* Don't take longer than 3 days.

Nutropin

Nutropin is an artificial form of the hormone that stimulates the growth of bones, muscles, and organs.

Why it's prescribed

Doctors prescribe Nutropin to treat chronic growth failure in children whose bodies don't produce enough growth hormone and in children with poor growth due to kidney failure who are awaiting kidney transplant. Nutropin is available only by injection. Doctors usually prescribe the following amounts for children.

▶ **For poor growth due to lack of growth hormone,** by injection.

▶ **For poor growth in children with kidney failure, awaiting transplant,** by injection.

How to take Nutropin

• Follow your doctor's directions for treatment with Nutropin.

• Don't shake the vial to mix; gently roll the vial in your hand.

• Use only one dose per vial. Discard any leftover drug.

• Rotate injection sites to decrease irritation.

• You will be given a puncture-resistant container to place your used needles in.

NUTROPIN'S OTHER NAMES

Nutropin's generic name is somatropin. Another brand name is Humatrope.

 SIDE EFFECTS

Call your doctor if you have any of these possible drug side effects. Call *immediately* about any labeled "serious."

Serious: pancreatitis (nausea, vomiting, abdominal pain)

Common: none reported

Other: mildly high blood sugar (increased thirst, hunger, urination), resistance to growth hormone (no response to therapy), swelling in arms or legs, enlarged breast

 DRUG INTERACTIONS

Combining certain drugs may alter their action or produce unwanted side effects. Tell your doctor about other drugs you're taking.

• Store in the refrigerator; do not freeze vials.

If you miss a dose

Consult your doctor.

 If you suspect an overdose

Consult your doctor.

 Warnings

• Make sure your doctor knows your child's medical history. The child may not be able to take Nutropin if he or she has another problem, such as brain injury, diabetes, or underactive thyroid, or if the child is allergic to this or other drugs.

• Be aware that children with growth hormone deficiency may dislocate hip joints more often. Check with your doctor if you notice a limp in a child who's taking Nutropin.

• Be aware that if Nutropin is given to children or adults who don't need growth hormone, it may cause diabetes, abnormal growth of bones and internal organs, hardening of the arteries, and high blood pressure.

KEEP IN MIND...

∗ Given only by injection.

∗ Harmful for children or adults who don't need growth hormones.

∗ Hip joints may slip more often while taking drug; watch for limping.

∗ Rotate injection sites.

Ocuflox

Ocuflox is an antibiotic that stops disease-causing bacteria from reproducing and spreading.

Why it's prescribed

Doctors prescribe Ocuflox to treat eye inflammation and infection (conjunctivitis) that's caused by some types of bacteria. It comes in eyedrops. Doctors usually prescribe the following amounts for adults and children.

▶ **For conjunctivitis**, 1 to 2 drops inside lower eyelid every 2 to 4 hours for first 2 days, and then four times a day for up to 5 more days.

How to use Ocuflox

• Use Ocuflox only as your doctor directs.
• Wash your hands before and after using this drug.
• Don't touch tip of the dropper to eye or surrounding tissue when applying, to prevent contamination.
• Pull lower eyelid gently away from eye and place drops in the space that's created. Then gently close eyes without blinking.
• Press lightly on the inside corners of your closed eyes for 1 minute after taking the drops.
• Discard leftover drug; don't use for a new eye infection.

OCUFLOX'S OTHER NAME

Ocuflox's generic name is ofloxacin.

 SIDE EFFECTS

Call your doctor if you have any of these possible drug side effects. Call *immediately* about any labeled "serious."

Serious: allergic reaction (stinging, redness, itching)

Common: temporary burning or discomfort
Tip: Dab eye with a tissue; do not rub.

Other: stinging, redness, itching, sensitivity to light, excessive tearing or eye dryness, dizziness (rare)
Tip: Avoid bright light and wear sunglasses outdoors.

 DRUG INTERACTIONS

Combining certain drugs may alter their action or produce unwanted side effects. Tell your doctor about other drugs you're taking.

If you miss a dose

Use the missed dose as soon as possible. However, if it's almost time for your next dose, skip the missed dose and go back to your regular schedule. Don't use a double dose.

 If you suspect an overdose

Consult your doctor.

X Warnings

• Make sure your doctor knows your medical history. You may not be able to use Ocuflox if you're allergic to this drug or its ingredients, or to other drugs.
• Tell your doctor if you're pregnant or breast-feeding before you begin using Ocuflox.

• If your condition doesn't improve after 7 days of treatment, check with your doctor. Overuse may cause other infection-causing organisms, such as fungi, to flourish.

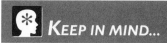 **KEEP IN MIND...**

* Wash hands before and after using.
* Don't allow dropper to touch eye or other surface.
* If no improvement after 7 days, stop using and tell doctor.
* Don't use longer than prescribed, to prevent new infection.
* Discard leftover medicine.

Ocupress

Ocupress reduces pressure in the eyes, although how it works isn't fully understood.

Why it's prescribed

Doctors prescribe Ocupress to treat glaucoma and high pressure in the eyes. It comes in eyedrops. Doctors usually prescribe the following amounts for adults.

▶ **For glaucoma and high pressure in the eyes,** 1 drop inside lower lid of the affected eye twice a day.

How to use Ocupress

• Use Ocupress only as your doctor directs.
• Wash your hands before and after using this drug.
• Don't touch tip of dropper to eye or surrounding tissue.
• Pull lower eyelid gently away from eye and place drops in the space that's created. Then gently close eyes without blinking.
• Press lightly on the inside corners of your closed eyes for 1 minute after taking the drops. This prevents the drug from being absorbed into the body.

If you miss a dose

Apply the missed dose as soon as possible. However, if it's almost time for your next dose, skip the missed dose and go back to your regular schedule. Don't apply a double dose.

 If you suspect an overdose

Contact your doctor *immediately.* Signs that too much Ocupress is be-

OCUPRESS' OTHER NAME

Ocupress' generic name is carteolol hydrochloride.

 SIDE EFFECTS

Call your doctor if you have any of these possible drug side effects. Call *immediately* about any labeled "serious."

Serious: trouble breathing, palpitations, low blood pressure (dizziness, weakness)

Common: temporary eye irritation, burning, tearing, inflammation, or swelling
Tip: Dab the eye with a tissue; do not rub.

Other: blurred and cloudy vision, sensitivity to light, poor night vision, other eye disorders, slow or irregular heartbeat, palpitations, headache, sleeplessness, sinus irritation, taste perversion

 DRUG INTERACTIONS

Combining certain drugs may alter their action or produce unwanted side effects. Tell your doctor about other drugs you're taking, especially:
• beta blockers (heart drugs)
• catecholamine-depleting agents (such as reserpine)
• other eyedrops (use at least 10 minutes before or after using Ocupress).

ing absorbed into the body include nervousness, burning or prickling feeling, change in taste, chest pain, clumsiness, confusion, depression, coughing, wheezing, troubled breathing, decreased sexual ability, diarrhea, dizziness, drowsiness, hair loss, hallucinations, headache, muscle or joint pain, nausea or vomiting, red areas of skin; irregular, slow, or pounding heartbeat; trouble sleeping, unusual tiredness or weakness; runny, stuffy, or bleeding nose; rash, hives, or itching; and swelling of feet or legs.

 Warnings

• Make sure your doctor knows your medical history. You may not be able to use Ocupress if you have other medical problems, especially asthma, lung or heart disease, bron-

chial spasm, diabetes, or overactive thyroid, or if you're allergic to the drug, its ingredients, or other drugs.
• Tell your doctor if you're pregnant or breast-feeding before you begin using Ocupress eyedrops.

KEEP IN MIND...

* Wash hands before and after using.

* Don't allow dropper to touch eye or other surface.

* Press on inside corners of closed eyes after using.

* Use any other eyedrops 10 minutes before or after Ocupress.

Ogen

Ogen is an artificial form of the female hormones called estrogens.

Why it's prescribed

Doctors prescribe Ogen to treat degeneration of the vulva and vagina, failure to ovulate, or osteoporosis (bone disease) and to relieve symptoms of menopause such as hot flashes, sweating, or chills. Ogen comes in tablets and a vaginal cream. Doctors usually prescribe the following amounts for women.

▶ **For vulva and vagina degeneration,** 0.625 to 5 milligrams (mg) orally per day in cycle of 3 weeks on, 1 week off, or 2 to 4 grams (g) of vaginal cream applied each day.

▶ **For ovary failure, decreased sex hormone levels after hysterectomy,** 1.25 to 7.5 mg orally each day for 3 weeks, followed by a rest period of 8 to 10 days. If bleeding does not occur by the end of the rest period, cycle is repeated.

▶ **For menopause symptoms,** 0.625 to 5 mg orally each day in cycle of 3 weeks on, 1 week off.

▶ **To prevent osteoporosis,** 0.625 mg orally each day for 25 days of a 31-day cycle.

How to take Ogen

• Take Ogen only as your doctor directs.

If you miss a dose

Take the missed dose as soon as possible. However, if it's almost time

OGEN'S OTHER NAMES

Ogen's generic name is estropipate. Another brand name is OrthoEST.

SIDE EFFECTS

Call your doctor if you have any of these possible drug side effects. Call *immediately* about any labeled "serious."

Serious: abdominal pain, blood clots (stiffness or numbness in legs or buttocks, chest pain, shortness of breath), severe headaches, vision problem, breast lumps, swollen hands or feet, liver problems (yellow-tinged skin or eyes, dark urine, light-colored stools)

Common: dizziness, water retention (decreased urination, swelling, weight gain), nausea, vomiting, headache

Other: depression, abdominal cramps, bloating, weight change, endometriosis, abnormal or absent menstruation, hairiness, blotchy skin, hair loss, breast engorgement or enlargement, changed sex drive

DRUG INTERACTIONS

Combining certain drugs may alter their action or produce unwanted side effects. Tell your doctor about other drugs you're taking, especially:

• anticoagulants (blood thinners) such as Coumadin
• corticosteroids such as Decadron and Kenacort
• Nolvadex, Parlodel, Rifadin, Sandimmune
• Solfoton, Tegretol.

for your next dose, skip the missed dose and go back to your regular schedule. Don't take a double dose.

If you suspect an overdose

Consult your doctor. Although overdose of this drug has not been reported, nausea would probably be a sign of overdose.

Warnings

• Make sure your doctor knows your medical history. You may not be able to take Ogen if you have other medical problems, especially blood clots, cancer, genital bleeding, heart or artery disease, asthma, depression, bone disease, migraine, seizures, or liver or kidney dysfunction; or if you have a family history of breast cancer.

• Don't take Ogen during pregnancy. If you think you may be pregnant, stop using this drug immediately.

• Examine your breasts regularly and schedule regular checkups.

KEEP IN MIND...

∗ Don't take if pregnant.
∗ Perform monthly breast self-exam.
∗ Take only as directed.

Omnipen

Omnipen is an antibiotic related to penicillin. It kills bacteria by preventing them from multiplying.

Why it's prescribed

Doctors prescribe Omnipen to treat bacterial infections. It comes in capsules and a liquid. Doctors usually prescribe the following amounts for adults; children's dosages appear in parentheses.

▶ **For body-wide infections and urinary tract infections,** 250 to 500 milligrams (mg) every 6 hours. (Children weighing 45 pounds [lb] or more: same as adults. Children weighing 45 lb or less: 50 to 100 mg for each 2.2 lb of body weight, divided into four equal doses taken every 6 hours.)

▶ **For gonorrhea,** 3.5 grams (g) along with 1 g of probenecid taken as a single dose. (Children weighing over 100 lb: same as adults.)

How to take Omnipen

- To keep a steady level of this drug in your blood, space doses throughout the day and night.
- Take Omnipen with a full glass (8 ounces) of water on an empty stomach.
- Swallow capsules whole; don't break, chew, or crush them.
- If you're taking the liquid, use a specially marked measuring spoon.

OMNIPEN'S OTHER NAMES

Omnipen's generic name is ampicillin. Other brand names include D-Amp, Polycillin, Principen, Nu-Ampi, Totacillin; and, in Canada, Apo-Ampi and Novo Ampicillin.

 ## SIDE EFFECTS

Call your doctor if you have any of these possible drug side effects. Call *immediately* about any labeled "serious."

Serious: severe allergic reaction (difficulty breathing, rash, hives, itching, wheezing), blood problems (fatigue, bleeding, bruising, fever, chills, increased risk of infection)

Common: nausea, diarrhea

Other: vomiting, swollen or inflamed tongue, infection by bacteria not susceptible to Omnipen

 ## DRUG INTERACTIONS

Combining certain drugs may alter their action or produce unwanted side effects. Tell your doctor about other drugs you're taking, especially:
- antibiotics called aminoglycosides, such as Garamycin or Tobrex
- Augmentin
- Benemid
- birth control pills that contain estrogen (use different or additional birth control method when taking Omnipen)
- Mexate
- Zyloprim.

If you miss a dose

Take the missed dose as soon as possible. If you take three or more doses a day, space the missed dose and the next dose 2 to 4 hours apart. Then go back to your regular schedule. Don't take a double dose.

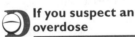 ### If you suspect an overdose

Contact your doctor *immediately.* Excessive Omnipen can cause seizures.

Warnings

- Make sure your doctor knows your medical history. You may not be able to take Omnipen if you're allergic to other penicillins or to antibiotics called cephalosporins, or if you have other medical problems, especially mononucleosis, congestive heart failure, kidney problems, or digestive problems.
- If you're breast-feeding, tell your doctor before taking Omnipen.
- If you have diabetes, Omnipen may cause false test results with some urine sugar tests.

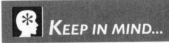 ### KEEP IN MIND...

* Space doses evenly throughout day and night.
* Take with water on empty stomach.
* Supplement birth control pills.

Opticrom

Opticrom relieves redness, swelling, congestion, and itchy, watering eyes by stopping the release of substances in the body called histamines.

Why it's prescribed

Doctors prescribe Opticrom to relieve symptoms of asthma, bronchial spasm, allergic reactions affecting the eyes, and severe allergic hives. Opticrom comes in capsules (for oral solution), aerosol spray, nose drops, solution for inhalant, and eyedrops. Doctors usually prescribe the following amounts for adults; children's dosages appear in parentheses.

▶ **For eye allergy symptoms,** 1 to 2 drops in each eye four to six times a day. (Children age 4 and older: same dosage as adults.)

▶ **For bronchial asthma,** 2 metered sprays using inhaler four times a day. Or, 20 milligrams (mg) inhaled using nebulizer four times a day. (Children age 5 and older: same dosage as adults.)

▶ **To prevent and treat stuffy or inflamed nose,** 1 spray in each nostril three or four times a day, up to six times a day. (Children age 5 and older: same dosage as adults.)

▶ **To prevent exercise-induced bronchial spasm,** 2 sprays inhaled 1 hour or less before exercise. (Children age 5 and older: same dosage as adults.)

OPTICROM'S OTHER NAMES

Opticrom's generic name is cromolyn sodium. Other brand names include Gastrocrom, Intal, Nalcrom, Nasalcrom, and, in Canada, Rynacrom.

SIDE EFFECTS

Call your doctor if you have any of these possible drug side effects. Call *immediately* about any labeled "serious."

Serious: bronchial spasm after inhaling dry powder, severe hives

Common: irritated throat and heartburn, cough, pneumonia
Tip: Relieve heartburn by taking antacids or a glass of milk.

Other: dizziness, headache, stuffy nose, nausea, absent or frequent urination, wheezing, rash, hives, joint swelling and pain, runny eyes, swollen glands

DRUG INTERACTIONS

Combining certain drugs may alter their action or produce unwanted side effects. Tell your doctor about other drugs you're taking.

▶ **For severe allergic hives,** 200 mg orally four times a day before meals and at bedtime. (Children over age 12: same dosage as adults. Children age 2 to 12: 100 mg orally four times a day 30 minutes before meals or at bedtime.)

How to use Opticrom

• Use Opticrom only as your doctor directs. Use this drug only when asthma attack has been controlled, your airway is clear, and you can inhale on your own.
• Dissolve powder in capsules for oral liquid in hot water and further dilute with cold water before drinking. Do not mix with fruit juice, milk, or food.

If you miss a dose

Take the missed dose as soon as possible. Then go back to your regular schedule. Don't take a double dose.

 If you suspect an overdose

Consult your doctor.

Warnings

• Make sure your doctor knows your medical history. You may not be able to use Opticrom if you have other medical problems, especially asthma, heart or artery disease, or irregular heartbeats, or if you're allergic to this or other drugs.
• Tell your doctor if you're pregnant or breast-feeding before you begin using Opticrom.

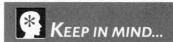 **KEEP IN MIND...**

* Use when asthma attack is under control.
* Don't mix powder with fruit juice, milk, or food.
* Relieve heartburn with antacids or milk.

Optimine

Optimine prevents—but does not reverse—the release of substances in the body called histamines. These substances cause congestion, itching, swelling, and other allergic reactions.

Why it's prescribed

Doctors prescribe Optimine to relieve stuffy or runny nose, chronic hives, and other allergic reactions. It comes in tablets and syrup. Doctors usually prescribe the following amounts for adults; children's dosage appears in parentheses.

▶ **For allergy symptoms,** 1 to 2 milligrams (mg) twice a day. Maximum dosage is 4 mg a day. (Children age 12 and older: same dosage as adults.)

How to take Optimine

• Take Optimine only as your doctor directs. This drug begins to take effect within 15 to 60 minutes. Effects last for 12 hours.
• If you feel this drug is no longer working, check with your doctor. You may need a different drug because you've built up tolerance to Optimine.

If you miss a dose

If you're taking this drug on a regular schedule, take the missed dose as soon as possible. However, if it's almost time for your next dose, skip the missed dose and go back to your regular schedule. Don't take a double dose.

OPTIMINE'S OTHER NAME

Optimine's generic name is azatadine maleate.

 ## SIDE EFFECTS

Call your doctor if you have any of these possible drug side effects.

Serious: none reported

Common: drowsiness or dizziness (especially in older people), dry mouth and throat
Tips: Avoid activities that require alertness until you know how this drug affects you; coffee or tea may reduce drowsiness. Sugarless gum, sugarless hard candy, or ice chips may relieve dry mouth.

Other: feeling of spinning or other sensation, disturbed coordination, low blood pressure (dizziness, weakness), palpitations, drastic appetite and weight loss, nausea, vomiting, heartburn, inability to urinate, blood problems (unusual weakness, bleeding or bruising, sore throat, fever), thick bronchial secretions, hives, rash
Tip: Take doses with food or milk to reduce stomach upset.

 ## DRUG INTERACTIONS

Combining certain drugs may alter their action or produce unwanted side effects. Tell your doctor about other drugs you're taking, especially:
• alcohol and other drugs that relax you or make you sleepy, such as sedatives or sleeping pills
• drugs for depression called MAO inhibitors.

 ### If you suspect an overdose

Contact your doctor *immediately.* Excessive Optimine can cause sedation, reduced alertness, breathing interruption, heart and blood circulation failure, sleeplessness, hallucinations, tremor, or seizures. Dry mouth, flushed skin, fixed and enlarged pupils, seizures, and post-seizure depression are common, especially in children.

Warnings

• Make sure your doctor knows your medical history. You may not be able to take Optimine if you have asthma, pressure in the eyes, overactive thyroid, heart or kidney disease, high blood pressure, inability to urinate, prostate problem, bladder obstruction, or ulcer, or if you're allergic to this or other drugs.
• Tell your doctor if you're pregnant or breast-feeding before you begin taking Optimine.
• Stop taking Optimine 4 days before allergy skin tests to make sure results are accurate.

 ## KEEP IN MIND...

∗ Take with food or milk to reduce stomach upset.

∗ Stop taking 4 days before allergy skin tests, as directed.

∗ Sugarless gum, hard candy, or ice chips may relieve dry mouth.

Orap

Orap is thought to reduce uncontrollable behavior by blocking the effects of certain substances in the brain and nervous system.

Why it's prescribed

Doctors prescribe Orap to treat the symptoms of Tourette syndrome, such as vocal outbursts and uncontrollable, repeated body movements. It comes in tablets. Doctors usually prescribe the following amounts for adults and children over age 12.

▶ **For Tourette syndrome**, at first, 1 to 2 milligrams(mg) each day in divided doses, increased every other day as needed. Maximum dosage is 10 mg a day.

How to take Orap

- Take Orap only as your doctor directs. Don't use more drug than prescribed or take it more often than recommended.
- Don't stop taking this drug suddenly.

If you miss a dose

Take the missed dose as soon as possible. Then take any remaining doses for the day at regularly spaced intervals. Don't take a double dose.

If you suspect an overdose

Contact your doctor *immediately*. Excessive Orap can cause severe extrapyramidal reactions, low blood pressure (dizziness, weakness, fainting), shallow breathing, coma, and abnormal heartbeat.

ORAP'S OTHER NAME

Orap's generic name is pimozide.

SIDE EFFECTS

Call your doctor if you have any of these possible drug side effects. Call *immediately* about any labeled "serious."

Serious: seizures, difficulty breathing, fast pulse, high fever, heavy sweating, severe muscle stiffness, loss of bladder control, extreme fatigue, difficulty speaking or swallowing, loss of balance, mood changes, muscle spasms or unusual body movements

Common: uncontrollable rhythmic movements of the tongue, lips, jaw, or other body parts; sedation; dry mouth; constipation
Tips: Don't drive or perform other activities that require alertness until you know how this drug affects you. Sugarless hard candy, gum, and liquids may relieve dry mouth.

Other: increased reflexes, eyes looking up, decreased muscle tone, muscle quivering, low blood pressure (dizziness, weakness, fainting), vision disturbances, impotence, rigid muscles

DRUG INTERACTIONS

Combining certain drugs may alter their action or produce unwanted side effects. Tell your doctor about other drugs you're taking, especially:
- alcohol and drugs that relax you or make you sleepy, such as sleeping pills and many cold and flu medicines
- phenothiazines, tricyclic antidepressants, heart rhythm drugs
- other drugs for depression, mental illness, and stomach or abdominal cramps
- seizure drugs.

Warnings

- Make sure your doctor knows your medical history. You may not be able to take Orap if you have breast cancer, glaucoma, prostate problem, seizure disorder, or heart, kidney, or liver disease; if you're allergic to this or other drugs; or if you've ever had tics other than those caused by Tourette syndrome.
- If you're pregnant, check with your doctor before taking Orap.
- Be aware that older adults may be especially prone to side effects from Orap.
- Before you have surgery, dental work, or emergency care, tell the doctor you're taking Orap.

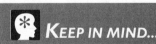 KEEP IN MIND...

- Don't use more or take more often than prescribed.
- Don't stop taking suddenly, to avoid withdrawal symptoms.
- Be aware that older adults may be more prone to side effects.

Oretic

Oretic is a diuretic (water pill). It rids the body of excess water by increasing urination. This, in turn, helps lower blood pressure.

Why it's prescribed

Doctors prescribe Oretic to treat high blood pressure and swelling (edema). It comes in tablets. Doctors usually prescribe the following amounts for adults.

▶ **For high blood pressure,** 25 to 50 milligrams (mg) every day as a single dose or divided into equal doses, increased or decreased according to blood pressure.

▶ **For swelling,** 25 to 200 mg a day or intermittently. Usual dose is 75 to 100 mg daily. Maximum dose is 100 mg twice a day.

How to take Oretic

• To avoid waking up to urinate, take Oretic in the morning. If you're taking more than one daily dose, take the last dose before 6 p.m.

• If you're taking Oretic for high blood pressure, don't stop taking it suddenly even if you feel well.

If you miss a dose

Take the missed dose as soon as possible. But if it's almost time for the next dose, skip the missed dose and take the next dose as scheduled. Don't take a double dose.

ORETIC'S OTHER NAMES

Oretic's generic name is hydrochlorothiazide. Other brand names include Esidrix, Hydrochlor, Hydro-D, HydroDIURIL; and, in Canada, Apo-Hydro, Diuchlor H, Neo-Codema, Novo-Hydrazide, and Urozide.

 SIDE EFFECTS

Call your doctor if you have any of these possible drug side effects. Call *immediately* about any labeled "serious."

Serious: blood problems (fatigue), infection, abnormal bleeding, liver problems with resulting brain disease (confusion, slurred speech, lethargy, tremor)

Common: none reported

Other: dehydration (thirst, dry skin), dizziness, appetite loss, nausea, stomach pain, excessive or frequent urination, sensitivity to sunlight, shortness of breath, cough, fever, rash, ill feeling, difficulty waking, muscle weakness and cramps, increased thirst and hunger, gout

 DRUG INTERACTIONS

Combining certain drugs may alter their action or produce unwanted side effects. Tell your doctor about other drugs you're taking, especially:
• alcohol
• barbiturates
• blood pressure drugs
• Colestid, Questran (take at least 1 hour before Oretic)
• Crystodigin, Lanoxin
• diabetes drugs
• Lithobid
• narcotic pain relievers
• nonsteroidal anti-inflammatory drugs such as Advil.

 If you suspect an overdose

Contact your doctor *immediately.* Excessive Oretic can cause diarrhea, vomiting, increased urination, sluggishness, and possibly coma.

 Warnings

• Make sure your doctor knows your medical history. You may not be able to take Oretic if you have other medical problems.

• If you're pregnant or breast-feeding, tell your doctor before you start taking Oretic.

• If you're diabetic, be aware that Oretic may interfere with the results of sugar tests.

• Eat potassium-rich foods, take a potassium supplement, and decrease your salt intake, as directed by your doctor. Call your doctor if you have muscle weakness or cramps.

KEEP IN MIND...

∗ Take last dose before 6 p.m.

∗ Take with food if stomach upset occurs.

∗ Eat foods high in potassium.

O rinase stimulates the pancreas to produce more insulin and regulates the amount of sugar in the bloodstream.

Why it's prescribed

Doctors prescribe Orinase to help control — but not cure — type II (or non-insulin-dependent) diabetes. It comes in tablets. Doctors usually prescribe the following amounts for adults.

▶ **For diabetes,** at first, 1 to 2 grams (g) each day as a single dose or divided into two or three equal doses. Dosage is adjusted, if necessary, to maximum of 3 g a day; however, the manufacturer of this drug states that little benefit occurs with doses greater than 2 g a day.

▶ **To change from insulin use,** if insulin dosage is less than 20 units a day, insulin is stopped and Orinase is started at 1 to 2 g a day. If insulin dosage is 20 to 40 units a day, insulin is reduced by 30% to 50% and Orinase is started as above. If insulin dosage is over 40 units a day, insulin is reduced by 20% and Orinase is started as above. Further reductions in insulin are based on the person's response to oral therapy.

How to take Orinase

• Take Orinase only as your doctor directs. This drug begins to take effect within 1 hour. Effects last for 6 to 12 hours.
• Take each dose with food. If you're taking one dose a day, take it

SIDE EFFECTS

Call your doctor if you have any of these possible drug side effects. Call *immediately* about any labeled "serious."

Serious: severe allergic reactions (diarrhea, yellow-tinged skin and eyes, skin lesions), blood disorders (fatigue, bleeding, bruising, chills, fever, and increased risk of infection) low blood sugar (confusion, weakness, fainting)

Common: weakness, tingling in fingers or toes

Other: nausea, heartburn, rash, itching, flushing

DRUG AND FOOD INTERACTIONS

Combining certain drugs and foods may alter drug action or produce unwanted side effects. Tell your doctor about your diet and other drugs you're taking, especially:

• alcohol, foods and medicines that contain alcohol
• anabolic steroids such as Teslac
• anticoagulants (blood thinners) such as Coumadin
• aspirin
• Atromid-S
• beta blockers such as Inderal and Lopressor
• Butazolidin
• Catapres
• Chloromycetin
• diet pills
• diuretics (water pills) such as Vaseretic and HydroDIURIL
• drugs for asthma, colds, or allergies
• Ismelin
• Laniazid, Rifadin
• MAO inhibitors, such as Marplan, Nardil, and Parnate
• seizure drugs
• sulfa drugs such as Bactrim.

ORINASE'S OTHER NAMES

Orinase's generic name is tolbutamide. Other brand names include Apo-Tolbutamide and, in Canada, Mobenol and Novo-Butamide.

with breakfast. If you're taking two doses a day, take one dose with breakfast and the second dose with your evening meal.
• Keep taking this drug, even if you feel well. Also, don't change your dosage without your doctor's consent.

If you miss a dose

Take the missed dose as soon as possible. But if it's almost time for your next dose, skip the missed dose and take your next dose as scheduled. Don't take a double dose.

If you suspect an overdose

Contact your doctor *immediately.* Excessive Orinase can cause low blood sugar, which can cause drowsiness, headache, nervousness,

Continued on next page ▶

cold sweats, and confusion. If these symptoms occur, eat or drink something sweet, such as orange juice, and call your doctor. Other signs of overdose may include tingling of lips and tongue, hunger, nausea, lethargy, yawning, confusion, agitation, nervousness, fast pulse, sweating, tremor, seizures, stupor, and coma.

Warnings

• Make sure your doctor knows your medical history. You may not be able to take Orinase if you have type I diabetes (insulin-dependent) or diabetes that can be controlled by diet or have type II diabetes complicated by surgery, infection, or injury (trauma); if you have other problems, such as a disorder that affects the liver, kidneys, adrenal glands, pituitary gland, or thyroid gland; or if you're allergic to this or other drugs.

• Tell your doctor if you're pregnant or breast-feeding before you begin taking Orinase.
• Be aware that older people may be especially sensitive to Orinase's side effects.
• Follow your doctor's instructions for testing your blood or urine for sugar. Also, closely follow your prescribed diet and exercise regimen.
• Carry candy or other sugar sources to treat mild low blood sugar during treatment. Severe low blood sugar may require hospital treatment.
• When switching from insulin to Orinase, you may need to have your blood sugar level tested at least three times a day before meals. You may have to be hospitalized during the transition.
• Wear a medical identification bracelet that tells others you have diabetes and lists the drugs you are taking.

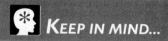

KEEP IN MIND...

* Take with food.
* Continue taking as prescribed, even when feeling well.
* Follow diet and exercise plan.
* Carry sugar source to treat mild low blood sugar.
* Wear a medical identification bracelet.

Orlaam

Orlaam is similar to methadone and acts as a substitute for addictive narcotic drugs in the body.

Why it's prescribed

Doctors prescribe Orlaam to ease some of the symptoms of withdrawal from narcotics, such as tearing, runny nose, sneezing, yawning, sweating, restlessness, and high blood pressure. It comes in an oral liquid. Doctors usually prescribe the following amounts for adults.

▶ **For narcotic addiction,** at first, 20 to 40 milligrams (mg) every 48 to 72 hours, increased by 5 to 10 mg at 48- to 72-hour intervals until the desired response is reached, usually within 1 to 2 weeks. Most people are stable on 60 to 90 mg three times a week.

How to take Orlaam

- Take Orlaam only as your doctor directs.
- Effects last for 48 to 72 hours.

If you miss a dose

Consult your doctor.

 If you suspect an overdose

Contact your doctor *immediately.* Never take Orlaam on a daily basis because of the risk of fatal overdose. Signs of an overdose are slowed and shallow breathing, muscle weak-

ORLAAM'S OTHER NAME

Orlaam's generic name is levo-methadyl acetate hydrochloride.

 SIDE EFFECTS

Call your doctor if you have any of these possible drug side effects.

Serious: none reported

Common: abdominal pain, diarrhea, constipation, dry mouth, nausea, vomiting, impotence, difficulty with ejaculation, cough, rash, sweating
Tip: Increase fluids and high-fiber foods to prevent constipation.

Other: drowsiness, sedation, slow pulse, water retention (decreased urination, swelling, weight gain), heart rhythm change, blurred vision, stuffy or runny nose, yawning, joint pain, weakness, back pain, chills, flulike symptoms, malaise, abstinence syndrome with sudden withdrawal (tearing, runny nose, sneezing, yawning, sweating, restlessness, high blood pressure, headache, blurred vision)

DRUG INTERACTIONS

Combining certain drugs may alter their action or produce unwanted side effects. Tell your doctor about other drugs you're taking, especially:
- carbamazepine, phenobarbital, Dilantin, rifampin
- naloxone, pentazocine, or other opioid agonist-antagonists
- Tagamet, erythromycin, ketoconazole.

ness, cold and clammy skin, and low blood pressure (dizziness).

 Warnings

- Make sure your doctor knows your medical history. You may not be able to take Orlaam if you have other problems, such as a heart, liver, or kidney disorder, or if you're allergic to this or other drugs.
- Tell your doctor if you're pregnant or breast-feeding before you begin taking Orlaam. Your treatment will be changed if you become pregnant.
- Orlaam is dispensed only by licensed and approved clinics. By law, take-home doses are forbidden.

KEEP IN MIND...

* Eases symptoms of withdrawal from addictive narcotic drugs.

* Stable response usually reached within 1 to 2 weeks.

* Effects last 48 to 72 hours after taking.

* Never take daily; risk of fatal overdose.

* Only given by licensed and approved clinics.

Orthoclone OKT3 stops organ rejection by suppressing the person's immune system; this prevents white blood cells from attacking the organ.

Why it's prescribed

Doctors prescribe Orthoclone OKT3 to stop the body from rejecting a transplanted organ, such as a kidney, or other tissue. It comes only in an injectable form. Doctors usually prescribe the following amounts for adults.

▶ **For organ transplant rejection,** by injection for 10 to 14 days.

How to take Orthoclone OKT3

- Orthoclone OKT3 is given only by injection.
- This drug begins to take effect almost immediately. Effects dwindle within 1 week after treatment ends.
- Treatment is usually not repeated, to avoid severe side effects.

If you miss a dose

Consult your doctor.

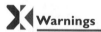

If you suspect an overdose

Consult your doctor.

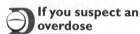

Warnings

- Make sure your doctor knows your medical history. You may not

ORTHOCLONE OKT3'S OTHER NAME

Orthoclone OKT3's generic name is muromonab-CD3.

SIDE EFFECTS

Call your doctor if you have any of these possible drug side effects. Call *immediately* about any labeled "serious."

Serious: seizures, fluid in lungs (shortness of breath, cough, moist cough), infection, severe allergic reaction (swelling of face and throat, difficulty breathing, chest pain, anxiety)

Common: tremor, chest pain, nausea, vomiting, difficulty breathing, fever, chills

Tips: Most side effects develop within $\frac{1}{2}$ to 6 hours after the first dose; these subside as treatment progresses. A fever-reducing drug is given to prevent fever and chills. Other drugs are given to reduce other side effects.

Other: headache, fast pulse, diarrhea

DRUG INTERACTIONS

Combining certain drugs may alter their action or produce unwanted side effects. Tell your doctor about other drugs you're taking, especially:
- Indocin
- live-virus vaccines
- other drugs that suppress the immune system.

---

be able to take Orthoclone OKT3 if you're allergic to this or other drugs or to rodents (because this drug is grown in living cells from mice) or if you have other medical problems, especially a history of seizures.
- Tell your doctor if you're pregnant or breast-feeding before you receive this drug.
- While you're taking Orthoclone OKT3, avoid being vaccinated with any live-virus vaccines. These may infect people whose immune systems are depressed, such as after organ transplant.
- Your doctor may prescribe additional drugs to relieve any side effects.

KEEP IN MIND...

- *Stops organ rejection by suppressing immune system.
- *Given by injection only.
- *Report allergy to rodents (mice or rats).
- *Not recommended during pregnancy or breast-feeding.
- *Most side effects ease as treatment progresses.

Ortho-Novum

O rtho-Novum is a birth control pill used to suppress ovulation by inhibiting hormones that cause ovualtion.

Why it's prescribed

Doctors prescribe Ortho-Novum to prevent pregnancy. It comes in tablets. Doctors usually prescribe the following amounts for adults.
▶ **For contraception,** one-phase pills: 1 tablet once a day, beginning on day 1 of menstrual cycle.

How to take Ortho-Novum

• Take Ortho-Novum only as your doctor directs.
• Take tablets at the same time each day; take at night to avoid nausea and headaches.

If you miss a dose

Adjust your schedule as follows:
• If you miss 1 tablet, take it as soon as you remember or take 2 tablets the next day; then continue your regular schedule.
• If you miss 2 consecutive days, take 2 tablets a day for 2 days; then resume your normal schedule. Use an additional method of birth control for 7 days.
• If you miss 3 or more days, discard the remaining tablets and use a different birth control method.

 SIDE EFFECTS

Call your doctor if you have any of these possible drug side effects. Call *immediately* about any labeled "serious."

Serious: blood clots (numbness, stiffness, or pain in legs or buttocks; chest pain), severe skin reaction, high blood pressure (headache, blurred vision), blood sugar change, migraine

Common: headache, dizziness, nausea, vomiting, diarrhea, breast tenderness, breakthrough bleeding, sensitivity to sunlight, rash

Other: depression, lethargy, bloating, vision disturbances, constipation, weight loss or gain, cervical secretions, vaginal yeast infection, menstrual change, oily skin, breast changes, sex drive change, abdominal pain

 DRUG INTERACTIONS

Combining certain drugs may alter their action or produce unwanted side effects. Tell your doctor about other drugs you're taking, especially:
• corticosteroids such as Decadron and Kenacort
• Nolvadex, Parlodel, Sandimmune
• oral anticoagulants (blood thinners) such as Coumadin
• Rifadin, Solfoton, Tegretol
• tobacco.

ORTHO-NOVUM'S OTHER NAMES

Ortho-Novum's generic name is norethindrone and mestranol. Brand names include Genora 1/50, Nelova 1/50M, Norethin 1/50M, Norinyl 1+50; and, in Canada, Norinyl 1/50.

• If your next menstrual period doesn't begin on time, check with your doctor to rule out pregnancy before starting a new dosing cycle.

 If you suspect an overdose

Consult your doctor.

 Warnings

• Make sure your doctor knows your medical history. You may not be able to take Ortho-Novum if you have a blood clotting disorder, blood vessel or heart disease, migraines, seizures, asthma, cancer, kidney or liver disease, or vaginal bleeding.

• Stop taking the pills and call your doctor if you think you may be pregnant; don't take them if you're breast-feeding.
• The hormones in birth control pills may affect treatment for diabetes.
• Examine breasts monthly as directed.

KEEP IN MIND...

* Take at same time each day.
* Many side effects go away after 3 to 6 months.
* Examine breasts monthly.

Orudis

Orudis is one of a large group of drugs called non-steroidal anti-inflammatory drugs (NSAIDs). Orudis reduces inflammation, pain, and swelling, possibly by reducing the body's production of substances called prostaglandins, which cause these symptoms.

Why it's prescribed

Doctors prescribe Orudis to reduce fever, pain, swelling, and joint stiffness with some types of arthritis (including osteoarthritis), and mild to moderate pain, as in painful menstruation. It comes in sustained-release tablets, enteric-coated tablets (which dissolve after reaching the intestine), capsules, extended-release capsules, and suppositories. Doctors usually prescribe the following amounts for adults.

▶ **For arthritis,** 75 milligrams (mg) orally three times a day, 50 mg four times a day, or 200 mg sustained-release tablet once a day. Maximum dosage is 300 mg a day. Or 100 mg rectal suppository twice a day or 1 suppository at bedtime (with oral forms during the day).

▶ **For mild to moderate pain,** 25 to 50 mg orally every 6 to 8 hours as needed.

How to take Orudis

• Take Orudis only as your doctor directs. Overuse can aggravate side

ORUDIS' OTHER NAMES

Orudis' generic name is ketoprofen. Other brand names include Oruvail and, in Canada, Apo-Keto, Novo-Keto-EC, and Rhodis.

 SIDE EFFECTS

Call your doctor if you have any of these possible drug side effects. Call *immediately* about any labeled "serious."

Serious: ulcer (signs of bleeding such as bloody or tarry stools, severe nausea, coffee ground–like vomit, heartburn, or indigestion); liver problems (yellow-tinged skin and eyes); blood disorder (fatigue, bleeding, bruising, fever, chills, increased risk of infection); bronchial spasm; swelling in breathing passage of throat; severe skin rash, hives, or peeling; other allergic reaction (wheezing, difficulty breathing, puffy eyes)

Common: headache, nervousness, nausea, abdominal pain, diarrhea, constipation, gas
Tips: These symptoms usually disappear as your body adjusts to the drug. Take with food to avoid nausea. Increase fluid and high-fiber foods to avoid constipation.

Other: dizziness, decreased level of wakefulness, ringing in ears, vision disturbances, drastic appetite and weight loss, vomiting, inflamed tongue, sensitivity to light
Tip: Wear sunscreen and protective clothing in the sun.

 DRUG INTERACTIONS

Combining certain drugs may alter their action or produce unwanted side effects. Tell your doctor about other drugs you're taking, especially:
• alcohol
• anticoagulants (blood thinners) such as Coumadin
• Anturane, Depakene, Geocillin, Persantine
• aspirin and aspirin-containing products
• blood pressure drugs such as Catapres and Inderal
• Calan, Dilantin, Procardia
• corticosteroids such as Kenacort and Orasone
• Eskalith, Mexate
• hydrochlorothiazide, other diuretics (water pills), such as Aldactone and Lasix
• insulin and oral diabetes drugs such as Micronase
• other NSAIDs such as Motrin
• probenecid
• Tylenol.

effects. Pain relief begins within 1 to 2 hours and lasts for 3 to 4 hours. Onset and duration of relief are not known for arthritis; full effect may be delayed for 2 to 4 weeks; for best results, keep taking regularly.

• Take Orudis capsules with a full glass (8 ounces) of water either 30 minutes before or 2 hours after meals. If this drug upsets your stomach, you may take it with milk or meals.

• Avoid lying down for 15 to 30 minutes after you take Orudis capsules, to reduce the chance of stomach upset.

If you miss a dose

Take the missed dose as soon as possible. But if it's almost time for your next dose, skip the missed dose and take the next one as scheduled. Don't take a double dose.

If you suspect an overdose

Contact your doctor. Excessive Orudis can cause nausea and drowsiness.

Warnings

• Make sure your doctor knows your medical history. You may not be able to take Orudis if you have another problem, such as an ulcer, kidney dysfunction, high blood pressure, heart failure, or fluid retention, or if you're overly sensitive to this or other drugs (for example, if you have had aspirin- or NSAID-induced asthma, hives, or other allergic reactions).

• If you're pregnant or breast-feeding, check with your doctor before taking this drug. Orudis is not recommended during third trimester of pregnancy.

• Be aware that older adults may be especially susceptible to side effects when taking Orudis.

• During long-term treatment, have regular checkups so your doctor can make sure your kidneys and liver are functioning well.

• Tell your doctor if you're on a special diet; Orudis may contain sugar or sodium.

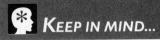

KEEP IN MIND...

∗ Don't take during third trimester of pregnancy.

∗ For arthritis, relief may take 2 to 4 weeks to begin.

∗ Take capsules on empty stomach, or with milk or meals to avoid stomach upset.

∗ Signs of overdose include nausea and drowsiness.

∗ Most side effects subside as body adjusts to drug.

∗ Have regular checkups with long-term treatment.

Ovcon interferes with ovulation, stops sperm movement, and prevents fertilized eggs from attaching in the uterus.

Why it's prescribed

Doctors prescribe Ovcon to prevent pregnancy. It comes in tablets. Doctors usually prescribe the following amounts for adults.

▶ **For contraception,** 1 tablet once a day, beginning on the first day of menstrual flow.

How to take Ovcon

• Take Ovcon only as directed.
• Take tablets at the same time each day; take at night to avoid nausea and headaches.

If you miss a dose

Adjust your schedule as follows:
• If you miss 1 tablet, take it as soon as you remember or take 2 tablets the next day; then continue your regular schedule.
• If you miss 2 consecutive days, take 2 tablets a day for 2 days; then resume your normal schedule. Use an additional method of birth control for 7 days.
• If you miss 3 or more days, discard the remaining tablets in the monthly package and substitute a different birth control method.
• If your next menstrual period doesn't begin on time, check with

OVCON'S OTHER NAMES

Ovcon's generic name is norethindrone and ethinyl estradiol. Brand names include Brevicon, Jenest-28, Modicon, Ovcon-35, Ortho-Novum 7/7/7, Tri-Norinyl; and, in Canada, Brevicon 0.5/35, Ortho 0.5/35, and Synphasic.

 SIDE EFFECTS

Call your doctor if you have any of these possible drug side effects. Call *immediately* about any labeled "serious."

Serious: blood clots (numbness, stiffness, or pain in legs or buttocks; chest pain), severe skin reaction, high blood pressure (headache, blurred vision), blood sugar change, migraine

Common: headache, dizziness, nausea, vomiting, diarrhea, breast tenderness, breakthrough bleeding, swelling. lethargy, rash

Other: depression, vision disturbances, constipation, weight loss or gain, cervical secretions, vaginal yeast infection, menstrual change, oily skin, darkening skin color, breast changes, sex drive change, abdominal pain, sensitivity to sunlight

 DRUG INTERACTIONS

Combining certain drugs may alter their action or produce unwanted side effects. Tell your doctor about other drugs you're taking, especially:
• corticosteroids such as Decadron and Kenacort
• Nolvadex, Parlodel, Sandimmune
• oral anticoagulants (blood thinners) such as Coumadin
• Rifadin, Solfoton, Tegretol
• tobacco.

your doctor to rule out pregnancy before starting a new dosing cycle. If your menstrual period begins, start a new dosing cycle 7 days after you took the last tablet.

 If you suspect an overdose

Consult your doctor.

 Warnings

• Make sure your doctor knows your medical history. You may not be able to take Ovcon if you have a blood clotting disorder, heart disease, blood clots in eyes (double vision), migraine, seizures, asthma, breast cancer or other cancer, kidney or liver disease, or vaginal bleeding.

• Stop taking the pills and call your doctor if you think you may be pregnant; don't take them if you're breast-feeding.
• Ovcon may help protect against cancer of the ovaries or uterus, but may increase the risk of cervical cancer.
• The hormones in Ovcon may affect treatment for diabetes.
• Examine breasts monthly.

 KEEP IN MIND...

* Take at same time each day.
* Many side effects go away after 3 to 6 months.
* Examine breasts monthly.

Oxsoralen

Oxsoralen, along with light treatment from a special type of lamp that emits ultraviolet light, acts on the skin's color pigments to produce inflammation and reduce symptoms such as pigment loss. This drug is very potent.

Why it's prescribed

Doctors prescribe Oxsoralen to treat psoriasis and vitiligo, a disease that causes skin pigment loss. It comes in a lotion. Doctors usually prescribe the following amounts for adults; children's dosages appear in parentheses.

▶ **For vitiligo or psoriasis,** lotion applied to small, well-defined spots that have lost pigment. For best effect, applied about 1 to 2 hours before exposure to ultraviolet light for a limited time. After light exposure, wash area with soap and water and protect area with sunblock. Manufacturer recommends weekly treatment. (Children over age 12: same dosage as adults. Children under age 12: treatment is individualized by doctor.)

How to use Oxsoralen

• Use Oxsoralen only as your doctor directs.
• Protect yourself from exposure during light treatments by wearing sunblock, protective clothing, and sunglasses.

OXSORALEN'S OTHER NAME

Oxsoralen's generic name is topical methoxsalen.

SIDE EFFECTS

Call your doctor if you have any of these possible drug side effects. Call *immediately* about any labeled "serious."

Serious: potential for severe burns

Common: none reported

Other: water retention (decreased urination, swelling, weight gain), redness, painful blistering, burning, peeling, itching
Tip: Avoid excessive exposure to sunlight during treatment.

DRUG INTERACTIONS

Combining certain drugs may alter their action or produce unwanted side effects. Tell your doctor about other drugs you're taking, especially:
• other drugs that cause sensitivity to light.

If you miss a dose

Apply the missed dose as soon as possible. However, if it's almost time for your next dose, skip the missed dose and go back to your regular treatment schedule. Don't apply a double dose.

If you suspect an overdose

Contact your doctor *immediately.* Signs of overdose or overexposure to ultraviolet light include serious burning and blistering of skin.

Warnings

• Make sure your doctor knows your medical history. You may not be able to use Oxsoralen if you have other problems, such as diseases that cause sensitivity to light (such as porphyria or lupus), any form of skin cancer, stomach or intestinal disorders or a chronic infection, or if you're allergic to this or other drugs.

• Tell your doctor if you're pregnant or breast-feeding before you begin using Oxsoralen.
• Schedule regular checkups during treatment for vitiligo (especially at beginning of treatment), so your doctor can monitor your progress and check for side effects.

KEEP IN MIND...

* Used with ultraviolet light treatment.

* Check with doctor before treatment during pregnancy or while breast-feeding.

* Protect eyes and lips from light during ultraviolet light treatments.

* Avoid excessive sunlight during treatment to prevent serious burns and blisters.

* Schedule regular checkups during treatment.

Pamelor

Pamelor is a tricyclic antidepressant, which increases the amount of natural antidepressants in the body.

Why it's prescribed

Doctors prescribe Pamelor to relieve the symptoms of depression. It comes in tablets, capsules, and an oral liquid. Doctors usually prescribe the following amounts for adults.

▶ **For depression,** 25 milligrams(mg) three or four times a day, gradually increased to maximum of 150 mg a day. Entire dosage may be taken at bedtime.

How to take Pamelor

• Take Pamelor only as your doctor directs. This drug is thought to take 2 to 4 weeks or longer to take effect.
• To reduce stomach upset, take Pamelor with food unless your doctor tells you to take it on an empty stomach.
• If you're taking the oral liquid, use the dropper provided to carefully measure each dose. Dilute with about half a glass (4 ounces) of water, milk, or orange juice before drinking.
• Don't suddenly stop taking this drug. Check with your doctor about gradually stopping.

If you miss a dose

Adjust your schedule as follows:
• If you take one dose a day at bedtime, don't take the missed dose

 SIDE EFFECTS

Call your doctor if you have any of these possible drug side effects. Call *immediately* about any labeled "serious."

Serious: seizures, fast or changed heartbeat, high blood pressure (headache, blurred vision)

Common: drowsiness, dizziness, blurred vision, constipation, inability to urinate, sweating
Tip: Avoid activities that require alertness and coordination if you become dizzy or drowsy; these effects usually subside after a few weeks.

Other: excitement, tremor, weakness, confusion, headache, nervousness, extrapyramidal reactions (increased reflexes, eyes looking up, decreased muscle tone, muscle quivering), ringing in the ears, enlarged pupils, dry mouth, nausea, vomiting, drastic appetite and weight loss, intestinal disorder, rash, hives, sensitivity to light, allergic reaction; after abruptly stopping long-term treatment: nausea, headache, malaise

 DRUG INTERACTIONS

Combining certain drugs may alter their action or produce unwanted side effects. Tell your doctor about other drugs you're taking, especially:
• alcohol
• Aldomet, Catapres, Inderal, Ismelin, Lopressor
• Antabuse
• anticoagulants (blood thinners) such as Coumadin
• atropine sulfate
• Darvon, Haldol
• drugs that make you relaxed or sleepy, such as pain relievers, barbiturates (Solfoton), narcotics, and tranquilizers (Xanax)
• nasal sprays and antihistamines, such as Allerest and Brofedrol
• Persantine, Procan SR, Quinaglute Dura-tabs
• Sinemet
• thyroid drugs
• tobacco.

the next morning; it may cause side effects during waking hours. Check with your doctor about what to do.
• If you take more than one dose a day, take the missed dose as soon as possible. If it's almost time for your next dose, skip the missed dose and take your next dose as scheduled. Don't take a double dose.

 If you suspect an overdose

Contact your doctor *immediately.* Excessive Pamelor can cause agitation, confusion, seizures, decreased urine output, constipation, decreased body temperature, slowed breathing, and low blood pressure (dizziness, weakness).

✕ Warnings

- Make sure your doctor knows your medical history. You may not be able to take Pamelor if you have other problems, such as glaucoma, suicidal tendency, urine retention, seizures, heart disease, or overactive thyroid; if you're allergic to this or other drugs; or if you've recently had a heart attack.
- If you're pregnant or breast-feeding, don't use Pamelor unless you've discussed the risks and benefits with your doctor.

- Be aware that children and older adults are especially prone to Pamelor's side effects.
- Follow your doctor's recommendations to drink extra fluids and to use a stool softener or high-fiber diet, as needed, during treatment.
- Report mood changes and other signs of mental change to your doctor so that your dosage can be adjusted.
- If you'll be having surgery, tell your doctor so that your dosage of Pamelor can be gradually reduced.

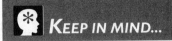

KEEP IN MIND...

- * Takes effect in 2 to 4 weeks or longer.
- * Take Pamelor with food or on empty stomach as directed.
- * Carefully measure oral liquid; mix with water, milk, or orange juice.
- * Drink extra fluids and eat high-fiber diet as directed.
- * Don't suddenly stop taking this drug.
- * Report mood changes to doctor.

Panadol

Panadol relieves mild pain by blocking pain impulses. It also relieves fever, probably by acting on the heat-regulating center of the brain. Unlike aspirin and similar drugs, Panadol does not reduce inflammation.

Why it's taken

Panadol is taken to reduce mild pain and fever. It comes in tablets, chewable tablets, drops, and solution. The following amounts are usually recommended for adults; children's dosages follow.

▶ **For mild pain or fever,** 325 to 650 milligrams (mg) every 4 to 6 hours or 1 gram (g) three or four times a day, as needed. Maximum dosage is 4 g a day.
• Children over age 11: same as adults.
• Children age 11: 480 mg every 4 to 6 hours.
• Children ages 9 to 10: 400 mg every 4 to 6 hours.
• Children ages 6 to 8: 320 mg every 4 to 6 hours.
• Children ages 4 to 5: 240 mg every 4 to 6 hours.
• Children ages 2 to 3: 160 mg every 4 to 6 hours.
• Children ages 12 to 23 months: 120 mg every 4 to 6 hours.
• Children ages 4 to 11 months: 80 mg every 4 to 6 hours.

PANADOL'S OTHER NAMES

Panadol's generic name is acetaminophen. Other brand names include Aceta, Anacin-3, Banesin, Genapap, Genebs, Liquiprin Infants' Drops, Neopap, St. Joseph Aspirin-Free Fever Reducer for Children, Suppap-120, Tempra, and Tylenol.

SIDE EFFECTS

Call your doctor if you have any of these possible drug side effects. Call *immediately* about any labeled "serious."

Serious: severe liver damage with excessive doses (yellow-tinged skin and eyes, rash, hives)

Common: none reported

Other: reduced blood sugar (confusion, weakness, dizziness), blood problems (fatigue, bleeding, bruising, fever, chills, increased risk of infection), rash, hives
Tips: Avoid contact sports and other activities that increase your risk of bleeding or bruising. To prevent infection, avoid people who are ill or have an infection.

DRUG INTERACTIONS

Combining certain drugs may alter their action or produce unwanted side effects. Tell your doctor about other drugs you're taking, especially:
• alcohol
• Anturane
• aspirin and other nonsteroidal anti-inflammatory drugs
• barbiturates
• caffeine
• Coumadin
• Dolobid
• nonprescription drugs containing acetaminophen (count acetaminophen content toward daily acetaminophen total)
• Retrovir (AZT)
• Rifadin and tetracycline antibiotics
• seizure drugs called hydantoins
• Tegretol.

• Children under age 3 months: 40 mg every 4 to 6 hours.

How to take Panadol

• Carefully follow the precautions listed on the package label.
• You can take a dose of Panadol every 4 hours as needed, but don't exceed the total that's recommended on the package.

If you miss a dose

Take the missed dose as soon as possible. However, if it's almost time for your next dose, skip the missed dose and take your next dose as scheduled. Don't take a double dose.

 If you suspect an overdose

Contact your doctor *immediately.* Excessive Panadol can cause bluish skin, yellow-tinged skin and eyes, fever, vomiting, delirium, coma, seizures, and death.

Warnings

• Make sure your doctor knows your medical history. You may not be able to take Panadol if you're allergic to it; if you have diabetes, kidney or liver problems, viral infection, heart disease, phenylketonuria, or a blood disorder; or if you have a history of chronic alcohol abuse.

• Don't use Panadol if you have a high fever (over 103° F [39.5° C], a fever that lasts longer than 3 days, or a fever that recurs. Instead, talk with your doctor.

• Don't use Panadol for arthritis or other rheumatic conditions without your doctor's consent. Panadol may reduce the pain of these conditions, but not the other symptoms.

• Consult a doctor before giving this drug to a child under age 2.

• Use a liquid form of Panadol for children and for anyone who has trouble swallowing.

• If you're diabetic, check your sugar levels carefully. Panadol may produce false-positive decreases in blood sugar levels on home monitoring kits. Call your doctor if you notice a change.

• If you need high doses of Panadol for a long time, your doctor will probably want to test your blood and your kidney and liver function from time to time.

• Contact your doctor if Panadol doesn't relieve your pain after 10 days (5 days for children), if you have new symptoms, if the pain gets worse, or if the pain site appears red and swollen.

• Call the doctor if Panadol doesn't eliminate your fever within 3 days, if the fever returns or rises, or if new symptoms, redness, or swelling occurs.

• Check with the doctor or pharmacist before taking any nonprescription drugs. Many contain acetaminophen that must count toward your total daily dosage.

• Keep in mind that large doses of Panadol may cause liver damage. Call the doctor if you develop a rash or hives or if your skin turns yellowish.

• Don't drink alcoholic beverages when taking Panadol because this combination may cause liver damage, especially if you take Panadol regularly for a long time.

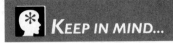

KEEP IN MIND...

* Don't take more than total dosage recommended on package.

* If pain or fever don't subside in a few days, call the doctor.

* Don't take with aspirin or other nonsteroidal anti-inflammatory drugs.

* If you're diabetic, check sugar levels carefully.

Parlodel

Parlodel is used to regulate certain hormones in the treatment of menstrual problems and infertility.

Why it's prescribed

Doctors prescribe Parlodel to treat menstrual or fertility problems. It's also used to treat Parkinson's disease and overproduction of growth hormone (acromegaly). Parlodel comes in tablets and capsules. Doctors usually prescribe the following amounts for adults.

▶ **For menstrual and fertility disorders,** 1.25 to 2.5 milligrams (mg) a day, increased by 2.5 mg a day at 3- to 7-day intervals until desired effect occurs. Therapeutic dosage is 2.5 to 5 mg per day.

▶ **For Parkinson's disease,** 1.25 mg twice a day with meals, increased every 14 to 28 days, up to 100 mg a day, as needed.

▶ **For acromegaly,** 1.25 to 2.5 mg with bedtime snack for 3 days, increased until benefit occurs. Maximum dosage is 100 mg a day.

How to take Parlodel

• If Parlodel upsets your stomach, take with meals or milk.

If you miss a dose

Take the missed dose as soon as possible if you remember within 4 hours. If more than 4 hours have passed, skip the missed dose and resume your normal schedule. Don't take a double dose.

PARLODEL'S OTHER NAME

Parlodel's generic name is bromocriptine mesylate.

 SIDE EFFECTS

Call your doctor if you have any of these possible drug side effects. Call *immediately* about any labeled "serious."

Serious: seizures, fluid in lungs (moist cough, shortness of breath), chest pain, severe nausea and vomiting, high blood pressure (headache, blurred vision), stroke (weakness)

Common: low blood pressure (dizziness, weakness, fainting), abdominal cramps
Tips: Avoid dizziness and fainting by sitting up and standing slowly.

Other: confusion, hallucinations, uncontrollable movements, fatigue, mania, delusions, nervousness, depression, stuffy nose, ringing in ears, dry mouth, nausea, vomiting, constipation, diarrhea, inability to urinate, frequent urination, cool and pale fingers and toes

 DRUG INTERACTIONS

Combining certain drugs may alter their action or produce unwanted side effects. Tell your doctor about other drugs you're taking, especially:
• alcohol
• Aldomet, Haldol, Loxitane, Reglan, Serpasil, Sinemet
• birth control pills, estrogens, progestins
• blood pressure drugs
• MAO inhibitors, such as Eldepryl and Parnate
• phenothiazines, such as Taractan and Thorazine.

 If you suspect an overdose

Contact your doctor *immediately.* Excessive Parlodel can cause nausea, vomiting, and severe low blood pressure (severe dizziness and weakness).

 Warnings

• Make sure your doctor knows your medical history. You may not be able to take Parlodel if you have high blood pressure, kidney or liver problems, irregular heartbeats, a drug allergy, or a history of heart attack or of toxemia during pregnancy.

• Tell your doctor if you're pregnant or breast-feeding before you begin taking Parlodel.
• Be aware that Parlodel may increase your chance of pregnancy, and that menstruation may take 6 to 8 weeks or longer to return to normal.

KEEP IN MIND...

* Take with meals or milk.
* Take with other drugs as directed.
* May cause increased fertility.

Parnate

Parnate, an MAO inhibitor, blocks the action of a chemical substance called monoamine oxidase in the nervous system.

Why it's prescribed

Doctors prescribe Parnate to treat depression. It comes in tablets. Doctors usually prescribe the following amounts for adults.

▶ **For depression,** 10 milligrams (mg) three times a day, increased as needed.

How to take Parnate

• Don't suddenly stop taking Parnate. Your dosage will usually be reduced to a minimum maintenance level as soon as possible.

If you miss a dose

Take the missed dose as soon as possible. If it's within 2 hours of your next dose, skip the missed dose and go back to your regular schedule. Don't take a double dose.

If you suspect an overdose

Contact your doctor immediately. Excessive Parnate can cause severe anxiety, confusion, dizziness, drowsiness, fast and irregular heartbeat, fever, hallucinations, headache, high blood pressure (headache, blurred vision), low blood pressure (dizziness, weakness), muscle stiffness, sweating, trouble breathing, sleeplessness, irritability, and cool, clammy skin.

Warnings

• Make sure your doctor knows your medical history. You may not

PARNATE'S OTHER NAME

Parnate's generic name is tranylcypromine sulfate.

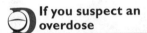 SIDE EFFECTS

Call your doctor if you have any of these possible drug side effects. Call *immediately* about any labeled "serious."

Serious: fast pulse, high blood pressure (headache, blurred vision), palpitations, liver problems (yellow-tinged skin or eyes)

Common: dizziness, drastic appetite and weight loss

Other: feeling of spinning, headache, overstimulation, numbness, tingling, tremor, confusion, memory loss, blurred vision, ringing in ears, dry mouth, nausea, diarrhea, constipation, abdominal pain, impotence, inability to urinate, rash, water retention (decreased urination, swelling, weight gain), muscle spasm, chills

FOOD AND DRUG INTERACTIONS

Combining certain drugs and certain foods may alter drug action or produce unwanted effects. Tell your doctor about your diet and other drugs you're taking, especially:

• alcohol, caffeine, foods high in tryptophan or tyramine (aged cheese, Chianti wine, beer, avocados, chicken livers, chocolate, bananas, soy sauce, meat tenderizers, salami, and bologna)
• amphetamines (diet pills), antihistamines (Actifed, Benadryl), nasal spray, Ritalin, many cold remedies
• antiparkinsonian drugs such as Sinemet
• barbiturates (such as Solfoton), narcotics, Levoprome, sedatives (Ativan, Xanax), tricyclic antidepressants (Elavil, Pamelor)
• blood pressure drugs
• BuSpar, Welbutrin
• Desyrel, Prozac, Zoloft
• insulin, oral diabetes drugs such as Micronase
• other MAO inhibitors such as Eldepryl.

be able to take Parnate if you have heart or vascular disease, high blood pressure, headaches, kidney disease, diabetes, seizures, Parkinson's disease, or overactive thyroid; if you're allergic to it; or if you're at risk for suicide.
• Follow your doctor's instructions for stopping treatment 14 days before surgery.

• Make sure your doctor knows if you're pregnant or breast-feeding.
• Be aware that this drug can mask warning signs of angina (chest pain).

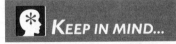 KEEP IN MIND...

∗ Don't suddenly stop taking.
∗ Go for regular checkups.
∗ Parnate may hide signs of angina.

Paxil

P axil increases natural anti-depressants in the brain.

Why it's prescribed

Doctors prescribe Paxil to relieve the symptoms of depression. It comes in tablets. Doctors usually prescribe the following amounts for adults.

▶ **For depression,** at first, 20 milligrams (mg) per day, increased by 10 mg a day at weekly intervals, to a maximum of 50 mg a day, as needed. For older or sickly adults or those with severe liver or kidney disease: at first, 10 mg per day, increased by 10 mg a day at weekly intervals, to a maximum of 40 mg a day, as needed.

How to take Paxil

• Take Paxil only as your doctor directs. This drug usually begins to take effect within 1 to 4 weeks.
• Take Paxil in the morning for best results.

If you miss a dose

Take the missed dose as soon as possible. However, if it's almost time for your next dose, skip the missed dose and go back to your regular schedule. Don't take a double dose.

 ## If you suspect an overdose

Contact your doctor *immediately*. Excessive Paxil can cause severe drowsiness, dry mouth, irritability, enlarged pupils, severe nausea and vomiting, racing pulse, and severe tremor.

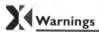 **Warnings**

• Make sure your doctor knows your medical history. You may not be able to take Paxil if you have

PAXIL'S OTHER NAME

Paxil's generic name is paroxetine hydrochloride.

 ## SIDE EFFECTS

Call your doctor if you have any of these possible drug side effects. Call *immediately* about any labeled "serious."

Serious: palpitations, low blood pressure (dizziness, weakness)

Common: sleepiness, dizziness, sleeplessness, tremor, nervousness, dry mouth, nausea, constipation, diarrhea, decreased appetite, weakness, sweating

Tip: Don't drive or perform other activities that require alertness and coordination until you know how this drug affects you.

Other: blurred vision, anxiety, tingling, confusion, tightness in throat, increased appetite, gas, vomiting, stomach upset, erection or ejaculation problem, frequent urination, rash, blood problems (fatigue, bleeding, bruising, fever, chills), pinpoint pupils, muscle pain, weakness, decreased sex drive, yawning

 ## FOOD AND DRUG INTERACTIONS

Combining certain drugs and foods may alter drug action or produce unwanted side effects. Tell your doctor about your diet and other drugs you're taking, especially:
• Coumadin
• Digoxin
• Dilantin, Solfoton
• foods containing tryptophan (aged cheese, Chianti wine, beer, avocados, chicken livers, chocolate, bananas, soy sauce, meat tenderizers, salami, and bologna)
• Kemadrin
• MAO inhibitors such as Eldepryl and Parnate (allow at least 2 weeks after stopping Paxil use before starting treatment with an MAO inhibitor)
• Tagamet.

other medical problems, especially a severe illness, are allergic to this or other drugs, or have a history of seizure disorders or mania.
• Tell your doctor if you're pregnant or breast-feeding before you begin taking Paxil.
• Record your mood changes and report them regularly during treatment so that your doctor can monitor your progress and dosage.
• Because tryptophan can worsen Paxil's side effects, ask your doctor for a list of foods containing it.

 ## KEEP IN MIND...

* Takes effect within 1 to 4 weeks.
* Take in the morning for best results.
* Record and report mood changes.
* Avoid foods containing tryptophan.

Paxipam

Paxipam is one of a group of drugs called central nervous system depressants, which reduce symptoms by slowing down the nervous system.

Why it's prescribed

Doctors prescribe Paxipam to relieve nervousness, tension, and anxiety. It comes in tablets. Doctors usually prescribe the following amounts for adults; children's dosage appears in parentheses.

▶ **For anxiety,** 20 to 40 milligrams (mg) three or four times a day. For older adults, 20 mg one or two times a day. (Children: dosage is individualized by doctor.)

How to take Paxipam

• Take Paxipam only as your doctor directs, in the amount prescribed. Overuse could lead to dependency and increased risk of overdose.
• Don't suddenly stop taking Paxipam; to avoid withdrawal symptoms, follow your doctor's instructions for gradually decreasing your dosage.

If you miss a dose

Take the missed dose if you remember within an hour or so after the scheduled time. Otherwise, skip the missed dose and take the next dose as scheduled. Don't take a double dose.

If you suspect an overdose

Contact your doctor *immediately.* Excessive Paxipam can cause sleepiness, confusion, coma, slow reflexes, trouble breathing, low blood pressure (dizziness, weakness), slow pulse, slurred speech, and unsteady gait or poor coordination.

PAXIPAM'S OTHER NAME

Paxipam's generic name is halazepam.

 ## SIDE EFFECTS

Call your doctor if you have any of these possible drug side effects. Call *immediately* about any labeled "serious."

Serious: prolonged confusion, severe drowsiness, difficulty breathing, slow pulse, slurred speech, staggering, severe weakness

Common: drowsiness, dizziness, difficulty thinking clearly, a hangover-type feeling, nausea, vomiting, dry mouth

Tips: Side effects usually subside as your body adjusts to the drug. If drowsiness or dizziness occur, avoid driving or other activities that require alertness. To minimize dizziness, rise slowly after sitting or lying down. Relieve dry mouth with sugarless hard candy or gum, ice chips, mouthwash, or a saliva substitute. (Mouth dryness that lasts more than 2 weeks increases your risk of tooth and gum problems; check with doctor or dentist for advice.)

Other: none reported

 ## DRUG INTERACTIONS

Combining certain drugs may alter their action or produce unwanted side effects. Tell your doctor about other drugs you're taking, including:
• alcohol.

Warnings

• Make sure your doctor knows your medical history. You may not be able to take Paxipam if you have other problems, such as a mental disorder, glaucoma, epilepsy or other seizure disorder, or heart, lung, liver, or kidney disease; if you're allergic to this or other drugs; or if you have a history of drug or alcohol abuse.
• Tell your doctor if you're pregnant or breast-feeding before you begin taking Paxipam.
• Be aware that children and older adults may be more prone to side effects and may need lower dosages. Check with your doctor.

KEEP IN MIND...

* Dosage for children under age 18 is determined by doctor.

* Overuse could lead to dependency and overdose.

* Don't suddenly stop taking Paxipam, to avoid withdrawal symptoms.

PCE Disperstab

PCE Disperstab is a form of the antibiotic erythromycin, which fights infection by preventing bacteria from reproducing.

Why it's prescribed

Doctors prescribe PCE Disperstab to treat infections. It comes in tablets. Doctors usually prescribe the following amounts for adults; children's dosages appear in parentheses.

▶ **To treat infections,** one PCE 333 milligrams (mg) every 8 hours, or one PCE 500 mg every 12 hours. Dosage may be increased for more severe infections.

▶ **To prevent endocarditis (heart valve infection) after dental procedures,** 1 gram by mouth 1 hour before the procedure, then 500 mg 6 hours later.

How to take PCE Disperstab

• Take all of the drug exactly as prescribed; no more, no less.
• Take with a full glass (8 ounces) of water 1 hour before meals or 2 hours after.
• If the tablets are coated or the drug upsets your stomach, take the drug with food or milk. But don't take it with fruit juice.

PCE DISPERSTAB'S OTHER NAMES

PCE Disperstab's generic name is oral erythromycin base. Other brand names include ERYC, Ery-Tab; and, in Canada, Apo-Erythro, Erybid, Erythromid, and Novo-rythro Encap.

 SIDE EFFECTS

Call your doctor if you have any of these possible drug side effects. Call *immediately* about any labeled "serious."

Serious: severe allergic reaction (swelling in face and throat, difficulty breathing), rash, itchy skin

Common: abdominal pain and cramping, nausea, vomiting, diarrhea

Other: hives

 DRUG INTERACTIONS

Combining certain drugs may alter their action or produce unwanted side effects. Tell your doctor about other drugs you're taking, especially:
• antibiotics, such as Cleocin and Lincocin
• anticoagulants (blood thinners) such as Coumadin
• Halcion, Tegretol, Theo-Dur
• Hismanal, Seldane
• Sandimmune.

If you miss a dose

Don't take a double dose. Take the missed dose as soon as possible. Adjust your schedule as follows:
• If it's almost time for your next dose, and you take two doses a day, space the missed dose and the next one 5 to 6 hours apart.
• If you take three or more doses a day, space the missed dose and the next one 2 to 4 hours apart. Then resume your regular schedule.

 If you suspect an overdose

Consult your doctor.

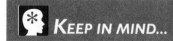 **Warnings**

• Make sure your doctor knows your medical history. You may not be able to take PCE Disperstab if you have liver disease or if you're allergic to any antibiotic or other drug or to any food.
• Tell the doctor that you're taking PCE Disperstab before you have medical tests because the drug may interfere with some test results.

KEEP IN MIND...

* Take entire prescription, even if you feel better.
* Take with water 1 hour before or 2 hours after meals.
* Tell your doctor if you have a rash or trouble breathing.

Pediazole

Pediazole is a combination of two antibiotics that kill infection-causing bacteria.

Why it's prescribed

Doctors prescribe Pediazole to treat children's ear infections. Pediazole is not normally used by adults or teenagers. It comes in an oral liquid. Doctors usually prescribe the following amounts for children.

▶ **For ear infection,** for children age 2 months and older, dosage is based on body weight. Children under 18 pounds (lb), dose is determined by doctor. Children weighing 18 to 35 lb, ½ teaspoon (tsp), or 2.5 milliters (ml) every 6 hours for 10 days. Children weighing 35 to 53 lb, 1 tsp (5 ml) every 6 hours for 10 days. Children weighing 53 to 100 lb, 1½ tsp (7.5 ml) every 6 hours for 10 days. Children weighing more than 100 lb, 2 tsp (10 ml) every 6 hours for 10 days.

How to take Pediazole

• Give your child Pediazole only as your doctor directs.
• Use a specially marked measuring spoon to measure each dose.
• Give Pediazole with food or water, and have your child drink extra water throughout the day.
• Pediazole works best if there's a constant amount in the blood, so give it to your child in evenly spaced doses during the day and night. If four doses a day are given,

PEDIAZOLE'S OTHER NAME

Pediazole is a combination of the generic drugs erythromycin and sulfisoxazole.

SIDE EFFECTS

Call your doctor if you have any of these possible drug side effects. Call *immediately* about any labeled "serious."

Serious: difficulty breathing, persistent fever, sore throat, joint pain

Common: none reported

Other: abdominal pain, nausea, vomiting, diarrhea

DRUG INTERACTIONS

Combining certain drugs may alter their action or produce unwanted side effects. Tell your doctor about other drugs you're taking, especially:
• oral anticoagulants (blood thinners) such as Coumadin
• Seldane
• Theo-Dur.

schedule the doses 6 hours apart. Check with your doctor if this schedule cannot be followed.
• Continue to give this drug to your child as directed, even if the child starts to feel better in a few days. If you stop giving it too soon, your child's infection may return.

If you miss a dose

Give your child the missed dose as soon as possible unless it's almost time for the next dose. In that case (if giving three or more doses a day), space the missed dose and the next dose 2 to 4 hours apart. Then return to the regular schedule. Don't give the child a double dose.

 If you suspect an overdose

Consult your doctor.

 Warnings

• Make sure your doctor knows your child's medical history. The child may not be able to take Pediazole if he or she is allergic to this or other drugs (especially sulfa drugs or erythromycin).
• Have your child drink lots of extra water to prevent kidney stones or other side effects.
• If taken by an adult, Pediazole can decrease the effectiveness of birth control pills. If necessary, switch to a barrier type of birth control while taking this drug.

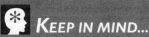 KEEP IN MIND...

* Use specially marked measuring spoon to measure each dose.
* Give with food or water.
* Give at evenly spaced intervals, day and night.
* Give as directed, even if child starts to feel better, to keep infection from coming back.

Penetrex

P enetrex, an antibiotic, works by stopping the spread of and killing infection-causing bacteria.

Why it's prescribed

Doctors prescribe Penetrex to treat urinary tract infections and uncomplicated gonorrhea. It comes in tablets. Doctors usually prescribe the following amounts for adults.

▶ **For uncomplicated urinary tract infections,** 200 milligrams (mg) every 12 hours for 7 days.

▶ **For severe or complicated urinary tract infections,** 400 mg every 12 hours for 14 days.

▶ **For uncomplicated gonorrhea (urethral or endocervical),** 400 mg as a single dose. Treatment with other drugs for other infections (chlamydia) may follow if necessary. For people with kidney failure, depending on response, treatment is started with usual initial dose, but doses that follow are decreased by half.

How to take Penetrex

• Take Penetrex only as your doctor directs.
• Take 2 hours after a meal, on empty stomach.

If you miss a dose

Take the missed dose as soon as possible to keep a constant amount of drug in body. However, if it's almost time for your next dose, skip the missed dose and go back to your regular schedule. Don't take a double dose.

PENETREX'S OTHER NAME

Penetrex's generic name is enoxacin.

 SIDE EFFECTS

Call your doctor if you have any of these possible drug side effects. Call *immediately* about any labeled "serious."

Serious: seizures, blood problems (fatigue, bleeding bruising, increased risk for infection, fever, chills), kidney problems (decreased urine output), liver problems (yellow-tinged skin or eyes)
Tips: Avoid people who are ill or infected. Avoid strenuous physical activity.

Common: nausea, diarrhea, rash

Other: headache, restlessness, tremor, light-headedness, confusion, hallucinations, vomiting, abdominal pain or discomfort, yeast infection in mouth (thrush), sensitivity to light, cough

 FOOD AND DRUG INTERACTIONS

Combining certain drugs and foods may alter drug action or produce unwanted side effects. Tell your doctor about your diet and other drugs you're taking, especially:
• antacids containing magnesium hydroxide or aluminum hydroxide, oral iron supplements, Carafate (take at least 2 hours before or after Penetrex)
• anticoagulants (blood thinners) such as Coumadin
• caffeine-containing beverages
• cyclosporine, Sandimmune, Theo-Dur.

 If you suspect an overdose

Consult your doctor.

Warnings

• Make sure your doctor knows your medical history. You may not be able to take Penetrex if you have central nervous system disorders (such as severe hardening of the arteries to the brain or seizure disorders) or poor kidney or liver function, or if you're allergic to any drugs (especially antibiotics).

• Tell your doctor if you're pregnant or breast-feeding before you begin taking Penetrex.
• Drink lots of extra fluids while taking Penetrex, to avoid kidney and urine problems.

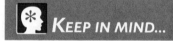 **KEEP IN MIND...**

∗ Drink lots of extra fluids.

∗ Don't take a double dose if you miss a dose.

∗ Don't drink caffeine-containing beverages.

Pen Vee K

Pen Vee K, a natural penicillin, kills bacteria or stops them from growing.

Why it's prescribed

Doctors prescribe Pen Vee K to treat or prevent bacterial infections. It comes in tablets, film-coated tablets, capsules, and liquid. Doctors usually prescribe the following amounts for adults; children's dosages appear in parentheses.

▶ **For mild to moderate infections,** 250 to 500 milligrams (mg) (400,000 to 800,000 units) every 6 hours. (Children: 15 to 50 mg for each 2.2 pounds [lb] of body weight [25,000 to 90,000 units for each 2.2 lb] a day, divided into equal doses given every 6 to 8 hours.)

▶ **To prevent heart infection before dental surgery,** 2 grams (g) 30 to 60 minutes before procedure, then 1 g 6 hours afterward. (Children weighing under 66 lb: half the adult dose.)

How to take Pen Vee K

• Take this drug exactly as your doctor directs for the full time prescribed, even if you feel well after a few days.

• Take it on a full or an empty stomach, but don't take it with fruit juice or a carbonated beverage.

PEN VEE K'S OTHER NAMES

Pen Vee K's generic name is penicillin V potassium. Other brand names include Beepen-VK, Betapen-VK, Ledercillin VK, Pen Vee, V-Cillin-K, Veetids; and, in Canada, Apo-Pen-VK, Nadopen-VK, Novo-Pen-VK, Nu-Pen-VK, and PVF K.

SIDE EFFECTS

Call your doctor if you have any of these possible drug side effects. Call *immediately* about any labeled "serious."

Serious: allergic reactions (facial swelling, chills, fever, shortness of breath, rash)

Common: stomach upset, nausea

Other: muscle weakness, vomiting, diarrhea, blood problems (fatigue, bruising); numbness, tingling, or pain in arms or legs
Tip: Diarrhea drugs may worsen diarrhea. Check with doctor before taking.

DRUG INTERACTIONS

Combining certain drugs may alter their action or produce unwanted side effects. Tell your doctor about other drugs you're taking, especially:
• birth control pills containing estrogen.

• Measure liquid doses with a specially marked measuring spoon, not a household teaspoon.
• Take at evenly spaced times, day and night.
• Discard leftover penicillin.

If you miss a dose

Take the missed dose as soon as possible. However, if it's almost time for your next dose, skip the missed dose and take your next dose as scheduled. Don't take a double dose.

If you suspect an overdose

Contact your doctor *immediately.* Excessive Pen Vee K can cause seizures, muscle spasms and weakness, and pain or tingling in arms or legs.

Warnings

• Make sure your doctor knows your medical history. You may not be able to take Pen Vee K if you have other problems, especially allergies, heart failure, kidney disease, or stomach or intestinal disease, or if you've ever had an unusual reaction to any antibiotic.

• If you're breast-feeding, tell your doctor before you start taking Pen Vee K.

• If you're diabetic, this drug may cause false test results with some urine sugar tests. Check with your doctor before changing your diet or the dosage of your diabetes medicine.

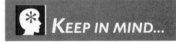

KEEP IN MIND...

* Take with full glass of water.
* Keep taking for full time prescribed.
* Don't take diarrhea drug unless doctor approves.

Pepcid

Pepcid decreases the amount of acid produced by the stomach.

Why it's prescribed

Doctors prescribe Pepcid to treat ulcers, heartburn, excess stomach acid, and acid reflux disease (in which the stomach contents flow backward into the esophagus). You can buy Pepcid without a prescription. It comes in tablets and a powder for oral liquid. It's also available in an injectable form. Doctors usually prescribe the following amounts for adults.

▶ **For duodenal ulcers,** initially, 40 milligrams (mg) once a day at bedtime or 20 mg twice a day. Usual dosage is 20 mg once a day.

▶ **For stomach ulcers,** 40 mg once a day for 8 weeks.

▶ **To prevent heartburn,** 10 mg 1 hour before meals.

▶ **For excess stomach acid,** 20 to 160 mg every 6 hours.

▶ **For acid reflux disease,** 20 mg twice a day for up to 6 weeks. For esophageal inflammation, 20 to 40 mg twice a day for up to 12 weeks.

How to take Pepcid

• Take this drug exactly as your doctor directs. If you're treating yourself, follow the package instructions.

• You may take Pepcid with a snack if you wish.

• If you're taking one dose a day, take it at bedtime unless your doc-

PEPCID'S OTHER NAMES

Pepcid's generic name is famotidine. The brand name of the nonprescription form is Pepcid AC.

SIDE EFFECTS

Call your doctor if you have any of these possible drug side effects. Call *immediately* about any labeled "serious."

Serious: abnormal bleeding (easy bruising and bleeding, bleeding gums)

Common: headache
Tip: If headache persists or is severe, call your doctor.

Other: dizziness, hallucinations, diarrhea, constipation, nausea, gas, acne, itching, rash

DRUG INTERACTIONS

Combining certain drugs may alter their action or produce unwanted side effects. Tell your doctor about other drugs you're taking or using, especially:

• antacids (take 30 minutes to one hour before taking Pepcid)

• tobacco (don't smoke after taking last dose of the day).

tor directs otherwise. If you're taking two doses a day, take one dose in the morning and one at bedtime. If you're taking more than two doses a day, take with meals and at bedtime for best results.

• It may be several days before Pepcid begins to relieve your stomach pain. Meanwhile, unless your doctor tells you otherwise, you can take antacids to help relieve pain.

If you miss a dose

Take the missed dose as soon as possible. However, if it's almost time for your next dose, skip the missed dose and take your next dose as scheduled. Don't take a double dose.

If you suspect an overdose

Consult your doctor.

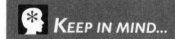

Warnings

• Make sure your doctor knows your medical history. You may not be able to take Pepcid if you have other problems, especially kidney or liver disease.

• If you're pregnant or breast-feeding, check with your doctor before you start taking Pepcid.

• Older adults may be especially prone to Pepcid's side effects.

• Contact your doctor if your ulcer pain continues or gets worse.

KEEP IN MIND...

* Don't smoke, especially after last dose of day.

* Take last daily dose at bedtime.

* Call doctor about persistent or worsening ulcer pain or headache.

Pepto-Bismol

Pepto-Bismol eliminates toxins and extra water from the bowel and forms a protective coating on the intestinal lining.

Why it's taken

Pepto-Bismol is taken to treat diarrhea or upset stomach. You can buy Pepto-Bismol without a prescription. It comes in chewable tablets and an oral liquid. The following amounts are usually recommended for adults; children's dosages appear in parentheses.

▶ **For mild diarrhea,** 2 tablets or 30 milliliters (ml) every 30 to 60 minutes to maximum of eight doses daily for no more than 2 days. (Children age 13 and older: same as adults. Children ages 9 to 12: 15 ml (1 tablespoon) or 1 tablet every 30 to 60 minutes. Children ages 6 to 8: 10 ml (2 teaspoons) or $^2/_3$ tablet every 30 to 60 minutes. Children ages 3 to 5: 5 ml (1 teaspoon) or $^1/_3$ tablet every 30 to 60 minutes. Maximum dosage for all age-groups is eight doses daily.)

How to take Pepto-Bismol

• If you're treating yourself, carefully follow the directions on the label. If your doctor prescribed Pepto-Bismol, follow the doctor's instructions exactly.
• Chew the tablets well before swallowing. If you're using the liquid, shake the bottle well before measuring your dose.

PEPTO-BISMOL'S OTHER NAME

Pepto-Bismol's generic name is bismuth subsalicylate.

SIDE EFFECTS

Call your doctor if you have any of these possible drug side effects. Call *immediately* about any labeled "serious."

Serious: ringing in ears

Common: none reported

Other: nausea, vomiting (with high doses); temporary darkening of tongue and stools

DRUG INTERACTIONS

Combining certain drugs may alter their action or produce unwanted side effects. Tell your doctor about other drugs you're taking, especially:
• anticoagulants (blood thinners) such as Coumadin
• aspirin and other salicylates
• Benemid
• oral diabetes medicines
• tetracycline (take at least 2 hours before or after Pepto-Bismol).

If you miss a dose

If you're taking this drug on a regular schedule, take the missed dose as soon as possible. However, if it's almost time for your next dose, skip the missed dose and take your next dose as scheduled. Don't take a double dose.

If you suspect an overdose

Contact your doctor *immediately*. Excessive Pepto-Bismol can cause fever and ringing in the ears.

Warnings

• Consult your doctor before taking Pepto-Bismol if you have other problems, especially kidney disease, stomach ulcer, dysentery, gout, or bleeding problems (such as hemophilia), or if you've ever had a bad reaction to a salicylate, such as aspirin, or to other nonnarcotic pain relievers, such as Advil or Naprosyn.
• If you're pregnant or breast-feeding, tell your doctor before you start taking Pepto-Bismol.
• Consult your doctor before giving Pepto-Bismol to children or adolescents who have — or are recovering from — the flu or chickenpox.
• Don't give this drug to children under age 3 because they may develop severe health problems from the fluid loss caused by diarrhea. Call the doctor instead.

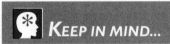

* Don't take if allergic to aspirin.
* Chew tablets well or shake liquid before pouring dose.
* Stop taking if you have ringing in ears.

Percocet

Percocet is a pain reliever containing both a narcotic and acetaminophen. For many people, this combination relieves pain better than either drug would if used alone, and it allows lower doses of each drug. Percocet changes a person's perception of pain and emotional response to it.

Why it's prescribed

Doctors prescribe Percocet for moderate to moderately severe pain. It comes in tablets. Doctors usually prescribe the following amounts for adults.

▶ **For pain,** 1 tablet every 6 hours, as needed.

How to take Percocet

• Take this drug exactly as your doctor directs. Take with food or a full glass (8 ounces) of water. Store Percocet at room temperature.

• Don't take more of this drug than directed; doing so could cause an overdose or lead to drug dependence.

• Don't suddenly stop taking Percocet after taking it for several weeks; doing so could cause withdrawal symptoms. Call your doctor, who will tell you how to reduce your dosage gradually.

If you miss a dose

Take the missed dose as soon as possible. However, if it's almost time

PERCOCET'S OTHER NAMES

Percocet's generic name is acetaminophen with oxycodone. Other brand names include Roxicet, Tylox; and, in Canada, Endocet and Oxycocet.

SIDE EFFECTS

Call your doctor if you have any of these possible drug side effects. Call *immediately* about any labeled "serious."

Serious: decreased and shallow breathing, extreme tiredness, drug dependence, seizures, shortness of breath, slow pulse, cold and clammy skin

Common: dizziness, nausea, vomiting
Tip: When lying or sitting, get up slowly to avoid dizziness.

Other: constipation, inability to urinate
Tip: Drink liquids to avoid constipation.

DRUG INTERACTIONS

Combining certain drugs may alter their action or produce unwanted side effects. Tell your doctor about other drugs you're taking, especially:
• alcohol
• antidepressants called MAO inhibitors, such as Nardil and Parnate
• eyedrops that enlarge pupils such as Timoptic drops
• Tylenol and other acetaminophen-containing drugs
• Xanax and other tranquilizers.

for your next dose, skip the missed dose and take your next dose as scheduled. Don't take a double dose.

If you suspect an overdose

Contact your doctor *immediately.* Excessive Percocet can cause confusion, nervousness, restlessness, seizures, shortness of breath or difficulty breathing, and severe weakness, dizziness, and drowsiness.

Warnings

• Make sure your doctor knows your medical history. You may not be able to take Percocet if you have other problems, especially seizures, heart disease, brain disease, head injury, asthma or another chronic lung disease, colitis, hepatitis or other liver disease, kidney disease,

an underactive thyroid, gallbladder disease or gallstones, or a history of drug or alcohol dependence.

• If you're pregnant or breast-feeding, tell your doctor before taking Percocet. Overuse of narcotics during pregnancy can cause drug dependence in your fetus.

• Be aware that older adults may be especially prone to Percocet's side effects.

• Before surgery (including dental surgery) or emergency treatment, tell your doctor or dentist that you're taking Percocet.

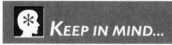

* Take only as prescribed.

* Don't take with alcohol.

* Don't stop taking suddenly.

Percodan

Percodan is a pain reliever that contains both a narcotic and aspirin. It works by changing a person's perception of and emotional response to pain.

Why it's prescribed

Doctors prescribe Percodan for moderate to moderately severe pain. It comes in tablets. Doctors usually prescribe the following amounts for adults.

▶ **For moderate to moderately severe pain,** 1 tablet every 6 hours, as needed.

How to take Percodan

• Take this drug exactly as directed. To prevent possible stomach upset, take it with food or a full glass (8 ounces) of water.
• Percodan can be habit-forming. Don't take more than the prescribed amount. If the drug isn't relieving your pain, call your doctor; don't increase the dose.
• If you've been taking Percodan regularly for a few weeks or more, don't stop taking it suddenly because this could cause withdrawal symptoms. Consult your doctor, who may want you to reduce the amount you're taking gradually before stopping.

If you miss a dose

Take the missed dose as soon as possible. However, if it's almost time

PERCODAN'S OTHER NAMES

Percodan's generic name is aspirin with oxycodone. Other brand names include Roxiprin and, in Canada, Endodan and Oxycodan.

 SIDE EFFECTS

Call your doctor if you have any of these possible drug side effects. Call *immediately* about any labeled "serious."

Serious: decreased and shallow breathing, extreme tiredness, drug dependence, ringing in ears, hearing problems, fast pulse, rash

Common: dizziness, shortness of breath, constipation, nausea, vomiting

Other: vision changes, urination problems, dry mouth, restlessness, appetite loss, headache

 DRUG INTERACTIONS

Combining certain drugs may alter their action or produce unwanted side effects. Tell your doctor about other drugs you're taking, especially:
• alcohol
• anticoagulants (blood thinners) such as Coumadin
• antidepressants called MAO inhibitors, such as Nardil and Parnate
• aspirin or aspirin-containing products
• Benemid
• diabetes drugs, such as DiaBeta and Micronase
• Retrovir (AZT)
• Tylenol and other products containing acetaminophen.

for your next dose, skip the missed dose and take your next dose as scheduled. Don't take a double dose.

If you suspect an overdose

Contact your doctor *immediately.* Excessive Percodan can cause cold and clammy skin, itching, confusion, seizures, severe dizziness or drowsiness, increased sweating or thirst, slow heartbeat, severe stomach pain, constipation, ringing in ears, shallow breathing, vision problems, and weakness.

Warnings

• Make sure your doctor knows your medical history. You may not be able to take Percodan if you

have other problems, especially brain, kidney, liver, heart, or gallbladder disease; asthma; colitis; an enlarged prostate; seizures; emphysema; thyroid problems; anemia; gout; or bleeding problems.
• If you're pregnant or breast-feeding, check with your doctor before you start taking Percodan.
• If you're diabetic, this drug may cause false urine sugar test results.

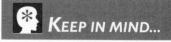 **KEEP IN MIND...**

∗ Don't increase dose unless doctor approves.

∗ Don't stop taking suddenly after using for several weeks.

∗ Don't take with alcohol.

Periactin

Periactin is an antihistamine. It works by blocking the effects of histamine, a natural substance that causes itching, sneezing, running nose, and watery eyes and that can make the throat close up.

Why it's prescribed

Doctors prescribe Periactin to relieve allergy symptoms. It comes in tablets and a syrup. Doctors usually prescribe the following amounts for adults; children's dosages appear in parentheses.

▶ **For allergy symptoms or itching,** 4 to 20 milligrams (mg) a day, divided into equal doses. Maximum dosage is 0.5 mg for each 2.2 pounds of body weight a day. (Children ages 7 to 14: 4 mg two or three times a day. Maximum dosage is 16 mg a day. Children ages 2 to 6: 2 mg two or three times a day. Maximum dosage is 12 mg a day.)

How to take Periactin

• Take this drug exactly as your doctor directs. To prevent possible stomach upset, take it with food or milk.

If you miss a dose

If you're taking this drug regularly, take the missed dose as soon as possible. However, if it's almost time for your next dose, skip the missed dose and take your next dose as scheduled. Don't take a double dose.

PERIACTIN'S OTHER NAME

Periactin's generic name is cyproheptadine.

 SIDE EFFECTS

Call your doctor if you have any of these possible drug side effects.

Serious: none reported

Common: drowsiness, dry mouth
Tips: Until you know how this drug affects you, don't drive or do anything else that requires you to be fully alert. To relieve dry mouth, use ice chips or sugarless gum or hard candy.

Other: headache, fatigue, nausea, vomiting, stomach upset, inability to urinate, rash, weight gain

 DRUG INTERACTIONS

Combining certain drugs may alter their action or produce unwanted side effects. Tell your doctor about other drugs you're taking, especially:
• antidepressants called MAO inhibitors such as Marplan (don't take within 14 days of taking Periactin)
• drugs that slow down the nervous system, such as other cold and allergy drugs, sedatives, tranquilizers, narcotic pain relievers, barbiturates, seizure drugs, and muscle relaxants.

 If you suspect an overdose

Contact your doctor *immediately*. Excessive Periactin can cause dry mouth, flushed skin, enlarged pupils, stomach discomfort, difficulty sleeping, hallucinations, tremor, seizures, stopped breathing, heart failure, and blood vessel collapse.

Warnings

• Make sure your doctor knows your medical history. You may not be able to take Periactin if you have other problems, especially glaucoma, a blockage in the urinary tract, difficulty urinating, an enlarged prostate, heart or blood vessel disease, an overactive thyroid, high blood pressure, or asthma.

• If you're pregnant or breast-feeding, tell your doctor before you start taking Periactin.
• Children and older adults may be especially prone to Periactin's side effects. Children under age 14 should use this drug only if directed by a doctor.
• Before you have skin tests for allergy, tell the doctor you're taking Periactin.

 KEEP IN MIND...

∗ Take with food or milk.

∗ Don't drive until you know how you react to drug.

∗ To relieve dry mouth, use ice chips or sugarless gum or hard candy.

Peridex

Peridex is a dental rinse that destroys the bacteria growing in the plaque that forms on the teeth.

Why it's prescribed

Doctors prescribe Peridex to reduce gum inflammation and swelling and to decrease gum bleeding caused by gum disease (gingivitis). It comes in an oral rinse. Doctors usually prescribe the following amounts for adults; children's dosages determined by dentist or doctor.

▶ **For gum disease,** 15 milliliters (ml) (1 tablespoon) as a mouthwash for 30 seconds twice a day.

How to use Peridex

• Use this drug exactly as your doctor or dentist directs. Use it after you've brushed and flossed your teeth. Make sure you've rinsed all the toothpaste from your mouth before using Peridex.

• Measure the adult dose by filling the cap on the original container to the "fill" line (15 ml). Don't mix or dilute the drug with water.

• Swish Peridex around in your mouth for 30 seconds; then spit it out. Don't swallow it.

• Even though Peridex may have a bitter aftertaste, don't rinse your mouth after using it. This will only worsen the bitterness and make the drug less effective.

PERIDEX'S OTHER NAME

Peridex's generic name is chlorhexidine.

SIDE EFFECTS

Call your doctor if you have any of these possible drug side effects.

Serious: none reported

Common: stained teeth, changed taste perception, calcium deposits under gums

Tips: Changes in the way foods taste should diminish with time. To reduce staining and tartar caused by Peridex, brush with a tartar-control toothpaste and floss teeth daily.

Other: irritated gums

DRUG INTERACTIONS

Combining certain drugs may alter their action or produce unwanted side effects. Tell your doctor about other drugs you're taking.

• Don't eat or drink for several hours after using Peridex.

If you miss a dose

Take the missed dose as soon as possible. However, if it's almost time for your next dose, skip the missed dose and take your next dose as scheduled. Don't take a double dose.

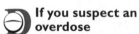

If you suspect an overdose

Contact your doctor *immediately*. Excessive Peridex can cause nausea and vomiting. A child who accidentally drinks Peridex may show signs of alcohol intoxication (slurred speech, sleepiness, or staggering).

Warnings

• Make sure your doctor knows your medical history. You may not be able to use Peridex if you have other problems, especially other gum problems. Also mention if you have front tooth fillings because Peridex may stain your teeth permanently.

• If you're breast-feeding, tell your doctor before you start using Peridex.

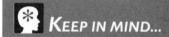

KEEP IN MIND...

* Use after brushing and flossing teeth.

* Don't mix or dilute with water.

* Don't swallow rinse.

* Don't rinse mouth with water after using.

* Don't eat or drink for several hours after using.

Peritrate

Peritrate works by widening the blood vessels, reducing the heart's oxygen needs, and increasing blood flow throughout the heart.

Why it's prescribed

Doctors prescribe Peritrate to prevent chest pain (angina). However, it's not meant to relieve an angina attack in progress. Peritrate comes in tablets, sustained-release tablets, and sustained-release capsules. Doctors usually prescribe the following amounts for adults.

▶ **To prevent angina,** 10 to 20 milligrams (mg) three or four times a day, increased gradually as needed to 40 mg four times a day; or 30 to 80 mg sustained-release form twice a day.

How to take Peritrate

• Take this drug exactly as your doctor directs. Take it with a full (8-ounce) glass of water 1 hour before or 2 hours after meals.
• Swallow the sustained-release forms whole. Don't crush or chew them.
• Keep container sealed tightly and store in a cool, dry place.
• Don't stop taking this drug suddenly because this could cause a serious heart problem. Call your doctor, who will tell you how to gradually reduce the amount you take before stopping.

PERITRATE'S OTHER NAMES

Peritrate's generic name is pentaerythritol tetranitrate. Other brand names include Duotrate, Pentylan, Peritrate SA, P.E.T.N.; and, in Canada, Peritrate Forte.

 SIDE EFFECTS

Call your doctor if you have any of these possible drug side effects. Call *immediately* about any labeled "serious."

Serious: blurred vision, dry mouth, rash

Common: headache (which may be throbbing), dizziness
Tips: Take aspirin or Tylenol for headache. Call the doctor if your headache is persistent or severe. To help prevent dizziness, stand up slowly, and be careful when exercising in hot weather and when using stairs.

Other: weakness, fast pulse, flushing, palpitations, fainting, nausea, vomiting

 DRUG INTERACTIONS

Combining certain drugs may alter their action or produce unwanted side effects. Tell your doctor about other drugs you're taking, especially:
• alcohol (may increase dizziness)
• blood pressure drugs, such as Cardizem, Corgard, Lopressor, and nitroglycerin
• Ergostat
• phenothiazines, such as Phenergan and Thorazine.

If you miss a dose

Take the missed dose as soon as possible. However, if it's within 2 hours of your next dose (or within 6 hours if you take a sustained-release form), skip the missed dose and take your next dose as scheduled. Don't take a double dose.

If you suspect an overdose

Contact your doctor *immediately.* Excessive Peritrate can cause fainting, weakness, palpitations, extreme headache, difficulty breathing, bluish lips or hands, weak pulse, paralysis, and seizures.

Warnings

• Make sure your doctor knows your medical history. You may not be able to take Peritrate if you have other medical problems, especially glaucoma, diarrhea, kidney or liver disease, or severe anemia, or if you've recently had a heart attack or stroke.
• Notify your doctor if you see undigested sustained-release tablets in your stools.

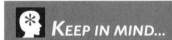 **KEEP IN MIND...**

* Take with full glass of water.
* Don't crush or chew sustained-release forms.
* Don't use to stop angina attack in progress.
* Avoid alcohol.
* Don't stop taking suddenly.

Permax

Permax increases the concentration of dopamine, a chemical that's deficient in people with Parkinson's disease. This improves body movements.

Why it's prescribed

Doctors prescribe Permax along with other drugs to manage the symptoms of Parkinson's disease. It comes in tablets. Doctors usually prescribe the following amounts for adults.

▶ **For Parkinson's disease,** 0.05 milligrams (mg) a day for first 2 days, increased by 0.1 to 0.15 mg every third day over 12 days. If needed, dosage increased by 0.25 mg every third day until desired response occurs. Drug usually is divided into three equal doses.

How to take Permax

• Take this drug exactly as your doctor directs. To prevent stomach upset, take it with meals.
• The full effects of this drug may take several weeks to develop. Don't stop taking it or reduce your dosage without consulting your doctor.

If you miss a dose

Take the missed dose as soon as possible. However, if it's almost time for your next dose, skip the missed dose and take your next dose as scheduled. Don't take a double dose.

PERMAX'S OTHER NAME

Permax's generic name is pergolide mesylate.

 SIDE EFFECTS

Call your doctor if you have any of these possible drug side effects. Call *immediately* about any labeled "serious."

Serious: palpitations, heart attack (arm and chest pain, anxiety)

Common: inability to perform voluntary body movements, dizziness, hallucinations, sleepiness, nausea, constipation

Tip: Avoid driving and other activities that require full alertness and coordination until you know how this drug affects you.

Other: headache, weakness, muscle spasms, confusion, anxiety, depression, tremor, abnormal dreams, strange behavior, abnormal gait, agitation, poor coordination, paralyzed muscles, speech disorder, fainting, runny nose, abnormal vision, dry mouth, taste abnormalities, abdominal pain, diarrhea, stomach upset, appetite loss, vomiting, frequent urination, urinary tract infection, rash, sweating, numbness or tingling sensations, flulike symptoms, joint and muscle pain, bursitis; pain in jaw, neck, chest, back, or pelvis

 DRUG INTERACTIONS

Combining certain drugs may alter their action or produce unwanted side effects. Tell your doctor about other drugs you're taking, especially:
• drugs for psychosis, such as Haldol, Navane, and Taractan
• other dopamine antagonists
• phenothiazines, such as Phenergan and Thorazine
• Reglan.

 If you suspect an overdose

Contact your doctor *immediately.* Excessive Permax can cause vomiting, hallucinations, involuntary body movements, palpitations, irregular heartbeats, and low blood pressure (dizziness, weakness).

 Warnings

• Make sure your doctor knows your medical history. You may not be able to take Permax if you have other problems, especially heart disease or mental problems.

• If you're breast-feeding, tell your doctor before you start taking Permax. This drug may reduce your flow of milk.

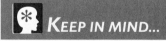 **KEEP IN MIND...**

∗ Take Permax with meals.
∗ Don't stop taking or reduce dosage unless doctor approves.
∗ Don't drive if dizziness or sleepiness occurs.
∗ Call doctor about chest pain.

Persantine

Persantine interferes with the activity of platelets, the blood cells essential for blood clotting.

Why it's prescribed

Doctors prescribe Persantine to prevent blood clots after heart valve replacement surgery or to treat lack of blood flow to the heart and some other heart and blood vessel disorders. It comes in tablets. It's also available in an injectable form. Doctors usually prescribe the following amounts for adults.

▶ **To prevent blood clots,** 75 to 100 milligrams orally four times a day.

How to take Persantine

• Take this drug exactly as your doctor directs. Persantine works best when taken in regularly spaced doses.
• Take each dose with a full glass (8 ounces) of water at least 1 hour before or 2 hours after meals. If the drug upsets your stomach, your doctor may tell you to take it with food or milk.
• If your doctor tells you to take Persantine with aspirin, take only the amount of aspirin prescribed.

If you miss a dose

Take the missed dose as soon as possible. However, if it's within 4 hours of your next scheduled dose,

PERSANTINE'S OTHER NAMES

Persantine's generic name is dipyridamole. Other brand names include Dipridacot, I.V. Persantine; and, in Canada, Apo-Dipyridamole and Novodipiradol.

 SIDE EFFECTS

Call your doctor if you have any of these possible drug side effects. Call *immediately* about any labeled "serious."

Serious: low blood pressure (dizziness, weakness)
Tip: If Persantine makes you dizzy when rising, get up slowly. If this problem continues or gets worse, check with your doctor.

Common: headache, nausea, rash

Other: flushing, vomiting, diarrhea, itching, chest pain, liver problems (nausea, vomiting, yellow-tinged eyes and skin, bloating, swelling)

 DRUG INTERACTIONS

Combining certain drugs may alter their action or produce unwanted side effects. Tell your doctor about other drugs you're taking, especially:
• Adenocard
• anticoagulants (blood thinners) such as Coumadin
• aspirin-containing products
• Cefobid
• Depakene
• Mandol
• Mithracin
• nonsteroidal anti-inflammatory drugs, such as Advil and Indocin.

skip the missed dose and take your next dose as scheduled. Don't take a double dose.

If you suspect an overdose

Contact your doctor *immediately*. Excessive Persantine can widen blood vessels, which causes low blood pressure (dizziness, weakness).

Warnings

• Make sure your doctor knows your medical history. You may not be able to take Persantine if you have other problems, especially chest pain or low blood pressure.

• If you're pregnant or breast-feeding, tell your doctor before you start taking Persantine.

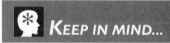 **KEEP IN MIND...**

* Take with full glass of water on empty stomach.
* Rise slowly to avoid dizziness.
* Don't take aspirin unless doctor orders this.

Pfizerpen

Pfizerpen, a natural penicillin, causes bacterial cell walls to rupture, killing the bacteria or preventing their growth.

Why it's prescribed

Doctors prescribe Pfizerpen to treat infections that affect various parts of the body. It comes in tablets and an oral liquid. It's also available in an injectable form. Doctors usually prescribe the following amounts for adults; children's dosages appear in parentheses.

▶ **For moderate to severe infections,** 1.6 to 3.2 million units orally a day, divided into equal doses given every 6 hours. (Children: 25,000 to 100,000 units for each 2.2 pounds of body weight orally a day, divided into equal doses given every 6 hours.)

How to take Pfizerpen

• Take this drug exactly as your doctor directs. Take it 1 to 2 hours before or 2 to 3 hours after meals.
• Measure liquid doses with a specially marked measuring spoon, not a household teaspoon.
• For best results, take doses at evenly spaced times day and night.

If you miss a dose

Take the missed dose as soon as possible. However, if it's almost time for your next dose, skip the missed dose and take your next dose as scheduled. Don't take a double dose.

PFIZERPEN'S OTHER NAMES

Pfizerpen's generic name is penicillin G potassium. A Canadian brand name is Megacillin.

 ## SIDE EFFECTS

Call your doctor if you have any of these possible drug side effects. Call *immediately* about any labeled "serious."

Serious: anemia (fatigue); inflamed, peeling skin; allergic reaction (facial swelling or puffiness, chills, fever, shortness of breath, rash, hives, itching, red, scaly skin); blood problems (bruising, bleeding, increased risk of infection)

Common: none reported

Other: diarrhea
Tip: Check with doctor before taking diarrhea drugs; they may worsen diarrhea.

 ## DRUG AND FOOD INTERACTIONS

Combining certain drugs and foods may alter drug action or produce unwanted side effects. Tell your doctor about your diet and other drugs you're taking, especially:
• antibiotics, such as Amikin, Garamycin, Myciguent, and Netromycin
• Colestid (take 1 hour after or 4 hours before taking Pfizerpen)
• diuretics (water pills), such as Aldactone, Dyrenium, and Midamor
• fruit juices and other acidic beverages (don't drink within 1 hour of taking Pfizerpen).

 ## If you suspect an overdose

Contact your doctor *immediately.* Excessive Pfizerpen can cause changes in sensations, pain in arms and legs, muscle spasms, seizures, or coma.

Warnings

• Make sure your doctor knows your medical history. You may not be able to take Pfizerpen if you have other problems, especially allergies (asthma or hay fever) and kidney, stomach, or intestinal disease, or if you've ever had a bad reaction to any antibiotic.

• If you're pregnant or breast-feeding, tell your doctor before you start taking Pfizerpen.
• If you're diabetic, this drug may cause false test results with some urine sugar tests. Before changing your diet or the dosage of your diabetes drug, consult your doctor.

 ## KEEP IN MIND...

* Take on empty stomach at evenly spaced times day and night.

* Don't drink fruit juices within 1 hour of taking Pfizerpen.

* Don't take diarrhea drugs unless doctor approves.

Phenergan

Phenergan, an antihistamine, blocks the effects of histamine, which causes itching, sneezing, runny nose, and watery eyes. Phenergan also prevents motion sickness.

Why it's prescribed

Doctors prescribe Phenergan to prevent motion sickness, relieve nausea, cause sedation, and treat allergy symptoms. It comes in tablets, a syrup, and suppositories. It's also available in an injectable form. Doctors usually prescribe the following amounts for adults; children's dosages appear in parentheses.

▶ **To prevent motion sickness,** 25 milligrams (mg) orally twice a day. (Children: 12.5 to 25 mg orally or rectally twice a day.)

▶ **For nausea,** 12.5 to 25 mg orally or rectally every 4 to 6 hours, as needed. (Children: 12.5 to 25 mg rectally every 4 to 6 hours, as needed.)

▶ **For allergy symptoms,** 12.5 mg orally four times a day, or 25 mg at bedtime. (Children: 6.25 to 12.5 mg orally three times a day, or 25 mg orally or rectally at bedtime.)

▶ **For sedation,** 25 to 50 mg by mouth at bedtime or as needed. (Children: 12.5 to 25 mg orally or rectally at bedtime.)

 SIDE EFFECTS

Call your doctor if you have any of these possible drug side effects. Call *immediately* about any labeled "serious."

Serious: blood problems (fever, chills, bruising, bleeding, infection)

Common: sedation, drowsiness, dry mouth
Tips: Avoid driving and other hazardous activities until you know how this drug affects you. To relieve dry mouth, use ice chips or sugarless gum or hard candy.

Other: confusion, restlessness, tremor, dizziness, weakness, temporary near-sightedness, stuffy nose, appetite loss, nausea, vomiting, constipation, inability to urinate, skin sensitivity to sunlight
Tips: To help prevent dizziness, exercise cautiously, stand up slowly, and use stairs carefully. Use sunscreen and wear protective clothing outdoors, and avoid prolonged exposure to intense sunlight to protect skin.

 DRUG INTERACTIONS

Combining certain drugs may alter their action or produce unwanted side effects. Tell your doctor about other drugs you're taking or using, especially:

• alcohol and other drugs that slow down the nervous system, such as cold and allergy drugs, sedatives, tranquilizers, narcotic pain relievers, barbiturates, seizure drugs, and muscle relaxants
• antidepressants, such as Elavil and Eldepryl
• Aramine
• beta blockers such as Inderal
• Dopastat
• drugs for cramps or spasms of the abdomen or stomach
• Larodopa
• Lithobid
• MAO inhibitors, such as Furoxone and Matulane
• Parlodel
• phenothiazines (used for anxiety, nausea, vomiting, or psychosis) such as Thorazine
• Primatene Mist.

How to take Phenergan

• Take this drug exactly as your doctor directs. To prevent stomach upset, take it with food or milk.

• If you're using Phenergan to prevent motion sickness, take the first dose 30 to 60 minutes before your trip. On every travel day, take one dose when you wake up and one dose with your evening meal.

• Store this drug in a tight, light-resistant container, preferably between 59° and 86° F.

If you miss a dose

Take the missed dose as soon as possible. However, if it's almost time for your next dose, skip the missed dose and take your next dose as scheduled. Don't take a double dose.

 If you suspect an overdose

Contact your doctor *immediately*. Excessive Phenergan can cause sedation, difficulty sleeping, reduced alertness, hallucinations, tremor, seizures, stopped breathing, and extremely low blood pressure (severe dizziness and weakness).

Warnings

• Make sure your doctor knows your medical history. You may not be able to take Phenergan if you have other problems, especially bowel or urinary tract blockage, an enlarged prostate, seizures, heart or blood vessel disease, glaucoma, a blood disorder, or liver disease, or are pregnant or breast-feeding.

• Children and older adults may be especially prone to Phenergan's side effects. Don't give this drug to a child who has a family history of sudden infant death syndrome or to a child who has Reye's syndrome (vomiting, violent headaches, stiff arms and legs, disturbed breathing).

• Stop taking this drug 4 days before allergy skin tests. Phenergan may affect the results.

• If you're diabetic, be aware that Phenergan may affect the results of glucose tolerance tests. Make sure your doctor knows you're taking this drug before you undergo this test.

• Avoid drinking alcohol when you're taking Phenergan; drinking could make you more drowsy.

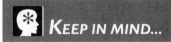 **KEEP IN MIND...**

∗ Take with food or milk.

∗ For motion sickness, take 30 to 60 minutes before traveling.

∗ Don't drive if this drug makes you drowsy.

∗ Use ice chips or sugarless gum or hard candy to relieve dry mouth.

Phillips' Milk of Magnesia is a laxative and an antacid. It draws water into the bowel from surrounding tissues, producing a soft stool. The drug also neutralizes stomach acid.

Why it's taken

Phillips' Milk of Magnesia is taken to relieve constipation or to treat heartburn and indigestion. You can buy Phillips' Milk of Magnesia without a prescription. It comes in an oral liquid. The following amounts are usually recommended for adults; children's dosages appear in parentheses.

▶ **For constipation,** 30 to 60 milliliters (ml), or 2 to 4 tablespoons, a day as a single dose or divided into equal doses. (Children ages 13 and older: same as adults. Children ages 6 to 12: 15 to 30 ml a day as a single dose or divided into equal doses. Children ages 2 to 5: 5 to 15 ml a day as a single dose or divided into equal doses.)

▶ **For heartburn and indigestion,** 5 to 15 ml three or four times a day.

How to take Phillips' Milk of Magnesia

• If you're treating yourself, read the label carefully.
• If your doctor prescribed this drug or gave you special instructions on how to use it, follow those instructions.

PHILLIPS' MILK OF MAGNESIA'S OTHER NAME

Phillips' Milk of Magnesia's generic name is magnesium hydroxide.

 SIDE EFFECTS

Call your doctor if you have any of these possible drug side effects.

Serious: none reported

Common: abdominal cramps, nausea, diarrhea

Other: laxative dependence (with long-term or excessive use), increased thirst, confusion, dizziness or light-headedness, irregular heartbeat, muscle cramps, unusual tiredness or fatigue

 DRUG INTERACTIONS

Combining certain drugs may alter their action or produce unwanted side effects. Tell your doctor about other drugs you're taking, especially:
• any oral drug (don't take within one hour of this drug).

• Shake the bottle well and take your dose with a full glass (8 ounces) of fruit juice or water.
• Schedule your dose so that the bowel movement it produces won't interfere with your sleep or activities. Phillips' Milk of Magnesia usually produces a watery stool in 3 to 6 hours. However, it may take longer if you take a small dose with food.

If you miss a dose

Not applicable because this drug is taken only as needed.

 If you suspect an overdose

Consult your doctor.

 Warnings

• Consult your doctor before taking Phillips' Milk of Magnesia if you have other problems, especially appendicitis (abdominal pain, nausea, vomiting), fecal impaction, an ileostomy or a colostomy, rectal bleeding, a blockage in the bowel, heart or kidney disease, high blood pressure, or diabetes.
• If you're breast-feeding, tell your doctor before you start taking Phillips' Milk of Magnesia.
• Don't give this drug to a child under age 6 unless directed by the doctor.
• Don't take this or any other laxative regularly; you could become dependent on it. And don't take it if you've missed a bowel movement for only 1 or 2 days.
• Don't take this drug for more than 1 week unless directed by your doctor.

KEEP IN MIND...

∗ Shake liquid well; take with full glass of fruit juice or water.

∗ Schedule dose so bowel movement won't interfere with sleep or activities.

∗ Don't take regularly or for a long time.

Phosphaljel

Phosphaljel is a phosphate supplement. It increases the body's supply of this essential element by causing less phosphate to be eliminated in stools.

Why it's taken

Phosphaljel is taken to correct a phosphate deficiency, such as from kidney disease, malnutrition, malabsorption, or an overactive parathyroid gland. You can buy Phosphaljel without a prescription. It comes in an oral liquid. The following amounts are usually recommended for adults.

▶ **To reduce elimination of phosphate in stools,** 15 to 30 milliliters undiluted every 2 hours between meals and at bedtime.

How to take Phosphaljel

• If you're treating yourself, follow the directions on the label. If the doctor has prescribed Phosphaljel, take it exactly as directed.
• Shake the bottle well. You may take Phosphaljel alone or with a small amount of milk or water.
• The doctor may want you to alternate Phosphaljel with an antacid that contains magnesium.

If you miss a dose

Take the missed dose 2 hours after your next meal or at bedtime. Don't take a double dose.

PHOSPHALJEL'S OTHER NAME

Phosphaljel's generic name is aluminum phosphate.

 SIDE EFFECTS

Call your doctor if you have any of these possible drug side effects.

Serious: none reported

Common: constipation
Tip: To avoid constipation, eat a high-fiber diet and increase the amount of fluids you drink. Good sources of dietary fiber include bran and other cereals and fresh fruits and vegetables.

Other: bowel blockage
Tip: If you notice a change in your bowel elimination pattern after you've been taking this drug for some time, consult your doctor.

 DRUG INTERACTIONS

Combining certain drugs may alter their action or produce unwanted side effects. Tell your doctor about other drugs you're taking, especially:
• antibiotics, such as Cipro, Penetrex, Maxaquin, Noroxin, Floxin, and tetracycline (take 1 to 2 hours before or after taking Phosphaljel)
• anticoagulants (blood thinners) such as Coumadin
• aspirin
• Chenix
• delayed-release drugs (take at least 1 hour before or after taking Phosphaljel)
• digoxin
• iron supplements
• Librium
• Thorazine
• Valium.

 If you suspect an overdose

Consult your doctor.

 Warnings

• You may not be able to take Phosphaljel if you have other problems, especially chronic kidney disease. Consult your doctor.
• Don't take Phosphaljel indiscriminately.

 KEEP IN MIND...

* Shake the bottle well.
* Take Phosphaljel alone or with milk or water.
* Don't take indiscriminately.
* Don't take at same time as antibiotic or delayed-release drug.

Phospholine Iodide

Phospholine Iodide contracts the pupils and reduces fluid pressure in the eye.

Why it's prescribed

Doctors prescribe Phospholine Iodide to treat some types of glaucoma. It comes in eyedrops. Doctors usually prescribe the following amounts for adults and children.
▶ **For glaucoma or eye fluid obstruction,** 1 drop a day instilled in sac behind lower eyelid. Maximum dosage is 1 drop twice a day.

How to use Phospholine Iodide

• Use this drug exactly as your doctor directs.
• Always wash your hands before and after using this drug.
• Don't touch the applicator tip to your eye or any other surface.
• After instilling the drops, apply light finger pressure to the inner corner of the eye for 1 or 2 minutes to help the eye absorb the drug.
• You can store eyedrops in the refrigerator for up to 6 months.

If you miss a dose

Adjust your schedule as follows:
• If you use one dose a day, apply the missed dose as soon as possible. However, if you don't remember until the next day, skip the missed dose and apply your next dose as scheduled.
• If you use one dose every other day, apply the missed dose as soon as possible. But if you don't remember until the next day, use it at that

time. Then skip a day and apply your next dose as scheduled.

 If you suspect an overdose

Contact your doctor *immediately*. Excessive Phospholine Iodide can cause tremors, fainting, headache, slow pulse, irregular heartbeat, diarrhea, nausea, vomiting, abdominal pain, excessive salivation, urinary incontinence, difficulty breathing, dizziness, and weakness.

⟫⟨ Warnings

• Make sure your doctor knows your medical history. You may not be able to take Phospholine Iodide

if you have other problems, especially seizures, asthma, high blood pressure, heart disease, myasthenia gravis, an overactive thyroid, Parkinson's disease, stomach ulcer, urinary tract blockage, or another eye problem, or if you're pregnant or breast-feeding.

 SIDE EFFECTS

Call your doctor if you have any of these possible drug side effects. Call *immediately* about any labeled "serious."

Serious: wheezing, closing up of throat

Common: none reported

Other: fatigue, tingling sensations, headache, slow pulse, dizziness, eye redness or swelling, cataracts, eye cysts, blurred vision, eye or brow pain, eyelid twitching, unusual eye sensitivity to light, clouding of eye lens, excessive tearing, retinal detachment, diarrhea, nausea, vomiting, abdominal pain or cramps, increased salivation and urination, profuse sweating

✶ DRUG INTERACTIONS

Combining certain drugs may alter their action or produce unwanted side effects. Tell your doctor about other drugs you're taking or may be exposed to, especially:
• adrenocorticoids for eyes, such as Decadron and Maxidex
• cholinergics, such as Antilirium, Cognex, Mestinon, Mytelase, Prostigmin, and Tensilon
• drugs to treat abdominal or stomach cramps or spasms
• eye drugs, such as atropine sulfate, Cyclogyl, and Pilocar
• insecticides and pesticides, such as malathion, parathion, Systox, and Trolene.

PHOSPHOLINE IODIDE'S OTHER NAME

Phospholine Iodide's generic name is echothiophate iodide.

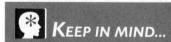 **KEEP IN MIND...**

∗ Wash hands before and after using.

∗ Don't touch applicator tip to eye or other surface.

∗ Store drops in refrigerator.

Pilocar

Pilocar contracts the pupils, relaxes the vessels, and reduces fluid pressure in the eye.

Why it's prescribed

Doctors prescribe Pilocar for glaucoma. It comes in eyedrops, an eye gel, and an eye insert. Doctors usually prescribe the following amounts for adults and children.

▶ **For long-term treatment of glaucoma,** 1 or 2 drops every 4 to 12 hours; or a $\frac{1}{3}$-inch ribbon of gel applied at bedtime; or one insert applied every 7 days.

▶ **For emergency treatment of glaucoma,** 1 drop every 5 to 10 minutes for three to six doses, followed by 1 drop every 1 to 3 hours until pressure in eye is controlled.

How to use Pilocar

• Use this drug exactly as directed by your doctor. Don't use more of it or take it more often than prescribed.

• Always wash your hands before and after using this drug.

• Apply Pilocar at bedtime because it will blur your vision.

• If you're using the eye insert, read the label instructions carefully. If the insert falls out of your eye during sleep, wash your hands, rinse the insert in cool tap water, and reposition it in your eye. Never use an insert that's deformed.

• Don't touch the applicator tip to your eye or any other surface.

PILOCAR'S OTHER NAMES

Pilocar's generic name is pilocarpine hydrochloride. Other brand names include Adsorbocarpine, Ocusert Pilo, Pilopine HS, P.V. Carpine Liquifilm; and, in Canada, Miocarpine.

 SIDE EFFECTS

Call your doctor if you have any of these possible drug side effects. Call *immediately* about any labeled "serious."

Serious: wheezing, closing up of throat, fluid buildup in lungs (shortness of breath, anxiety)

Common: near-sightedness, blurred vision, brow pain
Tip: Avoid hazardous activities, such as driving, until your vision clears.

Other: headache, eye irritation and tearing, vision changes, nausea, vomiting, abdominal cramps, diarrhea, increased salivation, allergic reaction (irritation, redness, itching, and swelling in or around eye)

 DRUG INTERACTIONS

Combining certain drugs may alter their action or produce unwanted side effects. Tell your doctor about other drugs you're taking, especially:
• eye drugs, such as atropine sulfate, Cyclogyl, Isopto Carbachol, Isopto Frin, Isopto Hyoscine, Phospholine Iodide, and scopolamine hydrobromide.

If you miss a dose

If you forget to use the drops or gel, apply the missed dose as soon as possible. But if it's almost time for your next dose, skip the missed dose and apply your next dose as scheduled. If you forget to replace the eye insert on time, replace it as soon as possible. Then return to your regular schedule.

If you suspect an overdose

Contact your doctor *immediately*. Excessive Pilocar can cause vomiting, flushed skin, slow pulse, wheezing, sweating, tearing, involuntary urination, tremor, dizziness, and weakness.

Warnings

• Make sure your doctor knows your medical history. You may not be able to use Pilocar if you have other problems, especially other eye problems, asthma, heart disease, difficulty urinating, stomach ulcers, an overactive thyroid, or Parkinson's disease.

• If you're breast-feeding, tell your doctor before you start using Pilocar.

KEEP IN MIND...

* Wash hands before and after using.

* Apply at bedtime because drug will blur vision.

* Don't touch applicator tip to eye or other surface.

* Don't drive until vision clears.

* Never use a deformed eye insert.

Pitressin

Pitressin, a natural hormone, decreases the amount of urine that the body produces by increasing the amount of fluid that the kidneys absorb.

Why it's prescribed

Doctors prescribe Pitressin to treat diabetes insipidus (water diabetes), which causes water loss, frequent urination, and increased thirst. It comes as a nasal solution. It's also available in an injectable form. Doctors usually prescribe the following amounts for adults and children.

▶ **For diabetes,** as nasal spray or applied to cotton balls in individualized dosage based on person's response.

How to use Pitressin

• Use this drug exactly as your doctor directs.

• Spray the dose into your nostrils, or spray a small amount on a cotton ball and insert the cotton ball slightly into your nostril.

• For best results, follow your dose with one or two glasses of water to prevent nausea.

If you miss a dose

Apply the missed dose as soon as possible. However, if it's almost time for your next dose, skip the missed dose and apply your next dose as scheduled. Don't apply a double dose.

PITRESSIN'S OTHER NAME

Pitressin's generic name is vasopressin (also called antidiuretic hormone).

 ## SIDE EFFECTS

Call your doctor if you have any of these possible drug side effects. Call *immediately* about any labeled "serious."

Serious: slow or irregular pulse; wheezing; closing up of throat; rash; hives; itching; swelling of face, lips, hands, or feet; difficulty breathing; water intoxication (drowsiness, listlessness, headache, confusion, weight gain, seizures, coma)

Common: none reported

Other: tremor, dizziness, chest pain, abdominal cramps, nausea, vomiting, diarrhea, inability to urinate, pale skin around mouth, uterine cramps, sweating

 ## DRUG INTERACTIONS

Combining certain drugs may alter their action or produce unwanted side effects. Tell your doctor about other drugs you're taking, especially:
• alcohol
• Atromid-S
• Declomycin
• Diabinese
• Florinef
• Liquaemin Sodium
• Lithobid
• Tegretol
• tricyclic antidepressants, such as Asendin and Elavil.

 ### If you suspect an overdose

Contact your doctor *immediately.* Excessive Pitressin can cause drowsiness, listlessness, headache, confusion, inability to urinate, and weight gain.

Warnings

• Make sure your doctor knows your medical history. You may not be able to take Pitressin if you have seizures, migraine headache, asthma, heart or blood vessel disease, heart failure, or kidney disease.

• Be aware that children and older adults may be especially prone to Pitressin's side effects.

 ## KEEP IN MIND...

* Follow dose with one or two glasses of water.

* Call doctor if you have trouble breathing; swelling of face, hands, or feet; or slow or irregular pulse.

* Don't apply a double dose if you miss a dose.

Plaquenil

Plaquenil kills or inhibits the growth of parasites that cause malaria. In arthritis and lupus, it reduces inflammation by inhibiting the effects of certain substances in the body.

Why it's prescribed

Doctors prescribe Plaquenil to prevent and treat malaria and to relieve symptoms of arthritis and lupus. It comes in tablets. Doctors usually prescribe the following amounts for adults; children's dosages appear in parentheses.

▶ **To prevent malaria,** up to 400 milligrams (mg) taken weekly on same day of week, beginning 2 weeks before entering malaria-prone area and continuing for 8 weeks after leaving area. (Children: 5 mg for each 2.2 pounds [lb] of body weight but not more than 400 mg.) If started after malaria exposure, initial dose is 800 mg for adults (10 mg for each 2.2 lb for children) divided into two equal doses given 6 hours apart.

▶ **For malarial attacks,** at first, 800 mg, then 400 mg after 6 to 8 hours, then 400 mg a day for 2 days (total 2 grams). (Children: 13 mg for each 2.2 lb, then 6.5 mg for each 2.2 lb 6 hours later, then 6.5 mg for each 2.2 lb a day for 2 days.)

▶ **To control lupus,** 400 mg once or twice a day, continued for several weeks or months, depending on response. Usual long-term dosage is 200 to 400 mg a day.

▶ **To relieve rheumatoid arthritis,** at first, 400 to 600 mg a day, then reduced when good response occurs.

PLAQUENIL'S OTHER NAME

Plaquenil's generic name is hydroxychloroquine.

 SIDE EFFECTS

Call your doctor if you have any of these possible drug side effects. Call *immediately* about any labeled "serious."

Serious: blood problems (fever and bleeding ulcers of mouth, rectum, vagina), fatigue, headache, paleness, shortness of breath, rapid pulse, seizures, vision changes, abnormal bleeding

Common: none reported

Other: irritability, incoordination, dizziness, muscle weakness, ringing in ears, appetite loss, abdominal cramps, diarrhea, vomiting, changes in hair or skin color, hair loss

Tips: Don't perform hazardous activities until you know how this drug affects you. Take it with meals or milk to avoid vomiting.

 DRUG INTERACTIONS

Combining certain drugs may alter their action or produce unwanted side effects. Tell your doctor about other drugs you're taking, especially:
- Kaopectate and drugs containing magnesium or aluminum (such as some antacids) (take at least 2 hours before or after Plaquenil)
- Tagamet.

How to take Plaquenil

- Take this drug exactly as your doctor directs.

If you miss a dose

Take the missed dose as soon as possible. But if it's almost time for your next dose, skip the missed dose and take your next dose as scheduled. Don't take a double dose.

 If you suspect an overdose

Contact your doctor *immediately.* Excessive Plaquenil can cause headache, drowsiness, vision changes, seizures, and respiratory and cardiac arrest.

 Warnings

- Make sure your doctor knows your medical history. You may not be able to take Plaquenil if you have other problems, especially an eye disorder or vision problem; liver, brain, nerve, bowel, or stomach disease; porphyria; psoriasis; or G6PD deficiency.
- If you're pregnant or breast-feeding, tell your doctor before taking Plaquenil.
- Call your doctor if your symptoms don't improve or if they get worse.

 KEEP IN MIND...

* Take with meals or milk.
* Call doctor immediately about vision changes.
* Don't drive until you know how drug affects you.

Plendil is one of several drugs called calcium channel blockers. It blocks calcium from entering the heart muscle, thereby slowing heart contractions. It also widens the heart's blood vessels, allowing more oxygen-carrying blood to reach and nourish the heart.

Why it's prescribed

Doctors prescribe Plendil for high blood pressure. It comes in tablets and extended-release tablets. Doctors usually prescribe the following amounts for adults.

▶ **For high blood pressure,** at first, 5 milligrams (mg) a day, adjusted according to person's response, usually at intervals of at least 2 weeks. Usual dosage is 5 to 10 mg a day; maximum recommended dosage is 20 mg a day.

How to take Plendil

• Take this drug exactly as your doctor directs. If you're taking the extended-release tablets, swallow them whole, without breaking, crushing, or chewing the tablet.
• Keep taking Plendil even if you feel well. You may have to take this drug for the rest of your life.

If you miss a dose

Take the missed dose as soon as possible. However, if it's almost time for your next dose, skip the missed dose and take your next dose as

PLENDIL'S OTHER NAMES

Plendil's generic name is felodipine. A Canadian brand name is Renedil.

 SIDE EFFECTS

Call your doctor if you have any of these possible drug side effects.

Serious: none reported

Common: swelling of lower legs or feet, flushed skin

Other: headache, dizziness, numbness or tingling sensations, weakness, chest pain, palpitations, fast pulse, runny nose, sore throat, stomach upset, abdominal pain, nausea, constipation, diarrhea, upper respiratory tract infection, cough, rash, muscle cramps, back pain, gum problems

Tips: To help prevent swelling, bleeding, or tenderness of the gums, brush and floss your teeth carefully and see your dentist regularly. If you have severe or persistent headaches, call your doctor.

 DRUG INTERACTIONS

Combining certain drugs may alter their action or produce unwanted side effects. Tell your doctor about other drugs you're taking, especially:
• Lanoxin
• Lopressor
• seizure drugs
• Tagamet.

scheduled. Don't take a double dose.

If you suspect an overdose

Contact your doctor *immediately.* Excessive Plendil can widen blood vessels, causing a slow pulse and low blood pressure (dizziness, weakness).

Warnings

• Make sure your doctor knows your medical history. You may not be able to take Plendil if you have other problems, especially other heart or blood vessel diseases, irregular heartbeats, Parkinson's disease, kidney or liver disease, or depression.

• If you're pregnant or breast-feeding, tell your doctor before you start taking Plendil.
• Older adults may be especially prone to Plendil's side effects.
• To help control your blood pressure, follow any special diet (such as a low-salt diet) the doctor prescribes.

 KEEP IN MIND...

* Swallow extended-release tablets whole.

* Follow prescribed diet.

* Keep taking even if you feel well.

* Brush and floss teeth carefully.

* Call doctor about severe or persistent headaches.

Polaramine

Polaramine is an antihistamine. It works by impeding the effects of histamine, a natural substance that causes itching, sneezing, runny nose, and watery eyes and that can make the throat close up.

Why it's prescribed

Doctors prescribe Polaramine to control or prevent allergy symptoms and similar reactions to irritants. It comes in tablets, timed-release tablets, and a syrup. Doctors usually prescribe the following amounts for adults and children.

▶ **For allergy or irritant reactions,** 2 milligrams (mg) every 4 to 6 hours but not more than 12 mg a day; or 4 to 6 mg timed-release tablets two or three times a day. (Children over age 12: same as adults. Children ages 6 to 12: 1 mg every 4 to 6 hours but not more than 6 mg a day; or 4 mg timed-release tablet at bedtime. Children ages 2 to 5: 0.5 mg every 4 to 6 hours but not more than 3 mg a day.)

How to take Polaramine

• Take this drug exactly as your doctor directs. To avoid stomach upset, take it with food, water, or milk.

If you miss a dose

Take the missed dose as soon as possible. However, if it's almost time

POLARAMINE'S OTHER NAMES

Polaramine's generic name is dexchlorpheniramine. Other brand names include Dexchlor, Poladex T.D., and Polaramine Repetabs.

 SIDE EFFECTS

Call your doctor if you have any of these possible drug side effects.

Serious: none reported

Common: drowsiness, agitation, dry mouth
Tip: To relieve dry mouth, use ice chips or sugarless gum or hard candy.

Other: dizziness, nausea, increased urination, pain on urination, inability to urinate
Tip: Don't drive or do anything else that could be dangerous if dizziness occurs.

 DRUG INTERACTIONS

Combining certain drugs may alter their action or produce unwanted side effects. Tell your doctor about other drugs you're taking, especially:
• antidepressants called MAO inhibitors such as Marplan
• drugs that slow down the nervous system, such as cold and allergy drugs, sedatives, tranquilizers, narcotic pain relievers, barbiturates, seizure drugs, and muscle relaxants.

for your next dose, skip the missed dose and take your next dose as scheduled. Don't take a double dose.

 If you suspect an overdose

Contact your doctor *immediately.* Excessive Polaramine can cause dry mouth, flushed skin, enlarged pupils, stomach upset, sedation, reduced alertness, hallucinations, seizures, tremor, difficulty sleeping, stopped breathing, heart failure, irregular heartbeat, and low blood pressure (dizziness, weakness).

Warnings

• Make sure your doctor knows your medical history. You may not be able to take Polaramine if you have other problems, especially asthma, glaucoma, an enlarged prostate, difficulty urinating, urinary tract blockage, irregular heartbeat, an overactive thyroid, heart or blood vessel disease, or kidney disease.

• If you're pregnant or breast-feeding, tell your doctor before you start taking Polaramine.

• Children and older adults may be especially prone to Polaramine's side effects. Don't give this drug to children under age 6 unless directed by a doctor; children should not take the timed-release tablets.

 KEEP IN MIND...

* Take with food, water, or milk.

* Don't drive if dizziness occurs.

* Use ice chips or sugarless gum or hard candy to relieve dry mouth.

Pondimin

Pondimin is an appetite suppressant. This drug affects chemical activity in the brain that helps control appetite and may increase the body's use of sugar.

Why it's prescribed

Doctors prescribe Pondimin, with diet and exercise, as a short-term treatment for obesity. It comes in tablets. Doctors usually prescribe the following amounts for adults.
► **To suppress appetite,** 1 tablet three times a day. Maximum dosage is 40 mg three times a day, adjusted according to person's response.

How to take Pondimin

• Take Pondimin exactly as your doctor directs. Don't increase your dosage or take this drug more often than prescribed because it can become habit-forming. Usually it is taken for several weeks, until new eating habits are established.
• Take Pondimin before meals.
• Don't stop taking Pondimin suddenly. Consult your doctor first.

If you miss a dose

Take the missed dose as soon as possible. However, if it's almost time for your next dose, skip the missed dose and take your next dose on schedule. Don't take a double dose.

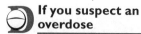 **If you suspect an overdose**

Contact your doctor *immediately*. Excessive Pondimin can cause jaw tremor, confusion, sweating, abdomi-

PONDIMIN'S OTHER NAME

Pondimin's generic name is fenfluramine hydrochloride.

 SIDE EFFECTS

Call your doctor if you have any of these possible drug side effects. Call *immediately* about any labeled "serious."

Serious: chest pain, low blood pressure (dizziness, weakness), high blood pressure (headache, blurred vision), palpitations

Common: drowsiness, dizziness, incoordination, difficulty sleeping, rash, eye irritation, constipation, dry mouth, change in sex drive, difficulty urinating

Tips: Don't drive or do anything else that could be dangerous if your vision is blurry or you're not fully alert. To avoid constipation, add fluids and high-fiber foods to your diet. Try ice chips or sugarless candy or gum to relieve dry mouth.

Other: nausea, sweating, fever, chills, abdominal pain, weakness, fatigue, impotence

 DRUG INTERACTIONS

Combining certain drugs may alter their action or produce unwanted side effects. Tell your doctor about other drugs you're taking, especially:
• alcohol and other drugs that make you feel relaxed or sleepy, such as tranquilizers (Valium, Xanax) and sleeping pills (Halcion)
• Aldomet
• MAO inhibitors, such as Nardil and Parnate
• insulin
• Ismelin
• Serpasil.

nal pain, rapid breathing, abnormal eye movements, palpitations, seizures, and decreased consciousness.

 Warnings

• Make sure your doctor knows your medical history. You may not be able to take Pondimin if you have high blood pressure, heart disease, diabetes, depression, or alcoholism or if you're pregnant or breast-feeding.
• Older adults may be especially prone to Pondimin's side effects.
• Don't start any new medications without first checking with your doctor.

• Before having surgery (including dental surgery), tell your doctor or dentist that you're taking this drug.
• See your doctor regularly so your progress and drug effects can be monitored.

KEEP IN MIND...

* Don't exceed recommended dosage.
* Take before meals.
* Don't stop taking abruptly.
* Avoid alcohol.

Ponstel

Ponstel is a nonsteroidal anti-inflammatory drug (NSAID). It reduces inflammation and pain by inhibiting production of a hormone called prostaglandin and by impeding the action of other substances in the body.

Why it's prescribed

Doctors prescribe Ponstel to relieve pain and menstrual discomfort. It comes in capsules. Doctors usually prescribe the following amounts for adults and children over age 14.

▶ **For mild to moderate pain,** at first, 500 milligrams (mg), then 250 mg every 6 hours, as needed, for up to 1 week.

How to take Ponstel

• Take this drug exactly as your doctor directs. Don't take for more than 1 week at a time unless directed by your doctor. Take each dose with a full glass (8 ounces) of water.
• To avoid stomach upset, take Ponstel with food or an antacid, then stay upright for 15 to 30 minutes.

If you miss a dose

If you're taking Ponstel regularly, take the missed dose as soon as possible. But if it's almost time for your next dose, skip the missed dose and take your next dose as scheduled. Don't take a double dose.

PONSTEL'S OTHER NAMES

Ponstel's generic name is mefenamic acid. A Canadian brand name is Ponstan.

SIDE EFFECTS

Call your doctor if you have any of these possible drug side effects. Call *immediately* about any labeled "serious."

Serious: diarrhea, heartburn, indigestion, stomach pain, bloating, nausea, vomiting, restlessness, mottled skin, irregular or rapid heartbeat, fever, infection, unusual bleeding, weakness, fatigue, headache, pale skin, shortness of breath, yellow-tinged skin and eyes, cold and clammy arms and legs

Common: none reported

Other: drowsiness, dizziness, nervousness, headache, blurred vision, eye irritation, painful urination, blood in urine, swelling, rash, hives
Tip: Don't drive or do anything else that could be dangerous if your vision is blurry or you're not fully alert.

DRUG INTERACTIONS

Combining certain drugs may alter their action or produce unwanted side effects. Tell your doctor about other drugs you're taking, especially:
• alcohol
• anticoagulants (blood thinners) such as Coumadin
• aspirin
• blood pressure drugs such as diuretics (water pills)
• oral diabetes drugs such as Diabinese
• steroids.

If you suspect an overdose

Contact your doctor *immediately*. Excessive Ponstel can cause restlessness, agitation, irrational behavior, and seizures.

Warnings

• Make sure your doctor knows your medical history. You may not be able to take Ponstel if you have a stomach or intestinal problem; hemorrhoids or bleeding problem; frequent infections; high blood pressure; water retention; liver, kidney, or heart disease; diabetes; Parkinson's disease; mental illness; asthma; seizures; or blood disorder or if you've ever had an unusual reaction to aspirin, Advil, or any other pain reliever.
• If you're pregnant or breast-feeding, tell your doctor before taking Ponstel.

KEEP IN MIND...

* Take with full glass of water, plus food or antacid.

* Stay upright for 15 to 30 minutes after taking.

* Don't take for more than 1 week.

Pravachol

Pravachol reduces the amount of fat in the blood and interferes with the body's production of cholesterol, a fatlike substance that can clog blood vessels.

Why it's prescribed

Doctors prescribe Pravachol to reduce high cholesterol levels. It comes in tablets. Doctors usually prescribe the following amounts for adults.

▶ **To reduce cholesterol levels,** at first, 10 or 20 milligrams (mg) once a day at bedtime. Dosage is adjusted every 4 weeks based on the person's tolerance and response. Maximum dosage is 40 mg a day.

How to take Pravachol

• Take this drug exactly as your doctor directs.
• For best results, take Pravachol in the evening with food. If you take more than one dose a day, take it with a snack or meal to avoid nausea and heartburn.

If you miss a dose

Skip the missed dose and take your next dose as scheduled. Don't take a double dose.

 If you suspect an overdose

Consult your doctor.

PRAVACHOL'S OTHER NAME

Pravachol's generic name is pravastatin sodium.

 SIDE EFFECTS

Call your doctor if you have any of these possible drug side effects. Call *immediately* about any labeled "serious."

Serious: muscle pain, rust-colored urine, decreased urine output

Common: none reported

Other: headache, fatigue, dizziness, chest pain, runny nose, vomiting, diarrhea, heartburn, nausea, cough, rash, flulike symptoms, kidney failure (tiredness, low or absent urine output), pain, inflammation, weakness, wasting of muscles

 DRUG INTERACTIONS

Combining certain drugs may alter their action or produce unwanted side effects. Tell your doctor about other drugs you're taking, especially:
• alcohol
• Atromid-S
• Colestid and Questran (take 1 hour after or 4 hours before taking Pravachol)
• drugs that affect the body's steroids, such as Tagamet, Nizoral, and Aldactone
• drugs that may cause liver damage, such as Tylenol, Cordarone, or methotrexate
• drugs that suppress the immune system such as Sandimmune
• E-Mycin
• Lopid
• niacin (in doses of 1 gram or more per day).

 Warnings

• Make sure your doctor knows your medical history. You may not be able to take Pravachol if you have other medical problems, especially liver disease.
• Don't take Pravachol if you're pregnant or breast-feeding. Discuss other options with your doctor.
• Pravachol is not recommended for children under age 18.
• Follow any special diet, exercise, or smoking cessation program your doctor recommends.

• See your doctor regularly so your progress can be checked and dosage adjusted.

KEEP IN MIND...

* Take in evening with food.
* Follow prescribed diet.
* Don't take if pregnant or breast-feeding
* Follow any recommended diet, exercise, and smoking cessation programs.

Precose

Precose lowers and controls the amount of sugar in the blood by slowing the body's digestion of foods that contain sugar and starches.

Why it's prescribed

Doctors prescribe Precose to manage non-insulin-dependent (type II) diabetes. It comes in tablets. Doctors usually prescribe the following amounts for adults and children.

▶ **For controlling diabetes**, at first, 25 milligrams (mg) three times a day at the beginning of each meal. Dosage is adjusted every 4 to 8 weeks, depending on the person's tolerance and response. Maintenance dosage is usually 50 to 100 mg three times a day.

How to take Precose

• Take Precose only as your doctor directs.
• Take with the first bite of food at each of your three main meals of the day.

If you miss a dose

Take the missed dose as soon as possible. But if it's almost time for your next dose, skip the missed dose and go back to your regular schedule. Don't take a double dose.

 If you suspect an overdose

Consult your doctor. Although no overdose of Precose has been reported, likely symptoms would be increased gas, diarrhea, and stomach pain that later subsides.

PRECOSE'S OTHER NAME

Precose's generic name is acarbose.

 SIDE EFFECTS

Call your doctor if you have any of these possible drug side effects. Call *immediately* about any labeled "serious."

Serious: severe stomach pain or increase in size of abdomen

Common: gas, diarrhea, abdominal discomfort

Other: none reported

 DRUG INTERACTIONS

Combining certain drugs may alter their action or produce unwanted side effects. Tell your doctor about other drugs you're taking, especially:
• amylase, pancreatin (digestive drugs)
• calcium channel blockers (heart and blood pressure drugs)
• corticosteroids
• Duvoid
• insulin and oral diabetes drugs, such as DiaBeta and Micronase
• isoniazid (INH)
• Isopto Carpine
• phenothiazines, such as Primazine and Thorazine
• thiazide and other diuretics (water pills)
• thyroid drugs, hormone treatment (estrogens), birth control pills.

Warnings

• Make sure your doctor knows your medical history. You may not be able to take Precose if you have a drug allergy, kidney or liver disease, a bowel or intestinal disorder, or an ulcer.
• Tell your doctor if you're pregnant or breast-feeding before you take Precose.
• Follow your doctor's advice about diet, weight loss, and exercise.
• Have your blood or urine sugar levels checked regularly during treatment so your dosage may be adjusted if necessary.
• Carry sugar pills or another source of sugar with you at all times in case of sudden attacks of low blood sugar (fatigue, weakness, shakiness), especially when taking other diabetes drugs. Call your doctor if you experience any of these symptoms.
• Check with your doctor if your body is under stress due to fever, trauma, infection, or surgery, for example; you may need insulin temporarily to control blood sugar levels.

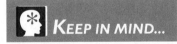 **KEEP IN MIND...**

* Take three times a day at start of each meal.

* Follow diet, weight, and exercise programs.

* Check blood or urine sugar levels regularly.

* You may need insulin during pregnancy or physical stress.

Premarin

Premarin is an estrogen — a female hormone essential for normal sexual development and regulation of the menstrual cycle. Premarin is used to replace the body's estrogen supply after menopause, when the ovaries start to produce less.

Why it's prescribed

Doctors prescribe Premarin to relieve menopausal symptoms such as hot flashes, to treat some breast cancers, to prevent osteoporosis, and to treat some types of prostate cancer in men. It comes in tablets and a vaginal cream. It's also available in an injectable form. Doctors usually prescribe the following amounts for adults.

▶ **For breast cancer in men and in women who've been menopausal for at least 5 years,** 10 milligrams (mg) orally three times a day for 3 months or more.

▶ **For ovary failure (infertility),** 1.25 mg orally a day in cycles (3 weeks on, 1 week off).

▶ **For osteoporosis,** 0.625 mg orally a day in cycles (3 weeks on, 1 week off).

▶ **For slowed sexual development,** 2.5 mg orally two or three times a day for 20 consecutive days each month.

▶ **For hot flashes,** 0.3 to 1.25 mg orally a day in cycles (3 weeks on, 1 week off).

▶ **For vaginal or vulval tissue shrinkage,** 2 to 4 grams applied to

---

PREMARIN'S OTHER NAMES

Premarin's generic name is conjugated estrogen. A brand name in Canada is C.E.S.

 ## SIDE EFFECTS

Call your doctor if you have any of these possible drug side effects. Call *immediately* about any labeled "serious."

Serious: blood clots (sudden or severe headache, sudden incoordination, vision changes, shortness of breath, numbness or stiffness in legs, pain in chest, groin, or legs), stroke (headache, vomiting, mental impairment, seizures, fever, stiff neck, disorientation, coma), pulmonary embolism (labored breathing, chest pain, fast pulse, productive cough, slight fever), heart attack

Common: nausea

Other: headache, dizziness, involuntary rapid movements, (grimacing, flexing of fingers), depression, sluggishness, high blood pressure (headache, blurred vision), swelling, vision change, intolerance of contact lenses, vomiting, abdominal cramps, bloating, diarrhea, constipation, change in appetite, weight change, inflammation of pancreas (stomach pain, vomiting, rigid abdomen, restlessness, mottled skin, irregular heartbeats, fever, cold, sweaty arms and legs), yellow-tinged skin and eyes, hives, acne, darkening of facial skin, oily or scaly skin, unusual hair growth (especially on face), hair loss, breast changes (tenderness, enlargement, or secretion), leg cramps, high blood sugar level (increased thirst, hunger, and urination), folic acid deficiency, change in sex drive; in women — vaginal inflammation, altered or absent menstruation, menstrual discomfort, altered cervical secretions, enlargement of fibrous uterine tumors (abdominal pain or swelling), vaginal yeast infection; in men — enlarged breasts, shrinkage of testicles, impotence

Tips: Call your doctor right away if you experience rapid weight gain; swelling, pain, or a lump in your breast; or unusual vaginal bleeding. If you're using the vaginal cream, call your doctor if your vaginal area becomes swollen, red, or itchy.

 ## DRUG INTERACTIONS

Combining certain drugs may alter their action or produce unwanted side effects. Tell your doctor about other drugs you're taking, especially:
- anticoagulants (blood thinners) such as Coumadin
- drugs that can damage the liver such as Dantrium
- drugs for seizures, such as Barbita and Tegretol
- Parlodel
- Rifadin
- Sandimmune
- steroids
- Tamofen.

the vagina once a day in cycles (3 weeks on, 1 week off).

▶ **For prostate cancer,** 1.25 to 2.5 mg orally three times a day.

How to take Premarin

• Take this drug exactly as your doctor directs. For best results, take at the same time each day.

• Take tablets with food to avoid nausea.

• Apply vaginal cream at bedtime for better absorption. If you apply it at a different time, lie down for 30 minutes after use.

If you miss a dose

If you miss a tablet, take it as soon as possible. However, if it's almost time for your next dose, skip the missed dose and take your next dose as scheduled. Don't take a double dose. If you forget to apply a dose of vaginal cream and don't remember until the next day, skip the missed dose and apply your next dose as scheduled.

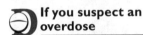 **If you suspect an overdose**

Consult your doctor. Excessive Premarin can cause nausea and vomiting

Warnings

• Make sure your doctor knows your medical history. You may not be able to take Premarin if you have other problems, especially breast disease, cancer, diabetes, high blood pressure, porphyria, gynecologic problems, diseases of major organs, a blood clot, or a stroke, or if anyone in your family has had breast cancer or cancer of the sex organs.

• If you're pregnant or breast-feeding, don't use Premarin. If you think you may have become pregnant, stop taking it immediately and call your doctor.

• If you have diabetes, Premarin may affect your blood sugar level. Check with your doctor if you notice any changes.

• Keep all appointments for follow-up care so your doctor can check your progress and monitor drug effects.

• Perform monthly breast self-exams and see your doctor for routine breast exams.

• Stop using Premarin at least 1 month before you undergo surgery that will keep you in bed for a long time, such as hip or knee surgery.

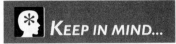 **KEEP IN MIND...**

∗ Take tablets with food to control nausea.

∗ Apply vaginal cream at bedtime.

∗ Examine breasts regularly.

∗ Call doctor if you have symptoms of a blood clot, such as sudden or severe headache, loss of coordination, vision changes, shortness of breath, numbness or stiffness in legs, or pain in chest, groin, or legs.

Prevacid

Prevacid blocks the formation of stomach acid, helping to relieve symptoms of stomach ulcers, such as heartburn and indigestion.

Why it's prescribed

Doctors prescribe Prevacid for stomach ulcers and related conditions. It comes in delayed-release capsules. Doctors usually prescribe the following amounts for adults.

▶ **For duodenal ulcer,** 15 milligrams (mg) a day for 4 weeks.

▶ **For inflammation of the esophagus,** 30 mg a day for up to 8 weeks. If healing doesn't occur, drug may be taken for an additional 8 weeks.

▶ **For chronic excess stomach acid,** at first, 60 mg a day, increased as needed. Daily dosages of more than 120 mg are divided into equal doses.

How to take Prevacid

• Take this drug exactly as your doctor directs. For best results, take it before eating.

• Swallow the capsules whole. Don't break, crush, or chew them.

If you miss a dose

Take the missed dose as soon as possible. But if it's almost time for your next dose, skip the missed dose and go back to your regular schedule. Don't take a double dose.

 If you suspect an overdose

Consult your doctor.

PREVACID'S OTHER NAME

Prevacid's generic name is lansoprazole.

 SIDE EFFECTS

Call your doctor if you have any of these possible drug side effects. Call *immediately* about any labeled "serious."

Serious: shock (extremely low blood pressure, severe dizziness and weakness), paralysis of one side of body, chest pain, stroke (headache, vomiting, mental impairment, seizures, fever, rigidity at back of neck, disorientation, coma), high blood pressure (headache, blurred vision), black tarry stools, gallstones (acute pain in upper right abdomen that spreads to back or front of chest), vomiting of blood, rectal bleeding, difficulty breathing

Common: diarrhea, nausea, abdominal pain

Other: headache, anxiety, confusion, depression, dizziness, hallucinations, hostility, decreased sex drive, numbness or tingling sensations, swelling, palpitations, vision problems, deafness, eye pain, middle ear infection, ringing in ears, bad breath, appetite loss, constipation, dry mouth, difficulty swallowing, discolored stools, increased salivation, mouth sores, bloody urine, kidney stones (lower back pain), anemia (weakness, fatigue, pale skin), swollen thyroid (goiter), high blood sugar levels (increased thirst, hunger, and urination), low blood sugar levels (tremor, restlessness, clammy skin), gout, weight gain or loss, arthritis, joint or muscle pain, asthma, bronchitis, nosebleeds, coughing up of blood, pneumonia, itching, rash, flulike symptoms, infection, abnormal menstruation, breast enlargement or tenderness

 DRUG INTERACTIONS

Combining certain drugs may alter their action or produce unwanted side effects. Tell your doctor about other drugs you're taking, especially:

• ampicillin esters, such as Omnipen-N and Polycillin
• Carafate (take 30 minutes after taking Prevacid)
• iron salts, such as Feosol and Feostat
• Lanoxin
• Nizoral
• Theo-Dur.

 Warnings

• Make sure your doctor knows if you have other medical problems, especially liver or kidney disease.
• If you're pregnant or breast-feeding, tell your doctor before you start taking Prevacid.
• Don't give Prevacid to children under age 18.

KEEP IN MIND...

* Take before eating.
* Swallow capsules whole.
* Don't take a double dose if you miss a dose.

Prilosec

Prilosec is used to treat ulcers, heartburn, and other problems involving excess stomach acid. It works by blocking the formation of stomach acid.

Why it's prescribed

Doctors prescribe Prilosec for stomach ulcers, inflammation of the esophagus, gastroesophageal reflux disease (GERD, or backward flow of stomach contents into the esophagus), and other conditions in which stomach acid is excessive. Prilosec comes in delayed-release capsules. Doctors usually prescribe the following amounts for adults.

▶ **For ulcers,** 20 milligrams (mg) a day for 4 to 8 weeks.

▶ **For esophageal inflammation or GERD,** 20 mg a day for 4 to 8 weeks.

▶ **For chronic excess stomach acid,** at first, 60 mg a day, adjusted according to person's response. Daily dosage is 80 mg divided into equal doses.

How to take Prilosec

• Take this drug exactly as your doctor directs. Don't break, chew, or crush the capsules; swallow them whole.

• Several days of treatment may pass before you experience pain relief. Until then, you can take antacids with Prilosec, unless your doctor advises otherwise.

PRILOSEC'S OTHER NAME

Prilosec's generic name is omeprazole.

SIDE EFFECTS

Call your doctor if you have any of these possible drug side effects.

Serious: none reported

Common: none reported

Other: headache, dizziness, diarrhea, abdominal pain, nausea, vomiting, constipation, gas, cough, rash, back pain

Tip: Consult your doctor if Prilosec's side effects become bothersome.

DRUG INTERACTIONS

Combining certain drugs may alter their action or produce unwanted side effects. Tell your doctor about other drugs you're taking, especially:
• Antabuse
• Coumadin
• Dilantin
• iron derivatives, such as Feosol and Feostat
• Nizoral
• Omnipen-N, Polycillin
• Sandimmune
• Valium.

• Take Prilosec for the full treatment period, even if you feel better.

If you miss a dose

Take the missed dose as soon as possible. However, if it's almost time for your next dose, skip the missed dose and take your next dose as scheduled. Don't take a double dose.

If you suspect an overdose

Consult your doctor.

Warnings

• Make sure your doctor knows your medical history. You may not be able to take Prilosec if you have other problems, especially liver disease, or if you're allergic to any drugs or other substances, such as foods or dyes.

• If you're pregnant or breast-feeding, tell your doctor before you start taking Prilosec.

• Keep appointments for follow-up checkups so your doctor will know when you can stop taking this drug.

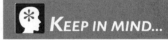

KEEP IN MIND...

* Swallow capsules whole.

* Take antacids for first few days if doctor approves.

* Take Prilosec for full treatment period.

Primatene Mist

Primatene Mist is one of a group of drugs called bronchodilators. It stimulates the nervous system so that air passages in the lungs open to ease breathing.

Why it's used

Primatene Mist is used to treat asthma attacks, wheezing, closing of the throat, and other allergic reactions. Although you can buy this drug without a prescription, don't use it unless a doctor tells you to. It comes in an aerosol inhaler and a nebulizer inhaler. It's also available in an injectable form. The following amounts are usually recommended for adults and children age 4 and over.

▶ **For asthma attacks,** 160 to 250 micrograms (if using metered aerosol) or 1 inhalation. Repeat once, if necessary, after at least 2 minutes; subsequent doses at least 3 hours apart. Or 1 to 3 deep inhalations by hand-bulb nebulizer, repeated every 3 hours, as needed.

How to use Primatene Mist

• Use this drug exactly as your doctor directs. Also, read the instructions carefully before using the inhalant.
• Don't use solution if it looks pink, brown, or cloudy.

PRIMATENE MIST'S OTHER NAMES

Primatene Mist's generic name is epinephrine. Other brand names include Adrenalin, Adrenalin Chloride, AsthmaHaler Mist, Bronitin Mist, Bronkaid Mist, EpiPen Auto-Injector, Medihaler-Epi, Sus-Phrine; and, in Canada, Bronkaid Mistometer.

SIDE EFFECTS

Call your doctor if you have any of these possible drug side effects. Call *immediately* about any labeled "serious."

Serious: suicidal thoughts, high blood pressure (headache, blurred vision), fast pulse, life-threatening irregular pulse (dizziness), stroke (headache, vomiting, mental impairment, seizures, fever, rigidity at back of neck, disorientation, coma), fluid in lungs (shortness of breath, anxiety), high blood sugar level (increased thirst, hunger, and urination)

Common: nervousness, headache, palpitations, chest pain, dry mouth and throat
Tip: To ease dry mouth and throat, rinse your mouth with water after each dose.

Other: tremor, unusual feeling of well-being, anxiety, cold arms and legs, feeling of spinning or other sensation, fainting, sweating, disorientation, agitation, difficulty breathing, pale skin

DRUG INTERACTIONS

Combining certain drugs may alter their action or produce unwanted side effects. Tell your doctor about other drugs you're taking, especially:
• alpha blockers, such as Cardura and Minipress
• antidepressants (tricyclics and MAO inhibitors), such as Elavil, Nardil, Pamelor, and Parnate
• antihistamines such as Benadryl
• beta blockers, such as Inderal and Lopressor
• Crystodigin, Lanoxin
• Dibenzyline
• Dopram, Mazanor, Ritalin
• Ergomar
• ergot alkaloids such as Cafergot
• Ergotrate Maleate
• Hydergine
• Hylorel, Ismelin
• Larodopa
• Medihaler Ergotamine
• Methergine
• Regitine
• Sanorex
• Sinemet
• thyroid hormones.

• When taking Primatene Mist by aerosol inhaler, keep the spray away from your eyes. Don't take more than 2 inhalations at any one time unless directed by your doctor. Wait at least 2 minutes after the first inhalation to make sure you need a second.

• When using the aerosol inhaler along with a steroid or an ipratropium inhaler (such as Atrovent), use Primatene Mist first, then wait about 5 minutes before using the steroid or ipratropium inhaler to help the second drug work better.

• You should start to feel relief 3 to 5 minutes after using the inhaler. If you still have difficulty breathing after taking this drug, call your doctor at once.

If you miss a dose

If you use this drug regularly, take the missed dose as soon as possible. However, if it's almost time for your next dose, skip the missed dose and take your next dose as scheduled. Don't take a double dose.

 ## If you suspect an overdose

Contact your doctor *immediately*. Excessive Primatene Mist can cause high blood pressure (headache, blurred vision), severe anxiety, irregular pulse, severe nausea or vomiting, severe breathing problems, large pupils, pale and cold skin, fluid buildup in the lungs (shortness of breath), and kidney failure (decreased urination).

Warnings

• Make sure your doctor knows your medical history. You may not be able to use Primatene Mist if you have other problems, especially glaucoma, brain damage, irregular heartbeats, high blood pressure, heart or blood vessel disease, diabetes, seizures, an overactive thyroid, Parkinson's disease, or mental disease, or if you're allergic to sulfites.

• If you're pregnant or breast-feeding, tell your doctor before you start taking Primatene Mist.

• Children may be especially sensitive to Primatene's effects.

• If you have diabetes, be aware that Primatene Mist may worsen it. Your doctor may need to change the dosage of your diabetes drugs.

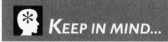 KEEP IN MIND...

* Don't use unless you've been diagnosed with asthma.

* Keep spray from aerosol inhaler out of eyes.

* Don't take more than two inhalations unless directed by doctor.

* Don't use if solution is pink, brown, or cloudy.

Prinivil

Prinivil is a blood-pressure drug. It reduces blood pressure by causing blood vessels to relax.

Why it's prescribed

Doctors prescribe Prinivil to reduce high blood pressure. It's also used with other drugs to treat heart failure. It comes in tablets. Doctors usually prescribe the following amounts for adults.

▶ **For high blood pressure,** at first, 10 milligrams (mg) a day when not taking a diuretic (water pill); dosage increased as needed, usually to 20 to 40 mg a day as a single dose.

▶ **For heart failure,** at first, 5 mg a day, increased as needed to a maximum of 20 mg a day.

How to take Prinivil

• Take this drug exactly as the doctor orders, even if you feel well.
• Don't stop taking abruptly.

If you miss a dose

Take the missed dose as soon as possible. But, if it's almost time for your next dose, skip the missed dose and take your next dose as scheduled. Don't take a double dose.

If you suspect an overdose

Consult your doctor.

 Warnings

• Make sure your doctor knows your medical history. You may not

PRINIVIL'S OTHER NAMES

Prinivil's generic name is lisinopril. Another brand name is Zestril.

 SIDE EFFECTS

Call your doctor if you have any of these possible drug side effects. Call *immediately* about any labeled "serious."

Serious: swelling of head, face, neck, or internal organs; difficulty breathing, blood problems (fever, chills, increased risk of infection)

Common: dizziness, headache, fatigue, light-headedness, nasal congestion, diarrhea, muscle cramps, dry, persistent, tickling cough

Tips: To relieve light-headedness, get up slowly from a sitting or lying position. Sit and dangle your legs for a few minutes before getting out of bed. If you faint, stop taking Prinivil and call your doctor right away.

Other: depression, sleepiness, tingling or numbness, low blood pressure (dizziness, weakness), chest pain, nausea, stomach upset, altered taste, impotence, rash, decreased sex drive, increased thirst

 DRUG AND FOOD INTERACTIONS

Combining certain drugs or foods may alter drug action or produce unwanted side effects. Tell your doctor about your diet and other drugs you're taking, especially:
• Colestid
• diuretics (water pills), especially potassium-sparing and thiazide diuretics, such as Aldactone and HydroDIURIL
• drugs or diet supplements containing potassium
• Eskalith
• heart drugs called digitalis glycosides such as Lanoxin
• Indocin
• insulin and oral diabetes drugs, such as Diabinese and Orinase
• Questran
• salt substitutes.

be able to take Prinivil if you're allergic to it or to related drugs, if you've recently had a heart attack or stroke, or if you have kidney problems, lupus, diabetes, or high potassium levels.

• Tell your doctor right away if you think you're pregnant or if you plan to breast-feed.

• While taking this drug, monitor your blood pressure regularly, if your doctor orders. See your doctor routinely for blood tests.

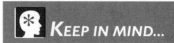 **KEEP IN MIND...**

∗ Take drug exactly as ordered, even if you feel well.

∗ Don't stop taking abruptly.

∗ Stand up slowly to avoid dizziness.

Privine

Privine is a decongestant that relieves stuffy nose by narrowing blood vessels inside the nose. This reduces blood flow and relieves the swelling caused by inflammation. It also helps drain the sinuses.

Why it's used

Privine is used to relieve nasal congestion. You can buy Privine without a prescription. It comes in nose drops and a nasal spray. The following amounts are usually recommended for adults; children's dosages appear in parentheses.

▶ **For stuffy nose,** 2 drops or sprays in each nostril every 3 to 4 hours. (Children age 12 and over: same as adults. Children ages 6 to 12: 1 to 2 drops or sprays in each nostril every 3 to 6 hours, as needed, but for no longer than 5 days.)

How to use Privine

• If you're treating yourself, follow the instructions on the label. If your doctor has prescribed Privine, use it exactly as directed. Don't take more than the recommended dosage.

• To use the nose drops, tilt your head back as far as possible, instill the drops in one nostril, and then lean your head forward while inhaling. Repeat the procedure for the other nostril.

SIDE EFFECTS

Call your doctor if you have any of these possible drug side effects. Call *immediately* about any labeled "serious."

Serious: very low blood pressure (severe dizziness and weakness)

Common: none reported

Other: recurrence of stuffy nose (with excessive or long-term use), sneezing, stinging, dryness of lining of nostril, sedation, and sleepiness, slow heart rate, and slow breathing in children after excessive or long-term use

DRUG INTERACTIONS

Combining certain drugs may alter their action or produce unwanted side effects. Tell your doctor about other drugs you're taking, especially:
• MAO inhibitors (antidepressants), such as Nardil and Parnate.

• To use the nasal spray, hold the spray container and your head upright. Don't shake the container.
• Privine starts to work within 10 minutes; its effects last 2 to 6 hours.

If you miss a dose

Take the missed dose as soon as possible. However, if it's almost time for your next dose, skip the missed dose and go back to your regular dosing schedule. Don't take a double dose.

If you suspect an overdose

Contact your doctor *immediately*. Excessive Privine can cause reduced alertness, sluggishness, sweating, decreased body temperature, cardiovascular collapse (which can cause slow pulse, dizziness, and weakness), and decreased breathing.

Warnings

• Make sure your doctor knows your medical history. You may not be able to use Privine if you have other problems, especially an overactive thyroid, heart disease, high blood pressure, or diabetes.
• Make sure your doctor knows if you're pregnant or breast-feeding before you begin taking Privine.
• Don't give Privine to children under age 6 unless your doctor tells you to do so.
• Contact your doctor if your nose is still stuffy after 5 days.
• Don't share this product with family members or friends because this could spread infection.

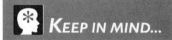
KEEP IN MIND...

* Don't take more than recommended dosage.

* Call doctor if stuffy nose persists after 5 days.

* Don't share drug with family or friends.

PRIVINE'S OTHER NAMES

Privine's generic name is naphazoline hydrochloride. Other brand names include Allerest and Allergy Drops.

Pro-Banthine

Pro-Banthine is used to treat spasms or cramps of the stomach, bowels, and bladder. It works by decreasing bowel action, reducing stomach acid, and decreasing bladder movement.

Why it's prescribed

Doctors prescribe Pro-Banthine to treat ulcers and other conditions. It comes in tablets. Doctors usually prescribe the following amounts for adults.

▶ **For ulcers,** 15 milligrams (mg) three times a day before meals and 30 mg at bedtime. Older adults: 7.5 mg three times a day before meals.

How to take Pro-Banthine

• Take Pro-Banthine exactly as directed 30 to 60 minutes before meals. Take bedtime dose at least 2 hours after your last meal of the day.
• Swallow the tablets whole; don't chew or crush them.

If you miss a dose

Take the missed dose as soon as possible. But if it's almost time for your next dose, skip the missed dose and take your next dose as scheduled. Don't take a double dose.

If you suspect an overdose

Contact your doctor *immediately.* Excessive Pro-Banthine can cause respiratory paralysis, headache, large pupils, blurred vision, dry mucous membranes, difficulty swal-

PRO-BANTHINE'S OTHER NAMES

Pro-Banthine's generic name is propantheline bromide. A Canadian brand name is Propanthel.

SIDE EFFECTS

Call your doctor if you have any of these possible drug side effects.

Serious: none reported

Common: confusion or excitement (in older adults), palpitations, blurred vision, dry mouth, difficulty urinating, inability to urinate

Other: headache, difficulty sleeping, drowsiness, dizziness, nervousness, weakness, fast pulse, large pupils, increased pressure in eyes, light sensitivity, difficulty swallowing, constipation, heartburn, loss of taste, nausea, vomiting, bowel problems, impotence, decreased sweating, skin problems, fever, allergic reaction (hives, rash)

Tips: Don't drive or do anything else that could be dangerous if your vision isn't clear or if you're not fully alert. Drink plenty of fluids to avoid constipation.

DRUG INTERACTIONS

Combining certain drugs may alter their action or produce unwanted side effects. Tell your doctor about other drugs you're taking, especially:
• antacids (take 2 to 3 hours before or after taking Pro-Banthine)
• antihistamines
• Cardioquin, Lanoxin, Norpace, Procan SR
• Demerol
• Doriden
• drugs for Parkinson's disease such as Symmetrel
• Nizoral
• phenothiazines such as Thorazine
• tricyclic antidepressants, such as Elavil and Pamelor.

lowing, fever, inability to urinate, fast pulse, fast breathing, high blood pressure (headache and blurred vision), and flushed, hot, dry skin.

Warnings

• Make sure your doctor knows your medical history. You may not be able to take Pro-Banthine if you have other problems, especially glaucoma, an overactive thyroid, high blood pressure, an enlarged prostate, difficulty urinating, myasthenia gravis, or a disorder of the digestive tract, heart, liver, or kidneys.

• If you're pregnant or breast-feeding, check with your doctor before you start taking Pro-Banthine.
• To avoid heatstroke, don't exercise in hot weather.

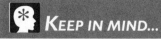

* Take bedtime dose at least 2 hours after last meal.

* Don't drive if vision isn't clear or you're not fully alert.

* Don't exercise in hot weather.

Procan SR

P rocan SR is used to regulate an overactive heart. It makes heart tissues less sensitive, which helps the heart work more efficiently.

Why it's prescribed

Doctors prescribe Procan SR to treat potentially life-threatening irregular heartbeats. It comes in tablets, sustained-release tablets, and capsules. It's also available in an injectable form. Doctors usually prescribe the following amounts for adults.
▶ **For irregular heartbeats,** 500 milligrams to 1 gram every 6 hours.

How to take Procan SR

• Take this drug exactly as your doctor directs at evenly spaced times day and night.
• Take Procan SR with a glass of water 1 hour before or 2 hours after meals. If it upsets your stomach, take it with food or milk.
• Swallow sustained-release tablets whole. Don't break, crush, or chew them.
• Don't stop taking this drug suddenly, even if you feel well, because this could cause a serious heart problem.

If you miss a dose

Take the missed dose if you remember within 2 hours (4 hours if you're taking sustained-release tablets). However, if you don't remember until later, skip the missed dose and take your next dose as scheduled. Don't take a double dose.

PROCAN SR'S OTHER NAMES

Procan SR's generic name is procainamide. Other brand names include Promine, Pronestyl, and Pronestyl-SR.

 SIDE EFFECTS

Call your doctor if you have any of these possible drug side effects. Call *immediately* about any labeled "serious."

Serious: seizures, extremely low blood pressure (severe dizziness and weakness), potentially fatal irregular pulse (palpitations, weakness, fainting), fever, hemolytic anemia (fatigue), bleeding ulcers of mouth, rectum, and vagina.

Common: slow pulse, rash, lupuslike syndrome (muscle aches, weakness, fatigue, weight loss, red rash, sensitivity to light)

Other: hallucinations confusion depression, dizziness, heart dysfunction (irregular pulse, weakness), nausea, vomiting, appetite loss, diarrhea, bitter taste (with high doses), abnormal bleeding, infection

Tip: Don't drive or do anything else that could be dangerous if you're dizzy.

 DRUG INTERACTIONS

Combining certain drugs may alter their action or produce unwanted side effects. Tell your doctor about other drugs you're taking, especially:
• Cordarone
• drugs for cramps or spasms of the stomach or abdomen
• glaucoma drugs such as Pilocar
• myasthenia gravis drugs, such as Prostigmin and Regonol
• Tagamet.

 If you suspect an overdose

Contact your doctor *immediately.* Excessive Procan SR can cause extremely low blood pressure (severe dizziness and weakness), potentially fatal irregular heartbeats and other heart problems, decreased urination, confusion, lethargy, nausea, and vomiting.

Warnings

• Make sure your doctor knows your medical history. You may not be able to take Procan SR if you have other problems, especially liver or kidney disease, asthma, myasthenia gravis, a blood disorder, bone marrow suppression, or lupus.
• If you're pregnant or breast-feeding, tell your doctor before you start taking Procan SR.

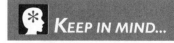 **KEEP IN MIND...**

* Space doses evenly throughout day and night.
* Swallow sustained-release tablets whole.
* Don't stop taking suddenly.

Procardia

Procardia is one of several drugs called calcium channel blockers. It blocks calcium from entering the heart muscle, thereby slowing heart contractions, widening the heart's blood vessels, and allowing more oxygen-carrying blood to reach and nourish the heart.

Why it's prescribed

Doctors prescribe Procardia for chest pain or high blood pressure. It comes in extended-release tablets and capsules. Doctors usually prescribe the following amounts for adults.

▶ **For chest pain,** at first, 10 milligrams (mg) three times a day. Usual effective range is 10 to 20 mg three times a day. Some people may require up to 30 mg four times a day. Maximum dosage is 180 mg a day.

▶ **For high blood pressure,** 30 or 60 mg extended-release capsules once a day, adjusted over 7 to 14 days.

How to take Procardia

• Take this drug exactly as your doctor directs. Keep taking it even when you feel well and don't have chest pain. Don't switch to another brand without consulting your doctor (not all brands have the same effects).

• Swallow tablets or capsules whole. Don't break, crush, or chew

PROCARDIA'S OTHER NAMES

Procardia's generic name is nifedipine. Other brand names include Adalat CC, Procardia XL; and, in Canada, Adalat FT, Adalat P.A., and Nu-Nifed.

 SIDE EFFECTS

Call your doctor if you have any of these possible drug side effects.

Serious: none reported

Common: increased chest pain, dizziness, light-headedness, flushing, headache, nausea, heartburn

Tip: Chest pain may increase when you start taking Procardia or increase dosage; although this is usually temporary, report it immediately to the doctor.

Other: weakness, muscle cramps, fainting, swollen feet or ankles, heart palpitations, stuffy nose, diarrhea, difficulty breathing

 DRUG INTERACTIONS

Combining certain drugs may alter their action or produce unwanted side effects. Tell your doctor about other drugs you're taking, especially:

• beta blockers such as Inderal
• ulcer drugs, such as Tagamet and Zantac.

them. (Don't be alarmed if the empty shell appears in your stool.)

• Don't stop taking Procardia suddenly because your previous problem could return. Your doctor will tell you how to reduce your dosage gradually before stopping.

If you miss a dose

Take the missed dose as soon as possible. However, if it's almost time for your next dose, skip the missed dose and take your next dose as scheduled. Don't take a double dose.

 If you suspect an overdose

Contact your doctor *immediately*. Excessive Procardia can cause widening of the blood vessels and low blood pressure (dizziness and weakness).

X Warnings

• Make sure your doctor knows your medical history. You may not

be able to take Procardia if you have other problems, especially other heart or blood vessel disorders or kidney or liver disease.

• Make sure your doctor knows if you're pregnant or breast-feeding before you begin taking Procardia.

• Follow any special diet or exercise program the doctor prescribes.

• See your doctor regularly so your progress can be checked.

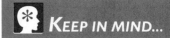 KEEP IN MIND...

∗ Don't break, crush, or chew tablets or capsules.

∗ Don't stop taking unless doctor approves.

∗ Follow special diet and exercise programs.

Prograf is an immune system suppressant. It works by inhibiting white blood cells, which play an important role in immunity.

Why it's prescribed

Doctors prescribe Prograf to prevent organ rejection in people who've received liver transplants. It comes in capsules and an injectable form. Doctors usually prescribe the following amounts.

▶ **To prevent transplant organ rejection,** first oral dose (given 8 to 12 hours after injections stop), 0.15 to 0.3 milligrams (mg) for each 2.2 pounds (lb) of body weight a day divided into two equal doses every 12 hours. (Children: after injections stop, 0.3 mg for each 2.2 lb a day orally on adult schedule, adjusted as needed.)

How to take Prograf

• Take this drug as your doctor directs on an empty stomach.

If you miss a dose

Take the missed dose as soon as possible. But if it's almost time for your next dose, skip the missed dose and go back to your regular dosing schedule. Don't take a double dose.

If you suspect an overdose

Consult your doctor.

Warnings

• Make sure your doctor knows your medical history. You may not be able to take Prograf if you have kidney disease or other problems.
• Make sure your doctor knows if you're pregnant before you begin taking Prograf. Don't breast-feed while taking this drug.

PROGRAF'S OTHER NAME

Prograf's generic name is tacrolimus.

SIDE EFFECTS

Call your doctor if you have any of these possible drug side effects. Call *immediately* about any labeled "serious."

Serious: blood problems (increased bleeding, bruising, chance of infection, fatigue), fluid buildup in lungs (fever, chest pain, difficulty breathing, cough) *Tip:* Avoid people who are ill or infected.

Common: headache, tremor, high blood pressure (headache, blurred vision), diarrhea, nausea, kidney dysfunction (decreased urination), increased blood sugar level (increased thirst, hunger, and urination), pain, fever, weakness

Other: difficulty sleeping, numbness or tingling sensations, swelling of feet or lower legs, constipation, appetite loss, vomiting, abdominal pain, electrolyte imbalances (nausea, diarrhea, muscle weakness, tremor, and tiredness), urinary tract infection (pain on urination), back pain, fluid buildup in abdomen

DRUG INTERACTIONS

Combining certain drugs may alter their action or produce unwanted side effects. Tell your doctor about other drugs you're taking, especially:
• antifungal drugs, such as Diflucan, Lotrimin Cream, and Nizoral
• Barbita, Dilantin, Tegretol
• Biaxin, E-Mycin
• Calan, Cardene, Cardizem
• Danocrine
• drugs that can damage the kidneys, such as Amikin, Fungizone, Garamycin, Myciguent, Netromycin, Platinol, and streptomycin
• Medrol
• Mycobutin
• other drugs that suppress the immune system (except adrenal steroids)
• Parlodel
• Reglan, Tagamet
• Rifadin
• Sandimmune
• viral vaccines.

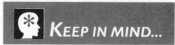

* Avoid people with infections.
* Call doctor if you have an infection or high blood sugar.

Prolastin

Prolastin is made from human blood and is used to replace a certain protein in people with emphysema, whose bodies produce too little of the protein.

Why it's prescribed

Doctors prescribe Prolastin for emphysema caused by too little of the essential protein alpha$_1$-antitrypsin. It's available in an injectable form. Doctors usually prescribe the following amounts for adults.

▶ **For emphysema,** 60 milligrams for each 2.2 pounds of body weight injected into a vein once weekly.

How to take Prolastin

• To make sure this drug works properly, you must get weekly injections.
• You may need to receive this drug regularly for a long time.

If you miss a dose

Reschedule a missed injection as soon as possible.

 If you suspect an overdose

Contact your doctor *immediately*. Excessive Prolastin can cause decreased breathing and slow heart rate.

PROLASTIN'S OTHER NAME

Prolastin's generic name is alpha$_1$-proteinase inhibitor.

 SIDE EFFECTS

Call your doctor if you have any of these possible drug side effects. Call *immediately* about any labeled "serious."

Serious: virus
Tip: This drug is tested for viruses, such as hepatitis B and human immunodeficiency virus, and is treated to reduce the risk of virus transmission. Still, it's a good idea to get the hepatitis B vaccine before you start taking Prolastin, although sometimes there may not be enough time for the hepatitis vaccine to take effect before you receive Prolastin. Be aware that you also may be given hepatitis B immune globulin at the same time as the hepatitis B vaccine. Talk to your doctor about this.

Common: none reported

Other: chills, fever, dizziness, light-headedness
Tip: Chills and fever may occur several hours after you receive Prolastin but are usually mild and only temporary. A fever up to 102° F may occur up to 12 hours after you receive Prolastin and will disappear within 24 hours. If these side effects continue or are bothersome, call your doctor if you develop any of these symptoms.

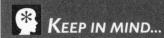 **DRUG INTERACTIONS**

Combining certain drugs may alter their action or produce unwanted side effects. Tell your doctor about other drugs you're using, especially:
• nicotine (don't smoke during Prolastin treatment).

 Warnings

• Make sure your doctor knows your medical history. You may not be able to take Prolastin if you have other medical problems, especially an immune system disorder or an allergy to this type of drug, to other drugs, or to preservatives and dyes.
• If you're pregnant or breast-feeding, tell your doctor before you start taking Prolastin.

KEEP IN MIND...

∗ Get injections regularly.
∗ Get hepatitis B vaccine before starting drug.
∗ Don't smoke while taking this drug.
∗ Consult your doctor if you develop a fever, chills, dizziness, or light-headedness.

Prolixin

Prolixin is used to treat some mental and emotional disorders. It affects the brain, causing sedation and reducing psychosis (mental illness).

Why it's prescribed

Doctors prescribe Prolixin to treat mental or emotional disorders, anxiety, and nausea or vomiting. Prolixin comes in tablets, an elixir, and an oral concentrate. It's also available in an injectable form. Doctors usually prescribe the following amounts for adults.

▶ **For mental or emotional disorders,** at first, 1.25 to 10 milligrams (mg) orally a day divided into equal doses given every 6 to 8 hours, increased cautiously as needed to 20 mg. Maintenance dosage is 1 to 5 mg a day. Older adults should take lower dosages (1 to 2.5 mg a day).

How to take Prolixin

• Follow your doctor's instructions exactly. To avoid stomach upset, take Prolixin with food or a full glass (8 ounces) of water or milk.
• Measure liquid doses with a special dropper. Dilute it in a half glass (4 ounces) of orange juice, grapefruit juice, or water. Don't spill the drug on your skin; it can cause irritation and a rash.
• Several weeks may pass before you notice the full effects of this drug.

SIDE EFFECTS

Call your doctor if you have any of these possible drug side effects. Call *immediately* about any labeled "serious."

Serious: severe muscle stiffness, fever, unusual tiredness or weakness, fast pulse, difficulty breathing, increased sweating, loss of bladder control, seizures, blood problems (increased risk of infection, fever, bleeding ulcers of mouth, rectum, and vagina), rash, anxiety, appetite and weight loss
Tips: Avoid people who may have an infection or be ill. Also avoid contact sports and other activities that pose a high risk of injury.

Common: drowsiness, restlessness, tardive dyskinesia (uncontrolled movements of tongue, mouth, cheeks, jaw, or arms and legs), dizziness (especially when standing up), blurred vision, dry mouth, constipation, inability to urinate, skin sensitivity to sunlight
Tips: Don't drive or do anything else that could be dangerous if your vision isn't clear or if you're not fully alert. Use ice chips or sugarless gum or candy to relieve dry mouth. To prevent skin reactions from sunlight, avoid sun exposure and apply a sunblock and wear protective clothing before going outdoors. To prevent dizziness when standing up, rise slowly to your feet.

Other: sedation; slow, shuffling walk; rigid muscles; tremors; difficulty swallowing, speaking, or chewing; dark urine; menstrual abnormalities; enlarged breasts; ejaculation problems; unusual milk secretion; allergic reaction (rash, fever, swelling, yellow-tinged skin and eyes); weight gain; increased appetite

DRUG INTERACTIONS

Combining certain drugs may alter their action or produce unwanted side effects. Tell your doctor about other drugs you're taking, especially:
• alcohol and other drugs that slow down the nervous system, such as cold and allergy drugs, sedatives, tranquilizers, narcotic pain relievers, barbiturates, seizure drugs, and muscle relaxants
• antacids (take at least 2 hours before or after taking Prolixin)
• blood pressure drugs, such as Aldomet and Catapres
• drugs for abdominal or stomach cramps or spasms
• Lithobid.

PROLIXIN'S OTHER NAMES

Prolixin's generic name is fluphenazine. Other brand names include Permitil, Permitil Concentrate; and, in Canada, Apo-Fluphenazine, Modecate Concentrate, Moditen Enanthate, Moditen HCl, and Moditen HCI-H.P.

• Don't stop taking this drug suddenly because this may make your condition worse. Your doctor may tell you to gradually reduce your dosage before stopping.

If you miss a dose

If you take one dose a day, take the missed dose as soon as possible, then take your next dose as sched-

Continued on next page ▶

uled. However, if you don't remember until the next day, skip the missed dose and take your next dose as scheduled. If you take more than one dose a day, take the missed dose as soon as possible. However, if you don't remember within an hour or so, skip the missed dose and take your next dose as scheduled. Don't take a double dose.

If you suspect an overdose

Contact your doctor *immediately*. Excessive Prolixin can cause very deep sleep, possibly coma, rapidly changing high blood pressure (headache, blurred vision) or low blood pressure (dizziness, weakness), restlessness, muscle spasms, involuntary muscle movements, agitation, seizures, irregular pulse, and fever or low body temperature.

Warnings

• Make sure your doctor knows your medical history. You may not be able to take Prolixin if you have other problems, especially heart or blood vessel disease, lung disease, seizures, Parkinson's disease, stomach ulcers, liver disease, pheochromocytoma, an enlarged prostate, difficulty urinating, blood disease, breast cancer, glaucoma, or a history of alcohol abuse.
• If you're pregnant or breast-feeding, check with your doctor before you start taking Prolixin.
• Be aware that older adults may be especially prone to Prolixin's side effects.
• Before surgery (including dental surgery) or emergency care, tell the doctor or dentist that you're taking Prolixin.
• See your doctor regularly so your progress and drug effects can be monitored.

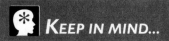

KEEP IN MIND...

* Take with food or full glass of water or milk.
* Stand up slowly to avoid dizziness.
* Don't spill liquid form on skin.
* Don't stop taking suddenly.
* Don't drive if your vision isn't clear or you're not fully alert.

Propacet 100

Propacet 100 is a combination drug prescribed for relief of pain when nonprescription pain relievers are ineffective. Propacet 100 contains a narcotic. Although the complete action of the drug is unknown, it seems to block pain impulses from reaching the brain, leading to pain relief.

Why it's prescribed

Doctors prescribe Propacet 100 for mild pain relief with or without fever. It comes in tablets. Doctors usually prescribe the following amounts for adults.

▶ **For mild pain relief,** 1 tablet every 4 hours as needed. Maximum recommended dosage is 6 tablets in 24 hours.

How to take Propacet 100

• Take Propacet 100 exactly as prescribed by your doctor. Don't increase the amount or frequency without speaking to your doctor.
• Store the drug at room temperature away from heat, light, and moisture.

If you miss a dose

Not applicable because this drug is taken only as needed.

PROPACET 100'S OTHER NAMES

Propacet 100 is a combination of the generic drugs acetaminophen and propoxyphene napsylate. Another brand name is Darvocet-N 100. This drug also comes as Darvocet-N 50, containing half the amount of acetaminophen and propoxyphene napsylate.

 SIDE EFFECTS

Call your doctor if you have any of these possible drug side effects. Call *immediately* about any labeled "serious."

Serious: slow and shallow breaths; extreme tiredness; physical and psychological dependence; seizures; cold, clammy skin; shortness of breath; slow heartbeat

Common: dizziness, nausea, vomiting, drowsiness
Tips: When lying or sitting, get up slowly to avoid dizziness. Take with food to avoid nausea. Avoid driving or other activities that require alertness until you know how Propacet 100 affects you.

Other: constipation, inability to urinate
Tip: Increase fluids to avoid constipation.

 DRUG INTERACTIONS

Combining certain drugs may alter their action or produce unwanted side effects. Tell your doctor about other drugs you're taking, especially:
• alcohol
• antidepressants, such as Eldepryl, Pamelor and Parnate
• tranquilizers, such as Ativan and Xanax
• Tylenol and other products containing acetaminophen (can cause liver damage).

If you suspect an overdose

Contact your doctor *immediately*. Excessive Propacet 100 can cause shallow, slow breathing; deep sleep; and slow or difficult waking.

Warnings

• Make sure your doctor knows your medical history. You may not be able to take Propacet 100 if you have other medical problems. Don't take it if you have a history of depression, suicidal thoughts, or drug addiction. As a narcotic pain reliever, it can depress your mood and become habit-forming.
• Don't take this drug if you're allergic to Tylenol.

• If you're pregnant or breast-feeding, tell your doctor before taking Propacet 100.
• Be aware that older adults may be especially prone to this drug's side effects.

 KEEP IN MIND...

∗ Take only as prescribed.
∗ Avoid alcohol and acetaminophen.
∗ Can cause drowsiness.
∗ Can be habit-forming.

Propine

Propine is an eye medication. It enlarges the pupils and paralyzes the eye's fine-focusing muscles. It also decreases aqueous humor (a fluid in the eye) and reduces pressure within the eye, relieving glaucoma.

Why it's prescribed

Doctors prescribe Propine for glaucoma. It comes in eyedrops. Doctors usually prescribe the following amounts for adults.

▶ **For glaucoma,** at first, 1 drop of 0.1% solution every 12 hours, adjusted according to person's response.

How to use Propine

• Use this drug exactly as your doctor directs.

• Always wash your hands before and after using the eyedrops.

• Don't touch the dropper tip to your eye or any other surface.

• After instilling the drops, apply light finger pressure to the inner corner of your eye for 1 or 2 minutes to help your eye absorb the drug.

• If your container has a compliance cap (C cap), make sure the number 1 or the correct day of the week appears in the window on the cap before you start using the drug. When replacing the cap, rotate the bottle until the cap clicks to the next position.

If you miss a dose

Instill the missed dose as soon as possible. However, if it's almost

PROPINE'S OTHER NAME

Propine's generic name is dipivefrin.

SIDE EFFECTS

Call your doctor if you have any of these possible drug side effects.

Serious: none reported

Common: none reported

Other: fast pulse, high blood pressure (headache, blurred vision), eye burning or stinging

DRUG INTERACTIONS

Combining certain drugs may alter their action or produce unwanted side effects. Tell your doctor about other drugs you're taking, especially:

• Crystodigin, Lanoxin
• Daranide, Neptazane
• Diamox
• eye drugs, such as Betoptic, Blocadren, OptiPranolol, and Timoptic
• general anesthetics.

time for your next dose, skip the missed dose and instill your next dose as scheduled. Don't use a double dose.

If you suspect an overdose

Contact your doctor *immediately.* Accidental ingestion of Propine can cause high blood pressure (headache, blurred vision), a fast or slow pulse, irregular heartbeats, chest pain, anxiety, nervousness, difficulty sleeping, muscle tremor, bleeding in the brain (headache, vision change, vomiting, lethargy), seizures, decreased consciousness, appetite loss, nausea, vomiting, and kidney failure (decreased urination).

Warnings

• Make sure your doctor knows your medical history. You may not be able to use Propine if you have other medical problems, especially

other eye problems, asthma, or heart or blood vessel disease, or if you've ever had an unusual reaction to a medicine containing epinephrine.

• Make sure your doctor knows if you're pregnant or breast-feeding before you begin taking Propine.

• If you're having surgery with general anesthesia, tell your doctor you take Propine. The combination of Propine and certain anesthetics can cause an irregular pulse.

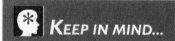

* Wash hands before and after using.

* Don't touch dropper to eye or other surface.

* After each dose, rotate bottle until compliance cap clicks to next position.

Propulsid

Propulsid is used to treat certain stomach conditions and intestinal problems. It increases the release of acetylcholine, a substance produced in the intestine's lining that causes increased contractions and movements of the stomach and intestines.

Why it's prescribed

Doctors prescribe Propulsid to relieve heartburn and other symptoms that occur when stomach contents flow backward into the esophagus (a condition called gastroesophageal reflux disease). It comes in tablets. Doctors usually prescribe the following amounts for adults.

▶ **For gastroesophageal reflux disease (GERD),** at first, 10 milligrams (mg) four times a day, increased to 20 mg four times a day, as needed.

How to take Propulsid

• Take this drug exactly as your doctor directs; usually, with a beverage 15 minutes before meals and at bedtime.

If you miss a dose

Take the missed dose as soon as possible. However, if it's almost time for your next dose, skip the missed dose and take your next dose as scheduled. Don't take a double dose.

PROPULSID'S OTHER NAME

Propulsid's generic name is cisapride.

 SIDE EFFECTS

Call your doctor if you have any of these possible drug side effects.

Serious: none reported

Common: headache, diarrhea, abdominal pain

Other: fast pulse, nausea, constipation, gas, frequent or urgent urination, vaginal infection, runny nose, sinus inflammation, cough, rash, itching, flulike symptoms, pain, fever

Tip: Drink extra fluids and eat high-fiber foods, such as whole grains, fruits, and vegetables, to avoid constipation.

 DRUG INTERACTIONS

Combining certain drugs may alter their action or produce unwanted side effects. Tell your doctor about other drugs you're taking, especially:

• alcohol
• anticoagulants (blood thinners) such as Coumadin
• antifungal drugs, such as Monistat I.V., Nizoral, and Sporanox
• drugs for abdominal or stomach cramps or spasms
• tranquilizers and sleeping pills
• Troleandomycin
• ulcer drugs, such as Tagamet and Zantac.

 If you suspect an overdose

Contact your doctor immediately. Excessive Propulsid can cause retching; rumbling, gurgling, or tinkling bowel sounds; gas; and more frequent passage of stool and urine.

Warnings

• Make sure your doctor knows your medical history. You may not be able to take Propulsid if you have other problems, especially stomach or abdominal bleeding, a blockage in the bowel, seizures, or kidney or liver disease.

• If you're pregnant or breast-feeding, tell your doctor before you start taking Propulsid.

• Be aware that older adults may be especially prone to Propulsid's side effects.

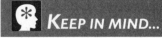 **KEEP IN MIND...**

∗ Take 15 minutes before meals and at bedtime.

∗ Consult doctor about drinking alcohol.

∗ Drink extra fluids and eat high-fiber foods to avoid constipation.

Propylthiouracil

Propylthiouracil controls overactive thyroid, a condition in which the thyroid gland produces too much thyroid hormone.

Why it's prescribed

Doctors prescribe Propylthiouracil to treat overactive thyroid and related conditions and to prepare the thyroid for surgery. It comes in tablets. Doctors usually prescribe the following amounts for adults; children's dosages appear in parentheses.

▶ **For overactive thyroid,** 100 to 150 milligrams (mg) three times a day. Maintenance dosage is 100 to 150 mg a day divided into three equal doses. (Children over age 10: 150 to 300 mg a day divided into three equal doses. Children ages 6 to 10: 50 to 150 mg a day divided into three equal doses. Maintenance dosage depends on response.)

▶ **For emergency treatment of uncontrolled thyroid hormone release or before surgery,** 200 mg every 4 to 6 hours on first day; once symptoms are fully controlled, dosage gradually reduced to usual maintenance levels. (Children: same as adults.)

How to take Propylthiouracil

• Take this drug exactly as your doctor directs. Take it with meals to prevent stomach upset.
• Don't stop taking this drug without consulting your doctor.

PROPYLTHIOURACIL'S OTHER NAME

Propylthiouracil is this drug's generic name. A brand name in Canada is Propyl-Thyracil.

 SIDE EFFECTS

Call your doctor if you have any of these possible drug side effects. Call *immediately* about any labeled "serious."

Serious: blood problems (fever, chills, infection, bleeding, and bruising); liver damage (yellow-tinged skin and eyes, nausea, vomiting)

Common: nausea, vomiting

Other: headache, drowsiness, vertigo, blood vessel inflammation, vision disturbances, diarrhea, enlarged salivary glands, loss of taste, rash, hives, itching, joint and muscle pain, underactive thyroid (depression, cold intolerance, hard swelling)

DRUG INTERACTIONS

Combining certain drugs may alter their action or produce unwanted side effects. Tell your doctor about other drugs you're taking, especially:
• certain steroids, such as Cortef, Decadron, Orasone, and Prelone
• Lithobid
• SSKI (saturated solution of potassium iodide).

If you miss a dose

Take the missed dose as soon as possible. But if it's almost time for your next dose, take both doses together, then go back to your regular schedule. If you miss more than one dose, consult your doctor.

 If you suspect an overdose

Contact your doctor *immediately.* Excessive Propylthiouracil can cause nausea, vomiting, stomach upset, fever, headache, joint pain, itching, swelling, and blood problems (fatigue, bleeding, bruising, infection, chills, and fever).

 Warnings

• Make sure your doctor knows your medical history. You may not be able to take Propylthiouracil if you have other medical problems.
• If you're pregnant or breast-feeding, check with your doctor before using this drug.
• Avoid iodine-containing foods, such as iodized salt and shellfish, while taking this drug.

KEEP IN MIND...

* Take with meals to prevent stomach upset.

* Don't stop taking unless doctor approves.

* Avoid eating iodine-containing foods.

* Call doctor about injury, infection, or illness.

Proscar

Proscar is one of several drugs called enzyme inhibitors. It blocks an enzyme that causes noncancerous prostate gland enlargement in men.

Why it's prescribed

Doctors prescribe Proscar to reduce the size of an enlarged prostate. It comes in tablets. Doctors usually prescribe the following amounts for adults.

▶ **For enlarged prostate,** 5 milligrams a day.

How to take Proscar

• Take this drug exactly as your doctor directs, preferably at the same time each day. You may crush the tablets to make them easier to swallow.

• You may need to take Proscar for 6 months to find out if it will improve your condition.

• Proscar decreases the size of your prostate only as long as you take it. Don't stop taking it without consulting your doctor.

If you miss a dose

Take the missed dose as soon as possible. However, if it's almost time for your next dose, skip the missed dose and take your next dose as scheduled. Don't take a double dose.

 If you suspect an overdose

Consult your doctor.

PROSCAR'S OTHER NAME

Proscar's generic name is finasteride.

 SIDE EFFECTS

Call your doctor if you have any of these possible drug side effects.

Serious: none reported

Common: none reported

Other: impotence, decreased amount of ejaculate, reduced sex drive
Tip: Although Proscar may decrease the amount of your ejaculate, it shouldn't impair your normal sexual function.

 DRUG INTERACTIONS

Combining certain drugs may alter their action or produce unwanted side effects. Tell your doctor about other drugs you're taking, especially:

• amphetamines
• antihistamines such as Benadryl
• drugs for asthma (such as Theo-Dur), colds, or sinus problems
• Norpace
• Phenergan
• Pro-Banthine
• Pronestyl
• Quinidine
• Symmetrel
• Tegretol.

Warnings

• Make sure your doctor knows your medical history. You may not be able to take Proscar if you have other problems, especially liver disease.

• If your female sexual partner is pregnant or planning to become pregnant, don't allow her to handle crushed Proscar tablets or come in contact with your semen. This drug can cause abnormal genitals in male infants of women exposed to this drug.

• Keep all scheduled doctor's appointments. Your doctor will need to check you regularly for changes in prostate size.

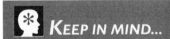 **KEEP IN MIND...**

＊ Crush tablets to make them easier to swallow.

＊ Keep taking drug to keep prostate size down.

＊ Don't expose pregnant women (or women attempting to become pregnant) to this drug.

ProSom

ProSom is one of several drugs called benzodiazepines. It slows down the nervous system, causing a calming effect or inducing sleep.

Why it's prescribed

Doctors prescribe ProSom to induce sleep in people with insomnia. It comes in tablets. Doctors usually prescribe the following amounts for adults.

▶ **For insomnia,** 1 milligram (mg) at bedtime. Some people may require 2 mg.

How to take ProSom

• Take ProSom exactly as directed. Taking too much can lead to dependence or make the drug ineffective.

• Call your doctor if you think the drug isn't working well, especially if you've been taking it every night for several weeks.

If you miss a dose

Skip the missed dose and take your next dose as scheduled. Don't take a double dose.

 If you suspect an overdose

Contact your doctor *immediately.* Excessive ProSom can cause sleepiness, confusion, decreased reflexes, decreased or absent breathing, low blood pressure (dizziness, weakness), impaired coordination, slurred speech, seizures, or coma.

PROSOM'S OTHER NAME

ProSom's generic name is estazolam.

 SIDE EFFECTS

Call your doctor if you have any of these possible drug side effects.

Serious: none reported

Common: daytime drowsiness, sleepiness, lack of energy, reduced muscle activity
Tip: Until you know how this drug affects you, don't drive or do anything else that could be dangerous if you're not fully alert.

Other: fatigue, dizziness, headache; after you stop taking ProSom, stomach upset, irritability, nervousness, trouble sleeping

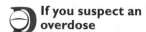 **DRUG INTERACTIONS**

Combining certain drugs may alter their action or produce unwanted side effects. Tell your doctor about other drugs you're taking, especially:
• alcohol and other drugs that slow down the nervous system, such as cold and allergy drugs, sedatives, tranquilizers, narcotic pain relievers, barbiturates, seizure drugs, and muscle relaxants
• Antabuse
• birth control pills (use different birth control method while taking ProSom)
• Laniazid
• Rifadin
• Tagamet
• Theo-Dur
• tobacco.

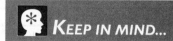 **Warnings**

• Make sure your doctor knows your medical history. You may not be able to take ProSom if you have other problems, especially a brain disorder, asthma or another lung disease, kidney or liver disease, myasthenia gravis, seizures, breathing problems while sleeping, depression, or a history of alcohol or drug dependence.
• If you're pregnant or breast-feeding, check with your doctor before you start taking ProSom.
• Be aware that older adults may be especially prone to ProSom's side effects.

• Check with your doctor at least every 4 months to find out if you need to keep taking ProSom.

KEEP IN MIND...

* Take only as much and as often as prescribed.

* Don't drive if you're not fully alert.

* Don't use birth control pills for contraception while taking ProSom.

P rostaphlin is a penicillin-type antibiotic that fights bacterial infection by rupturing cells of the bacteria. This kills the bacteria or prevents their growth.

Why it's prescribed

Doctors prescribe Prostaphlin for bacterial infections throughout the body. It comes in capsules and an oral solution. It's also available in an injectable form. Doctors usually prescribe the following amounts for adults; children's dosages appear in parentheses.

▶ **For bacterial infections,** 500 milligrams (mg) orally every 4 to 6 hours. (Children weighing over 80 pounds [lb]: same as adults. Children weighing 80 lb or less: 50 to 100 mg for each 2.2 lb of body weight orally, divided into equal doses given every 6 hours.)

How to take Prostaphlin

• Take this drug exactly as your doctor directs for the full time prescribed. Take it with a full glass (8 ounces) of water 1 hour before or 2 to 3 hours after meals.
• For best results, take doses at evenly spaced times day and night.

If you miss a dose

Take the missed dose as soon as possible. However, if it's almost time for your next dose, skip the missed

dose and take your next dose as scheduled. Don't take a double dose.

 If you suspect an overdose

Contact your doctor *immediately.* Excessive Prostaphlin can cause seizures, pain, tingling, and loss of sensation.

 Warnings

• Make sure your doctor knows your medical history. You may not be able to take Prostaphlin if you have other problems, especially heart failure, asthma, hay fever, hives, kidney disease, or

stomach or intestinal disease, or if you've ever had an unusual reaction to penicillin or any other antibiotic.
• If you're pregnant or breast-feeding, tell your doctor before you start taking Prostaphlin.

 SIDE EFFECTS

Call your doctor if you have any of these possible drug side effects. Call *immediately* about any labeled "serious."

Serious: seizures, blood problems (fatigue, increased risk of infection, fever, and chills), serious allergic reaction (hives, itching, closing of throat, shock, swelling of face, lips, hands, and feet), liver problems (yellow-tinged skin and eyes, nausea, vomiting, diarrhea)
Tip: Avoid people who are ill or infected.

Common: diarrhea
Tip: Don't take a drug for diarrhea without consulting your doctor. Doing so may cause your diarrhea to worsen.
Other: muscle weakness or spasms, changes in sensations, pain, mouth sores, kidney problems (bloody or absent urine, fever), white patches on tongue or mouth

DRUG INTERACTIONS

Combining certain drugs may alter their action or produce unwanted side effects. Tell your doctor about other drugs you're taking, especially:
• antibiotics, such as Amikin, Garamycin, Myciguent, Netromycin, and streptomycin
• Rifadin.

PROSTAPHLIN'S OTHER NAMES

Prostaphlin's generic name is oxacillin sodium. Another brand name is Bactocill.

KEEP IN MIND...

∗ Take with full glass of water.
∗ Don't take diarrhea medicine unless doctor approves.
∗ Avoid people who are ill or infected.

Prostigmin is used to treat myasthenia gravis, a disorder in which the muscles become weak and easily fatigued. The drug works by increasing amounts of acetylcholine, a substance in the nervous system.

Why it's prescribed

Doctors prescribe Prostigmin to improve myasthenia gravis symptoms. It comes in tablets. It's also available in an injectable form. Doctors usually prescribe the following amounts for adults; children's dosages appear in parentheses.

▶ **For myasthenia gravis,** 15 to 30 milligrams (mg) orally three times a day. (Children: 7.5 to 15 mg orally three or four times a day.) Dosage is highly individualized, depending on the person's response. Treatment may be required day and night and continue for the person's entire life.

How to take Prostigmin

• Take this drug exactly as directed. To avoid stomach upset, take it with food or milk.

If you miss a dose

Take the missed dose as soon as possible. But if it's almost time for your next dose, skip the missed dose and take your next dose as scheduled. Don't take a double dose.

PROSTIGMIN'S OTHER NAME

Prostigmin's generic name is neostigmine.

SIDE EFFECTS

Call your doctor if you have any of these possible drug side effects. Call *immediately* about any labeled "serious."

Serious: decreased and shallow breathing, wheezing and closing of throat

Common: nausea, vomiting, diarrhea, abdominal cramps, muscle cramps

Other: dizziness, headache, muscle weakness or twitching, confusion, jitters, sweating, slow pulse, small pupils, excessive tearing, blurred vision, excessive salivation, frequent urination, rash

DRUG INTERACTIONS

Combining certain drugs may alter their action or produce unwanted side effects. Tell your doctor about other drugs you're taking, especially:
• antibiotics, such as Amikin, Garamycin, Myciguent, Netromycin, and streptomycin
• atropine sulfate
• drugs for abdominal or stomach cramps or spasms
• Procan
• Quinaglute Dura-tabs
• steroids.

If you suspect an overdose

Contact your doctor *immediately.* Excessive Prostigmin can cause headache, nausea, vomiting, diarrhea, blurred vision, small pupils, excessive tearing, wheezing and closing up of the throat, poor coordination, excessive sweating, muscle weakness and twitching, cramps, paralysis, slow or fast pulse, excessive salivation, restlessness, agitation, and low blood pressure (dizziness, weakness).

Warnings

• Make sure your doctor knows your medical history. You may not be able to take Prostigmin if you have other problems, especially bowel or urinary tract blockage, stomach ulcer, urinary tract infection, asthma, slow pulse, seizures, irregular heartbeats, or an overactive thyroid.
• If you're pregnant, tell your doctor before you start taking Prostigmin.

 KEEP IN MIND...

* Take with food or milk.
* Carry medical identification stating that you have myasthenia gravis.

Protropin

Protropin is an artificial human growth hormone. This hormone stimulates normal growth in children. It replaces the hormone and stimulates the growth of bones, muscles, and organs.

Why it's prescribed

Doctors prescribe Protropin to stimulate growth in children whose bodies don't produce enough growth hormone. It comes in a powder that is reconstituted into an injectable solution. Doctors usually prescribe the following amounts for children.

▶ **For long-term treatment of growth hormone deficiency,** by injection three times a week.

How to take Protropin

• If you're giving your child injections at home, closely follow your doctor's instructions.
• Don't use cloudy solution; it has begun to deteriorate.
• When reconstituting the drug, swirl the vial gently to dissolve the medicine. Don't shake the vial.
• Store the reconstituted vial in the refrigerator. Be sure to use it within 7 days.

If you miss a dose

This drug is usually given every other day. Administer a missed dose as soon as possible.

PROTROPIN'S OTHER NAME

Protropin's generic name is somatrem.

 SIDE EFFECTS

Call your doctor if you have any of these possible drug side effects.

Serious: none reported

Common: none reported

Other: underactive thyroid (depression, cold intolerance, hard swelling), high blood sugar level (fatigue, frequent urination, excessive thirst, dry skin), headache, nausea, vomiting, allergic reaction (itching, rash), failure to respond to treatment and lack of bone growth, limp, pain or swelling at injection site, pain in hip or knee

 DRUG INTERACTIONS

Combining certain drugs may alter their action or produce unwanted side effects. Tell your doctor about other drugs you're taking, especially:
• anabolic steroids
• estrogens
• glucocorticoids, such as Beclovent, Decadron, and Medrol
• thyroid hormones

 If you suspect an overdose

Contact your doctor *immediately.* Excessive Protropin can cause too much growth (gigantism) in children. If taken by people whose bodies produce normal amounts of growth hormone, Protropin can cause enlarged bones of the face, jaw, arms, and legs; enlarged organs; diabetes; hardening of the arteries; and high blood pressure (headache, blurred vision).

 Warnings

• Make sure your doctor knows your child's medical history. The child may not be able to take Protropin if he or she has other problems, especially an underactive thyroid, which can interfere with the effects of growth hormone.
• Have your child see the doctor regularly to check his or her progress and monitor for side effects.
• Keep this drug out of the reach of children to prevent the serious side effects that can result when Protropin is taken by people with normal growth.

 KEEP IN MIND...

* Have child see doctor regularly.
* Store reconstituted vial in refrigerator.
* Give drug only by injection.

Proventil

Proventil is a bronchodilator that relaxes muscles in the lung passages.

Why it's prescribed

Doctors prescribe Proventil to prevent and treat bronchospasm (closing of the throat) such as in asthma. It comes in an aerosol inhaler, solution for inhalation, capsules for inhalation, tablets, sustained-release tablets, and a syrup. Doctors usually prescribe the following amounts.

▶ **To prevent or treat bronchospasm,** in adults and children age 12 and older: 1 or 2 puffs of aerosol inhaler every 4 to 6 hours; or 2.5 milligrams (mg) of solution for inhalation three or four times a day by nebulizer; or 200 to 400 micrograms (mcg) of capsules for inhalation every 4 to 6 hours; or 1 to 3 tablets three or four times a day; or 1 or 2 sustained-release tablets every 12 hours; or (adults under age 65 and children over age 14) 2 to 4 teaspoons (tsp) syrup three or four times a day.
• Children ages 6 to 12: 1 tablet three or four times a day.
• Children ages 6 to 13 and adults over age 65: 1 tsp syrup three or four times a day.
• Children ages 2 to 5: 0.1 mg syrup for each 2.2 pounds of body weight three times a day.

▶ **To prevent exercise-induced asthma in adults,** 2 inhalations 15 minutes before exercise.

How to take Proventil

• Take this drug exactly as your doctor orders. Don't take more than recommended.

PROVENTIL'S OTHER NAMES

Proventil's generic name is albuterol. Another brand name is Ventolin.

SIDE EFFECTS

Call your doctor if you have any of these possible drug side effects. Call *immediately* about any labeled "serious."

Serious: bronchospasm (wheezing, closing of throat), rapid heartbeat, palpitations, high blood pressure (headache, blurred vision)
Tip: Repeated use of Proventil can sometimes *cause* bronchospasm. If it does, stop using the drug and call your doctor right away.

Common: tremor, nervousness, dizziness, headache, insomnia

Other: drying and irritation of nose, mouth, and throat; heartburn; nausea; vomiting; muscle cramps
Tip: Use a cool-mist humidifier to prevent dryness.

DRUG INTERACTIONS

Combining certain drugs may alter their action or produce unwanted side effects. Tell your doctor about other drugs you're taking, especially:
• central nervous system stimulants, such as caffeine and amphetamines (diet pills)
• drugs for depression, such as MAO inhibitors and tricyclic antidepressants
• Inderal and other beta blockers
• Larodopa.

• If you're using an aerosol inhaler and take more than 1 inhalation, wait at least 2 minutes between doses.
• If you're also using a steroid inhaler, use Proventil first; then wait at least 5 minutes before using the steroid.

If you miss a dose

Take the missed dose as soon as possible. If you have more doses scheduled for that day, space them at equal intervals. Don't take a double dose.

If you suspect an overdose

Contact your doctor *immediately.* Excessive Proventil can cause angina (chest pain), high blood pressure (headache, blurred vision), and seizures.

Warnings

• Make sure your doctor knows your medical history. You may not be able to take Proventil if you have heart or blood vessel problems, an overactive thyroid, diabetes, or a drug allergy.
• If you have trouble breathing after using Proventil, call your doctor.

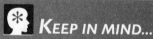

KEEP IN MIND...

∗ Use inhaler properly.
∗ Call doctor if breathing doesn't improve.
∗ Wait at least 2 minutes between inhalations.

Provera

Provera is a progestin (female hormone) that suppresses ovulation, causes cervical mucus to thicken, and regulates menstruation. It may also inhibit cancers of the uterus and kidneys.

Why it's prescribed

Doctors prescribe Provera to regulate the menstrual cycle; to treat endometriosis, abnormal uterine bleeding caused by hormonal imbalance, and some cancers of the uterus and kidneys; and to prevent pregnancy. It comes in tablets. It's also available in an injectable form. Doctors usually prescribe the following amounts for adults.

▶ **For abnormal uterine bleeding,** 5 to 10 milligrams (mg) orally a day for 5 to 10 days, starting on day 16 of menstrual cycle. In women who also have received estrogen, 10 mg a day for 10 days, starting on day 16 of cycle.

▶ **For absent menstruation,** 5 to 10 mg orally a day for 5 to 10 days.

▶ **For birth control,** 150 mg injected into a muscle once every 3 months.

How to take Provera

• Take this drug exactly as your doctor directs. Don't take more of it and don't take it longer than ordered.

If you miss a dose

Take the missed dose as soon as possible (unless you're taking Provera

PROVERA'S OTHER NAMES

Provera's generic name is medroxyprogesterone acetate. Other brand names include Amen, Curretab, and Cycrin.

 ## SIDE EFFECTS

Call your doctor if you have any of these possible drug side effects. Call *immediately* about any labeled "serious."

Serious: blood clot in lung (labored breathing, chest pain, rapid pulse, productive cough, slight fever), high blood pressure (headache; sudden slurring of speech, blurred vision; weakness, numbness, or pain in arm or leg)

Common: none reported

Other: dizziness, migraines, lethargy, depression, swelling, nausea, vomiting, abdominal cramps, changes in menstrual cycle, abnormal vaginal secretions, fibrous uterine growth, vaginal yeast infection, tan or brown pigmentation of face, rash or abscesses, high blood sugar level (fatigue, increased thirst and urination), decreased sex drive; breast tenderness, enlargement, or secretion

 ## DRUG INTERACTIONS

Combining certain drugs may alter their action or produce unwanted side effects. Tell your doctor about other drugs you're taking, especially:

• Cytadren
• Parlodel
• Rifadin.

for birth control). But if it's almost time for your next dose, skip the missed dose and take your next dose as scheduled. Don't take a double dose.

 ## If you suspect an overdose

Consult your doctor.

 ## Warnings

• Make sure your doctor knows your medical history. You may not be able to take Provera if you have a history of blood clots, severe liver disease, breast or genital cancer, or abnormal vaginal bleeding.

• Don't take Provera if you're pregnant or breast-feeding. If you become pregnant while taking Provera, stop using the drug *immediately* because it may harm the fetus.

• Contact your doctor if your menstrual period doesn't start within 45 days of your last period or if vaginal bleeding lasts an unusually long time.

KEEP IN MIND...

∗ Call doctor if menstrual period doesn't start within 45 days of last period.

∗ Call doctor if you develop symptoms of blood clot.

∗ Stop taking Provera at once if you become pregnant.

Prozac

Prozac is used to treat depression and other mental disorders. It's thought to work by increasing the level of serotonin, an important chemical in the brain.

Why it's prescribed

Doctors prescribe Prozac to help relieve depression and to treat obsessive-compulsive disorder. It comes in pulvules (which resemble capsules) and an oral solution. Doctors usually prescribe the following amounts for adults.

► **For depression or obsessive-compulsive disorder,** at first, 20 milligrams (mg) in the morning, increased according to person's response. May be taken twice a day (morning and noon). Maximum dosage is 80 mg a day.

How to take Prozac

• Take this drug exactly as prescribed. Avoid taking it in the afternoon because it may cause nervousness and difficulty sleeping.
• Four weeks or more may pass before you begin to notice the effects of this drug.

If you miss a dose

Skip the missed dose and take your next dose as scheduled. Don't take a double dose.

 ## If you suspect an overdose

Contact your doctor *immediately*. Excessive Prozac can cause agitation, restlessness, expansive mood, hyperactivity, nausea, and vomiting.

PROZAC'S OTHER NAME

Prozac's generic name is fluoxetine.

 ## SIDE EFFECTS

Call your doctor if you have any of these possible drug side effects. Call *immediately* about any labeled "serious."

Serious: palpitations, rash, hives, itching, difficulty breathing

Common: nervousness, anxiety, difficulty sleeping, headache, drowsiness, dizziness, weakness, tremors, nausea, diarrhea, dry mouth, appetite loss, weight loss

Tips: Don't drive or do anything else that could be dangerous if you're dizzy or drowsy. To relieve dry mouth, use ice chips or sugarless gum or candy.

Other: abnormal dreams, flushed skin, slow pulse, stuffy nose, sore throat, cough, sinus inflammation, vision disturbances, ringing in ears, constipation, abdominal pain, vomiting, taste change, gas, increased appetite, sexual dysfunction, inability to urinate, upper respiratory tract infection, flulike symptoms, muscle pain, weight loss, swelling, swollen glands, sweating

DRUG AND FOOD INTERACTIONS

Combining certain drugs and foods may alter drug action or produce unwanted side effects. Tell your doctor about your diet and other drugs you're taking, especially:
• antidepressants called MAO inhibitors, such as Nardil and Parnate (don't take within 14 days of Prozac)
• Coumadin, Serozone
• Dilantin, Tegretol
• foods high in tryptophan, including meats, poultry, fish, liver, kidney, eggs, nuts, peanut butter, broad beans, and wheat germ
• insulin and oral diabetes drugs
• Lithobid
• Tambocor
• tricyclic antidepressants, such as Elavil and Pamelor
• Velban.

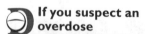 **Warnings**

• Make sure your doctor knows your medical history. You may not be able to take Prozac if you have other problems, especially diabetes, kidney or liver disease, or seizures.
• If you're breast-feeding, check with your doctor before you start taking Prozac.

 ## KEEP IN MIND...

* Take in morning.
* Avoid foods high in tryptophan.
* Don't drive if you feel dizzy or drowsy.

Pulmozyme

Pulmozyme, a respiratory drug, thins the mucus in the lungs and makes it more elastic. This eases breathing in people with cystic fibrosis, in which thick mucus blocks the airways.

Why it's prescribed

Doctors prescribe Pulmozyme to make breathing easier and to help prevent respiratory infections in people with cystic fibrosis. It comes in a solution for inhalation. Doctors usually prescribe the following amounts for adults and children age 5 and older.

▶ **To improve respiratory function and ward off respiratory infections in cystic fibrosis,** 1 ampule (2.5 milligrams) inhaled once a day.

How to take Pulmozyme

• Take this drug exactly as your doctor directs. Make sure you understand how to use this drug in the nebulizer.
• Look at the drug closely. If it looks cloudy or discolored, discard it.
• If you receive this drug in containers called ampules, insert an ampule into the nebulizer. Then put the mouthpiece in your mouth, squeeze the nebulizer, and inhale. This will spray the drug into your mouth so it can flow into your lungs. Read the label directions to see how many times to squeeze the nebulizer.
• Breathe only through your mouth when using the nebulizer. If this is difficult, use a nose clip.

PULMOZYME'S OTHER NAME

Pulmozyme's generic name is dornase alfa recombinant.

SIDE EFFECTS

Call your doctor if you have any of these possible drug side effects. Call *immediately* about any labeled "serious."

Serious: chest pain

Common: sore throat

Other: voice changes, hoarseness, pinkeye, rash, hives

DRUG INTERACTIONS

Combining certain drugs may alter their action or produce unwanted side effects. Tell your doctor about other drugs you're taking.

• If you begin coughing during treatment, turn off the nebulizer without spilling the drug. To resume treatment, turn on the nebulizer and keep breathing through the mouthpiece until the nebulizer cup is empty or mist is no longer produced.
• Use only the following nebulizers and compressors with Pulmozyme: Hudson T Up-draft II disposable jet nebulizer, Marquest Acorn II disposable jet nebulizer used with the Pulmo-Aide compressor, or PARI LC Je⁺ reusable nebulizer used with the PARI PRONEB compressor.
• To gain the full benefits, use Pulmozyme every day. But remember that the drug's full effects may not occur for weeks or months.

If you miss a dose

Take the missed dose as soon as possible. However, if it's almost time for your next dose, skip the missed dose and take your next dose as scheduled. Don't take a double dose.

If you suspect an overdose

Contact your doctor *immediately*. Excessive Pulmozyme can cause severe high blood pressure (headache, blurred vision).

Warnings

• Make sure your doctor knows your medical history. You may not be able to take Pulmozyme if you have any drug allergies.
• If you're pregnant or breast-feeding, tell your doctor before you start taking Pulmozyme.
• Keep Pulmozyme refrigerated. Throw out the opened ampule after you take the prescribed dose.

KEEP IN MIND...

* Breathe only through mouth when using nebulizer.
* Use only designated nebulizers and compressors.
* Don't use if drug looks cloudy or discolored.

Purinethol

Purinethol is a cancer-fighting drug that interferes with the growth of cancer cells, eventually causing their destruction.

Why it's prescribed

Doctors prescribe Purinethol to treat some cancers, especially leukemias. It comes in tablets. Doctors usually prescribe the following amounts for adults; children's dosages appear in parentheses (except for acute lymphoblastic leukemia).

▶ **For acute myeloblastic leukemia or chronic myelocytic leukemia,** 80 to 100 milligrams (mg) per square meter (m^2) of body surface area once a day as a single dose, up to 5 mg for each 2.2 pounds (lb) of body weight a day. (Children: 70 mg per m^2 once a day.) Maintenance dosage is 1.5 to 2.5 mg for each 2.2 lb daily.

▶ **For acute lymphoblastic leukemia in children,** 70 mg per m^2 once a day. Maintenance dosage is 1.5 to 2.5 mg for each 2.2 lb daily.

How to take Purinethol

• Take this drug exactly as your doctor directs. Don't take more or less of it than ordered.
• If you vomit shortly after taking a dose, call your doctor, who will tell you whether to take the dose again.

If you miss a dose

Don't take the missed dose and don't double the next dose. In-

PURINETHOL'S OTHER NAME

Purinethol's generic name is mercaptopurine.

stead, call your doctor and return to your regular dosage schedule.

 If you suspect an overdose

Contact your doctor *immediately*. Excessive Purinethol can cause fatigue, bleeding, bruising, chills, fever, nausea, vomiting, yellow-tinged skin and eyes, clay-colored stools, and frothy, dark urine.

 Warnings

• Make sure your doctor knows your medical history. You may not be able to take Purinethol if you have other problems, such as shingles, gout, kidney disease or kidney stones, liver disease, or infection.
• Before starting Purinethol, tell your doctor if you're pregnant or breast-feeding or if you intend to have children. This drug may cause birth defects if taken at conception by the father or mother or if taken

during pregnancy. Use an effective birth control method during Purinethol therapy.
• Don't get any immunizations without your doctor's approval. This drug may reduce your resistance to infection, causing you to get the infection the immunization is meant to prevent. Also, try to avoid contact with people who've just received the oral polio vaccine. If you can't avoid them, wear a protective mask.

 SIDE EFFECTS

Call your doctor if you have any of these possible drug side effects. Call *immediately* about any labeled "serious."

Serious: blood problems (abnormal bleeding, bruising, fatigue, increased risk of infection), liver problems (yellow-tinged skin and eyes, clay-colored stools, frothy, dark urine)

Common: nausea, vomiting, appetite loss

Other: painful mouth sores, rash, skin darkening

DRUG INTERACTIONS

Combining certain drugs may alter their action or produce unwanted side effects. Tell your doctor about other drugs you're taking, especially:
• anticoagulants (blood thinners) such as Coumadin
• drugs that damage the liver such as Tylenol
• Zyloprim.

KEEP IN MIND...

∗ Don't get immunizations unless doctor approves.

∗ Use effective birth control method during therapy.

∗ Call doctor if you have an infection or abnormal bleeding.

Pyridium

Pyridium eases the pain of an infected or irritated urinary tract. It works by reducing sensitivity to pain within the lining of the urinary tract.

Why it's prescribed

Doctors prescribe Pyridium to relieve symptoms of urinary tract irritation or infection, such as pain and burning. You can buy some brands of this drug without a prescription. It comes in tablets. Doctors usually prescribe the following amounts for adults; children's dosages appear in parentheses.

▶ **For pain caused by urinary tract irritation or infection,** 200 milligrams (mg) three times a day. (Children: 12 mg for each 2.2 pounds of body weight once a day divided into three equal doses.)

How to take Pyridium

- Take this drug exactly as your doctor directs.
- If you bought Pyridium without a prescription, read the package instructions carefully before taking it.
- Stop taking the drug after 3 days if your pain is gone, unless your doctor gives you other instructions.

PYRIDIUM'S OTHER NAMES

Pyridium's generic name is phenazopyridine. Other brand names include Azo-Standard, Baridium, Eridium, Geridium, Phenazodine, Pyrazodine, Pyridiate, Urodine, Urogesic; and, in Canada, Phenazo, and Pyronium.

 SIDE EFFECTS

Call your doctor if you have any of these possible drug side effects.

Serious: none reported

Common: none reported

Other: headache, vertigo, nausea, rash
Tip: To prevent nausea, take the tablets with meals or a snack.

 DRUG INTERACTIONS

Combining certain drugs may alter their action or produce unwanted side effects. Tell your doctor about other drugs you're taking.

If you miss a dose

Take the missed dose as soon as possible. However, if it's almost time for your next dose, skip the missed dose and take your next dose as scheduled. Don't take a double dose.

If you suspect an overdose

Contact your doctor *immediately*. Excessive Pyridium can cause bluish skin, kidney problems (decreased urination), and liver problems (nausea, vomiting, itching, and yellow-tinged skin and eyes).

✕ Warnings

- You may not be able to take Pyridium if you have other problems, such as G6PD deficiency, hepatitis, or kidney disease. Consult your doctor.
- If you're diabetic, be aware that this drug may cause false results with urine sugar or urine ketone tests. Check with your doctor for

more information, especially if your diabetes isn't well controlled.
- Call your doctor if your symptoms become worse while you're taking Pyridium.
- Don't be surprised if the drug turns your urine reddish orange. This is expected and won't cause any harm. Pyridium may also may stain your clothing.
- Don't wear soft contact lenses while taking this drug because Pyridium may permanently discolor them.
- If you get a urinary tract problem in the future, don't use leftover Pyridium without checking with your doctor.

 KEEP IN MIND...

* Take with meals or snacks.
* Call doctor if symptoms get worse.
* Don't use leftover drug for future infection.
* Expect drug to turn urine reddish orange.

Quarzan

Quarzan blocks the action of acetylcholine, an important chemical. The drug helps to decrease bowel action and stomach acid, easing conditions caused by excess stomach acid.

Why it's prescribed

Doctors prescribe Quarzan to treat stomach ulcers. It comes in capsules. Doctors usually prescribe the following amounts for adults.

▶ **For stomach ulcers,** 2.5 to 5 milligrams three or four times a day before meals and at bedtime.

How to take Quarzan

• Take this drug exactly as directed. Unless your doctor tells you otherwise, take it 30 to 60 minutes before meals and at bedtime. Make sure to take the bedtime dose at least 2 hours after your last meal of the day.

• Don't stop taking Quarzan suddenly. Instead, call your doctor, who may want you to reduce the amount you're taking gradually.

If you miss a dose

Take the missed dose as soon as possible. But if it's almost time for your next dose, skip the missed dose and take your next dose as scheduled. Don't take a double dose.

If you suspect an overdose

Contact your doctor *immediately*. Excessive Quarzan can cause difficulty breathing, enlarged pupils,

---

QUARZAN'S OTHER NAME

Quarzan's generic name is clidinium bromide.

 SIDE EFFECTS

Call your doctor if you have any of these possible drug side effects.

Serious: none reported

Common: confusion or excitability (in older adults), palpitations, blurred vision, dry mouth, bowel problems, constipation, difficulty urinating, inability to urinate

Other: headache, difficulty sleeping, drowsiness, dizziness, nervousness, weakness, fast pulse, enlarged pupils, increased eye pressure (headache, eye pain), unusual eye sensitivity to light, difficulty swallowing, heartburn, loss of taste, nausea, vomiting, impotence, decreased sweating, fever, allergic reaction (hives, itching, difficulty breathing)

Tip: Decreased sweating may cause your body temperature to rise. To avoid heatstroke, use caution during exercise and hot weather, and avoid hot baths and saunas.

 DRUG INTERACTIONS

Combining certain drugs may alter their action or produce unwanted side effects. Tell your doctor about other drugs you're taking, especially:
• antacids (take 2 to 3 hours before or after taking Quarzan)
• antihistamines (drugs for colds and hay fever)
• Demerol
• Doriden
• drugs for Parkinson's disease
• Levoprome
• Nizoral
• Norpace, Procan, Quinaglute Dura-tabs
• phenothiazines (used for anxiety, nausea, vomiting, or psychosis)
• Symmetrel
• tricyclic antidepressants such as Elavil.

---

blurred vision, dry mucous membranes, difficulty swallowing, inability to urinate, fever, fast pulse, high blood pressure (headache, blurred vision), and hot, flushed, dry skin.

Warnings

• Make sure your doctor knows your medical history. You may not be able to take Quarzan if you have other medical problems.

• If you're pregnant or breast-feeding, tell your doctor before you start taking Quarzan.

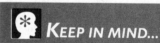 KEEP IN MIND...

∗ Take 30 to 60 minutes before meals and at bedtime.

∗ Take bedtime dose at least 2 hours after last meal.

∗ Don't take within 2 to 3 hours of taking antacid.

Questran

Questran works by removing bile (which promotes fat absorption) from the digestive system. This reduces the amount of fat absorbed from food and lowers the blood's cholesterol level.

Why it's prescribed

Doctors prescribe Questran to lower the blood's cholesterol level and to remove bile acids from the body. It comes as a powder and a chewable bar. Doctors usually prescribe the following amounts for adults.

▶ **For high blood fat levels or severe itching caused by too much bile acid,** 4 grams (g) once or twice a day. Maintenance dosage is 8 to 16 g once a day. Maximum dosage is 24 g once a day.

How to take Questran

• Take this drug exactly as your doctor directs. Don't stop taking it without consulting your doctor.
• If you're taking the powder form, first mix it with liquid. Never take it in its dry form because you might choke. To mix it, place the prescribed dose in 2 ounces (60 milliliters) of any beverage and stir thoroughly. Add 2 to 4 more ounces of the beverage and again mix thoroughly (it won't dissolve). Drink all the liquid. Then rinse the glass with a little more liquid and drink that too.
• If you're using the chewable bar, chew each bite well before swallowing.

QUESTRAN'S OTHER NAMES

Questran's generic name is cholestyramine. Other brand names include Cholybar and Questran Light.

 SIDE EFFECTS

Call your doctor if you have any of these possible drug side effects. Call *immediately* about any labeled "serious."

Serious: intestinal obstruction (severe abdominal pain)

Common: constipation, abdominal discomfort, nausea, rash, deficiency of vitamin A, D, E, or K

Tips: To help prevent constipation, drink extra fluids and eat high-fiber foods, such as whole wheat crackers and bran cereal. If severe constipation develops, call your doctor.

Other: fecal impaction, hemorrhoids, gas, vomiting, frothy and foul-smelling stools, irritation of skin, tongue, and area around anus

 DRUG INTERACTIONS

Combining certain drugs may alter their action or produce unwanted side effects. Take this drug at least 2 hours before or after taking any other drug. Tell your doctor about other drugs you're taking, especially:
• beta blockers such as Calan
• Crystodigin, Lanoxin
• fat-soluble vitamins (A, D, E, and K)
• iron preparations
• some anticoagulants (blood thinners)
• some diuretics (water pills)
• steroids such as Decadron
• thyroid hormones
• Tylenol and other drugs containing acetaminophen.

If you miss a dose

Take the missed dose as soon as possible. But if it's almost time for your next dose, skip the missed dose and take your next dose as scheduled. Don't take a double dose.

 If you suspect an overdose

Consult your doctor.

 Warnings

• Make sure your doctor knows your medical history. You may not be able to take Questran if you have other medical problems or certain allergies.
• If you're pregnant or breast-feeding, check with your doctor before you start taking Questran.

 KEEP IN MIND...

* Drink extra fluids and eat high-fiber foods.
* Never take powder in dry form.
* Chew each bite of bar well before swallowing.

Quinaglute Dura-tabs

Quinaglute Dura-tabs make the heart less responsive and slow the flow of impulses throughout the heart, helping it work more efficiently.

Why it's prescribed

Doctors prescribe Quinaglute Dura-tabs to steady an irregular heartbeat or to slow an overactive heart. The drug comes in extended-release tablets. Doctors usually prescribe the following amounts for adults; children's dosage is based on weight.

▶ **For irregular heartbeat,** 2 tablets every 8 hours, or 1 tablet every 8 to 12 hours. Or 1 tablet every 8 hours for 2 days, then 2 tablets every 12 hours for 2 days, then 2 tablets every 8 hours for up to 4 days.

How to take Quinaglute Dura-tabs

• Take Quinaglute Dura-tabs exactly as your doctor directs.
• To make sure your body absorbs the drug properly, take your dose with a full glass (8 ounces) of water on an empty stomach 1 hour before or 2 hours after meals.
• Swallow the tablets whole; don't chew, crush, or break them.
• Don't stop taking this drug, even if you feel well, without first checking with your doctor.

If you miss a dose

If you remember the missed dose within 2 hours, take it as soon as

 SIDE EFFECTS

Call your doctor if you have any of these possible drug side effects. Call *immediately* about any labeled "serious."

Serious: irregular heartbeat, dizziness, weakness, aggravated congestive heart failure (shortness of breath, fatigue), blood problems (fatigue, weakness, easy bruising and bleeding), liver problems (nausea, vomiting, yellow-tinged skin and eyes), stopped breathing

Common: headache, heart block (dizziness, fainting, fatigue), fast pulse, diarrhea, fever, ringing in ears, deafness

Other: confusion, restlessness, cold sweats, pallor, fainting, dementia, excessive salivation, blurred vision, appetite loss, stomach pain, acute asthma attack, rash, tiny red spots on insides of cheeks, itching, swelling of face, hands, and feet

 DRUG INTERACTIONS

Combining certain drugs may alter their action or produce unwanted side effects. Tell your doctor about other drugs you're taking, especially:
• Alka Seltzer, antacids, Tagamet
• barbiturates, Dilantin
• calcium channel blockers, such as Calan and Procardia
• diuretics (water pills), such as Diamox, Diuril, and HydroDIURIL
• other drugs for irregular heartbeat such as Cordarone
• Rifadin.

possible. But if you don't remember until later, skip the missed dose and take your next dose as scheduled. Don't take a double dose.

 If you suspect an overdose

Contact your doctor *immediately.* Excessive Quinaglute can cause extremely low blood pressure (severe weakness, dizziness), possibly fatal irregular heartbeats, seizures, breathing problems, incoordination, or hallucinations.

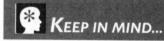 **Warnings**

• Make sure your doctor knows your medical history. You may not be able to take this drug if you have other medical problems.
• If you're pregnant or breast-feeding, check with your doctor before taking this drug.

KEEP IN MIND...

∗ Don't crush, chew, or break tablets.

∗ Take with full glass of water on an empty stomach.

∗ Don't stop taking without doctor's approval.

Reglan

Reglan increases bowel and stomach movements and acts on the brain center that controls vomiting. These actions relieve nausea, vomiting, and some other stomach problems.

Why it's prescribed

Doctors prescribe Reglan to treat certain digestive tract disorders, to prevent nausea and vomiting after treatment with cancer-fighting drugs, and to help relieve nausea, vomiting, and bloating after meals. It comes in tablets and a syrup. It's also available in an injectable form. Doctors usually prescribe the following amounts for adults.

▶ **For diabetic gastroparesis (paralysis of the stomach),** 10 milligrams (mg) orally for mild symptoms before meals and at bedtime for 2 to 8 weeks, depending on person's response.

▶ **For backward flow of stomach acid into the esophagus,** 10 to 15 mg orally four times a day, as needed, before meals and at bedtime.

How to take Reglan

- Take this drug exactly as your doctor directs. Unless instructed otherwise, take doses 30 minutes before meals and at bedtime.

REGLAN'S OTHER NAMES

Reglan's generic name is metoclopramide. Other brand names include Clopra, Maxolon, Octamide, Octamide PFS, Reclomide; and, in Canada, Apo-Metoclop, Emex, and Maxeran.

 SIDE EFFECTS

Call your doctor if you have any of these possible drug side effects.

Serious: none reported

Common: restlessness, anxiety, drowsiness, listlessness
Tip: For 2 hours after each dose, avoid driving and other activities that might be dangerous if you're not fully alert.

Other: fatigue; difficulty sleeping; headache; dizziness; urge to keep moving; fine, wormlike movements of tongue or other uncontrollable movements of mouth, tongue, cheeks, jaws, arms, and legs; spastic movements; sedation; high blood pressure (headache, blurred vision); nausea; diarrhea; rash; fever; unusual milk secretion; decreased sex drive

 DRUG INTERACTIONS

Combining certain drugs may alter their action or produce unwanted side effects. Tell your doctor about other drugs you're taking, especially:
- alcohol and other drugs that slow down the nervous system, such as cold and allergy drugs, sedatives, tranquilizers, narcotic pain relievers, barbiturates, seizure drugs, and muscle relaxants
- drugs for anxiety, nausea, vomiting, or psychosis, such as Haldol
- other drugs for abdominal or stomach cramps or spasms.

If you miss a dose

Take the missed dose as soon as possible. But if it's almost time for your next dose, skip the missed dose and take your next dose as scheduled. Don't take a double dose.

 If you suspect an overdose

Contact your doctor *immediately*. Excessive Reglan can cause drowsiness, seizures, muscle spasms, and an urge to keep moving.

Warnings

- Make sure your doctor knows your medical history. You may not be able to take Reglan if you have other problems, such as stomach bleeding, breast cancer, blockage of the bowel, pheochromocytoma, seizures, Parkinson's disease, high blood pressure, severe kidney or liver disease, or depression.
- If you're pregnant or breast-feeding, tell your doctor before you start taking this drug.

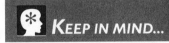 **KEEP IN MIND...**

- Take doses 30 minutes before meals and at bedtime.
- Don't drive for 2 hours after each dose.

Relafen

Relafen is a nonsteroidal anti-inflammatory drug (NSAID). These drugs seem to reduce pain and inflammation by inhibiting the production of certain hormones.

Why it's prescribed

Doctors prescribe Relafen to reduce joint pain, swelling, and stiffness from arthritis. It comes in tablets. Doctors usually prescribe the following amounts for adults.

▶ **For rheumatoid arthritis or osteoarthritis,** initially, 1,000 milligrams (mg) a day as a single dose or divided into two equal doses. Maximum dosage is 2,000 mg a day.

How to take Relafen

• Take this drug exactly as your doctor directs. If Relafen gives you heartburn, check with your doctor to see if you may take it with food or an antacid.
• Keep taking this drug even if your symptoms don't get better right away. Relafen may take about 1 month to achieve its full effect.

If you miss a dose

Take the missed dose as soon as possible. However, if it's almost time for your next dose, skip the missed dose and take your next dose as scheduled. Don't take a double dose.

 If you suspect an overdose

Consult your doctor.

RELAFEN'S OTHER NAME

Relafen's generic name is nabumetone.

 SIDE EFFECTS

Call your doctor if you have any of these possible drug side effects. Call *immediately* about any labeled "serious."

Serious: bleeding in stomach or bowel (severe stomach pain or burning; black, tarry stools; severe, persistent heartburn or nausea; vomiting of blood or material that looks like coffee grounds)

Common: dizziness, headache, ringing in ears, heartburn, diarrhea, abdominal pain, constipation, gas, nausea, rash, itching, swelling
Tips: Until you know how this drug affects you, don't drive or do anything else that could be dangerous if you're dizzy. Abdominal pain, headache, heartburn, gas, nausea, and vomiting usually go away as your body adjusts to the drug.

Other: fatigue, increased sweating, difficulty sleeping, nervousness, sleepiness, dry mouth, gastritis (indigestion, cramps), ulcers, mouth sores, vomiting, difficulty breathing, lung inflammation (dry cough)

 DRUG INTERACTIONS

Combining certain drugs may alter their action or produce unwanted side effects. Tell your doctor about other drugs you're taking, especially:
• alcohol
• Coumadin
• diuretics (water pills).

 Warnings

• Make sure your doctor knows your medical history. You may not be able to take Relafen if you're allergic to aspirin or if you have other problems, such as bowel disease, stomach ulcers, diabetes, hemorrhoids, rectal irritation, low white blood cell count, mental illness, Parkinson's disease, porphyria, lupus, anemia, asthma, seizures, swelling of the lower legs or feet, high blood pressure, bleeding problems, liver or kidney disease, or heart or blood vessel disease.
• If you're pregnant or breast-feeding, tell your doctor before you start taking Relafen.

• Be aware that older adults may be more prone to side effects.
• If you take this drug for a long time, have regular checkups.
• Before having surgery (including dental surgery), tell your doctor or dentist that you take Relafen.

KEEP IN MIND...

* Take with food or antacid to help prevent heartburn.
* Keep taking drug even if symptoms don't improve right away.
* Call doctor immediately if you have symptoms of digestive tract bleeding.

Respbid

Respbid relaxes the muscles in the lower airways and blood vessels of the lungs.

Why it's prescribed

Doctors prescribe Respbid to help treat and prevent the symptoms of asthma, such as wheezing and closing of the throat (bronchospasm). It comes in sustained-release tablets. Doctors usually prescribe the following amounts.

▶ **For symptoms of asthma,** initially, 16 milligrams (mg) for each 2.2 pounds of body weight or 400 mg a day (whichever is less), divided into equal doses taken every 8 to 12 hours, increased as needed.

How to take Respbid

• Follow your doctor's instructions.
• Take at the same time every day.
• Take Respbid ½ to 1 hour before meals or 2 hours after meals, or take it with food. Whichever you decide, take all doses the same way.
• Don't crush, break, or chew the tablets.

If you miss a dose

Take the missed dose as soon as possible. But if it's almost time for your next dose, skip the missed dose and take your next dose on schedule. Don't take a double dose.

 If you suspect an overdose

Contact your doctor *immediately.* Excessive Respbid can cause vomiting, rapid heartbeat, and seizures.

RESPBID'S OTHER NAMES

Respbid's generic name is theophylline anhydrous. Other brand names include Quibron-T/SR, Theolair-SR, Theo-Time, and Uniphyl.

 SIDE EFFECTS

Call your doctor if you have any of these possible drug side effects. Call *immediately* about any labeled "serious."

Serious: seizures, fast breathing, dizziness, weakness, rapid pulse

Common: dizziness, restlessness, nausea, vomiting, appetite loss
Tip: You may experience some dizziness, especially at the start of therapy and especially if you're an older adult. Change positions slowly and move about carefully until you get used to Respbid's effects.

Other: headache, light-headedness, muscle twitching, flushing, bitter aftertaste, stomach upset, diarrhea, hives
Tip: Call the doctor right away if you develop diarrhea.

 DRUG AND FOOD INTERACTIONS

Combining certain drugs and foods may alter drug action or produce unwanted side effects. Tell your doctor about your diet and other drugs you're taking, especially:
• antibiotics, such as Cipro and E-Mycin
• barbiturates, such as Solfoton
• beta blockers, such as Corgard and Inderal
• birth control pills
• caffeine (found in tea, coffee, colas, and chocolate), char-broiled foods
• marijuana and tobacco
• seizure drugs, such as Dilantin and Tegretol
• tuberculosis drugs such as Rifaden
• ulcer drugs such as Tagamet.

Warnings

• Make sure your doctor knows your medical history. You may not be able to take Respbid if you're allergic to sulfites, caffeine, asthma drugs, or the drug theobromine; if you've recently had a heart attack; if you have heart or circulatory problems, angina, diabetes, glaucoma, high blood pressure, an overactive thyroid, seizures, ulcers or indigestion, or lung, kidney, or liver problems; or if you're pregnant or breast-feeding.
• Older adults may be especially prone to side effects.

• An older adult or a person with congestive heart failure or liver disease needs a lower dosage. A regular smoker of tobacco or marijuana needs a higher dosage.
• Call your doctor right away if you develop a fever or the flu. They can increase your risk of developing side effects.

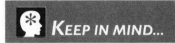 **KEEP IN MIND...**

* Take at same time each day.
* Don't crush or chew tablets.
* Avoid caffeine and char-broiled foods.

Restoril

Restoril is one of several drugs called benzodiazepines, which decrease anxiety and induce sleep. It seems to act on the brain areas that help govern emotions and wakefulness.

Why it's prescribed

Doctors prescribe Restoril to help induce sleep. It comes in capsules. Doctors usually prescribe the following amounts for adults.

▶ **For difficulty sleeping,** 7.5 to 30 milligrams at bedtime.

How to take Restoril

• Take this drug exactly as your doctor directs. Don't increase your dosage, even if you think your current one isn't effective. Instead, call your doctor.
• Don't take Restoril if your schedule won't allow you to get a full night's sleep. Otherwise, you'll feel drowsy during the day.

If you miss a dose

Not applicable because this drug is taken only as needed.

If you suspect an overdose

Contact your doctor *immediately*. Excessive Restoril can cause sleepiness, confusion, decreased reflexes, shortness of breath, low blood pressure (dizziness, weakness), a

---

RESTORIL'S OTHER NAME

Restoril's generic name is temazepam.

SIDE EFFECTS

Call your doctor if you have any of these possible drug side effects.

Serious: none reported

Common: drowsiness, dizziness, lethargy
Tips: Until you know how this drug affects you, don't drive or do anything else that could be dangerous if you're dizzy or drowsy. If the drug makes you feel extremely drowsy or dizzy or if you feel hungover the day after you've taken it, your dose may be too high. Call your doctor so your dosage can be adjusted.

Other: poor coordination, daytime sedation, confusion, appetite loss, diarrhea

DRUG INTERACTIONS

Combining certain drugs may alter their action or produce unwanted side effects. Tell your doctor about other drugs you're taking, especially:
• alcohol and other drugs that slow down the nervous system, such as cold and allergy drugs, sedatives, tranquilizers, narcotic pain relievers, barbiturates, seizure drugs, and muscle relaxants.

---

slow pulse, slurred speech, poor coordination, and coma.

Warnings

• Make sure your doctor knows your medical history. You may not be able to take Restoril if you have other problems, such as glaucoma, depression, myasthenia gravis, Parkinson's disease, asthma, emphysema, chronic bronchitis, sleep apnea (temporary stoppage of breathing during sleep), kidney or liver disease, porphyria, or a history of drug or alcohol abuse.
• Don't take Restoril if you think you might be pregnant or if you're breast-feeding.
• Be aware that older adults may be more sensitive to Restoril's side

effects. Older adults are especially likely to feel drowsy during the day.
• Because Restoril can be habit-forming, don't take it longer than your doctor recommends. Check with the doctor every month to make sure you still need to take this drug.

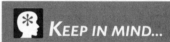

KEEP IN MIND...

* Don't increase dosage without doctor's approval.

* Don't drive until you know how drug affects you.

* Call doctor about severe drowsiness, dizziness, tiredness, or next-day hangover.

Retin-A

Retin-A inhibits the formation of blackheads by speeding the turnover of skin cells.

Why it's prescribed

Doctors prescribe Retin-A for acne or to treat fine wrinkles due to sun damage. It comes in a cream, a gel, and a solution for topical use. Doctors usually prescribe the following amounts for adults and children.

▶ **For acne,** applied lightly to affected area once a day at bedtime.

How to use Retin-A

• Use this drug exactly as your doctor directs. First wash your skin with a mild, nonallergenic soap and water. Gently pat your skin dry, and then wait 20 to 30 minutes to allow your skin to dry completely.
• If you're applying the cream or gel, use enough to cover the affected areas and rub in gently.
• If you're applying the solution, use your fingertips, a gauze pad, or a cotton swab to cover the affected areas.
• Avoid applying Retin-A close to your eyes or mouth, in the angles of your nose, on your mucous membranes, in an open wound, or to windburned or sunburned skin.

If you miss a dose

Skip the missed dose and apply your next dose as scheduled. Don't apply a double dose.

RETIN-A'S OTHER NAMES

Retin-A's generic name is tretinoin. A Canadian brand name is Stieva-A.

 SIDE EFFECTS

Call your doctor if you have any of these possible drug side effects.

Serious: none reported

Common: stinging, redness, warmth, peeling, chapping, swelling, blistering, or crusting of skin; temporary lightening or darkening of skin
Tips: Retin-A makes your skin more sensitive to sunlight, wind, and cold temperatures. To protect yourself, wear a sunblock and cover all exposed skin when you go out. If your face becomes sunburned, stop using the drug until the burn heals.

Other: severe skin burning or redness

 DRUG INTERACTIONS

Combining certain drugs may alter their action or produce unwanted side effects. Tell your doctor about other drugs you're taking, especially:
• topical preparations containing resorcinol, salicylic acid (such as Aspercream), or sulfur.

 If you suspect an overdose

Rinse off drug and consult your doctor.

Warnings

• Make sure your doctor knows your medical history. You may not be able to use Retin-A if you have other problems, such as eczema or sunburn, or if you're allergic to vitamin A or retinoic acid.
• If you're pregnant or breast-feeding, tell your doctor before you start using Retin-A.
• During Retin-A treatment, don't use any of the following, unless your doctor tells you otherwise: abrasive or perfumed soaps or cleansers, cosmetics or soaps that dry the skin, medicated cosmetics, or other skin drugs. However, you may wear unmedicated cosmetics.
• To keep your skin from drying out, don't wash your face more than three times a day.

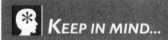 **KEEP IN MIND...**

∗ Keep drug away from eyes, mouth, angles of nose, mucous membranes, and open wounds.

∗ Don't use abrasive, drying, or perfumed soaps, cleansers, or cosmetics or other topical skin products.

∗ Protect skin from sun, wind, and cold temperatures.

Retrovir

etrovir is an antiviral drug that stops human immuno-deficiency virus (HIV) from reproducing, thus slowing its destruction of the immune system.

Why it's prescribed

Doctors prescribe Retrovir to treat HIV infection. It comes in capsules, a syrup, and an injectable form. Doctors usually prescribe the following amounts for adults; children's dosages appear in parentheses.

▶ **For HIV infection in people with symptoms,** 100 milligrams (mg) orally every 4 hours around the clock. (Children age 13 and older: same as adults. Children ages 3 months to 12 years: 180 mg per square meter of body surface area [m^2] orally every 6 hours [720 mg per m^2 a day], but not more than 200 mg every 6 hours.)

▶ **For HIV infection in people without symptoms,** 100 mg orally every 4 hours while awake (500 mg a day). (Children age 13 and older: same as adults. Children ages 3 months to 12 years: 180 mg per m^2 orally every 6 hours [720 mg per m^2 a day], but not more than 200 mg every 6 hours.)

▶ **To reduce risk of HIV transmission from infected mothers to their newborns,** 100 mg orally initially taken between 14 and 34 weeks' gestation and continued throughout pregnancy. (Newborns:

RETROVIR'S OTHER NAMES

Retrovir's generic name is zidovudine (also called AZT). Canadian brand names include Apo-Zidovudine and Novo-AZT.

2 mg for each 2.2 pounds of body weight orally [syrup] every 6 hours for 6 weeks, starting 8 to 12 hours after birth.)

▶ **For AIDS or advanced AIDS-related complex in people with a history of *Pneumocystis carinii* pneumonia or a low T-cell count,** 200 mg orally every 4 hours around the clock after treatment is started by intravenous injection.

SIDE EFFECTS

Call your doctor if you have any of these possible drug side effects. Call *immediately* about any side effects labeled "serious."

Serious: seizures, poor coordination, involuntary rapid eye movements, blood problems (weakness, fatigue, pale skin, fever, sore throat, abnormal bleeding), liver toxicity (abdominal discomfort, nausea, decreased appetite, general feeling of illness)

Common: headache, nausea, rash

Other: numbness, agitation, overall feeling of illness, difficulty sleeping, confusion, anxiety, abdominal pain, itching, muscle ache, sweating, fever, taste abnormalities, sore throat, sinus inflammation, difficulty urinating, flulike symptoms, chest pain, potential for infection and delayed healing

DRUG INTERACTIONS

Combining certain drugs may alter their action or produce unwanted side effects. Tell your doctor about other drugs you're taking, especially:
- antifungal drugs, such as Ancobon and Fungizone
- Ativan, Valium
- Avlosulfon
- Bactrim
- Benemid
- Biaxin
- cancer drugs such as Ganciclovir
- morphine
- NebuPent
- Ribavirin
- some pain relievers, such as aspirin, Indocin, and Tylenol
- Tagamet
- Zovirax.

How to take Retrovir

- Take this drug only as directed, at the same times every day.
- Measure a dose of syrup in a specially marked spoon, not a household teaspoon.

If you miss a dose

Take the missed dose as soon as possible. But if it's almost time for your next dose, skip the missed dose and take your next dose as scheduled. Don't take a double dose.

If you suspect an overdose

Contact your doctor *immediately*. Excessive Retrovir can cause seizures, poor coordination, severe nausea and vomiting, fever, increased bleeding or bruising, and involuntary rapid eye movements.

✗ Warnings

• Make sure your doctor knows your medical history. You may not be able to take Retrovir if you have anemia, other blood problems, or liver disease.

• If you're pregnant or breast-feeding, let your doctor know at once.

• Make sure your doctor knows you take Retrovir if you're about to start radiation therapy. Your dosage may need to be adjusted.

• Tell your dentist that you take Retrovir; you may be prone to delayed healing and thus have a greater risk of developing infections.

• Be aware that your doctor may want to perform blood tests regularly to monitor your progress during Retrovir therapy. Be sure to keep all medical appointments.

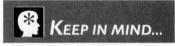

* Take exactly as directed, at the same time every day.

* Measure syrup with specially marked spoon.

* Tell your dentist that you take Retrovir.

ReVia

R eVia is one of several drugs called narcotic antagonists, which block the effects of narcotics (especially the "high" feeling) by acting on specific parts of the brain.

Why it's prescribed

Doctors prescribe ReVia as part of a program to help former narcotic addicts remain drug-free and to treat alcohol dependence. It comes in tablets. Doctors usually prescribe the following amounts for adults.

▶ **To help maintain a narcotic-free state in people who've gone through withdrawal from narcotics,** at first, 25 milligrams (mg). If no withdrawal signs occur in 1 hour, an additional 25 mg is given. After person has been started on 50 mg every 24 hours, maintenance dosage ranges from 50 to 150 mg once a day.

▶ **For alcohol dependence,** 50 mg once a day.

How to take ReVia

• Take this drug exactly as your doctor directs.

• Because ReVia causes severe withdrawal symptoms in people who are physically dependent on narcotics, it isn't given until you've been detoxified and are no longer drug dependent. Before you start taking it, tell your doctor if you think you're still having withdrawal symptoms.

REVIA'S OTHER NAME

ReVia's generic name is naltrexone.

 SIDE EFFECTS

Call your doctor if you have any of these possible drug side effects.

Serious: none reported

Common: difficulty sleeping, anxiety, nervousness, headache, nausea, vomiting, abdominal pain, muscle and joint pain

Other: depression, appetite loss, yellow-tinged skin and eyes

 DRUG INTERACTIONS

Combining certain drugs may alter their action or produce unwanted side effects. Tell your doctor about other drugs you're taking, especially:
• drugs used to treat coughs, colds, pain, or diarrhea that contain narcotics, such as codeine, or alcohol, such as Benylin (ask pharmacist for names of drugs that are free of narcotics and alcohol).

If you miss a dose

Adjust your schedule as follows:
• If you take one dose a day, take the missed dose as soon as possible. However, if you don't remember until the next day, skip the missed dose and take your next dose as scheduled. Don't take a double dose.
• If you're on a flexible drug regimen (such as 1 dose every weekday and 2 tablets on Saturday, or 2 tablets every other day), consult your doctor or pharmacist.

 If you suspect an overdose

Consult your doctor.

 Warnings

• Make sure your doctor knows your medical history. You may not be able to take ReVia if you have other problems, such as hepatitis or another liver disease.
• If you're pregnant or breast-feeding, tell your doctor before you start taking ReVia.
• See your doctor regularly so your progress can be monitored and side effects can be checked.
• Carry medical identification stating that you take ReVia. Tell your other doctors, dentists, and pharmacists that you take this drug.

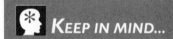 KEEP IN MIND...

* Don't take if you're physically dependent on narcotics or having withdrawal symptoms.

* Use only nonnarcotic cough, cold, pain, or diarrhea drugs.

* Carry medical identification stating that you take ReVia.

Rheumatrex

Rheumatrex is one of several drugs called antimetabolites. The exact way the drug helps treat arthritis is unknown, but it may affect the immune system.

Why it's prescribed

Doctors prescribe Rheumatrex to treat psoriasis and rheumatoid arthritis that resist conventional treatment. It's also used to treat some types of cancer. (For instructions on taking Rheumatrex for cancer, see Mexate.) Rheumatrex comes in tablets. It's also available in an injectable form. Doctors usually prescribe the following amounts for adults.

▶ **For rheumatoid arthritis,** at first, 7.5 milligrams (mg) orally as a single weekly dose, or 2.5 mg every 12 hours for three doses once a week. Gradually increased to maximum of 20 mg a week.

▶ **For psoriasis,** 10 to 25 mg orally as a single weekly dose.

How to take Rheumatrex

• Take this drug exactly as your doctor directs. Carefully check the prescription label. Take only the prescribed amount.
• If you vomit shortly after taking a dose, ask the doctor whether you should take the dose again or wait until the next scheduled dose.

If you miss a dose

Don't take the missed dose or double the next dose. Instead, call your doctor and resume your regular schedule.

RHEUMATREX'S OTHER NAMES

Rheumatrex's generic name is methotrexate. Other brand names include Folex PFS and Mexate-AQ.

 ## SIDE EFFECTS

Call your doctor if you have any of these possible drug side effects. Call *immediately* about any labeled "serious."

Serious: bleeding and inflammation of bowel lining (bloody or black vomit or stools), bowel perforation (diarrhea, stomach pain), blood problems (fatigue, shortness of breath, dizziness, headache, increased risk of infection, abnormal bleeding), lung problems (cough, shortness of breath), liver problems (yellow-tinged skin and eyes, nausea, vomiting)

Tips: Avoid people with infections. Call your doctor right away if you have symptoms of infection, such as fever, chills, or a sore throat. To prevent abnormal bleeding, take care when using a toothbrush, dental floss, or a razor. Also, avoid situations in which injury or bruising could occur. Call your doctor immediately if you notice unusual bruising or bleeding, such as black tarry stools, bloody stools or urine, or pinpoint red spots on your skin.

Common: mouth sores, diarrhea, nausea, vomiting, kidney damage (decreased urination), hives

Other: hair loss, sore throat, gum disease, lung inflammation (dry cough), itching, rash, skin darkening, worsening of psoriasis after sun exposure, unusual skin sensitivity to sun, too much uric acid in blood (swollen, painful joints)

Tips: Avoid sun exposure during treatment, especially if you have psoriasis. When going outdoors, apply a sunblock and wear protective clothing. Normal hair growth should return after you finish Rheumatrex treatment.

 ## DRUG INTERACTIONS

Combining certain drugs may alter their action or produce unwanted side effects. Tell your doctor about other drugs you're taking, especially:
• Benemid
• Dilantin
• drugs for pain and inflammation, such as Advil, aspirin, and Butazone
• drugs for urinary tract infections, such as Bactrim, Gantrisin, and Microsulfon
• folic acid such as Folvite
• Lanoxin
• vaccines.

 ### If you suspect an overdose

Contact your doctor *immediately.* Excessive Rheumatrex can cause bone marrow suppression (dizziness, pale skin, headache, bleeding, bruising, increased risk of infection), nausea, vomiting, skin in-

Continued on next page ▶

flammation, hair loss, and black, tarry stools.

✕ Warnings

• Make sure your doctor knows your medical history. You may not be able to take Rheumatrex if you have other problems, such as a stomach ulcer, colitis, an immune system disease, an infection, liver or kidney disease, or a blood disorder.

• If you're pregnant, don't take this drug. Rheumatrex may cause birth defects if the mother or father takes it at the time of conception or if the mother takes it during pregnancy. If you think you've become pregnant during Rheumatrex treatment, call your doctor right away. Practice birth control during treatment and for at least 3 months afterward.

• If you're breast-feeding, check with your doctor before you start taking Rheumatrex. It could cause serious side effects in your baby.

• Be aware that older adults may be especially prone to side effects of Rheumatrex.

• See your doctor regularly so your progress and drug effects can be monitored.

• Don't get immunizations during treatment except with your doctor's approval. This drug lowers your resistance, so you could get the infection the immunization is meant to prevent. Also, try to avoid people who've just received the oral polio vaccine because they could pass the polio virus to you. If you can't avoid them, wear a protective mask.

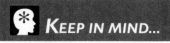

KEEP IN MIND...

∗ Call doctor if you vomit after taking dose.

∗ Avoid sun during treatment.

∗ Call doctor if you have symptoms of infection or unusual bleeding.

∗ Don't get immunizations without doctor's approval.

Rhinocort

Rhinocort is a nasal steroid that relieves symptoms of allergies and some other conditions. It seems to ease nasal inflammation by inhibiting the actions of the cells and substances involved in allergies.

Why it's prescribed

Doctors prescribe Rhinocort for allergies and other nasal conditions that cause stuffy nose or nasal irritation. It comes in a nasal spray. Doctors usually prescribe the following amounts for adults and children age 6 and older.

▶ **For symptoms of hay fever and other allergies,** 2 sprays in each nostril in the morning and evening, or 4 sprays in each nostril in the morning. Maintenance dosage is the fewest number of sprays needed to control symptoms.

How to use Rhinocort

• Use this drug exactly as your doctor directs. Don't use it more often than ordered because you may absorb the drug through the lining of your nose, which can cause unwanted effects.
• Make sure you understand how to use the special inhaler. Before using it, blow your nose. Then shake the container and insert the nosepiece into your nostril. Holding your other nostril closed, aim the spray toward the inner corner of your eye, breathe in gently, and spray. Repeat for the other nostril.
• For Rhinocort to work properly, use it regularly. Be aware that you

RHINOCORT'S OTHER NAME

Rhinocort's generic name is budesonide.

 ## SIDE EFFECTS

Call your doctor if you have any of these possible drug side effects.

Serious: none reported

Common: nasal irritation, nosebleeds, sore throat, cough

Other: nervousness, impaired sense of smell, nasal pain, hoarseness, bad taste, dry mouth, nausea, respiratory yeast infection (wheezing, shortness of breath), muscle ache, allergic reaction (facial swelling, rash, itching, peeling, redness)

Tip: Use a cool mist humidifier to help relieve dry mouth, nasal pain, and hoarseness.

 ## DRUG INTERACTIONS

Combining certain drugs may alter their action or produce unwanted side effects. Tell your doctor about other drugs you're taking, especially:
• steroid drugs such as prednisone.

may not feel the full effects of this drug for 3 weeks.

If you miss a dose

Take the missed dose as soon as possible if you remember within an hour. However, if you don't remember until later, skip the missed dose and take your next dose as scheduled. Don't take a double dose.

 ## If you suspect an overdose

Consult your doctor.

Warnings

• Make sure your doctor knows your medical history. You may not be able to use Rhinocort if you have other problems, such as glaucoma, tuberculosis, untreated infections, herpes infection of the eye, amebiasis, liver disease, or an underactive thyroid, or if you have recently had nose surgery or injury to your nose.

• If you're pregnant or breast-feeding, tell your doctor before you start using Rhinocort.
• This drug may slow a child's growth. Before your child starts using it, discuss its risks and benefits with the doctor.
• To prevent the spread of infection, don't share this drug with family members or friends.
• Don't use this drug for nasal problems other than the one for which the doctor prescribed it.
• Contact the doctor if your symptoms don't improve in 3 weeks or if they get worse.

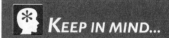 KEEP IN MIND...

* Blow nose before using inhaler.
* Use drug regularly to get full benefits.
* Don't share drug with anyone.

RID is a pediculicide — a drug used to kill lice. It disrupts the nervous system of the louse, causing it to become paralyzed and die.

Why it's used

RID is used to treat lice infestations. You can buy RID without a prescription. It comes in a shampoo, a gel, and a topical solution. The following amounts are usually recommended for adults and children.

▶ **For head, body, or pubic (crab) lice,** apply to hair, scalp, or other infested areas until entirely wet, leave on affected area for 10 minutes, then wash off with warm water and soap or shampoo. Remove dead lice and eggs (nits) with fine-toothed comb. Repeat treatment, if necessary, in 7 to 10 days to kill newly hatched lice. No more than two applications within 24 hours.

How to use RID

• Carefully read and follow the package instructions.
• Keep RID away from your eyes, mouth, and nose. Apply it in a well-ventilated room so you don't inhale the vapors.
• Wash your hands right after using RID.

RID's OTHER NAMES

RID is a combination of the generic drugs pyrethrins and piperonyl butoxide. Other brand names include A-200 Pyrinate, Barc, Blue Gel, Pronto, Pyrinyl, R&C, Tisit, and Triple X.

SIDE EFFECTS

Call your doctor if you have any of these possible drug side effects.

Serious: none reported

Common: skin irritation with repeated use

Other: none reported

DRUG INTERACTIONS

Combining certain drugs may alter their action or produce unwanted side effects. Tell your doctor about other drugs you're taking.

If you miss a dose

No applicable because drug is used as needed.

If you suspect an overdose

Consult your doctor.

Warnings

• Make sure your doctor knows your medical history. You may not be able to use RID if you have other problems, such as ragweed allergy, hay fever, or severe skin inflammation.
• If you're pregnant or breast-feeding, tell your doctor before you apply RID.
• To prevent the spread of lice and possible reinfestation, machine-wash all clothing, bedding, towels, and washcloths in very hot water. Then dry them using the hot cycle of a dryer for at least 20 minutes. Clothing or bedding that can't be washed should be dry-cleaned and sealed in a plastic bag for 2 weeks.
• Wash all hairbrushes and combs in very hot soapy water for 5 to 10 minutes.
• Thoroughly vacuum upholstered furniture, rugs, and floors.
• Have all members of your household checked for lice. Anyone who's infested should be treated.

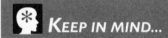
KEEP IN MIND...

* Leave on hair or skin for exactly 10 minutes.
* Wash hands right after using.
* Keep drug away from eyes, mouth, and nose.
* Launder clothing, bedding, and towels in hot water and dry in hot cycle for 20 minutes.
* Wash hairbrushes and combs in hot, soapy water.

Ridaura

Ridaura is a gold compound. It eases inflammation and other symptoms of arthritis, possibly by inhibiting the release of certain enzymes and altering the body's immune response.

Why it's prescribed

Doctors prescribe Ridaura to relieve arthritis symptoms, such as pain and inflammation. It comes in capsules. Doctors usually prescribe the following amounts for adults.

▶ **For rheumatoid arthritis,** 6 milligrams (mg) once a day or 3 mg twice a day. After 6 months, may be increased to 9 mg a day.

How to take Ridaura

• Take this drug exactly as your doctor directs. Never take more than ordered because this could cause serious unwanted effects.
• Keep taking Ridaura as prescribed even if you think it isn't working. You may not feel the effects of the drug until you've been taking it regularly for 3 to 6 months.

If you miss a dose

Adjust your schedule as follows:
• If you take one dose a day, take the missed dose as soon as possible. However, if you don't remember until the next day, skip the missed dose and take your next dose as scheduled. Don't take a double dose.
• If you take more than one dose a day, take the missed dose as soon as possible. However, if it's almost time for your next dose, skip the missed dose and take your next dose as scheduled. Don't take a double dose.

If you suspect an overdose

Consult your doctor.

Warnings

• Make sure your doctor knows your medical history. You may not be able to take Ridaura if you have other problems, such as colitis or another bowel disorder, lupus, a skin disease, blood or blood vessel disease, kidney disease, or Sjögren's syndrome.
• See your doctor monthly for blood and urine tests.

RIDAURA'S OTHER NAME

Ridaura's generic name is auranofin.

SIDE EFFECTS

Call your doctor if you have any of these possible drug side effects. Call *immediately* about any labeled "serious."

Serious: blood problems (abnormal bleeding, weakness, fatigue, pale skin, shortness of breath, headache, rapid pulse, fever, sore throat, bruising, bleeding sores of mouth, rectum, and vagina), skin inflammation (redness, itching, peeling)
Tip: Contact your doctor immediately if you see blood in your stool. Avoid physical activity that could cause bleeding or bruising.

Common: diarrhea, abdominal pain, nausea, vomiting, rash, itching, skin sensitivity to sunlight
Tips: Stop taking Ridaura and call your doctor immediately if you develop a rash or other skin problem. To protect your skin, avoid direct sunlight, apply a sunblock, and wear protective clothing.

Other: mouth sores, bowel inflammation (severe abdominal pain or cramping, bloody or black vomit or stools), appetite loss, metallic taste, stomach upset, gas, blood in urine, kidney problems (bloody or cloudy urine, decreased urination, flank pain), liver problems (yellow-tinged skin and eyes, itching), lung inflammation (cough, shortness of breath)

DRUG INTERACTIONS

Combining certain drugs may alter their action or produce unwanted side effects. Tell your doctor about other drugs you're taking, especially:
• Dilantin.

KEEP IN MIND...

* Keep taking drug even if it doesn't seem to be working; effects may be delayed for several months.

* Avoid sun exposure.

* Stop taking drug and call doctor if rash or other skin problem occurs.

Rifadin

Rifadin is a tuberculosis drug that impairs the genetic material of the bacteria that cause tuberculosis, resulting in death of the bacteria.

Why it's prescribed

Doctors prescribe Rifadin to treat tuberculosis, to prevent the spread of meningitis, and for certain other infections. It comes in capsules. It's also available in an injectable form. Doctors usually prescribe the following amounts for adults; children's dosages appear in parentheses.

▶ **For tuberculosis of the lungs,** 600 milligrams (mg) orally once a day in single dose 1 hour before or 2 hours after meals. (Children over age 5: 10 to 20 mg for each 2.2 pounds [lb] of body weight orally once a day in a single dose 1 hour before or 2 hours after meals. Maximum dosage is 600 mg a day.)

▶ **To prevent meningitis carriers from spreading the bacteria to others,** 600 mg orally twice a day for 2 days, or 600 mg orally once a day for 4 days. (Children ages 1 month to 12 years: 10 mg for each 2.2 lb orally twice a day for 2 days, not to exceed 600 mg a day, or 10 to 20 mg for each 2.2 lb once a day for 4 days. Newborns: 5 mg for each 2.2 lb orally twice a day for 2 days.)

▶ **To prevent *Haemophilus influenzae* type b,** 20 mg for each 2.2 lb orally once a day for 4 days, but not more than 600 mg a day. (Children: same as adults.)

RIFADIN'S OTHER NAMES

Rifadin's generic name is rifampin. Other brand names include Rimactane and, in Canada, Rofact.

 ## SIDE EFFECTS

Call your doctor if you have any of these possible drug side effects. Call *immediately* about any labeled "serious."

Serious: blood problems (fatigue, weakness, easy bruising and bleeding, increased risk of infection), serious liver damage (nausea, vomiting, confusion, yellow-tinged skin and eyes)

Tips: Avoid people with known infections. Call your doctor immediately if you have symptoms of infection, such as fever, sore throat, or fatigue. To help prevent bleeding, take precautions when using a toothbrush, dental floss, or a razor. Also, avoid contact sports and other activities in which bruising or injury can occur. Call the doctor if you have symptoms of bleeding, such as easy bruising, nosebleeds, bleeding gums, and black, tarry stools.

Common: drowsiness

Other: headache, dizziness, numbness, appetite loss, nausea, vomiting, abdominal pain, diarrhea, gas, sore mouth and tongue, itching, hives, rash, flulike symptoms, reddish orange urine, saliva, sweat, tears, sputum, and stools

 ## DRUG INTERACTIONS

Combining certain drugs may alter their action or produce unwanted side effects. Tell your doctor about other drugs you're taking, especially:
- alcohol
- anticoagulants (blood thinners) such as Coumadin
- Atromid-S
- barbiturates (used for sedation or seizures)
- Benemid
- birth control pills
- Chloromycetin
- drugs for high blood pressure, irregular heartbeats, and other heart conditions, such as Calan, Crystodigin, Inderal, Lanoxin, Mexitil, Norpace, Quinaglute Dura-tabs, and other beta blockers
- drugs for menstrual problems and uterine bleeding, such as Norlutin and Provera
- narcotic pain relievers, methadone
- Nizoral and P.A.S. Sodium (take 8 to 12 hours before or after taking Rifadin)
- oral diabetes drugs
- Sandimmune
- steroids
- Theo-Dur
- Valium.

How to take Rifadin

• Take this drug exactly as your doctor directs.

• Take Rifadin with a full glass (8 ounces) of water 1 hour before or 2 hours after meals. However, if it upsets your stomach, your doctor may tell you to take it with food.

• If you can't swallow the capsules, open them and mix the contents with applesauce or jelly. Or ask your pharmacist to prepare an oral liquid form of this drug.

• To help clear up your infection, keep taking this drug even after you start to feel well. Take Rifadin for the full time prescribed. You may have to take it every day for 2 years or even longer.

If you miss a dose

Take the missed dose as soon as possible. However, if it's almost time for your next dose, skip the missed dose and take your next dose as scheduled. Don't take a double dose.

If you suspect an overdose

Contact your doctor *immediately*. Excessive Rifadin can cause lethargy, nausea, vomiting, liver damage (yellow-tinged skin and eyes, itching), loss of consciousness, and orange discoloration of the skin, urine, sweat, saliva, tears, and stools.

Warnings

• Make sure your doctor knows your medical history. You may not be able to take Rifadin if you have other problems, such as liver disease or alcoholism.

• If you're pregnant or breast-feeding, don't use this drug without careful discussion with your doctor. Avoid becoming pregnant while taking Rifadin because the drug can cause birth defects. Because Rifadin makes birth control pills (oral contraceptives) less effective, use another birth control method while taking this drug.

• See your doctor regularly so your progress and the drug effects can be monitored.

• Call your doctor if your symptoms seem worse or don't subside after 2 to 3 weeks of therapy. But remember that you'll probably have to take Rifadin for a long time to defeat the disease.

• Rifadin causes body fluids (saliva, sweat, urine, tears) to turn reddish orange or reddish brown. These fluids can permanently stain clothing and soft contact lenses. If possible, avoid wearing soft contact lenses during treatment.

• Your doctor will probably want to monitor your progress closely while you're taking Rifadin. Be sure to keep all follow-up medical appointments.

• If you have dental problems, check with your doctor. You may need to delay dental work until the end of therapy.

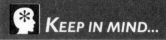

KEEP IN MIND...

* Take with full glass of water or, if directed, with food to prevent stomach upset.

* If necessary, mix contents of capsules with applesauce or jelly.

* Take for full time prescribed, even if you start to feel better.

* Use a nonhormonal birth control method while taking Rifadin.

Riopan

Riopan reduces the amount of acid in the digestive tract, decreases the activity of a stomach enzyme called pepsin, and strengthens the stomach lining. These actions relieve heartburn and acid indigestion.

Why it's taken

Riopan is taken to relieve heartburn or the symptoms of a stomach or duodenal ulcer. You can buy Riopan without a prescription. It comes in tablets, chewable tablets, and a liquid. The following amounts are usually recommended for adults.

▶ **As an antacid,** 540 to 1,080 milligrams (mg) (5 to 10 milliliters) of the liquid with water between meals and at bedtime; or 480 to 960 mg tablets (1 to 2 tablets) with water between meals and at bedtime; or 480 to 960 mg chewable tablets (1 to 2 tablets), chewed before swallowing, between meals and at bedtime.

How to take Riopan

- If you're treating yourself, carefully follow the instructions on the label.
- If your doctor prescribed this drug or gave you special dosage instructions, follow those instructions carefully.
- If you're using the chewable tablets, chew them completely before swallowing. Drink a glass of milk or water afterward.

RIOPAN'S OTHER NAMES

Riopan's generic name is magaldrate. Other brand names include Lowsium and, in Canada, Antiflux.

 SIDE EFFECTS

Call your doctor if you have any of these possible drug side effects.

Serious: none reported

Common: none reported

Other: mild constipation or diarrhea

 DRUG INTERACTIONS

Combining certain drugs may alter their action or produce unwanted side effects. Tell your doctor about other drugs you're taking. Don't take Riopan within 1 to 2 hours of taking any of these drugs:
- antibiotics
- Cuprimine
- Dolobid
- enteric-coated drugs
- iron
- Laniazid
- Lanoxin
- phenothiazines (used for anxiety, nausea, vomiting, or psychosis)
- Quinaglute Dura-tabs
- Zyloprim.

- If you're using the liquid, shake the bottle well before pouring your dose. Sip water or juice after taking the drug.

If you miss a dose

If you're taking this drug on a regular schedule, take the missed dose as soon as possible. However, if it's almost time for your next dose, skip the missed dose and take your next dose as scheduled. Don't take a double dose.

 If you suspect an overdose

Consult your doctor.

 Warnings

- Consult your doctor before taking Riopan if you have other medical problems.
- If you're pregnant, tell your doctor before you start taking Riopan.
- Don't take this drug for more than 2 weeks unless directed by your doctor.

KEEP IN MIND...

* Chew chewable tablets completely before swallowing.
* Shake the bottle of liquid well.
* Don't take for more than 2 weeks unless doctor approves.

Risperdal

Risperdal reduces stimulation to the brain stem, causing sedation. It also seems to block certain crucial receptors in the brain. These actions probably ease symptoms of psychosis.

Why it's prescribed

Doctors prescribe Risperdal for psychosis. It comes in tablets. Doctors usually prescribe the following amounts for adults; dosages for older adults and seriously ill people appear in parentheses.

▶ **For symptoms of psychosis,** initially, 1 milligram (mg) twice a day, increased by 1 mg twice a day on second and third days to target dose of 3 mg twice a day. At least 1 week must pass before dosage is changed further. (Older adults, seriously ill people, and those with low blood pressure or severe kidney or liver disorders: initially, 0.5 mg twice a day, increased by 0.5 mg twice a day on second and third days to target dose of 1.5 mg twice a day. At least 1 week must pass before dosage is increased further.)

How to take Risperdal

• Take this drug exactly as your doctor directs.
• Take this drug with food to help prevent nausea.

If you miss a dose

Take the missed dose as soon as possible. But if it's almost time for your next dose, skip the missed dose and take your next dose as scheduled. Don't take a double dose.

RISPERDAL'S OTHER NAME

Risperdal's generic name is risperidone.

 SIDE EFFECTS

Call your doctor if you have any of these possible drug side effects. Call *immediately* about any labeled "serious."

Serious: neuroleptic malignant syndrome (severe muscle stiffness, fever, unusual tiredness or weakness, fast pulse, difficulty breathing, increased sweating, loss of bladder control, seizures)

Common: sleepiness or difficulty sleeping, restlessness, urge to keep moving, headache, agitation, anxiety, constipation, nausea, vomiting, stomach upset
Tip: If this drug makes you sleepy, don't drive or perform any other activity that could be dangerous.

Other: tardive dyskinesia (uncontrollable movements of tongue, mouth, cheeks, jaws, arms, and legs), aggressiveness, fast pulse, chest pain, dizziness when standing up, runny nose, coughing, upper respiratory tract infection, sore throat, sinus inflammation, abnormal vision, rash, dry skin, skin sensitivity to sunlight, joint pain, back pain, fever
Tips: To help prevent dizziness when standing up, rise slowly to your feet. Avoid sun exposure, use sunblock, and wear protective clothing.

 DRUG INTERACTIONS

Combining certain drugs may alter their action or produce unwanted side effects. Tell your doctor about other drugs you're taking, especially:
• alcohol
• Clozaril
• Larodopa
• Tegretol.

 If you suspect an overdose

Contact your doctor *immediately.* Excessive Risperdal can cause drowsiness, sedation, seizures, a fast pulse, dizziness, confusion, weakness, lethargy, restlessness, and an urge to keep moving.

 Warnings

• Make sure your doctor knows your medical history. You may not be able to take Risperdal if you

have other problems, such as heart or blood vessel disease or seizures.
• Tell your doctor if you're pregnant or breast-feeding or if you plan to become pregnant.

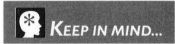 **KEEP IN MIND...**

* Don't drive until you know how you react to drug.

* Avoid sun exposure.

* Rise slowly to your feet to avoid dizziness.

Ritalin

Ritalin is one of several drugs called central stimulants. It probably works by aiding the transmission of nerve impulses in the brain. In children who are hyperactive, have poor concentration, and are easily distracted, this effect increases attention and eases restlessness.

Why it's prescribed

Doctors prescribe Ritalin to treat attention deficit hyperactivity disorder (ADHD) in children and occasionally to treat narcolepsy (sudden episodes of sleeping) in adults. It comes in tablets and sustained-release tablets. Doctors usually prescribe the following amounts.

▶ **For ADHD in children age 6 and older,** initially, 5 to 10 milligrams (mg) a day, divided into equal doses before breakfast and lunch, with weekly increases of 5 to 10 mg as needed, up to 60 mg a day.

▶ **For narcolepsy in adults,** 10 mg two or three times a day, 30 to 45 minutes before meals.

How to take Ritalin

• Take Ritalin exactly as the doctor directs. To help the drug work better, take it 30 to 45 minutes before meals. However, if the drug causes loss of appetite, take it after meals.

• If you're using the regular tablets, take the last dose before 6 p.m., if possible, to reduce the risk of sleep disturbances.

RITALIN'S OTHER NAME

Ritalin's generic name is methylphenidate.

 SIDE EFFECTS

Call your doctor if you have any of these possible drug side effects. Call *immediately* about any labeled "serious."

Serious: seizures, skin inflammation (redness, itching, peeling)

Common: nervousness, difficulty sleeping, palpitations
Tip: Take the last dose of the day 6 hours before bedtime so it won't cause difficulty sleeping.

Other: Tourette syndrome (uncontrollable vocal outbursts and movements), dizziness, restlessness, agitation, chest pain, high blood pressure (headache, blurred vision), fast pulse, dry throat, nausea, abdominal pain, appetite loss, weight loss, abnormal bleeding, tiny purple or red spots on skin, rash, hives, delayed growth in children
Tips: Don't perform activities requiring alertness or good coordination until you know how this drug affects you. To prevent unnecessary bleeding, use a soft toothbrush and be careful when using a razor. To help prevent delayed growth, the doctor may recommend drug-free periods for children.

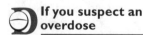 **DRUG AND FOOD INTERACTIONS**

Combining certain drugs and foods may alter drug action or produce unwanted side effects. Tell your doctor about your diet and other drugs you're taking, especially:
• anticoagulants (blood thinners) such as Coumadin
• antidepressants called MAO inhibitors (don't take within 14 days of taking Ritalin)
• certain blood pressure drugs, such as Aldomet and Catapres
• foods and beverages that contain caffeine, such as coffee, tea, cola, and chocolate
• seizure drugs, such as Dilantin and Solfoton
• tricyclic antidepressants, such as Elavil and Pamelor.

• If the doctor has prescribed the sustained-release tablets, make sure you swallow the tablets whole. Don't break, crush, or chew them.
• Don't stop taking Ritalin suddenly. With long-term Ritalin therapy, the doctor may want to reduce the dosage gradually.
• Some children with ADHD can tolerate a lower dosage in times of reduced stress, such as school holidays and summer vacation. Discuss this possibility with your doctor.

If you miss a dose

Take the missed dose as soon as possible; then take the remaining doses for that day at regularly spaced times. Don't take a double dose.

If you suspect an overdose

Contact your doctor *immediately.* Excessive Ritalin can cause an unusual sense of well-being, confusion, delirium, strange behavior, self-injury, agitation, headache, vomiting, dry mouth, enlarged pupils, fever, sweating, tremor, increased reflexes, muscle twitching, seizures, flushed skin, high blood pressure (headache, blurred vision), fast or irregular pulse, and coma.

Warnings

• Make sure the doctor knows your medical history. You may not be able to take Ritalin if you have other problems, such as seizures, Tourette syndrome, glaucoma, high blood pressure, psychosis, severe anxiety, agitation, depression, or tics, or if you're prone to drug abuse or dependence.

• Tell your doctor if you're pregnant or breast-feeding before you start taking Ritalin.

• Be aware that children are more likely than adults to develop stomach pain, trouble sleeping, and loss of appetite and weight during Ritalin therapy.

• If you have diabetes, the doctor may need to adjust the dosage of your diabetes drug.

• Be aware that Ritalin can be habit forming. Call your doctor if you notice symptoms of mental or physical dependence, such as a strong need or desire to keep taking the drug, a need to increase the dosage to get the same effects, or withdrawal side effects (unusual weakness or tiredness, strange behavior, or depression).

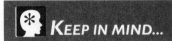

KEEP IN MIND...

* Take 30 to 45 minutes before meals; if drug decreases appetite, take after meals.

* Take last dose of day 6 hours before bedtime.

* Swallow sustained-release tablets whole.

* Avoid foods and beverages that contain caffeine.

* Don't stop taking drug abruptly.

Robaxin

Robaxin is a muscle relaxant that acts on the central nervous system to relax injured muscles. The drug works by causing sedation and altering the perception of pain.

Why it's prescribed

Doctors prescribe Robaxin to relax muscles and to relieve pain and discomfort caused by muscle injury, such as sprains and strains. It comes in tablets. It's also available in an injectable form. Doctors usually prescribe the following amounts for adults.

▶ **For acute, painful musculoskeletal conditions (along with other drugs),** 1.5 grams (g) orally four times a day for 2 to 3 days, then 1 g orally four times a day, repeated every 8 hours, as needed.

How to take Robaxin

• Take this drug exactly as your doctor directs. To prevent stomach upset, take it with meals or milk.
• If you have trouble swallowing the tablets, crush them and mix them with food or a liquid.

If you miss a dose

Take the missed dose if you remember within 1 hour or so. Otherwise, skip the missed dose and take your next dose as scheduled. Don't take a double dose.

If you suspect an overdose

Contact your doctor *immediately.* Excessive Robaxin can cause extreme drowsiness, nausea, vomiting, and irregular pulse.

Warnings

• Make sure your doctor knows your medical history. You may not be able to take Robaxin if you have other problems, such as allergies, kidney disease, seizures, or a blood disease caused by an allergy to another drug. Also tell the doctor if you've ever abused or been dependent on drugs.

• If you're breast-feeding, check with your doctor before you start taking Robaxin.
• If you're taking Robaxin for more than a few weeks, have regular medical checkups so the doctor can evaluate your progress and detect unwanted drug effects.
• Follow your doctor's recommendations for physical activity.

SIDE EFFECTS

Call your doctor if you have any of these possible drug side effects.

Serious: none reported

Common: none reported

Other: drowsiness, dizziness, fainting, weakness, headache, nausea, appetite loss, stomach upset, metallic taste, discolored urine, hives, itching, rash, flushed skin, blood clots (leg pain, difficulty breathing), fever

Tips: Until you know how Robaxin affects you, don't drive or do anything else that could be dangerous if you're dizzy or drowsy. Once you stop taking the drug, urine discoloration will go away.

DRUG INTERACTIONS

Combining certain drugs may alter their action or produce unwanted side effects. Tell your doctor about other drugs you're taking, especially:
• alcohol and other drugs that slow down the nervous system, such as cold and allergy drugs, sedatives, tranquilizers, narcotic pain relievers, barbiturates, seizure drugs, and muscle relaxants.

ROBAXIN'S OTHER NAMES

Robaxin's generic name is methocarbamol. Other brand names include Delaxin, Marbaxin-750, Robomol-500, and Robomol-750.

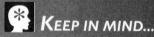

KEEP IN MIND...

∗ Take with meals or milk.

∗ If necessary, crush tablets and mix with food or liquid.

∗ Don't drive until you know how you react to drug.

Robinul

Robinul blocks the action of a substance called acetylcholine, which decreases bowel action and the production of stomach acid.

Why it's prescribed

Doctors prescribe Robinul to treat stomach ulcers and ease cramps and spasms of the stomach and intestines. It comes in tablets. It's also available in an injectable form. Doctors usually prescribe the following amounts for adults.

▶ **For stomach or other digestive disorders (along with other drugs),** dosage varies depending on person, but usually 1 to 2 milligrams (mg) orally three times a day. Maximum dosage is 8 mg a day.

How to take Robinul

• Take this drug exactly as your doctor directs. Unless your doctor tells you otherwise, take it 30 minutes to 1 hour before meals.
• Don't stop taking this drug suddenly; doing so may cause withdrawal symptoms, such as dizziness and vomiting. Call your doctor for instructions on reducing your dosage gradually.

If you miss a dose

Take the missed dose as soon as possible. But if it's almost time for your next dose, skip the missed dose and take your next dose as scheduled. Don't take a double dose.

 If you suspect an overdose

Contact your doctor *immediately*. Excessive Robinul can cause en-

ROBINUL'S OTHER NAME

Robinul's generic name is glycopyrrolate.

 SIDE EFFECTS

Call your doctor if you have any of these possible drug side effects.

Serious: none reported

Common: enlarged pupils, blurred vision, constipation, dry mouth, difficulty urinating or inability to urinate, bronchial plugging (thick mucus, difficulty breathing)

Other: disorientation, irritability, incoherence, weakness, nervousness, drowsiness, dizziness, headache, confusion or excitability (in older adults), palpitations, fast or slow pulse, unusual eye sensitivity to light, increased eye pressure, difficulty swallowing, nausea, vomiting, bloated abdomen, stomach upset, impotence, hives, decreased sweating, skin problems, fever, loss of taste

Tips: To help prevent heatstroke, don't get overheated during exercise or hot weather; avoid hot baths or saunas while taking this drug.

 DRUG INTERACTIONS

Combining certain drugs may alter their action or produce unwanted side effects. Tell your doctor about other drugs you're taking, especially:
• antacids (take 2 to 3 hours before or after taking Robinul)
• antihistamines, such as nonprescription cold and hay fever drugs
• Demerol
• Doriden
• drugs for Parkinson's disease
• Levoprome
• Nizoral
• Norpace, Procan, Quinaglute Dura-tabs
• phenothiazines (used for anxiety, nausea, vomiting, or psychosis)
• tricyclic antidepressants, such as Elavil and Pamelor.

larged pupils, blurred vision, dry mucous membranes, difficulty swallowing, inability to urinate, fever, fast pulse and breathing, high blood pressure (headache, blurred vision), and flushed, hot, dry skin.

 Warnings

• Make sure your doctor knows your medical history. You may not be able to take Robinul if you have other medical problems.

• If you're pregnant or breast-feeding, tell your doctor before you start taking Robinul.

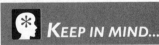 **KEEP IN MIND...**

* Take 2 to 3 hours before or after antacids.
* Don't get overheated.
* Don't stop taking suddenly.

Robitussin

Robitussin is an expectorant, a drug that loosens mucus or phlegm in the lungs. This, in turn, relieves coughs due to colds. However, the drug isn't helpful for long-term coughs, such as those caused by asthma, emphysema, or smoking.

Why it's taken

Robitussin is taken to help relieve a dry, hacking cough. You can buy Robitussin without a prescription. It comes in tablets, capsules, extended-release tablets and capsules, and an oral solution. The following amounts are usually recommended for adults; children's dosages appear in parentheses.

▶ **To relieve cough,** 200 to 400 milligrams (mg) every 4 hours, or 600 to 1,200 mg extended-release form every 12 hours. Maximum dosage is 2,400 mg a day. (Children over age 12: same as adults. Children ages 6 to 12: 100 to 200 mg every 4 hours. Maximum dosage is 1,200 mg a day. Children ages 2 to 5: 50 to 100 mg every 4 hours. Maximum dosage is 600 mg a day.)

How to take Robitussin

• Although Robitussin is available without a prescription, follow your

ROBITUSSIN'S OTHER NAMES

Robitussin's generic name is guaifenesin. Other brand names include Anti-Tuss, Baytussin, Breonesin, Cremacoat 2, Gee-Gee, GG-CEN, Glyate, Glycotuss, Glytuss, Guiatuss, Halotussin, Humibid L.A., Hytuss, Naldecon Senior EX, Nortussin, Robafen, S-T Expectorant; and, in Canada, Balminil Expectorant, Neo-Spec, and Resyl.

SIDE EFFECTS

Call your doctor if you have any of these possible drug side effects.

Serious: none reported

Common: none reported

Other: drowsiness; stomach pain, diarrhea, vomiting, nausea (with large doses)

Tip: Don't drive, operate machinery, or perform other activities requiring alertness until you know how you respond to this drug.

DRUG INTERACTIONS

Combining certain drugs may alter their action or produce unwanted side effects. Tell your doctor about other drugs you're taking, especially:
• Liquaemin Sodium (a blood thinner).

doctor's suggestions, if any, for the proper dosage for your condition.
• If you're treating yourself, carefully read and follow the directions and precautions on the product label. Don't take more than the recommended total daily dosage.
• Swallow the extended-release tablets or extended-release capsules whole. Don't crush, break, or chew them.
• Drink a full glass (8 ounces) of water with each dose to help loosen phlegm.
• Don't take this drug longer than the directions recommend, unless your doctor tells you otherwise.

If you miss a dose

If you're taking Robitussin regularly, take the missed dose as soon as possible. However, if it's almost time for the next dose, skip the missed dose and take your next dose as scheduled. Don't take a double dose.

If you suspect an overdose

Consult your doctor.

Warnings

• If you're pregnant or breast-feeding, or if you think you may be pregnant, check with your doctor before you start taking this drug.
• If your cough doesn't improve within 7 days or if you develop a fever, rash, persistent headache, or sore throat, check with your doctor.

KEEP IN MIND...

∗ Drink full glass of water with each dose.

∗ Swallow extended-release tablets or capsules whole.

∗ Don't drive until you know how you react to drug.

∗ Call doctor if cough doesn't improve within 7 days.

Rocaltrol is a potent form of vitamin D. It promotes calcium absorption from the intestine and calcium movement from bones to the blood. These effects increase the amount of calcium in the blood.

Why it's prescribed

Doctors prescribe Rocaltrol for people with too little calcium in the blood, such as some people undergoing kidney dialysis and those with conditions that cause the body to use calcium improperly. The drug comes in capsules. Doctors usually prescribe the following amounts for adults and children age 1 and older.

▶ **For calcium deficiency in people undergoing kidney dialysis,** initially, 0.25 micrograms (mcg) once a day, increased by 0.25 mcg a day at intervals of 4 to 8 weeks. Usual dosage is 0.25 mcg every other day, up to 1.25 mcg a day.

▶ **For calcium deficiency due to parathyroid hormone disorders,** initially, 0.25 mcg a day, increased every 2 to 4 weeks. Usual dosage is 0.25 to 2 mcg a day.

How to take Rocaltrol

• Take this drug exactly as your doctor directs.

If you miss a dose

Adjust your schedule as follows:
• If you take one or more doses a day, take the missed dose as soon as possible. Don't take a double dose.

ROCALTROL'S OTHER NAME

Rocaltrol's generic name is calcitriol.

SIDE EFFECTS

Call your doctor if you have any of these possible drug side effects. Call *immediately* about any labeled "serious."

Serious: vitamin D intoxication associated with excessive calcium in blood (headache, sleepiness, pinkeye, unusual eye sensitivity to light, runny nose, nausea, vomiting, constipation, metallic taste, dry mouth, appetite loss, increased urination, weakness, bone and muscle pain)

Common: none reported

Other: none reported

DRUG INTERACTIONS

Combining certain drugs may alter their action or produce unwanted side effects. Tell your doctor about other drugs you're taking, especially:
• antacids that contain magnesium
• Colestid, Questran, and other drugs that lower cholesterol levels
• Crystodigin, Lanoxin
• mineral oil (excessive amounts)
• nonprescription drugs or dietary supplements that contain calcium, vitamin D, or phosphorus
• steroids.

• If you take one dose every other day, take the missed dose as soon as possible. However, if you don't remember until the next day, take it at that time. Then skip a day and return to your regular schedule.

If you suspect an overdose

Contact your doctor *immediately.* Excessive Rocaltrol can cause too much calcium in the blood (weakness, vomiting, appetite loss, and bone and muscle pain).

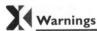
Warnings

• Make sure your doctor knows your medical history. You may not be able to take Rocaltrol if you have other medical problems.

• If you're pregnant or breast-feeding, tell your doctor before you start taking Rocaltrol.

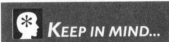

* Don't take antacids or other nonprescription drugs that contain magnesium.

* Call doctor if you have weakness, nausea, vomiting, dry mouth, constipation, muscle or bone pain, or metallic taste.

Roferon-A

Roferon-A is a synthetic version of interferon — a naturally occurring substance that helps fight infections and tumors. The drug is thought to prevent viral cells from reproducing, to stop tumor cells from multiplying, and to enhance the body's immunity.

Why it's prescribed

Doctors prescribe Roferon-A to treat some leukemias and AIDS-related Kaposi's sarcoma. It comes in an injectable form. Doctors usually prescribe the following amounts for adults.

▶ **For hairy-cell leukemia,** initially, 3 million units injected under the skin or into a muscle daily for 16 to 24 weeks. Usual dosage is 3 million units injected three times a week.

▶ **For AIDS-related Kaposi's sarcoma,** initially, 36 million units injected under the skin or into a muscle daily for 10 to 12 weeks. Usual dosage is 36 million units injected three times a week.

How to take Roferon-A

• If you're taking this drug at home, carefully follow your doctor's directions. If Roferon-A makes you feel extremely tired, inject it at bedtime to reduce daytime fatigue.

• Read the instruction sheet that comes with each package of Roferon-A.

ROFERON-A'S OTHER NAME

Roferon-A's generic name is recombinant interferon alfa-2a (RIFN-A).

SIDE EFFECTS

Call your doctor if you have any of these possible drug side effects. Call *immediately* about any labeled "serious."

Serious: congestive heart failure (shortness of breath, cough), blood problems (infection, abnormal bleeding), hepatitis (nausea, vomiting, yellow-tinged skin and eyes, appetite loss, dark urine, clay-colored stools), wheezing and closing of throat
Tips: Avoid people with known infections. Call your doctor immediately if you have symptoms of infection, such as fever, sore throat, or fatigue. To help prevent bleeding, take precautions when using a toothbrush, dental floss, or a razor. Avoid activities in which bruising or injury can occur. Call the doctor if you have symptoms of bleeding, such as easy bruising, nosebleeds, bleeding gums, or black, tarry stools.

Common: dizziness, appetite loss, nausea, diarrhea, rash, itching
Tips: Until you know how this drug affects you, don't drive or do anything else that could be dangerous if you're dizzy. If nausea or diarrhea becomes bothersome, call your doctor.

Other: weakness, sleepiness, apathy, vertigo, incoordination, fainting, swelling, dry or inflamed throat, sinus inflammation, pinkeye, eye irritation, earache, vomiting, abdominal fullness or pain, gas, constipation, bad taste in mouth, coughing, difficulty breathing, flushed or dry skin, partial hair loss, flulike symptoms (fever, chills, fatigue, headache), hot flashes, excessive salivation, bluish skin, increased sweating
Tips: Any hair lost during treatment should return once you stop taking this drug. To offset fluid loss from heavy sweating, drink extra fluids, unless the doctor tells you otherwise. If you develop flulike symptoms, take Tylenol, as instructed by your doctor.

DRUG INTERACTIONS

Combining certain drugs may alter their action or produce unwanted side effects. Tell your doctor about other drugs you're taking, especially:
• drugs that slow down the nervous system, such as cold and allergy drugs, sedatives, tranquilizers, narcotic pain relievers, barbiturates, seizure drugs, and muscle relaxants
• live-virus vaccines (don't get vaccinations without your doctor's approval)
• Theo-Dur.

If you miss a dose

Don't take the missed dose and don't double the next one. Call your doctor for instructions.

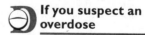
If you suspect an overdose

Consult your doctor.

✕ Warnings

• Make sure your doctor knows your medical history. You may not be able to take Roferon-A if you have other problems, such as heart, kidney, liver, lung, or thyroid disease; seizures; diabetes; bleeding problems; or mental problems; or if you've recently had a heart attack.

• If you're pregnant or breast-feeding, tell your doctor before you start taking Roferon-A.

• Be aware that older adults may be especially prone to side effects of Roferon-A.

• Also be aware that teenage girls who take this drug may experience changes in their menstrual cycle.

• See your doctor regularly so your progress and the drug effects can be monitored.

• Store this drug in the refrigerator.

• Avoid contact with people who've just received the oral polio vaccine because they could pass the polio virus to you. If you can't avoid them, wear a protective mask.

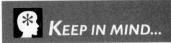

✱ KEEP IN MIND...

∗ Drink extra fluids.

∗ Inject at bedtime to reduce tiredness during day.

∗ Call doctor about symptoms of infection or bleeding.

∗ Don't drive until you know how drug affects you.

∗ Avoid people with infections and those who've just received oral polio vaccine.

Rogaine

R ogaine is a hair growth stimulant. Researchers suspect it works by changing the metabolism of the male hormone androgen in the scalp or by enhancing the circulation around the hair follicles.

Why it's prescribed

Doctors prescribe Rogaine to stimulate hair growth in men and women with a certain type of baldness. You can also buy Rogaine without a prescription. It comes in a topical solution that's used with an applicator or a spray pump. Doctors usually prescribe the following amounts for adults.

▶ **For male-pattern baldness of the crown and scalp,** 1 milliliter (ml) of 2% solution applied to affected area twice a day. Maximum dosage is 2 ml a day.

How to use Rogaine

• Use this drug exactly as your doctor directs. If you bought Rogaine without a prescription, carefully follow the package instructions.
• Apply the drug once in the morning and again at bedtime. Before applying the morning dose, make sure you shampoo your hair and dry it thoroughly with a towel. Then, starting at the center of the bald area, spread the drug with the applicator.
• Don't use a hair dryer after applying Rogaine.
• After applying your bedtime dose, let the solution dry for at least 30 minutes.

ROGAINE'S OTHER NAME

Rogaine's generic name is minoxidil.

 SIDE EFFECTS

Call your doctor if you have any of these possible drug side effects.

Serious: none reported

Common: none reported

Other: headache, dizziness, swelling, chest pain, palpitations, sinus inflammation, bronchitis, skin irritation, unusual growth of body hair, dry flaking skin or scalp

Tip: Red, dry, or flaky skin and increased hair growth usually go away as your body adjusts to the drug. Check with your doctor if they persist or become bothersome.

 DRUG INTERACTIONS

Combining certain drugs may alter their action or produce unwanted side effects. Tell your doctor about other drugs you're taking, especially:
• Ismelin
• topical steroids, Vaseline, and other drugs that enhance skin absorption.

• If you're spraying Rogaine on your hair, avoid inhaling the spray or getting it in your eyes.
• If you apply Rogaine by hand, wash your hands thoroughly when you're finished.
• If your scalp becomes irritated or sunburned, stop using Rogaine temporarily and consult your doctor.
• You must use Rogaine every day. If you stop using it, hair growth will stop and you'll lose any new hair within a few months.
• It may take 4 or more months before you see results.

If you miss a dose

Apply the missed dose as soon as possible; then resume your regular schedule. However, if it's almost time for your next dose, skip the missed dose and apply the next dose as scheduled. Don't apply the drug twice.

If you suspect an overdose

Contact your doctor *immediately*. Excessive Rogaine can cause a fast pulse, headache, and flushed skin.

Warnings

• You may not be able to use Rogaine if you have other medical problems. Consult your doctor.
• If you're pregnant or breast-feeding, tell your doctor before you start using Rogaine.

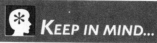

* Apply in morning and at bedtime.
* After applying bedtime dose, let drug dry for at least 30 minutes.
* Don't use hair dryer during treatment.

Rolaids

Rolaids is an antacid. It neutralizes stomach acid and strengthens the stomach lining. These effects relieve acid indigestion and heartburn.

Why it's taken

Rolaids is taken to relieve sour stomach, heartburn, and indigestion. You can buy Rolaids without a prescription. It comes in tablets. The following amounts are usually recommended for adults.

▶ **As an antacid,** 1 to 2 tablets as needed.

How to take Rolaids

• Take this drug exactly as the package directs. Chew the tablets well.
• Don't take Rolaids for more than 2 weeks unless directed by your doctor.

If you miss a dose

If you're taking Rolaids regularly, take the missed dose as soon as possible. But if it's almost time for your next dose, skip the missed dose and take your next dose as scheduled. Don't take a double dose.

 If you suspect an overdose

Consult your doctor.

 Warnings

• Consult your doctor before taking Rolaids if you have other problems, such as colitis, constipation,

ROLAIDS' OTHER NAME

Rolaids' generic name is dihydroxyaluminum sodium carbonate.

 SIDE EFFECTS

Call your doctor if you have any of these possible drug side effects.

Serious: none reported

Common: constipation
Tip: If constipation occurs, take a laxative or stool softener, or alternate Rolaids with an antacid that contains magnesium. However, if you have kidney disease, don't take a magnesium-containing antacid.

Other: appetite loss, intestinal blockage (abdominal pain and bloating, unrelieved constipation)

 DRUG INTERACTIONS

Combining certain drugs may alter their action or produce unwanted side effects. Tell your doctor about other drugs you're taking, especially the following (take them 1 to 2 hours before or after taking Rolaids):
• antibiotics
• Cuprimine
• Dolobid
• enteric-coated drugs
• iron
• Laniazid
• Lanoxin
• phenothiazines (used for anxiety, nausea, vomiting, or psychosis)
• Quinaglute Dura-tabs
• Zyloprim.

hemorrhoids, intestinal or rectal bleeding, a colostomy or an ileostomy, swelling of the feet or lower legs, underactive parathyroid, sarcoidosis, or heart, liver, or kidney disease. Don't take Rolaids if you have symptoms of an inflamed bowel or appendicitis, such as pain in your stomach or lower abdomen, bloating, nausea, vomiting, or cramping.
• If you're pregnant, tell your doctor before you start taking Rolaids. The drug's high salt content may cause problems if you retain water.
• If you take this drug in large doses or for a long time, see your doctor regularly so your progress and the drug effects can be monitored.

• Rolaids contains a lot of salt. If you're on a low-salt diet, consult your doctor before taking it.
• If your condition doesn't improve, call your doctor.

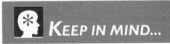 **KEEP IN MIND...**

* Chew tablets well.
* Don't take for more than 2 weeks unless doctor approves.
* Don't take if you have symptoms of inflamed bowel or appendicitis.

Rowasa

Rowasa reduces inflammation and other symptoms of bowel disease. Researchers think it works by inhibiting the production of hormones called prostaglandins in the bowel.

Why it's prescribed

Doctors prescribe Rowasa to treat inflammatory bowel diseases, such as ulcerative colitis. It comes in delayed-release tablets, controlled-release capsules, a rectal suspension, and rectal suppositories. Doctors usually prescribe the following amounts for adults.

▶ **For ulcerative colitis, inflammation of the rectum and anus, or inflammation of the rectum and sigmoid colon,** 800 milligrams (mg) of tablets three times a day for 6 weeks; or 1 gram (g) of capsules four times a day for up to 8 weeks; or 4 g of suspension as an enema once a day; or 500 mg by rectal suppository two times a day.

How to take Rowasa

• Take Rowasa only as directed.
• If your doctor has prescribed the rectal suspension form, take it as an enema once a day, preferably at bedtime. You may need to continue the routine for up to 6 weeks. Just before taking the enema, empty your bowels. Then shake the suspension well and administer the enema. Be sure to retain the enema for at least 8 hours.

ROWASA'S OTHER NAMES

Rowasa's generic name is mesalamine. Other brand names include Asacol and Pentasa.

• Keep taking Rowasa for the full treatment time prescribed by your doctor, even if you feel better within several days. Don't miss doses.
• Store this drug away from heat and direct light. Keep the suppositories at room temperature. Don't allow the rectal suspension to freeze.

If you miss a dose

If you remember the same night, take the missed dose as soon as possible. If you don't remember until the next morning, skip the missed dose and resume your regular schedule.

 If you suspect an overdose

Consult your doctor.

 SIDE EFFECTS

Call your doctor if you have any of these possible drug side effects. Call *immediately* about any labeled "serious."

Serious: rash, wheezing, itching, hives, severe stomach or abdominal pain or cramps, fever, bloody diarrhea, severe headache

Common: pancolitis (severe pain, cramping, bloody diarrhea)

Other: headache, dizziness, fatigue, hair loss, stomach pain and cramps, gas, diarrhea, rectal irritation (pain, bleeding, burning, itching), nausea, allergic reaction (itching, rash, hives)

Tips: Call your doctor as soon as possible if you develop symptoms of rectal irritation after you start using the enema form of the drug. Relieve these symptoms by applying zinc oxide or A&D ointment to the anal area. Mild headache and stomach discomfort usually go away as your body adjusts to the drug. Check with your doctor if they persist or become bothersome.

 DRUG INTERACTIONS

Combining certain drugs may alter their action or produce unwanted side effects. Tell your doctor about other drugs you're taking.

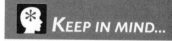 **Warnings**

• Make sure your doctor knows your medical history. You may not be able to take Rowasa if you're allergic to aspirin or have kidney disease.
• Have regular medical checkups so the doctor can evaluate your progress.

KEEP IN MIND...

* Keep taking for full treatment time prescribed.

* Take rectal suspension as enema at bedtime.

* Call doctor about sudden rectal pain, bleeding, burning, or itching.

Roxicet

Roxicet is a pain reliever containing both a narcotic and acetaminophen. For many people, this combination relieves pain better than either drug used alone, and it allows lower doses of each drug. Roxicet changes a person's perception of and response to pain.

Why it's prescribed

Doctors prescribe Roxicet for moderate to moderately severe pain. It comes in tablets and a solution. Doctors usually prescribe the following amounts for adults.

▶ **For pain,** 1 tablet or 1 tablespoon of solution every 6 hours, as needed.

How to take Roxicet

- Take this drug exactly as your doctor directs. Take with food or a full glass (8 ounces) of water. Store Roxicet at room temperature.
- Don't take more of this drug than directed; doing so could cause an overdose or lead to drug dependence.
- Don't stop taking Roxicet suddenly after regular use because doing so could cause withdrawal symptoms. Call your doctor, who will tell you how to reduce your dosage gradually.

If you miss a dose

Take the missed dose as soon as possible. But if it's almost time for your

SIDE EFFECTS

Call your doctor if you have any of these possible drug side effects. Call *immediately* about any labeled "serious."

Serious: slow and shallow breaths, extreme tiredness, physical or psychological dependence, seizures, shortness of breath, slow pulse, cold, clammy skin

Common: dizziness, nausea, vomiting
Tip: When lying or sitting, get up slowly to avoid dizziness.

Other: constipation, inability to urinate
Tip: Drink liquids to avoid constipation.

DRUG INTERACTIONS

Combining certain drugs may alter their action or produce unwanted side effects. Tell your doctor about other drugs you're taking, especially:

- alcohol
- antidepressants called MAO inhibitors, such as Parnate and Nardil
- eyedrops that enlarge pupils such as Timoptic
- Tylenol and other acetaminophen-containing drugs
- Xanax and other tranquilizers.

next dose, skip the missed dose and take your next dose as scheduled. Don't take a double dose.

If you suspect an overdose

Contact your doctor *immediately.* Excessive Roxicet can cause confusion, nervousness, restlessness, seizures, shortness of breath or difficulty breathing, and severe weakness, dizziness, and drowsiness.

Warnings

- Make sure your doctor knows your medical history. You may not be able to take Roxicet if you have seizures, heart disease, brain disease, head injury, asthma or another chronic lung disease, colitis, hepatitis or other liver disease, kidney disease, an underactive thyroid, gallbladder disease or

gallstones, or a history of drug or alcohol dependence.

- If you're pregnant or breast-feeding, tell your doctor before starting Roxicet. Overuse of narcotics during pregnancy can cause drug dependence in your baby.
- Children and older adults may be especially prone to Roxicet's side effects.
- Before surgery (including dental surgery) or emergency treatment, tell your doctor or dentist that you're taking Roxicet.

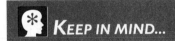

KEEP IN MIND...

* Take only as prescribed.
* Don't take with alcohol.
* Can cause drowsiness.

ROXICET'S OTHER NAMES

Roxicet is a combination of the generic drugs acetaminophen and oxycodone. Other brand names include Percocet, Tylox; and, in Canada, Endocet and Oxycocet.

Roxicodone

Roxicodone is a narcotic pain reliever. It acts on opiate receptors in the brain, changing the way a person perceives and responds to pain.

Why it's prescribed

Doctors prescribe Roxicodone to help relieve pain. It comes in tablets, an oral solution, and suppositories. Doctors usually prescribe the following amounts for adults; children's dosages appear in parentheses.

▶ **For moderate to severe pain,** 5 milligrams (mg) orally every 6 hours, as needed. Or 1 to 3 suppositories rectally a day, as needed. (Children age 13 and older: 2.44 mg orally every 6 hours, as needed. Children ages 6 to 12: 1.22 mg orally three or four times a day, as needed.)

How to take Roxicodone

• Take this drug exactly as your doctor directs.
• Don't take more of the drug than directed; this could cause an overdose or lead to drug dependence.
• Check with your doctor before you stop taking this drug. Stopping suddenly could cause withdrawal symptoms.

If you miss a dose

Take the missed dose as soon as possible. But if it's almost time for your next dose, skip the missed dose and

ROXICODONE'S OTHER NAMES

Roxicodone's generic name is oxycodone. A Canadian brand name is Supeudol.

 SIDE EFFECTS

Call your doctor if you have any of these possible drug side effects. Call *immediately* about any labeled "serious."

Serious: shallow breathing, seizures (with large doses)

Common: sleepiness, clouded thinking, unusual sense of well-being, dizziness, weakness, nausea, vomiting, constipation, inability to urinate
Tips: Until you know how this drug affects you, don't drive or do anything else that could be dangerous if you're dizzy or not fully alert. To prevent or relieve nausea, take Roxicodone after meals or with milk.

Other: slow pulse, intestinal blockage (abdominal pain and bloating, unrelieved constipation), physical drug dependence

 DRUG INTERACTIONS

Combining certain drugs may alter their action or produce unwanted side effects. Tell your doctor about other drugs you're taking, especially:
• alcohol and other drugs that slow down the nervous system, such as cold and allergy drugs, sedatives, tranquilizers, narcotic pain relievers, barbiturates, seizure drugs, and muscle relaxants
• anticoagulants (blood thinners)
• drugs used for depression (including MAO inhibitors and tricyclic antidepressants).

take your next dose as scheduled. Don't take a double dose.

 If you suspect an overdose

Contact your doctor *immediately*. Excessive Roxicodone can cause seizures, shallow or arrested breathing, small pupils, decreased level of consciousness, slow pulse, low blood pressure (dizziness, weakness), low body temperature, and fluid buildup in the lungs (difficulty breathing).

Warnings

• Make sure your doctor knows your medical history. You may not be able to take Roxicodone if you have other medical problems.
• If you're pregnant or breast-feeding, check with your doctor before you start taking Roxicodone.

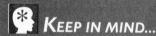 **KEEP IN MIND...**

* Take after meals or with milk to prevent stomach upset.

* To prevent withdrawal symptoms, don't stop taking suddenly.

* Don't drive until you know how drug affects you.

Rythmol

Rythmol is an antiarrhythmic drug — one that corrects an irregular heartbeat. It slows nerve impulses in the heart and makes heart tissues less sensitive, which helps to change an irregular heartbeat to a normal rhythm.

Why it's prescribed

Doctors prescribe Rythmol to convert a dangerous irregular heartbeat to a normal heart rhythm. It comes in tablets. Doctors usually prescribe the following amounts for adults.

▶ **For suppression of dangerous irregular heartbeat,** initially, 150 milligrams (mg) every 8 hours, increased every 3 to 4 days to 225 mg every 8 hours, if needed, or to 300 mg every 8 hours. Maximum dosage is 900 mg a day.

How to take Rythmol

• Take this drug exactly as your doctor directs, preferably at evenly spaced times day and night.
• Keep taking Rythmol as prescribed, even if you feel well.

If you miss a dose

If you remember within 4 hours, take the missed dose as soon as possible. However, if you don't remember until later, skip the missed dose and take your next dose as scheduled. Don't take a double dose.

RYTHMOL'S OTHER NAME

Rythmol's generic name is propafenone.

SIDE EFFECTS

Call your doctor if you have any of these possible drug side effects. Call *immediately* about any labeled "serious."

Serious: heart failure (shortness of breath, swelling), new irregular heartbeat or worsening of existing one

Common: none reported

Other: appetite loss, anxiety, incoordination, dizziness, weakness, drowsiness, fatigue, headache, difficulty sleeping, fainting, tremor, slow pulse, palpitations, chest pain, swelling, blurred vision, abdominal pain or cramps, constipation, diarrhea, stomach upset, gas, nausea, vomiting, dry mouth, unusual taste, joint pain

Tip: Call your doctor immediately if you have chest pain, palpitations, an irregular heartbeat, or difficulty breathing. Make sure you know how you react to Rythmol before you drive or perform other activities that require alertness, good coordination, and clear vision.

DRUG INTERACTIONS

Combining certain drugs may alter their action or produce unwanted side effects. Tell your doctor about other drugs you're taking, especially:
• local anesthetics such as Lanacane
• other drugs used to treat heart problems or high blood pressure, such as Crystodigin and Lanoxin
• Rifadin
• Tagamet.

If you suspect an overdose

Contact your doctor *immediately.* Excessive Rythmol can cause a slow pulse, fast and irregular heartbeat, low blood pressure (dizziness, weakness), sleepiness, and seizures.

Warnings

• Make sure your doctor knows your medical history. You may not be able to take Rythmol if you have other medical problems.

• If you're pregnant, check with your doctor before you start taking this drug.

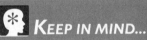

KEEP IN MIND...

* Space doses evenly throughout day and night.

* Don't drive until you know how drug affects you.

* Call doctor immediately if you have chest pain, a fast or irregular pulse, or difficulty breathing.

Sandimmune

Sandimmune is one of several drugs called immunosuppressants. It inhibits the body's infection-fighting system.

Why it's prescribed

Doctors prescribe Sandimmune to prevent rejection in people who've received an organ transplant. It comes in a liquid and capsules. It's also available in an injectable form. Doctors usually prescribe the following amounts for adults and children.

▶ **To prevent organ rejection,** 15 milligrams (mg) for each 2.2 pounds (lb) of body weight orally 4 to 12 hours before transplantation, continued daily for 1 to 2 weeks after surgery. Then dosage reduced by 5% each week to reach a level of 5 to 10 mg for each 2.2 lb a day.

How to take Sandimmune

• Take this drug exactly as your doctor directs. Take your dose at the same time each day, preferably in the morning.
• If you wish, mix your dose in a glass container with fruit juice (preferably at room temperature) or milk to make it taste better. Stir it well and drink it immediately. Then rinse the glass with a little more liquid and drink that, too.
• Remember that the capsules come in two strengths: 25 mg and 100 mg. You may be taking some of both strengths to obtain an exact dose. Swallow the capsules whole; don't chew or open them.
• Don't stop taking this drug without consulting your doctor.

SANDIMMUNE'S OTHER NAME

Sandimmune's generic name is cyclosporine.

SIDE EFFECTS

Call your doctor if you have any of these possible drug side effects. Call *immediately* about any labeled "serious."

Serious: kidney problems (decreased urination), liver problems (yellow-tinged skin and eyes, itching), blood problems (abnormal bleeding, fatigue, increased risk of infection, black, tarry stools), high blood pressure (headache, blurred vision)

Common: tremor, headache, unusual hair growth on face and body; swollen, tender, or bleeding gums

Other: white patches inside mouth and on tongue, nausea, vomiting, diarrhea, flushed skin, acne, sinus inflammation, increased cholesterol level
Tip: If Sandimmune causes nausea, take it with meals.

DRUG INTERACTIONS

Combining certain drugs may alter their action or produce unwanted side effects. Tell your doctor about other drugs you're taking, especially:
• antibiotics, antifungal drugs, and other drugs used to treat infections
• Calan, Cardizem
• certain pain relievers, such as Advil and aspirin
• Cytoxan, Imuran
• Laniazid, Rifadin
• Reglan, Tagamet
• seizure drugs, such as Barbita, Dilantin, and Tegretol
• steroids
• vaccines.

If you miss a dose

If you forget a dose or if you vomit soon after taking it, call your doctor right away. Follow the doctor's instructions for getting back on schedule. Don't take a double dose.

If you suspect an overdose

Contact your doctor *immediately.* Excessive Sandimmune can cause nausea, vomiting, and tremor.

Warnings

• Make sure your doctor knows your medical history. You may not be able to take Sandimmune if you have other medical problems.
• If you're pregnant or breast-feeding, check with your doctor before you start taking Sandimmune.

KEEP IN MIND...

* Take dose at same time each day.
* Take with meals if drug causes nausea.
* Call doctor about symptoms of infection or bleeding.

Sandoglobulin

Sandoglobulin boosts the body's immunity to several diseases and increases the number of platelets, the blood cells required for clotting.

Why it's prescribed

Doctors prescribe Sandoglobulin to prevent or treat certain illnesses that result from an immune system deficiency, such as agammaglobulinemia. This drug is also used to build up the body's platelet count and prevent bleeding in a blood disorder called idiopathic thrombocytopenic purpura (ITP). Sandoglobulin comes in an intravenous form. Doctors usually prescribe the following amounts.

▶ **For an immune system deficiency in adults and children,** 200 milligrams (mg) for each 2.2 pounds (lb) of body weight once a month. If response is poor, dosage may be increased up to 800 mg for each 2.2 lb and frequency may be increased to twice a month.

▶ **For ITP in adults,** 400 mg for each 2.2 lb every day for 5 days, then repeated as needed.

How to take Sandoglobulin

• Follow your doctor's instructions for receiving this drug.
• A health care professional will administer Sandoglobulin to you, usually through a vein in the arm.
• If you're taking Sandoglobulin for ITP, be aware that the rise in platelet count usually lasts from several days to several weeks; on

SANDOGLOBULIN'S OTHER NAME

Sandoglobulin's generic name is immune globulin intravenous (IGIV).

SIDE EFFECTS

Call your doctor if you have any of these possible drug side effects. Call *immediately* about any labeled "serious."

Serious: allergic reaction (fever, chills, vomiting, chest tightness, sweating, dizziness, wheezing), difficulty breathing, fast pulse, blue-tinged lips, stiff neck, severe headache, sensitivity to bright light

Common: general feeling of illness, backache, muscle or joint pain

Other: rash, redness, or pain at injection site

DRUG INTERACTIONS

Combining certain drugs may alter their action or produce unwanted side effects. Tell your doctor about other drugs you're taking, especially:
• live-virus vaccines, such as measles, mumps, and rubella (consult your doctor before being immunized during Sandoglobulin treatment).

rare occasions, it may last 1 year or longer.

If you miss a dose

Consult your doctor.

If you suspect an overdose

Consult your doctor. Signs and symptoms of an overdose may include dizziness, fever, chills, sweating, vomiting, trouble breathing, blue-tinged lips, chest tightness, fast pulse, stiff neck, severe headache, and sensitivity to bright light.

Warnings

• Make sure your doctor knows your medical history. You may not be able to take Sandoglobulin if you have other problems, such as an allergy to this or other immune globulin drugs, allergy to foods or dyes, heart problems, or certain immune deficiencies (depending on how recently you received treatment, side effects may be worse).

• Before you start taking Sandoglobulin, tell your doctor if you're pregnant or breast-feeding.
• If you're taking Sandoglobulin for ITP and are prone to bleeding, remember to brush your teeth gently, use an electric shaver, wear a seatbelt, and avoid cuts and falls.
• If you're taking Sandoglobulin for ITP, your doctor may want to take a blood sample regularly to check your platelet count.
• Be advised that Sandoglobulin does not contain the hepatitis B virus or the human immunodeficiency virus (HIV).

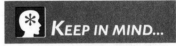
KEEP IN MIND...

∗ Don't take if you're pregnant or breast-feeding.
∗ Report any side effects.
∗ Delay vaccinations until doctor approves.

Sanorex

Sanorex is an appetite suppressant thought to reduce appetite by decreasing the levels of two important brain chemicals.

Why it's prescribed

Doctors prescribe Sanorex as part of an overall treatment plan to help obese people lose weight. It comes in tablets. Doctors usually prescribe the following amounts for adults.

▶ **For short-term use in treating some types of obesity,** 1 milligram (mg) three times a day 1 hour before meals, or 2 mg 1 hour before lunch in a single dose each day. Lowest effective dosage should be used.

How to take Sanorex

• Take this drug exactly as your doctor directs. Don't take more of it or take it more often than prescribed.

• Because this drug may cause difficulty sleeping, take your last dose of the day 4 to 6 hours before bedtime if you take the 1-mg tablet, or 10 to 14 hours before bedtime if you take the 2-mg tablet.

If you miss a dose

Take the missed dose with the next meal. Don't take a double dose.

 If you suspect an overdose

Contact your doctor *immediately*. Excessive Sanorex can cause fever,

SANOREX'S OTHER NAMES

Sanorex's generic name is mazindol. Another brand name is Mazanor.

 SIDE EFFECTS

Call your doctor if you have any of these possible drug side effects.

Serious: none reported

Common: nervousness, difficulty sleeping, palpitations, fast pulse

Other: dizziness, overall feeling of illness, depression, drowsiness, tremor, headache, dry mouth, nausea, constipation, diarrhea, difficulty urinating, impotence, low blood sugar level (clammy or pale skin, tremor), rash, shivering, sweating, change in sex drive

Tip: Until you know how this drug affects you, don't drive or do anything else that could be dangerous if you're dizzy or drowsy.

 DRUG AND FOOD INTERACTIONS

Combining certain drugs and foods may alter drug action or produce unwanted side effects. Tell your doctor about your diet and other drugs you're taking, especially:

• antidepressants called MAO inhibitors (don't take within 14 days of taking Sanorex)

• certain blood pressure drugs, such as Aldomet and Catapres

• foods and beverages containing caffeine, such as coffee, tea, cola, and chocolate

• insulin and oral diabetes drugs.

restlessness, tremor, increased reflexes, fast breathing, dizziness, nausea, vomiting, diarrhea, cramps, high blood pressure (headache, blurred vision), and fast pulse.

 Warnings

• Make sure your doctor knows your medical history. You may not be able to take Sanorex if you have other problems, such as glaucoma, high blood pressure, heart or blood vessel disease, seizures, an overactive thyroid, kidney disease, diabetes, mental illness, or a history of drug or alcohol abuse.

• If you're pregnant or breast-feeding, tell your doctor before you start taking Sanorex.

• Children under age 12 shouldn't take this drug.

• If you're diabetic, be aware that you may need to change the amount of diabetes drug you take during Sanorex treatment.

KEEP IN MIND...

* Take last dose of day well before bedtime.

* Don't give to children under age 12.

* Don't drive until you know how drug affects you.

Santyl

Santyl is an enzyme that helps remove dirt, damaged tissue, and cell debris from burns and wounds.

Why it's prescribed

Doctors prescribe Santyl to help clean wounds and thereby prevent infection and promote healing. It comes in an ointment. Doctors usually prescribe the following amounts for adults and children.

▶ **To promote healing of severe burns and skin ulcers (including bedsores),** a small amount applied directly to wound once every other day.

How to use Santyl

• Use this drug exactly as your doctor directs. Don't apply it near the eyes.
• Wash your hands thoroughly before and after applying Santyl.
• Before each application, gently clean the wound with a gauze pad saturated with 0.9% sodium chloride solution or hydrogen peroxide to remove dead tissue.
• Remove any excess ointment at the time of each dressing change.
• Use a sterile wooden tongue depressor to apply Santyl directly to a deep wound. For a shallow wound, first apply the ointment to a sterile gauze pad, and then apply the gauze to the wound and secure it.
• Take care not to get the ointment on any healthy surrounding skin.

SANTYL'S OTHER NAME

Santyl's generic name is collagenase.

 SIDE EFFECTS

Call your doctor if you have any of these possible drug side effects.
Serious: none reported
Common: pain and burning at application site, slight redness of surrounding tissue
Tip: Do not apply to healthy surrounding skin.

 DRUG INTERACTIONS

Combining certain drugs may alter their action or produce unwanted side effects. Tell your doctor about other drugs you're using, especially:
• Burow's solution
• detergents
• Furacin
• Mercurochrome II
• phisoHex
• tincture of iodine.

• Applying a protectant, such as zinc oxide paste, to the area around the wound may minimize skin irritation. Discuss this with your doctor.
• Don't store Santyl at temperatures higher than 98.6° F (37° C).

If you miss a dose

Apply the missed dose as soon as possible. Don't apply a double dose.

 If you suspect an overdose

Consult your doctor.

Warnings

• Make sure your doctor knows your medical history. You may not be able to use Santyl if you are allergic to it.

• Before you start using Santyl, tell your doctor if you're pregnant or breast-feeding.
• If you get Santyl in your eyes, flush them immediately with lots of water.

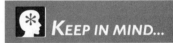 **KEEP IN MIND...**

∗ Wash hands before and after using.
∗ Clean wound thoroughly, as directed.
∗ Don't apply on healthy skin around wound.

Sectral

Sectral is a beta blocker — a drug that interferes with the action of a specific part of the nervous system. This, in turn, steadies the heartbeat and lowers high blood pressure.

Why it's prescribed

Doctors prescribe Sectral to help control high blood pressure or to correct an irregular heartbeat. It comes in capsules. Doctors usually prescribe the following amounts for adults.

▶ **For high blood pressure,** 400 milligrams (mg) a day in a single dose or divided into two equal doses. Maximum dosage is 1,200 mg a day.

▶ **To suppress irregular heartbeats known as premature ventricular contractions,** 400 mg a day divided into two equal doses, increased as needed. Usual dosage is 600 to 1,200 mg a day. Older adults may require a lower dosage; they should not take more than 800 mg a day.

How to take Sectral

• Take this drug exactly as your doctor directs. Don't break, chew, or crush the capsules. Swallow them whole.

• Always check your pulse before taking Sectral. If it's under 50 beats a minute, call your doctor and don't take the drug.

• Don't stop taking Sectral abruptly. Doing so could lead to heart problems.

SECTRAL'S OTHER NAMES

Sectral's generic name is acebutolol. A Canadian brand name is Monitan.

 SIDE EFFECTS

Call your doctor if you have any of these possible drug side effects. Call *immediately* about any labeled "serious."

Serious: wheezing, closing of throat

Common: fatigue, dizziness, weakness
Tip: Until you know how this drug affects you, don't drive or do anything else that could be dangerous if you're dizzy.

Other: headache, difficulty sleeping, chest pain, swelling, slow pulse, nausea, constipation, diarrhea, stomach upset, difficulty breathing or shortness of breath, rash, fever, increased sensitivity to cold
Tip: Avoid prolonged exposure to cold, and dress warmly in cold weather.

 DRUG INTERACTIONS

Combining certain drugs may alter their action or produce unwanted side effects. Tell your doctor about other drugs you're taking, especially:
• Crystodigin, Lanoxin
• insulin and oral diabetes drugs
• nonsteroidal anti-inflammatory drugs, such as Advil and Naprosyn

If you miss a dose

Take the missed dose as soon as possible. But if it's within 4 hours of your next dose, skip the missed dose and take your dose as scheduled. Don't take a double dose.

 If you suspect an overdose

Contact your doctor *immediately.* Excessive Sectral can cause severe low blood pressure (dizziness and weakness), a slow pulse, wheezing and closing of the throat, and heart failure (fatigue, swelling, shortness of breath).

 Warnings

• Make sure your doctor knows your medical history. You may not be able to take Sectral if you have other problems, such as heart or blood vessel disease, unusually slow heartbeat, chronic lung disease, diabetes, kidney or liver disease, myasthenia gravis, thyroid problems, or depression, or if you're allergic to certain drugs, foods, preservatives, or dyes.

• If you're pregnant or breast-feeding, tell your doctor before you start taking Sectral.

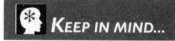 **KEEP IN MIND...**

* Swallow capsules whole; don't break, chew, or crush them.

* Check pulse before taking.

* Dress warmly in cold weather.

Seldane is an antihistamine, and Seldane-D is an antihistamine and decongestant combination. The antihistamine impedes the effects of histamine, a natural substance that causes itching, sneezing, runny nose, and watery eyes. This action dries up secretions of the nose, throat, and eyes and relieves itching. The decongestant in Seldane-D narrows blood vessels in the nose, easing nasal congestion.

Why it's prescribed

Doctors prescribe Seldane to relieve allergy symptoms and Seldane-D to relieve a runny nose, stuffy nose, and sneezing caused by colds or hay fever. These drugs come in tablets and a liquid. Doctors usually prescribe the following amounts for adults and children age 12 and older.

▶ **For runny nose and other allergy symptoms,** 60 milligrams twice a day.

How to take Seldane or Seldane-D

• Take these drugs exactly as your doctor directs. Don't take more than the recommended dose, even if your symptoms don't subside. Don't crush or chew tablets.

SELDANE'S AND SELDANE-D'S OTHER NAMES

Seldane's generic name is terfenadine. Seldane-D is a combination of the generic drugs terfenadine and pseudoephedrine.

 SIDE EFFECTS

Call your doctor if you have any of these possible drug side effects. Call *immediately* about any labeled "serious."

Serious: irregular heartbeat

Common: headache
Tip: If Seldane or Seldane-D causes a headache, take Tylenol or another mild pain reliever. If the headache is severe, call your doctor.

Other: fatigue, dizziness, sleepiness, dry throat, stuffy nose, stomach upset, nausea, dry mouth, hair loss, yellow-tinged skin, rash, hives; with Seldane-D, nervousness, restlessness, difficulty sleeping
Tip: If Seldane-D makes you nervous or restless or causes difficulty sleeping, take the last daily dose a few hours before bedtime.

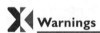 **DRUG INTERACTIONS**

Combining certain drugs may alter their action or produce unwanted side effects. Tell your doctor about other drugs you're taking, especially:
• antibiotics, such as Cipro, E-Mycin, and TAO
• antifungal drugs, such as Nizoral and Sporanox
• Tagamet.

• Drink plenty of fluids, especially if you're congested, to prevent your mucus from becoming thick and difficult to cough up.

If you miss a dose

Take the missed dose as soon as possible. But if it's almost time for your next dose, skip the missed dose and take your next dose as scheduled. Don't take a double dose.

 If you suspect an overdose

Contact your doctor *immediately.* Excessive Seldane or Seldane-D can cause mild headache, nausea, confusion, and an irregular heartbeat.

 Warnings

• Make sure your doctor knows your medical history. You may not be able to take Seldane or Seldane-D if you have other medical problems.
• If you're pregnant or breast-feeding, check with your doctor before taking either drug.

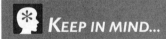 **KEEP IN MIND...**

∗ Take last daily dose of Seldane-D a few hours before bedtime.

∗ Drink lots of fluids.

∗ Call doctor about severe headache.

Senokot

Senokot is a laxative that promotes bowel movements by acting on the intestinal wall and enhancing the muscle contractions that cause the stool to move through the bowel. It also increases fluid accumulation in the bowel.

Why it's taken

Senokot is taken to treat constipation. You can buy Senokot without a prescription. It comes in tablets, granules, a syrup, and suppositories. The following amounts are usually recommended for adults; children's dosages appear in parentheses.

▶ **For acute constipation,** 1 to 8 tablets or ½ to 4 teaspoons of granules added to liquid orally, or 1 to 2 suppositories rectally at bedtime, or 1 to 4 teaspoons of syrup orally at bedtime. (Children ages 6 to 12: 1 tablet or 1 teaspoon granules once a day. Children ages 2 to 5: ½ tablet or ½ teaspoon granules once a day.)

How to take Senokot

• If you're treating yourself, follow the package instructions carefully.
• If your doctor gave you special instructions on how to take this drug, follow the instructions exactly.
• For faster results, take Senokot on an empty stomach.

SENOKOT'S OTHER NAMES

Senokot's generic name is senna. Other brand names include Black-Draught, Fletcher's Castoria, Lax-Senna, Senexon, and Senolax.

 SIDE EFFECTS

Call your doctor if you have any of these possible drug side effects.

Serious: none reported

Common: nausea, abdominal cramps (especially in people with severe constipation)

Other: vomiting, diarrhea, loss of normal bowel function (with excessive use), constipation after bowel movement, yellow or yellow-green tinge to stools, darkening of rectal lining (with long-term use), laxative dependence (with excessive use), red-pink or yellow-brown urine discoloration, too little potassium in blood (muscle weakness, cramps)
Tip: To help prevent laxative dependence or loss of normal bowel function, don't get into the habit of taking laxatives.

 DRUG INTERACTIONS

Combining certain drugs may alter their action or produce unwanted side effects. Tell your doctor about other drugs you're taking.

If you miss a dose

Not applicable because drug is taken only as needed.

If you suspect an overdose

Consult your doctor.

Warnings

• Consult your doctor before taking Senokot if you have other medical problems, such as bowel disease or blockage, rectal bleeding, a colostomy or an ileostomy, heart disease, high blood pressure, or diabetes. Don't take this drug if you have symptoms of an inflamed bowel or appendicitis, such as pain in your stomach or lower abdomen, cramping, bloating, nausea, or vomiting. Instead, call your doctor promptly.

• If you're pregnant or breast-feeding, tell your doctor before you start taking Senokot.
• Children under age 6 shouldn't take a laxative unless it's prescribed by the doctor.
• Drink six to eight glasses of water daily to soften your stools.

 KEEP IN MIND...

* For fast results, take on empty stomach.

* Drink six to eight glasses of fluids daily to soften stools.

* Don't get into laxative habit.

* Call doctor about symptoms of inflamed bowel or appendicitis.

Ser-Ap-Es

Ser-Ap-Es is a combination of three drugs used to treat high blood pressure. One drug controls nerve impulses that act on the heart and blood vessels to decrease blood pressure. Another drug relaxes blood vessels, increases blood flow to the heart, and lowers the heart's workload. The third drug, a diuretic (water pill), lowers blood pressure by increasing urine flow, which rids the body of excess water.

Why it's prescribed

Doctors prescribe Ser-Ap-Es to reduce high blood pressure. It comes in tablets. Doctors usually prescribe the following amounts for adults and children.

▶ **For high blood pressure,** dosage depends on the person but may be up to 0.25 milligrams a day.

How to take Ser-Ap-Es

• Take this drug exactly as your doctor directs.

• Ser-Ap-Es may cause you to urinate more frequently. Scheduling your doses can help prevent this side effect from affecting your sleep. If you take one dose a day, take it in the morning after breakfast. If you take more than one dose a day, take the last dose before 6 p.m., unless your doctor gives you other instructions.

SER-AP-ES'S OTHER NAMES

Ser-Ap-Es is a combination of the generic drugs reserpine, hydralazine, and hydrochlorothiazide. Other brand names include Cam-Ap-Es, Cherapas, Ser-A-Gen, Seralazide, Serpazide, Tri-Hydroserpine, and Unipres.

 SIDE EFFECTS

Call your doctor if you have any of these possible drug side effects. Call *immediately* about any labeled "serious."

Serious: extreme tiredness, impotence, depression, inability to concentrate, black stools, seizures, irregular pulse, difficulty sleeping, potassium deficiency (muscle weakness, cramps)
Tips: Tiredness should subside once your body adjusts to the drug. Eat foods that are high in potassium, such as bananas and oranges.

Common: dry mouth, moodiness, diarrhea, stomach upset, appetite loss
Tips: To relieve dry mouth, use ice chips or sugarless gum or candy. Brush your teeth and rinse with water frequently. If the tablets upset your stomach, take them with food or milk.

Other: constipation, skin sensitivity to sunlight, swelling, eye irritation, drowsiness, dizziness, increased urination
Tips: Avoid constipation by drinking more liquids and eating high-fiber foods. To protect your skin, avoid sun exposure, apply a sunblock, and wear protective clothing when going outdoors. Until you know how this drug affects you, don't drive or do anything else that could be dangerous if you're not fully alert. To prevent dizziness when standing up, rise slowly from a sitting or lying position.

 DRUG INTERACTIONS

Combining certain drugs may alter their action or produce unwanted side effects. Tell your doctor about other drugs you're taking, especially:
• alcohol and other drugs that slow down the nervous system, such as cold and allergy drugs, sedatives, tranquilizers, narcotic pain relievers, barbiturates, seizure drugs, and muscle relaxants
• Aldomet, Isuprel, Quinaglute Dura-tabs
• antidepressants called MAO inhibitors
• insulin
• Lanoxin
• Lithobid
• nonsteroidal anti-inflammatory drugs, such as Advil and Naprosyn
• Questran
• steroids
• tricyclic antidepressants, such as Elavil and Pamelor.

• Keep taking this drug as long as prescribed. You may have to take it for the rest of your life to control your blood pressure.

If you miss a dose

Take the missed dose as soon as possible. However, if it's almost time

Continued on next page ▶

for your next dose, skip the missed dose and take your next dose as scheduled. Don't take a double dose.

If you suspect an overdose

Contact your doctor *immediately*. Excessive Ser-Ap-Es can cause difficulty breathing, difficulty waking, low blood pressure (dizziness and weakness), low body temperature, diarrhea, headache, and fast pulse.

✗ Warnings

• Make sure your doctor knows your medical history. You may not be able to take Ser-Ap-Es if you have other problems, such as asthma, allergies, diabetes, seizures, stomach ulcers, gallstones, gout, depression, ulcerative colitis, Parkinson's disease, pheochromocytoma, lupus, kidney or liver disease, mitral valve disease, coronary artery disease, or rheumatic heart disease.

• If you're pregnant or breast-feeding, don't take Ser-Ap-Es without discussing the risks and benefits with your doctor.

• Be aware that older adults may be especially prone to side effects of Ser-Ap-Es.

• If you're diabetic, be aware that this drug may raise your blood sugar level. Call your doctor if you notice a change.

• Before surgery (including dental surgery) or emergency treatment, tell the doctor or dentist that you're taking this drug.

• Ser-Ap-Es may cause your body to lose potassium. To help prevent this, consume high-potassium foods and beverages, such as bananas and orange juice. Also, ask your doctor about taking a potassium supplement. If you become ill with severe vomiting or diarrhea, call your doctor at once. These conditions may make you lose even more potassium and fluid.

• Follow any special diet the doctor prescribes, such as a low-salt diet.

• See your doctor regularly so your progress and the drug effects can be monitored.

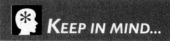

KEEP IN MIND...

* Take with meals or milk.

* To prevent nighttime urination, take last daily dose before 6 p.m.

* Follow prescribed diet.

* Eat high-potassium foods, such as bananas and citrus fruits.

* Wear protective clothing when outdoors.

Serax

Serax is a benzodiazepine, a drug that slows down the nervous system. Researchers suspect it relieves anxiety by inhibiting excitation in the brain.

Why it's prescribed

Doctors prescribe Serax to relieve anxiety and to cause sleepiness during withdrawal from alcohol. It comes in tablets and capsules. Doctors usually prescribe the following amounts for adults.

▶ **For mild to moderate anxiety,** 10 to 15 milligrams (mg) three or four times a day.

▶ **For severe anxiety,** 15 to 30 mg three or four times a day.

▶ **For alcohol withdrawal,** 15 to 30 mg three or four times a day.

How to take Serax

• Take this drug exactly as your doctor directs. Serax can become habit-forming.

• If you've been taking Serax for a long time, don't stop taking it suddenly; this could cause withdrawal symptoms. Call your doctor, who may want you to reduce the amount you're taking gradually before stopping completely.

If you miss a dose

Take the missed dose if you remember within an hour. However, if you don't remember until later, skip the missed dose and take your next dose as scheduled. Don't take a double dose.

SERAX'S OTHER NAMES

Serax's generic name is oxazepam. Canadian brand names include Apo-Oxazepam, Novoxapam, Ox-Pam, and Zapex.

 ## SIDE EFFECTS

Call your doctor if you have any of these possible drug side effects. Call *immediately* about any labeled "serious."

Serious: increased risk of infection, liver problems (yellow-tinged skin and eyes, nausea, vomiting, itching, swelling)
Tips: Avoid people with known infections. Call your doctor immediately if you have symptoms of infection, such as fever, sore throat, and fatigue.

Common: drowsiness, sluggishness, "hangover" feeling

Other: fainting, dizziness, weakness, nausea, vomiting, abdominal discomfort
Tip: Until you know how this drug affects you, don't drive or do anything else that could be dangerous if you're dizzy, drowsy, or weak.

 ## DRUG INTERACTIONS

Combining certain drugs may alter their action or produce unwanted side effects. Tell your doctor about other drugs you're taking, especially:
• alcohol and other drugs that slow down the nervous system, such as cold and allergy drugs, sedatives, tranquilizers, narcotic pain relievers, barbiturates, seizure drugs, and muscle relaxants
• Lanoxin
• Tagamet
• tobacco.

 ## If you suspect an overdose

Contact your doctor *immediately.* Excessive Serax can cause sleepiness, confusion, decreased reflexes, shortness of breath or difficulty breathing, low blood pressure (dizziness and weakness), slow pulse, slurred speech, staggering, poor coordination, and coma.

Warnings

• Make sure your doctor knows your medical history. You may not be able to take Serax if you have other problems, such as chronic lung disease (including emphysema or asthma), seizures, kidney or liver disease, myasthenia gravis, porphyria, sleep apnea, depression, severe mental illness, or a history of drug or alcohol abuse.

• Don't use this drug if you're pregnant or breast-feeding because it could harm the fetus or baby.

 ## KEEP IN MIND...

∗ Take exactly as prescribed; drug can be habit-forming.

∗ Don't stop taking suddenly.

∗ Don't drive until you know how drug affects you.

Serentil

Serentil is one of several drugs called phenothiazines, which are used to treat anxiety or psychosis (a type of mental illness).

Why it's prescribed

Doctors prescribe Serentil for anxiety, psychosis, and other mental, emotional, and nervous disorders and to help manage alcoholism. It comes in tablets and a concentrated liquid. It's also available in an injectable form. Doctors usually prescribe the following amounts for adults and children over age 12.

▶ **For anxiety,** 10 milligrams (mg) orally three times a day, to maximum of 150 mg a day.

▶ **For schizophrenia,** initially 50 mg orally three times a day, to maximum of 400 mg a day.

▶ **For alcoholism,** 25 mg orally twice a day, to maximum of 200 mg a day.

▶ **For behavioral problems caused by organic mental syndrome,** 25 mg orally three times a day, to maximum of 300 mg a day.

How to take Serentil

• Take this drug exactly as your doctor directs. To help prevent stomach upset, take it with a full glass of water or with food.
• Don't stop taking Serentil suddenly without consulting your doctor, who may want you to reduce the amount you're taking gradually before stopping completely.

 ## SIDE EFFECTS

Call your doctor if you have any of these possible drug side effects. Call *immediately* about any labeled "serious."

Serious: blood problems (fever, sore throat, mouth sores, increased risk of infection), neuroleptic malignant syndrome (severe muscle stiffness, fever, unusual tiredness, fast pulse, difficulty breathing, increased sweating, loss of bladder control, seizures), liver problems (yellow-tinged skin and eyes)

Common: fine, wormlike movements of tongue or other uncontrollable movements of mouth, tongue, cheeks, jaw, arms, or legs; dizziness, sleepiness, blurred vision, dry mouth, constipation, inability to urinate, unusual skin sensitivity to sunlight
Tips: Call your doctor if you have symptoms of tardive dyskinesia (listed above). To prevent dizziness when standing up, rise slowly to your feet. Until you know how this drug affects you, don't drive or do anything else that could be dangerous if your vision is blurred or you're not fully alert. To relieve dry mouth, use ice chips or sugarless gum or hard candy.

Other: restlessness, an urge to keep moving, fast pulse, disease of the retina (flashing light, floaters, visual disturbances), dark urine, menstrual abnormalities, unusual milk secretion, allergic reaction (rash, fever, hives), weight gain, increased appetite; (in men) enlarged breasts, inhibited ejaculation
Tip: Consult your doctor if you notice any vision changes.

 ## DRUG INTERACTIONS

Combining certain drugs may alter their action or produce unwanted side effects. Tell your doctor about other drugs you're taking, especially:
• alcohol and other drugs that slow down the nervous system, such as cold and allergy drugs, sedatives, tranquilizers, narcotic pain relievers, barbiturates, seizure drugs, and muscle relaxants
• antacids (don't take within 2 hours of taking Serentil)
• drugs for abdominal or stomach cramps or spasms.

SERENTIL'S OTHER NAMES

Serentil's generic name is mesoridazine. The brand name of the liquid form is Serentil Concentrate.

If you miss a dose

Take the missed dose as soon as possible if you remember within an hour. However, if you don't remember until later, skip the missed dose and take your next dose as scheduled. Don't take a double dose.

 ## If you suspect an overdose

Contact your doctor *immediately.* Excessive Serentil can cause extremely high blood pressure (headache, blurred vision) or low blood pressure (dizziness, weakness), abnormal muscle movements, drowsiness, confusion, dry mouth, nasal congestion, vomiting, enlarged pupils, agitation, seizures, irregular pulse, or fever or low body temperature.

✗ Warnings

• Make sure your doctor knows your medical history. You may not be able to take Serentil if you have other problems, such as lung disease, seizures, blood disease, difficulty urinating, an enlarged prostate, breast cancer, liver disease, stomach ulcers, Reye's syndrome, glaucoma, heart or blood vessel disease, or Parkinson's disease.

• If you're pregnant or breast-feeding, tell your doctor before you start taking Serentil.

• Be aware that children and older adults may be especially prone to Serentil's side effects.

• Don't get the liquid form on your skin or clothing because it may cause a rash.

• Know that you may notice the effects of this drug for several weeks.

• See your doctor regularly so your progress can be checked and your dosage changed, if necessary.

• Before surgery (including dental surgery), tell the doctor or dentist that you're taking this drug.

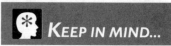

KEEP IN MIND...

* Don't stop taking suddenly.

* Don't get liquid form on skin or clothing.

* Rise slowly to avoid dizziness.

* Don't drive until you know how drug affects you.

* Call doctor about any vision changes.

Serevent

Serevent is a bronchodilator, a drug that widens the air passages and makes breathing easier. It also blocks the release of substances in the respiratory tract that are involved in allergic reactions.

Why it's prescribed

Doctors prescribe Serevent to help prevent and relieve asthma. It comes in an inhalation aerosol. Doctors usually prescribe the following amounts for adults and children over age 12.

▶ **For long-term treatment of asthma or to prevent acute asthma attacks,** 2 inhalations twice a day, one in the morning and one in the evening.

▶ **To prevent wheezing and closing of the throat caused by exercise,** 2 inhalations at least 30 to 60 minutes before exercise.

How to use Serevent

• Use this drug with an inhaler, exactly as your doctor directs. Follow the directions carefully on how to use your inhaler.

• Shake the container well before using it.

• For best results, space doses about 12 hours apart. Take Serevent even when you're feeling better.

• Don't take Serevent more than the recommended twice a day. If you're still having breathing problems, call your doctor.

• If you're taking Serevent to prevent breathing problems during ex-

SEREVENT'S OTHER NAME

Serevent's generic name is salmeterol.

SIDE EFFECTS

Call your doctor if you have any of these possible drug side effects. Call *immediately* about any labeled "serious."

Serious: wheezing and closing of throat

Common: none reported

Other: headache, sinus headache, tremor, fast pulse, respiratory tract infection, sore throat, nasal cavity or sinus problems, stomachache, cough, allergic reaction (rash, hives)

DRUG INTERACTIONS

Combining certain drugs may alter their action or produce unwanted side effects. Tell your doctor about other drugs you're taking, especially:

• antidepressants called MAO inhibitors (don't take within 14 days of taking Serevent)

• beta blockers such as Inderal

• other bronchodilators, such as Bronkaid and Primatene Mist

• tricyclic antidepressants.

ercise, take it 30 to 60 minutes before you exercise.

If you miss a dose

Take the missed dose as soon as possible. But if it's almost time for your next dose, skip the missed dose and take your next dose as scheduled. Don't take a double dose.

If you suspect an overdose

Contact your doctor *immediately*. Excessive Serevent can cause a fast or irregular pulse, potassium deficiency (irritability, confusion, decreased reflexes, speech changes, difficulty breathing, muscle cramps), high blood sugar (fatigue, frequent thirst and urination), tremor, and headache.

Warnings

• Make sure your doctor knows your medical history. You may not be able to take Serevent if you have other medical problems.

• If you're pregnant or breast-feeding, tell your doctor before you start taking Serevent.

• If you have an asthma attack, use your asthma attack drug, not Serevent.

KEEP IN MIND...

* Shake container well before using.

* Space doses 12 hours apart.

* Don't use for acute asthma attacks.

Seromycin

Seromycin is an antibiotic that's used to treat tuberculosis. It prevents the growth of the bacteria that cause tuberculosis.

Why it's prescribed

Doctors prescribe Seromycin along with other drugs to treat tuberculosis. It comes in capsules. Doctors usually prescribe the following amounts for adults.

▶ **For tuberculosis,** initially, 250 milligrams (mg) every 12 hours for 2 weeks, increased to 250 mg every 8 hours for 2 weeks, if needed, and again to 250 mg every 6 hours. Maximum dosage is 1 gram a day.

How to take Seromycin

• Take this drug exactly as your doctor directs.
• Take doses at evenly spaced times throughout the day and night, such as every 12 hours if you're taking two doses a day.
• Keep taking Seromycin for the full time prescribed, even if you feel better after a few weeks. You may have to take it for several years to clear up your infection completely.

If you miss a dose

Take the missed dose as soon as possible. However, if it's almost time for your next dose, skip the missed dose and take your next dose as scheduled. Don't take a double dose.

SEROMYCIN'S OTHER NAME

Seromycin's generic name is cycloserine.

SIDE EFFECTS

Call your doctor if you have any of these possible drug side effects. Call *immediately* about any labeled "serious."

Serious: seizures, suicidal tendencies
Tip: If you start having thoughts of suicide, call your doctor, who will probably change your drug.

Common: nervousness, hallucinations, depression

Other: drowsiness, headache, tremor, speech problems, dizziness, confusion, memory loss, strange behavior, increased irritability, numbness or tingling sensations, slight paralysis, increased reflexes, allergic reaction (redness, rash), stomach upset
Tips: Until you know how this drug affects you, don't drive or do anything else that could be dangerous if you're drowsy. If the drug upsets your stomach, take it after meals.

DRUG INTERACTIONS

Combining certain drugs may alter their action or produce unwanted side effects. Tell your doctor about other drugs you're taking, especially:
• alcohol
• other drugs for tuberculosis, such as Laniazid and Trecator-SC.

If you suspect an overdose

Contact your doctor *immediately*. Excessive Seromycin can cause a decreased level of consciousness, dizziness, increased reflexes, seizures, and confusion.

Warnings

• Make sure your doctor knows your medical history. You may not be able to take Seromycin if you have other problems, such as seizures, severe anxiety, psychosis, kidney disease, depression, or history of alcohol abuse.
• If you're breast-feeding, tell your doctor before you start taking Seromycin.

• See your doctor regularly so your progress can be checked and the level of Seromycin in your blood can be measured.
• If your symptoms don't improve in 2 or 3 weeks or if they get worse, consult your doctor.

KEEP IN MIND...

* Take after meals.

* Space doses evenly.

* Keep taking for full time prescribed.

* Call doctor if symptoms don't improve in a few weeks or if suicidal thoughts arise.

Serpalan

Serpalan is used to treat high blood pressure. It relaxes blood vessels so blood can flow through them more easily. It also slows the heartbeat and decreases the amount of blood pumped by the heart.

Why it's prescribed

Doctors prescribe Serpalan to reduce high blood pressure. It comes in tablets. Doctors usually prescribe the following amounts for adults; children's dosages appear in parentheses.

▶ **For mild to moderate high blood pressure,** 0.1 to 0.25 milligrams a day. (Children: 5 to 20 micrograms for each 2.2 pounds of body weight a day.)

How to take Serpalan

• Take this drug exactly as your doctor directs. Keep taking it even if you feel well.
• Don't stop taking Serpalan suddenly without consulting your doctor.

If you miss a dose

Don't take the missed dose. Instead, take your next dose as scheduled. Don't take a double dose.

 If you suspect an overdose

Contact your doctor *immediately.* Excessive Serpalan can cause low blood pressure (dizziness and weak-

SERPALAN'S OTHER NAMES

Serpalan's generic name is reserpine. Other brand names include Serpasil and, in Canada, Novoreserpine.

 SIDE EFFECTS

Call your doctor if you have any of these possible drug side effects.

Serious: none reported

Common: drowsiness, nervousness, anxiety, nightmares, depression, dizziness, slow pulse, fainting, stuffy nose, nausea, vomiting, dry mouth, impotence, weight gain

Tips: Call your doctor if you have symptoms of depression, such as unusually vivid nightmares or early-morning sleeplessness. To help prevent dizziness when standing up, rise to your feet slowly and avoid sudden position changes. To relieve dry mouth, use ice chips or sugarless gum or hard candy. Weigh yourself daily, and call your doctor if you gain more than 5 pounds. Until you know how this drug affects you, don't drive or do anything else that could be dangerous if you're drowsy. If Serpalan upsets your stomach, take it with meals or milk.

Other: confusion, glaucoma, rash, itching, dark or bloody vomit or stools

 DRUG INTERACTIONS

Combining certain drugs may alter their action or produce unwanted side effects. Tell your doctor about other drugs you're taking, especially:
• antidepressants called MAO inhibitors
• Crystodigin, Lanoxin.

ness), a slow pulse, decreased level of consciousness, coma, slow breathing, low body temperature, diarrhea, vomiting, flushed skin, small pupils, leg pain, and tremors.

 Warnings

• Make sure your doctor knows your medical history. You may not be able to take Serpalan if you have other problems, such as asthma, allergies, a seizure disorder, stomach ulcers, depression, Parkinson's disease, pheochromocytoma, or heart or kidney disease.
• If you're pregnant or breast-feeding, tell your doctor before you start taking Serpalan.

• Older adults may be especially prone to Serpalan's side effects.
• Before surgery (including dental surgery), or emergency treatment, tell the doctor or dentist that you're taking Serpalan.

KEEP IN MIND...

* Take with meals or milk if drug upsets stomach.

* Don't drive until you know how you react to drug.

* Call doctor if you gain more than 5 pounds.

Serzone

Serzone acts in the brain and central nervous system. It helps to maintain levels of the brain chemicals serotonin and norepinephrine, which relieve the symptoms of depression.

Why it's prescribed

Doctors prescribe Serzone to help treat depression. It comes in tablets of varying strengths. Doctors usually prescribe the following amounts for adults.

▶ **For depression,** initially, 200 milligrams (mg) a day divided into two equal doses. Dosage increased weekly by 100 to 200 mg a day, as needed. Usual dosage is 300 to 600 mg a day.

How to take Serzone

• Take Serzone exactly as your doctor prescribes.
• To prevent nausea, take Serzone with food.
• Be advised that Serzone may not achieve its full antidepressant effect for several weeks. Once you start feeling better, don't stop taking the drug without your doctor's permission.

If you miss a dose

Take the missed dose as soon as you remember. However, if it's almost time for your next dose, skip the missed dose and take your next dose as scheduled. Don't take a double dose.

SERZONE'S OTHER NAME

Serzone's generic name is nefazodone hydrochloride.

 SIDE EFFECTS

Call your doctor if you have any of these possible drug side effects.

Serious: none reported

Common: sleepiness, low blood pressure (dizziness, weakness), loss of strength, confusion, blurred or abnormal vision, dry mouth, nausea, constipation, increased or decreased urination, urinary tract infection
Tips: Avoid activities that require full alertness or coordination until you know how Serzone affects you. To reduce constipation, drink plenty of water and increase fiber-rich foods in your diet.

Other: headache, impaired memory, numness and tingling sensations, abnormal dreams, decreased concentration, loss of balance and coordination, altered taste sensation, tremor, swollen ankles and hands, ringing in ears, diarrhea, increased appetite, vomiting, sore throat, cough, itchiness, rash, infection, flulike symptoms (chills, fever, sore throat), vaginal irritation, insomnia

 DRUG INTERACTIONS

Combining certain drugs may alter their action or produce unwanted side effects. Tell your doctor about other drugs you're taking, especially:
• alcohol and other drugs that slow down the central nervous system
• antihistamines, such as Hismanal and Seldane
• Coumadin
• Halcion
• Lanoxin
• MAO inhibitors
• Xanax.

 If you suspect an overdose

Contact your doctor *immediately.* Excessive Serzone can cause nausea, vomiting, and extreme tiredness.

 Warnings

• Make sure your doctor knows your medical history. You may not be able to take Serzone if you're overly sensitive to it or to similar antidepressants, have taken an antidepressant called an MAO inhibitor within 14 days, are taking

Seldane or Hismanal, or have heart disease, low blood pressure, or a history of manic episodes.
• If you think you're pregnant, or intend to become pregnant during therapy, tell your doctor.

✳ KEEP IN MIND...

* Avoid alcohol.
* Full effect occurs only after several weeks.
* Don't stop taking without doctor's permission.

Silvadene

Silvadene is a topical sulfa drug that kills certain bacteria and fungi.

Why it's prescribed

Doctors prescribe Silvadene to help prevent or treat infections in second- and third-degree burns. It comes in a cream. Doctors usually prescribe the following amounts for adults and children.

▶ **To prevent and treat infections from burns,** cream applied once or twice a day.

How to use Silvadene

• Use Silvadene exactly as your doctor directs.
• Don't use Silvadene cream that has darkened. Instead, discard it and get new cream.
• Before applying Silvadene cream, clean your burn wound carefully, as directed by your doctor. Be sure to remove all dead or burned skin.
• Apply Silvadene cream using sterile technique, as instructed by your doctor.
• Spread a thin film of the cream over the entire burned surface.
• Keep the burn covered by Silvadene cream at all times.
• Keep the cream away from unburned areas as much as possible. Don't get it in your eyes or on mucous membranes.
• Use Silvadene for as long as your doctor has prescribed it.

SILVADENE'S OTHER NAMES

Silvadene's generic name is silver sulfadiazine. Other brand names include Flamazine, Flint SSD, Sildimac, SSD, and Thermazene.

 SIDE EFFECTS

Call your doctor if you have any of these possible drug side effects. Call *immediately* about any labeled "serious."

Serious: blood problems, such as a low white blood cell count (increased susceptibility to infection), especially if you need widespread application

Common: mild burning sensation
Tip: Contact your doctor if the medicated area burns or becomes very painful.

Other: rash, itchiness, increased sensitivity to sun, skin discoloration
Tip: Avoid exposure to intense sunlight; if you do go outdoors, wear a sunscreen and protective clothing, including a hat.

 DRUG INTERACTIONS

Combining certain drugs may alter their action or produce unwanted side effects. Tell your doctor about other drugs you're taking, especially:
• Panafil ointment
• Travase ointment.

If you miss a dose

Apply the missed dose as soon as possible. However, if it's almost time for your next dose, skip the missed dose and apply your next dose as scheduled. Don't apply a double dose.

 If you suspect an overdose

Consult your doctor. To treat over-application, clean the area thoroughly.

 Warnings

• Make sure your doctor knows your medical history. You may not be able to use Silvadene cream if you're overly sensitive to it or to other sulfa drugs, if you're pregnant and nearly ready to give birth, or if you have liver or kidney disease.

• The doctor probably won't prescribe Silvadene cream for infants less than 2 months old because the cream could cause them to develop jaundice.
• Be sure to bathe every day, if possible.
• Your doctor may want to do periodic tests to see how your kidneys and liver are functioning.

KEEP IN MIND...

* Don't use darkened cream.
* Clean the burn carefully before applying cream.
* Apply cream in sterile manner.
* Keep cream on the burn at all times.
* Use Silvadene for as long as prescribed.

Sinemet

Sinemet is a combination of two drugs, both of which increase brain levels of dopamine, a substance that helps to control motor activity problems present in Parkinson's disease.

Why it's prescribed

Doctors prescribe Sinemet to treat several types of Parkinson's disease, which is thought to be caused by low dopamine levels. Sinemet comes in tablets and slow-release tablets. Doctors usually prescribe the following amounts for adults.

▶ **For Parkinson's disease or parkinson-like symptoms resulting from an overdose of carbon monoxide or manganese,** 1 tablet of 25 milligrams (mg) carbidopa and 100 mg levodopa twice a day followed by an increase of 1 tablet every day or every other day as necessary to a maximum daily dosage of 8 tablets. If necessary to obtain the best response, the doctor may substitute tablets with 25 mg carbidopa and 250 mg levodopa or 10 mg carbidopa and 100 mg levodopa. Most effective daily dosage differs for each person.

How to take Sinemet

• Take Sinemet only as your doctor prescribes.

SINEMET'S OTHER NAMES

Sinemet is a combination of two generic drugs: levodopa and carbidopa. The brand name of the slow-release form is Sinemet CR.

SIDE EFFECTS

Call your doctor if you have any of these possible drug side effects. Call *immediately* about any labeled "serious."

Serious: mental changes (depression, suicidal thoughts), difficulty urinating, involuntary movements, seizures, fluttering in chest, nausea, vomiting, dizziness, anemia (unusual tiredness), stomach pain

Common: dizziness, anxiety, nervousness, confusion
Tips: If you experience some dizziness at the start of therapy, change positions slowly and dangle your legs before getting out of bed. Wearing elastic stockings may also help reduce this sensation. Avoid activities that require full alertness or coordination until you know how Sinemet affects you.

Other: constipation, trouble sleeping, muscle twitching or cramps, nightmares, euphoria, dry mouth, bitter taste, hiccups, gas, burning sensation on tongue, weight gain or loss, dark-colored perspiration
Tips: To avoid constipation, increase fluids and high-fiber foods. Use sugarless candy or gum to help relieve dry mouth or burning tongue. Wear underarm garment protectors to prevent staining clothes if perspiration becomes dark.

DRUG INTERACTIONS

Combining certain drugs may alter their action or produce unwanted side effects. Tell your doctor about other drugs you're taking, especially:
• blood pressure drugs such as Aldomet
• Dilantin
• MAO inhibitors, such as Nardil and Parnate
• Cerebid
• phenothiazines such as Thorazine
• tricyclic antidepressants, such as Elavil and Pamelor.

• If you switch from regular tablets to slow-release tablets, your dosage will change as well. Follow your doctor's directions.
• Don't chew or crush the slow-release tablets.
• About 15 minutes after taking Sinemet, eat something to lessen stomach upset.
• You may not notice this drug's effects for several weeks. If you don't think it's working, don't stop taking it; call your doctor. Also, don't increase the dosage or frequency if your symptoms continue or get worse; check with the doctor.

If you miss a dose

Take the missed dose as soon as possible. However, if your next scheduled dose is within 2 hours, skip the missed dose and take your next dose as scheduled. Don't take a double dose.

Continued on next page ▶

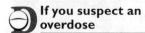

If you suspect an overdose

Contact your doctor *immediately*. Early signs of a Sinemet overdose include twitching muscles or eyelids and fluttering in the chest.

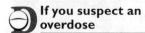

Warnings

• Make sure your doctor knows your medical history. You may not be able to take Sinemet if you're overly sensitive to it, if you've taken an antidepressant called an MAO inhibitor within 14 days, or if you have angle-closure glaucoma, melanoma, undiagnosed skin lesions, heart disease, liver or kidney problems, endocrine abnormalities, lung problems, a history of stomach ulcer or heart attack, irregular heartbeats, mental illness, bronchial asthma, or emphysema.

• If you're pregnant or breast-feeding, check with your doctor before taking Sinemet.

• Be aware that older adults may be especially prone to Sinemet's side effects.

• If you have diabetes, your doctor may need to adjust your dosage of insulin or other diabetes drugs. Also, you may need to switch to another type of urine glucose test.

• This drug may interfere with the results of urine ketone tests. Ask your doctor if you should change to another type of urine ketone test.

• Increase your physical activites gradually so your body can adjust to your changing balance, coordination, and circulation.

• If you've taken levodopa alone and you're switching to Sinemet, your doctor will probably ask you to stop taking the levodopa for at least 8 hours before starting your new medication.

• Your doctor may need to change your dosage, possibly several times, to find the right amount for you to take.

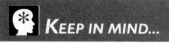

KEEP IN MIND...

* Eat something 15 minutes after taking drug.

* Don't expect the full effect for several weeks.

* Warn family members that you may experience mental changes.

* Don't stop taking without doctor's approval.

Sine-Off Nasal Spray

Sine-Off Nasal Spray probably works by causing the small arteries in the nasal passages to constrict, thus reducing blood flow and swelling.

Why it's taken

Sine-Off is taken to relieve a stuffy nose caused by allergies, hay fever, or a cold. You can buy this drug without a prescription. It comes in nasal spray and nose drops. The following amounts are usually recommended for adults; children's dosages appear in parentheses.

▶ **For nasal congestion,** 2 to 3 drops or sprays of 0.1% solution in each nostril every 8 to 10 hours. (Children age 12 and over: same as adults. Children ages 2 to 11: 2 to 3 drops of 0.05% solution in each nostril every 8 to 10 hours. Children ages 6 months to 1 year: 1 drop of 0.05% solution in each nostril every 6 hours, as needed.)

How to use Sine-Off Nasal Spray

• To use the spray, hold your head upright so that the drug doesn't run down your throat. Then sniff as you spray the drug briskly into your nose.
• To use the drops, sit in a reclining position and tilt your head back and toward the affected side. Then, with the tip of the dropper

SINE-OFF NASAL SPRAY'S OTHER NAMES

Sine-Off's generic name is xylometazoline hydrochloride. Other brand names include Neo-Synephrine II Long Acting Nasal Spray Adult Strength and Otrivin Nasal Spray.

pointed in toward your eye, squeeze 2 or 3 drops into your nostril.
• Don't use more than the recommended dose. And don't use Sine-Off for more than 5 days.

If you miss a dose

Apply the missed dose as soon as possible. However, if it's almost time for your next dose, skip the missed dose and apply your next dose as scheduled. Don't apply a double dose.

If you suspect an overdose

Call your doctor *immediately*. Excessive Sine-Off can cause blurred vision, headache, light-headedness, nervousness, pounding or irregular heartbeat, and trouble sleeping.

Warnings

• Make sure your doctor knows your medical history. You may not

be able to use Sine-Off Nasal Spray if you're overly sensitive to it or if you have angle-closure glaucoma, an overactive thyroid, heart disease, high blood pressure, or diabetes.
• To prevent the spread of infection, don't share this drug with friends or family members.

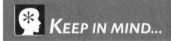

* Don't share drug with family or friends.
* Use for no more than 5 days.
* Don't exceed recommended dosage.
* After stopping drug, expect increased congestion briefly.

SIDE EFFECTS

Call your doctor if you have any of these possible drug side effects.

Serious: none reported

Common: increased nasal congestion (after stopping drug)
Tip: When you stop using Sine-Off, especially if you used it excessively or for a long time, your nose may become congested again. This is temporary and will subside as your body gets used to not having the drug.

Other: sneezing and burning, stinging, or dryness inside nose
Tip: Use a cool-mist humidifier to help relieve nasal dryness.

DRUG INTERACTIONS

Combining certain drugs may alter their action or produce unwanted side effects. Tell your doctor about other drugs you're taking.

Sinequan

Sinequan is one of a group of drugs known as tricyclic antidepressants. It elevates mood by increasing levels of the brain chemicals norepinephrine and serotonin, which help relieve symptoms of depression.

Why it's prescribed

Doctors prescribe Sinequan to relieve symptoms of depression. It also helps treat symptoms of anxiety, fear, and sleep disturbances. It comes in capsules and an oral concentrate. Doctors usually prescribe the following amounts for adults.

▶ **For depression, anxiety, or both,** initially, 25 to 75 milligrams (mg) a day divided into equal doses taken throughout the day, increased to a maximum of 300 mg a day. Or one dose of no more than 150 mg a day.

How to take Sinequan

• Take Sinequan only as your doctor has prescribed.
• Sinequan is one of the more sedating drugs in its class. Don't take any more of it than your doctor prescribes. And don't stop taking it abruptly.
• If you're taking the oral concentrate, dilute it with 4 ounces of water, milk, or juice (orange, grapefruit, tomato, prune, or pineapple). Don't mix it with carbonated beverages.

SINEQUAN'S OTHER NAMES

Sinequan's generic name is doxepin hydrochloride. Other brand names include Adapin and, in Canada, Novo-Doxepin and Triadapin.

SIDE EFFECTS

Call your doctor if you have any of these possible drug side effects. Call *immediately* about any labeled "serious."

Serious: seizures, heart problems (palpitations, chest pain, rapid pulse)

Common: drowsiness, dizziness, fainting, blurred vision, dry mouth, swollen tongue, constipation, difficulty urinating, profuse sweating

Tips: Avoid activities that require full alertness or coordination until you know how Sinequan affects you. Drowsiness and dizziness usually subside after a few weeks. Stand up slowly to avoid dizziness. When getting out of bed, sit up slowly and dangle your legs over the side of the bed for several minutes before standing. Relieve dry mouth with sugarless hard candy or gum, ice chips, or saliva substitutes. If you have trouble urinating or you become constipated, drink more water and eat more fiber-rich foods. If you're still constipated, ask your doctor about using a stool softener.

Other: excitability, tremor, weakness, confusion, headache, nervousness, changes in muscle tone or function, high blood pressure (headache, blurred vision), ringing in ears, enlarged pupils, indigestion, nausea, vomiting, appetite and weight loss, intestinal blockage (abdominal pain and bloating, unrelieved constipation), skin sensitivity to sun, allergic reaction (fever, swelling, hives, rash), changes in sex drive, breast enlargement in males and females

Tip: To prevent skin reactions, use a sunscreen, wear protective clothing, and avoid prolonged exposure to the sun.

DRUG INTERACTIONS

Combining certain drugs may alter their action or produce unwanted side effects. Tell your doctor about other drugs you're taking, especially:
• alcohol
• antiarrhythmic drugs, such as Quinaglute Dura-tabs, Rythmol, and Tambocor
• anticoagulants (blood thinners) such as Coumadin
• antihistamines, such as Benadryl and Insomnal
• blood pressure drugs, such as Catapres and Serpalan
• drugs found in nasal sprays, such as ephedrine, epinephrine, and phenylephrine
• narcotics, such as Darvon and Dilaudid
• other antidepressants, such as Eldepryl, Nardil, Elavil, Pamelor, Prozac, and Zoloft
• phenothiazines such as Thorazine
• Tagamet
• Tolinase.

• The antianxiety effect will be felt before the antidepressant effect, which may take 2 to 3 weeks.

If you miss a dose

Take the missed dose as soon as possible. However, if it's almost time for your next dose, skip the missed dose and take your next dose as scheduled. Don't take a double dose.

If you suspect an overdose

Contact your doctor *immediately*. Excessive Sinequan can cause agitation, hallucinations, seizures, sleepiness, and irregular heartbeat.

✕ Warnings

• Make sure your doctor knows your medical history. You may not be able to take Sinequan if you're overly sensitive to it or other drugs or if you have other medical problems, such as glaucoma, difficulty urinating, asthma, blood problems, manic-depressive disorder or schizophrenia, seizures, an enlarged prostate, heart disease, kidney or liver problems, an overactive thyroid, or stomach or intestinal problems.

• Before you begin taking Sinequan, tell your doctor if you're pregnant or breast-feeding.
• Adolescents, older adults, and people who are ill or taking certain other drugs (especially some muscle relaxants) may need a reduced dosage of Sinequan.
• If you need surgery, your doctor will probably decrease your dosage gradually and then have you stop taking Sinequan temporarily.
• If you take liquid Sinequan as well as Dolophine syrup, you may mix both drugs together in lemonade, orange juice, sugar water, or water, but <u>not</u> in grape juice.

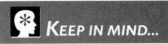

KEEP IN MIND...

∗ Don't mix oral solution with carbonated drinks.

∗ Don't stop taking Sinequan abruptly.

∗ Stand up slowly to avoid dizziness.

∗ Increase fluids and fiber in diet if you become constipated.

∗ Avoid alcohol.

∗ The drug's antianxiety effect will be felt before the antidepressant effect.

Slow-K

S low-K is a potassium supplement. It replaces the body's potassium and maintains a normal level of potassium in the blood.

Why it's prescribed

Doctors prescribe Slow-K to increase the potassium level in people who don't get enough potassium in their regular diet or have lost much potassium due to illness or certain drugs. Slow-K comes in extended-release tablets. Doctors usually prescribe the following amounts for adults.

▶ **For potassium deficiency,** 40 to 100 milliequivalents (mEq) a day divided into three or four equal doses. Further dosages depend on blood potassium level.

▶ **To prevent potassium deficiency,** 20 mEq a day.

How to take Slow-K

• Take this drug exactly as your doctor directs.
• Swallow the tablets whole. Don't crush or chew them.

If you miss a dose

Take the missed dose as soon as possible if you remember within 2 hours. However, if you don't re-

 SIDE EFFECTS

Call your doctor if you have any of these possible drug side effects. Call *immediately* about any labeled "serious."

Serious: life-threatening low blood pressure and heart block (extreme dizziness, weakness, fainting), fluttering in chest, reduced urination, cold or graying skin

Common: nausea, vomiting, stomach pain
Tip: To prevent possible stomach upset, take the drug with or after meals with a full glass (8 ounces) of water or fruit juice.

Other: numbness, prickling, or tingling sensations in arms and legs; listlessness; confusion; weakness or heaviness of limbs; muscle paralysis; diarrhea; stomach ulcers

 DRUG AND FOOD INTERACTIONS

Combining certain drugs and foods may alter drug action or produce unwanted side effects. Tell your doctor about your diet and other drugs you're taking, especially:
• diuretics (water pills) that decrease potassium excretion, such as Aldactone, Dyrenium, and Midamor
• drugs used to treat high blood pressure or heart failure, particularly Accupril, Altace, Capoten, Lotensin, Monopril, Prinivil, Vasotec, and Zestril
• salt substitutes containing potassium, low-sodium foods, and milk containing potassium

member until later, skip the missed dose and take the next dose as scheduled. Don't take a double dose.

 If you suspect an overdose

Contact your doctor *immediately.* Excessive Slow-K can cause life-threatening heart problems (slowing or stopping of heartbeat), weakness, muscle paralysis, and difficulty breathing and swallowing.

 Warnings

• Make sure your doctor knows your medical history. You may not

be able to take Slow-K if you have other medical problems.
• Be aware that older adults may be more prone to high blood levels of potassium when taking Slow-K.

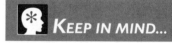 **KEEP IN MIND...**

* Take with or after meals with full glass of fluid.

* Avoid salt substitutes and low-sodium foods.

* Older adults may be more prone to high potassium levels.

Slow-Mag

Slow-Mag is used to increase or maintain the body's magnesium level. Because a magnesium deficiency can contribute to serious problems throughout the body, Slow-Mag may be necessary as a dietary supplement.

Why it's prescribed

Doctors prescribe Slow-Mag to provide dietary magnesium. You can buy this drug without a prescription. It comes in slow-release tablets. Doctors usually prescribe the following amounts for adults.

▶ As a magnesium supplement, 1 64-milligram tablet twice a day.

How to take Slow-Mag

• Swallow the tablets whole. Don't crush or chew them.

If you miss a dose

Missing one or more doses of Slow-Mag should not be harmful. However, it's important to take your supplement as recommended or as your doctor prescribed. Don't take a double dose.

 If you suspect an overdose

Contact your doctor *immediately*. Excessive magnesium can cause fainting, slow pulse, difficulty breathing, and coma.

SLOW-MAG'S OTHER NAME

Slow-Mag's generic name is magnesium chloride.

 SIDE EFFECTS

Call your doctor if you have any of these possible drug side effects. Call *immediately* about any labeled "serious."

Serious: calcium deficiency (difficulty swallowing, muscle spasms, palpitations, tingling and numbness in fingers), irregular heartbeat (fluttering sensation in chest), slow or difficult breathing

Common: weak reflexes, low blood pressure (dizziness, weakness)

Other: diarrhea, drowsiness, low body temperature, slow pulse, profuse sweating

Tips: Take Slow-Mag with meals to avoid diarrhea. Avoid activities that require full alertness until you know how this drug affects you.

 DRUG INTERACTIONS

Combining certain drugs may alter their action or produce unwanted side effects. Tell your doctor about other drugs you're taking, especially:

• antacids, such as Alka-Seltzer and Riopan
• Calcibind
• Cytotec
• Didronel
• diuretics (water pills), such as Diamox and Lasix
• Kayexalate
• Lanoxin
• laxatives, such as Dialose and Dulcolax
• Macrodantin
• other magnesium-containing drugs, including enemas
• penicillamine (Cuprimine)
• tetracyclines such as Achromycin.

 Warnings

• Make sure your doctor knows your medical history. You may not be able to take Slow-Mag if you have heart disease or kidney problems.

• If you're pregnant or breast-feeding, tell your doctor before you start taking Slow-Mag.

KEEP IN MIND...

* Take with food to avoid diarrhea.

* Don't chew or crush slow-release tablets.

* Avoid activities that require full alertness until you know how Slow-Mag affects you.

Sofarin

Sofarin is an anticoagulant (blood thinner) that helps treat certain heart, lung, and blood vessel disorders. It works by reducing the blood's clotting tendency. This, in turn, helps prevent dangerous clots from blocking veins and arteries and causing a heart attack or stroke.

Why it's prescribed

Doctors prescribe Sofarin to prevent blood clots in people with heart, lung, and blood vessel disorders. Sofarin comes in tablets. Doctors usually prescribe the following amounts for adults.

▶ **To prevent blood clots,** 10 to 15 milligrams (mg) for 2 to 4 days, adjusted according to person's response. Usual long-term dosage is 2 to 10 mg once a day.

How to take Sofarin

• Take Sofarin exactly as your doctor directs. Don't take more or less of it than prescribed, and don't take it more often or longer than directed.
• Take Sofarin at the same time each day.

If you miss a dose

Take the missed dose as soon as possible. Then go back to your regular schedule. If you don't remember until the next day, don't take the missed dose at all. Never take a double dose; this may cause bleeding.

 ## SIDE EFFECTS

Call your doctor if you have any of these possible drug side effects. Call *immediately* about any labeled "serious."

Serious: hemorrhage (with excessive dosage), severe infection (chills, fever, sore throat), pain or swelling in joints or stomach, unusual backache, diarrhea, constipation, dizziness, headache, bleeding problems (bleeding gums, bruises or purplish marks on skin, nosebleeds, heavy bleeding or oozing from cuts or wounds, excessive or unexpected menstrual bleeding, blood in urine or sputum, dark or bloody vomit or stools), allergic reaction (fever, rash)

Common: none reported

Other: drastic appetite and weight loss, nausea, vomiting, cramps, mouth sores, liver problems (yellow-tinged skin and eyes, nausea), hives, hair loss
Tip: Take Sofarin with food to prevent nausea.

 ## DRUG AND FOOD INTERACTIONS

Combining certain drugs and foods may alter drug action or produce unwanted side effects. Tell your doctor about your diet and other drugs you're taking, especially:
• alcohol
• anabolic steroids, corticosteroids
• Antabuse
• antiarrhythmics, such as Cordarone and Quinaglute Dura-tabs
• antibiotics and antifungal drugs, such as Achromycin, Bactrim, Cipro, E-Mycin, Flagyl, Keflex, Monistat, Rifadin Tapazole, and Unipen
• Anturane, heparin
• Atromid-S, Mevacor
• barbiturates, tricyclic antidepressants (Elavil), sedatives
• birth control pills containing estrogen
• Carafate, Tagamet
• Danocrine, Nolvadex
• diuretics (water pills), such as Aldactone, Edecrin, and HydroDIURIL
• flu vaccine
• nonsteroidal anti-inflammatory drugs such as Advil
• Tegretol
• thyroid drugs such as PTU
• Trental
• Tylenol
• vitamin E, vitamin K, calcium (including foods that contain these vitamins or minerals).

If you suspect an overdose

Contact your doctor *immediately*. Excessive Sofarin can cause bruising, bleeding gums, blood in stools or urine, or nosebleeds.

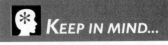

Warnings

• Make sure your doctor knows your medical history. You may not be able to take Sofarin if you have other medical problems, especially a bleeding tendency, ulcers or other intestinal or stomach problems, high blood pressure or blood disorders, vitamin K deficiency, or heart, liver, or kidney disease. Also, make sure your doctor knows if you've recently undergone eye, brain, or spinal cord surgery or if you have drainage tubes in place.
• Make sure your doctor knows if you're pregnant or breast-feeding before you begin taking Sofarin. Discuss the need to delay pregnancy while taking Sofarin to avoid harming yourself or the baby.
• Sofarin is not recommended for children under age 18.
• To reduce the risk of injuring yourself while taking Sofarin, always wear shoes, place a nonskid mat in your bathtub, shave with an electric razor, and use a soft toothbrush. Check with your doctor before beginning any strenuous exercise programs, and avoid risky activities, such as roughhousing with children and pets.

• Keep all appointments for follow-up blood tests. If test results show that your blood isn't clotting correctly, your doctor may decrease the amount of Sofarin you take.
• Be sure to let other doctors and your dentist know that you're taking Sofarin; carry medical identification that lets others know you're using Sofarin.
• Ask your doctor how to handle mild pain, such as headache or back pain. You'll probably be told to use Tylenol. Don't use aspirin or Advil.
• Tell your doctor if menstruation is heavier than usual; your dosage may need to be changed.
• Don't change your diet without talking to your doctor. Doing so could affect your Sofarin dosage.
• Eat the same daily amount of leafy green vegetables, which contain vitamin K. Eating different amounts daily could change Sofarin's effect.
• Read all food labels. Foods and supplements that contain vitamin K can interfere with how well Sofarin works.
• Ask your doctor to provide you with an educational guide about Sofarin.

Solfoton

Solfoton acts in the central nervous system to make seizures harder to start. Although it's not known exactly how the drug works, it's thought to act as a sedative, depressing the central nervous system.

Why it's prescribed

Doctors prescribe Solfoton to prevent seizures caused by epilepsy and other disorders. It's also used as a sedative to produce relaxation — for example, before surgery. Solfoton comes in tablets, capsules, oral solution, and elixir. It's also available in an injectable form. Doctors usually prescribe the following amounts for adults; children's dosages appear in parentheses.

▶ **For epilepsy and fever-induced seizures,** 60 to 200 milligrams (mg) a day orally divided into three equal doses or taken once a day at bedtime. (Children: 3 to 6 mg for each 2.2 pounds [lb] of body weight orally daily, usually divided into two equal doses taken every 12 hours or entire daily dose taken once a day, usually at bedtime.)

▶ **For sedation,** 30 to 120 mg a day orally divided into two or three equal doses. (Children: 3 to 5 mg for each 2.2 lb orally daily divided into three equal doses.)

▶ **For insomnia,** 100 to 200 mg orally at bedtime.

SIDE EFFECTS

Call your doctor if you have any of these possible drug side effects. Call *immediately* about any labeled "serious."

Serious: shortness of breath or slowed breathing, fever, white spots in mouth, painful sores, low blood pressure (dizziness, weakness), slow pulse, fainting, sudden burnlike rash, swelling of face, tongue, and throat

Common: drowsiness, sluggishness, "hangover" feeling
Tip: Avoid activities that require full alertness or coordination until you know how Solfoton affects you.

Other: excitability (in older adults), nausea, vomiting, hives, worsening of porphyria

DRUG INTERACTIONS

Combining certain drugs may alter their action or produce unwanted side effects. Tell your doctor about other drugs you're taking, especially:
• alcohol and other drugs that make you feel relaxed or sleepy, including tranquilizers (Valium), narcotic pain relievers, sleeping pills, and cold and allergy drugs
• anticoagulants (blood thinners) such as Coumadin
• Chloromycetin
• corticosteroids
• Crystodigin
• estrogen-containing drugs such as birth control pills
• Grisactin
• MAO inhibitors such as Parnate
• narcotics, such as Darvon and Dilaudid
• other seizure drugs, such as Depakene, Mebaral, and Mysoline
• phenothiazines such as Thorazine
• Rifadin
• tricyclic antidepressants, such as Elavil and Sinequan
• Vibramycin.

SOLFOTON'S OTHER NAMES

Solfoton's generic name is phenobarbital. Other brand names include Ancalixir and Barbita. Phenobarbital sodium is available under the brand name Luminal.

How to take Solfoton

• Take this drug exactly as your doctor directs. Don't increase your dose.
• If you're taking capsules or tablets, swallow them whole; don't chew or crush them.
• If you're taking this drug for epilepsy, take it every day in regularly spaced doses, as prescribed.

• Don't stop taking Solfoton abruptly.

If you miss a dose

Take the missed dose as soon as possible. However, if it's almost time for your next dose, skip the missed dose and take your next dose as scheduled. Don't take a double dose.

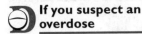 **If you suspect an overdose**

Contact your doctor *immediately*. Excessive Solfoton can cause severe drowsiness, weakness, and confusion; slurred speech; and difficulty breathing.

Warnings

• Make sure your doctor knows your medical history. You may not be able to take Solfoton if you're overly sensitive to it or to other barbiturates or if you have asthma, lung disease, porphyria, depression, chronic pain, or kidney or liver disease.
• If you're pregnant or breast-feeding, tell your doctor.
• Be aware that older adults may be especially sensitive to Solfoton's side effects.
• Be aware that you may not feel the drug's full effect for 2 to 3 weeks.
• Before you have medical tests, tell the doctor you're taking Solfoton.

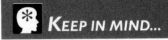 **KEEP IN MIND...**

* Avoid alcohol.
* Don't chew or crush tablets or capsules.
* Don't expect full effect for 2 to 3 weeks.
* Don't stop taking abruptly.

Soma

Soma works in the central nervous system to alter pain perception.

Why it's prescribed

Doctors prescribe Soma to relax muscles and relieve the pain and discomfort of strains, sprains, and other muscle injuries. It comes in tablets. Doctors usually prescribe the following amounts for adults.

▶ **For pain relief in acute, painful musculoskeletal conditions,** 350 milligrams three times a day and at bedtime.

How to take Soma

- Follow the directions on the drug label exactly.
- Take Soma with food to help prevent nausea.
- To avoid withdrawal effects, don't stop taking the drug abruptly.

If you miss a dose

Take the missed dose right away if you remember within an hour or so. If you don't remember until later, skip the missed dose and take your next dose as scheduled. Don't take a double dose.

If you suspect an overdose

Contact your doctor *immediately*. Excessive Soma can cause stupor, shock, and coma.

SOMA'S OTHER NAME

Soma's generic name is carisoprodol.

SIDE EFFECTS

Call your doctor if you have any of these possible drug side effects. Call *immediately* about any labeled "serious."

Serious: blood problems (increased risk of infection), skin eruptions, low blood pressure (dizziness, weakness), rapid pulse, severe allergic reaction (facial and throat swelling, trouble breathing, tightness in chest)

Common: drowsiness, dizziness
Tip: Avoid activities that require full alertness or coordination until you know how Soma affects you.

Other: vertigo, loss of balance, tremor, agitation, irritability, headache, depression, insomnia, facial flushing, nausea, vomiting, hiccups, cramps, diarrhea, fever, rash, hives, itching, redness

DRUG INTERACTIONS

Combining certain drugs may alter their action or produce unwanted side effects. Tell your doctor about other drugs you're taking, especially:
- alcohol
- antipsychotics, such as Mellaril and Thorazine
- MAO inhibitors, such as Nardil and Parnate
- narcotics, such as codeine, Darvocet, Dilaudid, and morphine
- tranquilizers, such as Librium and Valium
- tricyclic antidepressants, such as Elavil and Pamelor.

Warnings

- Make sure your doctor knows your medical history. You may not be able to take Soma if you're allergic to this or other drugs or if you have porphyria or kidney or liver problems.
- If you become pregnant while taking Soma, tell your doctor.
- If you're breast-feeding, be aware that Soma passes into breast milk and can cause drowsiness and stomach upset in breast-feeding infants. Discuss its use with your doctor.
- If you're taking this drug for more than a few weeks, see your doctor regularly to check your progress.
- Be sure to follow your doctor's advice about resting and getting physical therapy.

KEEP IN MIND...

- ✳ Don't stop taking Soma abruptly.
- ✳ Avoid alcohol.
- ✳ Follow your doctor's directions about rest and physical therapy.

Sorbitrate

Sorbitrate relaxes the blood vessels, which boosts the supply of blood and oxygen to the heart and eases the heart's workload.

Why it's prescribed

Doctors prescribe Sorbitrate to treat attacks of angina (chest pain) and other heart conditions. It comes in tablets, chewable tablets, sublingual (under-the-tongue) tablets, and capsules. Doctors usually prescribe the following amounts for adults.

▶ **For acute chest pain,** 2.5 to 5 milligrams (mg) sublingual tablets.

▶ **For chronic chest pain,** 5 to 20 mg two or three times a day, increased up to 40 mg a day as needed.

▶ To prevent chest pain in situations in which it's likely to occur, 5 mg chewable tablets 15 minutes before activity.

How to take Sorbitrate

• Take this drug exactly as your doctor directs.

• At the first sign of chest pain, place a sublingual tablet under your tongue and let it dissolve. Don't chew or swallow it.

• Chew a chewable tablet well and hold it in your mouth for about 2 minutes before swallowing.

• If you still have chest pain after taking three sublingual or chew-

SIDE EFFECTS

Call your doctor if you have any of these possible drug side effects. Call *immediately* about any labeled "serious."

Serious: palpitations, fainting

Common: headache, dizziness, fast pulse, swollen ankles, flushing
Tip: If you get a headache, call your doctor, who may reduce the dosage temporarily.

Other: weakness, nausea, vomiting, allergic reaction (rash, hives)

DRUG INTERACTIONS

Combining certain drugs may alter their action or produce unwanted side effects. Tell your doctor about other drugs you're taking, especially:
• alcohol
• blood pressure drugs.

SORBITRATE'S OTHER NAMES

Sorbitrate's generic name is isosorbide dinitrate. Other brand names include Dilatrate-SR, Iso-Bid, Isonate, Isorbid, Isordil, Isotrate; and, in Canada, Apo-ISDN, Cedocard-SR, Coradur, Coronex, and Novosorbide.

---

able tablets in 15 minutes, seek emergency care.

• Take oral forms of the drug with 8 ounces of water on an empty stomach (30 minutes before or 1 to 2 hours after a meal).

• The sublingual and chewable tablets take effect in 2 to 5 minutes and work for 1 to 2 hours; other oral forms take effect in 15 to 40 minutes and work for 1 to 2 hours.

• Don't suddenly stop using this drug if you've been taking it regularly. Doing so could trigger an angina attack.

If you miss a dose

Take the missed dose as soon as possible. But, if it's within 2 hours of the next dose, skip the missed dose and take the next dose as scheduled. Don't take a double dose.

 If you suspect an overdose

Contact your doctor *immediately.* Excessive Sorbitrate can cause persistent throbbing headache, confusion, fever, vertigo, palpitations, vi-

sion disturbances, vomiting, fainting, difficulty breathing, sweating, slow pulse, seizures, and death.

Warnings

• Make sure your doctor knows your medical history. You may not be able to take Sorbitrate if you have other medical problems or are pregnant.

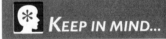

* Place sublingual tablet under tongue at first sign of chest pain.

* Seek emergency care if chest pain persists after three sublingual or chewable tablets in 15 minutes.

* Don't suddenly stop taking.

Sparine

Sparine helps maintain levels of dopamine, a substance that affects the transmission of nerve impulses in the brain.

Why it's prescribed

Doctors prescribe Sparine to treat nervous, mental, and emotional disorders. It comes in tablets. Doctors usually prescribe the following amounts for adults; children's dosages appear in parentheses.
► For psychosis, 10 to 200 milligrams (mg) every 4 to 6 hours, increased as needed up to 1 gram daily. (Children over age 12: 10 to 25 mg every 4 to 6 hours.)

How to take Sparine

• Follow your doctor's directions exactly.
• Take each dose with food or a full glass (8 ounces) of water or milk.
• Don't stop taking drug abruptly.

If you miss a dose

Take the missed dose right away if you remember within 1 hour or so. But if you don't remember until later, skip it and take your next dose on schedule. Don't take a double dose.

If you suspect an overdose

Contact your doctor *immediately*. Excessive Sparine can cause seizures, a coma, and other problems.

SPARINE'S OTHER NAMES

Sparine's generic name is promazine hydrochloride. Other brand names include Primazine and Prozine-50.

SIDE EFFECTS

Call your doctor if you have any of these possible drug side effects. Call *immediately* about any labeled "serious."

Serious: severe blood problems (fatigue, bleeding, bruising, increased risk of infection, fever, chills), severe headache

Common: unusual movements, dizziness, dry mouth, constipation, inability to urinate, skin sensitivity to sun

Other: rapid pulse, blurred vision, menstrual irregularities, breast enlargement and inhibited ejaculation in men, yellow-tinged skin and eyes, weight gain, increased appetite; after abruptly stopping long-term therapy, gastritis (indigestion, cramps), nausea, vomiting, dizziness, tremors, feeling of warmth or cold, profuse sweating, rapid heartbeat, headache, insomnia

DRUG INTERACTIONS

Combining certain drugs may alter their action or produce unwanted side effects. Tell your doctor about other drugs you're taking, especially:
• alcohol and other drugs that make you feel relaxed or sleepy, such as tranquilizers (Valium), sleeping pills, antidepressants (Nardil, Elavil), barbiturates (Solfoton), and muscle relaxants
• antacids
• anticoagulants (blood thinners) such as Coumadin
• blood pressure drugs, such as Aldomet and Catapres
• drugs for Parkinson's disease such as Sinemet
• Eskalith, Lithobid.

Warnings

• Make sure your doctor knows your medical history. You may not be able to take Sparine if you have bone marrow problems, brain damage, heart or blood problems, glaucoma, respiratory problems, low calcium levels, an enlarged prostate, seizures, severe reactions to insulin, Parkinson's disease, or kidney, lung, or liver problems or if you've recently been exposed to extreme heat or cold or certain pesticides.

• If you're pregnant or breast-feeding, check with your doctor before taking Sparine.
• Children and older adults are especially prone to Sparine's side effects.

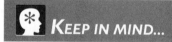 KEEP IN MIND...

∗ Take with food or liquids.
∗ Avoid alcohol.
∗ Don't stop taking abruptly.

Spectrobid

Spectrobid is an antibiotic related to penicillin.

Why it's prescribed

Doctors prescribe Spectrobid to help fight susceptible infections throughout the body. It comes in tablets and liquid. Doctors usually prescribe the following amounts for adults; children's dosages appear in parentheses.

▶ **For certain infections of the upper respiratory tract, ear, urinary tract, and skin,** 400 milligrams (mg) every 12 hours. (Children weighing more than 55 pounds (lb): same as adults. Children weighing 55 lb or less: 25 mg for each 2.2 lb of body weight daily, divided into equal doses and taken every 12 hours.)

▶ **For lower respiratory tract and other severe infections,** 800 mg every 12 hours. (Children weighing more than 55 lb: same as adults. Children weighing 55 lb or less: 50 mg for each 2.2 lb daily, divided into equal doses and taken every 12 hours.)

▶ **For gonorrhea,** 1.6 grams as a single dose.

How to take Spectrobid

• Unlike many antibiotics, Spectrobid tablets can be taken with meals to reduce stomach upset.

• Take the liquid with a full glass (8 ounces) of water at least 1 hour before or 2 hours after a meal, unless your doctor says otherwise.

SPECTROBID'S OTHER NAMES

Spectrobid's generic name is bacampicillin hydrochloride. Another brand name is Penglobe.

 ## SIDE EFFECTS

Call your doctor if you have any of these possible drug side effects. Call *immediately* about any labeled "serious."

Serious: blood problems (fatigue, bleeding, bruising, increased risk of infection, fever, chills), allergic reaction (rash, fever, chills), severe allergic reaction (swelling of face and throat, trouble breathing, chest pain, anxiety)

Common: nausea, diarrhea

Tip: If you develop severe diarrhea, don't take a drug for diarrhea without consulting your doctor.

Other: vomiting, tongue or mouth inflammation

 ## DRUG INTERACTIONS

Combining certain drugs may alter their action or produce unwanted side effects. Tell your doctor about other drugs you're taking, especially:

• Antabuse
• Benemid
• Zyloprim.

• Space your doses evenly throughout the day and night, and try not to miss any doses.

• Take all of the prescribed drug, even if you feel better before the prescription is finished.

If you miss a dose

Take the missed dose as soon as possible. But if it's almost time for your next dose, skip the missed dose and take your next dose as scheduled. Don't take a double dose.

 ### If you suspect an overdose

Contact your doctor *immediately.* Excessive Spectrobid can cause seizures.

 ## Warnings

• Make sure your doctor knows your medical history. You may not be able to take Spectrobid if you're overly sensitive to it or to other penicillins or antibiotics or if you have mononucleosis.

• If you're pregnant or breast-feeding, tell your doctor before taking Spectrobid.

• If you're a diabetic, be aware that Spectrobid may alter your blood sugar tests. Check with your doctor before changing your diet or your diabetes drugs.

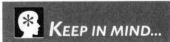 ## KEEP IN MIND...

∗ Space doses evenly through day and night.

∗ Take entire amount prescribed, even if you feel better.

∗ Take liquid with a full glass of water.

∗ Call doctor if you have signs of infection or allergic reaction.

Sporanox

Sporanox weakens or kills fungi that infect the body.

Why it's prescribed

Doctors prescribe Sporanox to treat fungal infections involving various parts of the body. It comes in capsules. Doctors usually prescribe the following amounts for adults.

▶ **For blastomycosis and histoplasmosis,** 200 milligrams (mg) a day, increased as needed in 100-mg increments to a maximum of 400 mg a day, probably divided into two equal doses. In life-threatening illness, therapy may start with 200 mg three times a day for 3 days.

▶ **For aspergillosis,** 200 to 400 mg a day.

How to take Sporanox

• If you have a reduced level of stomach acid, your doctor may advise you to take Sporanox with an acidic drink (such as cranberry juice).

• Take Sporanox with food to improve the drug's absorption.

• Make sure you take the full amount prescribed. Treatment for blastomycosis or histoplasmosis lasts for at least 3 months.

If you miss a dose

Take the missed dose as soon as possible. However, if it's almost time for your next dose, skip the missed

SPORANOX'S OTHER NAME

Sporanox's generic name is itraconazole.

SIDE EFFECTS

Call your doctor if you have any of these possible drug side effects. Call *immediately* about any labeled "serious."

Serious: high blood pressure (headache, blurred vision), liver problems (appetite loss, dark urine, pale stools, unusual fatigue, yellow-tinged skin and eyes)

Common: none reported

Other: nausea, vomiting, diarrhea, abdominal pain, appetite loss, rash, itchiness, swelling, fatigue, fever, overall feeling of illness, depression, insomnia, decreased sex drive, impotence

DRUG INTERACTIONS

Combining certain drugs may alter their action or produce unwanted side effects. Tell your doctor about other drugs you're taking, especially:
• antacids
• anticoagulants (blood thinners) such as Coumadin
• antihistamines, such as Hismanal and Seldane
• Dilantin
• Lanoxin
• oral diabetes drugs
• Sandimmune
• tuberculosis drugs, such as Laniazid and Rifadin
• ulcer drugs, such as Axid and Pepcid.

dose and take your next dose as scheduled. Don't take a double dose.

If you suspect an overdose

Consult your doctor.

Warnings

• Make sure your doctor knows your medical history. You may not be able to take Sporanox of you are overly sensitive to it, are breast-feeding, have reduced stomach acid, or are infected with HIV.

• Your doctor will probably want you to have regular liver tests to make sure Sporanox isn't harming your liver.

KEEP IN MIND...

* Take drug with acidic drink if ordered.

* Take with food.

* Take full amount prescribed.

* Report signs of liver damage.

Stadol NS

Stadol NS acts on the brain to alter how people perceive and respond to pain.

Why it's prescribed

Doctors prescribe Stadol NS to relieve pain. It comes in a nasal spray. It's also available in an injectable form. Doctors usually prescribe the following amounts for adults.

▶ **For moderate to severe pain,** 1 spray every 3 to 4 hours.

How to use Stadol NS

• Use Stadol NS exactly as prescribed. Don't increase your dose without your doctor's permission.
• To achieve the prescribed dose, spray Stadol NS once into each nostril.
• If the pain doesn't subside, you can repeat the spray in 60 to 90 minutes.

If you miss a dose

Take the missed dose as soon as possible. However, if it's almost time for your next dose, skip the missed dose and take your next dose as scheduled. Don't take a double dose.

 If you suspect an overdose

Consult your doctor.

 Warnings

• Make sure your doctor knows your medical history. You may not

STADOL NS'S OTHER NAME

Stadol NS's generic name is butorphanol tartrate.

 SIDE EFFECTS

Call your doctor if you have any of these possible drug side effects. Call *immediately* about any labeled "serious."

Serious: slow or shallow breathing, change in mental status, palpitations, fluctuating blood pressure (dizziness, headache)

Common: sedation, headache, vertigo, floating sensation, confusion, nasal congestion, dry mouth, nausea, vomiting, constipation, clammy skin, sweating

Tips: Avoid activities that require full alertness or coordination until you know how Stadol NS affects you. To reduce constipation, drink plenty of fluids and eat fiber-rich foods.

Other: sluggishness, nervousness, unusual dreams, agitation, euphoria, hallucinations, flushing, blurred or double vision, rash, hives

 DRUG INTERACTIONS

Combining certain drugs may alter their action or produce unwanted side effects. Tell your doctor about other drugs you're taking, especially:
• alcohol and other drugs that make you feel relaxed or sleepy, such as tranquilizers (Valium), sleeping pills (Halcion), antihistamines (Benadryl), and narcotic pain relievers
• Dilantin
• Lanoxin
• oral diabetes drugs
• phenothiazines, such as Primazine and Thorazine
• Rifadin
• Sandimmune
• Seldane
• Tagamet
• tricyclic antidepressants, such as Elavil and Pamelor.

be able to use Stadol NS if you're overly sensitive to it or to certain preservatives; if you've recently had a heart attack or head injury; or if you have a narcotic addiction, heart or respiratory disease, or kidney or liver problems.
• Tell your doctor right away if you are pregnant or intend to breastfeed your baby.
• Be aware that older adults are usually more prone to this drug's side effects. If you're an older adult, your doctor will probably start you

on a lower dose than the one listed above.

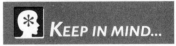 **KEEP IN MIND...**

∗ Don't increase dose without doctor's permission.

∗ Increase fluids and fiber in diet.

∗ Avoid activities that require full alertness until you know how Stadol NS affects you.

Sudafed

Sudafed constricts small blood vessels in the respiratory tract.

Why it's taken

Sudafed is taken to relieve nasal or sinus stuffiness and ear congestion. You can buy Sudafed without a prescription. It comes in tablets, syrup, oral solution, and extended-release tablets and capsules. The following amounts are usually recommended for adults; children's dosages appear in parentheses.

▶ **For nasal and eustachian tube decongestion,** 60 milligrams (mg) every 4 hours to maximum of 240 mg a day. (Children over age 12: 120 mg every 12 hours. Children ages 6 to 12: 30-mg tablet every 4 to 6 hours to maximum of 120 mg a day. Children ages 2 to 5: 15-mg tablet every 4 to 6 hours to maximum of 60 mg a day).

▶ **For relief of nasal congestion,** 120 mg every 12 hours.

How to take Sudafed

• Follow package instructions carefully.

SUDAFED'S OTHER NAMES

Sudafed's generic name is pseudoephedrine hydrochloride. Other brand names include Cenafed, Children's Sudafed Liquid, Decofed, Dorcol Children's Decongestant, Drixoral, Efidac/24, Eltor 120, Genaphed, Halofed, Halofed Adult Strength, Maxenal, Myfedrine, Novafed, PediaCare Infants' Oral Decongestant Drops, Pseudo, Pseudogest, Robidrine, and Sufedrin.

 SIDE EFFECTS

Call your doctor if you have any of these possible drug side effects.

Serious: none reported

Common: anxiety, nervousness, restlessness, palpitations, trouble sleeping

Other: temporary excitability, tremor, dizziness, headache, irregular or rapid heartbeat, appetite loss, nausea, vomiting, dry mouth, difficulty urinating, difficulty breathing, pale skin

 DRUG INTERACTIONS

Combining certain drugs may alter their action or produce unwanted side effects. Tell your doctor about other drugs you're taking, especially:
• beta blockers, such as Corgard and Lopressor
• blood pressure drugs, such as Aldomet, Inversine, and Serpasil
• caffeine, diet pills
• MAO inhibitors such as Marplan
• tricyclic antidepressants, such as Elavil and Pamelor.

• Swallow extended-release tablets or capsules whole; don't chew, crush, or break them.
• To prevent trouble sleeping, take your last dose at least 2 hours before bedtime.

If you miss a dose

If you remember within 1 hour or so, take the missed dose right away. If you don't remember until later, skip the missed dose and take your next dose on schedule. Don't take a double dose.

 If you suspect an overdose

Contact your doctor *immediately.* Excessive Sudafed can cause nausea and vomiting, seizures, and irregular heartbeat.

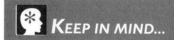 **Warnings**

• Consult your doctor before taking Sudafed if you're overly sensitive to it or if you have high blood pressure, heart disease, an overactive thyroid, diabetes, glaucoma, an enlarged prostate, or difficulty urinating.
• If you're pregnant or breast-feeding, check with your doctor before taking Sudafed.

KEEP IN MIND...

∗ Don't break or crush extended-release formulas.

∗ Don't take within 2 hours of bedtime.

∗ Don't take a double dose.

Sular

Sular blocks calcium from entering the heart. This slows heart contractions and widens blood vessels, making it easier for the heart to pump oxygen-rich blood through the body.

Why it's prescribed

Doctors prescribe Sular to lower blood pressure. It comes in extended-release tablets. Doctors usually prescribe the following amounts for adults.

▶ **For high blood pressure**, at first, 20 milligrams (mg) once a day (or 10 mg for people over 65 or with liver problems). Increased by 10 mg every week or less often, as needed. Usual dosage is 20 to 40 mg once a day. Maximum dosage is 60 mg a day.

How to take Sular

• Take Sular only as your doctor directs.
• Swallow extended-release tablets whole; don't chew, divide, or crush them.
• Don't take Sular with high-fat foods, which decrease this drug's effectiveness, or with grapefruit, which increases the amount of drug the body uses and poses a risk of an overdose.
• Keep taking Sular, even when you're feeling well.

If you miss a dose

Take the missed dose as soon as possible. However, if it's almost time

SULAR'S OTHER NAME

Sular's generic name is nisoldipine.

 SIDE EFFECTS

Call your doctor if you have any of these possible drug side effects. Call *immediately* about any labeled "serious."

Serious: chest pain (especially at beginning of treatment or after dosage increase), heart attack (chest and arm pain, anxiety, shortness of breath)

Common: headache, swelling of hands, feet, or face
Tip: Elevate your legs when sitting to relieve swelling.

Other: dizziness, flushing, palpitations, nausea, inflamed throat or sinuses, rash

 DRUG INTERACTIONS

Combining certain drugs may alter their action or produce unwanted side effects. Tell your doctor about other drugs you're taking, especially:
• Quinaglute Dura-tabs
• Tagamet.

for your next dose, skip the missed dose and go back to your regular dosing schedule. Don't take a double dose.

If you suspect an overdose

Consult your doctor. No cases of Sular overdose have been reported.

Warnings

• Make sure your doctor knows your medical history. You may not be able to take Sular if you have a drug allergy or heart, lung, or liver disease.
• Make sure your doctor knows if you're pregnant or breast-feeding before you start taking Sular. This drug is not recommended for pregnant or breast-feeding women.

• Schedule periodic follow-up visits during treatment so your doctor can evaluate your progress and check for side effects.

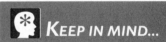 **KEEP IN MIND...**

* Take as directed, even when feeling well.

* Don't chew, divide, or crush tablets.

* Don't take with high-fat foods or grapefruit.

* Don't take while pregnant or breast-feeding.

Sumycin

Sumycin kills many different types of bacteria by not allowing them to reproduce.

Why it's prescribed

Doctors prescribe Sumycin to help treat infections. It comes in tablets, capsules, and liquid. Doctors usually prescribe the following amounts for adults; children's dosages appear in parentheses.

▶ **For infections caused by sensitive bacteria (including *Rickettsia, Chlamydia, Mycoplasma,* and organisms that cause trachoma),** 250 to 500 milligrams (mg) every 6 hours. (Children over age 8: 25 to 50 mg for each 2.2 pounds of body weight daily, divided into equal doses and taken every 6 hours.)

▶ **For uncomplicated urethral, cervical, or rectal infections caused by *Chlamydia,*** 500 mg four times a day for at least 7 days.

▶ **For brucellosis,** 500 mg every 6 hours for 3 weeks, combined with 1 gram (g) of streptomycin injected every 12 hours for the first week and once a day for the second week.

▶ **For gonorrhea in adults sensitive to penicillin,** initially, 1.5 g, then 500 mg every 6 hours for a total dose of 9 g.

▶ **For syphilis in adults sensitive to penicillin,** a total of 30 to 40 g, divided into equal doses over 10 to 15 days.

▶ **For acne in adults and adolescents,** initially, 250 mg every 6

SIDE EFFECTS

Call your doctor if you have any of these possible drug side effects. Call *immediately* about any labeled "serious."

Serious: pericarditis (fever, chest pain, shortness of breath), blood problems (bleeding, sore throat, fatigue, fever), allergic reaction (itching, swelling, difficulty breathing), behavioral changes, increased pressure in skull (headache, irritability, lethargy)

Common: stomach upset, nausea, diarrhea, kidney problems (increased thirst and urination); in children under age 8, permanent discoloration of teeth, enamel defects, delayed bone growth

Other: dizziness, headache, swollen tongue or mouth, difficult or painful swallowing, appetite loss, vomiting, mouth infections, colitis (cramping, diarrhea), lesions around anus or genitals, blood problems, rash, hives, increased sensitivity to sun, darker skin color

Tips: To avoid infections in your mouth, practice excellent oral hygiene while taking Sumycin. To protect your skin, limit your exposure to the sun and wear a sunscreen and protective clothing when you go out.

DRUG AND FOOD INTERACTIONS

Combining certain drugs and foods may alter drug action or produce unwanted side effects. Tell your doctor about your diet and other drugs you're taking, especially:

- anticoagulants (blood thinners) such as Coumadin
- birth control pills
- diarrhea drugs containing bismuth subsalicylate, kaolin, or pectin
- Eskalith
- iron supplements such as Feosol
- laxatives and antacids containing aluminum, calcium, magnesium, or sodium bicarbonate
- methoxyflurane
- milk and other dairy products
- penicillins.

---

hours, then 125 to 500 mg a day or every other day.

How to take Sumycin

- Take this drug 1 hour before or 2 hours after meals because food can decrease your body's ability to absorb the drug.
- Don't take Sumycin with dairy products or iron supplements.

- To help prevent stomach irritation, drink a full glass (8 ounces) of water with each dose. To avoid irritating your esophagus, take your last dose of the day at least 1 hour before bedtime.
- Take your entire prescription, even if you feel better before it's finished.

If you miss a dose

Take the missed dose as soon as possible. But if it's almost time for your next dose, adjust your schedule as follows:

• If you're taking one dose a day, make up a missed dose the following day by leaving a 12-hour space between doses. (For example, take your regularly scheduled dose at 7 a.m. and a makeup dose at 7 p.m.)

• If you're taking two doses a day, space the missed dose and the next one 5 to 6 hours apart.

• If you're taking three or more doses a day, space the missed dose and the next one 2 to 4 hours apart. Then resume your regular dosing schedule. Don't take a double dose.

If you suspect an overdose

Contact your doctor *immediately.* Excessive Sumycin can cause increased stomach distress.

Warnings

• Make sure your doctor knows your medical history. You may not be able to take Sumycin if you are overly sensitive to it or have diabetes or liver or kidney problems.

• Sumycin is not recommended for women who are more than 4 months' pregnant because it may permanently stain infants' teeth.

• Children under age 8 should not take Sumycin because it may delay bone growth.

• Sumycin may reduce the effectiveness of birth control pills. Use an additional form of birth control while taking this drug.

• Don't use old or expired Sumycin. It may cause added side effects.

• Don't expose Sumycin to heat or light.

✻ KEEP IN MIND...

* Take with water 1 hour before or 2 hours after meals.

* Don't take with dairy products or iron supplements.

* Practice excellent oral hygiene.

* Don't take Sumycin after 4th month of pregnancy.

* Wear a sunscreen and protective clothes outside.

Suprax

Suprax kills certain bacteria by preventing their cell walls from growing.

Why it's prescribed

Doctors prescribe Suprax to treat certain infections. It comes in tablets and a powder that's mixed with water. Doctors usually prescribe the following amounts for adults; children's dosages appear in parentheses.

▶ **For some urinary tract infections, ear infections, pharyngitis, tonsillitis, and bronchitis,** 400 milligrams (mg) a day as a single 400-mg tablet or 200 mg every 12 hours. (Children over age 12 or weighing over 110 pounds [lb]: same as adults. Children age 12 and younger or weighing 110 lb or less: 8 mg for each 2.2 lb of body weight daily as a single liquid dose or 4 mg for each 2.2 lb every 12 hours.)

▶ **For gonorrhea,** 400 mg as a single dose.

How to take Suprax

• If you're using the liquid form, add half the required amount of water to the powder and shake well. Then add the remaining water and shake again.

• After mixing, the liquid will last for 14 days. You don't need to refrigerate it, but keep the container tightly closed and shake it well before using.

• Keep a steady level of the drug in your blood by spacing doses evenly throughout the day and night.

SUPRAX'S OTHER NAME

Suprax's generic name is cefixime.

 ## SIDE EFFECTS

Call your doctor if you have any of these possible drug side effects. Call *immediately* about any labeled "serious."

Serious: blood problems (fatigue), burnlike rash, severe diarrhea, allergic reaction (fever, increased risk of infection), difficulty breathing, swelling of face and throat, chest pain, anxiety

Common: diarrhea
Tip: If diarrhea becomes bothersome, call your doctor.

Other: headache, dizziness, nervousness, fatigue, sleepiness, insomnia, abdominal pain, nausea, vomiting, heartburn, gas, genital itching or infection, temporary kidney or liver problems (decreased urination, nausea, vomiting, yellow-tinged eyes and skin), itchiness, rash, hives
Tip: Eating yogurt that contains active cultures may help prevent genital itching and infection.

 ## DRUG INTERACTIONS

Combining certain drugs may alter their action or produce unwanted side effects. Tell your doctor about other drugs you're taking, especially:

• aspirin and other products containing salicylates
• Benemid.

• Take the full amount prescribed, even if you feel better before it's finished.

If you miss a dose

Take the missed dose as soon as possible. However, if it's almost time for your next dose, skip the missed dose and take your next dose as scheduled. Don't take a double dose.

 ### If you suspect an overdose

Consult your doctor.

Warnings

• Make sure your doctor knows your medical history. You may not be able to take Suprax if you're overly sensitive to it or drugs like it or if you have kidney or liver problems.

• If you're diabetic, keep in mind that Suprax may cause false-positive results on Clinitest. Clinistix and Tes-Tape results aren't affected.

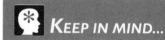 ### KEEP IN MIND...

* Space doses evenly throughout day and night.

* Reconstituted liquid lasts 14 days.

* Report burnlike rash to doctor.

* Finish entire prescription.

Surfak

Surfak is a laxative that softens stool by increasing its water content.

Why it's taken

Surfak is taken to treat constipation, especially when it's important not to strain, such as after some types of surgery. You can buy this drug without a prescription. It comes in capsules. The following amounts are usually recommended for adults and children over age 12.

▶ **For constipation,** 50 to 500 mg daily until bowel movements are normal.

How to take Surfak

• If your doctor prescribed Surfak, take it exactly as prescribed. If you're treating yourself, follow the package instructions carefully.
• If you're taking other drugs, take them at least 2 hours before or after taking Surfak because Surfak may interfere with the desired actions of the other drugs.
• Don't take Surfak for more than 1 week unless your doctor has prescribed a special schedule for you. This is true even if you continue to have constipation.

If you miss a dose

Because this drug is taken once a day, postpone a missed dose until early the next day. Don't take a double dose.

SURFAK'S OTHER NAMES

Surfak's generic name is docusate calcium. Another brand name is Pro-Cal-Sof.

 SIDE EFFECTS

Call your doctor if you have any of these possible drug side effects.

Serious: none reported

Common: none reported

Other: throat irritation, mild abdominal cramping, diarrhea, laxative dependence (with long-term or excessive use)
Tip: If Surfak causes bothersome side effects, especially severe cramping, call your doctor.

 DRUG INTERACTIONS

Combining certain drugs may alter their action or produce unwanted side effects. Tell your doctor about other drugs you're taking, especially:
• mineral oil.

 If you suspect an overdose

Consult your doctor.

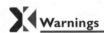 **Warnings**

• Consult your doctor before taking Surfak if you are overly sensitive to it or have abdominal pain or rectal bleeding from an unknown cause, a colostomy or ileostomy, or a blocked intestine.
• Don't use Surfak (or any other laxative) if you have symptoms of appendicitis or an inflamed bowel, such as stomach or lower abdominal pain, cramping, bloating, soreness, nausea, or vomiting. Call your doctor as soon as possible.
• If you're pregnant, check with your doctor before taking Surfak.
• If your constipation represents a sudden change in your bowel habits and lasts longer than 2 weeks or keeps recurring from time to time, check with your doctor.

• Drink at least six 8-ounce glasses of water or other liquids daily, eat plenty of fiber-rich foods, and get adequate exercise.
• Use Surfak only occasionally and never for more than 1 week without a doctor's prescription. Otherwise, you may become dependent on it to produce a bowel movement. In severe cases, overuse of laxatives can damage the nerves, muscles, and other tissues of the bowel.

 KEEP IN MIND...

* Don't take for more than 1 week.

* Don't take mineral oil with Surfak.

* Call doctor if you develop severe abdominal cramps.

* Increase fluids and fiber in diet.

* Tell doctor about sudden changes in bowel habits.

Surmontil

Surmontil is one of a group of drugs called tricyclic antidepressants. It improves a person's mood by increasing or maintaining levels of the chemicals norepinephrine and serotonin in the central nervous system.

Why it's prescribed

Doctors prescribe Surmontil to treat symptoms of depression. It comes in capsules. Doctors usually prescribe the following amounts for adults.

▶ **For depression,** 75 to 100 milligrams (mg) taken once a day or divided into equal doses. Maximum daily dosage is 200 mg.

How to take Surmontil

• Take Surmontil with food or milk to reduce stomach upset.
• To prevent dizziness, lie down for about 30 minutes after each dose.
• To avoid sleepiness during the day, ask your doctor if you can take your full dose at bedtime.
• Don't stop taking Surmontil abruptly, even if you're feeling better. Doing so could cause nausea, headache, and an overall feeling of illness.

If you miss a dose

Adjust your schedule as follows:
• If you take one dose a day at bedtime and you miss a dose, check with your doctor. Don't take your

SURMONTIL'S OTHER NAMES

Surmontil's generic name is trimipramine maleate. Other brand names include Apo-Trimip, Novo-Tripramine, and Rhotrimine.

 ## SIDE EFFECTS

Call your doctor if you have any of these possible drug side effects. Call *immediately* about any labeled "serious."

Serious: seizures, tremor or difficulty moving, fast or irregular pulse, difficulty urinating, mood changes
Tips: Call your doctor if you experience mood changes, movement problems, or suicidal thoughts. Also report a fast pulse or difficulty urinating.

Common: drowsiness, dizziness, light-headedness, blurred vision, dry mouth, constipation, inability to urinate, profuse sweating
Tips: Avoid activities that require full alertness or coordination until you know how Surmontil affects you. Drowsiness and dizziness usually subside in a few weeks. To reduce dizziness and light-headedness when you wake in the morning, sit up slowly and dangle your legs before getting out bed. Relieve dry mouth with sugarless hard candy or gum. Saliva substitutes may be necessary. Relieve constipation by drinking more water and eating more fiber-rich foods. If you're still constipated, ask your doctor about a stool softener.

Other: excitability, weakness, confusion, headache, nervousness, high blood pressure (headache, blurred vision), ringing in ears, dilated pupils, nausea, vomiting, appetite loss, prolonged constipation, abdominal pain, increased skin sensitivity to sun, allergic reaction (rash, hives, fever, swelling); after abruptly stopping long-term therapy, nausea, headache, and overall feeling of illness
Tip: To protect your skin, avoid exposure to intense sunlight, and wear a sunblock, a hat, and protective clothes when you go outdoors.

 ## DRUG INTERACTIONS

Combining certain drugs may alter their action or produce unwanted side effects. Tell your doctor about other drugs you're taking, especially:
• alcohol
• barbiturates such as Solfoton
• Bronkaid Mist
• Catapres
• Ismelin
• MAO inhibitors, such as Nardil and Parnate
• Paxil, Prozac
• phenothiazines, such as Primazine and Thorazine
• Quinaglute Dura-tabs, Rythmol, Tambocor
• Tagamet
• thyroid drugs
• tricyclic antidepressants, such as Elavil and Pamelor.

missed dose in the morning because it could cause side effects.
• If you take more than one dose a day, take the missed dose as soon as possible. However, if it's almost time for your next dose, skip the missed dose and take your next dose as scheduled. Don't take a double dose.

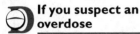

If you suspect an overdose

Contact your doctor *immediately*. Excessive Surmontil can cause agitation, confusion, hallucinations, seizures, low blood pressure (dizziness, weakness), drowsiness, restlessness, coma, hyperactive reflexes, stiff muscles, rapid pulse, difficulty breathing, vomiting, and profuse sweating.

Warnings

• Make sure your doctor knows your medical history. You may not be able to take Surmontil if you are overly sensitive to it, have heart disease or had a heart attack recently, have taken other types of antidepressants within the last 2 weeks, or have stomach or intestinal problems, angle-closure glaucoma, an overactive thyroid, asthma, an enlarged prostate, an inability to urinate, schizophrenia, a history of seizures, or kidney or liver problems.
• If you are ill, a teenager, or an older adult, your doctor will probably start you on a lower dosage than usual.
• Be aware that you may have to take Surmontil for several weeks before you begin to feel better.
• If you're scheduled for surgery, your doctor will probably have you reduce your dosage and then stop taking Surmontil before the procedure. Afterward, you can resume taking the drug.

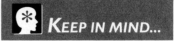

KEEP IN MIND...

* Lie down for 30 minutes after taking.
* Don't stop Surmontil abruptly.
* Avoid alcohol.
* Sit and stand slowly to reduce dizziness.

Symmetrel

Symmetrel probably works by blocking influenza A virus from penetrating susceptible cells. In Parkinson's disease, its action is unknown.

Why it's prescribed

Doctors prescribe Symmetrel to prevent or treat type A influenza (flu) and to treat Parkinson's disease and the stiffness and shaking caused by some other drugs. It comes in capsules and syrup. Doctors usually prescribe the following amounts.

▶ **To prevent and treat influenza type A in adults,** 200 milligrams (mg) once a day or divided into two equal doses.

▶ **To prevent and treat influenza type A in children ages 1 to 9,** 4.4 to 8.8 mg for each 2.2 pounds (lb) of body weight as a single dose or divided into two equal doses. Maximum dosage is 150 mg daily.

▶ **To prevent and treat influenza type A in adults over age 64,** 100 mg once a day.

▶ **For drug-induced parkinson-like reactions in adults,** 100 mg twice a day, increased to 300 or 400 mg a day divided into equal doses. Dosages over 200 mg must be closely supervised.

▶ **For Parkinson's disease in adults,** 100 mg twice a day. For those who are seriously ill or taking other drugs for Parkinson's disease, 100 mg a day for at least 1 week, then 100 mg twice a day if needed.

SYMMETREL'S OTHER NAMES

Symmetrel's generic name is amantadine hydrochloride. Another brand name is Symadine.

 ## SIDE EFFECTS

Call your doctor if you have any of these possible drug side effects. Call *immediately* about any labeled "serious."

Serious: congestive heart failure (shortness of breath, chest pain, anxiety), low blood pressure (dizziness, weakness)

Common: dizziness, distractibility, irritability, difficulty sleeping, purplish lacy spots on skin (with long-term use)
Tips: Avoid activities that require full alertness or coordination until you know how Symmetrel affects you. To reduce dizziness, dangle your legs before getting out of bed and get up slowly.

Other: depression, fatigue, confusion, strange behavior, hallucinations, anxiety, loss of balance, weakness, headache, light-headedness, difficulty concentrating, swelling of ankles or hands, appetite loss, nausea, constipation, vomiting, dry mouth, inability to urinate
Tips: Contact the doctor immediately if you faint, become nauseous, feel confused or anxious, become depressed, have difficulty urinating, or experience hallucinations. Reduce mouth dryness by using sugarless hard candy or gum, ice chips, or a saliva substitute. If dryness persists after 2 weeks, check with your doctor.

 ## DRUG INTERACTIONS

Combining certain drugs may alter their action or produce unwanted side effects. Tell your doctor about other drugs you're taking, especially:
- alcohol
- certain muscle relaxants, such as Cogentin and Trihexare
- Dyrenium
- HydroDIURIL
- Mellaril
- stimulant drugs, such as caffeine and diet pills.

How to take Symmetrel

- Follow your doctor's directions exactly.
- If you're taking the syrup, use a measuring spoon — not a household teaspoon — to get an accurate dose.
- Take the doses at regular intervals both day and night, for example, 8 a.m. and 8 p.m.
- If you have trouble sleeping, take your last dose 2 hours before bedtime.

- To avoid making symptoms worse, don't stop taking Symmetrel suddenly.
- If you're taking Symmetrel to prevent or treat the flu, finish the entire prescription. If you stop taking it too soon, your symptoms may recur.

If you miss a dose

Take the missed dose as soon as possible. However, if you're within 4 hours of your next dose, skip the missed dose and take your next

dose as scheduled. Don't take a double dose.

If you suspect an overdose

Contact your doctor *immediately*. Excessive Symmetrel can cause slurred speech, vomiting, seizures, high blood pressure (headache, blurred vision), irregular or rapid heartbeat, difficulty breathing, anxiety, aggressive behavior, tremor, confusion, disorientation, hallucinations, and coma.

Warnings

• Make sure your doctor knows your medical history. You may not be able to take Symmetrel if you're overly sensitive to it or if you have seizures, congestive heart failure, fluid buildup in hands and feet, mental illness, a rash, low blood pressure, or kidney or liver problems.

• If you're pregnant or breast-feeding, notify your doctor.

• Be aware that older adults may be especially prone to Symmetrel's side effects.

• If you're taking this drug to prevent or treat the flu and your symptoms continue or worsen within a few days, contact your doctor.

• If you think Symmetrel is losing its effectiveness, call your doctor. Don't change the dosage on your own.

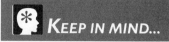
KEEP IN MIND...

* Take doses at regular intervals day and night.

* Take last dose 2 hours before bedtime if you have trouble sleeping.

* Stand up slowly to avoid dizziness.

* Don't stop taking abruptly.

* Finish entire prescription.

Synalar stimulates the production of chemicals in the body that decrease inflammation.

Why it's prescribed

Doctors prescribe Synalar to help relieve redness, swelling, itching, and other types of skin discomfort. It comes in a cream, an ointment, and a topical solution. Doctors usually prescribe the following amounts for adults.

▶ **For inflammation associated with certain skin problems,** cream, ointment, or topical solution applied sparingly two to four times a day.

How to use Synalar

• Follow your doctor's directions exactly.
• Wash your hands before and after applying Synalar.
• Wash the area to be treated; then use your finger to gently apply a thin layer of Synalar. When treating a hairy site, part the hair and apply Synalar to the skin.
• Don't bandage or wrap the area being treated unless your doctor directs you to do so. If the doctor does tell you to apply an occlusive dressing (an airtight covering, such as plastic wrap or a special patch), be sure to get complete directions for doing so.
• If you're applying Synalar to a child's diaper area, avoid using tight-fitting diapers or plastic pants, which could increase absorp-

SIDE EFFECTS

Call your doctor if you have any of these possible drug side effects. Call *immediately* about any labeled "serious."

Serious: congestive heart failure (shortness of breath), suppressed immune system (risk of infection)

Common: new infection, tiny bumps caused by blocked sweat ducts
Tip: If your skin condition gets worse or you develop a new infection, contact your doctor; you may need a different drug.

Other: burning, itching, irritation, dryness, redness, skin color or texture change, infected hair follicles, excessive hair growth, loss of pigmentation, acnelike eruptions, rash around mouth, allergic contact dermatitis (reddened, itchy rash), changes in blood sugar levels (increased thirst, hunger, and urination)

DRUG INTERACTIONS

Combining certain drugs may alter their action or produce unwanted side effects. Tell your doctor about other drugs you're taking.

tion of the drug through the skin and possibly cause side effects.
• Don't apply this drug near your eyes, on mucous membranes, in your ear canal, or on your breasts before breast-feeding. If you get any in your eye, flush it immediately with water.

If you miss a dose

Apply the missed dose as soon as possible. However, if it's almost time for your next dose, skip the missed dose and apply your next dose as scheduled. Don't apply a double dose.

If you suspect an overdose

Consult your doctor.

Warnings

• Make sure your doctor knows your medical history. If you have other medical problems, you may

need to change your medication while you're using Synalar.
• If you become pregnant while using Synalar, consult your doctor.
• Be aware that older adults may be especially prone to certain side effects.
• Don't use leftover Synalar for other skin problems without first consulting your doctor.

KEEP IN MIND...

* Apply gently and sparingly.
* Keep away from eyes, ears, and mucous membranes.
* Don't bandage treated area unless doctor directs.
* Call doctor if skin condition worsens.

SYNALAR'S OTHER NAMES

Synalar's generic name is fluocinolone acetonide. Other brand names include Fluocet, Fluonid, Flurosyn, and Synemol.

Synthroid

Synthroid is a thyroid hormone that stimulates the body's metabolism.

Why it's prescribed

Doctors prescribe Synthroid to supplement the amount of hormone produced by the thyroid gland. It comes in tablets. Doctors usually prescribe the following amounts.

▶ **For thyroid hormone replacement in adults,** 0.025 to 0.05 milligrams (mg) a day, increased by 0.025 mg every 2 to 4 weeks until desired response occurs. Usual dosage is 0.1 to 0.4 mg a day.

▶ **For thyroid hormone replacement in adults over age 65,** 0.0125 to 0.025 mg a day, increased by 0.025 mg every 3 to 8 weeks, as needed.

▶ **For thyroid hormone replacement in children,** 0.025 to 0.05 mg in children younger than age 1. Or 3 to 5 micrograms a day for each 2.2 pounds of body weight in children age 1 and older, gradually increased by 0.025 to 0.05 mg every 2 to 4 weeks, as needed.

▶ **For cretinism in children under age 1,** 0.025 to 0.05 mg a day, increased by 0.05 mg every 4 to 6 weeks, as needed.

How to take Synthroid

• Take Synthroid exactly as your doctor directs. Don't take more or less of it, and don't take it more often than prescribed. The doctor may have to adjust the dosage repeatedly.

SYNTHROID'S OTHER NAMES

Synthroid's generic name is levothyroxine sodium. Other brand names include Eltroxin, Levothroid, and Levoxyl.

SIDE EFFECTS

Call your doctor if you have any of these possible drug side effects. Call *immediately* about any labeled "serious."

Serious: chest pain, fast pulse, palpitations, high blood pressure (headache, blurred vision), shortness of breath, dizziness

Tip: If you have heart disease, Synthroid may cause you to develop chest pain or shortness of breath when you exert yourself. If this occurs, reduce your physical exercise.

Common: nervousness, insomnia, tremor

Other: appetite change, nausea, diarrhea, headache, leg cramps, weight loss, sweating, heat intolerance, fever, menstrual irregularities, hair loss, rash, itching

DRUG INTERACTIONS

Combining certain drugs may alter their action or produce unwanted side effects. Tell your doctor about other drugs you're taking, especially:

• allergy and cold drugs
• amphetamines
• anticoagulants (blood thinners) such as Coumadin
• aspirin and aspirin-containing drugs
• asthma and other respiratory drugs
• birth control pills and other estrogen-containing drugs
• blood pressure drugs such as Tenormin
• Colestid
• diet pills
• epinephrine and similar drugs
• insulin and oral diabetes drugs, such as Micronase and Orinase
• Kayexalate
• Maalox and other aluminum-containing drugs
• Protropin
• Questran
• seizure drugs such as Dilantin.

• Take this drug at the same time each morning, preferably before breakfast, to maintain constant hormone levels and avoid insomnia.

• Once you've achieved the correct dosage, don't change brand names.

• Don't stop taking this drug without first talking with your doctor.

If you miss a dose

Take the missed dose as soon as possible. However, if it's almost time for your next dose, skip the missed dose and take your next dose as scheduled. Don't take a double dose. If you miss two or more doses in a row, call your doctor.

Continued on next page ▶

If you suspect an overdose

Contact your doctor *immediately.* Excessive Synthroid can cause chest pain, nervousness, trouble sleeping, hand tremor, rapid pulse or palpitations, nausea, headache, fever, sweating, shortness of breath, heat intolerance, irregular menstrual periods, weight loss, increased appetite, diarrhea, and abdominal cramps.

Warnings

• Make sure your doctor knows your medical history. You may not be able to take Synthroid if you're overly sensitive to it; if you've recently had a heart attack or stroke; or if you have diabetes, coronary artery disease, angina, high blood pressure, lung problems, untreated Graves' disease, an underactive adrenal or pituitary gland, myxedema (severely underactive thyroid), or kidney problems.

• Call your doctor if you become pregnant or start breast-feeding while taking Synthroid.
• If you're taking Synthroid for an underactive thyroid gland, realize that it may take several weeks before you notice any change in your condition.
• If your infant is on formula, be aware that infant formulas containing soybean flour may alter the effectiveness of Synthroid. Consult your child's doctor before giving the child this drug.

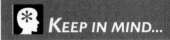 KEEP IN MIND...

* Take at same time each morning, before breakfast.
* Don't change dosage or stop taking without doctor's approval.
* Don't change brand names.
* Don't expect full effect for several weeks.

Tacaryl

Tacaryl is an antihistamine. It blocks histamine, which causes such symptoms as a runny nose and watery eyes.

Why it's prescribed

Doctors prescribe Tacaryl to help reduce the signs and symptoms of allergy, such as runny nose, congestion, and itching. It comes in tablets and syrup. Doctors usually prescribe the following amounts for adults; children's dosages appears in parentheses.

▶ **For runny nose, congestion, and itching caused by allergy,** 8 milligrams (mg) two to four times a day. (Children over age 3: 4 mg two to four times a day.)

How to take Tacaryl

• If Tacaryl causes stomach upset, take it with food or milk.

If you miss a dose

Take the missed dose as soon as possible. However, if it's almost time for your next dose, skip the missed dose and take your next dose as scheduled. Don't take a double dose.

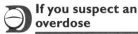 If you suspect an overdose

Contact your doctor *immediately*. Excessive Tacaryl can cause sedation, seizures, stopped breathing, and cardiovascular collapse (irregular heartbeat, fainting, drop in blood pressure).

TACARYL'S OTHER NAME

Tacaryl's generic name is methdilazine hydrochloride.

 SIDE EFFECTS

Call your doctor if you have any of these possible drug side effects.

Serious: none reported

Common: drowsiness, dry mouth and throat
Tips: Avoid activities that require full alertness or coordination until you know how Tacaryl affects you. To reduce drowsiness, try drinking some coffee or tea. To relieve dry mouth, try sugarless gum or hard candy or ice chips.

Other: dizziness, headache, nausea, inability to urinate, rash, yellow-tinged skin and eyes

 DRUG INTERACTIONS

Combining certain drugs may alter their action or produce unwanted side effects. Tell your doctor about other drugs you're taking, especially:
• drugs that make you relaxed or sleepy, such as tranquilizers (Valium, Xanax) and sleeping pills (Halcion)
• epinephrine
• MAO inhibitors, such as Nardil and Parnate
• phenothiazines, such as Primazine and Thorazine.

 Warnings

• Make sure your doctor knows your medical history. You may not be able to take Tacaryl if you're overly sensitive to it, or if you have other medical problems, especially acute asthma attacks, angle-closure glaucoma, an enlarged prostate, heart or lung disease, a stomach ulcer or obstruction, an overactive thyroid, or high blood pressure.
• Before taking Tacaryl, tell your doctor if you're breast-feeding.
• If you're scheduled for allergy tests, your doctor will probably tell you to stop taking Tacaryl about 4 days before the tests because Tacaryl could affect the results.

• Tell your doctor if you feel that Tacaryl is becoming less effective. It may be necessary to switch you to a different antihistamine.

KEEP IN MIND...

* Stop taking Tacaryl about 4 days before allergy tests.

* Relieve dry mouth with sugarless gum or hard candy or with ice chips.

* Tell doctor if drug seems less effective.

* Relieve drowsiness with coffee or tea.

TACE

TACE is a type of estrogen, a female hormone, that's used to replace decreasing levels of estrogen in the body.

Why it's prescribed

Doctors prescribe TACE to battle prostate cancer, offset poorly functioning ovaries, and treat bothersome symptoms of menopause. It comes in capsules. Doctors usually prescribe the following amounts for adults.

▶ **For prostate cancer,** 12 to 25 milligrams (mg) a day.

▶ **For poorly functioning ovaries,** 12 to 25 mg for 21 days, followed by one injection of progesterone (100 mg) or 5 days of oral progestogen given together with the last 5 days of TACE.

▶ **For menopausal symptoms,** 12 to 25 mg a day for 30 days or cyclic therapy that includes 3 weeks on and 1 week off.

How to take TACE

• Take TACE exactly as your doctor directs.

If you miss a dose

Take the missed dose as soon as possible. However, if it's almost time for your next dose, skip the missed dose and take your next dose as scheduled. Don't take a double dose.

 ## If you suspect an overdose

Excessive TACE can cause nausea. If you suspect an overdose or have questions, consult your doctor.

TACE's OTHER NAME

TACE's generic name is chlorotrianisene.

 ## SIDE EFFECTS

Call your doctor if you have any of these possible drug side effects. Call *immediately* about any labeled "serious."

Serious: blood clots (pain, redness, swelling in arm, leg, or buttock), stroke (slurred speech, loss of sensation, headache, blurred vision), pulmonary embolism and heart attack (chest pain, shortness of breath, anxiety), high blood pressure (headache, blurred vision)

Common: nausea; in men, breast enlargement, smaller testicles, and impotence

Other: headache, dizziness, uncontrollable hand motions, migraine, depression, swelling of ankles and hands, vision changes, intolerance of contact lenses, vomiting, abdominal cramps, bloating, diarrhea, constipation, increased or decreased appetite, weight changes, pancreatitis (abdominal pain, vomiting, fever), altered or absent menstrual flow, abnormal cervical secretions, enlargement of uterine fibromas (pain, bleeding), yellow-tinged skin and eyes, darker skin color, hives, acne, oily skin, hair growth or loss, leg cramps, breast changes (tenderness, enlargement, secretion), increased thirst and urination, increased calcium levels (muscle weakness, confusion), folic acid deficiency (diarrhea, red swollen tongue or mouth), changes in sex drive, vaginal bleeding, discharge, or infection

Tip: Monitor your weight closely because estrogen therapy may cause fluid retention and swelling. If necessary, reduce the amount of salt in your diet.

 ## DRUG INTERACTIONS

Combining certain drugs may alter their action or produce unwanted side effects. Tell your doctor about other drugs you're taking, especially:
• anticoagulants (blood thinners) such as Coumadin
• corticosteroids
• Dilantin
• Dantrium
• Mysoline
• Nolvadex
• Parlodel
• Rifadin
• Sandimmune
• Solfoton
• Tegretol.

 ## Warnings

• Make sure your doctor knows your medical history. You may not be able to take TACE if you have blood clots; cancer of the breast or reproductive organs; a family history (mother, grandmother, sister) of breast cancer, breast nodules, or

fibrocystic disease; an abnormal mammogram; undiagnosed genital bleeding; heart or blood vessel disease; asthma; bone disease; migraines; seizures; liver or kidney problems; or increased calcium levels.

• Tell your doctor if you're pregnant before taking TACE or if you become pregnant while taking it.

• Be aware that older adults are more prone to this drug's side effects.

• If you're diabetic, tell your doctor if your blood sugar levels rise. Your diabetes drugs may need adjustment.

• Your doctor will probably want you to have a complete physical before starting estrogen therapy.

• While taking TACE, be sure to have routine physicals and do routine breast self-examinations.

• To reduce the risk of blood clots, your doctor will probably want you to stop taking TACE at least a month before you have surgical procedures known to cause lengthy immobilization, such as knee or hip surgery.

• If you are on cyclic therapy for menopausal symptoms, you may bleed during the week you aren't taking the drug. However, you can't get pregnant because you haven't ovulated.

• TACE contains an additive that may cause you to have an allergic reaction if you're sensitive to aspirin. If you are aspirin-sensitive or have ever had an allergic reaction to aspirin, consult your doctor before taking this drug.

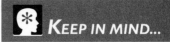

KEEP IN MIND...

* Have routine physicals and perform routine breast exams.

* Tell doctor right away if you think you're pregnant.

* Reduce salt in your diet if you retain water.

* If you're sensitive to aspirin, consult doctor before taking drug.

* Consult doctor before taking drug if you're sensitive to aspirin.

Tagamet

Tagamet reduces secretion of stomach acid.

Why it's prescribed

Doctors prescribe Tagamet to treat ulcers and prevent their return. It may also be used to treat Zollinger-Ellison syndrome, in which the stomach makes too much acid. You can buy Tagamet without a prescription. It comes in tablets and liquid. Doctors usually prescribe the following amounts.

▶ **For duodenal ulcer (short-term treatment) in adults and children age 16 and over,** 800 milligrams (mg) a day, or 400 mg twice a day, or 300 mg four times a day. Usual treatment time is 4 to 6 weeks. Usual dosage is 400 mg a day.

▶ **For active benign gastric ulcers (stomach ulcers) in adults,** 800 mg a day or 300 mg four times a day for up to 8 weeks.

▶ **For conditions characterized by excessive gastric acid secretion (such as Zollinger-Ellison syndrome, systemic mastocytosis, and multiple endocrine adenomas) in adults and children age 16 and over,** 300 mg four times a day, adjusted as needed. Maximum dosage is 2,400 mg a day.

▶ **For gastroesophageal reflux (heartburn) in adults,** 800 mg twice a day or 400 mg four times a day.

How to take Tagamet

• If your doctor prescribed Tagamet, take it exactly as directed.

TAGAMET'S OTHER NAME

Tagamet's generic name is cimetidine. The brand name of the nonprescription form is Tagamet-HB.

SIDE EFFECTS

Call your doctor if you have any of these possible drug side effects. Call *immediately* about any labeled "serious."

Serious: severe blood problems (rare), such as fatigue, bleeding, bruising, infection, chills, fever

Common: mild diarrhea
Tip: Although you may develop diarrhea, it should be temporary. If it lingers or becomes severe, call your doctor.

Other: confusion, dizziness, headaches, agitation, anxiety, depression, hallucinations, disorientation, tingling in hands and feet, slower heartbeat, yellow-tinged skin and eyes (rare), acnelike rash, hives, allergic reaction (difficulty breathing or swallowing, swelling of face, itching), muscle pain, mild breast enlargement (with use for 1 month or more)
Tip: If you develop signs of an allergic reaction, seek emergency medical help immediately.

DRUG INTERACTIONS

Combining certain drugs may alter their action or produce unwanted side effects. Tell your doctor about other drugs you're taking, especially:
• antacids (wait 1 hour before taking Tagamet)
• certain kinds of sedatives
• certain tranquilizers and sleeping pills
• Coumadin
• Dilantin
• Inderal
• Librium
• lidocaine
• Nizoral
• Procardia
• Theo-Dur
• tobacco
• Valium.

If you're treating yourself, carefully follow the package instructions.
• If you're taking this drug once a day, take it at bedtime unless otherwise directed. If you're taking two doses a day, take one in the morning and one at bedtime. If you're taking more than two doses a day, take them with meals and at bedtime for best results. If you're taking this drug for heartburn, take it before meals and at bedtime.

If you miss a dose

Take the missed dose as soon as possible. However, if it's almost time for your next dose, skip the missed dose and take your next dose as scheduled. Don't take a double dose.

If you suspect an overdose

Contact your doctor *immediately*. Signs and symptoms of a Tagamet overdose may include difficulty breathing, fast pulse, and unresponsiveness.

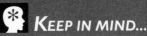

Warnings

• Make sure your doctor knows your medical history. You may not be able to take Tagamet if you're overly sensitive to it or if you have liver or kidney disease.
• If you're pregnant or breast-feeding, talk to your doctor before you use Tagamet.
• Be aware that older adults may be especially prone to Tagamet's side effects.

• Be aware that several days may pass before Tagamet begins to relieve your stomach pain. In the meantime, you may take antacids unless your doctor has told you not to use them.
• Tell your doctor if your stomach pain continues or worsens while taking Tagamet.
• Tell the doctor that you're taking Tagamet before you have skin tests for allergies or tests to determine how much acid your stomach produces.
• Contact your doctor *immediately* if you develop signs and symptoms of infection or bleeding.
• If you have arthritis or joint pain, consult your doctor before taking Tagamet because this drug may worsen your symptoms.

KEEP IN MIND...

* Take Tagamet with meals and at bedtime.
* Relief make take several days.
* Don't take antacids within 1 hour of Tagamet.
* Avoid smoking.
* Consult doctor if pain continues or if you develop signs of infection or bleeding.

Talwin-Nx

Talwin-Nx is a narcotic that alters the brain's perception of pain.

Why it's prescribed

Doctors prescribe Talwin-Nx to relieve pain. It comes in tablets. It's also available in an injectable form. Doctors usually prescribe the following amounts for adults.

▶ **For moderate to severe pain,** 50 to 100 milligrams (mg) orally every 3 to 4 hours, as needed. Maximum oral dosage is 600 mg a day.

How to take Talwin-Nx

- Follow your doctor's directions.
- Don't take more of this drug than directed or use it for a longer time than specified because it may become habit-forming.
- Don't stop taking Talwin-Nx suddenly without checking first with your doctor. Your doctor may want you to reduce your dosage gradually.

If you miss a dose

Take the missed dose as soon as possible. However, if it's almost time for your next dose, skip the missed dose and take your next dose as scheduled. Don't take a double dose.

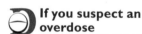 If you suspect an overdose

Contact your doctor *immediately*. Excessive Talwin-Nx can cause seizures; confusion; severe nervousness, restlessness, dizziness, weakness, or drowsiness; and slowed or difficult breathing.

TALWIN-NX'S OTHER NAME

Talwin-Nx is a combination of the generic drugs pentazocine and naloxone hydrochloride.

SIDE EFFECTS

Call your doctor if you have any of these possible drug side effects. Call *immediately* about any labeled "serious."

Serious: slowed and shallow breathing, severe allergic reaction (shortness of breath, swelling of face and throat, difficulty breathing)

Common: sedation, dizziness, light-headedness, euphoria, nausea, vomiting

Other: visual disturbances, hallucinations, drowsiness, confusion, headache, low blood pressure (dizziness, weakness), dry mouth, altered taste, constipation, difficulty urinating, physical and psychological dependence

Tips: To relieve dry mouth, try sugarless gum or hard candy, ice chips, or a saliva substitute. To relieve constipation, increase the fluids and fiber in your diet. Avoid activities that require full alertness or coordination until you know how Talwin-Nx affects you.

DRUG INTERACTIONS

Combining certain drugs may alter their action or produce unwanted side effects. Tell your doctor about other drugs you're taking, especially:
- alcohol and other drugs that make you feel relaxed or sleepy, such as sleeping pills, tranquilizers, and cold and allergy drugs
- Darvon and other narcotic pain relievers.

✕ Warnings

- Make sure your doctor knows your medical history. You may not be able to take Talwin-Nx if you are overly sensitive to it, are under age 12, have recently had a heart attack, or have lung disease, colitis, heart disease, liver or kidney problems, head injury, increased pressure in your head (headache, nausea, vomiting, tiredness, double or blurred vision), slowed and shallow breathing, or a history of seizures, emotional problems, or alcohol or drug abuse.
- If you're pregnant or breast-feeding, check with your doctor before using Talwin-Nx.

- Older adults may be especially prone to Talwin-Nx's side effects.
- If you think this drug isn't helping your pain, check with your doctor.

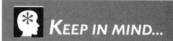 KEEP IN MIND...

* Don't increase dosage without doctor's permission.
* Don't stop taking abruptly.
* Avoid alcohol.
* Increase fluids and fiber in diet.
* Ease dry mouth with sugarless gum or hard candy, ice chips, or a saliva substitute.

Tambocor

Tambocor is one of several drugs called antiarrhythmics that slow electrical impulses in the heart.

Why it's prescribed

Doctors prescribe Tambocor to help stabilize various types of irregular heartbeats (arrhythmias). It comes in tablets. Doctors usually prescribe the following amounts for adults.

▶ **For paroxysmal supraventricular tachycardia or paroxysmal atrial fibrillation or flutter in people without structural heart disease,** 50 milligrams (mg) every 12 hours, increased in increments of 50 mg twice a day every 4 days. Maximum dosage is 300 mg a day. Initial dosage for anyone with kidney problems is 100 mg once a day or 50 mg twice a day.

▶ **For life-threatening ventricular arrhythmias, such as sustained ventricular tachycardia,** 100 mg every 12 hours, increased in increments of 50 mg twice a day every 4 days, if necessary. Maximum dosage is 400 mg a day for most people. Initial dosage for anyone with congestive heart failure is 50 mg every 12 hours.

How to take Tambocor

• Take two doses a day, 12 hours apart in the morning and evening, unless ordered otherwise.
• If you've been taking this drug regularly for several weeks, don't suddenly stop taking it. Your doctor will have you reduce the dosage gradually.

TAMBOCOR'S OTHER NAME

Tambocor's generic name is flecainide acetate.

 ## SIDE EFFECTS

Call your doctor if you have any of these possible drug side effects. Call *immediately* about any labeled "serious."

Serious: congestive heart failure (shortness of breath, anxiety, chest pain), irregular heartbeat, swelling in feet or lower legs, trembling or shaking, cardiac arrest

Common: dizziness, headache, blurred vision and other visual disturbances

Tips: Avoid activities that require full alertness or coordination until you know how Tambocor affects you. To reduce dizziness, stand up and change positions slowly.

Other: fatigue, tremor, nausea, constipation, abdominal pain, swelling of hands, rash

 ## DRUG INTERACTIONS

Combining certain drugs may alter their action or produce unwanted side effects. Tell your doctor about other drugs you're taking, especially:
• beta blocker drugs such as Inderal
• Cordarone
• digitalis glycosides such as Lanoxin
• Tagamet
• urine-acidifying and alkalinizing agents, such as sodium bicarbonate and vitamin C.

• You may not feel Tambocor's full effect for 3 to 5 days.

If you miss a dose

Take the missed dose as soon as possible if you remember within 6 hours of your regularly scheduled dose. If it's later than that, skip the missed dose and resume your normal dosage schedule. Don't take a double dose.

 ### If you suspect an overdose

Contact your doctor *immediately*. Excessive Tambocor can cause serious heartbeat abnormalities.

 ## Warnings

• Make sure your doctor knows your medical history. You may not be able to take Tambocor if you recently had a heart attack, have liver or kidney problems or a pacemaker, or are pregnant or breast-feeding.

KEEP IN MIND...

* Take doses morning and evening, 12 hours apart.
* Don't expect drug effect for 3 to 5 days.
* Don't stop taking suddenly.

Tapazole

Tapazole reduces the thyroid gland's ability to form thyroid hormones.

Why it's prescribed

Doctors prescribe Tapazole to treat an overactive thyroid gland. It comes in tablets. Doctors usually prescribe the following amounts for adults; children's dosages appear in parentheses.

▶ **For an overactive thyroid,** if mild, 15 milligrams (mg) a day; if moderately severe, 30 to 45 mg a day; if severe, 60 mg a day. Daily dosage is divided into three equal doses and taken at 8-hour intervals. Maintenance dosage is 15 mg a day. (Children: 0.4 mg for each 2.2 pounds [lb] of body weight a day, divided into equal doses and taken every 8 hours. Maintenance dosage is 0.2 mg for each 2.2 lb a day, divided into equal doses and taken every 8 hours.)

How to take Tapazole

• Carefully follow your doctor's directions.

• If the doctor has prescribed more than one dose a day, take the doses at evenly spaced intervals throughout the day and night.

• Take this drug at the same time every day in relation to meals — for example, either take all doses with meals or take all doses on an empty stomach.

• If this drug upsets your stomach, you may want to take it with meals.

TAPAZOLE'S OTHER NAME

Tapazole's generic name is methimazole.

 SIDE EFFECTS

Call your doctor if you have any of these possible drug side effects. Call *immediately* about any labeled "serious."

Serious: severe rash, enlarged lymph nodes in neck, nausea, vomiting (may be dose-related), jaundice and other liver problems (yellow-tinged skin and eyes), severe blood problems (bleeding, bruising, fatigue, heightened proneness to infection, chills and fever), underactive thyroid (depression, cold intolerance, swelling of legs or arms that becomes hard)

Common: none reported

Other: headache, drowsiness, vertigo, loss of taste, diarrhea, enlarged salivary glands, hives, skin discoloration, joint and muscle pain, drug-induced fever, swollen lymph nodes

 DRUG AND FOOD INTERACTIONS

Combining certain drugs and foods may alter drug action or produce unwanted side effects. Tell your doctor about your diet and other drugs you're taking, especially:

• Eskalith
• Pima
• shellfish, iodized salt, and nonprescription drugs containing iodine such as cough remedies.

• Tapazole may take several weeks to work. Don't stop taking it in the meantime.

If you miss a dose

Take the missed dose as soon as possible. However, if it's almost time for your next dose, take both doses together; then resume your regular dosage schedule. If you miss two or more doses, check with your doctor.

If you suspect an overdose

Contact your doctor *immediately*. Excessive Tapazole can cause vomiting, fever, joint pain, and blood problems (bleeding, bruising, extreme fatigue).

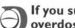 **Warnings**

• Make sure your doctor knows your medical history. You may not be able to take Tapazole if you are overly sensitive to it, have other medical problems such as an infection or liver disease, or are pregnant or breast-feeding.

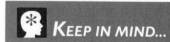 **KEEP IN MIND...**

∗ Take with food if the drug upsets your stomach.

∗ Avoid iodine in shellfish, salt, and nonprescription drugs.

Tavist

Tavist, an antihistamine, blocks the body's response to histamine, which causes runny nose and watery eyes.

Why it's prescribed

Doctors prescribe Tavist to relieve symptoms of hay fever or other allergies. You can also buy this drug without a prescription. It comes in tablets and syrup. Doctors usually prescribe the following amounts for adults.

▶ **For runny nose, congestion, and allergy symptoms,** 1 tablet (prescription) a day; dose may be increased. Maximum daily dose is 3 tablets. Or, 1 tablet of Tavist-1 (nonprescription) twice a day; dose may be increased. Maximum daily dose is 6 tablets.

How to take Tavist

• Take Tavist exactly as directed on your prescription label.

If you miss a dose

Take the missed dose as soon as possible. However, if it's almost time for your next dose, skip the missed dose and take your next dose as scheduled. Don't take a double dose.

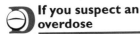

If you suspect an overdose

Contact your doctor *immediately*. Excessive Tavist can cause severe sleepiness, hallucinations, seizures, and cardiovascular collapse.

TAVIST'S OTHER NAME

Tavist's generic name is clemastine fumarate.

SIDE EFFECTS

Call your doctor if you have any of these possible drug side effects. Call *immediately* about any labeled "serious."

Serious: severe blood problems (bleeding, bruising, fatigue, fever, chills, infection), low blood pressure (dizziness, weakness), palpitations, rapid heartbeat

Common: sleepiness, drowsiness, dry mouth
Tips: Avoid activities that require full alertness or coordination until you know how Tavist affects you. To reduce drowsiness, try some coffee or tea. To relieve dry mouth, try using sugarless hard candy or gum, ice chips, or a saliva substitute. If it lasts for more than 2 weeks, check with your doctor or dentist.

Other: nausea, appetite loss, vomiting, constipation, difficulty urinating, thick phlegm, rash, hives
Tips: Take with food, water, or milk to avoid nausea. Increase fluids and fiber to avoid constipation.

DRUG INTERACTIONS

Combining certain drugs may alter their action or produce unwanted side effects. Tell your doctor about other drugs you're taking, especially:
• alcohol and other drugs that make you feel relaxed or sleepy, such as sleeping pills, tranquilizers, and cold and allergy drugs
• antidepressants called MAO inhibitors such as Marplan
• aspirin (high doses).

Warnings

• Make sure your doctor knows your medical history. You may not be able to take Tavist if you're overly sensitive to it or similar antihistamines or if you have asthma, glaucoma, an enlarged prostate, bladder problems, difficulty urinating, heart disease, high blood pressure, an overactive thyroid, diabetes, or stomach ulcers.
• If you're pregnant or breast-feeding, don't use Tavist unless your doctor tells you otherwise.
• Older adults are especially prone to Tavist's side effects.

• If you're scheduled to have allergy tests, stop taking Tavist 4 days beforehand to ensure the tests' accuracy.

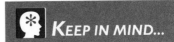

KEEP IN MIND...

* Take with food, water, or milk.

* Report fever, dizziness, or bleeding to doctor.

* Ease dry mouth with sugarless gum or hard candy, ice chips, or a saliva substitute.

* Stop taking Tavist 4 days before allergy tests.

Tegison

Tegison is thought to block an enzyme that regulates cell growth. It may also block white blood cell migration under the skin.

Why it's prescribed

Doctors prescribe Tegison when other treatments for the skin disorder psoriasis have failed. This drug comes in capsules. Doctors usually prescribe the following amounts for adults.

▶ **For severe psoriasis unresponsive to standard therapy,** initially, 0.75 to 1 milligram (mg) for each 2.2 pounds (lb) of body weight, divided into equal doses and taken throughout the day. Maximum initial dosage is 1.5 mg for each 2.2 lb a day. Maintenance dosage is 0.5 to 0.75 mg for each 2.2 lb a day.

How to take Tegison

• Take the exact amount that your doctor prescribed.
• Take Tegison with milk or fatty foods to enhance your body's absorption of the drug.

If you miss a dose

Take the missed dose as soon as possible. However, if it's almost time for your next dose, skip the missed dose and take your next dose as scheduled. Don't take a double dose.

If you suspect an overdose

Consult your doctor.

TEGISON'S OTHER NAME

Tegison's generic name is etretinate.

SIDE EFFECTS

Call your doctor if you have any of these possible drug side effects. Call *immediately* about any labeled "serious."

Serious: blood problems (bleeding, bruising, heightened susceptibility to infection, fatigue), blood clots (shortness of breath, pain in legs or chest), hepatitis (yellow-tinged skin and eyes, nausea, vomiting, itching)

Common: benign intracranial hypertension (headache, nausea, vomiting, vision changes), eye pain, dry eyes, appetite change, sore tongue, chapped lips, dry mouth, dry or peeling skin, itching, bone pain, contact lens intolerance

Tip: To relieve dry mouth, use ice chips or sugarless hard candy or gum; check with your dentist if it continues for more than 2 weeks.

Other: fatigue, dizziness, lethargy, swelling, sensitivity to sun, decreased night vision

DRUG INTERACTIONS

Combining certain drugs may alter their action or produce unwanted side effects. Tell your doctor about other drugs you're taking, especially:
• alcohol
• Rheumatrex and other drugs toxic to the liver
• tetracyclines
• vitamin A preparations.

Warnings

• Make sure your doctor knows your medical history. You may not be able to take Tegison if you have other medical problems, especially diabetes, obesity, a history of high cholesterol, heart disease, or a family history of alcohol abuse.
• Don't take Tegison if you are pregnant, ever intend to become pregnant, or are unwilling to use reliable contraception before, during, and after treatment. This drug causes severe birth defects. Significant amounts of Tegison have been found in the blood nearly 3 years after the end of treatment. Consequently, no one knows how long after treatment that pregnancy becomes safe.
• If you're diabetic, monitor your blood sugar levels closely. Your doctor may need to adjust your diabetes drug dosage.
• Your psoriasis may get a little worse after you start therapy; it will get better eventually.

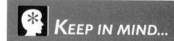

* Take with milk or fatty foods.
* Prevent pregnancy during and after treatment.
* Avoid alcoholic beverages and vitamin A supplements.

Tegopen

Tegopen is an antibiotic, a type of penicillin that stops bacteria from multiplying, especially bacteria that resist other penicillins.

Why it's prescribed

Doctors prescribe Tegopen to treat bacterial infections known as staph infections. It comes in liquid. Doctors usually prescribe the following amounts for adults; children's dosages appear in parentheses.

▶ **For staph infections,** 250 to 500 milligrams (mg) every 6 hours. (Children weighing more than 44 pounds [lb]: same dosage as adults. Children weighing 44 lbs or less: 50 to 100 mg for each 2.2 lb of body weight each day, divided into equal doses given every 6 hours.)

How to take Tegopen

• Take Tegopen only as your doctor directs.
• If you're taking the liquid, use a dropper or specially marked measuring spoon — not a household teaspoon — to measure each dose accurately.
• Take your dose with a full glass (8 ounces) of water on an empty stomach, either 1 hour before or 2 hours after meals. Don't take with fruit juice or carbonated drinks, which could stop Tegopen from working.

 SIDE EFFECTS

Call your doctor if you have any of these possible drug side effects. Call *immediately* about any labeled "serious."

Serious: allergic reaction (difficulty breathing, rash, hives, itching, or wheezing), liver problems (yellow-tinged skin and eyes), blood problems (bleeding, bruising, fever, chills, increased infection, fatigue)

Common: nausea, heartburn, diarrhea

Other: vomiting, other infections

 DRUG INTERACTIONS

Combining certain drugs may alter their action or produce unwanted side effects. Tell your doctor about other drugs you're taking, especially:
• other antibiotics (take at least 1 hour after taking Tegopen, or as your doctor directs)
• Probalan.

• Take Tegopen for the entire time prescribed, even after you start to feel better, to prevent your infection from coming back.
• Discard any leftover drug.

If you miss a dose

Take the missed dose as soon as possible. But if it's almost time for your next dose, adjust your dosage schedule as follows:
• If you take two doses a day, space the missed dose and the next dose 5 to 6 hours apart. Then resume your regular schedule.
• If you take three or more doses a day, space the missed dose and the next dose 2 to 4 hours apart. Then resume your regular schedule.

 If you suspect an overdose

Contact your doctor *immediately.* Excessive Tegopen can cause seizures.

 Warnings

• Make sure your doctor knows your medical history. You may not be able to take Tegopen if you're allergic to penicillin or other antibiotics or if you have kidney disease, mononucleosis, or stomach and bowel problems.
• If you're pregnant or breast-feeding, check with your doctor before taking Tegopen.

TEGOPEN'S OTHER NAMES

Tegopen's generic name is cloxacillin sodium. Other brand names include Cloxapen and, in Canada, Apo-Cloxi, Novocloxin, Nu-Cloxi, and Orbenin.

KEEP IN MIND...

* Don't break, chew, or crush capsules.
* Take with water, on empty stomach, 1 hour before or 2 hours after meals.
* Don't take with acidic fruit juices or carbonated drinks.

Tegretol

Tegretol limits seizure activity probably by altering the movement of sodium and stopping impulses at the place where a seizure begins.

Why it's prescribed

Doctors prescribe Tegretol to control some types of seizures. It's also used to treat pain from trigeminal neuralgia. It comes in tablets, slow-release tablets, chewable tablets, and a liquid suspension. Doctors usually prescribe the following amounts for adults; children's dosages appear in parentheses.

▶ **For generalized tonic-clonic and complex partial seizures (mixed seizure patterns),** initially, 200 milligrams (mg) in tablets twice a day or 1 teaspoon (tsp) of liquid suspension four times a day. May be increased at weekly intervals by 200 mg a day, divided into equal doses and taken at 6- to 8-hour intervals. Dosage adjusted to minimum effective level when seizures are controlled. Maximum dosage is 1.2 grams (g) a day. (Children over age 15: same as adults; children ages 12 to 15: same as adults except for maximum dosage, which is 1 g. Children under age 12: initially, 100 mg twice a day or ½ tsp of liquid suspension four times a day, increased at weekly intervals by 100 mg a day. Maximum dosage is 1 g a day.)

▶ **For pain of trigeminal neuralgia in adults,** initially, 100 mg twice a

TEGRETOL'S OTHER NAMES

Tegretol's generic name is carbamazepine. Other brand names includeApo-Carbamazepine, Epitol, and Novocarbamaz.

 ## SIDE EFFECTS

Call your doctor if you have any of these possible drug side effects. Call *immediately* about any labeled "serious."

Serious: infection (fever, sore throat, chills, cough), blood problems (bleeding, bruising, fatigue, increased risk of infection), worsening of seizures (usually in people who have mixed seizure types), congestive heart failure (shortness of breath, anxiety, chest pain), hepatitis (yellow-tinged skin and eyes), Stevens-Johnson syndrome (reddened, burnlike rash), altered blood pressure (dizziness and weakness or headache and blurred vision), aggravation of coronary artery disease (chest pain), water intoxication (change in mental status), mouth sores, rash

Common: dizziness, drowsiness, clumsiness
Tip: Avoid activities that require full alertness or coordination until you know how Tegretol affects you.

Other: fatigue, pinkeye, dry mouth and throat, blurred or double vision, uncontrolled eye movements, abdominal pain, diarrhea, appetite loss, inflamed mouth or tongue, increased urination, difficulty urinating, impotence, kidney problems (sugar or protein in urine), liver problems (yellow-tinged skin and eyes)

 ## DRUG INTERACTIONS

Combining certain drugs may alter their action or produce unwanted side effects. Tell your doctor about other drugs you're taking, especially:
- alcohol and other drugs that make you feel relaxed or sleepy, such as tranquilizers, sleeping pills, and cold and allergy drugs
- antidepressants called MAO inhibitors such as Marplan
- birth control pills
- Calan
- Cardizem
- Coumadin
- Danocrine
- Darvon
- erythromycin and similar antibiotics such as Vibramycin
- Eskalith, Haldol
- Laniazid
- seizure drugs, such as Depakene, Dilantin, Mysoline, and Solfoton
- Tagamet
- Theo-Dur.

day or ½ tsp of liquid suspension four times a day with meals; may be increased by 100 mg every 12 hours for tablets or ½ tsp of liquid suspension four times a day until pain subsides. Maximum dosage is 1.2 g a day. Maintenance dosage is 200 to 400 mg twice a day.

How to take Tegretol

• Take Tegretol with meals, exactly as prescribed.

• If you're taking the liquid suspension, shake the bottle well before measuring the dose.

• Store tablets in the original container. Keep the container tightly closed and away from moisture.

• If you're taking Tegretol for seizures, don't stop using it without consulting your doctor, who may reduce the dosage gradually.

If you miss a dose

Take the missed dose as soon as possible. However, if it's almost time for your next dose, skip the missed dose and take your next dose as scheduled. Don't take a double dose. If you miss more than one dose a day, check with your doctor.

If you suspect an overdose

Contact your doctor *immediately*. Excessive Tegretol can cause a change in appetite, irregular breathing, rapid heartbeat, seizures, and coma.

Warnings

• Make sure your doctor knows your medical history. You may not be able to take Tegretol if you're overly sensitive to it or to certain antidepressants, if you've taken an MAO inhibitor (a type of antidepressant) during the past 14 days, or if you have a history of bone marrow suppression.

• If you're pregnant or breast-feeding, consult your doctor before taking Tegretol.

• If you're diabetic, monitor your blood sugar levels carefully. Tegretol may alter them.

• Have regular checkups so the doctor can monitor your progress and make dosage changes. Also have regular eye exams during treatment.

• As a pain reliever, Tegretol works only for certain kinds of pain. Don't take it for other types of discomfort.

• If you're taking Tegretol for trigeminal neuralgia, your doctor will probably try to decrease your dosage or withdraw the drug every 3 months.

• Before medical tests, surgery, dental work, or emergency treatment, tell your doctor or dentist that you're taking Tegretol.

• Carry or wear medical identification that says you're taking Tegretol.

• Appetite changes or loss may indicate too much Tegretol in your blood.

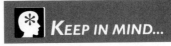

KEEP IN MIND...

* Take with meals.

* Store in tightly closed container away from moisture.

* Don't stop taking abruptly.

* Have regular eye and medical exams.

Temaril

Temaril blocks the action of the chemical histamine, which causes allergy symptoms, such as itching.

Why it's prescribed

Doctors prescribe Temaril to reduce itching. It comes in tablets, slow-release capsules, and a syrup. Doctors usually prescribe the following amounts for adults; children's dosages are in parentheses.

▶ **For itching,** 2.5 milligrams (mg) four times a day, or 5 mg slow-release capsules twice a day. (Children age 3 and over: 2.5 mg one to three times a day, as needed. Children ages 6 months to 2 years: 1.25 mg one to three times a day, as needed.)

How to take Temaril

• If you're taking one dose a day, take it at bedtime.

If you miss a dose

Take the missed dose as soon as possible. However, if it's almost time for your next dose, skip the missed dose and take your next dose as scheduled. Don't take a double dose.

If you suspect an overdose

Contact your doctor *immediately*. Excessive Temaril can cause low blood pressure (dizziness, weakness), large pupils that are unresponsive to light, flushing of the skin, dry mouth, nausea, vomiting, sleepiness, hallucinations, seizures, unconsciousness, and coma.

TEMARIL'S OTHER NAMES

Temaril's generic name is trimeprazine tartrate. Another brand name is Panectyl.

SIDE EFFECTS

Call your doctor if you have any of these possible drug side effects. Call *immediately* about any labeled "serious."

Serious: severe blood problems (bleeding, bruising, chills, fever, fatigue, increased risk of infection), low blood pressure (dizziness, weakness), palpitations, rapid heartbeat, severe sensitivity to the sun

Common: dry mouth and throat, increased sensitivity to sun
Tips: To relieve dry mouth, try sugarless gum or hard candy or ice chips. For protection from the sun, wear a sunscreen, a hat, and protective clothing when you go outdoors.

Other: drowsiness, dizziness, confusion, headache, restlessness, tremors, irritability, insomnia, excitability in children, appetite loss, nausea, vomiting, increased urination, difficulty urinating, hives, rash
Tip: Avoid activities that require full alertness or coordination until you know how Temaril affects you. To avoid nausea, take doses with food.

◼ DRUG INTERACTIONS

Combining certain drugs may alter their action or produce unwanted side effects. Tell your doctor about other drugs you're taking, especially:
• alcohol and other drugs that make you feel relaxed or sleepy, such as tranquilizers, sleeping pills, and cold and allergy drugs
• antidepressants, such as Elavil and Parnate
• Arlidin
• Eskalith
• Larodopa
• narcotics, such as codeine and Demerol
• oral contraceptives
• progesterone such as Femotrone
• Serpalan.

✕ Warnings

• Make sure your doctor knows your medical history. You may not be able to take Temaril if you have a drug allergy, asthma, a depressed central nervous system, bone marrow depression, angle-closure glaucoma, an enlarged prostate, a stomach ulcer, or a bowel blockage.
• If you're on long-term therapy, your doctor may want to test your blood from time to time.

• Consult your doctor before having any allergy tests or other diagnostic tests.

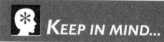 KEEP IN MIND...

∗ Take doses with food.
∗ Consult doctor before diagnostic tests.
∗ Expect periodic blood tests.

Temovate

Temovate is a powerful corticosteroid. It constricts blood vessels to reduce itching and inflammation and is used when other drugs are not effective.

Why it's prescribed

Doctors prescribe Temovate to treat areas of inflamed skin. It comes in a cream, a lotion, and an ointment. Doctors usually prescribe the following amounts for adults.

▶ **For inflamed skin,** apply a thin layer to affected area twice a day, morning and evening, for no more than 14 days.

How to use Temovate

• Wash the affected area gently before applying Temovate. To prevent skin damage, rub the drug in gently, leaving a thin coat. When treating hairy sites, part the hair and apply Temovate directly to the skin.
• Don't use Temovate near your eyes, and don't get it on mucous membranes or in your ear canals.
• Don't cover or bandage the treated area unless your doctor tells you to.
• If you're using Temovate on a child's diaper area, don't cover the area with plastic pants or a tight-fitting diaper.
• Don't refrigerate this drug.

If you miss a dose

Apply the missed dose as soon as possible. However, if it's almost

TEMOVATE'S OTHER NAMES

Temovate's generic name is clobetasol propionate. Another brand name is Dermovate.

 SIDE EFFECTS

Call your doctor if you have any of these possible drug side effects. Call *immediately* about any labeled "serious."

Serious: hypothalamic-pituitary-adrenal axis suppression, a depression of the body's own steroids; the body is unable to handle stress, such as infection or surgery (weak pulse, fainting, vomiting, diarrhea), allergic contact dermatitis (burning, itching, irritation)

Common: none reported

Other: dry or red skin, inflamed hair follicles, dermatitis around mouth, loss of pigmentation, excessive facial hair growth, acnelike reaction, Cushing's syndrome (raised blood pressure, headache, blurred vision, obesity, increased thirst, hunger, and urination), increased blood sugar (sugar in urine, increased thirst, hunger, and urination)

 DRUG INTERACTIONS

Combining certain drugs may alter their action or produce unwanted side effects. Tell your doctor about other drugs you're taking.

time for your next dose, skip the missed dose and apply your next dose as scheduled. Don't apply a double dose.

If you suspect an overdose

Consult your doctor.

Warnings

• Make sure your doctor knows your medical history. You may not be able to use Temovate if you're overly sensitive to it or to related drugs or if you have other medical problems, especially glaucoma, cataracts, diabetes, tuberculosis, or an infection or sores in the area needing treatment.
• Keep in mind that the longer you use Temovate, the less effective it will become.

• If you have an infection that needs to be treated with an antibiotic or an antifungal drug, your doctor will probably ask you to stop using Temovate until your other infection is under control.
• Don't use leftover Temovate for other skin problems without your doctor's permission.

KEEP IN MIND...

* Keep drug away from eyes, ears, and mucous membranes.
* Don't cover or bandage treated area.
* Don't refrigerate Temovate.
* Don't use for more than 14 days.

Tenex

Tenex is a blood pressure drug (antihypertensive) that probably works by dilating blood vessels and decreasing the amount of blood the heart has to pump.

Why it's prescribed

Doctors prescribe Tenex to control high blood pressure. It comes in tablets. Doctors usually prescribe the following amounts for adults.
▶ **For high blood pressure,** initially, 1 milligram (mg) a day, increased to 2 mg after 3 to 4 weeks, as needed. Dosage further increased to 3 mg after an additional 3 to 4 weeks, as needed. Average dosage is 1 to 3 mg a day.

How to take Tenex

• Your doctor may prescribe Tenex alone or with a diuretic. Take it exactly as prescribed — no more, no less.
• Take Tenex at bedtime to avoid daytime drowsiness.
• Don't stop taking Tenex abruptly because your blood pressure could rise dangerously high.

If you miss a dose

Take the missed dose as soon as possible. However, if it's almost time for your next dose, skip the missed dose and take your next dose as scheduled. Don't take a double dose. If you miss taking Tenex for more than 2 days in a row, call your doctor.

 If you suspect an overdose

Contact your doctor *immediately*. Excessive Tenex can cause extreme

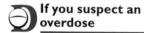 **TENEX'S OTHER NAME**

Tenex's generic name is guanfacine hydrochloride.

 SIDE EFFECTS

Call your doctor if you have any of these possible drug side effects. Call *immediately* about any labeled "serious."

Serious: slow heartbeat, low blood pressure (dizziness, weakness), high blood pressure if therapy is stopped abruptly (headache, blurred vision)

Common: drowsiness, slight dizziness, constipation
Tips: The higher your dosage of Tenex, the more likely you are to experience side effects. Avoid activities that require full alertness or coordination until you know how Tenex affects you.

Other: fatigue, confusion, depression, headache, insomnia, diarrhea, nausea, abdominal pain, itching, shortness of breath, leg cramps, decreased sex drive, dry mouth, dry or burning eyes, altered taste, incontinence, testicular changes
Tip: To relieve dry mouth, use sugarless gum or hard candy or ice chips.

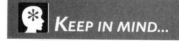 **DRUG INTERACTIONS**

Combining certain drugs may alter their action or produce unwanted side effects. Tell your doctor about other drugs you're taking, especially:
• alcoholic beverages and other drugs that make you relaxed or sleepy, such as sleeping pills and cold and allergy drugs
• barbiturates such as Solfoton
• Dilantin
• narcotic pain relievers.

---

dizziness, difficulty breathing, weakness, and a slow heartbeat.

Warnings

• Make sure your doctor knows your medical history. You may not be able to take Tenex if you've recently had a heart attack or a stroke or if you have severe heart disease or chronic kidney or liver disease.
• Follow any prescribed diet. You may need to lose weight or reduce salt in your diet.
• Store Tenex away from heat, light, and children's reach.
• Have your blood pressure checked often to track the drug's effect.

• You may have to take a blood pressure drug for the rest of your life.
• Before any surgical, dental, or emergency procedure, tell the doctor or dentist that you're taking Tenex.

KEEP IN MIND...

∗ Take at bedtime.
∗ Follow prescribed diet.
∗ Check blood pressure often.
∗ Ease dry mouth with sugarless gum or hard candy or ice chips.
∗ Don't stop taking abruptly.

Tenormin

Tenormin is one of several heart drugs called beta blockers. It reduces the amount of blood your heart pumps, decreases the force it needs to pump, and reduces the amount of oxygen the heart muscle needs.

Why it's prescribed

Doctors prescribe Tenormin to treat high blood pressure, to relieve chest pain caused by angina, and to prevent another heart attack in recent heart attack victims. Tenormin comes in tablets. Doctors usually prescribe the following amounts for adults.

▶ **For high blood pressure,** initially, 50 milligrams (mg) once a day, increased to 100 mg once a day after 7 to 14 days, as needed. Dosages above 100 mg unlikely to produce further benefit.

▶ **For angina pectoris,** 50 mg once a day, increased as needed to 100 mg a day after 7 days for optimal effect. Maximum dosage is 200 mg a day.

How to take Tenormin

• Your doctor may tell you to check your pulse rate before and after taking Tenormin. If it's much slower than usual, call the doctor before taking the next dose.
• Swallow tablets whole; don't crush, break, or chew them.
• Take Tenormin at the same time every day.

TENORMIN'S OTHER NAMES

Tenormin's generic name is atenolol. A Canadian brand name is Apo-Atenolol.

 SIDE EFFECTS

Call your doctor if you have any of these possible drug side effects. Call *immediately* about any labeled "serious."

Serious: congestive heart failure (shortness of breath, anxiety), asthmalike attacks (wheezing, tightness in chest), slow pulse, low blood pressure (dizziness, weakness), slow pulse
Tip: To minimize dizziness from low blood pressure, sit up and dangle your legs before getting out of bed in the morning.

Common: none reported

Other: fatigue, lethargy, intermittent leg cramps, nausea, vomiting, diarrhea, rash, fever
Tips: If these symptoms persist or become severe, contact your doctor. Avoid activities that require full alertness or coordination until you know how Tenormin affects you.

 DRUG INTERACTIONS

Combining certain drugs may alter their action or produce unwanted side effects. Tell your doctor about other drugs you're taking, especially:
• allergy and cold drugs
• allergy shots or skin tests (tell your doctor that you're taking Tenormin)
• antidepressants called MAO inhibitors such as Marplan
• caffeine-containing drugs
• calcium channel blockers, such as Calan and Cardizem
• Catapres
• Choledyl
• digitalis glycosides such as Lanoxin
• Eskalith
• Indocin
• insulin and oral diabetes drugs
• Lufyllin
• Somophyllin and Somophyllin-T
• Wytensin.

• Try not to miss any doses. Some conditions become worse when this medication isn't taken regularly.
• Don't suddenly stop taking this drug because your condition may worsen. Your doctor may gradually reduce the amount you're taking.

If you miss a dose

Take the missed dose as soon as possible. However, if it's within 8 hours of your next dose, skip the missed dose and take your next

Continued on next page ▶

dose as scheduled. Don't take a double dose.

If you suspect an overdose

Contact your doctor *immediately*. Excessive Tenormin can cause very low blood pressure (extreme dizziness and weakness, fainting), very slow heartbeat, and heart failure.

Warnings

• Make sure your doctor knows your medical history. You may not be able to take Tenormin if you're overly sensitive to it or if you have serious heart or blood vessel problems, an unusually slow heartbeat, breathing problems or bronchitis, emphysema, gout, lupus, an inflamed pancreas, diabetes, kidney or liver disease, depression, allergies, myasthenia gravis, psoriasis, or an overactive thyroid.

• Contact your doctor right away if you become pregnant while taking Tenormin.

• Be aware that older adults are especially prone to this drug's side effects.

• If you're diabetic, check your blood sugar levels carefully. Tenormin can mask the symptoms of low blood sugar levels.

• If you have allergies to certain drugs, foods, preservatives, or dyes, this drug may worsen allergic reactions and make them harder to treat.

• Your dosage may need adjustment if you have kidney problems.

• If you're taking Tenormin for high blood pressure, your doctor may recommend some diet restrictions, such as reduced sodium (salt) and fats. Follow these recommendations carefully.

• You may have to take a blood pressure drug for the rest of your life.

• Monitor your blood pressure carefully to be sure the drug is working properly.

• Contact your doctor *immediately* if you have trouble breathing, swollen ankles, or a sudden weight gain of 3 pounds or more (signs that you're retaining water) or if your blood pressure rises.

• Tenormin may mask chest pain brought on by exercise and activity; discuss with your doctor an appropriate level of physical activity.

• Don't take any other prescription or nonprescription drugs (especially cold and allergy drugs) without your doctor's knowledge.

• Before you have any surgical or dental procedure, emergency treatment, or medical tests, tell the doctor or dentist that you're taking Tenormin.

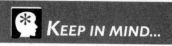
KEEP IN MIND...

* Swallow tablets whole; don't break, crush, or chew them.

* Take at same time each day.

* Check blood pressure and pulse regularly.

* Follow prescribed diet and exercise restrictions.

* If you're diabetic, check sugar levels carefully.

Tensilon

Tensilon improves muscle strength in people who have a disease called myasthenia gravis. This disease causes progressive muscle weakness.

Why it's prescribed

Doctors prescribe Tensilon as a test to diagnose myasthenia gravis. If the disease is present, muscle strength will improve after injection of Tensilon. This drug comes in an injectable form only. Doctors usually prescribe the following amounts for adults; children's dosages appear in parentheses.

▶ **To diagnose myasthenia gravis,** 1 to 2 milligrams (mg) injected into a vein (intravenous, or I.V.), then 8 mg if muscle strength doesn't increase. (Children weighing more than 75 pounds [lb]: 2 mg I.V.; if no response, 1 mg I.V. every 45 seconds up to 10 mg. Children weighing less than 75 lb: 1 mg I.V.; if no response, 1 mg every 45 seconds up to 5 mg. Infants: 0.5 mg I.V.)

How to take Tensilon

• A doctor or nurse will give you Tensilon.

If you miss a dose

Not applicable because Tensilon is given only during testing.

If you suspect an overdose

Tell your doctor *immediately* if you think you've received too much of

TENSILON'S OTHER NAMES

Tensilon's generic name is edrophonium chloride. Another brand name is Enlon.

SIDE EFFECTS

Tell your doctor if you have any of these possible drug side effects. Call *immediately* about any labeled "serious."

Serious: difficulty breathing, wheezing, tightness in chest, unusual weakness, low blood pressure (dizziness, weakness, fainting), palpitations, slow heartbeat

Common: nausea, vomiting, diarrhea

Other: muscle cramps

DRUG INTERACTIONS

Combining certain drugs may alter their action or produce unwanted effects. Tell your doctor about other drugs you're taking, especially:

• corticosteroids, such as Decadron and Kenalog
• Lanoxin
• Procan SR
• Quinaglute Dura-tabs.

the drug. Excessive Tensilon can cause muscle weakness, nausea, vomiting, blurred vision, wheezing, low blood pressure (dizziness, weakness, fainting), sweating, cramps, fast or slow heartbeat, incoordination, and weakness.

Warnings

• Make sure your doctor knows your medical history. You may not be able to take Tensilon if you have an allergy to Tensilon or other medical problems, especially low blood pressure, intestinal or urinary tract blockage, an overactive thyroid, heart disease (including slow heartbeat), or asthma.
• Tell your doctor if you're pregnant or breast-feeding before you receive Tensilon.
• Before you receive Tensilon, tell your doctor if you've ever had a reaction to the drug atropine. This

drug may be given during the testing for myasthenia gravis to counteract the side effects of Tensilon.
• Be aware that older adults may be especially prone to Tensilon's side effects.

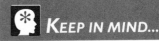
KEEP IN MIND...

* This drug is for diagnosis only.

* Before test, inform doctor of any drug allergies, especially to atropine.

* Don't breast-feed while receiving Tensilon.

* Most side effects are temporary.

Tenuate

Tenuate appears to decrease the senses of smell and taste, which decreases appetite.

Why it's prescribed

Doctors prescribe Tenuate as a short-term measure to treat obesity. It comes in tablets, slow-release tablets, and slow-release capsules. Doctors usually prescribe the following amounts for adults.

▶ **For short-term treatment of obesity,** 25 milligrams (mg) three times a day or 75 mg slow-release tablet or capsule once a day.

How to take Tenuate

• Follow your doctor's directions exactly.
• Don't break, crush, or chew slow-release tablets — swallow them whole.
• If you're taking the regular tablets three times a day, take them before meals. If you're taking the slow-release tablets or capsules, take them in midmorning.
• Take the last dose of the day about 4 to 6 hours before bedtime to help prevent insomnia.
• Don't stop taking this drug suddenly without first checking with your doctor. Your doctor may want to decrease your dose gradually to prevent withdrawal symptoms.

If you miss a dose

Consult your doctor.

TENUATE'S OTHER NAMES

Tenuate's generic name is diethylpropion hydrochloride. Other brand names include Tenuate Dospan and Tepanil Ten-Tab.

 SIDE EFFECTS

Call your doctor if you have any of these possible drug side effects. Call *immediately* about any labeled "serious."

Serious: abnormally high pressure in the pulmonary circulation (shortness of breath, rapid heartbeat, chest pain, fainting), increased blood pressure (headache, blurred vision)

Common: nervousness, palpitations

Other: headache, dizziness, blurred vision, dry mouth, nausea, abdominal cramps, diarrhea, constipation, impotence, decreased blood sugar level (weakness, tremor, fast pulse, clammy skin), hives, altered sex drive, menstrual changes, restlessness, tremor, anxiety, insomnia, unpleasant taste, muscle pain, hair loss, and increased and painful urination.

Tips: Avoid activities that require full alertness or coordination until you know how Tenuate affects you. Call your doctor if symptoms persist or become severe. To relieve dry mouth, use sugarless gum or hard candy or ice chips.

 DRUG INTERACTIONS

Combining certain drugs may alter their action or produce unwanted side effects. Tell your doctor about other drugs you're taking, especially:
• amphetamines
• antidepressants called MAO inhibitors such as Marplan
• asthma drugs
• caffeine, diet pills
• Cesamet
• Cylert
• insulin and oral diabetes drugs
• Ismelin
• Ritalin
• Symmetrel
• Ulone.

 If you suspect an overdose

Contact your doctor *immediately*. Excessive Tenuate can cause confusion, hallucinations, seizures, and coma.

Warnings

• Make sure your doctor knows your medical history. You may not be able to take Tenuate if you're overly sensitive to it or to sympathomimetic amines, if you've taken an MAO inhibitor (a type of antidepressant) within 14 days, or if you have an overactive thyroid, moderate to severe high blood pressure, heart disease, diabetes, glaucoma, seizures, or a history of agitation or drug abuse.

• If you're pregnant or breast-feeding, don't take this drug without your doctor's approval.

• If you have diabetes, check your sugar levels carefully. If you notice a change in the results of your urine or blood sugar tests, call your doctor.

• If you're taking insulin for your diabetes, consult your doctor before taking Tenuate. You may need to adjust your insulin dosage.

• If your doctor recommends a weight-loss diet, follow it carefully.

• See your doctor regularly to rule out unwanted effects from Tenuate.

• If you've taken Tenuate for a long time and think you may be dependent on it, check with your doctor. Signs of dependence include a strong desire or need to continue taking Tenuate, a need to increase the dose, or withdrawal side effects when you stop taking it.

• Before having any kind of surgery, dental treatment, or emergency treatment, tell the doctor or dentist that you're taking Tenuate.

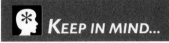

KEEP IN MIND...

* Don't crush or chew slow-release form.

* If you're diabetic, check sugar levels carefully.

* Follow prescribed weight-loss diet.

* Avoid caffeine.

* Don't stop taking drug suddenly.

Teramine

Teramine is an appetite suppressant that is chemically related to amphetamines; however, it has fewer side effects and less addictive potential than the amphetamines.

Why it's prescribed

Doctors prescribe Teramine as a short-term aid in weight reduction for obese people. It comes in tablets, capsules, and slow-release capsules. Doctors usually prescribe the following amounts for adults.

▶ **For weight reduction,** 1 capsule a day.

How to take Teramine

- Take Teramine exactly as your doctor prescribes. Don't increase the amount you take or take it more frequently.
- Take Teramine at least 6 hours before bedtime to avoid interfering with your sleep. For best results, take it 2 hours after breakfast.
- Intermittent therapy (6 weeks on, 4 weeks off) works as well as continuous therapy.

If you miss a dose

Take the missed dose as soon as possible. However, if it's almost time for your next dose, skip the missed dose and take your next dose as scheduled. Don't take a double dose.

TERAMINE'S OTHER NAMES

Teramine's generic name is phentermine hydrochloride. Other brand names include Adipex-P, Fastin, Obe-Nix, Obephen, Phentrol, and Zantryl.

SIDE EFFECTS

Call your doctor if you have any of these possible drug side effects.

Serious: none reported

Common: insomnia, heart palpitations, rapid heartbeat

Other: overstimulation, euphoria, depression or anguish, dizziness, increased blood pressure (headache, blurred vision), dry mouth, altered taste, stomach upset, hives, impotence, altered sex drive

DRUG AND FOOD INTERACTIONS

Combining certain drugs and foods may alter drug action or produce unwanted side effects. Tell your doctor about your diet and other drugs you're taking, especially:

- ammonium chloride (diuretic or expectorant)
- antacids, baking soda
- antipsychotic drugs such as Haldol
- caffeine-containing beverages
- Diamox
- insulin and oral diabetes drugs
- MAO inhibitors and tricyclic antidepressants
- vitamin C.

If you suspect an overdose

Contact your doctor *immediately*. Excessive Teramine can cause restlessness, confusion, aggression, fatigue, depression, seizures, coma, and death.

Warnings

- Make sure your doctor knows your medical history. You may not be able to take Teramine if you have an overactive thyroid, moderate to severe high blood pressure, advanced artery disease, heart disease, or glaucoma; if you're extremely allergic to stimulant drugs; or if you're agitated or have taken certain antidepressants recently.
- Your doctor will probably prescribe Teramine in conjunction with a weight-reduction program.

- If you're diabetic, monitor your blood sugar level closely.
- After the first few weeks, you may develop a tolerance to Teramine and it won't work as well. Your doctor will probably stop your therapy for a while rather than increase the dosage.
- When you stop taking Teramine, you'll feel some fatigue and you may need more rest as the drug wears off.

KEEP IN MIND...

* Don't take more than prescribed.
* Avoid caffeine-containing beverages.
* Follow a weight-loss plan.

Terazol

Terazol appears to break down the cell walls of fungus, which kills them.

Why it's prescribed

Doctors prescribe Terazol to treat vaginal fungal infections. It comes in a cream and in vaginal suppositories. Doctors usually prescribe the following amounts for adults.

▶ **For vulvovaginal candidiasis,** one applicatorful of cream or one suppository inserted into vagina; 0.4% cream continued for 7 consecutive days; 0.8% cream or 80-mg vaginal suppositories continued for 3 consecutive days.

How to use Terazol

• Both forms of Terazol come with an applicator. Use the applicator to insert the drug into your vagina.
• Insert the drug at bedtime. If you're inserting a vaginal suppository, remain lying down for at least 30 minutes after each dose to allow the drug to be completely absorbed.
• Wear a menstrual pad to protect your clothes from leakage.
• Use the drug for the full number of nights prescribed by your doctor, even if your symptoms subside. If you stop too soon, your symptoms may return.

If you miss a dose

Apply the missed dose as soon as possible. However, if it's almost time for your next dose, skip the missed dose and apply your next

TERAZOL'S OTHER NAME

Terazol's generic name is terconazole.

 SIDE EFFECTS

Call your doctor if you have any of these possible drug side effects.

Serious: none reported

Common: itching

Other: headache, vaginal burning or irritation, fever, chills, body aches. *Tips:* Take Tylenol or another mild pain reliever for headache. For other symptoms, stop using the drug and call your doctor as soon as possible.

 DRUG INTERACTIONS

Combining certain drugs may alter their action or produce unwanted side effects. Tell your doctor about other drugs you're taking.

dose as scheduled. Don't apply a double dose.

 If you suspect an overdose

Consult your doctor.

Warnings

• Make sure your doctor knows your medical history. You may not be able to use Terazol if you are overly sensitive to it or to its ingredients.
• Tell your doctor if you've ever had an allergic reaction to any antifungal drug or if you're using a douche or another type of vaginal drug.
• Keep using Terazol even if your period starts. But don't use tampons because they could remove some of the drug from your vagina.
• If your symptoms don't subside or if they worsen after using the medication for several days, call your doctor.

• To help keep your infection from returning, wear cotton-crotch panties and pantyhose.
• It's possible to spread your infection to your sexual partner during intercourse. Also, your partner could be carrying the fungus and transmitting it to you. To keep from spreading the infection or becoming reinfected, abstain from sex or have your partner wear a condom during intercourse. If your partner becomes infected, tell him to consult a doctor about treatment.

 KEEP IN MIND...

* Don't stop using drug, even during your period.
* Don't use tampons; wear menstrual pad to protect clothes.
* Abstain from sex or have partner wear condom.
* If symptoms worsen, call doctor.

Teslac

Teslac is a drug that's pre-scibed to fight cancer. It's believed to work by changing the tumor's hormonal environment. Teslac is similar to the hormone testosterone but causes fewer side effects.

Why it's prescribed

Doctors prescribe Teslac to treat some forms of breast cancer in women. It comes in tablets. Doctors usually prescribe the following amounts.

▶ **For advanced breast cancer in postmenopausal women,** 250 milligrams four times a day, for a minimum of 3 months.

How to take Teslac

• Take Teslac exactly as prescribed. Don't take more of this drug than your doctor has ordered because higher-than-recommended doses will not have better effects.

If you miss a dose

Take the missed dose as soon as possible. However, if it's almost time for your next dose, skip the missed dose and take your next dose as scheduled. Don't take a double dose. If you miss two or more doses in a row, call your doctor.

 If you suspect an overdose

Consult your doctor.

TESLAC'S OTHER NAME

Teslac's generic name is testolactone.

 SIDE EFFECTS

Call your doctor if you have any of these possible drug side effects. Call *immediately* about any labeled "serious."

Serious: high blood pressure (headache, blurred vision)

Common: none reported

Other: nausea, vomiting, appetite loss, swelling or redness of tongue, numbness or pins-and-needles feeling in fingers, toes, or face, diarrhea, increased calcium level (increased thirst, increased urine, and constipation), hair loss, aches and swelling of legs and arms.

Tips: Call your doctor if you vomit shortly after taking a dose of Teslac. The doctor may want you to repeat the dose. You may experience nausea and vomiting while you're taking Teslac, but it's important that you keep taking the drug to give it time to work. Don't stop taking the drug without discussing it with your doctor first. Drink plenty of fluids to help your body get rid of excess calcium.

 DRUG INTERACTIONS

Combining certain drugs may alter their action or produce unwanted side effects. Tell your doctor about other drugs you're taking, especially:
• anticoagulants (blood thinners) such as Coumadin (your Coumadin dose may need to be adjusted).

Warnings

• Make sure your doctor knows your medical history. You may not be able to take Teslac if you're overly sensitive to it, are pregnant or breast-feeding, if you haven't yet reached menopause, or if you have a high calcium level or heart or kidney disease.
• This drug is not recommended for men who have breast cancer.
• Don't expect to see an improvement right after you start taking Teslac. In fact, doctors say that 3 months is an adequate trial for this drug.

• You doctor may want to check the calcium levels in your blood regularly while you're taking Teslac.

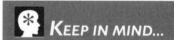 **KEEP IN MIND...**

* Keep taking Teslac even if it causes vomiting.
* Don't take more than pre-scribed.
* Drink plenty of fluids to rid body of excess calcium.
* Not recommended for men with breast cancer.

Tessalon

Tessalon suppresses the cough reflex by direct action on the cough center in the brain. It also acts as a local anesthetic.

Why it's prescribed

Doctors prescribe Tessalon for cough suppression. It comes in capsules. Doctors usually prescribe the following amounts for adults and children over age 10.

▶ **To relieve cough,** 100 milligrams (mg) three times a day, up to 600 mg a day, as needed.

How to take Tessalon

• Swallow the capsules promptly. Don't chew them or let them dissolve in your mouth.
• The drug takes effect in 15 to 20 minutes; the effect lasts for 3 to 8 hours.

If you miss a dose

Take the missed dose as soon as possible. However, if it's almost time for your next dose, skip the missed dose and take your next dose as scheduled. Don't take a double dose.

 ## If you suspect an overdose

Contact your doctor *immediately*. Excessive Tessalon can cause restlessness, tremors, and seizures.

TESSALON'S OTHER NAME

Tessalon's generic name is benzonatate.

 ## SIDE EFFECTS

Call your doctor if you have any of these possible drug side effects. Call *immediately* about any labeled "serious."

Serious: seizures

Common: none reported

Other: dizziness, drowsiness, headache, restlessness, nasal congestion, burning sensation in eyes, nausea, constipation, rash, chills, confusion, hallucinations

Tips: Drink plenty of water to help moisten the secretions in your lungs, which makes it easier to cough up moist secretions. If you're having trouble clearing fluid from your lungs, use a cold-mist vaporizer, and suck on sugarless hard candy to help increase saliva flow. Try not to talk or smoke.

DRUG INTERACTIONS

Combining certain drugs may alter their action or produce unwanted side effects. Tell your doctor about other drugs you're taking.

 ## Warnings

• Make sure your doctor knows your medical history. You may not be able to take Tessalon if you're overly sensitive to it or to certain anesthetics (such as procaine and tetracaine).
• Before you begin taking Tessalon, make sure your doctor knows if you're pregnant or breast-feeding.
• Your doctor won't prescribe Tessalon if your cough may help in diagnosing an illness or is beneficial to you, such as for clearing the lungs after chest surgery.
• Your doctor will prescribe Tessalon only if your cough is due to a cold, the flu, or another short-term problem. Tessalon is not appropriate for coughs resulting from smoking, asthma, or emphysema.

• Tessalon should not be used in infants and young children since numbness of the mouth, tongue, and throat can cause swallowing problems and choking.
• If your cough doesn't improve within 7 days, or if you have a high fever, skin rash, or continuing headache along with a cough, call your doctor right away.

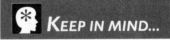

* Drink plenty of water.
* Don't chew the capsules or dissolve them in your mouth.
* If cough doesn't improve in a week, call the doctor.
* Don't use with infants or small children.

Testoderm

Testoderm provides a continuous dose of the hormone testosterone. This hormone is responsible for the development of the male sex organs and secondary sex characteristics (male hair distribution, muscle and fat distribution, and deepening voice).

Why it's prescribed

Doctors prescribe Testoderm for testosterone deficiency in males. It comes as a skin patch. Doctors usually prescribe the following amount for adults.

▶ **For testosterone deficiency,** 1 patch a day.

How to use Testoderm

• Use Testoderm only as your doctor has prescribed. Apply the patch to the skin of the scrotum because skin other than the scrotum won't absorb Testoderm as effectively.
• For best contact between the patch and skin, shave the area to receive the patch. Then, gently clean and dry the area before applying the patch.
• Wear each Testoderm patch for 22 to 24 hours.

If you miss a dose

Apply the missed patch as soon as possible. However, if it's almost time for your next patch, skip the missed patch and apply your next patch as scheduled. Never apply two patches at once.

TESTODERM'S OTHER NAME

Testoderm's generic name is testosterone.

SIDE EFFECTS

Call your doctor if you have any of these possible drug side effects. Call *immediately* about any labeled "serious."

Serious: excessive and frequent penile erections, liver tumors (nausea, vomiting, yellow-tinged skin and eyes), severe allergic reaction (swelling of face or throat, difficulty breathing)

Common: male pattern baldness, acne, nausea, headache

Others: anxiety, depression, decreased sex drive, decreased sperm count

DRUG INTERACTIONS

Combining certain drugs may alter their action or produce unwanted side effects. Tell your doctor about drugs you're taking, especially:
• anticoagulants (blood thinners) such as Coumadin
• insulin
• oxyphenbutazone.

If you suspect an overdose

Contact your doctor *immediately.* Excessive Testoderm can cause stroke (weakness on one side of the body or change of mental status).

Warnings

• Make sure your doctor knows your medical history. You may not be able to use Testoderm if you have breast or prostate cancer.
• You also may not be able to use Testoderm if you've had a reaction to it or to an anabolic steroid. Tell your doctor about this and any other allergies, including allergies to preservatives or dyes.
• Testoderm isn't given to females and isn't recommended for males under age 18.
• If you're planning to have children, discuss this with your doctor before you start using Testoderm.

You may experience a temporary decrease in sperm production during treatment.
• Be aware that older adults may be especially prone to Testoderm's side effects.
• In some cases, this drug can pass from you to your sexual partner. Tell your doctor if a female sexual partner develops unusual hair growth.
• Don't start any new medications without consulting your doctor first.

KEEP IN MIND...

∗ Apply to clean, dry, shaved scrotal skin.

∗ Wear for 22 to 24 hours unless otherwise directed.

∗ Not recommended for males under age 18 or for females.

Theo-Dur

Theo-Dur relaxes the muscles in the lower airways and blood vessels of the lungs.

Why it's prescribed

Doctors prescribe Theo-Dur to help treat and prevent the symptoms of asthma. It comes in tablets, extended-release capsules, and liquid. Doctors usually prescribe the following amounts for adults and children.

▶ **For acute bronchospasm in adult nonsmokers and children over age 16 not currently taking theophylline,** 6 milligrams (mg) for each 2.2 pounds (lb) of body weight, followed by 2 to 3 mg for each 2.2 lb every 6 hours, for a total of two doses. Maintenance dosage is 3 mg for each 2.2 lb every 8 hours.

▶ **For acute bronchospasm in otherwise healthy adult smokers and children over age 16 not currently taking theophylline,** 6 mg for each 2.2 lb, followed by 3 mg for each 2.2 lb every 6 hours for a total

THEO-DUR'S OTHER NAMES

Theo-Dur's generic name is theophylline anhydrous. Brand names for immediate-release liquids include Asmalix, Elixophyllin, Lanophyllin, and Theolair. Brand names for immediate-release tablets and capsules include Elixophyllin and Slo-Phyllin. Brand names for slow-release tablets include Quibron-T/SR, Respbid, Theolair-SR, Theo-Time, and Uniphyl. Brand names for slow-release capsules include Aerolate SR, Elixophyllin, Slo-bid Gyrocaps, Theo-24, Theobid Duracaps, Theochron, Theo-Dur, and Theovent Long-Acting.

 ## SIDE EFFECTS

Call your doctor if you have any of these possible drug side effects. Call *immediately* about any labeled "serious."

Serious: seizures, fast breathing, low blood pressure (dizziness, weakness), rapid heart rate (dizziness, fluttering in chest)

Common: restlessness, insomnia, nausea, vomiting, appetite loss, slight dizziness
Tip: You may experience some dizziness, especially at the start of therapy and especially if you're an older adult. Change positions slowly, and move about carefully until you get used to Theo-Dur's effects.

Other: headache, light-headedness, muscle twitching, flushing, bitter aftertaste, stomach upset, diarrhea, hives
Tips: If Theo-Dur upsets your stomach, ask your doctor if you can take it with a full glass of water after meals. This will alter the drug's absorption, but it should make your stomach feel better. Call the doctor right away if you develop diarrhea.

 ## DRUG AND FOOD INTERACTIONS

Combining certain drugs and certain foods may alter the drug's action or produce unwanted side effects. Tell your doctor about your diet and other drugs you're taking, especially:

- barbiturates such as Solfoton
- birth control pills
- caffeine (found in tea, coffee, colas, and chocolate)
- char-broiled foods
- ciprofloxacin and other quinolone antibiotics
- erythromycin and other macrolide antibiotics
- heart drugs known as beta blockers, such as Corgard and Inderal
- seizure medicines, such as Dilantin and Tegretol
- tobacco and marijuana
- tuberculosis drugs such as Reladen
- ulcer drugs such as Tagamet.

of three doses. Maintenance dosage is 3 mg for each 2.2 lb every 6 hours.

▶ **For acute bronchospasm in children ages 9 to 16,** 6 mg for each 2.2 lb in a single dose, followed by 3 mg for each 2.2 lb every 6 hours for a total of three doses. Maintenance dosage is 3 mg for each 2.2 lb every 6 hours.

▶ **For acute bronchospasm in children ages 6 months to 8 years,** 6 mg for each 2.2 lb in a single dose, followed by 4 mg for each 2.2 lb every 6 hours for a total of three doses. Maintenance dosage is 4 mg for each 2.2 lb every 6 hours.

▶ **For acute bronchospasm in adults and children currently tak-**

Continued on next page ▶

ing theophylline, some doctors recommend 2.5 mg of oral dose of rapid-acting theophylline for each 2.2 lb in an emergency, if the person has no obvious signs of theophylline toxicity.

▶ **For chronic bronchospasm in adults and children over age 16,** 16 mg for each 2.2 lb or 400 mg a day (whichever is less), divided into three or four equal doses and taken every 6 to 8 hours. Or, 12 mg for each 2.2 lb or 400 mg a day (whichever is less) of extended-release form, divided into two or three equal doses and taken every 8 to 12 hours. Dosage increased, as needed, every 2 or 3 days to maximum of 13 mg for each 2.2 lb or 900 mg a day (whichever is less).

▶ **For chronic bronchospasm in children ages 12 to 16,** 18 mg for each 2.2 lb a day.

▶ **For chronic bronchospasm in children ages 9 to 11,** 20 mg for each 2.2 lb a day.

▶ **For chronic bronchospasm in children under age 9,** 24 mg for each 2.2 lb a day.

How to take Theo-Dur

• Follow your doctor's instructions exactly. Don't take more or less, and don't take it more often or for longer than directed.

• Take your doses at the same time every day.

• Take Theo-Dur ½ to 1 hour before meals or 2 hours after meals, unless your doctor directs otherwise. Theo-Dur works best on an empty stomach.

• Make sure you know whether you're taking a regular-release or an extended-release form. (If you have acute bronchospasm, you probably won't be taking the extended-release form.)

• If you're taking the extended-release form of the medication, don't crush, break, or chew the tablets or capsules. Small children unable to swallow them can eat (without chewing) the contents of bead-filled capsules sprinkled over soft food.

If you miss a dose

For this drug to work properly, you need to take every dose on time. If you do miss a dose, though, take the missed dose as soon as possible. If it's almost time for your next dose, skip the missed dose and take your next dose on schedule. Don't take a double dose.

If you suspect an overdose

Contact your doctor *immediately.* Excessive Theo-Dur can cause vomiting, rapid heartbeat, and seizures.

✗❮ Warnings

• Make sure your doctor knows your medical history. You may not be able to take Theo-Dur if you're overly sensitive to it or to caffeine or the drug theobromine, have recently had a heart attack, or if you have heart or circulatory problems, angina, diabetes, glaucoma, high blood pressure, overactive thyroid, seizures, stomach ulcers, lung disease, kidney or liver problems, sensitivity to sulfites, or indigestion.

• Tell the doctor if you've ever had an allergic reaction to any drug for asthma.

• If you're pregnant or breast-feeding, check with your doctor before taking Theo-Dur.

• Older adults may be especially prone to Theo-Dur's side effects.

• If you're an older adult or have congestive heart failure or liver disease, you'll need a lower dosage because you'll metabolize the drug more slowly. If you smoke tobacco or marijuana regularly, you'll need a higher-than-normal dosage because smoking speeds up the drug's metabolism.

• Call your doctor right away if you develop a fever or feel as though you have the flu. These conditions could increase your risk of developing side effects.

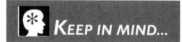

* Take on empty stomach at same time each day.

* Don't crush or chew extended-release form.

* Don't eat char-broiled foods often.

* Minimize caffeine.

* Don't take any other drugs without your doctor's knowledge.

Thorazine

Thorazine is one of a group of medicines called phenothiazines. These drugs affect levels of the neurotransmitter dopamine in the brain. Although the exact way it works is unknown, decreased levels of dopamine appear to lift a person's mood.

Why it's prescribed

Doctors prescribe Thorazine to treat psychosis, persistent hiccups, and nausea and vomiting. It comes in tablets, slow-release capsules, liquid concentrate, syrup, and suppositories. Doctors usually prescribe the following amounts for adults; children's dosages appear in parentheses.

▶ **For psychosis,** initially, 25 to 75 milligrams (mg) a day, divided into in two to four equal doses. Dosage increased by 20 to 50 mg twice a week, as needed, until symptoms are controlled. Some people may require up to 800 mg a day. (Children: 0.55 mg for each 2.2 pounds (lb) of body weight every 4 to 6 hours, or 1.1 mg for each 2.2 lb by suppository every 6 to 8 hours.)

▶ **For nausea and vomiting,** 10 to 25 mg every 4 to 6 hours, as needed, or 50 to 100 mg by suppository every 6 to 8 hours, as needed. (Children age 6 months and older:

THORAZINE'S OTHER NAMES

Thorazine's generic name is chlorpromazine hydrochloride. Other brand names include Chlorpromanyl-5, Chlorpromanyl-20, Chlorpromanyl-40, Novo-Chlorpromazine, Ormazine, and Thor-Prom.

SIDE EFFECTS

Call your doctor if you have any of these possible drug side effects. Call *immediately* about any labeled "serious."

Serious: severe blood disorders (bleeding and unusual bruising, heightened susceptibility to infection, chills, fever), jaundice (yellow-tinged skin and eyes), neuroleptic malignant syndrome (high fever, muscle rigidity, change in mental status, irregular sweating, fast heart rate, fluttering in chest), allergic reaction (fever, rash, swelling, difficulty breathing)

Common: sedation, low blood pressure (dizziness, weakness), dry mouth, constipation, difficulty urinating, sensitivity to sun, uncontrolled or repetitive muscle movements
Tips: Avoid activities that require full alertness or coordination until you know how Thorazine affects you. To relieve dry mouth, use ice chips or sugarless gum or hard candy. Call your doctor if you develop involuntary muscle movements, constipation, or trouble urinating. To protect skin, wear a sunscreen, a hat, and protective clothes when you go outdoors.

Other: blurred vision, menstrual irregularities, breast enlargement in men, inhibited ejaculation, nausea, vomiting, tremors (after abrupt withdrawal of long-term therapy)

DRUG INTERACTIONS

Combining certain drugs may alter their action or produce unwanted side effects. Tell your doctor about other drugs you're taking, especially:
- alcohol and other drugs that make you relaxed or sleepy, such as tranquilizers, sleeping pills, and cold and allergy drugs, such as Benadryl
- antacids
- anticoagulants (blood thinners) such as Coumadin
- antidepressants
- barbiturates such as Solfoton
- blood pressure drugs such as Inderal
- drugs for Parkinson's disease such as Sinemet
- Eskalith.

0.55 mg for each 2.2 lb every 4 to 6 hours, or 1.1 mg for each 2.2 lb by suppository every 6 to 8 hours.)
▶ **For chronic hiccups or acute intermittent porphyria (inborn metabolic abnormality),** 25 to 50 mg three or four times a day. For symptoms persisting 2 to 3 days, Thorazine can be given by injection.

How to take Thorazine

- Follow your doctor's directions exactly.
- Take oral forms with food, milk, or water to minimize stomach upset.

Continued on next page ▶

- Swallow slow-release capsules whole. Don't crush or chew them.
- If you're taking the concentrate, mix it in 2 to 4 ounces (50 to 125 milliliters) of water, soda, juice, milk, pudding, or applesauce just before taking it.
- Protect liquid concentrate from light. Wear gloves when preparing it, and prevent contact with skin and clothing. Thorazine liquid can cause dermatitis through contact.
- Don't stop taking Thorazine abruptly without your doctor's knowledge.

If you miss a dose

Adjust your schedule as follows:
- If you're taking one dose a day, take the missed dose as soon as you remember that day. If you don't remember until the next day, skip the dose you missed and take your next regular dose.
- If you're taking more than one dose a day and you remember within 1 hour or so of the scheduled time, take the missed dose right away. If you don't remember until later, skip the missed dose and take your next dose at the regular time. Don't take a double dose.

If you suspect an overdose

Contact your doctor *immediately*. Excessive Thorazine can cause seizures, unarousable sleep and, possibly, coma.

Warnings

- Make sure your doctor knows your medical history. You may not be able to take Thorazine if you're an older adult, very ill, or overly sensitive to the drug or if you have bone marrow or central nervous system depression (extreme fatigue, dulled senses), heart disease (irregular heartbeat, heart failure, chest pain, heart valve disease, or heart block), continual exposure to extreme heat or cold or to certain insecticides, breathing problems (such as asthma, emphysema), low calcium level, a history of seizures or severe reactions to insulin or electroconvulsive therapy, glaucoma, an enlarged prostate, kidney or liver problems, or a pacemaker.
- If you're pregnant or breast-feeding, tell your doctor before using Thorazine.
- Before surgery, dental work, or emergency treatment, tell the doctor or dentist that you're taking this drug.

KEEP IN MIND...

* Take oral forms with food, milk, or water.
* Don't crush or chew slow-release form.
* Immediately report jaundice, fever, sore throat, joint pain, or unusual bruising or bleeding.
* Don't stop taking Thorazine abruptly.
* Ask doctor before taking any other prescription or nonprescription drugs.

Thyroid USP Enseals

Thyroid USP Enseals stimulate the metabolism of all body tissues. Without enough thyroid hormones, the body's metabolism slows down.

Why it's prescribed

Doctors prescribe Thyroid USP Enseals when the thyroid gland isn't producing enough thyroid hormone or isn't producing any. This drug comes in tablets, beef-origin tablets, pork-origin tablets, coated tablets, strong tablets (50% stronger than thyroid USP and containing 0.3% iodine), and pork-origin capsules. Doctors usually prescribe the following amounts.

▶ **For mild hypothyroidism in adults,** initially, 60 milligrams (mg) a day, increased by 60 mg every 30 days until desired response occurs. Usual maintenance dosage is 60 to 180 mg a day.

▶ **For severe hypothyroidism in adults and congenital or severe hypothyroidism in children,** initially, 15 mg a day, increased by 30 mg a day after 2 weeks and to 60 mg a day 2 weeks later. After 2 months, dosage increased to 120 mg a day, as needed, for 2 months, then increased to 180 mg a day, as needed.

How to take Thyroid USP Enseals

• Take your dose at the same time each day, preferably before break-

THYROID USP ENSEALS' OTHER NAMES

Thyroid USP Enseals' generic name is thyroid USP (desiccated). Other brand names include Armour Thyroid, Thyrar, Thyroid Strong, and Westhroid.

 ## SIDE EFFECTS

Call your doctor if you have any of these possible drug side effects. Call *immediately* about any labeled "serious."

Serious: changes in heart rhythm, rapid heartbeat, increased blood pressure (headache, blurred vision), cardiac collapse (severe low blood pressure, extreme dizziness, fainting)

Common: nervousness, insomnia

Other: twitching, tremor, headache, fever, infection, chest pain, diarrhea, abdominal cramps, vomiting, weight loss, heat intolerance, sweating, menstrual irregularities

 ## DRUG INTERACTIONS

Combining certain drugs may alter their action or produce unwanted side effects. Tell your doctor about other drugs you're taking, especially:
• anticoagulants (blood thinners) such as Coumadin
• epinephrine and related drugs (sympathomimetics), such as Primatene Mist Suspension
• insulin and oral diabetes drugs, such as DiaBeta and Micronase
• Questran.

fast, to maintain constant hormone levels and to avoid insomnia.
• Don't store this drug in a warm, humid area.

If you miss a dose

Take the missed dose as soon as possible. However, if it's almost time for your next dose, skip the missed dose and take your next dose as scheduled. Don't take a double dose.

 ## If you suspect an overdose

Contact your doctor *immediately.* Excessive thyroid hormone can cause agitation, nervousness, heart palpitations, tremors, sweating, chest pain, and other symptoms.

 ## Warnings

• Make sure your doctor knows your medical history. You may not be able to take Thyroid USP Enseals if you're overly sensitive to it, if your hypothyroidism is related to a recent heart attack, or if you have untreated severe hypothyroidism, uncorrected adrenal insufficiency, angina, high blood pressure, heart or blood vessel disease, lung disease, diabetes, or kidney problems.
• Tell the doctor that you're taking Thyroid USP Enseals before having any thyroid function tests.
• Don't change brands.

 ## KEEP IN MIND...

∗ Take at same time each day, preferably before breakfast.

∗ Don't store in a warm, humid area.

∗ Don't change drug brands.

Ticlid

Ticlid is an antiplatelet agent that probably works by keeping the platelets from binding together. Platelets are the blood components that allow clotting.

Why it's prescribed

Doctors prescribe Ticlid to lower the risk of having a stroke. It comes in tablets. Doctors usually prescribe the following amounts for adults.

▶ **For reducing the risk of blood-clot-caused stroke in adults with a history of stroke or those who experience early symptoms of stroke (headache, weakness),** 250 milligrams twice a day.

How to take Ticlid

• Take Ticlid with meals to help your system absorb the drug and to reduce stomach upset.

If you miss a dose

Take the missed dose as soon as possible. However, if it's almost time for your next dose, skip the missed dose and take your next dose as scheduled. Don't take a double dose.

If you suspect an overdose

Consult your doctor.

Warnings

• Make sure your doctor knows your medical history. You may not be able to take Ticlid if you're overly sensitive to it or if you have a blood disorder, active bleeding (such as a stomach ulcer), or severe liver disease.

TICLID'S OTHER NAME

Ticlid's generic name is ticlopidine hydrochloride.

SIDE EFFECTS

Call your doctor if you have any of these possible drug side effects. Call *immediately* about any labeled "serious."

Serious: vasculitis (fever, extreme tiredness, achy joints, pale skin, hives, rash), severe kidney problems (decreased urine, bloody urine, pain), severe blood problems (fatigue, bleeding, bruising, chills, fever, heightened proneness to infection), serum sickness (joint pain, rash, fever), inadequate sodium in the blood (water intoxication), pneumonia

Common: diarrhea, stomach upset, pain, rash, increased cholesterol levels
Tips: Take with food to avoid stomach upset. Decrease cholesterol in your diet.

Other: dizziness, appetite loss, nosebleeds, bleeding of the mucous membranes of the eyes, vomiting, gas, light-colored stools, dark-colored urine, liver problems (yellow-tinged eyes and skin), allergic reaction (hives, itching), lupus, inflamed muscles, tingling or numbness in hands or feet
Tip: Call your doctor right away if you develop any of these symptoms.

DRUG INTERACTIONS

Combining certain drugs may alter their action or produce unwanted side effects. Tell your doctor about other drugs you're taking, especially:
• antacids
• anticoagulants (blood thinners) such as Coumadin
• aspirin and aspirin-containing products
• Lanoxin
• Tagamet
• Theo-Dur.

• Call your doctor right away if you're injured while taking this drug.
• Your doctor will probably want to do blood and liver function tests regularly while you're on Ticlid. Be sure to keep all appointments.
• Ticlid will prolong the amount of time you bleed before your blood clots; tell your doctor if you have any unusual or prolonged bleeding.
• Tell all doctors and your dentist that you're taking Ticlid before having tests, surgery, or dental work. Your doctor will probably have you stop taking Ticlid about 10 to 14 days before you have any surgical procedure.

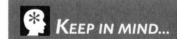

* Take with meals.
* Avoid aspirin and products containing aspirin.
* Report unusual bruising or bleeding.
* Keep appointments for blood tests.

Tigan

Tigan is a weak antihistamine that's used to treat extreme nausea. Its exact function is unknown, but it seems to indirectly send messages to the area of the brain that controls vomiting.

Why it's prescribed

Doctors prescribe Tigan to help treat nausea and vomiting. It comes in capsules and suppositories. Doctors usually prescribe the following amounts for adults.

▶ **For nausea and vomiting,** 250 milligrams (mg) three or four times a day, or 200 mg by suppository three or four times a day.

How to take Tigan

• Follow your doctor's instructions exactly. Don't use more of this drug or take it more often than your doctor has ordered.

If you miss a dose

Take the missed dose as soon as possible. However, if it's almost time for your next dose, skip the missed dose and take your next dose as scheduled. Don't take a double dose.

 If you suspect an overdose

Contact your doctor *immediately.* Excessive Tigan can cause seizures and coma.

TIGAN'S OTHER NAMES

Tigan's generic name is trimethobenzamide hydrochloride. Other brand names include Arrestin, Benzacot, Bio-Gan, Stemetic, Tebamide, Tegamide, T-Gen, Ticon, Triban, and Tribenzagan.

 SIDE EFFECTS

Call your doctor if you have any of these possible drug side effects. Call *immediately* about any labeled "serious."

Serious: seizures, liver problems (yellow-tinged skin and eyes)

Common: drowsiness

Tip: Avoid activities that require full alertness or coordination until you know how Tigan affects you.

Other: dizziness (high doses), low blood pressure (dizziness, weakness, fainting), diarrhea, worsening of preexisting nausea (with high doses), allergic reaction (reddened rash, itching, hives), blurry vision, headache, muscle cramps

Tip: Change positions slowly and move about carefully to minimize dizziness. When getting out of bed, dangle your legs over the side of the bed for several minutes.

 DRUG INTERACTIONS

Combining certain drugs may alter their action or produce unwanted side effects. Tell your doctor about other drugs you're taking, especially:

• alcohol and other drugs that make you relaxed or sleepy, such as tranquilizers, sleeping pills, and cold and allergy drugs.
• aspirin
• phenobarbitol

✗ Warnings

• Make sure your doctor knows your medical history. You may not be able to take Tigan if you're overly sensitive to it, or if you have a high fever, dehydration, or a bowel infection.
• If you're pregnant or breast-feeding, don't take Tigan without first talking with your doctor.
• Don't give Tigan to a child unless you know the cause of the vomiting and your doctor approves. When given to a child with a viral illness (a common cause of vomiting), this drug may lead to Reye's syndrome, which is a potentially fatal brain disorder.
• Refrigerate suppositories.

• Be aware that the suppository form contains a local anesthetic, benzocaine. If you've had a reaction to benzocaine or similar locat anesthetics, you should not use the suppository form of Tigan.

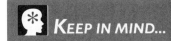 **KEEP IN MIND...**

* Tell your doctor about persistent vomiting.
* Don't give to a child when reason for vomiting is unknown.
* Refrigerate suppositories.
* Avoid alcohol.

Tilade

Tilade is an inhalant that reduces inflammation along the respiratory airways.

Why it's prescribed

Doctors prescribe Tilade to help prevent the wheezing and difficulty breathing that accompany asthma or bronchospasm. It comes in an aerosol to be inhaled. Doctors usually prescribe the following amounts for adults and children age 12 and over.

▶ **For regular maintenance in mild to moderate reversible obstructive airway disease,** two inhalations four times a day.

How to use Tilade

• Use Tilade at regular intervals as maintenance therapy.
• Make sure you know how to use your inhaler properly. Shake the Tilade canister well; then turn it over just before administering the inhalation.
• Clean your inhaler at least twice a week. Remove the drug canister before rinsing the inhaler in hot running water. Then allow the inhaler to air-dry overnight.
• You'll feel better if you use Tilade regularly. Most people say they feel better after 1 week of use; some require longer treatment before they notice any improvement.

If you miss a dose

Take the missed dose as soon as possible. However, if it's almost time

TILADE'S OTHER NAME

Tilade's generic name is nedocromil sodium.

 SIDE EFFECTS

Call your doctor if you have any of these possible drug side effects. Call *immediately* about any labeled "serious."

Serious: bronchospasm (wheezing, tightness in chest, difficulty breathing)

Common: unpleasant taste
Tip: Offset the bad taste with sugarless candy or gum and frequent mouth care.

Other: headache, nausea, vomiting, upper respiratory tract infection (mucous production, fever), stuffy or runny nose

 DRUG INTERACTIONS

Combining certain drugs may alter their action or produce unwanted side effects. Tell your doctor about other drugs you're taking.

for your next dose, skip the missed dose and take your next dose as scheduled. Don't take a double dose.

If you suspect an overdose

Consult your doctor. Using too much Tilade probably won't cause serious damage, but do your best to take it exactly as prescribed.

Warnings

• Make sure your doctor knows your medical history. You may not be able to use Tilade if you're overly sensitive to it or if you have an acute asthma attack or acute bronchospasm.
• Tell your doctor if you're pregnant or breast-feeding before you start taking Tilade.
• Keep in mind that Tilade can't replace the drug your doctor has

prescribed for use *during* an attack. Tilade is not a bronchodilator (it doesn't relax airways to make breathing easier). It may, however, reduce the need for bronchodilator and corticosteroid drugs. It may also reduce the number and severity of your asthma attacks.
• If your symptoms don't improve in 2 to 4 weeks, or if they get worse, call your doctor.

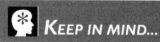 **KEEP IN MIND...**

* Use regularly, even if you're not having attacks.
* Know how to use your inhaler.
* Shake canister before using.
* Clean inhaler weekly.
* Call doctor if symptoms don't improve in 2 to 4 weeks.

Timoptic

Timoptic is a drug that's believed to reduce formation of the liquid in your eye and increase its outflow.

Why it's prescribed

Doctors prescribe Timoptic to lower the pressure in the eye. It comes in eyedrops. Doctors usually prescribe the following amounts for adults.

▶ **For chronic open-angle, secondary, and aphasic glaucomas and high pressure in the eye,** initially, 1 drop of 0.25% solution in affected eye twice a day, increased to 1 drop of 0.5% solution in affected eye twice a day, as needed. If pressure is controlled, maintenance dosage is 1 drop a day.

How to use Timoptic

• To avoid contaminating the drug, don't touch the dropper tip to your eye, the surrounding skin, or any other surface.
• After using the eyedrops, close your eyes and press a finger against the inside corner of each eye for 1 to 2 minutes. This keeps the drug in your eyes by preventing it from entering your tear ducts.
• Wash your hands after using Timoptic eyedrops.

If you miss a dose

Adjust your schedule as follows:
• If you use one dose a day, apply the missed dose as soon as possible. But if you don't remember until the next day, skip the missed dose and apply your next dose as scheduled. Don't apply a double dose.

TIMOPTIC'S OTHER NAME

Timoptic's generic name is timolol maleate.

 SIDE EFFECTS

Call your doctor if you have any of these possible drug side effects. Call *immediately* about any labeled "serious."

Serious: asthma attacks (wheezing, difficulty breathing), congestive heart failure (shortness of breath, chest, pain, anxiety)

Common: low blood pressure (dizziness, weakness), slow pulse, fainting

Other: headache, depression, fatigue, slightly lower resting pulse, minor eye irritation, decreased corneal sensitivity (with long-term use), appetite loss

 DRUG INTERACTIONS

Combining certain drugs may alter their action or produce unwanted side effects. Tell your doctor about other drugs you're taking, especially:
• calcium channel blockers such as Procardia
• Cardioquin
• Duragesic
• heart drugs called digitalis glycosides
• Inderal, Lopressor, and other beta blockers
• reserpine and other catecholamine-depleting drugs.

• If you use more than one dose a day, apply the missed dose as soon as possible. But if it's almost time for your next dose, skip the missed dose and apply your next dose as scheduled. Don't apply a double dose.

 If you suspect an overdose

Contact your doctor *immediately*. Excessive Timoptic can cause severely low blood pressure (extreme dizziness and weakness, fainting) and heart failure (shortness of breath, chest pain, anxiety).

 Warnings

• Make sure your doctor knows your medical history. You may not be able to use Timoptic if you are allergic to it; have a history of asthma, severe obstructive pulmonary disease, bronchospasm not caused by allergy, chronic bronchitis, emphysema, diabetes, heart or blood vessel disease, myasthenia gravis, kidney or liver disease, or an overactive thyroid; or if you are pregnant or breast-feeding.
• If you have diabetes, Timoptic may affect your blood sugar levels. If you notice a change in your blood or urine sugar tests, call your doctor.

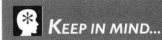 **KEEP IN MIND...**

* Don't touch dropper tip to eye, skin, or other surface.
* Press inside corners of eyes after using drops.
* If you're diabetic, check sugar levels carefully.

Tinactin

Tinactin interferes with the growth of certain fungi.

Why it's used

Tinactin is used to treat fungal skin infections. This nonprescription drug comes in cream, gel, powder, lotion, pump-spray liquid, and aerosol powder. The following amounts are usually recommended for adults and children.

▶ **For fungal infections of the skin,** ¼-inch to ½-inch ribbon of cream or 2 to 3 drops of solution to cover area about the size of one hand; same amount of cream or 2 to 3 drops of lotion to cover toes and area between toes on one foot; or gel, powder, or spray to cover affected area, all applied twice a day for 2 to 6 weeks.

How to use Tinactin

• Wash the affected area and dry it thoroughly. Then apply enough of the drug to cover the area.
• If you're using Tinactin powder on your feet, sprinkle it between your toes, on your feet, and in your socks and shoes.
• If you're using a pump-spray liquid, hold the container 4 to 6 inches away from the area and spray.
• If you're using the aerosol form, shake the can well. Then, holding it 6 to 10 inches away, spray the affected area. Don't inhale the vapor

or powder from the spray. Also, don't use it near heat or an open flame or while you're smoking.
• Massage drug gently into skin.
• Continue to use the drug for 2 weeks after burning, itching, and other symptoms have disappeared. This will help clear up the infection completely.

If you miss a dose

Apply the missed dose as soon as possible. Then return to your regular schedule. Don't apply a double dose.

 If you suspect an overdose

Consult your doctor.

 Warnings

• If you have any drug allergies, consult your doctor before using Tinactin.
• Don't use Tinactin on a child younger than age 2, unless your doctor orders otherwise.
• If you have a fungal infection of your hair or nails, see your doctor.

Tinactin alone won't cure these types of infections.
• If you're using the drug to treat athlete's foot and your symptoms haven't disappeared after 10 days, call your doctor. If you're treating another type of fungal infection and your symptoms persist or worsen after 4 weeks, call your doctor.
• To help prevent reinfection after you've finished your treatment, use the powder or aerosol powder each day after bathing, or sprinkle the powder or spray the aerosol inside your socks and shoes, as needed.

SIDE EFFECTS

Call your doctor if you have any of these possible drug side effects.

Serious: none reported

Common: none reported

Other: possible skin irritation

Tips: Check with your doctor or pharmacist if you develop skin irritation that wasn't present before you used this drug. If you're using the pump-spray form of Tinactin, you may experience a mild, temporary stinging sensation.

DRUG INTERACTIONS

Combining certain drugs may alter their action or produce unwanted side effects. Tell your doctor about other drugs you're taking.

TINACTIN'S OTHER NAMES

Tinactin's generic name is tolnaftate. Other brand names include Aftate, Dr. Scholl's Athlete's Foot Powder or Foot Spray, Footwork, Fungatin, Genaspor, NP-27, Ting, and Zeasorb-AF.

 KEEP IN MIND...

∗ Continue using for 2 weeks after symptoms subside.

∗ Check with your doctor if condition worsens.

∗ Don't use on children younger than age 2.

Tobrex

Tobrex is an antibiotic that kills a wide range of bacteria by preventing them from multiplying.

Why it's prescribed

Doctors prescribe Tobrex to treat eye infections. It comes in eyedrops and an ointment. Doctors usually prescribe the following amounts for adults and children.

▶ **For mild to moderate bacterial eye infection,** 1 or 2 drops in affected eye every 4 hours or a thin strip of ointment applied every 8 to 12 hours.

▶ **For severe bacterial eye infection,** 2 drops in affected eye every 30 to 60 minutes or a thin strip of ointment applied every 3 to 4 hours until condition improves; then the frequency is reduced.

How to use Tobrex

• Clean crusts and secretions from your eyes before using Tobrex.
• To avoid contaminating the drug, don't let the applicator tip touch your eye, the surrounding skin, or any other surface.
• After using eyedrops, press a finger against the inside corner of each eye for 1 minute. This keeps the drug in your eyes by preventing it from entering your tear ducts.
• If you're using the ointment, gently close your eye for 1 to 2 minutes after using it to let the drug spread.
• If your doctor has ordered another eye solution to be used with this one, wait at least 5 minutes before

TOBREX'S OTHER NAME

Tobrex's generic name is tobramycin.

 SIDE EFFECTS

Call your doctor if you have any of these possible drug side effects.

Serious: none reported

Common: none reported

Other: burning, stinging, or blurred vision after use, allergic reaction (constant swelling, itching, or burning eyelids)

 DRUG INTERACTIONS

Combining certain drugs may alter their action or produce unwanted side effects. Tell your doctor about other drugs you're taking, especially:
• eye drugs that contain tetracycline.

using the second drug. This will help keep the second drug from washing away the Tobrex.
• Use all of the drug as prescribed by your doctor, even if your symptoms improve after a few days.

If you miss a dose

Apply the missed dose as soon as possible. However, if it's almost time for your next dose, skip the missed dose and apply your next dose as scheduled. Don't apply a double dose.

 If you suspect an overdose

Contact your doctor *immediately*. Signs of overdose include an inflamed or painful cornea, red or swollen eyes, increased tearing, and lid itching.

 Warnings

• Make sure your doctor knows your medical history. You may not be able to use Tobrex if you're allergic to it or if you have a history of kidney disease, ringing in the ears, hearing loss, myasthenia gravis, Parkinson's disease, or low calcium levels.
• Your eyes may sting or burn for a few minutes after you apply the drops or ointment. Also expect your vision to blur briefly after applying the ointment.
• To avoid spreading the infection, never share your eye drug, washcloths, or towels with family members. If anyone develops similar symptoms, call the doctor.
• Call your doctor if your symptoms persist or get worse after a few days of treatment.

KEEP IN MIND...

∗ Finish drug even if you feel better after a few days.

∗ Don't share drug, towels, or washcloths.

∗ Call doctor if symptoms persist or worsen in a few days.

∗ Don't touch applicator tip to anything.

Tofranil

Tofranil is a tricyclic antidepressant that increases the amount of the mood-elevating chemicals norepinephrine, serotonin, or both in the brain.

Why it's prescribed

Doctors prescribe Tofranil to treat depression and childhood bed-wetting. It comes in tablets and capsules. Doctors usually prescribe the following amounts.

▶ **For depression in adults,** 75 to 100 milligrams (mg) divided into equal doses taken several times a day. Dosage increased in 25- to 50-mg increments, as needed, to maximum of 300 mg a day. Or entire dose at bedtime using Tofranil-PM.

▶ **For bed-wetting in children age 6 and over,** 25 mg 1 hour before bedtime. If no response within 1 week, increased to 50 mg if the child is under age 12 or to 75 mg if the child is over age 12. Maximum dosage is 2.5 mg for each 2.2 pounds a day.

How to take Tofranil

• Unless your doctor instructs otherwise, take Tofranil with food (even at bedtime) to reduce stomach upset.

• For an early-night bedwetter, ask your doctor about dividing the dosage in half and giving half at bedtime and half earlier in the day.

TOFRANIL'S OTHER NAMES

Tofranil's generic name is imipramine hydrochloride. Other brand names include Janimine, Norfranil, and Tipramine and, in Canada, Impril and Novopramine. The brand name of a similar drug, imipramine pamoate, is Tofranil-PM.

 SIDE EFFECTS

Call your doctor if you have any of these possible drug side effects. Call *immediately* about any labeled "serious."

Serious: seizures

Common: drowsiness, low blood pressure (dizziness, weakness), altered pulse, blurred vision, dry mouth, constipation, difficulty urinating, sweating

Tips: Avoid activities that require full alertness or coordination until you know how Tofranil affects you. Dizziness, drowsiness, headache, and sweating should go away as your body adjusts to the drug. To reduce dizziness, get up slowly from a sitting or lying position. If you have constipation, increase the amount of fluids and fiber in your diet.

Other: excitation, tremor, weakness, confusion, headache, nervousness, uncontrollable muscle movements, increased blood pressure (headache, blurred vision), ringing in ears, dilated pupils, nausea, vomiting, appetite loss, increased sensitivity to sun, allergic reaction (inability to urinate, dry mouth, rash, fever, swelling), difficulty sleeping

Tips: Call your doctor if you can't sleep or have uncontrollable lip, arm, or leg movements after you stop taking Tofranil. Limit your sun exposure. When you go outdoors, wear a sunscreen, a hat, and protective clothing.

 DRUG INTERACTIONS

Combining certain drugs may alter their action or produce unwanted side effects. Tell your doctor about other drugs you're taking, especially:
• alcohol and other drugs that make you feel relaxed or sleepy, such as tranquilizers, sleeping pills, or cold or allergy drugs
• antidepressants called MAO inhibitors such as Marplan
• barbiturates
• Catapres
• Dilantin
• epinephrine, norepinephrine
• Prozac
• Quinaglute Dura-tabs
• Ritalin
• Tagamet
• tricyclic antidepressants, such as Elavil and Pamelor.

• Don't stop taking Tofranil abruptly. Consult your doctor, who may decrease your dosage gradually to minimize withdrawal effects.

If you miss a dose

If you take one dose a day at bedtime, check with your doctor if you miss a dose. If you take more than one dose a day, take the missed dose as soon as possible. But if it's almost time for your next dose, skip the missed dose and resume your schedule. Don't take a double dose.

If you suspect an overdose

Contact your doctor *immediately*. Excessive Tofranil can cause seizures, confusion, severe drowsiness, restlessness, agitation, stiff muscles, difficulty breathing, vomiting, low blood pressure (dizziness, weakness), and a fast, slow, or irregular heartbeat. Be aware that children are more susceptible to an overdose than adults.

Warnings

• Make sure your doctor knows your medical history. You may not be able to take Tofranil if you are allergic to it, had a recent heart attack, are taking antidepressants called MAO inhibitors, or have suicidal thoughts, difficulty urinating, glaucoma, heart or blood vessel disease, kidney or liver problems, an overactive thyroid, or seizures.
• If you're pregnant or breast-feeding, check with your doctor before taking Tofranil.
• You'll probably take a reduced dose of Tofranil if you're very ill, an older adult, or an adolescent or if you have aggravated psychotic symptoms.
• If you're diabetic and Tofranil alters your sugar levels, call your doctor.

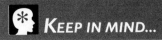

Keep in mind...

* Take with food unless doctor directs otherwise.
* Don't stop taking abruptly.
* Protect yourself from sun.
* Increase fluids and fiber in diet.

Tolectin

Tolectin, a nonsteroidal anti-inflammatory drug (NSAID), prevents the synthesis of prostaglandins, which reduces inflammation, pain, and fever.

Why it's prescribed

Doctors prescribe Tolectin to help control inflammation and pain. It comes in tablets and capsules. Doctors usually prescribe the following amounts.

▶ **For rheumatoid arthritis and osteoarthritis in adults,** 400 milligrams (mg) three or four times a day. Maximum dosage is 1.8 grams a day.

▶ **For juvenile rheumatoid arthritis in children age 2 and over,** initially, 20 mg for each 2.2 pounds (lb) of body weight a day, divided into several equal doses. Maintenance dosage is 15 to 30 mg for each 2.2 lb a day, divided into equal doses.

How to take Tolectin

• Take Tolectin with milk, meals, or an antacid to reduce stomach upset. If you use an antacid, choose one containing magnesium and aluminum hydroxide, such as Maalox.
• Drink a full glass (8 ounces) of water with each dose.
• Although Tolectin should begin working in 1 week, you may not feel its full effects for 2 to 4 weeks. If your pain persists or worsens, let your doctor know.

TOLECTIN'S OTHER NAME

Tolectin's generic name is tolmetin sodium.

SIDE EFFECTS

Call your doctor if you have any of these possible drug side effects. Call *immediately* about any labeled "serious."

Serious: stomach ulcer (abdominal pain, blood in stools), liver problems (yellow-tinged skin and eyes, nausea, vomiting), severe blood problems (fatigue, bleeding, bruising, fever, chills, increased risk of infection), severe allergic reaction (closing up of throat, difficulty breathing)
Tip: NSAIDs can damage your digestive tract without producing pain or other symptoms. When taking Tolectin, watch for bloody or black, tarry stools. If they occur, call your doctor right away.

Common: headache, weight gain

Other: dizziness, drowsiness, ringing in ears, visual disturbances, undetected blood loss (pale skin, weakness), rash, hives, itching, sodium retention (swelling in face, feet, or lower legs)
Tips: Call your doctor right away if you have vision or hearing changes, or swelling. Avoid activities that require full alertness or coordination until you know how Tolectin affects you.

DRUG INTERACTIONS

Combining certain drugs may alter their action or produce unwanted side effects. Tell your doctor about other drugs you're taking, especially:
• alcohol
• anticoagulants (blood thinners) such as Coumadin
• aspirin and other anti-inflammatory drugs
• Dilantin
• Rheumatrex
• thyroid drugs.

If you miss a dose

If your doctor has prescribed Tolectin on a regular schedule and you miss a dose, take the missed dose as soon as you remember. But if it's almost time for your next dose, skip the missed dose and take your next dose as scheduled. Don't take a double dose.

 ### If you suspect an overdose

Contact your doctor *immediately.* Excessive Tolectin can cause dizziness, drowsiness, confusion, and lethargy.

Warnings

• Make sure your doctor knows your medical history. You may not be able to take Tolectin if you're allergic to it; if you develop acute asthma attacks, hives, or cold symptoms when you take aspirin or other NSAIDs; or if you have heart or kidney disease, bleeding in your digestive tract, a history of stomach ulcers, high blood pressure, or a condition that makes you retain fluids.

• Consult your doctor if you're pregnant or breast-feeding before taking Tolectin.

• Tell your doctor if aspirin or any other anti-inflammatory drug has ever caused you to experience asthmalike symptoms, a runny nose, or itching.

• Tolectin can hide the symptoms of an infection. Therefore, if you have diabetes, you need to be especially careful about caring for your feet and watching for any abnormality that might be caused by an infection.

• Don't lie down for 15 to 30 minutes after taking Tolectin. This will help prevent irritation that could cause you to have difficulty swallowing.

• Tell the doctor that you're taking Tolectin before having any medical tests.

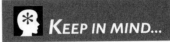

KEEP IN MIND...

* Take with milk, meals, or an antacid.

* Drink glass of water with each dose.

* Don't lie down for 15 to 30 minutes after taking Tolectin.

* Report bloody or black, tarry stools to doctor.

Tolinase

Tolinase is an oral diabetes drug called a sulfonylurea. It's believed to stimulate insulin release from the pancreas, reduce glucose (sugar) output by the liver, and increase your body's sensitivity to insulin.

Why it's prescribed

Doctors prescribe Tolinase to help control diabetes. It comes in tablets. Doctors usually prescribe the following amounts for adults.

▶ **To lower blood sugar levels in type II (non-insulin-dependent) diabetes,** initially, 100 milligrams (mg) a day if fasting blood sugar (FBS) is under 200 mg per deciliter (dl); 250 mg if FBS is over 200 mg per dl. Dosage adjusted once a week by 100 to 250 mg, as needed. Dosage for adults over age 65 is 100 mg once a day. Maximum dosage is 500 mg twice a day.

▶ **To switch from insulin to oral therapy,** if insulin dosage is under 20 units a day, insulin stopped and Tolinase started at 100 mg a day. If insulin dosage is 20 to 40 units a day, insulin stopped and Tolinase started at 250 mg a day. If insulin dosage is over 40 units a day, insulin decreased by 50% and Tolinase started at 250 mg a day. Dosage adjusted by 100 to 250 mg, as needed. Process may require hospitalization.

How to take Tolinase

• Take each dose with food at the same time every day.

 ## SIDE EFFECTS

Call your doctor if you have any of these possible drug side effects. Call *immediately* about any labeled "serious."

Serious: allergic reaction (difficulty breathing, itching, facial swelling), low blood sugar (drowsiness, headache, nervousness, cold sweats, confusion)

Tip: If a mild episode of low blood sugar occurs, eat or drink something sweet, such as candy or orange juice. Severe episodes may require hospitalization.

Common: none reported

Other: nausea, vomiting, rash, hives, facial flushing, sensitivity to sunlight
Tips: To prevent nausea, take Tolinase with food. Protect yourself from the sun by wearing protective clothing, a hat, and sunscreen when you go outdoors.

 ## DRUG INTERACTIONS

Combining certain drugs may alter their action or produce unwanted side effects. Tell your doctor about other drugs you're taking, especially:
• alcohol and other drugs that make you feel relaxed or sleepy, such as tranquilizers, sleeping pills, barbiturates, narcotic pain relievers, muscle relaxants, and cold and allergy drugs
• anabolic steroids or corticosteroids
• anticoagulants (blood thinners) such as Coumadin
• antidepressants called MAO inhibitors such as Marplan
• aspirin
• asthma drugs
• Atromid-S
• Benemid
• blood pressure drugs, such as Catapres, Ismelin, and Lopressor
• Butazolidin
• Chloromycetin
• diet pills
• glucagon
• lithium
• sulfa drugs
• thiazide diuretics (water pills)
• tuberculosis drugs such as Rifadin.

• If your doctor prescribes one dose a day, take it with breakfast. If you're taking two doses a day, take one dose with breakfast and the second dose with your evening meal.

• Don't change your dosage on your own. Instead, report abnormal sugar levels to your doctor.
• Keep taking the drug, even if you feel well. Tolinase doesn't cure dia-

betes; it only relieves the symptoms.

If you miss a dose

Take the missed dose as soon as possible. However, if it's almost time for your next dose, skip the missed dose and take your next dose as scheduled. Don't take a double dose.

If you suspect an overdose

Call your doctor *immediately*. Excessive Tolinase can cause low blood sugar (drowsiness, headache, nervousness, cold sweats, and confusion).

Warnings

• Make sure your doctor knows your medical history. You may not be able to take Tolinase if you're allergic to it, to other oral diabetes drugs, or to diuretics (water pills); if you have insulin-dependent diabetes; if your diabetes can be controlled with diet alone; or if you have severe infection, trauma, or a liver, kidney, adrenal gland, pituitary gland, or thyroid gland disorder.

• Before you begin taking Tolinase, tell your doctor if you're breastfeeding or pregnant.

• Follow your doctor's instructions for testing your blood or urine for sugar. Also closely follow your instructions for diet and exercise.

• Don't take any other drug, including nonprescription drugs, without asking your doctor.

• Always carry medical identification that lists diabetes and Tolinase.

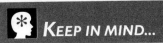

KEEP IN MIND...

* Take with food.
* Take at the same time each day.
* Don't change dosage without doctor's consent.
* Carry candy for mild episodes of low blood sugar.

Tonocard

Tonocard is a heart drug called an antiarrhythmic. It affects the passage of electrical impulses through the heart.

Why it's prescribed

Doctors prescribe Tonocard to correct an irregular heartbeat. It comes in tablets. Doctors usually prescribe the following amounts for adults.

▶ **For reduction of symptomatic life-threatening irregular heartbeats,** initially, 400 milligrams (mg) every 8 hours. Usual dosage is 1,200 to 1,800 mg a day, divided into three equal doses.

How to take Tonocard

• Take the exact amount of the drug prescribed by your doctor.
• Try to take your doses at the same times every day, and space them evenly throughout the day and night.
• Continue to take Tonocard as prescribed, even if you feel well.

If you miss a dose

If you remember your missed dose within 4 hours, take it as soon as possible. If you don't remember until later, skip the missed dose and take your next dose as scheduled. Don't take a double dose.

If you suspect an overdose

Contact your doctor *immediately.* Excessive Tonocard can cause dizziness, vomiting, and confusion.

TONOCARD'S OTHER NAME

Tonocard's generic name is tocainide hydrochloride.

 ## SIDE EFFECTS

Call your doctor if you have any of these possible drug side effects. Call *immediately* about any labeled "serious."

Serious: irregular heartbeat, congestive heart failure or pulmonary fibrosis (shortness of breath, difficulty breathing), blood problems (fatigue, bleeding, bruising, fever, chills, increased risk of infection)

Common: light-headedness, tremor, nausea, vomiting, heartburn
Tips: Avoid activities that require full alertness or coordination until you know how Tonocard affects you. If the drug causes nausea, take it with food or milk.

Other: restlessness, numbness or tingling, confusion, dizziness, low blood pressure (dizziness, weakness), blurred vision, constipation, diarrhea, appetite loss, hepatitis (yellow-tinged skin and eyes), rash
Tips: If you're an older adult, be careful when walking or first getting up out of a chair. Also, have someone take your arm while you're walking. You may be especially prone to dizziness, which could place you at risk for a fall. If any of these side effects become too bothersome, contact your doctor.

 ## DRUG INTERACTIONS

Combining certain drugs may alter their action or produce unwanted side effects. Tell your doctor about other drugs you're taking, especially:
• any new prescription or nonprescription drug
• beta blockers, such as Inderal and Lopressor.

Warnings

• Make sure your doctor knows your medical history. You may not be able to take Tonocard if you are allergic to it, have had an allergic reaction to an anesthetic (such as lidocaine), or have kidney or liver disease, a bone marrow disorder, congestive heart failure, or some other heart problem.
• If you're pregnant or breast-feeding, consult your doctor before taking Tonocard.

• Tell your doctor or dentist you're taking Tonocard before having any kind of surgery, dental work, or emergency treatment.

KEEP IN MIND...

* Take evenly spaced doses day and night.

* Take at same times each day.

* Take with food or milk if drug causes nausea.

* If you're older, have assistance while walking about.

Topicort

Topicort is a medium-strength corticosteroid that reduces inflammation and itching and constricts blood vessels.

Why it's prescribed

Doctors prescribe Topicort to relieve inflamed, itchy skin. It comes in a cream, a gel, and an ointment. Doctors usually prescribe the following amounts for adults and children.

▶ **For inflammation associated with certain skin reactions,** a small amount of cream, gel, or ointment applied twice a day.

How to use Topicort

• Before applying Topicort, gently wash and dry the area to be treated.
• To prevent skin damage, rub the drug in gently, leaving a thin coat. When treating hairy sites, part the hair and apply directly to the skin.
• Don't use Topicort near your eyes, and don't get it on mucous membranes or in your ear canals.
• Don't cover the treated area with a bandage unless your doctor tells you to. If your doctor tells you to use an airtight dressing, don't use it on infected areas or weeping sores, and don't leave it in place longer than 16 hours each day.
• If you're using a dressing and your skin is usually irritated by adhesive material, hold the dressing in place with gauze, elastic bandages, or stockings.
• If you're treating a baby's diaper area, don't cover it with rubber

pants or a tight diaper. The baby could absorb too much of the drug through the skin.
• Keep using Topicort for a few days after your skin clears up to prevent your infection from recurring.

If you miss a dose

Apply the missed dose as soon as possible. However, if it's almost time for your next dose, skip the missed dose and apply your next dose as scheduled. Don't apply a double dose.

If you suspect an overdose

Consult your doctor.

Warnings

• Make sure your doctor knows your medical history. You may not be able to use Topicort if you're allergic to it or if you have glaucoma, cataracts, diabetes, an infection or

sores in the area to be treated, or tuberculosis.
• If you're pregnant or breast-feeding, tell your doctor before you start using Topicort.
• If you're diabetic and the drug increases your sugar levels, call your doctor.
• Tell your doctor if you develop a fever, especially if you're using an airtight dressing.

SIDE EFFECTS

Call your doctor if you have any of these possible drug side effects. Call *immediately* about any labeled "serious."

Serious: decreased natural steroid level (inability to recover from surgery, infections, and other stress)

Common: skin breakdown, new infection, small bumps caused by blocked sweat ducts

Other: burning, itching, irritation, dryness or redness of skin; irritated hair follicles; hair growth; acnelike eruptions; inflammation around mouth; reduced pigmentation; Cushing's syndrome (unusual tiredness, irritability, round face, backache, irregular menstrual periods); increased sugar levels (increased thirst, hunger, and urination)

DRUG INTERACTIONS

Combining certain drugs may alter their action or produce unwanted side effects. Tell your doctor about other drugs you're taking.

KEEP IN MIND...

* Apply a thin coating to affected area.

* Don't use near eyes, on mucous membranes, or in ear canals.

* Bandage only if directed.

* Keep using for a few days after skin clears up.

TOPICORT'S OTHER NAME

Topicort's generic name is desoximetasone.

Toprol XL

Toprol XL reduces the heart's workload, slows the heart rate, lowers blood pressure, and reduces the amount of oxygen the heart consumes.

Why it's prescribed

Doctors prescribe Toprol XL to reduce high blood pressure (hypertension), ease chest pain (angina), and treat heart attack. It comes in slow-release tablets. Doctors usually prescribe these amounts for adults.

▶ **For high blood pressure,** initially, 50 milligrams (mg) twice a day or 100 mg once a day, up to 450 mg a day divided into two or three equal doses.

▶ **For angina,** initially, 100 mg a day as a single dose or divided into two equal doses, increased at weekly intervals, as needed, until adequate response or pronounced decrease in heart rate achieved.

▶ **For early treatment of heart attack,** initially, three doses given intravenously. Then, beginning 15 minutes after the last dose, 25 to 50 mg orally every 6 hours for 48 hours. Maintenance dosage is 100 mg twice a day for at least 3 months, possibly 1 to 3 years.

How to take Toprol XL

• Check your pulse before taking Toprol XL. If it's below 60 beats per

TOPROL **XL**'S OTHER NAMES

Toprol XL's generic name is metoprolol succinate. Brand names of a similar drug, metoprolol tartrate, include Lopressor; and, in Canada, Apo-Metoprolol, Apo-Metoprolol (Type L), Betaloc Durules, Lopresor, Lopresor SR, Novometoprol, and Nu-Metop.

SIDE EFFECTS

Call your doctor if you have any of these possible drug side effects. Call *immediately* about any labeled "serious."

Serious: congestive heart failure (shortness of breath, difficulty breathing), asthmalike attacks (wheezing, difficulty breathing)

Common: slow heartbeat, low blood pressure (dizziness, weakness)

Other: fatigue, lethargy, peripheral vascular disease, nausea, vomiting, diarrhea, rash, fever, joint pain

DRUG INTERACTIONS

Combining certain drugs may alter their action or produce unwanted side effects. Tell your doctor about other drugs you're taking, especially:
• barbiturates
• Calan
• Cardizem
• heart drugs called digitalis glycosides
• Indocin
• insulin and oral diabetes drugs
• Rifadin
• Tagamet
• Thorazine.

minute, call the doctor before taking your dose.
• Take the drug with meals.
• Don't stop taking Toprol XL abruptly.

If you miss a dose

Take the missed dose as soon as possible. However, if it's almost time for your next dose, skip the missed dose and take your next dose as scheduled. Don't take a double dose.

If you suspect an overdose

Contact your doctor *immediately.* Excessive Toprol XL can cause a slow or irregular heartbeat, dizziness, weakness, and difficulty breathing.

Warnings

• Let your doctor know your medical history. You may not be able to take Toprol XL if you are allergic to similar drugs or have certain types of heart disease, diabetes, or lung or liver disease.
• Tell your doctor if you're pregnant or wish to breast-feed.

KEEP IN MIND...

∗ Check pulse before taking.

∗ Take with food.

∗ Don't stop taking abruptly.

∗ If diabetic, monitor sugar levels carefully.

Toradol

Toradol is a nonsteroidal anti-inflammatory drug (NSAID) that prevents the synthesis of prostaglandins, which reduces inflammation and pain.

Why it's prescribed

Doctors prescribe Toradol to relieve pain on a short-term basis. It comes in tablets. Doctors usually prescribe the following amounts for adults.

▶ **For short-term (up to 15 days) pain relief,** 10 milligrams every 4 to 6 hours, as needed.

How to take Toradol

- Take Toradol exactly as your doctor directs.
- Drink a full glass (8 ounces) of water with each dose.
- Don't lie down for 15 to 30 minutes after taking Toradol to reduce the chance of irritating your esophagus.

If you miss a dose

Take the missed dose as soon as possible. However, if it's almost time for your next dose, skip the missed dose and take your next dose as scheduled. Don't take a double dose.

 If you suspect an overdose

Consult your doctor.

 Warnings

- Make sure your doctor knows your medical history. You may not

TORADOL'S OTHER NAME

Toradol's generic name is ketorolac tromethamine.

 SIDE EFFECTS

Call your doctor if you have any of these possible drug side effects.

Serious: none reported

Common: drowsiness, sedation, headache, stomach upset or pain
Tips: Avoid driving and other potentially hazardous activities until you know how Toradol affects you. To reduce stomach upset, take this drug with food or an antacid.

Other: sweating, high blood pressure (headache, blurred vision), diarrhea, stomach ulcer (black or bloody stools), increased bleeding time, unusual bruising
Tip: Toradol can damage your stomach without producing pain or discomfort. Call your doctor right away if you have bloody or black, tarry stools.

 DRUG INTERACTIONS

Combining certain drugs may alter their action or produce unwanted side effects. Tell your doctor about other drugs you're taking, especially:
- alcohol
- anticoagulants (blood thinners) such as Coumadin
- aspirin and other salicylates
- Benemid
- Cefobid, Cefotan
- Depakene
- diuretics (water pills) for high blood pressure
- Eskalith
- Mandol
- Mithracin
- Moxam
- Rheumatrex
- tobacco.

be able to take Toradol if you're allergic to it, aspirin, or other NSAIDs, or if you have liver or kidney problems, asthma, lupus, diabetes, a stomach ulcer or other serious digestive problems, heart disease, high blood pressure, a blood clotting problem, or swelling of the face, hands, or lower legs.
- Before you begin taking Toradol, tell your doctor if you're pregnant or you wish to breast-feed.

 KEEP IN MIND...

* Take with food or an antacid.
* Drink glass of water with each dose.
* Don't lie down for 15 to 30 minutes after taking a dose.
* Watch for black or bloody stools.

Torecan

Torecan is one of a group of drugs known as phenothiazines. It probably acts on the vomiting center in the brain, controlling nausea and vomiting.

Why it's prescribed

Doctors prescribe Torecan to treat nausea, vomiting, and sometimes dizziness (but not motion sickness). It comes in tablets. Doctors usually prescribe the following amounts for adults.

▶ **For nausea and vomiting,** 10 milligrams two or three times a day.

How to take Torecan

• Don't take more Torecan or take it more often than your doctor prescribes.

• Take each dose with food or with a full glass (8 ounces) of water to reduce stomach upset.

If you miss a dose

Take the missed dose as soon as possible. But if it's almost time for your next dose, skip the missed dose and take your next dose as scheduled. Don't take a double dose.

 If you suspect an overdose

Consult your doctor.

 Warnings

• Make sure your doctor knows your medical history. You may not be able to take Torecan if you're allergic to it, to other phenothiazines,

TORECAN'S OTHER NAMES

Torecan's generic name is thiethylperazine maleate. Another brand name is Norzine.

 SIDE EFFECTS

Call your doctor if you have any of these possible drug side effects. Call *immediately* about any labeled "serious."

Serious: blood problems (fatigue, bleeding, bruising, fever, chills, increased risk of infection), allergic reaction (fever, difficulty breathing, closing up of the throat)

Common: uncontrollable muscle movements, low blood pressure (dizziness, weakness), altered or blurred vision, dry mouth, constipation, inability to urinate, yellow-tinged skin and eyes, sensitivity to sun
Tips: To relieve dry mouth and throat, try sugarless gum or hard candy or ice chips. If dryness persists for 2 weeks or more, call your doctor. Wear sunscreen, a hat, and protective clothing outdoors.

Other: sleepiness, parkinson-like movements, confusion (especially in elderly patients), rapid or altered pulse, dark urine, menstrual irregularities, inhibited ejaculation, breast enlargement in men, weight gain, increased appetite

 DRUG INTERACTIONS

Combining certain drugs may alter their action or cause unwanted side effects. Tell your doctor about other drugs you're taking, especially:
• alcohol and other drugs that make you feel relaxed or sleepy, such as tranquilizers, sleeping pills, barbiturates, narcotic pain relievers, and cold and allergy drugs
• antidepressants and other drugs for mental illness
• atropine
• Levodopa
• Serpasil.

or to aspirin or if you have liver disease, a depressed central nervous system, asthma or other lung disease, heart or blood vessel disease, difficulty urinating, an enlarged prostate, glaucoma, Parkinson's disease, or seizures.

• Tell your doctor right away if you think you're pregnant.

• If you'll be taking Torecan for a long time, your doctor will probably want to see you regularly to check on your progress and to adjust your dosage if necessary.

• Tell the doctor you're taking Torecan before you have any medical test or procedure, especially if it involves an injection into the spinal cord.

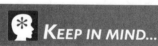 **KEEP IN MIND...**

* Take with food or full glass of water.

* Take only amount prescribed.

* Relieve dry mouth with sugarless gum or candy or ice chips.

* Protect yourself from sun.

Tornalate

Tornalate relaxes the muscles in the lower airways to permit easier breathing.

Why it's prescribed

Doctors prescribe Tornalate to relieve asthma and closing up of the throat (bronchospasm). It comes in an aerosol inhaler. Doctors usually prescribe the following amounts for adults and children over age 12.

▶ **To treat bronchial asthma and bronchospasm,** 2 inhalations separated by 2 to 3 minutes, followed by a 3rd inhalation after 2 to 3 minutes, if needed. Maximum dosage is 3 inhalations every 6 hours or 2 inhalations every 4 hours.

▶ **To prevent bronchospasm,** 2 inhalations every 8 hours. Maximum dosage is 3 inhalations every 6 hours or 2 inhalations every 4 hours.

How to take Tornalate

• Make sure you know how to use the inhaler properly.
• Don't take more Tornalate than prescribed; doing so could raise your heart rate.
• If you're also using a steroid inhaler, use Tornalate first, and then wait about 15 minutes before using the steroid inhaler. This way, Tornalate has a chance to open your air passages, which increases the steroid's effectiveness.
• Don't let the spray from your inhaler get in your eyes.
• Rinse your mouth after each dose to keep the drug from drying your mouth.

TORNALATE'S OTHER NAME

Tornalate's generic name is bitolterol mesylate.

 SIDE EFFECTS

Call your doctor if you have any of these possible drug side effects. Call *immediately* about any labeled "serious."

Serious: bronchospasm (wheezing, difficulty breathing), allergic reaction (bluish skin, severe dizziness, flushing, increased trouble breathing, hives, itching)

Common: tremor, changes in blood pressure (dizziness and weakness or headache and blurred vision)

Other: nervousness, light-headedness, palpitations, chest discomfort, rapid heartbeat, throat irritation, shortness of breath, cough, nausea

 DRUG INTERACTIONS

Combining certain drugs may alter their action or produce unwanted side effects. Tell your doctor about other drugs you're taking.

• After using your inhaler, rinse the plastic mouthpiece in warm water and dry it.
• Tornalate's beneficial effects last up to 8 hours.

If you miss a dose

Take the missed dose as soon as possible. Then take your remaining doses for that day at regularly spaced intervals. Don't take a double dose.

If you suspect an overdose

Contact your doctor *immediately.* Excessive Tornalate can cause a fast or irregular pulse, tremor, nausea, and vomiting.

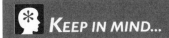 Warnings

• Make sure your doctor knows your medical history. You may not be able to take Tornalate if you're allergic to it or to similar drugs or if you have heart disease, high blood pressure, mental illness, an overactive thyroid, diabetes, or seizures.
• Tell your doctor right away if you think you're pregnant or wish to breast-feed.
• Call your doctor immediately if you still can't breathe 1 hour after using Tornalate, if your symptoms return within 4 hours, or if your breathing problem gets worse.

KEEP IN MIND...

∗ Don't use more than prescribed.
∗ Use inhaler properly.
∗ Call doctor if Tornalate doesn't control symptoms.
∗ Rinse mouth after each dose.
∗ Rinse and dry inhaler after each use.

Totacillin

Totacillin is an antibiotic related to penicillin. It kills bacteria by preventing them from multiplying.

Why it's prescribed

Doctors prescribe Totacillin to treat bacterial infections. It comes in capsules and a liquid. Another brand, Totacillin-N, comes in an injectable form. Doctors usually prescribe the following amounts for adults; children's dosages appear in parentheses.

▶ **For body-wide infections and acute and chronic urinary tract infections,** 250 to 500 milligrams (mg) orally every 6 hours. (Children weighing 44 pounds [lb] or more: same as adults. Children weighing 44 lb or less: 50 to 100 mg orally for each 2.2 lb of body weight, divided into four equal doses taken every 6 hours.)

▶ For gonorrhea, 3.5 grams (g) orally along with 1 g of probenecid taken as a single dose. (Children weighing over 99 lb: same as adults.)

▶ To prevent endocarditis (heart infection) during dental procedures, 1 to 2 g injected into a muscle or a vein along with 1.5 mg of gentamicin for each 2.2 lb of body weight (not to exceed 80 mg) ½ hour before the procedure; then, 1.5 g of amoxicillin orally 6 hours after the first dose. (Children: 50 mg for each 2.2 lb, injected into a muscle or a vein ½ hour before the procedure; then, 25 mg of amoxicillin orally for each 2.2 lb 6 hours after the first dose.)

TOTACILLIN'S OTHER NAMES

Totacillin's generic name is ampicillin. Other brand names include D-Amp, Polycillin, Principen, Nu-Ampi, Omnipen; and, in Canada, Apo-Ampi and Novo-Ampicillin.

SIDE EFFECTS

Call your doctor if you have any of these possible drug side effects. Call *immediately* about any labeled "serious."

Serious: severe allergic reaction (difficulty breathing, rash, hives, itching, wheezing), blood problems (fatigue, bleeding, bruising, fever, chills)

Common: nausea, diarrhea

Tip: Don't take any drug for diarrhea without first checking with your doctor; it could make your diarrhea worse or last longer.

Other: vomiting, swollen or inflamed tongue

DRUG INTERACTIONS

Combining certain drugs may alter their action or produce unwanted side effects. Tell your doctor about other drugs you're taking, especially:
- antibiotics
- birth control pills that contain estrogen (use different or additional birth control method when taking Totacillin)
- Mexate
- Zyloprim.

How to take Totacillin

- To keep a steady level of this drug in your blood, space doses throughout the day and night.
- Take Totacillin with 8 ounces of water on an empty stomach.
- Swallow capsules whole; don't break, chew, or crush them.
- If you're taking the liquid, use a specially marked measuring spoon.

If you miss a dose

Take the missed dose as soon as possible. If you take at least three a day, space the missed dose and the next dose 2 to 4 hours apart. Then go back to your regular schedule. Don't take a double dose.

If you suspect an overdose

Contact your doctor *immediately.* Excessive Totacillin can cause seizures.

Warnings

- Make sure your doctor knows your medical history. You may not be able to take Totacillin if you have allergies or other medical problems or are breast-feeding.
- If you have diabetes, Totacillin may cause false test results with some urine sugar tests.
- If your symptoms don't improve within a few days or if they become worse, check with your doctor.

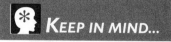

KEEP IN MIND...

- Space doses evenly throughout day and night.
- Take with water on empty stomach.
- Supplement birth control pills.

Trandate

Trandate is one of a group of heart drugs called beta blockers. These drugs reduce the heart's workload and help it beat more steadily by altering the body's response to certain nerve impulses.

Why it's prescribed

Doctors prescribe Trandate to control high blood pressure. It comes in tablets. Doctors usually prescribe the following amounts for adults.

▶ **For high blood pressure,** 100 milligrams (mg) twice a day, with or without a diuretic (water pill). Dosage increased by 100 mg twice a day every 2 to 4 days, as needed, until best response reached. Maintenance dosage is 200 to 400 mg twice a day.

How to take Trandate

• Take Trandate exactly as prescribed — no more, no less.
• Don't stop taking Trandate without your doctor's consent.

If you miss a dose

Take the missed dose as soon as possible. But if it's almost time for your next dose, skip the missed dose and take your next dose as scheduled. Don't take a double dose.

If you suspect an overdose

Contact your doctor *immediately.* Excessive Trandate can cause very low blood pressure (dizziness, weakness), slow pulse, heart failure, and asthmalike attacks.

TRANDATE'S OTHER NAMES

Trandate's generic name is labetalol. Another brand name is Normodyne.

SIDE EFFECTS

Call your doctor if you have any of these possible drug side effects.

Serious: none reported

Common: insomnia, weakness, tiredness, impotence, dizziness and light-headedness (especially early in treatment), cold fingers and toes
Tips: Avoid activities that require full alertness or coordination until you know how Trandate affects you. To reduce dizziness, stand up slowly and change positions carefully.

Other: vivid dreams, fatigue, headache, low blood pressure (dizziness, weakness), slow pulse, rash, tingling scalp (early in treatment), stuffy nose, low blood sugar (drowsiness, headache, nervousness, cold sweats, confusion), nausea, vomiting, stomach upset, difficulty urinating, yellow-tinged skin and eyes, wheezing

DRUG INTERACTIONS

Combining certain drugs may alter their action or produce unwanted side effects. Tell your doctor about other drugs you're taking, especially:
• alcohol and other drugs that make you feel relaxed or sleepy, such as tranquilizers, sleeping pills, and cold and allergy drugs
• allergy shots or skin tests
• antidepressants called MAO inhibitors such as Marplan
• caffeine-containing products
• calcium channel blockers
• Catapres
• Choledyl
• insulin and oral diabetes drugs
• Lufyllin or Theo-Dur
• Wytensin.

Warnings

• Make sure your doctor knows your medical history. You may not be able to take Trandate if you have heart or vascular disease, asthma, diabetes, or liver problems.
• Tell your doctor if you're pregnant or breast-feeding.
• Trandate won't cure high blood pressure; it will only control it.
• Be sure to follow any prescribed diet changes, especially sodium (salt) restriction and weight loss.
• Trandate may mask chest pain caused by overexertion. Talk to your doctor about a safe level of exercise.

✱ KEEP IN MIND...

∗ Don't stop taking abruptly.

∗ If prescribed, lose weight and reduce sodium (salt) in diet.

∗ Consult doctor about appropriate exercise level.

∗ Get up slowly until dizziness subsides.

Transderm-Scōp

Transderm-Scōp affects nerves in the inner ear that communicate with the part of the brain that controls vomiting.

Why it's prescribed

Doctors prescribe Transderm-Scōp to prevent nausea and vomiting caused by motion sickness. It comes in a small patch called a transdermal disk. Doctors usually prescribe the following amounts for adults.

▶ **To prevent nausea and vomiting from motion sickness,** 1 disk placed behind ear at least 4 hours before effect is desired and left in place for up to 3 days.

How to use Transderm-Scōp

• Follow your doctor's instructions exactly. Also, carefully read the directions that come with the disk.
• For best results, apply the disk about 12 hours before your trip. If necessary, however, you can apply it 4 hours beforehand.
• Wash your hands before and after applying the disk.
• Apply the disk to a dry, hairless area of skin behind your ear. Don't place it over any cuts or irritations on your skin.
• If the disk loosens, remove it and apply a new disk on another clean area behind the ear.
• When you no longer need the drug, remove and discard the disk. Wash your hands and the skin that was under the disk.
• The disk delivers the drug for up to 3 days (72 hours). Don't wear it for more than 3 days or you could experience unwanted effects.

TRANSDERM-SCŌP'S OTHER NAME

Transderm-Scōp's generic name is scopolamine.

 SIDE EFFECTS

Call your doctor if you have any of these possible drug side effects.

Serious: none reported

Common: dry mouth, constipation, vomiting, stomach upset
Tips: To relieve dry mouth, try sugarless gum or hard candy or ice chips. To reduce constipation, drink more fluids and eat plenty of fiber-rich foods.

Other: disorientation, restlessness, irritability, dizziness, drowsiness, headache, confusion, palpitations, slow pulse, unequally dilated pupils, blurred vision, sensitivity to light, increased pressure in eyes (headache, eye pain), difficulty swallowing, difficulty urinating, slow breathing, rash, flushing, dry skin, irritation under patch, fever, increased sensitivity to hot, humid environments

 DRUG INTERACTIONS

Combining certain drugs may alter their action or produce unwanted side effects. Tell your doctor about other drugs you're taking, especially:
• alcohol and other drugs that make you feel relaxed or sleepy, such as tranquilizers, sleeping pills, and cold and allergy drugs
• antacids
• drugs for depression called MAO inhibitors such as Marplan
• drugs for diarrhea
• Lanoxin
• Nizoral
• potassium supplements.

If you miss a dose

Not applicable because disk is only used as needed.

 If you suspect an overdose

Contact your doctor *immediately*. Excessive Transderm-Scōp can cause disorientation, hallucinations, and seizures.

 Warnings

• Make sure your doctor knows your medical history. You may not be able to use Transderm-Scōp if you're allergic to it or if you have glaucoma, asthma, lung or heart disease, high blood pressure, myasthenia gravis, hiatal hernia with reflux esophagitis, kidney or liver problems, an overactive thyroid, or bowel problems.
• If you're breast-feeding, check with your doctor before you use this disk.

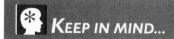 **KEEP IN MIND...**

* Apply 12 hours before trip to dry, hairless area behind ear.
* Wash hands before and after application.
* Don't wear disk more than 3 days.

Tranxene

Tranxene slows down the central nervous system, which slows the spread of seizures and decreases anxiety and symptoms of alcohol withdrawal.

Why it's prescribed

Doctors prescribe Tranxene to prevent seizures and to relieve extreme nervousness or tension. It comes in tablets and capsules. Doctors usually prescribe the following amounts for adults; where appropriate, children's dosages appear in parentheses.

▶ **For anxiety,** 15 to 60 milligrams (mg) a day.

▶ **For epilepsy,** initially, maximum of 7.5 mg three times a day, increased by no more than 7.5 mg a week. Maximum dosage is 90 mg a day. (Children over age 12: same as adults. Children ages 9 to 12: initially, maximum of 7.5 mg twice a day, increased by no more than 7.5 mg a week. Maximum dosage is 60 mg a day.)

▶ **For acute alcohol withdrawal,** first day, 30 mg initially, followed by 30 to 60 mg divided into equal doses. Second day, 45 to 90 mg divided into equal doses. Third day, 22.5 to 45 mg divided into equal doses. Fourth day, 15 to 30 mg divided into equal doses. Then, dosage gradually reduced to 7.5 to 15 mg a day until withdrawal is complete.

TRANXENE'S OTHER NAMES

Tranxene's generic name is clorazepate dipotassium. Other brand names include Gen-XENE; and, in Canada, Apo-Clorazepate and Novoclopate.

 SIDE EFFECTS

Call your doctor if you have any of these possible drug side effects.

Serious: none reported

Common: drowsiness, lethargy, "hangover" feeling

Other: fainting, restlessness, strange behavior, temporary low blood pressure (dizziness, weakness), visual disturbances, nausea, vomiting, abdominal discomfort, dry mouth, trouble urinating, reduced bladder control

Tip: To minimize dry mouth, try sugarless gum or hard candy or ice chips.

 DRUG INTERACTIONS

Combining certain drugs may alter their action or produce unwanted side effects. Tell your doctor about other drugs you're taking, especially:

• alcohol and other drugs that make you feel relaxed or sleepy, such as tranquilizers, sleeping pills, and cold and allergy drugs
• Lanoxin
• Tagamet
• tobacco.

How to take Tranxene

• Because this drug can be habit-forming, follow your doctor's instructions exactly.
• If you're taking Tranxene for seizures, take it in regularly spaced doses, day and night.
• If you've been taking this drug for a long time, don't stop abruptly.

If you miss a dose

Take the missed dose right away if you remember within an hour or so. If you don't remember until later, skip the missed dose and take your next dose as scheduled. Don't take a double dose.

 If you suspect an overdose

Contact your doctor *immediately.* Excessive Tranxene can cause slurred speech, confusion, staggering, and severe drowsiness.

Warnings

• Make sure your doctor knows your medical history. You may not be able to take Tranxene if you're allergic to it or if you have glaucoma, myasthenia gravis, Parkinson's disease, kidney or liver disease, or a history of mental illness or drug abuse.

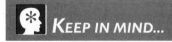 **KEEP IN MIND...**

∗ Take only as prescribed; drug is habit-forming.

∗ Don't stop taking abruptly.

∗ For seizures, space doses evenly throughout day and night.

∗ To relieve dry mouth, try sugarless gum or hard candy or ice chips.

Trental

Trental increases circulation by boosting the amount of blood that flows through blood vessels in the legs.

Why it's prescribed

Doctors prescribe Trental to reduce leg pain and cramps caused by poor circulation. It comes in slow-release tablets. Doctors usually prescribe the following amounts for adults.

▶ **For leg cramps caused by narrowed blood vessels,** 400 milligrams three times a day.

How to take Trental

• Swallow the tablets whole — don't chew, crush, or break them.
• Be aware that you may not feel better for several weeks.
• You'll need at least 8 weeks of therapy with Trental. In the meantime, don't stop taking it without first consulting your doctor.

If you miss a dose

Take the missed dose as soon as possible. However, if it's almost time for your next dose, skip the missed dose and take your next dose as scheduled. Don't take a double dose.

 If you suspect an overdose

Contact your doctor *immediately*. Excessive Trental can cause agita-

TRENTAL'S OTHER NAME

Trental's generic name is pentoxifylline.

 SIDE EFFECTS

Call your doctor if you have any of these possible drug side effects.
Serious: none reported
Common: none reported
Other: headache, dizziness, stomach upset, vomiting
Tips: Tell your doctor if you develop any of these symptoms. You may need a lower dosage. To lessen stomach upset, take your doses with meals or an antacid, unless your doctor tells you otherwise.

 DRUG INTERACTIONS

Combining certain drugs may alter their action or produce unwanted side effects. Tell your doctor about other drugs you're taking, especially:
• anticoagulants (blood thinners) such as Coumadin
• blood pressure drugs
• tobacco.

tion, fever, seizures, and loss of consciousness.

Warnings

• Make sure your doctor knows your medical history. You may not be able to take Trental if you're allergic to it, to caffeine, or to any foods or drugs or if you have liver or kidney problems, stomach ulcer, or recent bleeding in the brain or eye.
• Before you begin taking Trental, tell your doctor if you're pregnant or wish to breast-feed.
• Be aware that older adults may be especially prone to Trental's side effects.
• Your doctor may want to test your blood pressure and blood clotting time routinely while you're taking Trental, especially if you're also taking an anticoagulant

(blood thinner) or a drug for high blood pressure. Be sure to keep all follow-up appointments.
• Because nicotine can narrow your blood vessels and reduce circulation, cigarette smoking may worsen your condition. Therefore, if you smoke, you should try to quit.

 KEEP IN MIND...

∗ Don't crush or chew tablets.
∗ Take with meals or antacid.
∗ Don't stop taking abruptly.
∗ Quit smoking.
∗ Keep all doctor's appointments.

Triavil

Triavil is a combination of two drugs: a tranquilizer and an antidepressant. Triavil achieves its effects without dulling the senses.

Why it's prescribed

Doctors prescribe Triavil to treat moderate to severe depression, anxiety, and agitation, as well as other mental disorders. It comes in tablets. Doctors usually prescribe the following amounts for adults.

▶ **For moderate to severe depression, anxiety, or agitation,** 1 tablet three or four times a day, increased as needed. Maintenance dosage is 1 tablet two to four times a day.

How to take Triavil

- Follow your doctor's directions exactly.
- Take Triavil with food or right after meals, unless otherwise directed.
- Don't increase the dose or take the drug more often than prescribed.
- Triavil may take several weeks to produce its full effect.
- Don't stop taking this drug abruptly.

If you miss a dose

Take the missed dose as soon as possible. However, if you remember within 2 hours of your next dose, skip the missed dose and take your next dose as scheduled. Don't take a double dose.

TRIAVIL'S OTHER NAMES

Triavil is a combination of two generic drugs: amitriptyline and perphenazine. Other brand names include Etrafon; and, in Canada, Elavil Plus and PMS Levazine.

SIDE EFFECTS

Call your doctor if you have any of these possible drug side effects. Call *immediately* about any labeled "serious."

Serious: uncontrollable muscle movements, seizures, difficulty breathing, extreme tiredness, fast pulse, vision changes, bruising, bleeding, yellow-tinged eyes or skin

Common: drowsiness, dizziness, dry mouth, nasal congestion
Tips: Avoid activities that require full alertness or coordination until you know how Triavil affects you. Minimize dizziness by standing up slowly from a lying or sitting position and being careful while walking. To relieve dry mouth, suck on ice chips or hard candy, or chew sugarless gum.

Other: low blood pressure (dizziness, weakness), swelling of hands and feet, muscle weakness, mild insomnia, headache, allergic reaction (difficulty breathing, itching, rash, hives), increased sweating, menstrual irregularities, incontinence, fainting, confusion, constipation, heartburn, abdominal pain, appetite loss, nausea, vomiting, diarrhea, fever, hair loss, prolonged erection, decreased sex drive, ringing in ears
Tip: Avoid constipation by increasing fluids and high-fiber foods in your diet.

DRUG INTERACTIONS

Combining certain drugs may alter their action or produce unwanted side effects. Tell your doctor about other drugs you're taking, especially:
- alcohol and other drugs that make you relaxed or sleepy, such as tranquilizers, sleeping pills, and cold and allergy drugs
- amphetamines or diet pills
- antacids or drugs for diarrhea (take at least 2 hours before or after Triavil)
- blood pressure drugs, such as Aldomet and Desmer
- Cylert
- drugs for depression called MAO inhibitors, such as Marplan, and tricyclic antidepressants, such as Pamelor and Elavil
- drugs for seizures such as Dilantin
- dyes used in certain medical tests
- epinephrine
- Eskalith, Lithobid
- levodopa
- Orap
- Phenergan
- rauwolfia alkaloids such as Serpasil
- Reglan
- Tagamet
- Temaril
- thyroid drugs.

Continued on next page ▶

If you suspect an overdose

Contact your doctor *immediately*. Excessive Triavil can cause confusion, hallucinations, low body temperature, seizures, low blood pressure (dizziness, weakness), drowsiness, rapid heartbeat, dilated pupils, coma, rigid muscles, vomiting, and agitation.

Warnings

• Make sure your doctor knows your medical history. You may not be able to take Triavil if you're allergic to it or if you have glaucoma, trouble urinating, or a history of seizures.
• If you're pregnant or breast-feeding, talk to your doctor before taking Triavil.

• Triavil is not recommended for children.
• Be aware that older adults may be especially prone to Triavil's side effects.
• You may need to take a maintenance dosage, usually lower than the initial dosage, for a couple of weeks or months, depending on your condition.
• Triavil may raise your risk of heat stroke if you exercise too vigorously in the heat. So ask your doctor about a level of exercise that's safe for you.
• Before you have surgery, dental work, or emergency treatment, tell the doctor or dentist that you're taking Triavil.

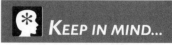

KEEP IN MIND...

* Take with food or right after meals.
* Don't take within 2 hours of antacids or drugs for diarrhea.
* Don't stop taking abruptly.
* Report any uncontrollable muscle movements.

Tridione

Tridione acts on the central nervous system to make it more difficult for seizures to start.

Why it's prescribed

Doctors prescribe Tridione to reduce the number of seizures in people with epilepsy. It comes in capsules, chewable tablets, and a liquid. Doctors usually prescribe the following amounts for adults; children's dosages appear in parentheses.

▶ **For absence seizures not responsive to other treatment,** initially, 300 milligrams (mg) three times a day, increased by 300 mg a day at weekly intervals, as needed, to maximum of 600 mg four times a day. (Children over age 13: same as adults. Children ages 6 to 13: 300 mg three times a day. Children ages 2 to 5: 200 mg three times a day. Children under age 2, 100 mg three times a day.)

How to take Tridione

• Take Tridione at evenly spaced intervals, as your doctor prescribes.
• If you prefer, ask your doctor if you can chew the tablets or crush them in a little water.
• Unless your doctor says otherwise, you can take Tridione with a little food or milk if it upsets your stomach.
• Don't stop taking Tridione abruptly; this could cause seizures.

If you miss a dose

Take the missed dose as soon as possible. However, if it's almost time for your next dose, skip the missed

TRIDIONE'S OTHER NAME

Tridione's generic name is trimethadione.

 SIDE EFFECTS

Call your doctor if you have any of these possible drug side effects. Call *immediately* about any labeled "serious."

Serious: blood problems (fatigue, bleeding, bruising, fever, chills, increased risk of infection), high blood pressure (headache, blurred vision), low blood pressure (dizziness, weakness), kidney problems (decreased urination), liver problems (yellow-tinged skin and eyes, nausea, vomiting), lupuslike syndrome (abdominal pain, difficulty swallowing, rash, fatigue), myasthenic syndrome (muscle weakness)

Common: drowsiness, overall feeling of illness, day blindness
Tips: Avoid activities that require full alertness or coordination until you know how Tridione affects you. If bright light blurs your vision, tell your doctor.

Other: insomnia, tingling or numbness, irritability, double vision, eye sensitivity to light, nosebleeds, bleeding in eye (impaired vision, floaters), nausea, vomiting, appetite loss, vaginal bleeding, hair loss, acne, skin sensitivity to sun, swollen glands
Tips: Wear a sunscreen, a hat, and protective clothing when you go outdoors. Avoid prolonged exposure to sunlight.

 DRUG INTERACTIONS

Combining certain drugs can alter their action or produce unwanted side effects. Tell your doctor about other drugs you're taking, especially:
• Mesantoin
• Phenurone.

dose and take your next dose as scheduled. Don't take a double dose.

 If you suspect an overdose

Contact your doctor *immediately.* Excessive Tridione can cause nausea, drowsiness, loss of balance, and coma.

Warnings

• Make sure your doctor knows your medical history. You may not be able to take Tridione if you're allergic to it or if you have diseases of the eye or optic nerve, porphyria, or severe blood or liver problems.

• Use a reliable form of birth control while taking Tridione. Tell your doctor right away if you think you're pregnant.

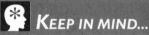 **KEEP IN MIND...**

* Take at evenly spaced intervals.
* May chew or crush tablets or take with food.
* Don't stop taking abruptly.
* Use reliable birth control.
* Wear sunscreen and protective clothing outdoors.

Trilafon

Trilafon is believed to block the use of dopamine in the brain. This action makes it effective in treating psychosis (mental illness), nausea, and vomiting.

Why it's prescribed

Doctors prescribe Trilafon to treat psychosis and to relieve severe nausea or vomiting. Trilafon comes in tablets and a concentrated liquid. It's also available in an injectable form. Doctors usually prescribe the following amounts for adults; where appropriate, children's dosages appear in parentheses.

▶ **For psychosis,** initially, 4 to 8 milligrams (mg) three times a day for nonhospitalized people, reduced as soon as possible to lowest effective dosage. In hospitalized people, 8 to 16 mg two, three, or four times a day, increased to 64 mg a day as needed. (Children over age 12: lowest adult dosage.)

▶ **For severe nausea and vomiting,** 8 to 16 mg a day, divided into several equal doses. Maximum dosage is 24 mg a day.

How to take Trilafon

• Dilute the concentrated oral solution in fruit juice, ginger ale, or semisolid food such as applesauce. Don't mix it with cola, coffee, tea, or grape or apple juice.

• You may not feel Trilafon's full effects for several weeks. Don't stop taking Trilafon without first checking with your doctor.

TRILAFON'S OTHER NAMES

Trilafon's generic name is perphenazine. Other brand names include PMS-Perphenazine and, in Canada, Apo-Perphenazine.

SIDE EFFECTS

Call your doctor if you have any of these possible drug side effects. Call *immediately* about any labeled "serious."

Serious: blood problems (fatigue, bleeding, bruising, fever, chills, increased risk of infection), neuroleptic malignant syndrome (high fever, muscle rigidity)

Common: uncontrollable movements of mouth, tongue, or other body parts; low blood pressure (dizziness, weakness); blurred vision; constipation; difficulty urinating; skin sensitivity to sun; dry mouth
Tips: Drink more fluids and eat high-fiber foods, such as fresh fruits and vegetables, if constipation is a problem. Wear a sunscreen, a hat, and protective clothing outdoors. To relieve dry mouth, try sugarless gum or hard candy or ice chips.

Other: sleepiness, dizziness, dark urine, menstrual changes, abnormal liver function (yellow-tinged skin and eyes), increased appetite, weight gain, nausea, vomiting, tremor, feeling of warmth or cold, sweating, fast pulse, headache, insomnia, breast enlargement in men, inhibited ejaculation
Tips: Avoid activities that require full alertness or coordination until you know how Trilafon affects you. Take this drug with food, water, or milk to prevent stomach upset.

DRUG AND FOOD INTERACTIONS

Combining certain drugs and foods may alter drug action or produce unwanted side effects. Tell your doctor about your diet and other drugs you're taking, especially:
• alcohol and other drugs that make you feel relaxed or sleepy, such as tranquilizers, sleeping pills, narcotic pain relievers, muscle relaxants, and cold and allergy drugs
• antacids and drugs for diarrhea (take at least 2 hours before or after Trilafon)
• appetite suppressants
• atropine
• caffeine
• drugs for depression called MAO inhibitors, such as Nardil and Parnate
• Eskalith, Lithobid
• Inderal, Lopressor
• levodopa, Sinemet
• Nitro-Dur
• nonprescription cold and allergy nasal sprays
• Norpace, Procan SR, Quinaglute Dura-tabs
• tobacco.

If you miss a dose

Adjust your schedule as follows:
• If you take one dose a day, take the missed dose as soon as possible. If you don't remember until the next day, skip it and go back to your regular schedule. Don't take a double dose.
• If you take more than one dose a day, take the missed dose within 1 hour of the scheduled time if you remember it. If not, skip the missed dose and go back to your regular dosage schedule. Don't take a double dose.

 If you suspect an overdose

Contact your doctor *immediately*. Excessive Trilafon can cause uncontrollable movements, seizures, unarousable sleep, and possibly a coma.

✕ Warnings

• Make sure your doctor knows your medical history. You may not be able to take Trilafon if you're allergic to it or to related drugs or if you have a depressed central nervous system (extreme tiredness), blood problems, bone marrow depression, liver or kidney problems, brain damage, alcohol withdrawal, depression, suicidal thoughts, or asthma, emphysema, or other breathing disorders.
• Tell your doctor if you're pregnant or wish to breast-feed.
• Before you have medical tests, tell the doctor that you're taking Trilafon.

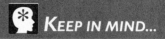 ### KEEP IN MIND...

* Take with food, water, or milk.
* Don't dilute concentrate in cola, coffee, tea, or grape or apple juice.
* Avoid alcohol and drugs that make you relaxed or sleepy.
* Don't stop taking unless doctor approves.
* Report any uncontrollable movements.

Tri-Levlen

Tri-Levlen changes the body's hormone balance. This inhibits ovulation, thus preventing pregnancy.

Why it's prescribed

Doctors prescribe Tri-Levlen as a form of oral birth control. It comes in tablets. Doctors usually prescribe the following amounts for adults.
▶ **To prevent pregnancy,** 1 tablet a day.

How to take Tri-Levlen

• Follow your doctor's orders exactly. To prevent pregnancy, you must take Tri-Levlen precisely on schedule.
• Take your pills at the same time each day, no more than 24 hours apart.
• Take your pills in the order that they're arranged in your package.

If you miss a dose

Adjust your schedule as follows:
• If you miss one dose, take it as soon as you remember. Then take the next dose at your regular time.
• If you miss two doses in a row during the first 2 weeks of your cycle, take two doses on the day you remember, followed by two doses the next day. Then resume your regular schedule.
• If you forget two doses during the second 2 weeks, or three doses any time during the month, check with your doctor.

TRI-LEVLEN'S OTHER NAMES

Tri-Levlen is a combination of two generic drugs: ethinyl estradiol and levonorgestrel. Another brand name is Triphasil.

 SIDE EFFECTS

Call your doctor if you have any of these possible drug side effects. Call *immediately* about any labeled "serious."

Serious: blood clots (shortness of breath, leg pain), redness, rash, high blood pressure (headache, blurred vision), liver tumor (yellow-tinged skin and eyes)

Common: headache, dizziness, nervousness, nausea, vomiting, breakthrough bleeding, increased vaginal secretions, hair loss
Tip: If you feel nauseous for the first few weeks of therapy, take your dose with food or just before bed.

Other: depression, lethargy, migraine headaches, swelling, worsening of near-sightedness or astigmatism, contact lens intolerance, vomiting, abdominal cramps, bloating, diarrhea, constipation, appetite change, weight gain, menstrual changes, enlargement of uterine fibromas, vaginal infection, gallbladder disease (abdominal pain, nausea, vomiting), acne, oily skin, darker skin color, breast changes, increased calcium level (drowsiness, weakness, nausea, headache, blurred vision), folic acid deficiency (fatigue, shortness of breath, palpitations, weakness, nausea, headache), altered sex drive

 DRUG INTERACTIONS

Combining certain drugs may alter their action or produce unwanted side effects. Tell your doctor about other drugs you're taking, especially:
• barbiturates, such as Seconal and Solfoton
• Butazolidin
• Dilantin
• Grisactin
• Omnipen
• Rifadin
• tetracyclines such as Achromycin.

 If you suspect an overdose

Consult your doctor. Excessive Tri-Levlen can cause nausea and excessive bleeding between periods.

 Warnings

• Make sure your doctor knows your medical history. You may not be able to take Tri-Levlen if you're allergic to it or to certain foods or dyes or if you have angina (chest pain), asthma, a history of blood clots, bone disease, fibrocystic breast disease, cancer, altered menstrual bleeding, endometriosis, seizures, gallbladder problems, heart or blood vessel disease, high cholesterol or blood pressure, jaundice, kidney or liver problems, depression, migraine headaches, stroke, tuberculosis, increased calcium level, or varicose veins.

• Tell your doctor right away if you think you're pregnant.

• Use another method of birth control during your first cycle of pills.

• Anytime you forget one or more pills, use another form of birth control. If you forget one dose, use another method of birth control for 7 days while you catch up with your schedule. If you forget two doses in a row, use another method until the start of your next cycle.

• You'll also need another method of birth control any time you take certain drugs, including many antibiotics, barbiturates, cortisone-like drugs, tranquilizers, and others.

Check with your doctor any time you get a new prescription.

• Always keep an extra month's supply of Tri-Levlen handy so you won't run out of pills.

• Tell the doctor or dentist that you're taking birth control pills before you have any surgical, dental, or emergency treatment.

• See your dentist for regular teeth cleanings because you may be prone to bleeding gums.

• If you smoke, try to quit; cigarette smoking increases the risk of serious side effects.

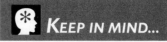

KEEP IN MIND...

* Take doses at same time each day, no more than 24 hours apart.

* Take in the proper package order.

* To reduce nausea, take with food or at bedtime.

* Use additional birth control if you miss doses or take certain other drugs.

Trilisate

Trilisate is a drug that's similar to aspirin. It's used to relieve pain and reduce fever and swelling.

Why it's prescribed

Doctors prescribe Trilisate to treat inflammation, fever, and pain. It comes in tablets and a liquid. Doctors usually prescribe the following amounts.

▶ **For rheumatoid arthritis, osteoarthritis, or other inflammatory conditions in adults,** initially, 1.5 to 2.5 grams (g) a day as a single dose or divided into two or three equal doses. Dosage adjusted according to person's response. Dosage range is 1 to 4.5 g a day.

▶ **For juvenile rheumatoid arthritis in children,** 60 to 110 mg for each 2.2 pounds (lb) of body weight a day, divided into equal doses taken every 6 to 8 hours.

▶ **For mild to moderate pain and fever in adults,** 2 to 3 g a day, divided into equal doses taken every 4 to 6 hours.

▶ **For mild to moderate pain and fever in children,** 10 to 15 mg for each 2.2 lb a day every 4 hours, up to 60 to 80 mg for each 2.2 lb a day.

How to take Trilisate

• Take Trilisate with food or a full glass (8 ounces) of water. If you prefer, you can mix it with fruit juice, but not with antacids.

• Trilisate causes less stomach upset than aspirin. However, if it does upset your stomach, take it before a

SIDE EFFECTS

Call your doctor if you have any of these possible drug side effects. Call *immediately* about any labeled "serious."

Serious: severe allergic reaction (shortness of breath, wheezing, closing up of throat)

Common: none reported

Other: ringing in ears, hearing loss, stomach upset, rash

DRUG INTERACTIONS

Combining certain drugs may alter their action or produce unwanted side effects. Tell your doctor about other drugs you're taking, especially:
• anticoagulants (blood thinners) such as Coumadin
• aspirin and products that contain aspirin
• corticosteroids
• Daranide, Miochol
• Depakene, Dilantin
• insulin and oral diabetes drugs, such as DiaBeta and Diabinese
• Mexate.

meal; then take an antacid about 2 hours after the meal.

• Don't take Trilisate that has a strong vinegar odor; this means the drug is breaking down.

If you miss a dose

Take the missed dose as soon as possible. However, if it's almost time for your next dose, skip the missed dose and take your next dose as scheduled. Don't take a double dose.

If you suspect an overdose

Contact your doctor *immediately.* Excessive Trilisate can cause seizures, loss of consciousness, and death.

Warnings

• Make sure your doctor knows your medical history. You may not be able to take Trilisate if you're al-

lergic to it or to other aspirin-like drugs or if you have hemophilia, stomach ulcers, bleeding problems, liver or kidney problems, gastritis, anemia, an overactive thyroid, asthma, gout, or G6PD deficiency.

• Tell your doctor if you think you're pregnant or you wish to breast-feed.

• To prevent potentially fatal Reye's syndrome, don't give Trilisate to a child or teenager who has chickenpox or a flulike illness.

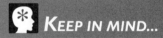

KEEP IN MIND...

* Take with food or a full glass of water.

* Don't give to child with chickenpox or flulike illness.

* Tell doctor if you're on low-salt (low-sodium) diet.

TRILISATE'S OTHER NAMES

Trilisate's generic name is choline magnesium trisalicylate. Another brand name is Tricusal.

Trimpex

Trimpex is an antibiotic that kills many types of bacteria.

Why it's prescribed

Doctors prescribe Trimpex to treat urinary tract infections. It comes in tablets. Doctors usually prescribe the following amounts for adults.

▶ **For urinary tract infections,** 200 milligrams a day as a single dose or divided into two equal doses taken every 12 hours for 10 days.

How to take Trimpex

• Trimpex is usually used along with another antibiotic. If your doctor prescribes both, take them exactly as ordered.
• Finish your entire prescription, even if you feel better sooner.

If you miss a dose

Take the missed dose as soon as possible. However, if it's almost time for your next dose, skip the missed dose and take your next dose as scheduled. Don't take a double dose.

If you suspect an overdose

Contact your doctor *immediately*. Excessive Trimpex can cause vomiting, headache, confusion, and bone marrow depression (anemia, bleeding, fatigue).

TRIMPEX'S OTHER NAMES

Trimpex's generic name is trimethoprim. Another brand name is Proloprim.

SIDE EFFECTS

Call your doctor if you have any of these possible drug side effects. Call *immediately* about any labeled "serious."

Serious: severe dermatitis (peeling skin), blood problems (fatigue, bleeding bruising, chills, fever, increased risk of infection)
Tips: Avoid contact sports or other activities that may increase your risk of bleeding or bruising. Avoid people with infections. Call your doctor right away if you develop symptoms of infection, such as a sore throat or fever, or unusual bleeding or bruising.

Common: nausea, vomiting, rash, itching
Tip: To prevent nausea, take Trimpex with food.

Other: swollen or inflamed tongue

DRUG INTERACTIONS

Combining certain drugs may alter their action or produce unwanted side effects. Tell your doctor about other drugs you're taking, especially:
• Dilantin.

Warnings

• Make sure your doctor knows your medical history. You may not be able to take Trimpex if you're allergic to it or if you have kidney or liver problems or megaloblastic anemia caused by a deficiency of folate.
• Tell your doctor if you're pregnant or breast-feeding.
• Trimpex is not recommended for children under age 12.
• Be aware that older adults may be especially prone to this drug's side effects.
• Don't take Trimpex for future infections without your doctor's consent, and don't share this drug with family or friends. If someone develops symptoms like yours, call the doctor.

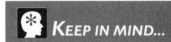

* Take with second antibiotic, as ordered.

* Finish entire prescription.

* Call doctor if you develop a sore throat, fever, or unusual bleeding or bruising.

* Don't share drug or keep for future use.

Triphasil

Triphasil changes the body's hormone balance. This inhibits ovulation, thus preventing pregnancy.

Why it's prescribed

Doctors prescribe Triphasil as a form of oral birth control. It comes in tablets. Doctors usually prescribe the following amounts for adults.

▶ **To prevent pregnancy,** 1 tablet a day.

How to take Triphasil

• Follow your doctor's orders exactly. To prevent pregnancy, you must take Triphasil precisely on schedule.

• Take your pills at the same time each day, no more than 24 hours apart.

• Take your pills in the order that they're arranged in your package.

If you miss a dose

Adjust your schedule as follows:

• If you miss one dose, take it as soon as you remember. Then take the next dose at your regular time.

• If you miss two doses in a row during the first 2 weeks of your cycle, take two doses on the day you remember, followed by two doses the next day. Then resume your regular schedule.

• If you forget two doses during the second 2 weeks, or three doses any time during the month, check with your doctor.

 SIDE EFFECTS

Call your doctor if you have any of these possible drug side effects. Call *immediately* about any labeled "serious."

Serious: blood clots (shortness of breath, leg pain), redness, rash, high blood pressure (prolonged headache, blurred vision), liver tumor (yellow-tinged skin and eyes)

Common: headache, dizziness, nausea, breakthrough bleeding
Tip: If you feel nauseous for the first few weeks of therapy, take your dose with food or just before bed.

Other: depression, lethargy, migraine headaches, swelling, worsening of near-sightedness or astigmatism, contact lens intolerance, vomiting, abdominal cramps, bloating, diarrhea, constipation, appetite change, weight gain, menstrual changes, vaginal infection, gallbladder disease (abdominal or back tenderness and pain, fever, sweating, vomiting, weight loss), acne, oily skin, increased pigmentation, breast changes, increased calcium level (abdominal or muscle pain, weakness, constipaton), folic acid deficiency (redness or swelling of tongue or mouth, diarrhea), altered sex drive

 DRUG INTERACTIONS

Combining certain drugs may alter their action or produce unwanted side effects. Tell your doctor about other drugs you're taking, especially:

• antibiotics, barbiturates, cortisone-like drugs, tranquilizers, and certain other drugs (use another birth control method)
• barbiturates, such as Seconal and Solfoton
• Butazolidin
• Dilantin
• Grisactin
• Omnipen
• Rifadin
• tetracyclines such as Achromycin.

TRIPHASIL'S OTHER NAMES

Triphasil is a combination of the generic drugs ethinyl estradiol and levonorgestrel. Another brand name is Tri-Levlen.

 If you suspect an overdose

Consult your doctor.

 Warnings

• Make sure your doctor knows your medical history. You may not be able to take Triphasil if you're allergic to it or to certain foods or dyes or if you have angina (chest pain), asthma, a history of blood clots, bone disease, fibrocystic breast disease, cancer, altered menstrual bleeding, endometriosis, seizures, gallbladder problems, heart or blood vessel disease, high cholesterol, high blood pressure, jaundice, kidney or liver problems, depression, migraine headaches, stroke, tuberculosis, increased calcium level, or varicose veins.

• Tell your doctor right away if you think you're pregnant.

• Use another method of birth control during your first cycle of pills.

• Any time you forget one or more pills, use another form of birth control. If you forget one dose, use another method of birth control for 7 days while you catch up with your schedule. If you forget two doses in a row, use another method until the start of your next cycle.

• You'll also need another method of birth control any time you take certain drugs, including many antibiotics, barbiturates, cortisone-like drugs, tranquilizers, and others. Check with your doctor any time you get a new prescription.

• Always keep an extra month's supply of Triphasil handy so you won't run out of pills.

• Tell the doctor or dentist that you're taking birth control pills before you have any surgical, dental, or emergency treatment.

• See your eye doctor for regular checkups because Triphasil can cause eye and vision changes.

• If you smoke, try to quit; cigarette smoking increases the risk of serious side effects.

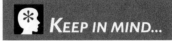

KEEP IN MIND...

* Take doses at same time each day, no more than 24 hours apart.

* Take in the proper package order.

* To reduce nausea, take with food or at bedtime.

* Use additional birth control if you miss doses or take certain other drugs.

Tums

Tums is an antacid that reduces acid levels in the stomach and intestines, reduces the stomach's pH, strengthens the mucous wall of the stomach, and strengthens the sphincter muscle between the stomach and the esophagus.

Why it's taken

Tums is taken to relieve heartburn and to provide a calcium supplement. It comes in tablets, chewable tablets, chewing gum, liquid, and lozenges. The following amounts are usually recommended for adults.

▶ **As an antacid and calcium supplement,** 350 milligrams to 1.5 grams or 2 pieces of chewing gum, as needed.

How to take Tums

• Take Tums with a full glass (8 ounces) of water or juice.
• Unless your doctor tells you otherwise, take Tums 60 to 90 minutes after a meal and at bedtime, as needed. If you take the liquid form of Tums, take it before meals.
• Avoid taking your calcium supplement within about 2 hours of taking other drugs or eating a large quantity of high-fiber food.

SIDE EFFECTS

Call your doctor if you have any of these possible drug side effects.

Serious: none reported

Common: constipation, nausea
Tip: To reduce constipation, drink plenty of water and increase your intake of fiber-rich foods.

Other: stomach bloating, gas

DRUG AND FOOD INTERACTIONS

Combining certain drugs and foods may alter drug action or produce unwanted side effects. Tell your doctor about your diet and other drugs you're taking, especially:
• antibiotics
• aspirin and other salicylates
• Calcibind or Ganite
• calcium-containing drugs
• Didronel
• enteric-coated drugs
• heart drugs called digitalis glycosides
• iron supplements
• Laniazid
• milk and other foods high in vitamin D
• seizure drugs such as Dilantin
• tobacco.

If you miss a dose

Not applicable because drug is taken only as needed.

If you suspect an overdose

Contact your doctor *immediately*. Excessive Tums can cause nausea, vomiting, headache, confusion, and appetite loss.

Warnings

• Make sure your doctor knows your medical history. You may not be able to take Tums if you have an abnormally high calcium level in your blood, sarcoidosis, or kidney or heart problems.

KEEP IN MIND...

* Take with a full glass of water or juice.

* Take 60 to 90 minutes after meals; take liquid form before meals.

* Don't take within 2 hours of other drugs or high-fiber foods.

Tylenol

Tylenol relieves mild pain by blocking the generation of pain impulses. It also relieves fever, probably by acting on the heat-regulating center of the brain. Unlike aspirin and similar drugs, Tylenol does not reduce inflammation.

Why it's taken

Tylenol is taken to reduce mild pain and fever. It comes in tablets, chewable tablets, capsules, slow-release caplets, various liquid forms, granules, powder for making solution, sprinkles, tablets for making solution, suppositories, and wafers. The following amounts are usually

TYLENOL'S OTHER NAMES

Tylenol's generic name is acetaminophen. Other brand names include Abenol, Aceta Elixir, Acetaminophen Uniserts, Aceta Tablets, Actamin, Actimol, Aminofen, Anacin-3, Apacet Capsules, Apo-Acetaminophen, Arthritis Pain Formula Aspirin Free, Atasol Caplets, Banesin, Dapa, Dapa XS, Datril XS, Dolanex, Dorcol Children's Fever and Pain Reducer, Exdol, Genapap Regular Strength Tablets, Genebs Regular Strength Tablets, Liquiprin Infants' Drops, Meda Cap, Myapap Elixir, Neopap, Oraphen-PD, Panadol, Panadol Maximum Strength Tablets, Panex, Panex-500, Redutemp, Ridenol Caplets, Robigesic, Rounox, Snaplets-FR, Stanback AF Extra Strength Powder, St. Joseph Aspirin-Free Fever Reducer for Children, Suppap-120, Tapanol Extra Strength Caplets, Tempra, and Valorin.

SIDE EFFECTS

Call your doctor if you have any of these possible drug side effects. Call *immediately* about any labeled "serious."

Serious: severe liver damage with excessive doses (yellow-tinged skin and eyes)

Common: none reported

Other: low blood sugar (drowsiness, headache, nervousness, cold sweats, confusion), blood problems (fatigue, bleeding, bruising, fever, chills, increased risk of infection), rash, hives

Tips: Avoid contact sports and other activities that increase your risk of bleeding or bruising. To prevent infection, avoid people who are ill or have an infection.

DRUG AND FOOD INTERACTIONS

Combining certain drugs and foods may alter drug action or produce unwanted side effects. Tell your doctor about your diet and other drugs you're taking, especially:
- alcohol
- Anturane
- aspirin and other nonsteroidal anti-inflammatory drugs
- barbiturates
- caffeine
- Coumadin
- Dolobid
- Retrovir
- Rifadin
- seizure drugs called hydantoins
- Tegretol
- tetracycline antibiotics (take at least 1 hour before or after taking Tylenol buffered effervescent granules).

recommended for adults; children's dosages appear in parentheses.

▶ **For mild pain or fever,** 325 to 650 milligrams (mg) every 4 to 6 hours or 1 gram (g) three or four times a day, as needed. Or 2 slow-release caplets every 8 hours. Maximum dosage is 4 g a day. (Children over age 11: same as adults. Children age 11: 480 mg orally or rectally every 4 to 6 hours. Children ages 9 and 10: 400 mg orally or rectally every 4 to 6 hours. Children ages 6 to 8: 320 mg orally or rectally every 4 to 6 hours. Children ages 4 and 5: 240 mg orally or rectally every 4 to 6 hours. Children ages 2 and 3: 160 mg orally or rectally every 4 to 6 hours. Children ages 12 to 23 months: 120 mg orally every 4 to 6 hours. Children ages 4 to 11 months: 80 mg orally every 4 to 6 hours. Children up to age 3 months: 40 mg orally every 4 to 6 hours.)

Continued on next page ▶

How to take Tylenol

• Carefully follow the precautions listed on the package label.

• You can take a dose of Tylenol every 4 hours as needed, but don't exceed the total that's recommended on the package.

• If you're using a suppository and it's too soft to insert, run cold water over it or refrigerate it briefly before removing the wrapper.

If you miss a dose

Take the missed dose as soon as possible. However, if it's almost time for your next dose, skip the missed dose and take your next dose as scheduled. Don't take a double dose.

If you suspect an overdose

Contact your doctor *immediately*. Excessive Tylenol can cause bluish skin, yellow-tinged skin and eyes, fever, vomiting, delirium, coma, seizures, and death.

Warnings

• Make sure your doctor knows your medical history. You may not be able to take Tylenol if you're allergic to it or if you have diabetes, kidney or liver problems, viral infection, heart disease, phenylketonuria, a blood disorder, or a history of chronic alcohol abuse.

• Don't use Tylenol if you have a high fever (over 103° F), a fever that lasts longer than 3 days, or a fever that recurs. Instead, talk with your doctor.

• Don't use Tylenol for arthritis or other rheumatic conditions without your doctor's consent. Tylenol may reduce the pain of these conditions, but not the other symptoms.

• Consult a doctor before giving this drug to a child under age 2.

• Use a liquid form of Tylenol for children and for anyone who has trouble swallowing.

• If you're diabetic, check your sugar levels carefully. Tylenol may produce false-positive decreases in blood sugar levels on home monitoring systems. Call your doctor if you notice a change.

• If you need high doses of Tylenol for a long time, your doctor will probably want to test your blood and your kidney and liver function from time to time.

• Contact your doctor if Tylenol doesn't relieve your pain after 10 days (5 days for children), if you have new symptoms, if the pain gets worse, or if the pain site appears red and swollen.

• Call the doctor if Tylenol doesn't eliminate your fever within 3 days, if the fever returns or rises, or if new symptoms, redness, or swelling occurs.

• Check with the doctor or pharmacist before taking any nonprescription drugs. Many contain acetaminophen that must count toward your total daily dosage.

• If you take Tylenol as buffered effervescent granules and you're on a salt-restricted diet, be sure to count the salt in this form of the drug.

• Keep in mind that large doses of Tylenol may cause liver damage. Call the doctor if you develop a rash or hives or if your skin turns yellowish.

• Don't drink alcoholic beverages when taking Tylenol because this combination may cause liver damage, especially if you take Tylenol regularly for a long time.

• Store suppositories in the refrigerator.

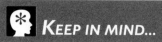

* Don't take more than total dosage recommended on package.

* If pain or fever doesn't subside in a few days, call your doctor.

* Don't take with aspirin or any nonsteroidal anti-inflammatory drugs.

* Don't use for arthritis or other inflammatory problems without doctor's approval.

* If you're diabetic, check sugar levels carefully.

Tylenol with Codeine

Tylenol with Codeine relieves pain by blocking the generation of pain impulses. Codeine is a stronger narcotic pain reliever.

Why it's prescribed

Doctors prescribe Tylenol with Codeine to relieve mild to moderately severe pain when nonprescription pain relievers are ineffective. It comes in tablets, capsules, and a liquid. Tablets are available as No. 2, No. 3, and No. 4; No. 2 contains 15 milligrams (mg) of codeine, No. 3 contains 30 mg, and No. 4 contains 60 mg. Doctors usually prescribe the following amounts for adults; children's dosages (for elixir) appear in parentheses.

▶ **To relieve mild to moderately severe pain using tablets or capsules,** up to 4,000 mg of acetaminophen with 360 mg of codeine a day.

▶ **To relieve mild to moderate pain using elixir,** 1 tablespoon every 4 hours, up to six doses a day. (Children ages 7 to 12: 2 teaspoons (tsp), every 6 to 8 hours, up to four doses a day. Children ages 3 to 6: 1

TYLENOL WITH CODEINE'S OTHER NAMES

Tylenol with Codeine is a combination of two generic drugs: acetaminophen and codeine phosphate. Other brand names include Aceta with Codeine, Capital with Codeine, M-Gesic, Myapap with Codeine, Phenaphen with Codeine, Proval, Pyregesic-C, Tylaprin with Codeine, Ty-Pap with Codeine; and, in Canada, Empracet, Emtec, Lenoltec with Codeine No. 4, and Rounox and Codeine.

 SIDE EFFECTS

Call your doctor if you have any of these possible drug side effects. Call *immediately* about any labeled "serious."

Serious: decreased and shallow breathing; shortness of breath; slow pulse; extreme tiredness; seizures; cold, clammy skin; allergic reaction (rash, difficulty breathing or swallowing)

Common: dizziness, nausea, vomiting, light-headedness, deep sleep
Tips: Avoid activities that require full alertness or coordination until you know how Tylenol with Codeine affects you. When lying or sitting, get up slowly to avoid dizziness. Increase the amount of rest you get. Take with meals or milk to avoid nausea.

Other: constipation, difficulty urinating
Tip: To avoid constipation, include plenty of fluids and fiber in your diet.

 DRUG AND FOOD INTERACTIONS

Combining certain drugs and food may alter drug action or produce unwanted side effects. Tell your doctor about your diet and other drugs you're taking, especially:

• alcohol and other drugs that make you feel relaxed or sleepy, such as tranquilizers, sleeping pills, narcotic pain relievers, muscle relaxants, and cold and allergy drugs
• anticholinergic drugs, such as atropine and Transderm-Scōp
• Anturane
• aspirin and other nonsteroidal anti-inflammatory drugs
• barbiturates
• caffeine
• Coumadin
• Dolobid
• drugs for depression, called MAO inhibitors, and tricyclic antidepressants
• nonprescription drugs that contain acetaminophen
• Retrovir
• Rifadin
• seizure drugs called hydantoins
• Tegretol
• tetracycline antibiotics.

tsp every 6 to 8 hours, up to four doses a day.)

How to take Tylenol with Codeine

• Take Tylenol with Codeine exactly as your doctor prescribes.

Don't increase the amount or frequency of this drug without speaking to your doctor.
• Usually, you may take this drug every 4 to 6 hours.

Continued on next page ▶

If you miss a dose

Not applicable because this drug is taken only as needed.

If you suspect an overdose

Contact your doctor *immediately*. Excessive Tylenol with Codeine can cause respiratory depression (shallow breathing, fewer breaths per minute) and decreased level of consciousness (difficulty awakening or inability to awaken).

Warnings

• Make sure your doctor knows your medical history. You may not be able to take Tylenol with Codeine if you are allergic to it or to morphine, other narcotics, or sulfites or if you have a history of head injury, severe headaches, diabetes, kidney or liver disease, or blood problems.

• If you're pregnant or breast-feeding, talk to your doctor before taking Tylenol with Codeine.
• Older adults may be especially prone to this drug's side effects.
• Because Tylenol with Codeine is a narcotic, it can be habit-forming. Take just the prescribed amount for only as long as directed.
• Check with the doctor or pharmacist before taking nonprescription drugs. Many contain acetaminophen and should be counted toward your total daily dosage. In normal amounts, Tylenol with Codeine is safe; in high doses, it can damage the liver.
• Don't drink alcohol while taking Tylenol with Codeine.
• Store the drug container away from direct light.
• Don't share this drug with anyone else; it's against federal law.

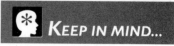

* Take with milk or meals.
* Don't increase dose without doctor's okay.
* Don't share drug with others.
* Avoid alcohol when taking Tylenol with Codeine.
* Increase fluids and fiber in diet.
* Be aware of potential for drowsiness.

Ultram

Ultram is a synthetic pain reliever. It's thought to affect levels of certain chemicals in the brain, which decreases the sensation of pain.

Why it's prescribed

Doctors prescribe Ultram to relieve pain. It comes in tablets. Doctors usually prescribe the following amounts for adults.

▶ **For moderate to moderately severe pain,** 50 to 100 milligrams (mg) every 4 to 6 hours, as needed. Maximum dosage is 400 mg a day.

How to take Ultram

• Take Ultram exactly as your doctor prescribes.
• Don't increase the dosage or take the drug more often than ordered. Ultram may become habit-forming.
• For best results, take Ultram before pain becomes intense. This drug begins to take effect within 2 to 3 hours and effects last 6 to 7 hours.

If you miss a dose

Take the missed dose as soon as possible. However, if it's almost time for your next dose, skip the missed dose and take your next dose as scheduled. Don't take a double dose.

If you suspect an overdose

Contact your doctor *immediately*. Excessive Ultram can cause slowed breathing and seizures.

ULTRAM'S OTHER NAME

Ultram's generic name is tramadol hydrochloride.

SIDE EFFECTS

Call your doctor if you have any of these possible drug side effects. Call *immediately* about any labeled "serious."

Serious: difficulty breathing, fast pulse, low blood pressure (dizziness, weakness)

Common: dizziness, vertigo, headache, drowsiness, nausea, constipation, vomiting

Tips: Until you know how Ultram affects you, don't drive or perform other activities that require you to be fully alert. To avoid dizziness when getting up from a lying position, sit up slowly and dangle your legs for a few minutes before you stand up. To reduce constipation, drink plenty of fluids and add fiber-rich foods to your diet. If necessary, talk to your doctor about using a stool softener or laxative.

Other: weakness, lack of energy, anxiety, confusion, incoordination, euphoria, nervousness, problems sleeping, visual disturbances, stomach upset, dry mouth, diarrhea, abdominal pain, appetite loss, gas, increased or decreased urination, menopausal symptoms, itchiness, sweating, rash, muscle spasm
Tip: To relieve dry mouth, try sugarless gum or hard candy or ice chips.

DRUG INTERACTIONS

Combining certain drugs may alter their action or produce unwanted side effects. Tell your doctor about other drugs you're taking, especially:
• drugs for depression called MAO inhibitors such as Marplan
• drugs that alter your mood or state of consciousness
• drugs that make you feel relaxed or sleepy, such as tranquilizers, sleeping pills, and cold and allergy drugs
• Tegretol.

✕ Warnings

• Make sure your doctor knows your medical history. You may not be able to take Ultram if you're allergic to it or other drugs; if you have a history of drug or alcohol dependence; or if you have seizures, respiratory problems, head injury, certain abdominal conditions, or kidney or liver problems.
• Make sure your doctor knows if you're pregnant or breast-feeding before you begin taking Ultram.

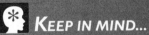 KEEP IN MIND...

* Take before pain becomes intense.

* Don't drive until you know how drug affects you.

* Increase fluids and fiber in diet.

* To relieve dry mouth, try sugarless gum or hard candy or ice chips.

Ultravate

Ultravate is a high-potency steroid-based drug that reduces skin redness, swelling, and itching.

Why it's prescribed

Doctors prescribe Ultravate to relieve some skin conditions. It comes in a cream and an ointment. Doctors usually prescribe the following amounts for adults; children's dosage appears in parentheses.

▶ **For inflamed skin,** cream or ointment applied to affected area once or twice a day for up to 2 weeks. Total dosage not more than 50 grams a week. (Children: small amount applied to affected area once or twice a day.)

How to use Ultravate

• Use this drug exactly as your doctor directs. Apply it sparingly, and rub it in gently and completely.
• Don't cover the treated area with a dressing unless your doctor directs you to.
• Don't use Ultravate on your face, groin, or armpits, and be sure to keep it out of your eyes and mouth.
• If you're using this drug on an infant's diaper area, don't cover it with plastic pants or a tight diaper.

If you miss a dose

Apply the missed dose as soon as possible. However, if it's almost time for your next dose, skip the missed dose and apply your next dose as scheduled.

If you suspect an overdose

Wash off any excess cream, and contact your doctor *immediately*. Excessive Ultravate can be absorbed through the skin into the body, possibly causing increased risk of infection (fever, sore throat) or increased blood sugar levels (increased thirst, hunger, and urination; weight loss).

Warnings

• Make sure your doctor knows your medical history. You may not be able to use Ultravate if you're allergic to it or to any of its components or if you have cataracts, glaucoma, diabetes, tuberculosis, or sores or an infection in the area to be treated.

• Tell your doctor if you're pregnant or breast-feeding before using Ultravate.
• Be aware that children are more prone to this drug's side effects.
• Report any burning, redness, or itching to your doctor.
• Don't use leftover Ultravate on future skin problems without your doctor's approval.

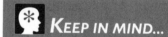

* Use sparingly.

* Don't apply to face, groin, or armpits.

* Don't cover treated area unless directed otherwise.

* Don't use for more than 2 weeks unless instructed otherwise.

ULTRAVATE'S OTHER NAME

Ultravate's generic name is halobetasol propionate.

SIDE EFFECTS

Call your doctor if you have any of these possible drug side effects. Call *immediately* about any labeled "serious."

Serious: hormonal problems (increased risk of infection)

Common: stinging, itching, burning

Other: dry skin, redness, rash, fluid-filled blisters, redness and swelling at hair follicles, increased hair growth, reduced skin pigmentation, acne, high blood sugar (increased thirst, hunger, and urination; weight loss)

DRUG INTERACTIONS

Combining certain drugs can alter their action or produce unwanted side effects. Tell your doctor about other drugs you're taking.

Univasc

U nivasc lowers blood pressure by stopping the body from producing a substance that narrows blood vessels. By widening blood vessels, the drug makes it easier for the heart to pump blood through the body.

Why it's prescribed

Doctors prescribe Univasc to lower and control blood pressure. It comes in tablets. Doctors usually prescribe the following amounts for adults.

▶ **For high blood pressure,** at first, 7.5 milligrams (mg) once a day before meals if person isn't taking a diuretic (water pill), increased or divided into several daily doses if blood pressure isn't controlled. Recommended dosage is 7.5 to 30 mg daily, divided into one or two equal doses. For the person who's taking a diuretic, at first, 3.75 mg once a day before meals, adjusted as needed.

How to take Univasc

• Take Univasc only as your doctor directs. Take it 1 hour before meals on an empty stomach; taking it with foods — particularly those that are high in fat — decreases the amount of the drug that the body can use.

If you miss a dose

Take the missed dose as soon as possible. However, if it's almost time

UNIVASC'S OTHER NAME

Univasc's generic name is moexipril hydrochloride.

 ## SIDE EFFECTS

Call your doctor if you have any of these possible drug side effects. Call *immediately* about any labeled "serious."

Serious: severe allergic reaction (difficulty breathing, swelling of face, arms, legs, eyes, lips, or tongue), blood problems (chills, fever, infection), fainting

Common: dizziness, dry, persistent, tickling, nonproductive cough
Tip: Stand up slowly to avoid dizziness.

Other: headache, fatigue, swelling of feet or hands, low blood pressure (dizziness, weakness), flushing, diarrhea, indigestion, nausea, frequent urination, rash, muscle pain, flu, upper respiratory infection

 ## DRUG INTERACTIONS

Combining certain drugs may alter their action or produce unwanted side effects. Tell your doctor about other drugs you're taking, especially:
• diuretics (water pills; stop 2 to 3 days before starting Univasc)
• Eskalith
• potassium supplements or salt substitutes containing potassium.

for your next dose, skip the missed dose and go back to your regular schedule. Don't take a double dose.

 ## If you suspect an overdose

Contact your doctor *immediately.* Although overdose of Univasc has not been reported, the most likely symptom would be very low blood pressure (dizziness, fainting).

⟨ Warnings

• Make sure your doctor knows your medical history. You may not be able to take Univasc if you have a drug allergy or kidney, heart, or blood vessel disease.
• Tell your doctor if you're pregnant or breast-feeding before you take Univasc. This drug isn't recommended during pregnancy—

especially during the second and third trimester—or for breast-feeding women. If pregnancy occurs during treatment, follow your doctor's instructions to stop taking this drug.
• This drug is less effective in black people than in other racial groups.
• Schedule periodic follow-up visits during treatment so that your doctor can check your progress.

 ## KEEP IN MIND...

∗ Take on empty stomach.

∗ Don't take if pregnant or breast-feeding.

∗ Avoid potassium supplements and salt substitutes that contain potassium.

Uracil Mustard Capsules

Uracil Mustard Capsules is a drug used to fight cancer. It prevents cancer cells from reproducing, which causes cell death.

Why it's prescribed

Doctors prescribe Uracil Mustard Capsules to treat leukemia, Hodgkin's disease, and other conditions. It comes in capsules. Doctors usually prescribe the following amounts for adults.

▶ **For cancer and other conditions,** 1 to 2 milligrams a day for 3 months or until desired response is achieved or side effects become intolerable. Maintenance dosage depends on person's response.

How to take Uracil Mustard Capsules

• Take this drug exactly as your doctor orders. Take it at bedtime to reduce nausea.
• Don't stop using Uracil Mustard Capsules without your doctor's knowledge, even if the drug makes you vomit or feel ill.
• If you vomit after taking a dose, check with your doctor to find out if you should repeat the dose.

If you miss a dose

Take the missed dose as soon as possible. However, if it's almost time for your next dose, skip the missed dose and take your next dose as scheduled. Don't take a double dose.

URACIL MUSTARD CAPSULES' OTHER NAME

Uracil Mustard Capsules' generic name is uracil mustard.

 ## SIDE EFFECTS

Call your doctor if you have any of these possible drug side effects. Call *immediately* about any labeled "serious."

Serious: blood problems (fatigue, bleeding, bruising, increased risk of infection)

Common: nausea, vomiting, diarrhea, stomach upset, irritability
Tip: Drink extra fluids while taking this drug to help reduce the kidney problems that may result from excess water loss.

Other: nervousness, confusion, depression, abdominal pain, appetite loss, itching, rash, darker skin, gout, hair loss

 ## DRUG INTERACTIONS

Combining certain drugs may alter their action or produce unwanted side effects. Tell your doctor about other drugs you're taking, especially:
• Ancobon
• anticoagulants (blood thinners) such as Coumadin
• Anturane, aspirin
• Benemid
• Chloromycetin
• colchicine
• Mithracin
• other cancer drugs, such as Imuran, Intron A, and Retrovir (AZT)
• thyroid drugs.

 ### If you suspect an overdose

Contact your doctor *immediately*. Excessive Uracil Mustard Capsules can cause fever, chills, nausea, and vomiting.

 ### Warnings

• Make sure your doctor knows your medical history. You may not be able to take Uracil Mustard Capsules if you're allergic to them or to aspirin or tartrazine dye; if you have a serious blood problem, shingles, an infection, gout, or liver or kidney problems; if you're undergoing radiation; or if you have or have recently been exposed to chickenpox.
• Talk with your doctor right away if you plan to get pregnant or think you might be. If appropriate, also discuss breast-feeding.

KEEP IN MIND...

* Take at bedtime to reduce nausea.

* Don't stop taking drug without doctor's approval.

* Don't take aspirin while taking this drug.

Urecholine

U recholine encourages urination by stimulating the bladder to empty.

Why it's prescribed

Doctors prescribe Urecholine to treat certain bladder or urinary tract disorders. It comes in tablets. Doctors usually prescribe the following amounts for adults.

▶ **For inability to urinate,** 10 to 50 milligrams (mg) two to four times a day. With close monitoring, up to 100 mg per dose may be prescribed.

How to take Urecholine

• Take this drug exactly as your doctor orders. Carefully follow the dosage directions on the prescription label.
• Unless your doctor directs otherwise, take Urecholine on an empty stomach (either 1 hour before or 2 hours after meals) to avoid nausea and vomiting.

If you miss a dose

If you remember within an hour or so, take the drug right away. But if you remember later, skip the dose you missed and resume your normal schedule. Don't take a double dose.

 If you suspect an overdose

Contact your doctor *immediately.* Excessive Urecholine can cause

URECHOLINE'S OTHER NAMES

Urecholine's generic name is bethanechol chloride. Other brand names include Duvoid and Urabeth.

 SIDE EFFECTS

Call your doctor if you have any of these possible drug side effects. Call *immediately* about any labeled "serious."

Serious: wheezing, difficulty breathing, severe or persistent abdominal cramps and diarrhea

Common: dizziness
Tip: To minimize dizziness and light-headedness, get up slowly from a sitting or lying position.

Other: headache, general feeling of illness, fast or slow pulse, increased eye tearing, small pupils, excessive salivation, nausea, vomiting, belching, audible stomach noises, throat spasms, phlegm in lungs, urinary urgency, flushing, sweating

 DRUG INTERACTIONS

Combining certain drugs may alter their action or produce unwanted side effects. Tell your doctor about other drugs you're taking, especially:
• Atropisol
• blood pressure drugs
• muscle relaxants
• Pro-Banthine
• Pronestyl
• Quinaglute Dura-tabs.

nausea, vomiting, abdominal cramps, uncontrolled diarrhea, sweating, and an altered heartbeat.

Warnings

• Make sure your doctor knows your medical history. You may not be able to take Urecholine if you're allergic to it or to any of its components; if you have a weakened bladder wall or urinary tract; or if you have an obstructed urinary or digestive passage or other digestive problem, a stomach ulcer, an overactive thyroid, asthma, slow pulse, low blood pressure, blood vessel problems, seizures, or Parkinson's disease.
• Tell your doctor if you become pregnant while taking Urecholine.

KEEP IN MIND...

∗ Take on an empty stomach.
∗ Call doctor if you develop breathing problems or severe diarrhea and cramps.
∗ Stand up slowly to avoid dizziness.

Urispas

Urispas helps relieve bladder spasms and may help reduce pain. It acts on a muscle in the bladder to increase the amount of urine the bladder can hold.

Why it's prescribed

Doctors prescribe Urispas to relieve painful urination, urinary frequency and urgency, nighttime urination, incontinence, and bladder pain. It comes in tablets. Doctors usually prescribe the following amounts for adults and children age 12 and over.

▶ **For urinary problems,** 100 to 200 milligrams three or four times a day.

How to take Urispas

• Take this drug exactly as your doctor orders.
• Try to take Urispas on an empty stomach. If it causes stomach upset, ask your doctor if you can take it with food or milk.

If you miss a dose

Take the missed dose as soon as possible. However, if it's almost time for your next dose, skip the missed dose and take your next dose as scheduled. Don't take a double dose.

 If you suspect an overdose

Contact your doctor *immediately*. Excessive Urispas can cause clumsi-

URISPAS'S OTHER NAME

Urispas's generic name is flavoxate hydrochloride.

 SIDE EFFECTS

Call your doctor if you have any of these possible drug side effects. Call *immediately* about any labeled "serious."

Serious: fast pulse, blood problems (infection, chills, fever)

Common: confusion (especially in older adults), dry mouth and throat, blurred vision, eye sensitivity to light, decreased sweating (may lead to heatstroke)

Tips: To help relieve dry mouth, try sugarless gum or hard candy or ice chips. If Urispas makes your eyes more sensitive to light, wear sunglasses or a hat to protect them. Avoid getting overheated to lower the risk of heatstroke.

Other: nervousness, dizziness, headache, drowsiness, difficulty concentrating, palpitations, difficulty focusing eyes, abdominal pain, constipation (with high doses), nausea, vomiting, hives, fever

Tip: Don't drive or perform activities that could be dangerous if you're not fully alert or your vision is blurry.

 DRUG INTERACTIONS

Combining certain drugs can alter their action or produce unwanted side effects. Tell your doctor about other drugs you're taking.

ness, drowsiness, fever, hallucinations, shortness of breath, nervousness, or restlessness.

 Warnings

• Make sure your doctor knows your medical history. You may not be able to take Urispas if you have a blocked or bleeding digestive tract, blocked urinary tract, glaucoma, or an enlarged prostate.
• Inform your doctor if you're pregnant or breast-feeding before you start taking this drug.
• Urispas is not recommended for children under age 12.

• Be aware that older adults may be more prone to this drug's side effects, especially confusion.
• Call your doctor if your symptoms don't improve.

✱ KEEP IN MIND...

✱ Take on empty stomach, if possible.

✱ Wear sunglasses in bright light.

✱ Relieve dry mouth with sugarless gum or hard candy or ice chips.

✱ Don't get overheated.

Vagistat

Vagistat is used to treat fungal infections of the vagina. It works by changing the cell walls of the fungus and killing it.

Why it's prescribed

Doctors prescribe Vagistat to treat vaginal fungal infections. It comes in an ointment. Doctors usually prescribe the following amounts for adults.

▶ **For fungal infection,** 1 applicatorful inserted into the vagina at bedtime.

How to use Vagistat

• Use this drug exactly as your doctor orders. Also, read the package instructions before using.
• To avoid contaminating the ointment, open the applicator just before using it.
• For best results, insert the drug high into the vagina.
• Be sure to use the entire amount prescribed. Don't miss any doses, and don't stop using the drug if your period starts or if you have sex during treatment.

If you miss a dose

Apply the missed dose as soon as possible. However, if it's almost time for your next dose, skip the missed dose and apply your next dose as scheduled. Don't use a double dose.

VAGISTAT'S OTHER NAME

Vagistat's generic name is tioconazole.

 SIDE EFFECTS

Call your doctor if you have any of these possible drug side effects.

Serious: none reported
Common: burning, itching
Other: vaginal discharge, swelling, or irritation

 DRUG INTERACTIONS

Combining certain drugs may alter their action or produce unwanted side effects. Tell your doctor about other drugs you're taking.

 If you suspect an overdose

Contact your doctor.

Warnings

• Make sure your doctor knows your medical history. You may not be able to use Vagistat if you're allergic to it or to similar antifungal drugs.
• If you're pregnant, check with your doctor before using the vaginal applicator.
• Tell your doctor if Vagistat irritates your skin.
• Wear a sanitary pad while using Vagistat so that the ointment doesn't stain your underwear.
• If you have recurring vaginal fungal infections, your doctor may want to check your blood sugar level because diabetes can cause this type of infection.
• To prevent reinfection, either don't have sex while you're using Vagistat or have your partner wear a condom. (Check with your doctor to make sure your partner can wear a latex condom; some antifungal drugs weaken latex.) Also suggest that your partner ask the doctor about treatment.
• To reduce the chance of reinfection, wear clean, cotton-crotch underwear and pantyhose.

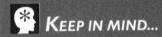 **KEEP IN MIND...**

* Use the entire amount prescribed.

* Open each applicator just before using it.

* Avoid sex during treatment, or have your partner wear a condom.

* Wear a small pad to protect your clothes.

* Always wear clean, cotton-crotch underwear and pantyhose.

Valium

Valium is one of the most commonly prescribed tranquilizers. It causes relaxation.

Why it's prescribed

Doctors prescribe Valium to treat severe tension or anxiety and muscle spasms. It also may be prescribed to control seizures. It comes in tablets, extended-release capsules, and an oral solution. Doctors usually prescribe the following amounts for adults; children's dosages appear in parentheses.

▶ **For anxiety,** 2 to 10 milligrams (mg) two to four times a day. (Children age 6 months and older: 1 to 2.5 mg three or four times a day, increased gradually as needed.)

▶ **For muscle spasms,** 2 to 10 mg two to four times a day.

▶ **For seizures,** 2 to 10 mg two to four times a day. (Children age 6 months and older: 1 to 2.5 mg three or four times a day, increased as tolerated and needed.)

How to take Valium

• Take this drug exactly as your doctor orders — no more, no less.
• Swallow extended-release capsules whole; don't crush, break, or chew them.
• To make the oral solution, dilute your dose in any liquid or soft food (such as applesauce or pudding).
• If you take Valium regularly, don't stop taking it abruptly without first asking your doctor.

VALIUM'S OTHER NAMES

Valium's generic name is diazepam. Other brand names include Diazepam Intensol, PMS Diazepam, T-Quil, Valrelease, Vazepam, Zetran; and, in Canada, Apo-Diazepam, Novodipam, and Vivol.

 SIDE EFFECTS

Call your doctor if you have any of these possible drug side effects. Call *immediately* about any labeled "serious."

Serious: acute withdrawal (sweating, agitation, fast pulse), extremely low blood pressure (dizziness, weakness)

Common: drowsiness, lethargy, loss of balance, dizziness, nausea
Tips: To reduce dizziness, change positions slowly. Don't drive or perform other activities that could be dangerous if you're not fully alert.

Other: fainting, depression, restlessness, memory loss, slurred speech, tremor, slow pulse, blurred or double vision, uncontrollable eye movements, vomiting, incontinence, inability to urinate, slow and shallow breathing, rash, hives, skin peeling, physical or psychological dependence

 DRUG INTERACTIONS

Combining certain drugs may alter their action or produce unwanted side effects. Tell your doctor about other drugs you're taking, especially:
• alcohol and other drugs that make you feel sleepy or relaxed, such as tranquilizers, sleeping pills, and cold and allergy drugs
• Lanoxin
• Solfoton
• Tagamet
• tobacco or nicotine.

If you miss a dose

Take the missed dose right away if you remember within 1 hour or so. However, if you remember later, skip the missed dose and take your next dose on schedule. Don't take a double dose.

 If you suspect an overdose

Contact your doctor *immediately*. Excessive Valium can cause sleepiness, confusion, shortness of breath, slow pulse, and slurred speech.

 Warnings

• Make sure your doctor knows your medical history. You may not be able to take Valium if you're allergic to it or if you have other medical problems, especially glaucoma, a muscle disorder, Parkinson's disease, liver or kidney problems, psychological problems, or a history of drug addiction.
• If you're pregnant or breastfeeding, call your doctor before taking.

 KEEP IN MIND...

∗ Don't stop taking abruptly.
∗ Don't drink alcohol or smoke.
∗ Swallow extended-release capsules whole.

Valtrex

Valtrex is used to treat shingles, a serious viral infection that can cause a painful, long-lasting rash in a patient whose immune system is unable to fight disease. Valtrex stops the disease-causing virus from multiplying and spreading through the body.

Why it's prescribed

Doctors prescribe Valtrex to treat shingles. It comes in caplets. Doctors usually prescribe the following amounts for adults.

▶ **For shingles,** 1 gram three times a day for 7 days. Dosage is adjusted for people with poor kidney function.

How to take Valtrex

• Take Valtrex only as your doctor directs.
• Check with your doctor right away if you have symptoms of shingles (such as rash, tingling, itching, and pain). Start taking Valtrex as soon as possible after symptoms appear; this drug is most effective when treatment begins within 48 hours.
• Take Valtrex with or without food.

If you miss a dose

Take the missed dose as soon as possible. However, if it's almost time

VALTREX'S OTHER NAME

Valtrex's generic name is valacyclovir hydrochloride.

 SIDE EFFECTS

Call your doctor if you have any of these possible drug side effects.

Serious: none reported

Common: headache, nausea
Tip: To prevent nausea, take this drug with food.

Other: dizziness, vomiting, diarrhea, constipation, abdominal pain, appetite loss, weakness

 DRUG INTERACTIONS

Combining certain drugs may alter their action or produce unwanted side effects. Tell your doctor about other drugs you're taking, especially:
• Benemid
• Tagamet.

for your next dose, skip the missed dose and go back to your regular schedule. Don't take a double dose.

 If you suspect an overdose

Contact your doctor *immediately.* Although overdoses of Valtrex have not been reported, the most likely symptom would be infrequent or absent urination.

Warnings

• Make sure your doctor knows your medical history. You may not be able to take Valtrex if you have any drug allergies, a depressed immune system, HIV infection, or liver or kidney problems.
• Tell your doctor if you're pregnant or breast-feeding before you take Valtrex.

• Don't give Valtrex to a child unless the doctor prescribes it. The drug's safety in children hasn't been established.
• The drug dosage may be different in older adults, depending on how well the person's kidneys are working.

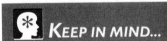 **KEEP IN MIND...**

∗ Take at first signs of shingles (rash, tingling, itching, and pain).

∗ Take with food to prevent nausea.

∗ Don't take if pregnant or breast-feeding.

∗ Don't give this drug to children unless prescribed.

Vancocin

Vancocin is an antibiotic that interferes with the growth and development of infection-causing bacteria.

Why it's prescribed

Doctors prescribe Vancocin to treat bacterial infections of the small intestine and colon. It comes in an oral liquid and capsules. Doctors usually prescribe the following amounts for adults; children's dosages appear in parentheses.

▶ **For intestinal infection,** 125 to 500 milligrams (mg) every 6 hours for 7 to 10 days. (Children: 40 mg for each 2.2 pounds of body weight daily, divided into four equal doses taken every 6 hours. Maximum dosage is 2 grams a day.)

How to take Vancocin

• Take this drug exactly as your doctor orders. Take the entire amount prescribed, even after you begin to feel better. Stopping too soon may allow the infection to return.

• If you're taking the oral liquid form of this drug, use a specially marked measuring spoon, not a household teaspoon, to measure each dose accurately.

• Store this drug in the refrigerator.

If you miss a dose

Take the missed dose as soon as possible. However, if it's almost time for your next dose, skip the missed dose and take your next dose as scheduled. Don't take a double dose.

If you suspect an overdose

Consult your doctor.

Warnings

• Make sure your doctor knows your medical history. You may not be able to take Vancocin if you're allergic to it or to other antibiotics or if you have liver or kidney problems, hearing loss, or an inflammatory bowel disorder.

• If you're pregnant or breast-feeding, check with your doctor before taking Vancocin.

• Be aware that older adults may be more prone to this drug's side effects.

SIDE EFFECTS

Call your doctor if you have any of these possible drug side effects. Call *immediately* about any labeled "serious."

Serious: severe allergic reaction (swelling of throat, wheezing, shortness of breath), kidney problems (decreased urine output), blood problems (fever, chills, increased risk of infection), ringing or feeling of fullness in ears

Common: nausea, vomiting

Other: hearing loss, rash or itching

Tip: With long-term treatment, have your hearing tested regularly.

DRUG INTERACTIONS

Combining certain drugs may alter their action or produce unwanted side effects. Tell your doctor about other drugs you're taking, especially:

• Amikin
• Colestid
• diarrhea drugs such as Kaopectate
• Fungizone
• NebuPent
• Platinol
• Questran.

VANCOCIN'S OTHER NAMES

Vancocin's generic name is vancomycin hydrochloride. Another brand name is Vancoled.

KEEP IN MIND...

* Take entire prescription, even if you feel better.

* Don't take a double dose if you miss a dose.

* With long-term treatment, have hearing tested regularly.

Vansil

Vansil is used to treat an infection that's caused by parasites called blood flukes. Although this infection is rare in North America, travelers to or immigrants from other parts of the world may have contracted it from contaminated water. This drug paralyzes the parasite that causes the infection.

Why it's prescribed

Doctors prescribe Vansil to treat a parasitic infection called schistosomiasis or snail fever. It comes in capsules. Doctors usually prescribe the following amounts.

▶ **For schistosomiasis occurring in the western hemisphere,** in adults and children weighing more than 66 pounds (lb): 15 milligrams (mg) for each 2.2 lb of body weight given as a single dose. Children under 66 lb: 10 mg for each 2.2 lb, followed by 10 mg for each 2.2 lb 2 to 8 hours later.

▶ **For schistosomiasis occurring in East or Central Africa,** 30 mg for each 2.2 lb as a single dose or divided into two equal doses and taken over 1 to 2 days.

▶ **For schistosomiasis occurring in Sudan, Uganda, or Zaire,** 40 mg for each 2.2 lb as a single dose or divided into two equal doses and taken over 1 to 2 days.

▶ **For schistosomiasis occurring in Egypt, South Africa, or Zimbabwe,** total dose of 60 mg for

VANSIL'S OTHER NAME

Vansil's generic name is oxamniquine.

SIDE EFFECTS

Call your doctor if you have any of these possible drug side effects. Call *immediately* about any labeled "serious."

Serious: seizures

Common: dizziness, drowsiness, headache, stomach upset
Tips: Don't drive or perform other activities that require you to be fully alert until you know how this drug affects you. Take Vansil just after eating a meal to reduce stomach upset.

Other: nausea, vomiting, abdominal pain, appetite loss, hives, urine color change
Tip: Don't be alarmed if your urine turns an orange or reddish color while taking Vansil. The color will return to normal when you stop taking the drug.

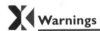

DRUG INTERACTIONS

Combining certain drugs may alter their action or produce unwanted side effects. Tell your doctor about other drugs you're taking.

---

each 2.2 lb taken as 15 mg for each 2.2 lb twice a day for 2 days or 20 mg for each 2.2 lb twice a day for 3 days.

How to take Vansil

• Take this drug exactly as your doctor orders. Take the entire amount prescribed, even if you start to feel better.

If you miss a dose

Take the missed dose as soon as possible. However, if it's almost time for your next dose, skip the missed dose and take your next dose as scheduled. Don't take a double dose.

If you suspect an overdose

Contact your doctor *immediately.* Excessive Vansil can cause blood

circulation, heart, and lung problems.

Warnings

• Make sure your doctor knows your medical history. You may not be able to take Vansil if you're allergic to it or if you have seizures.

KEEP IN MIND...

* Take entire amount prescribed.

* Take after meals to reduce side effects.

* Expect urine to turn orange or reddish while taking drug.

Vantin

Vantin is an antibiotic that kills various types of bacteria by destroying bacterial cell walls.

Why it's prescribed

Doctors prescribe Vantin to treat a variety of bacterial infections throughout the body. It comes in tablets and a liquid. Doctors usually prescribe the following amounts.

▶ **For pneumonia,** in adults and children age 13 and older, 200 milligrams (mg) orally every 12 hours for 14 days.

▶ **For bronchitis,** in adults and children age 13 and older, 200 mg orally every 12 hours for 10 days.

▶ **For gonorrhea,** in adults and children age 13 and older, 200 mg orally as a single dose.

▶ **For skin infections,** in adults and children age 13 and older, 400 mg orally every 12 hours for 7 to 14 days.

▶ **For ear infections,** in children age 6 months and over, 5 mg for each 2.2 pounds (lb) of body weight (but not more than 200 mg) orally every 12 hours for 10 days.

▶ **For throat infections,** in adults, 100 mg orally every 12 hours for 10 days. In children age 6 months and over, 5 mg for each 2.2 lb of body weight (but not more than 100 mg) orally every 12 hours for 10 days.

▶ **For urinary tract infections,** in adults, 100 mg orally every 12 hours for 7 days.

VANTIN'S OTHER NAME

Vantin's generic name is cefpodoxime proxetil.

 SIDE EFFECTS

Call your doctor if you have any of these possible drug side effects. Call *immediately* about any labeled "serious."

Serious: severe allergic reaction (wheezing, swelling of face and throat, difficulty breathing)

Common: diarrhea, headache, nausea

Other: vomiting, abdominal pain, vaginal fungal infections, rash

 DRUG INTERACTIONS

Combining certain drugs may alter their action or produce unwanted side effects. Tell your doctor about other drugs you're taking, especially:
• antacids
• Benemid.

How to take Vantin

• Take this drug exactly as your doctor orders. Take it with food to enhance the drug's effectiveness.
• To keep a steady level of the drug in your blood, space your doses evenly throughout the day and night, and don't skip any doses.
• Take the entire amount prescribed, even if you start to feel better.
• Shake the liquid form well before taking it. Store it in the refrigerator.

If you miss a dose

Take the missed dose as soon as possible. But if it's almost time for your next dose, skip the missed dose and take your next dose as scheduled. Don't take a double dose.

 If you suspect an overdose

Contact your doctor *immediately.* Excessive Vantin can cause nausea, vomiting, and diarrhea.

 Warnings

• Make sure your doctor knows your medical history. You may not be able to take Vantin if you're allergic to it or to other antibiotics. If you have kidney problems, you'll probably take a smaller dose.
• Tell your doctor if you're pregnant or breast-feeding.
• If you're diabetic and you use urine sugar tests, ask your doctor which one to use. Vantin can interfere with the results of Clinitest.
• Before having medical tests, tell the doctor you're taking Vantin.

KEEP IN MIND...

∗ Take entire amount prescribed.
∗ Take with food.
∗ Space doses evenly through day and night; don't skip doses.

Vaseretic

Vaseretic is a combination of a diuretic (water pill) and a drug that causes blood vessels to relax.

Why it's prescribed

Doctors prescribe Vaseretic to lower high blood pressure. This drug comes in tablets. Doctors usually prescribe the following amounts for adults.

▶ For high blood pressure, 1 or 2 tablets once a day.

How to take Vaseretic

• Take this drug exactly as your doctor orders.
• Vaseretic usually increases urination. If you take one dose a day, take it in the morning after breakfast. If you take two or more doses a day, take the last dose no later than 6:00 p.m. to prevent nighttime urination.

If you miss a dose

Take the missed dose as soon as possible. However, if it's almost time for your next dose, skip the missed dose and take your next dose as scheduled. Don't take a double dose.

If you suspect an overdose

Contact your doctor *immediately*. Excessive Vaseretic can cause dehydration (dry skin, weakness, thirst, fast pulse) and irregular heartbeats.

VASERETIC'S OTHER NAMES

Vaseretic is a combination of two generic drugs: enalapril maleate and hydrochlorothiazide.

SIDE EFFECTS

Call your doctor if you have any of these possible drug side effects. Call *immediately* about any labeled "serious."

Serious: angioedema (swelling of face, tongue, vocal cords), low blood pressure (dizziness, weakness), abdominal pain, chest pain, fast pulse, blood problems (fever, sore throat, joint pain, easy bleeding or bruising), muscle cramps, swelling of face, mouth, hands, ankles, or feet

Common: dizziness, tiredness, headache, skin sensitivity to sun
Tips: Prevent dizziness by standing up slowly and taking care while walking. If you're not fully alert, don't drive or perform other activities that could be dangerous. Protect yourself from the sun by wearing a sunscreen and protective clothing.

Other: nausea, vomiting, heartburn, gas, sleeplessness, cough
Tip: Take with food to avoid nausea.

DRUG INTERACTIONS

Combining certain drugs may alter their action or produce unwanted side effects. Tell your doctor about other drugs you're taking, especially:
• alcohol
• heart drugs, such as Aldomet, Apresoline, and nitroglycerin
• insulin or oral diabetes drugs such as Micronase
• lithium
• nonsteroidal anti-inflammatory drugs such as Motrin
• other diuretics such as Lasix
• steroids such as prednisone.

Warnings

• Make sure your doctor knows your medical history. You may not be able to take Vaseretic if you're allergic to it or if you have diabetes, immune diseases, pancreatitis, or kidney or liver disease.
• If you're pregnant, check with your doctor before taking this drug.
• If you have persistent diarrhea or vomiting, call your doctor right away. These problems can make you lose too much water, leading to low blood pressure.

• Follow your doctor's recommendation to follow a low-salt diet because too much salt can increase blood pressure.

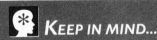 KEEP IN MIND...

∗ Take last dose no later than 6:00 p.m.

∗ Call doctor if you have fever or other signs of infection.

∗ Follow a low-salt diet, if prescribed.

Vasotec

Vasotec is used to reverse the action of a natural substance that narrows blood vessels. When the blood vessels relax, blood pressure decreases while the amount of blood and oxygen available to the heart increases.

Why it's prescribed

Doctors prescribe Vasotec to lower high blood pressure or, when used with other drugs, to treat heart conditions. It comes in tablets. Doctors usually prescribe the following amounts for adults.

▶ For high blood pressure, at first, 5 milligrams (mg) once a day, then adjusted according to response. Usual dosage is 10 to 40 mg a day as a single dose or divided into two equal doses.

How to take Vasotec

• Take this drug exactly as your doctor orders. Don't stop taking Vasotec suddenly without checking first with your doctor.

If you miss a dose

Take the missed dose as soon as possible. However, if it's almost time for your next dose, skip the missed dose and take your next dose as scheduled. Don't take a double dose.

 If you suspect an overdose

Contact your doctor *immediately*. Excessive Vasotec can cause low blood pressure (dizziness, weakness).

VASOTEC'S OTHER NAME

Vasotec's generic name is enalapril maleate.

 SIDE EFFECTS

Call your doctor if you have any of these possible drug side effects. Call *immediately* about any labeled "serious."

Serious: severe blood problems (fatigue, bleeding, bruising, chills, fever, increased risk of infection); swelling of face, eyes, lips, tongue, hands, or feet; difficulty swallowing or breathing; kidney problems (decreased urine output); light-headedness; low blood pressure (dizziness, weakness)

Common: headache, fatigue, tickle in throat, persistent dry cough
Tips: Headache and fatigue usually go away as your body adjusts to Vasotec; if not, check with your doctor. Don't drive or perform other activities that could be dangerous if you're not fully alert.

Other: sleeplessness, diarrhea, nausea, rash, heavy sweating
Tip: To prevent excessive fluid loss from sweating, avoid getting overheated.

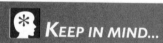 **DRUG INTERACTIONS**

Combining certain drugs may alter their action or produce unwanted side effects. Tell your doctor about other drugs you're taking, especially:
• Advil and other nonsteroidal anti-inflammatory drugs
• alcohol
• Eskalith
• insulin and oral diabetes drugs
• potassium supplements and some diuretics.

✗ Warnings

• Make sure your doctor knows your medical history. You may not be able to take Vasotec if you're allergic to it or to similar drugs; if you have kidney or liver problems, an immune disease, diabetes, heart or blood vessel disease, or lupus; or if you've recently had a heart attack or stroke.
• If you're pregnant or think you may be, check with your doctor before taking this drug.
• Follow the diet your doctor prescribes while taking Vasotec. You may need to restrict your intake of salt, but don't use salt substitutes or low-salt products unless your doctor tells you otherwise.

✳ KEEP IN MIND...

* Don't stop taking Vasotec abruptly.
* Don't drink alcohol without doctor's permission.
* Follow a low-salt diet if prescribed.
* Avoid getting overheated.

Veetids

Veetids is a natural penicillin that fights bacteria. It affects the bacteria's cell walls and stops them from growing.

Why it's prescribed

Doctors prescribe Veetids to treat internal bacterial infections. It comes in tablets, delayed-release tablets, and a liquid. Doctors usually prescribe the following amounts for adults; children's dosages appear in parentheses.

▶ **For mild to moderate infections,** 250 to 500 milligrams (mg) every 6 hours. (Children: 15 to 50 mg for each 2.2 pounds [lb] of body weight daily, divided into equal doses taken every 6 to 8 hours.)

▶ **To prevent heart infection after dental surgery,** 2 grams (g) 30 to 60 minutes before procedure, then 1 g 6 hours afterward. (Children who weigh 66 lb or more: same as adults. Children under 66 lb: half of adult dose.)

How to take Veetids

• Take this drug exactly as your doctor orders. Take it on an empty stomach (1 to 2 hours before or 3 to 4 hours after a meal).

• Take each dose with a full glass (8 ounces) of water (not fruit juice or carbonated drinks).

VEETIDS' OTHER NAMES

Veetids' generic name is penicillin V potassium. Other brand names include Beepen-VK, Betapen-VK, Ledercillin VK, Pen Vee, Robicillin VK, V-Cillin K, VC-K; and, in Canada, Apo-Pen-VK, Nadopen-V-200, NovoPen-VK, Nu-Pen VK, and PVF K.

 SIDE EFFECTS

Call your doctor if you have any of these possible drug side effects. Call *immediately* about any labeled "serious."

Serious: seizures (with high doses), severe blood problems (fatigue, bleeding, bruising, fever, chills, increased risk of infection), allergic reaction (rash, fever, chills, wheezing, swelling of face and throat, difficulty breathing)

Common: stomach upset, nausea

Other: numbness or tingling in hands or feet, vomiting, diarrhea
Tip: If you develop severe diarrhea, check with your doctor before taking a diarrhea drug.

 DRUG INTERACTIONS

Combining certain drugs may alter their action or produce unwanted side effects. Tell your doctor about other drugs you're taking, especially:
• aminoglycosides such as Gentamycin
• Anturane
• Benemid
• birth control pills (use an additional form of birth control while taking Veetids).

• Finish your entire prescription, even if you feel better. Discard leftover Veetids when treatment ends.

If you miss a dose

Take the missed dose as soon as possible. But if it's almost time for your next dose, skip the missed dose and take your next dose as scheduled. Don't take a double dose.

 If you suspect an overdose

Contact your doctor *immediately.* Excessive Veetids can cause seizures.

Warnings

• Make sure your doctor knows your medical history. You may not be able to take Veetids if you're allergic to it or to other antibiotics or if you have digestive problems.

• Tell your doctor if you're pregnant or breast-feeding.

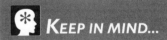 KEEP IN MIND...

* Take on an empty stomach, followed by a full glass of water.

* If you take birth control pills, use an extra form of birth control while taking Veetids.

* Don't use leftover Veetids for a new infection.

Ventolin

Ventolin eases breathing by relaxing muscles in the lung passages.

Why it's prescribed

Doctors prescribe Ventolin to prevent and treat the wheezing and throat closing (bronchospasm) of asthma and other breathing problems that temporarily restrict the lung passages. It comes in an aerosol inhaler, solution for inhalation, capsules for inhalation, tablets, sustained-release tablets, and syrup. Doctors usually prescribe the following amounts for adults; dosages for children and older adults appear in parentheses.

▶ **To prevent or treat bronchospasm,** 1 to 2 puffs of aerosol inhaler every 4 to 6 hours, or 2.5 milligrams (mg) of the solution for inhalation by nebulizer three or four times a day, or 200 micrograms (mcg) of capsules for inhalation using Rotahaler every 4 to 6 hours, or 2 to 4 mg of tablets three or four times a day to maximum of 8 mg four times a day.

• Children age 12 and older: same as adults or as follows.
• Children ages 6 to 13: 1 teaspoon (tsp) syrup three or four times a day.
• Children ages 2 to 5: 0.1 mg syrup for each 2.2 pounds of body weight three times a day to maximum of 1 tsp three times a day.
• Adults over age 65: 1 tsp three or four times a day.)

▶ **To prevent exercise-induced asthma,** 2 inhalations 15 minutes before exercise.

VENTOLIN'S OTHER NAMES

Ventolin's generic name is albuterol. Another brand name is Proventil.

 SIDE EFFECTS

Call your doctor if you have any of these possible drug side effects. Call *immediately* about any labeled "serious."

Serious: asthmalike attacks (bronchospasm), rapid pulse, palpitations, high blood pressure (headache, blurred vision)
Tip: Repeated use of Ventolin can sometimes *cause* bronchospasm. If it does, stop using the drug and call your doctor right away.

Common: tremor, nervousness, dizziness, headache, insomnia

Other: drying and irritation of nose, mouth, and throat; heartburn; nausea; vomiting; muscle cramps
Tip: Use a cool-mist humidifier to prevent dryness.

 DRUG INTERACTIONS

Combining certain drugs may alter their action or produce unwanted side effects. Tell your doctor about other drugs you're taking, especially:
• central nervous system stimulants, such as caffeine and amphetamines (diet pills)
• drugs for depression, such as MAO inhibitors and tricyclic antidepressants
• Inderal and other beta blockers
• Larodopa.

How to take Ventolin

• If you take more than 1 inhalation by aerosol inhaler, wait at least 2 minutes between doses.
• If you're also using a steroid inhaler, use Ventolin first; then wait at least 5 minutes before using the steroid.

If you miss a dose

Take the missed dose as soon as possible. If you have more doses scheduled that day, take at equal intervals. Don't take a double dose.

 If you suspect an overdose

Contact your doctor *immediately.* Excessive Ventolin can cause angina (chest pain), high blood pressure (headache, blurred vision), and seizures.

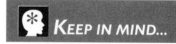 **Warnings**

• Make sure your doctor knows your medical history. You may not be able to take Ventolin if you're allergic to it or if you have heart or blood vessel problems, an overactive thyroid, or diabetes.
• If you have trouble breathing after using Ventolin, call your doctor.

KEEP IN MIND...

* Use your inhaler properly.
* Wait at least 2 minutes between inhalations.
* Call doctor if breathing doesn't improve.

VePesid

VePesid is a drug that fights cancer. It works by interfering with cell growth.

Why it's prescribed

Doctors usually prescribe VePesid to treat cancer of the testicles. It comes in capsules and is also available in an injectable form (to treat certain types of lung cancer). Doctors usually prescribe the following amounts for adults.

▶ **For testicular cancer,** 50 to 100 milligrams (mg) orally per square meter (m^2) of body surface area on 5 consecutive days every 3 to 4 weeks, or 100 mg per m^2 on days 1, 3, and 5 every 3 to 4 weeks.

How to take VePesid

• Take this drug exactly as your doctor orders. Continue taking it as prescribed, even if it makes you vomit or feel sick.
• If you vomit shortly after taking a dose, call your doctor to find out if you should repeat the dose.
• Store VePesid capsules in the refrigerator.

If you miss a dose

Don't take the missed dose. Skip it, call your doctor, and take your next dose as scheduled. Don't take a double dose.

 If you suspect an overdose

Contact your doctor *immediately*. Excessive VePesid can cause increased nausea, vomiting, bleed-

VEPESID'S OTHER NAME

VePesid's generic name is etoposide (also known as VP-16).

 SIDE EFFECTS

Call your doctor if you have any of these possible drug side effects. Call *immediately* about any labeled "serious."

Serious: severe blood problems (fatigue, bleeding, bruising, fever, chills, sore throat), severe allergic reaction (wheezing, throat and facial swelling, difficulty breathing)

Common: swollen or irritated mouth tissues, anemia (fatigue), reversible hair loss
Tip: Hair that is lost while taking VePesid will grow back when treatment ends. Meanwhile, wear a scarf, hat, or wig.

Other: occasional headache and fever, numbness or tingling in hands and feet, nausea and vomiting, appetite loss, abdominal pain

 DRUG INTERACTIONS

Combining certain drugs may alter their action or produce unwanted side effects. Tell your doctor about other drugs you're taking, especially:
• anticoagulants (blood thinners) such as Coumadin
• antiviral and antifungal drugs, such as Ancobon, Cytovene, Fungizone, and Retrovir (AZT)
• Chloromycetin
• colchicine
• Imuran (an immune system suppressant)
• other cancer drugs, such as Intron-A and Mitracin
• thyroid drugs.

ing, bruising, fatigue, fever, and chills.

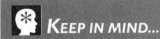 **Warnings**

• Make sure your doctor knows your medical history. You may not be able to take VePesid if you're allergic to it; if you've had previous chemotherapy or radiation therapy; if you have shingles, kidney or liver disease; or if you've recently been exposed to chickenpox.
• Tell your doctor right away if you're pregnant or you wish to breast-feed.

• While you're taking VePesid, don't get any vaccinations or let any family members get vaccinations without your doctor's knowledge.

KEEP IN MIND...

* Keep taking VePesid, even if it makes you feel sick.
* Store capsules in the refrigerator.
* Don't get vaccinations during treatment.

Vermox

Vermox interferes with the metabolism of parasitic worms.

Why it's prescribed

Doctors prescribe Vermox to treat pinworm, roundworm, whipworm, and hookworm. It comes in tablets and a liquid. Doctors usually prescribe the following amounts for adults and children over age 2.

▶ **For pinworms,** 100 milligrams (mg) as a single dose. If infection is still present 3 weeks later, treatment is repeated.

▶ **For roundworms, whipworms, and hookworms,** 100 mg twice a day for 3 days. If infection is still present 3 weeks later, treatment is repeated.

How to take Vermox

• Take Vermox exactly as your doctor orders.
• If you're taking the tablets, chew them, swallow them whole, or crush them.
• Take Vermox with meals. High-fat foods, such as ice cream and whole milk, help the drug work better. If you're on a low-fat diet, check with your doctor.

If you miss a dose

Take the missed dose as soon as possible. However, if it's almost time for your next scheduled dose and the doctor has prescribed two doses a day, space the missed dose and the next

VERMOX'S OTHER NAME

Vermox's generic name is mebendazole.

 SIDE EFFECTS

Call your doctor if you have any of these possible drug side effects. Call *immediately* about any labeled "serious."

Serious: fever, itching, rash, blood problems (sore throat, unusual weakness or fatigue)

Common: dizziness

Other: occasional abdominal pain and diarrhea (with large quantity of worms to expel)

 DRUG INTERACTIONS

Combining certain drugs may alter their action or produce unwanted side effects. Tell your doctor about other drugs you're taking, especially:
• seizure drugs, such as Dilantin and Tegretol.

dose 4 to 5 hours apart. Then resume your normal schedule.

 If you suspect an overdose

Contact your doctor *immediately.* Excessive Vermox can cause nausea, vomiting, confusion, and decreased alertness.

 Warnings

• Make sure your doctor knows your medical history. You may not be able to take Vermox if you're allergic to it or if you have liver disease or intestinal problems (Crohn's disease, ulcerative colitis).
• If you're pregnant, check with your doctor before taking this drug.
• If symptoms don't improve in a few days or if they get worse, call your doctor.
• To avoid spreading the infection, wash your hands often, especially before meals and after bowel move-

ments. Don't prepare food for other people while you're infected. Change your undergarments, pajamas, and bed linens daily while being treated. Handle bed linens gently; don't shake them. Vacuum or damp-mop floors daily.
• To prevent reinfection, members of your household may also need to take Vermox while you're being treated. To eliminate the infection, you may need a second treatment 2 to 3 weeks after the first.

KEEP IN MIND...

* Take Vermox with meals, preferably with high-fat foods.
* Wash hands often.
* Don't prepare other people's food while infected.
* Change undergarments, pajamas, and bed linens daily.

Vibramycin

Vibramycin is an antibiotic that kills bacteria by preventing them from reproducing.

Why it's prescribed

Doctors prescribe Vibramycin to treat bacterial infections, such as gonorrhea, syphilis, and others. Vibramycin comes in capsules, tablets, and an injectable form. Another form of the generic drug comes in a liquid. Doctors usually prescribe the following amounts for adults; children's dosages appear in parentheses.

▶ **For Lyme disease, chlamydia, and other infections,** 100 milligrams (mg) every 12 hours the first day, then 100 mg a day. (Children over 99 pounds [lb]: same as adults. Children over age 8 and under 99 lb: 4.4 mg for each 2.2 lb of body weight daily, divided into two equal doses taken every 12 hours the first day; then 2.2 to 4.4 mg for each 2.2 lb a day.)

▶ **For gonorrhea,** 200 mg initially, followed by 100 mg at bedtime and 100 mg twice a day for 3 days; or 300 mg initially, repeated in 1 hour.

▶ **For syphilis,** 300 mg a day, divided into several doses each day, for at least 10 days.

▶ **For urethral, cervical, or rectal infections,** 100 mg twice a day for at least 7 days.

VIBRAMYCIN'S OTHER NAMES

Vibramycin's generic name is doxycycline hyclate. The generic name for Vibramycin liquid is doxycycline calcium. Other brand names include Apo-Doxy, Doryx, Doxy-Caps, Monodox, Novodoxylin, Vibra-Tabs; and, in Canada, Doxycin and Novodoxylin.

 ## SIDE EFFECTS

Call your doctor if you have any of these possible drug side effects. Call *immediately* about any labeled "serious."

Serious: chest pain, increased pressure in head (confusion, sleepiness, headache), allergic reaction (severe headache, vision changes, hives, itching), severe allergic reaction (swelling, wheezing, difficulty breathing)

Common: stomach upset, nausea, diarrhea, sensitivity to sun, darker skin color
Tips: Limit your exposure to the sun. When you do go outdoors, wear a sunscreen, a hat, and protective clothing. Check with your doctor if the symptoms persist or become severe.

Other: sore throat, irritated tongue, trouble swallowing, appetite loss, vomiting, fungal infection in mouth, colitis, inflamed anus or genitals, tooth defects or discoloration, other infections, blood clots (sudden shortness of breath; pain, swelling, redness in legs)
Tips: Practice excellent oral hygiene during treatment. Call your doctor if you develop spots or patches in your mouth.

 ## DRUG INTERACTIONS

Combining certain drugs may alter their action or produce unwanted side effects. Tell your doctor about other drugs you're taking, especially:
• alcohol
• antacids (including sodium bicarbonate)
• anticoagulants (blood thinners) such as Coumadin
• birth control pills (use additional birth control method while taking Vibramycin)
• diarrhea drugs
• iron supplements
• laxatives containing aluminum, magnesium, or calcium
• penicillin
• seizure drugs, such as Solfoton and Tegretol.

▶ **To prevent malaria,** 100 mg a day starting 1 or 2 days before travel and continuing for 4 weeks after return. (Children over age 8: 2 mg for each 2.2 lb once a day. Dosage should not exceed adult dose.)

How to take Vibramycin

• Take this drug exactly as your doctor orders. Take your dose with food, milk, or a full glass (8 ounces) of water to prevent irritation of your esophagus or stomach.
• If you're taking the liquid form, use a specially marked spoon, not a household teaspoon, to measure each dose accurately.
• To avoid heartburn, don't take tablets or capsules within 1 hour of bedtime.

Continued on next page ▶

• Continue to take this drug even if you start to feel better after a few days. Stopping too soon may allow your infection to return.

• Store this drug away from heat and direct light. Don't keep it in the bathroom, near the kitchen sink, or in other damp places. Heat or moisture could cause the drug to break down. Keep the liquid form of the drug from freezing.

• If this drug has changed color, tastes or looks different, has become outdated, or has been stored incorrectly, don't use it; it could cause serious side effects. Discard the bottle and obtain a fresh supply.

If you miss a dose

Take the missed dose as soon as possible. But if it's almost time for your next dose, adjust your schedule as follows:

• If you take one dose a day, space the missed dose and the next dose 10 to 12 hours apart. Then resume your regular schedule.

• If you take two doses a day, space the missed dose and the next dose 5 to 6 hours apart. Then resume your regular schedule.

• If you take three or more doses a day, space the missed dose and the next dose 2 to 4 hours apart. Then resume your regular schedule.

If you suspect an overdose

Contact your doctor *immediately*. Excessive Vibramycin can cause nausea and vomiting.

Warnings

• Make sure your doctor knows your medical history. You may not be able to take Vibramycin if you're allergic to it or to other antibiotics (especially tetracyclines) or if you have liver or kidney disease.

• If you're pregnant or breast-feeding, check with your doctor before taking this drug. Vibramycin could stain your baby's teeth.

• Don't give this drug to children under age 8 because it can stain their teeth and slow down bone growth.

• If you're a diabetic, be aware that Vibramycin can produce false-positive readings on certain tests of urine sugar. Your doctor may instruct you to measure your sugar level another way.

• Because Vibramycin can interfere with the effectiveness of birth control pills, use another nonhormonal form of birth control, such as a diaphragm or condom, while you're taking this drug.

• If you have a job where you're exposed to the sun for long periods of time, notify your doctor, who may prescribe another antibiotic.

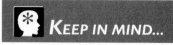 **KEEP IN MIND...**

* Take with food, milk, or water.

* Take full amount prescribed, even if you start to feel better.

* Don't give to children under age 8.

* Use a nonhormonal form of birth control during Vibramycin treatment.

* Don't drink alcohol while taking Vibramycin.

Vicodin

Vicodin is a combination of a narcotic pain reliever and acetaminophen (Tylenol). This combination reduces pain and fever and alters the perception of pain.

Why it's prescribed

Doctors prescribe Vicodin to relieve pain. It comes in tablets. Doctors usually prescribe the following amounts for adults.

▶ **For moderate or moderately severe pain,** 1 or 2 tablets every 4 to 6 hours, up to 8 tablets a day.

How to take Vicodin

• Take this drug exactly as your doctor orders. Don't take more of it than prescribed.
• If you take Vicodin regularly, don't stop taking it abruptly.

If you miss a dose

Take the missed dose as soon as possible. But if it's almost time for your next dose, skip the missed dose and take your next dose as scheduled. Don't take a double dose.

If you suspect an overdose

Contact your doctor *immediately.* Excessive Vicodin can cause unconsciousness, low blood sugar (drowsiness, cold sweats, nervousness, confusion, headache), decreased urine output, internal bleeding, nausea, vomiting, sweating, slow and shallow breathing, cold and clammy skin, and low

VICODIN'S OTHER NAMES

Vicodin is a combination of two generic drugs: acetaminophen and hydrocodone bitartrate.

 SIDE EFFECTS

Call your doctor if you have any of these possible drug side effects. Call *immediately* about any labeled "serious."

Serious: seizures

Common: dizziness, light-headedness, fainting, drowsiness, nausea, vomiting, tiredness, weakness
Tips: If you feel dizzy, light-headed, or nauseous, lie down for awhile after taking each dose. If you're not fully alert, don't drive or perform other activities that could be dangerous. To minimize dizziness and light-headedness, get up slowly after sitting or lying down.

Other: vision changes, constipation, dry mouth, headache, appetite loss, nervousness, sleeplessness, disturbing dreams
Tips: To reduce constipation, drink plenty of water and eat fiber-rich foods, such as whole grains, vegetables, and fruits. To relieve dry mouth, try sugarless gum or hard candy or ice chips. If your mouth stays dry for more than 2 weeks, tell your doctor or dentist.

 DRUG INTERACTIONS

Combining certain drugs may alter their action or produce unwanted side effects. Tell your doctor about other drugs you're taking, especially:
• alcohol and other drugs that make you feel relaxed or sleepy, such as tranquilizers, sleeping pills, and cold and allergy drugs
• drugs for depression, such as MAO inhibitors and tricyclic antidepressants
• other drugs that contain acetaminophen
• Retrovir (AZT)
• Tegretol
• Trexan.

blood pressure (dizziness, weakness).

X Warnings

• Make sure your doctor knows your medical history. You may not be able to take Vicodin if you're allergic to it or if you have a head injury, a digestive disorder, seizures, asthma or another chronic lung disease, liver or kidney problems, an underactive thyroid, an enlarged prostate, gallbladder disease, heart disease, alcohol or drug problems, or mental illness.

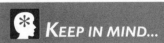

* Don't stop taking abruptly after regular use.

* Increase fluids and fiber in diet.

* Relieve dry mouth with sugarless gum or hard candy or ice chips.

Videx

Videx inhibits reproduction of the human immunodeficiency virus (HIV), which is the cause of AIDS.

Why it's prescribed

Doctors prescribe Videx for advanced HIV infection. It comes in chewable tablets and in a powder to make an oral solution or a children's oral solution. Doctors usually prescribe the following amounts for adults; children's dosages appear in parentheses.

▶ **For HIV,** in adults weighing 165 pounds (lb) and over, 300 mg every 12 hours or 375 mg of powder every 12 hours. In adults weighing 110 to 164 lb, 200 mg every 12 hours or 250 mg of powder every 12 hours. In adults weighing 77 to 109 lb, 125 mg every 12 hours or 167 mg of powder every 12 hours. (Children: 200 mg for each square meter of body surface area daily divided into two equal doses taken every 12 hours.)

How to take Videx

• Take this drug on an empty stomach.
• To use powder for oral solution, pour contents of single-dose packet into half a glass (4 ounces) of water (not fruit juice or other acidic beverages). Stir until the powder dissolves completely, and take the dose immediately.
• Chew the tablets thoroughly before swallowing, and drink water with each dose. Or crush the tablets and stir them thoroughly into an ounce of water; then drink the mixture immediately.

Videx's Other Name

Videx's generic name is didanosine (ddI).

Side Effects

Call your doctor if you have any of these possible drug side effects. Call *immediately* about any labeled "serious."

Serious: seizures, inflamed pancreas (nausea, vomiting, abdominal pain), high blood pressure (headache, blurred vision)

Common: headache, diarrhea, nausea, vomiting, numbness or tingling in hands or feet

Other: sleeplessness, dizziness, confusion, anxiety, abnormal thinking, swelling in hands or legs, dry mouth, gas, liver problems (yellow-tinged skin and eyes, unusual tiredness), rash, itchiness, weakness, muscle aches or spasms, muscle wasting, pain, arthritis, pneumonia, infection, cough, hair loss

Drug Interactions

Combining certain drugs may alter their action or produce unwanted side effects. Tell your doctor about other drugs you're taking, especially:
• antacids containing magnesium or aluminum hydroxides
• antibiotics (tetracyclines or fluoroquinolones such as Cipro)
• Nizoral
• Sporanox.

If you miss a dose

Take the missed dose as soon as possible. But if it's almost time for your next dose, skip the missed dose and take your next dose as scheduled. Don't take a double dose.

If you suspect an overdose

Consult your doctor *immediately.* Excessive Videx can cause nausea, vomiting, diarrhea, abdominal pain, pain in fingertips and toes, and yellow-tinged skin and eyes.

Warnings

• Make sure your doctor knows your medical history. You may not be able to take Videx if you're allergic to it or if you have an inflamed pancreas, liver or kidney problems, alcoholism, heart disease, high blood pressure, blood problems, gout, or swelling, numbness, or tingling in your hands or feet.
• Tell your doctor right away if you think you're pregnant or you wish to breast-feed.
• If you're on a low-sodium diet, include the sodium in Videx in your daily amount.

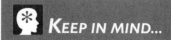

Keep in Mind...

* Take on empty stomach.
* Chew tablets thoroughly.
* If you're on a low-salt diet, include the sodium in Videx in your daily amount.

Vioform

Vioform is used to treat certain skin infections. It works by killing the infection-causing bacteria or fungi.

Why it's used

Vioform is used to treat bacterial or fungal infections of the skin. You can buy it without a prescription. It comes in a cream and an ointment. The following amounts are usually recommended for adults and children over age 2.

▶ **For inflamed skin conditions,** small amount applied two or three times a day.

How to use Vioform

• Apply Vioform in a thin layer and gently rub it in. Use it for as long as the package label directs, but not for more than 1 week. Or follow your doctor's recommendations.
• Don't use Vioform in or around your eyes.

If you miss a dose

Apply the missed dose as soon as possible. However, if it's almost time for your next dose, skip the

VIOFORM'S OTHER NAMES

Vioform's generic name is iodochlorhydroxyquin (also known as clioquinol). Other brand names include Ala-Quin, Corque, Cortin, and Torofor.

 SIDE EFFECTS

Call your doctor if you have any of these possible drug side effects. Call *immediately* about any labeled "serious."

Serious: unsteadiness, confusion

Common: burning, itching, acnelike eruptions

Other: itching, redness, rash

 DRUG INTERACTIONS

Combining certain drugs may alter their action or produce unwanted side effects. Tell your doctor about other drugs you're taking, especially:
• corticosteroids, such as Solu-Cortef and Solu-Medrol.

missed dose and apply your next dose as scheduled. Don't apply a double dose.

 If you suspect an overdose

Contact your doctor.

 Warnings

• You may not be able to use Vioform if you're allergic to it. Consult your doctor.
• Follow your doctor's recommendations to stop using Vioform at least 1 month before you have certain medical tests.
• Don't use Vioform to treat diaper rash or fungal infections of the scalp or nails.
• Be aware that Vioform may stain clothes or hair.

• If your skin condition doesn't improve or worsens after 1 week, call your doctor.

 KEEP IN MIND...

* Don't use in or around eyes.
* Don't use for more than 1 week unless prescribed by doctor.
* Call doctor if symptoms get worse or last more than 1 week.
* Don't use for diaper rash or fungal infections of nails or scalp.
* Don't get Vioform on clothing or in hair.

Visine

Visine reduces eye redness by narrowing blood vessels in the clear lining of the eye.

Why it's used

Visine is used to relieve eye redness and minor irritation. You can buy it without a prescription. It comes in eyedrops. The following amounts are usually recommended for adults and children over age 2.

▶ **For eye redness, irritation, and allergic reactions,** 1 to 2 drops instilled up to four times a day or as directed by doctor.

How to use Visine

- Use this drug exactly as the package instructions recommend. Don't use more of this drug than recommended. Overuse can increase redness.
- Wash your hands before and after using Visine.
- To avoid contaminating this drug, don't touch the dropper tip to your eye, the surrounding skin, or anything else.
- After using the drops, press a finger lightly against the inside corner of each eye for 1 or 2 minutes to prevent the drug from entering your tear ducts.

If you miss a dose

Instill the missed dose as soon as possible. However, if it's almost time for your next dose, skip the missed

VISINE'S OTHER NAMES

Visine's generic name is tetrahydrozoline hydrochloride. Other brand names include Murine Plus, Optigene, Soothe, and Tetrasine.

 SIDE EFFECTS

Call your doctor if you have any of these possible drug side effects. Call *immediately* about any labeled "serious."

Serious: altered heart rhythm, sleepiness, seizures, high blood pressure (headache, blurred vision)

Common: temporary stinging

Other: dizziness, headache, sleeplessness, tremor, anxiety, hallucinations, weakness, palpitations, sweating, temporary eye dryness, sneezing, increased redness (with long-term or excessive use), blurred vision, enlarged pupils, irritated eyes, tearing, sensitivity to light
Tip: Don't drive if you feel dizzy or if your vision is blurry.

 DRUG INTERACTIONS

Combining certain drugs may alter their action or produce unwanted side effects. Tell your doctor about other drugs you're taking, especially:
- drugs for depression, such as MAO inhibitors and tricyclic antidepressants
- Ismelin.

dose and instill your next dose as scheduled. Don't instill a double dose.

 If you suspect an overdose

Contact your doctor *immediately*. Excessive Visine can cause very low blood pressure (severe dizziness and weakness), sleepiness, and coma.

 Warnings

- Consult your doctor before using Visine if you're allergic to it or to any of its components or if you have glaucoma or another serious eye disease, an overactive thyroid, heart disease, high blood pressure, or diabetes.
- If you wear contact lenses, check with your doctor before using Visine.

- Stop using Visine and call your doctor if you experience eye pain or vision changes or if redness and irritation persist, get worse, or last more than 3 days.
- Don't share your eyedrops with anyone.

KEEP IN MIND...

* Don't allow dropper tip to touch anything.
* Wash hands before and after use.
* Call doctor if symptoms worsen or last more than 3 days.
* Press lightly on inside corners of eyes for 1 to 2 minutes after using drops.
* Don't share eyedrops.

Visine LR

Visine LR reduces eye redness by narrowing blood vessels in the clear lining of the eye.

Why it's prescribed

Doctors prescribe Visine LR to reduce eye redness caused by minor irritations. It comes in eyedrops. Doctors usually prescribe the following amounts for adults and children age 6 and over.

▶ **For eye redness,** 1 to 2 drops in lower eyelid two to four times a day (spaced at least 6 hours apart).

How to use Visine LR

• Use Visine LR exactly as your doctor directs.
• Wash your hands before and after using the drops.
• To avoid contaminating this drug, don't touch the dropper tip to your eye, the surrounding skin, or anything else. Discard solution that appears cloudy or discolored.
• After using the drops, press a finger lightly against the inside corner of each eye for 1 or 2 minutes to prevent the drug from entering your tear ducts.

If you miss a dose

Instill the missed dose as soon as possible. However, if it's almost time for your next dose, skip the

VISINE LR'S OTHER NAMES

Visine LR's generic name is oxymetazoline hydrochloride. Another brand name is OcuClear.

 SIDE EFFECTS

Call your doctor if you have any of these possible drug side effects. Call *immediately* about any labeled "serious."

Serious: eye pain, vision changes, redness and irritation that worsen or last more than 3 days

Common: temporary stinging

Other: blurred vision, increased redness (with excessive or prolonged use), palpitations, rapid or irregular heartbeat, headache, light-headedness, nervousness, trembling, sleeplessness

 DRUG INTERACTIONS

Combining certain drugs may alter their action or produce unwanted side effects. Tell your doctor about other drugs you're taking, especially:
• Ludiomil
• tricyclic antidepressants.

missed dose and instill your next dose as scheduled. Don't instill a double dose.

 If you suspect an overdose

Contact your doctor *immediately.* Excessive Visine LR can cause low blood pressure (dizziness, weakness), a slow pulse, and sleepiness.

 Warnings

• Make sure your doctor knows your medical history. You may not be able to use Visine LR if you're allergic to it or to any of its components or if you have glaucoma or another eye disease, an eye infection or injury, an overactive thyroid, heart disease, or high blood pressure.

• If you wear contact lenses, check with your doctor before using Visine LR.
• Don't share your eyedrops with anyone.

 KEEP IN MIND...

* Don't let dropper tip touch anything.

* Call doctor if symptoms worsen or last more than 3 days.

* Press lightly against inside corners of eyes for 1 to 2 minutes after using drops.

* Don't use cloudy or discolored solution.

Visken

V isken is one of a group of drugs called beta blockers. It reduces the heart's workload and its need for oxygen and relaxes blood vessels.

Why it's prescribed

Doctors prescribe Visken to treat high blood pressure. It comes in tablets. Doctors usually prescribe the following amounts for adults.
▶ **For high blood pressure,** at first, 5 milligrams (mg) twice a day, increased as needed and tolerated to a maximum of 60 mg a day.

How to take Visken

- Take this drug exactly as your doctor orders. Don't skip a dose, even if you feel well.
- Check your pulse before taking each dose of Visken. Call your doctor if your pulse is much slower or faster than usual.
- Don't stop taking Visken abruptly without your doctor's permission.

If you miss a dose

Take the missed dose as soon as possible. But if it's within 4 hours of your next dose, skip the missed dose and take your next dose as scheduled. Don't take a double dose.

If you suspect an overdose

Contact your doctor *immediately*. Excessive Visken can cause asthmalike attacks, severe low blood pressure (extreme dizziness and weakness, very slow pulse), and heart failure.

VISKEN'S OTHER NAMES

Visken's generic name is pindolol. Canadian brand names include Novo-Pindol and Syn-Pindolol.

SIDE EFFECTS

Call your doctor if you have any of these possible drug side effects. Call *immediately* about any labeled "serious."

Serious: congestive heart failure (shortness of breath, chest pain, anxiety)

Common: insomnia, fatigue, dizziness, nervousness, swelling, nausea, wheezing, muscle and joint pain, sensitivity to cold, exercise intolerance
Tips: Don't drive or perform other activities that could be dangerous if you're not fully alert. Dress warmly in cold weather.

Other: vivid dreams; hallucinations; lethargy; slow pulse; numbness or tingling in fingers, toes, or skin; low blood pressure (dizziness, weakness); vision disturbances; vomiting; diarrhea; rash

DRUG INTERACTIONS

Combining certain drugs may alter their action or produce unwanted side effects. Tell your doctor about other drugs you're taking, especially:
- allergy shots or tests
- caffeine-containing products
- calcium channel blockers, such as Calan and Cardizem
- Catapres
- Choledyl
- drugs for depression such as MAO inhibitors
- epinephrine
- heart drugs called digitalis glycosides
- Indocin
- insulin and oral diabetes drugs
- Lufyllin
- Somophyllin or Somophyllin-T
- Wytensin.

Warnings

- Make sure your doctor knows your medical history. You may not be able to take Visken if you're allergic to it or if you have asthma or other breathing problems, allergies, depression, diabetes, an overactive thyroid, a skin disorder, or heart, kidney, liver or muscle disease.
- Tell your doctor right away if you think you're pregnant or if you plan to breast-feed.

- Visken may affect blood sugar levels. If you're diabetic, monitor your sugar levels carefully.

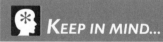

KEEP IN MIND...

* Take exactly as prescribed, even if you feel well.

* Take your pulse before each dose.

* Dress warmly in cold weather.

Vitamin D

Vitamin D helps the body absorb and use calcium and phosphate. It's needed for healthy bones and teeth.

Why it's prescribed

Doctors prescribe vitamin D to treat rickets (a bone disease) and other conditions caused by vitamin D deficiency. You can also buy vitamin D without a prescription. It comes in tablets, capsules, and a liquid. Doctors usually prescribe the following amounts.

▶ **For recommended daily allowance (RDA) of vitamin D,** in adults age 25 and over, 200 international units (IU). Infants age 6 months to adults age 24, 400 IU. Newborns and infants up to 6 months old, 300 IU. Pregnant or breast-feeding women, 400 IU.

▶ **For rickets and other diseases that affect bones,** in adults, at first 12,000 IU a day, increased, if needed, up to 500,000 IU a day. Children, 1,500 to 5,000 IU a day for 2 to 4 weeks, repeated if necessary.

▶ **For parathyroid gland disorder,** 50,000 to 200,000 IU a day, with calcium supplement.

▶ **For phosphate deficiency disease,** in adults, 10,000 to 80,000 IU a day.

How to take vitamin D

• Take this drug exactly as your doctor orders. If treating yourself, take no more than the amount recommended on the product's label.
• Swallow the tablets whole; don't chew or crush them.

VITAMIN D'S OTHER NAMES

Another generic name for vitamin D is ergocalciferol. Brand names include Calciferol, Deltalin Gelseals, and Drisdol.

SIDE EFFECTS

Call your doctor if you have any of these possible drug side effects. Call *immediately* about any labeled "serious."

Serious: seizures, impaired kidney function (decreased urine output), high calcium levels (muscle spasms), chest pain

Common: headache, dizziness, weakness, nausea, diarrhea

Other: sleepiness, decreased sex drive, runny nose, eye inflammation, sensitivity to light, ringing in ears, appetite loss, weight loss, frequent or nighttime urination, kidney stones, itchiness, bone and muscle pain

DRUG INTERACTIONS

Combining certain drugs may alter their action or produce unwanted side effects. Tell your doctor about other drugs you're taking, especially:
• antacids containing magnesium
• corticosteroids
• Dilantin
• heart drugs called digitalis glycosides, such as Lanoxin
• mineral oil
• nonprescription drugs or supplements with calcium, phosphorus, or vitamin D
• Questran
• Solfoton
• thiazide diuretics (water pills), such as Vaseretic.

If you miss a dose

If you're taking vitamin D as a dietary supplement, take the missed dose; then resume your normal schedule. If you're taking it for another reason, ask your doctor how to adjust your schedule.

If you suspect an overdose

Contact your doctor *immediately.* Excessive vitamin D can cause heart or kidney failure.

Warnings

• Make sure your doctor knows your medical history. You may not be able to take vitamin D if you have too much calcium, phosphorus, or vitamin A in your system or if you have kidney, heart, or blood vessel disease.
• Tell your doctor if you're pregnant or breast-feeding.

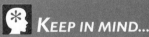

KEEP IN MIND...

* Swallow tablets whole.
* Don't take more than prescribed.
* Avoid antacids that contain magnesium.

Vivactil

Vivactil is a tricyclic antide-pressant. It elevates mood by increasing levels of certain chemicals in the brain.

Why it's prescribed

Doctors prescribe Vivactil to help treat depression. It comes in tab-lets. Doctors usually prescribe the following amounts for adults.

▶ **For depression,** 15 to 40 milli-grams (mg) a day, divided into sev-eral equal doses, increased to a maximum of 60 mg a day.

How to take Vivactil

• Take this drug exactly as your doctor orders. You may not feel bet-ter for several weeks.
• Take it with food or milk to avoid stomach upset.
• Don't stop taking it abruptly.
• To avoid sleeplessness, don't take Vivactil late in the day.

If you miss a dose

Take the missed dose as soon as possi-ble. But if it's early evening or almost time for your next dose, skip the miss-ed dose and take your next dose as scheduled. Don't take a double dose.

 ## If you suspect an overdose

Contact your doctor *immediately*. Excessive Vivactil can cause agita-tion, seizures, hallucinations, sleep-iness, and abnormal heartbeat.

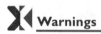 ## Warnings

• Make sure your doctor knows your medical history. You may not

VIVACTIL'S OTHER NAMES

Vivactil's generic name is pro-triptyline hydrochloride. Anoth-er brand name is Triptil.

 ## SIDE EFFECTS

Call your doctor if you have any of these possible drug side effects. Call *immediately* about any labeled "serious."

Serious: rapid or irregular heartbeat, seizures

Common: blurred vision, dry mouth, constipation, inability to urinate, sweating, headache, nausea, vomiting
Tips: To relieve dry mouth, try sugarless gum or hard candy or ice chips. To stop urination problems and constipation, drink plenty of water and eat fiber-rich foods, such as whole grains, vegetables, and fruits.

Other: tremor, weakness, confusion, nervousness, high blood pressure (headache, blurred vision), low blood pressure (dizziness, weakness), ringing in ears, dilated pupils, appetite loss, rash, hives, skin sensitivity to sunlight, allergic reaction (rash, tiredness, dry mouth)
Tips: If you're not fully alert, don't drive or perform other activities that may be dangerous. Wear a sunscreen, a hat, and protective cloth-ing when you go outside, and avoid strong sunlight.

 ## DRUG INTERACTIONS

Combining certain drugs may alter their action or produce unwanted side effects. Tell your doctor about other drugs you're taking, especially:
• alcohol and other drugs that make you feel relaxed or sleepy, such as tranquilizers, sleeping pills, and cold and allergy drugs
• barbiturates
• Catapres
• drugs for depression called MAO inhibitors such as Marplan
• epinephrine
• norepinephrine
• Ritalin
• Tagamet.

be able to take Vivactil if you're an older adult; if you're allergic to it; if you've had a recent heart attack; or if you have other medical prob-lems, especially a history of sei-zures, suicidal thoughts, inability to urinate, glaucoma, heart disease, or an overactive thyroid.
• Tell your doctor if you're preg-nant or breast-feeding before you begin taking Vivactil.
• Before surgery, make sure your surgeon knows that you're taking Vivactil.

 ## KEEP IN MIND...

∗ Take with food or milk.
∗ To avoid sleeplessness, don't take in evening.
∗ Increase fluids and fiber in diet.

Voltaren

Voltaren reduces inflammation, pain, and fever. It's thought to interfere with the body's production of substances called prostaglandins, which are involved in inflammation.

Why it's prescribed

Doctors prescribe Voltaren to relieve joint pain, swelling, and stiffness caused by arthritis. It comes in tablets, coated tablets, slow-release tablets, and suppositories. Doctors usually prescribe the following amounts for adults.

▶ **For severe joint disease,** 25 milligrams (mg) orally four times a day and at bedtime, as needed.

▶ **For osteoarthritis,** 50 mg orally two or three times a day, or 75 mg twice a day.

▶ **For rheumatoid arthritis,** 50 mg orally three or four times a day. Maximum dosage is 225 mg a day.

How to take Voltaren

• Take this drug exactly as your doctor orders. Take it with milk, meals, or a full glass (8 ounces) of water.

• Swallow the tablets whole; don't chew or break them.

If you miss a dose

Take the missed dose as soon as possible. However, if it's almost time for your next dose, skip the missed dose and take your next dose as scheduled. Don't take a double dose.

 If you suspect an overdose

Consult your doctor.

VOLTAREN'S OTHER NAME

Voltaren's generic name is diclofenac sodium.

 SIDE EFFECTS

Call your doctor if you have any of these possible drug side effects. Call *immediately* about any labeled "serious."

Serious: wheezing or shortness of breath, extremely low blood pressure (severe dizziness and weakness), ringing or buzzing in ears, severe abdominal pain, black tarry stools, severe nausea or heartburn, bloody or coffee ground-like vomit, bloody diarrhea, urination problems, burnlike rash, hives, itching

Common: headache, abdominal pain or cramps, constipation, diarrhea, indigestion, nausea, swelling, weight gain, esophagus irritation
Tip: To avoid irritating your esophagus, don't lie down for 15 to 30 minutes after taking this drug.

Other: anxiety, depression, dizziness, drowsiness, insomnia, muscle spasms, back or leg pain, migraine, high blood pressure (headache, blurred vision), gas, bloating, appetite change, change in amount of urine, liver problems (yellow-tinged skin and eyes, unusual tiredness), eye pain, night blindness, asthma, rash, hair loss, skin sensitivity to sunlight, weakness, tremor, clammy skin; swelling of lips, tongue, and throat

 DRUG INTERACTIONS

Combining certain drugs may alter their action or produce unwanted side effects. Tell your doctor about other drugs you're taking, especially:
• alcohol
• anticoagulants (blood thinners) such as Coumadin
• aspirin or Tylenol
• diuretics (water pills)
• Eskalith
• insulin and oral diabetes drugs
• Lanoxin
• Rheumatrex
• Sandimmune.

 Warnings

• Make sure your doctor knows your medical history. You may not be able to take Voltaren if you're allergic to it or to aspirin or similar drugs, or if you have asthma, hives, an ulcer, high blood pressure, fluid retention, or heart, liver, or kidney disease.

• Tell your doctor right away if you think you're pregnant or if you plan to breast-feed.

KEEP IN MIND...

* Take with food, milk, or water.

* Swallow the tablets whole. Don't chew or break them before swallowing.

* Don't lie down for 15 to 30 minutes after taking Voltaren.

Voltaren Ophthalmic

Voltaren Ophthalmic reduces eye inflammation. It's thought to interfere with the body's production of substances called prostaglandins, which are involved in inflammation.

Why it's prescribed

Doctors prescribe Voltaren Ophthalmic to reduce eye inflammation after cataract surgery. It comes in eyedrops. Doctors usually prescribe the following amounts for adults.

▶ **For eye inflammation,** 1 drop four times a day, beginning 24 hours after cataract surgery and continuing for 2 weeks.

How to use Voltaren Ophthalmic

• Use this drug exactly as your doctor orders. Don't use more than your doctor prescribes because this could slow the healing process. Take entire prescription, even if your symptoms subside.
• Wash your hands before and after using this drug.
• To avoid contamination, don't touch the dropper tip to your eye or any surface.
• Pull the lower lid away from each eye and instill 1 drop in the pouch that's created. Gently close eye and press a finger lightly against the inside corner of the eye for 1 minute to keep the drug from entering the tear duct.
• Don't use the drug if it's discolored or appears to contain sediment.

VOLTAREN OPHTHALMIC'S OTHER NAME

Voltaren Ophthalmic's generic name is diclofenac sodium 0.1%.

• Store the eyedrops away from heat and light.
• Discard any leftover eyedrops when you're finished with them. Don't use them for other eye problems.

If you miss a dose

Instill the missed dose as soon as possible. However, if it's almost time for your next dose, skip the missed dose and instill your next dose as scheduled. Don't instill a double dose.

 If you suspect an overdose

Consult your doctor.

 Warnings

• Make sure your doctor knows your medical history. You may not be able to use Voltaren Ophthalmic if you have a bleeding problem or if you're allergic to the drug, to

any of its components, or to aspirin or other drugs.
• Don't use this drug if you wear soft contact lenses.
• Tell your doctor right away if you think you're pregnant.
• Have your eyes examined regularly to check for glaucoma.
• If you or someone else in your household accidentally ingests this drug, drink fluids and call your doctor immediately.

 SIDE EFFECTS

Call your doctor if you have any of these possible drug side effects. Call *immediately* about any labeled "serious."

Serious: corneal irritation, continuous burning, increased pressure in eye (headache, eye pain), allergic eye reaction (redness, tearing)
Tip: If you develop signs of an allergic reaction, stop using the drug and call your doctor.

Common: temporary stinging and burning, delayed wound healing

Other: nausea, vomiting, viral infection
Tip: Antacids may relieve nausea.

DRUG INTERACTIONS

Combining certain drugs may alter their action or produce unwanted side effects. Tell your doctor about other drugs you're taking, especially:
• aspirin.

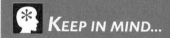 **KEEP IN MIND...**

* Don't allow dropper tip to touch anything.

* Wash hands before and after using drops.

* Don't use more than prescribed.

* Don't use if you're wearing soft contact lenses.

* Discard any leftover drug.

Vontrol

Vontrol is used to treat nausea, vomiting, and dizziness. It works in the inner ear where balance is regulated.

Why it's prescribed

Doctors prescribe Vontrol to prevent or control nausea, vomiting, and vertigo, a spinning sensation caused by disorders of the inner ear or central nervous system. It comes in tablets. Doctors usually prescribe the following amounts for adults; children's dosages appear in parentheses.

▶ **For vertigo,** 25 to 50 milligrams (mg) every 4 hours, as needed.
▶ **For nausea and vomiting,** 25 to 50 mg every 4 hours, as needed. (Children weighing more than 50 pounds [lb], 0.88 mg for each 2.2 lb of body weight every 4 hours, not to exceed 5.5 mg for each 2.2 lb in 24 hours. Usual dose is 25 mg.)

How to take Vontrol

• Take this drug exactly as your doctor orders.
• If you're taking Vontrol to *prevent* nausea and vomiting, take it with food, milk, or water to reduce stomach upset.
• If you're taking Vontrol because you *have* nausea and vomiting, take it on an empty stomach with only a little water.

 SIDE EFFECTS

Call your doctor if you have any of these possible drug side effects. Call *immediately* about any labeled "serious."

Serious: confusion, disorientation, hallucinations

Common: drowsiness
Tip: If you're not fully alert, don't drive or perform other activities that could be dangerous.

Other: dizziness, sleep disturbances, temporary low blood pressure (light-headedness), dry mouth, nausea, indigestion, heartburn, hives
Tip: Relieve dry mouth with sugarless gum or hard candy or ice chips.

 DRUG INTERACTIONS

Combining certain drugs may alter their action or produce unwanted side effects. Tell your doctor about other drugs you're taking.

VONTROL'S OTHER NAME

Vontrol's generic name is diphenidol hydrochloride.

If you miss a dose

Take the missed dose as soon as possible. However, if it's almost time for your next dose, skip the missed dose and take your next dose as scheduled. Don't take a double dose.

 If you suspect an overdose

Contact your doctor *immediately.* Excessive Vontrol can cause slow or shallow breathing and low blood pressure (dizziness, fainting).

Warnings

• Make sure your doctor knows your medical history. You may not be able to take Vontrol if you're allergic to it or to aspirin, if you're producing little or no urine, or if you have glaucoma,

digestive tract blockage or spasm, or an enlarged prostate.
• Notify your doctor if you're pregnant or breast-feeding before taking this drug.
• Don't give Vontrol to children weighing less than 50 pounds.

 KEEP IN MIND...

∗ To *prevent* nausea, take with food, milk, or water.

∗ To *control* nausea and vomiting, take on empty stomach.

∗ Relieve dry mouth with sugarless gum, hard candy, or ice chips.

∗ Don't drive or perform other hazardous activities if not fully alert.

Wellbutrin

Wellbutrin has a mild effect on chemicals in the brain that elevate a person's mood. The exact way this drug works is unknown.

Why it's prescribed

Doctors prescribe Wellbutrin to treat depression. It comes in tablets. Doctors usually prescribe the following amounts for adults.
▶ **For depression,** at first, 100 milligrams (mg) twice a day, increased after 3 days to 100 mg three times a day if needed. If no response occurs after several weeks of treatment, dosage increased to 150 mg three times a day.

How to take Wellbutrin

• Take this drug exactly as your doctor orders. Don't take more than prescribed. You may need to take Wellbutrin for several weeks before you begin to feel better.
• If Wellbutrin upsets your stomach, ask your doctor if you can take it with food.
• Don't stop taking Wellbutrin abruptly.

If you miss a dose

Take the missed dose as soon as possible. However, if it's within 4 hours of your next dose, skip the missed dose and take your next dose as scheduled. Don't take a double dose.

WELLBUTRIN'S OTHER NAME

Wellbutrin's generic name is bupropion hydrochloride.

 SIDE EFFECTS

Call your doctor if you have any of these possible drug side effects. Call *immediately* about any labeled "serious."

Serious: seizures, irregular or rapid heartbeat

Common: headache, agitation, confusion

Other: restlessness, anxiety, delusions, euphoria, sleeplessness, sleepiness, tremor, high blood pressure (headache, blurred vision), low blood pressure (dizziness, weakness), palpitations, blurred vision, dry mouth, increased appetite, constipation, nausea, vomiting, impotence, menstrual irregularities, frequent urination, decreased sex drive, itchiness, rash, arthritis, fever and chills

Tip: Restlessness, agitation, sleeplessness, and anxiety should subside after a while; check with your doctor if these side effects persist.

 DRUG INTERACTIONS

Combining certain drugs may alter their action or produce unwanted side effects. Tell your doctor about other drugs you're taking, especially:
• alcohol
• benzodiazepines such as Solfoton
• drugs for depression, such as Desyrel, Prozac, MAO inhibitors (Marplan), and tricyclic antidepressants (Elavil, Ludiomil)
• drugs for mental illness such as Eskalith
• Larodopa
• phenothiazines such as Thorazine.

 If you suspect an overdose

Contact your doctor *immediately*. Excessive Wellbutrin can cause labored breathing, salivation, an arched back, loss of balance, and seizures.

Warnings

• Make sure your doctor knows your medical history. You may not be able to take Wellbutrin if you're allergic to it; if you have a history of seizures, an eating disorder, or

heart, kidney, or liver disease; or if you've recently had a heart attack.
• Make sure your doctor knows if you're pregnant or breast-feeding before you begin taking Wellbutrin.

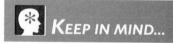 **KEEP IN MIND...**

* Take exactly as prescribed.
* Don't stop taking Wellbutrin abruptly.
* It may take several weeks before you feel better.

Wigraine

Wigraine contains ergotamine and caffeine. Ergotamine narrows the blood vessels, and caffeine helps the ergotamine to work faster.

Why it's prescribed

Doctors prescribe Wigraine to treat migraine, cluster, and vascular headaches. It comes in tablets and suppositories. Doctors usually prescribe the following amounts for adults.

▶ **To treat migraine, cluster, or vascular headache,** 2 tablets or 1 suppository at the first sign (aura) of headache. The maximum amount for a single headache attack is 6 tablets or 2 suppositories. For more than one headache attack per week, the maximum weekly amount is 10 tablets or 6 suppositories.

How to take Wigraine

• Take this drug exactly as your doctor has prescribed.
• For best results, take Wigraine at the first sign of a headache. Rest in a dark, quiet room.
• If you frequently experience nausea and vomiting with your headaches, use the suppositories rather than the tablets.
• If the suppository is too soft, moisten it with cold water before inserting it.
• If you've been using Wigraine regularly, don't stop taking it abruptly. Doing so may increase

WIGRAINE'S OTHER NAMES

Wigraine is a combination of the generic drugs ergotamine tartrate and caffeine. Another brand name is Cafergot.

 SIDE EFFECTS

Call your doctor if you have any of these possible drug side effects. Call *immediately* about any labeled "serious."

Serious: numbness, blistering, discoloration, or tingling in toes or fingers; weakness; chest pain; fast or slow pulse; swelling or itching; vision change

Common: diarrhea, dizziness, drowsiness
Tip: Prevent dizziness by standing up slowly and taking care when walking.

Other: nausea, vomiting, rectal ulcers

 DRUG INTERACTIONS

Combining certain drugs may alter their action or produce unwanted side effects. Tell your doctor about other drugs you're taking, especially:
• alcohol
• beta blockers such as Inderal
• nicotine.

the frequency and duration of headaches. Your doctor may want you to reduce the amount you take gradually.

If you miss a dose

Not applicable because this drug is taken only as needed.

 If you suspect an overdose

Contact your doctor *immediately.* Excessive Wigraine can cause drowsiness, tingling or numbness in your hands or feet, or high blood pressure (headache, blurred vision), or low blood pressure (dizziness, weakness, fainting).

Warnings

• Make sure your doctor knows your medical history. You may not be able to take Wigraine if you

have other problems, especially high blood pressure or diseases of the blood vessels, kidney, or liver.
• If you're pregnant or breast-feeding, don't take this drug.
• Use Wigraine only for migraine, cluster, or vascular headaches. It won't relieve the symptoms of tension headaches.
• Be aware that older adults may be especially prone to Wigraine's side effects.

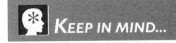 **KEEP IN MIND...**

∗ Take at first sign of headache.
∗ Rest in dark, quiet room for 2 hours after taking.
∗ Don't stop taking abruptly after regular use.
∗ Avoid alcohol.

Winstrol

Winstrol is a type of male hormone that rebuilds weakened tissues. It increases the level of a specific enzyme that decreases the frequency of angioedema attacks.

Why it's prescribed

Doctors prescribe Winstrol to treat angioedema, which causes swelling of the head, neck, hands, feet, genitals, or internal organs. Winstrol comes in tablets. Doctors usually prescribe the following amounts (although dosage tends to be individualized).

▶ **To prevent angioedema,** in adults, at first, 2 milligrams (mg) three times a day to 4 mg four times a day for 5 days, gradually reduced every 1 to 3 months to 2 mg a day.

▶ **For angioedema attacks,** in children ages 6 to 12, up to 2 mg a day. Children under age 6, 1 mg a day.

How to take Winstrol

• Take this drug exactly as your doctor orders.
• Take Winstrol just before or with meals to reduce stomach upset.
• If you have trouble swallowing the tablets, you may crush them or put them in soft foods, such as applesauce or pudding.

If you miss a dose

Adjust your schedule as follows:
• If you take one dose a day, take the missed dose as soon as you remember if it's on the same day; then go back to your usual schedule.

WINSTROL'S OTHER NAME

Winstrol's generic name is stanozolol.

 SIDE EFFECTS

Call your doctor if you have any of these possible drug side effects. Call *immediately* about any labeled "serious."

Serious: liver tumors (yellow-tinged skin and eyes, itching, swelling)

Common: none reported

Other: swelling, nausea, vomiting, constipation, diarrhea, change in appetite, bladder irritability (abdominal pain, spasm), muscle spasms, masculinizing effects in women (acne, water retention, hoarseness, clitoral enlargement, decrease in breast size, changes in sex drive, male-pattern baldness), low-estrogen effects in women (flushing, sweating, nervousness, emotional instability, menstrual irregularities, vaginal dryness, itching, burning, or bleeding), excessive hormonal effects in men (stunted growth, painful erection, and penile enlargement before puberty; under-developed testicles, low sperm count, decreased ejaculate, impotence, breast enlargement, and epididymitis after puberty)

 DRUG INTERACTIONS

Combining certain drugs may alter their action or produce unwanted side effects. Tell your doctor about other drugs you're taking, especially:
• Aldomet
• Antabuse
• antibiotics
• anticoagulants (blood thinners) such as Coumadin
• Aralen, Plaquenil
• cancer drugs, such as BiCNU, Cerubidine, Mexate, Mithracin, and Purinethol
• Cordarone
• Dantrium
• drugs harmful to liver such as Tylenol in high doses
• gold salts (type of arthritis drug)
• insulin and oral diabetes drugs
• malaria drugs
• male and female hormones, birth control pills (use an additional form of birth control while taking Winstrol)
• phenothiazines such as Thorazine
• seizure drugs, such as Depakene, Depakote, Dilantin, and Tegretol
• Tegison
• thyroid drugs
• Trexan (with high doses or prolonged use).

• If you don't remember the missed dose until the next day, skip it and go back to your usual schedule. If you take more than one dose a day, take the missed dose as soon as you remember. However, if it's almost time for your next dose, skip the missed dose and take your next

dose as scheduled. Don't take a double dose.

If you suspect an overdose

Consult your doctor.

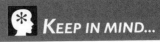

Warnings

• Make sure your doctor knows your medical history. You may not be able to take Winstrol if you're allergic to it or to similar drugs, if you have breast or prostate cancer, or if you have diabetes, seizures, migraine headaches, high blood pressure, excess calcium in your system, or kidney, liver, or heart disease.

• Make sure your doctor knows if you're pregnant or breast-feeding before you begin taking Winstrol or if you become pregnant during treatment.

• Be aware that older males may be more prone to this drug's side effects.

• Winstrol may lower blood sugar levels. If you have diabetes, check your sugar levels carefully, and call your doctor if they're low.

• Follow a low-salt diet and take diuretics (water pills), as your doctor directs, to reduce fluid retention.

• Unless your doctor tells you otherwise, follow a high-calorie, high-protein diet, and eat small meals throughout the day.

• Before undergoing any medical tests, tell the doctor that you're taking Winstrol.

• Have regular checkups so the doctor can monitor you for side effects.

• The doctor will probably want to check your cholesterol levels regularly.

• If you're taking an anticoagulant (blood thinner), call your doctor if you bruise or bleed.

• For children and adolescents, the doctor will probably order periodic X-rays of their wrists to check bone maturation. For boys under age 7, the doctor will watch for early development of adult male sexual characteristics. Semen evaluation may be needed every 3 or 4 months, especially for teenage boys.

• For young women, the doctor will probably prescribe a lower dosage to help reduce the drug's masculinizing side effects.

KEEP IN MIND...

* Take before or with meals to reduce stomach upset.

* Follow a high-calorie, high-protein diet, if prescribed.

* Eat small, frequent meals.

* Reduce salt in diet to minimize fluid retention.

* If you use birth control pills, use additional birth control method while taking Winstrol.

Wytensin

Wytensin helps control high blood pressure. It works by relaxing blood vessels, especially those in the arms and legs.

Why it's prescribed

Doctors prescribe Wytensin to reduce high blood pressure. It comes in tablets. Doctors usually prescribe the following amounts for adults.

▶ **For high blood pressure,** at first, 4 milligrams (mg) twice a day, increased by 4 to 8 mg a day every 1 to 2 weeks. Maximum dosage is 32 mg twice a day.

How to take Wytensin

• Take this drug exactly as your doctor orders. Don't stop taking it abruptly during treatment.
• To ensure adequate overnight blood pressure control, take your last dose of the day at bedtime.

If you miss a dose

Take the missed dose as soon as possible. However, if it's almost time for your next dose, skip the missed dose and take your next dose as scheduled. Don't take a double dose. If you miss two or more doses in a row, call your doctor.

If you suspect an overdose

Contact your doctor *immediately*. Excessive Wytensin can cause a very slow pulse, slow or absent breathing, and seizures.

WYTENSIN'S OTHER NAME

Wytensin's generic name is guanabenz acetate.

SIDE EFFECTS

Call your doctor if you have any of these possible drug side effects. Call *immediately* about any labeled "serious."

Serious: extremely high blood pressure (headache, blurred vision) if drug is stopped abruptly

Common: dry mouth
Tips: To relieve dry mouth, try sugarless gum or hard candy or ice chips. If your mouth feels dry for more than 2 weeks, tell your doctor.

Other: drowsiness, sleepiness, dizziness, weakness, headache, loss of balance, depression, impotence
Tips: If you're not fully alert, don't drive or perform other hazardous activities. To minimize dizziness when you get up from a sitting or lying position, change positions and get up slowly. Also, sit up and dangle your legs for a few minutes before getting out of bed.

DRUG INTERACTIONS

Combining certain drugs may alter their action or produce unwanted side effects. Tell your doctor about other drugs you're taking, especially:
• alcohol and other drugs that make you feel relaxed or sleepy, such as tranquilizers, sleeping pills, and cold and allergy drugs
• beta blockers (a type of heart drug)
• drugs for depression, such as MAO inhibitors and tricyclic antidepressants.

Warnings

• Make sure your doctor knows your medical history. You may not be able to take Wytensin if you're allergic to it, if you've recently had a heart attack, or if you have heart, blood vessel, kidney, or liver disease.
• Make sure your doctor knows if you're pregnant or breast-feeding before you begin taking Wytensin.
• Older adults may be especially prone to Wytensin's side effects.
• Lose weight and reduce the amount of salt in your diet as your doctor recommends. Follow diet carefully to help control your blood pressure.

KEEP IN MIND...

* Lose weight and reduce dietary salt as directed.
* Take last dose of the day at bedtime.
* Don't stop taking abruptly.
* Relieve dry mouth with sugarless gum or hard candy or ice chips.

Xanax

Xanax is used to treat anxiety. It's thought to have an effect on certain mood-related substances in the brain.

Why it's prescribed

Doctors prescribe Xanax to relieve anxiety or tension caused by unusual stress (not ordinary, everyday stress). It comes in tablets and a liquid. Doctors usually prescribe the following amounts for adults.

▶ **For anxiety,** usual initial dose is 0.25 to 0.5 milligrams (mg) three times a day. Elderly or very ill people or people with advanced liver disease, usual initial dose is 0.25 mg two or three times a day. Maximum dosage is 4 mg a day, divided into equal doses.

▶ **For panic disorders,** 0.5 mg three times a day, increased by no more than 1 mg at intervals of 3 to 4 days. Maximum dosage is 10 mg a day, divided into equal doses.

How to take Xanax

• Take this drug exactly as directed.
• Don't stop taking this drug abruptly without consulting your doctor.

If you miss a dose

Take the missed dose right away if it's within 1 hour or so of the scheduled time. If more than 1 hour has passed, skip the missed dose and take the next dose at the regular time. Don't take a double dose.

XANAX'S OTHER NAMES

Xanax's generic name is alprazolam. Canadian brand names include Apo-Alpraz, Novo-Alprazol, and Nu-Alpraz.

 SIDE EFFECTS

Call your doctor if you have any of these possible drug side effects. Call *immediately* about any labeled "serious."

Serious: slow or shallow breathing

Common: drowsiness, light-headedness
Tips: If you're not fully alert, don't drive or perform other hazardous activities. To ease light-headedness, get up slowly from a sitting or lying position.

Other: headache, confusion, hostility, memory loss, restlessness, mental problem, temporary low blood pressure (dizziness, weakness), rapid pulse, vision disturbances, dry mouth, nausea, vomiting, constipation, incontinence, inability to urinate, menstrual irregularities

 DRUG INTERACTIONS

Combining certain drugs may alter their action or produce unwanted side effects. Tell your doctor about other drugs you're taking, especially:
• alcohol and other drugs that make you feel relaxed or sleepy, such as tranquilizers, sleeping pills, and cold and allergy drugs
• Lanoxin
• nicotine, tobacco
• Tagamet
• tricyclic antidepressants.

 If you suspect an overdose

Contact your doctor *immediately.* Excessive Xanax can cause slurred speech, confusion, severe drowsiness, and staggering.

 Warnings

• Make sure your doctor knows your medical history. You may not be able to take Xanax if you're allergic to it or to similar drugs or if you have glaucoma, lung disease, or liver or kidney problems.
• Tell your doctor right away if you think you're pregnant or if you plan to breast-feed.

• Be aware that older adults may be more prone to Xanax's side effects.
• Before medical testing, tell the doctor that you're taking Xanax.
• See your doctor at least every 4 months to determine whether you need to keep taking this drug.

KEEP IN MIND...

∗ Don't stop taking Xanax abruptly.

∗ Don't drive or perform other dangerous activities if not fully alert.

∗ Stand up slowly to avoid dizziness.

Zantac

Zantac inhibits the action of histamine, a substance that causes increased secretion of stomach acid.

Why it's prescribed

Doctors prescribe Zantac to treat ulcers and to prevent them from recurring. It comes in tablets, effervescent tablets, granules, and a syrup. Doctors usually prescribe the following amounts for adults.

▶ **For ulcers (short-term treatment) and excess stomach acid,** 150 milligrams (mg) twice a day or 300 mg once a day at bedtime; maintenance treatment for duodenal ulcer is 150 mg at bedtime.

▶ **For stomach acid reflux disease,** 150 mg twice a day.

▶ **For severely inflamed esophagus,** 150 mg four times a day.

How to take Zantac

• Take this drug exactly as your doctor orders. Take the entire amount prescribed, even after you start to feel better.

• If you're taking one dose a day, take it at bedtime, unless otherwise directed.

• If you're taking two doses a day, take one in the morning and one at bedtime.

• If you're taking several doses a day, take them with meals and at bedtime for best results.

If you miss a dose

Take the missed dose as soon as possible. But if it's almost time for your next dose, skip the missed dose and

ZANTAC'S OTHER NAMES

Zantac's generic name is ranitidine hydrochloride. A Canadian brand name is Apo-Ranitidine.

 SIDE EFFECTS

Call your doctor if you have any of these possible drug side effects. Call *immediately* about any labeled "serious."

Serious: severe blood problems (bleeding, bruising, fever, chills, increased risk of infection), very slow pulse

Common: headache, malaise, nausea, constipation

Other: dizziness, confusion, liver problems or jaundice (yellow-tinged skin and eyes), rash

Tip: If you're not fully alert, don't drive or perform other hazardous activities.

 FOOD AND DRUG INTERACTIONS

Combining certain drugs and foods may alter drug action or produce unwanted side effects. Tell your doctor about your diet and other drugs you're taking, especially:

• antacids (take 30 minutes to 1 hour before or after Zantac)
• aspirin
• anticoagulants (blood thinners) such as Coumadin
• carbonated drinks, citrus fruits and juices, other acidic foods and beverages
• drugs to treat an irregular heartbeat
• muscle relaxants
• nicotine, tobacco
• oral diabetes drugs such as Glucotrol
• Procan SR
• Valium.

take your next dose as scheduled. Don't take a double dose.

 If you suspect an overdose

Consult your doctor.

Warnings

• Make sure your doctor knows your medical history. You may not be able to take Zantac if you're allergic to it or if you have kidney or liver problems.

• If you're pregnant or breast-feeding, check with your doctor before using Zantac.

• Older adults may be especially prone to Zantac's side effects.

KEEP IN MIND...

∗ Take entire amount prescribed, even if you feel better.

∗ Avoid foods and drinks that irritate your stomach.

∗ Don't take an antacid within 30 minutes of Zantac.

Zarontin

Zarontin is one of a group of drugs called anticonvulsants. It's thought to decrease seizures by affecting certain nerve transmissions in the brain.

Why it's prescribed

Doctors prescribe Zarontin to treat certain types of seizures. It comes in capsules and a syrup. Doctors usually prescribe the following amounts for adults; children's dosages appear in parentheses.

▶ **For seizures,** 500 milligrams (mg) a day. Ideal dose is 20 mg for each 2.2 pounds (lb) of body weight a day. (Children age 6 and older: same as adults. Children ages 3 to 5: 250 mg a day. Ideal dose is 20 mg for each 2.2 lb a day.)

How to take Zarontin

• Take Zarontin exactly as your doctor orders, at regularly spaced intervals.
• Take it with food to minimize stomach upset.
• Don't let the syrup form of this drug freeze.
• Don't stop taking Zarontin abruptly. Doing so could cause seizures.

If you miss a dose

Take the missed dose as soon as possible. However, if it's within 4 hours of your next dose, skip the missed dose and take your next dose as scheduled. Don't take a double dose.

ZARONTIN'S OTHER NAME

Zarontin's generic name is ethosuximide.

 SIDE EFFECTS

Call your doctor if you have any of these possible drug side effects. Call *immediately* about any labeled "serious."

Serious: blood problems (bleeding, bruising, fever, chills, fatigue, increased risk of infection)
Tip: Avoid contact with people who are ill or infected.

Common: drowsiness, headache, fatigue, dizziness, loss of balance, irritability, hiccups, euphoria, lethargy, depression, mental problems nausea, vomiting, diarrhea, weight loss, cramps, loss of appetite, stomach and abdominal pain
Tips: If you're not fully alert, don't drive or perform other hazardous activities. Avoid strenuous physical activity to prevent fatigue.

Other: nearsightedness, swollen tongue or gums, vaginal bleeding, frequent urination, hives, itchy or red rash, excessive hair growth

 DRUG INTERACTIONS

Combining certain drugs may alter their action or produce unwanted side effects. Tell your doctor about other drugs you're taking, especially:
• alcohol and other drugs that make you feel relaxed or sleepy, such as tranquilizers, sleeping pills, or cold and allergy drugs
• drugs to treat mental illness
• other seizure drugs.

 If you suspect an overdose

Contact your doctor *immediately.* Excessive Zarontin can cause stumbling, stupor, and coma.

Warnings

• Make sure your doctor knows your medical history. You may not be able to take Zarontin if you're allergic to this or other drugs or if you have a blood, liver, or kidney problem.
• Tell your doctor right away if you think you're pregnant or if you plan to breast-feed.

• If you take Zarontin regularly, you may need to undergo blood tests regularly to check your progress.
• Wear or carry medical identification that lets others know you have a seizure disorder and tells them which drugs you're taking.

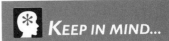 **KEEP IN MIND...**

∗ Take Zarontin at regularly spaced intervals.

∗ Take with food to minimize stomach upset.

∗ Don't stop taking abruptly.

Zaroxolyn

Zaroxolyn is one of a large group of drugs called diuretics (water pills). It helps the body get rid of excess sodium and water by increasing the amount of urine the body excretes.

Why it's prescribed

Doctors prescribe Zaroxolyn to treat high blood pressure and swelling in the lower legs from heart failure or kidney disease. Zaroxolyn comes in tablets. Doctors usually prescribe the following amounts for adults.

▶ **For swelling in congestive heart failure or kidney disease,** 5 to 20 milligrams (mg) a day.

▶ **For high blood pressure,** 2.5 to 5 mg a day. Maintenance dosage determined by blood pressure.

How to take Zaroxolyn

• Take this drug exactly as your doctor orders. Take only the prescribed amount. Keep taking it, even if you feel well.

• Take it in the morning to avoid nighttime urination.

• Store this drug at room temperature and away from light.

If you miss a dose

Take the missed dose as soon as possible. However, if it's almost time for your next dose, skip the missed dose and take your next dose as scheduled. Don't take a double dose.

 ## SIDE EFFECTS

Call your doctor if you have any of these possible drug side effects. Call *immediately* about any labeled "serious."

Serious: severe blood problems (fever, chills, increased risk of infection, rash, hives, unusual bleeding or bruising, bloody urine, or black, tarry stools)
Tip: Avoid contact with people who are ill or infected.

Common: fatigue, low blood pressure (dizziness, light-headedness, weakness), nausea
Tips: To prevent fatigue, avoid strenuous physical activity. To reduce dizziness, avoid sudden position changes and rise slowly from a sitting or lying position. Take this drug with food or milk if it causes nausea.

Other: headache, dehydration (dry skin, thirst, decreased urination, fast pulse), appetite loss, inflamed pancreas (abdominal pain, nausea, vomiting), nighttime or frequent urination, increased urination, liver problems (confusion, tremor), increased skin sensitivity to sun, rash, gout, increased blood sugar (thirst, hunger, weight loss), swelling, allergic reaction (rash, fever), irregular heartbeat, muscle pain or cramps, vomiting, unusual weakness, mood or mental changes
Tip: Wear a sunscreen, a hat, and protective clothing to protect yourself from the sun.

 ## DRUG INTERACTIONS

Combining certain drugs may alter their action or produce unwanted side effects. Tell your doctor about other drugs you're taking, especially:
• Advil, Anaprox, Indocin, and other nonsteroidal anti-inflammatory drugs
• alcohol and other drugs that make you feel relaxed or sleepy, such as tranquilizers, sleeping pills, narcotic pain relievers, and cold and allergy drugs
• asthma drugs
• barbiturates
• Colestid
• diazoxide
• heart drugs called digitalis glycosides such as Lanoxin
• lithium
• nonprescription drugs for appetite control
• Questran.

 ### If you suspect an overdose

Contact your doctor *immediately.* Excessive Zaroxolyn can cause digestive problems, increased urination, lethargy, drowsiness, low blood pressure (dizziness, weakness, fainting), and coma.

✕ Warnings

- Make sure your doctor knows your medical history. You may not be able to take Zaroxolyn if you're allergic to it or to similar drugs or if you have diabetes, gout, lupus, an inflamed pancreas, heart or blood vessel disease, or kidney or liver problems.
- Tell your doctor right away if you think you're pregnant or if you plan to breast-feed.
- Zaroxolyn is not recommended for children.
- Older adults may be especially prone to Zaroxolyn's side effects, especially dizziness and light-headedness. Older adults also may lose too much potassium when taking this drug.

- If you're diabetic, be sure to test your blood or urine sugar levels regularly. This drug may increase your blood sugar level.
- While taking this drug, follow any special diet the doctor orders, such as a low-salt, high-potassium diet. Foods rich in potassium include citrus fruits, tomatoes, bananas, dates, and apricots.
- Don't change to another brand of this drug without consulting your doctor. Other brands may work differently, requiring a change in your dosage.
- Weigh yourself weekly and notify your doctor if you gain more than 5 pounds in a short period.
- Keep all follow-up doctor's appointments. Your doctor will probably want to perform regular blood tests to monitor for side effects.
- Call your doctor if you experience joint pain.

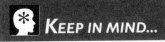

✱ KEEP IN MIND...

- ✱ Follow a low-salt, high-potassium diet if prescribed.
- ✱ Take Zaroxolyn in morning to avoid nighttime urination.
- ✱ Keep taking as directed, even if you feel well.
- ✱ Don't change brands of this drug.
- ✱ Notify doctor if you gain more than 5 pounds in a short time.

Zebeta

Zebeta is one of a group of drugs called beta blockers. It reduces the heart's workload, decreases the amount of blood and oxygen needed by the heart, and lowers blood pressure.

Why it's prescribed

Doctors prescribe Zebeta to reduce high blood pressure. It comes in tablets. Doctors usually prescribe the following amounts for adults.

▶ **For high blood pressure,** at first, 5 milligrams (mg) once a day. If response is inadequate, increased to 10 mg once a day or to 20 mg a day if needed. Maximum recommended dosage is 20 mg a day. In people with kidney or liver problems, initial dosage is 2.5 mg a day, adjusted for the individual.

How to take Zebeta

• Take Zebeta exactly as your doctor orders, even if you feel well.
• Don't stop taking this drug abruptly.

If you miss a dose

Take the missed dose as soon as possible. However, if it's almost time for your next dose, skip the missed dose and take your next dose as scheduled. Don't take a double dose.

 If you suspect an overdose

Contact your doctor *immediately*. Excessive Zebeta can cause as-

ZEBETA'S OTHER NAME

Zebeta's generic name is bisoprolol fumarate.

 SIDE EFFECTS

Call your doctor if you have any of these possible drug side effects. Call *immediately* about any labeled "serious."

Serious: slow pulse, chest pain
Tip: Zebeta may mask exercise-induced chest pain; ask your doctor to recommend a safe exercise program.

Common: increased sensitivity to cold, weakness, fatigue, dizziness, insomnia, nausea, vomiting
Tips: Dress warmly in cold weather. If you're not fully alert, don't drive or perform other hazardous activities.

Other: headache, numbness of fingers and toes, vivid dreams, depression, swelling of hands and lower legs, sore throat, runny nose, sinus congestion, diarrhea, dry mouth, cough, shortness of breath, sweating, joint pain

 DRUG INTERACTIONS

Combining certain drugs may alter their action or produce unwanted side effects. Tell your doctor about other drugs you're taking, especially:
• blood pressure drugs, such as Catapres, Ismelin, and Serpasil
• other beta blockers, such as Inderal and Lopressor.

thmalike attacks, a very slow pulse, and congestive heart failure (shortness of breath).

 Warnings

• Make sure your doctor knows your medical history. You may not be able to take Zebeta if you're allergic to it or if you have heart problems, asthma, diabetes, blood vessel disease, or thyroid disease.
• Make sure your doctor knows if you're pregnant or breast-feeding before you begin taking Zebeta.
• If you're diabetic, monitor your blood sugar levels carefully. Zebeta

may mask some signs of low blood sugar.
• While taking this drug, monitor your blood pressure frequently.

KEEP IN MIND...

* Take exactly as prescribed, even if you feel well.
* Don't stop taking abruptly.
* Monitor blood pressure regularly.
* Don't take other drugs without doctor's permission.
* Follow doctor's exercise recommendation.

Zerit

Zerit interferes with the growth and spread of the human immunodeficiency virus (HIV), which causes AIDS. Therefore, it may slow down the signs and symptoms of HIV.

Why it's prescribed

Doctors prescribe Zerit for advanced HIV infection in people who don't respond to, or can't tolerate, other drugs. This drug comes in capsules. Doctors usually prescribe the following amounts for adults.

▶ **For advanced HIV infection,** in people who weigh 130 pounds (lb) or more, 40 milligrams (mg) every 12 hours; in people who weigh less than 130 lb, 30 mg every 12 hours.

How to take Zerit

• Take this drug exactly as your doctor orders. Take it with meals or on an empty stomach, whichever you prefer.
• Store Zerit at room temperature in a tightly closed container.

If you miss a dose

Take the missed dose as soon as possible. However, if it's almost time for your next dose, skip the missed dose and take your next dose as scheduled. Don't take a double dose.

If you suspect an overdose

Consult your doctor.

ZERIT'S OTHER NAME

Zerit's generic name is stavudine.

SIDE EFFECTS

Call your doctor if you have any of these possible drug side effects. Call *immediately* about any labeled "serious."

Serious: pneumonia, tumors, blood problems (increased risk of infection, fever, chills, fatigue, bleeding, bruising), muscle pain, liver problems (yellow-tinged skin and eyes), abdominal pain
Tips: Avoid contact with people who are ill or have an infection. To minimize fatigue, avoid strenuous physical activity.

Common: nerve disorder (burning, tingling, aching, or numbness starting in hands or feet)

Other: headache, anxiety, sleeplessness, dizziness, confusion, tremor, rash, itching, change in vision, nausea, vomiting, weight loss, flulike syndrome

DRUG INTERACTIONS

Combining certain drugs may alter their action or produce unwanted side effects. Tell your doctor about other drugs you're taking, especially:
• bone marrow suppressants
• cancer drugs.

X Warnings

• Make sure your doctor knows your medical history. You may not be able to take Zerit if you're allergic to it or if you have other medical problems, especially kidney problems, a nerve disorder, or cancer.
• Tell your doctor right away if you think you're pregnant or if you plan to breast-feed.
• This drug is not recommended for children.
• Be aware that Zerit is not a cure for HIV infection and doesn't reduce the risk of transmitting HIV to others. Therefore, it's important that you abstain from sex or practice safe sex.

• While taking this drug, see your doctor regularly for blood tests to determine the drug's effectiveness, to monitor for side effects, and to check for other illnesses associated with HIV infection.
• Contact your doctor if you experience any signs or symptoms of a new infection or illness.

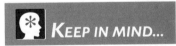 KEEP IN MIND...

∗ Take with food or on empty stomach.

∗ Tell doctor if you have tingling or numbness in hands or feet.

∗ Avoid contact with ill or infected people.

Zestril

Zestril is a drug for high blood pressure. It reduces blood pressure by causing blood vessels to relax.

Why it's prescribed

Doctors prescribe Zestril to reduce high blood pressure. It's also used with other drugs to treat heart failure. Zestril comes in tablets. Doctors usually prescribe the following amounts for adults.

▶ **For high blood pressure,** at first, 10 milligrams (mg) a day if person is not taking a diuretic (water pill); 5 mg a day if taking a diuretic. Usual dosage is 20 to 40 mg a day as a single dose.

▶ **For heart failure,** at first, 5 mg a day, increased as needed to a maximum of 20 mg a day.

How to take Zestril

• Take this drug exactly as the doctor orders, even if you feel well.
• Don't stop taking Zestril abruptly.

If you miss a dose

Take the missed dose as soon as possible. But if it's almost time for your next dose, skip the missed dose and take your next dose as scheduled. Don't take a double dose.

 If you suspect an overdose

Consult your doctor.

• Make sure your doctor knows your medical history. You may not

ZESTRIL'S OTHER NAMES

Zestril's generic name is lisinopril. Another brand name is Prinivil.

 SIDE EFFECTS

Call your doctor if you have any of these possible drug side effects. Call *immediately* about any labeled "serious."

Serious: angioedema (swelling of head, face, neck, or internal organs), difficulty breathing, blood problems (fever, chills, increased risk of infection)

Common: dizziness, headache, fatigue, light-headedness, nasal congestion, diarrhea, muscle cramps; dry, persistent, tickling cough
Tips: To relieve light-headedness, especially during the first few days of treatment, get up slowly from a sitting or lying position. Sit and dangle your legs for a few minutes before getting out of bed. If you faint, stop taking Zestril and call your doctor right away.

Other: depression, sleepiness, tingling or numbness, low blood pressure (dizziness, weakness), chest pain, nausea, stomach upset, altered taste, impotence, rash, decreased sex drive, increased thirst

DRUG AND FOOD INTERACTIONS

Combining certain drugs or foods may alter drug action or produce unwanted side effects. Tell your doctor about your diet and other drugs you're taking, especially:
• Colestid
• diuretics (water pills), especially potassium-sparing and thiazide diuretics
• drugs or supplements containing potassium
• Eskalith, Lithobid
• heart drugs called digitalis glycosides
• Indocin
• insulin and oral diabetes drugs
• Questran
• salt substitutes.

be able to take Zestril if you're allergic to it or to related drugs, if you've recently had a heart attack or stroke, or if you have kidney problems, lupus, diabetes, or high potassium levels.
• Tell your doctor right away if you think you're pregnant or if you plan to breast-feed.
• While taking this drug, monitor your blood pressure regularly, if your doctor orders. See your doctor regularly for blood tests.

 KEEP IN MIND...

∗ Take drug exactly as ordered, even if you feel well.

∗ Don't stop taking abruptly.

∗ Stand up slowly to avoid dizziness.

Zithromax

Zithromax is an antibiotic that works by destroying infection-causing bacteria.

Why it's prescribed

Doctors prescribe Zithromax to treat bacterial infections throughout the body. It comes in capsules. Doctors usually prescribe the following amounts for adults and children age 16 and over.

▶ **For throat, lung, and skin infections,** 500 milligrams (mg) as a single dose on day 1, followed by 250 mg a day on days 2 through 5. Total dose is 1.5 grams (g).

▶ **For chlamydia,** 1 g as a single dose.

How to take Zithromax

• Take this drug exactly as your doctor orders. Take it on an empty stomach, either 1 hour before or 2 hours after a meal.
• Take the entire amount prescribed, even if you feel better.

If you miss a dose

Take the missed dose as soon as possible. However, if it's almost time for your next dose, skip the missed dose and take your next dose as scheduled. Don't take a double dose.

If you suspect overdose

Consult your doctor.

ZITHROMAX'S OTHER NAME

Zithromax's generic name is azithromycin.

 SIDE EFFECTS

Call your doctor if you have any of these possible drug side effects. Call *immediately* about any labeled "serious."

Serious: kidney inflammation (decreased urination), angioedema (swelling of head, face, neck, and internal organs)

Common: nausea, vomiting, diarrhea, abdominal pain

Other: dizziness, spinning sensation, headache, fatigue, palpitations, chest pain, stomach upset, gas, jaundice (yellow-tinged skin and eyes), vaginal infection, rash, increased skin sensitivity to sunlight, black, tarry stools

DRUG INTERACTIONS

Combining certain drugs may alter their action or produce unwanted side effects. Tell your doctor about other drugs you're taking, especially:
• antacids containing aluminum or magnesium (don't take within 2 hours of taking Zithromax)
• anticoagulants (blood thinners) such as Coumadin
• Hismanal
• Lanoxin
• Seldane
• Theo-Dur.

Warnings

• Make sure your doctor knows your medical history. You may not be able to take Zithromax if you're allergic to it or to other antibiotics or if you have liver problems.
• Tell your doctor right away if your symptoms persist or worsen or if you develop signs of a different infection.
• If you're being treated for chlamydia, your doctor may also want to test you for syphilis and gonorrhea.

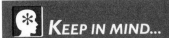 **KEEP IN MIND...**

∗ Take entire amount prescribed, even if you feel better.

∗ Take on an empty stomach.

∗ Don't take antacids that contain aluminum or magnesium within 2 hours of taking Zithromax.

∗ Tell your doctor about signs of persistent, worsening, or new infection.

Zocor

Zocor inhibits an enzyme that's needed for the body to form cholesterol. This lowers cholesterol levels.

Why it's prescribed

Doctors prescribe Zocor to reduce cholesterol levels when diet and nondrug treatments aren't effective. Zocor comes in tablets. Doctors usually prescribe the following amounts for adults.

▶ **For high cholesterol,** at first, 5 to 10 milligrams (mg) a day in the evening. Dosage may be adjusted every 4 weeks based on tolerance and response. Maximum daily dosage is 40 mg.

How to take Zocor

• Take this drug exactly as your doctor orders. Take it with your evening meal to enhance its absorption.
• If your cholesterol level drops too low, your dosage will probably be reduced.

If you miss a dose

Take the missed dose as soon as possible. However, if it's almost time for your next dose, skip the missed dose and take your next dose as scheduled. Don't take a double dose.

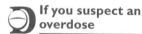 **If you suspect an overdose**

Consult your doctor.

ZOCOR'S OTHER NAME

Zocor's generic name is simvastatin.

 SIDE EFFECTS

Call your doctor if you have any of these possible drug side effects. Call *immediately* about any labeled "serious."

Serious: muscle inflammation (muscle aches or pain)

Common: stomach upset
Tip: Take with food to avoid stomach upset.

Other: headache, weakness, abdominal pain, constipation, diarrhea, gas, nausea, liver problems, cough, flulike symptoms

 DRUG INTERACTIONS

Combining certain drugs may alter their action or produce unwanted side effects. Tell your doctor about other drugs you're taking, especially:
• alcohol
• Aldactone
• anticoagulants (blood thinners) such as Coumadin
• Atromid-S
• drugs that harm the liver
• E-Mycin
• Lanoxin
• Lopid
• niacin
• Nizoral
• Sandimmune
• Tagamet.

 Warnings

• Make sure your doctor knows your medical history. You may not be able to take Zocor if you're allergic to it or if you have a blood or liver disorder.
• Tell your doctor immediately if you think you're pregnant.
• Follow a low-fat, low-cholesterol diet and take other steps to reduce heart disease risk factors, as your doctor recommends. These may include weight control, exercise, and smoking cessation.

• Your doctor will probably perform liver function tests periodically during Zocor therapy.

KEEP IN MIND...

∗ Take with evening meal.
∗ Follow low-fat, low-cholesterol diet.
∗ See doctor as scheduled for liver function tests.
∗ Tell doctor immediately if you think you're pregnant.

Zofran

Zofran helps prevent nausea and vomiting by affecting parts of the brain and nervous system.

Why it's prescribed

Doctors prescribe Zofran to prevent nausea and vomiting following surgery or drug therapy for cancer. It comes in tablets. Doctors usually prescribe the following amounts for adults; children's dosages appear in parentheses.

▶ **To prevent nausea and vomiting,** 8 milligrams (mg) 30 minutes before cancer drug therapy starts. Follow with 8 mg 4 and 8 hours after first dose. Then follow with 8 mg every 8 hours for 1 to 2 days. (Children age 12 and over: same as adults. Children ages 4 to 11: 4 mg 30 minutes before cancer drug therapy starts. Follow with 4 mg 4 and 8 hours after first dose. Then follow with 4 mg every 8 hours for 1 to 2 days.)

How to take Zofran

• Take this drug exactly as your doctor orders. You may take it with food or water.
• Store Zofran at room temperature and away from direct light.

If you miss a dose

Take the missed dose as soon as possible. However, if it's almost time for your next dose, skip the missed dose and take your next dose as

ZOFRAN'S OTHER NAME

Zofran's generic name is ondansetron hydrochloride.

 ## SIDE EFFECTS

Call your doctor if you have any of these possible drug side effects. Call *immediately* about any labeled "serious."

Serious: asthmalike attack (wheezing, difficulty breathing), chest pain, fast pulse

Common: drowsiness, dizziness, diarrhea, constipation
Tips: Avoid driving and other dangerous activities until you know how Zofran affects you. Increase fluids to avoid constipation and prevent dehydration.

Other: headache, rash, liver problems (nausea, vomiting, yellow-tinged skin and eyes), agitation, anxiety, itching

 ## DRUG INTERACTIONS

Combining certain drugs may alter their action or produce unwanted side effects. Tell your doctor about other drugs you're taking, especially:
• Solfoton
• Tagamet.

---

scheduled. Don't take a double dose.

 ## If you suspect an overdose

Contact your doctor *immediately.* Excessive Zofran can cause fainting and vision changes.

Warnings

• Make sure your doctor knows your medical history. You may not be able to take Zofran if you're allergic to it or if you have liver problems.
• Tell your doctor right away if you think you're pregnant or if you plan to breast-feed.
• Zofran is not used to treat children under age 3.

• If you're taking this drug on a regular basis, your doctor may want to perform blood tests periodically to check for side effects. Make sure you keep all doctor's appointments.

 ## KEEP IN MIND...

* Take 30 minutes before cancer drug therapy and as directed afterwards.

* Don't take a double dose if you miss a dose.

* Drink extra fluids if diarrhea occurs.

* Don't give to children under age 3.

Zoladex

Zoladex releases hormones that act on the pituitary gland to dramatically lower blood levels of sex hormones.

Why it's prescribed

Doctors prescribe Zoladex to treat the symptoms of advanced prostate cancer and endometriosis (in which tissues like the lining of the uterus grow anywhere outside the uterus). It comes as an implant that the doctor injects under the skin. Doctors usually prescribe the following amounts for adults.

▶ **For endometriosis or advanced prostate cancer,** 1 implant in upper abdominal wall every 28 days. Maximum duration of treatment for endometriosis is 6 months.

How to take Zoladex

• Report to your doctor every 28 days for a new implant.

If you miss a dose

Arrange to receive the missed dose as soon as possible.

If you suspect an overdose

Because of the way that Zoladex is given, an overdose is unlikely. However, if you have any concerns about the effects you may be experiencing, consult your doctor.

 Warnings

• Make sure your doctor knows your medical history. You may not be able to take Zoladex if you're allergic to it or to similar compounds or if you have risk factors for osteo-

ZOLADEX'S OTHER NAME

Zoladex's generic name is goserelin acetate.

 SIDE EFFECTS

Call your doctor if you have any of these possible drug side effects. Call *immediately* about any labeled "serious."

Serious: stroke, irregular heartbeat, heart failure (shortness of breath, anxiety), high blood pressure (headache, blurred vision), chest pain, fatigue

Common: lethargy, pain, dizziness, swelling, weight gain, nausea, vomiting, rash, sweating
Tip: Antacids may be taken to reduce nausea.

Other: sleeplessness, anxiety, depression, headache, chills, fever, emotional instability, diarrhea, constipation, ulcer, impotence, sexual dysfunction, decreased amount of urine, cloudy urine, difficult or painful urination, failure to menstruate, vaginal dryness, upper respiratory infection, hot flashes, gout, high blood sugar (frequent thirst and urination), weight increase, breast swelling and tenderness, change in breast size, brittle bones in women
Tips: Use water-soluble lubricant for vaginal dryness. Increase fluids and fiber in diet to treat constipation; good sources of fiber are whole grains, vegetables, and fruits.

 DRUG INTERACTIONS

Combining certain drugs may alter their action or produce unwanted side effects. Tell your doctor about other drugs you're taking, especially:
• corticosteroids
• seizure drugs.

porosis (degenerative bone disease), such as a history of smoking or chronic alcohol abuse or a family history of osteoporosis.
• Make sure your doctor knows if you're pregnant or breast-feeding before you begin taking Zoladex. Use a nonhormonal form of birth control while taking this drug. Serious birth defects can occur if you get pregnant while taking Zoladex.
• Menstruation should stop temporarily during treatment. If it continues or if occasional bleeding occurs, check with your doctor.
• This drug should not be used in women under age 18.

• Symptoms of prostate cancer may get worse initially, causing increased bone pain.

 KEEP IN MIND...

* Use a nonhormonal form of birth control during treatment.

* If you're at risk for osteoporosis, consult doctor before using Zoladex.

* Tell doctor if menstruation continues during therapy.

* Prostate cancer symptoms may worsen at first while taking drug.

Zoloft

Zoloft is a drug used to treat depression. It works by increasing the levels of a mood-related substance in the brain.

Why it's prescribed

Doctors prescribe Zoloft to treat depression. It comes in tablets. Doctors usually prescribe the following amounts for adults.

▶ **For depression,** 50 milligrams a day, adjusted weekly or less frequently as tolerated and as needed.

How to take Zoloft

• Take Zoloft exactly as your doctor orders. Don't take more of it than your doctor recommends. You may have to take Zoloft for several weeks before you begin to feel better.
• Take Zoloft once a day, either in the morning or evening.
• You may take Zoloft with or without food. Always take it in the same relation to food and snacks so that your body will absorb the drug the same way each time you take it.

If you miss a dose

Check with your doctor.

If you suspect an overdose

Consult your doctor.

Warnings

• Make sure your doctor knows your medical history. You may not

ZOLOFT'S OTHER NAME

Zoloft's generic name is sertraline hydrochloride.

SIDE EFFECTS

Call your doctor if you have any of these possible drug side effects. Call *immediately* about any labeled "serious."

Serious: high blood pressure (headache, blurred vision), low blood pressure (dizziness, weakness), rapid pulse

Common: headache, tremor, dizziness, sleeplessness, sleepiness, dry mouth, nausea, diarrhea, loose stools, stomach upset, sweating
Tips: If you're not fully alert, don't drive or perform other hazardous activities. To relieve dry mouth, try sugarless gum, hard candy, or ice chips. If dryness persists for more than 2 weeks, tell your doctor.

Other: fainting, numbness, twitching, confusion, loss of balance, palpitations, chest pain, light-headedness, swelling, circulation problems (pale, cold, or tingling hands or feet), uncontrollable eye movements, vomiting, increased or decreased appetite, abdominal pain, trouble swallowing, impotence, rash, acne, hair loss, itchiness, cold and clammy skin, dry skin, flushing, muscle pain

DRUG INTERACTIONS

Combining certain drugs may alter their action or produce unwanted side effects. Tell your doctor about other drugs you're taking, especially:
• alcohol and other drugs that make you feel relaxed or sleepy, such as tranquilizers, sleeping pills, and cold and allergy drugs
• Coumadin and other highly protein-bound drugs
• Orinase
• other antidepressants, such as MAO inhibitors (don't take Zoloft if you've taken an MAO inhibitor within the past 14 days)
• seizure drugs
• Tagamet.

be able to take Zoloft if you have suicidal thoughts, seizures, an emotional disorder, or a metabolic disorder.
• If you're pregnant or breast-feeding, inform your doctor before you start taking Zoloft.
• If you're an older adult, be aware that you may require a lower dosage of this drug.

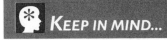 KEEP IN MIND...

* Take once a day in the morning or evening.

* Always take in the same relation to meals and snacks.

* Relieve dry mouth with sugarless gum, hard candy, or ice chips.

* It may take a few weeks before you notice drug's effects.

Zostrix

Zostrix relieves pain by making skin and joints insensitive to pain. How it does this is not exactly known.

Why it's prescribed

Doctors prescribe Zostrix to relieve pain due to shingles (a viral infection that causes a painful rash), surgery, osteoarthritis or rheumatoid arthritis, and other conditions that irritate nerves near the surface of your skin. It comes in a cream. Doctors usually prescribe the following amounts for adults and children over age 2.

▶ **For pain,** small amount applied to affected areas no more than four times a day.

How to use Zostrix

• Wash your hands before and after applying Zostrix. If you're using Zostrix for arthritis in your hands, don't wash them for at least 30 minutes after applying the drug.
• Rub a small amount of Zostrix into the skin over the painful area until the cream almost disappears. Do not apply a thick layer of cream.
• Don't get Zostrix in your eyes, and don't put it on broken skin.
• Don't cover the area with a tight bandage after applying the drug.

ZOSTRIX'S OTHER NAMES

Zostrix's generic name is capsaicin. Another brand name is Axsain.

SIDE EFFECTS

Call your doctor if you have any of these possible drug side effects.

Serious: none reported

Common: stinging or burning when cream is applied
Tip: Zostrix will burn or sting when you first apply it, especially early in treatment. This sensation should subside with regular use, but if you use Zostrix less than three times a day, it may continue to sting.

Other: skin redness; if inhaled, coughing or sneezing

DRUG INTERACTIONS

Combining certain drugs may alter their action or produce unwanted side effects. Tell your doctor about other drugs you're taking.

• Use Zostrix regularly, as prescribed. This drug may take from 1 week (for arthritis) to 6 weeks (for head and neck neuralgia) to relieve your pain.
• Store Zostrix at room temperature.

If you suspect an overdose

Consult your doctor.

Warnings

• Make sure your doctor knows your medical history. You may not be able to use Zostrix if you're allergic to it or if you've ever had an allergic reaction to hot peppers.
• Don't use Zostrix on children under age 2.
• Keep this cream away from children.

• If you're using Zostrix for pain related to shingles, wait until the blisters have healed before applying this drug.
• Call your doctor if your pain lasts 4 weeks or more.

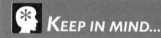

KEEP IN MIND...

* Don't apply Zostrix to broken skin or get it in eyes.

* Stinging and burning should subside with regular use of the drug.

* Don't cover treated area with tight bandage.

* Wash hands before and after using.

Zovirax

Zovirax interferes with the growth and spread of herpes viruses, thereby helping to fight the infections they cause.

Why it's prescribed

Doctors prescribe Zovirax to treat infections caused by herpes viruses, such as genital herpes and shingles. It's also given for chickenpox. Although this drug won't cure infection, it shortens the illness and eases discomfort. It comes in capsules, tablets, a liquid, and an ointment. Doctors usually prescribe the following amounts for adults and children.

▶ **For genital herpes,** 200 milligrams (mg) every 4 hours while awake for 5 to 10 days, or ointment applied thoroughly over all lesions every 3 hours, six times a day for 7 days. Dosage varies, depending on total lesion area.

▶ **For suppression of genital herpes,** 200 mg three times a day for up to 1 year.

▶ **For shingles,** 800 mg five times a day for 7 to 10 days.

▶ **For chickenpox,** 20 mg for each 2.2 pounds of body weight four times a day for 5 days.

How to take Zovirax

• Take this drug exactly as the doctor orders, in the amount prescribed.

• Start using Zovirax as soon as possible after the infection strikes. Then keep using it until your prescription is finished, even if your symptoms subside and you begin to feel better.

ZOVIRAX'S OTHER NAME

Zovirax's generic name is acyclovir.

SIDE EFFECTS

Call your doctor if you have any of these possible drug side effects.

Serious: none reported

Common: nausea, vomiting

Other: temporary burning and stinging, rash, itching, irritated vulva
Tips: Keep the affected areas clean and dry to avoid these effects. Also, wear loose-fitting clothing to avoid irritating the sores.

DRUG INTERACTIONS

Combining certain drugs may alter their action or produce unwanted side effects. Tell your doctor about other drugs you're taking.

• Take the capsule, tablet, or liquid forms of Zovirax with meals to minimize possible stomach upset.

• Use a specially marked measuring spoon to ensure that you measure each dose of liquid Zovirax accurately. Don't use a household teaspoon.

• Wear a disposable glove when applying Zovirax ointment to avoid spreading the infection to other parts of the body. Apply enough ointment to cover each herpes blister.

• Keep Zovirax ointment away from your eyes.

If you miss a dose

Take the missed dose as soon as possible. However, if it's almost time for your next dose, skip the missed dose and take your next dose as scheduled. Don't take a double dose.

If you suspect an overdose

Consult your doctor.

Warnings

• Make sure your doctor knows your medical history. You may not be able to take Zovirax if you're allergic to it.

• Inform your doctor if you're pregnant or breast-feeding before you start this drug.

• It's especially important for women with genital herpes to have annual Pap tests.

• Don't have sex if either you or your partner has genital herpes symptoms. Zovirax will not prevent the spread of herpes.

KEEP IN MIND...

* Start using Zovirax as soon as possible after infection starts.

* Take capsules, tablets, or liquid with food.

* Keep ointment away from eyes.

* Don't have sex if you or your partner has herpes symptoms.

Zyloprim

Zyloprim makes the body produce less uric acid.

Why it's prescribed

Doctors prescribe Zyloprim to treat chronic gout and excess uric acid caused by cancer or kidney disorders. It comes in tablets. Doctors usually prescribe the following amounts.

▶ **For gout,** in mild gout, 200 to 300 milligrams (mg) a day; in severe gout with large uric acid deposits, 400 to 600 mg a day divided into several equal doses a day.

▶ **To prevent gout attacks,** in adults, 100 mg daily, increased by 100 mg weekly up to 800 mg a day.

▶ **For excess uric acid caused by cancer,** in children under age 6, 50 mg three times a day; in children ages 6 to 10, 300 mg a day.

▶ **To prevent uric acid-related kidney damage during cancer drug therapy,** in adults, 600 to 800 mg a day for 2 to 3 days.

▶ **For kidney stones,** in adults, 200 to 300 mg a day in one or several equally divided doses.

How to take Zyloprim

• Take this drug exactly as your doctor orders and drink 10 to 12 full glasses (8 ounces each) of liquid every day for maximum effectiveness.
• Take Zyloprim after meals if it upsets your stomach.
• Keep taking Zyloprim, even if you take another drug for gout attacks.

If you miss a dose

Take the missed dose as soon as possible. But if it's almost time for your

ZYLOPRIM'S OTHER NAMES

Zyloprim's generic name is allopurinol. Another brand name is Lopurin.

 SIDE EFFECTS

Call your doctor if you have any of these possible drug side effects. Call *immediately* about any labeled "serious."

Serious: anemia and other severe blood problems (fatigue, bleeding, bruising, chills, fever, increased risk of infection), hepatitis (yellow-tinged skin and eyes), severe skin reactions (rash, skin ulcers, hives, itching), blood in urine, trouble breathing, chest tightness, weakness

Common: rash, drowsiness, diarrhea, nausea
Tip: If you're not fully alert, don't drive or perform other hazardous activities.

Other: headache, cataracts or other eye disorders, vomiting, abdominal pain, boils on nose

 DRUG INTERACTIONS

Combining certain drugs may alter their action or produce unwanted side effects. Tell your doctor about other drugs you're taking, especially:
• alcohol
• antibiotics, such as Amoxil, Spectrobid, and Totacillin
• anticoagulants (blood thinners) such as Coumadin
• cancer drugs such as Purinethol
• Diabinese
• diuretics (water pills) such as Edecrin
• Imuran
• Inversine
• urine-acidifying agents (ammonium chloride, ascorbic acid, potassium or sodium phosphate).

next dose, skip the missed dose and take your next dose as scheduled. Don't take a double dose.

 If you suspect an overdose

Consult your doctor.

 Warnings

• Make sure your doctor knows your medical history. You may not be able to take Zyloprim if you are allergic to it or if you have diabetes, high blood pressure, kidney problems, or impaired iron metabolism.

• If you're taking Zyloprim for recurrent kidney stones, eat less animal protein, sodium, refined sugers, calcium, and oxalate-rich foods (such as spinach and rhubarb).

KEEP IN MIND...

∗ Take after meals to avoid stomach upset.

∗ Drink plenty of fluids.

∗ Don't drive if not fully alert.

GUIDE TO SAFE DRUG USE, TREATMENTS, AND PREVENTION

Taking drugs safely

Taking drugs safely

To get the most benefit from the drug your doctor has prescribed, it's important that you take it properly. This section of the book shows you — step by step — how to best follow your doctor's instructions. It helps you use the right techniques for taking any type of drug.

The section begins with reminders about filling your prescription and taking and storing the drug as well as advice for staying on schedule. It proceeds to illustrated guidelines for taking, using, or giving every form of drug your doctor may prescribe: from simple tablets, capsules, and liquids to ointments, suppositories, bath products, aerosols, and injections (including how to self-administer insulins).

Also included are special tips on how to adapt your techniques to give drugs successfully to a child as well as how to self-administer drugs through a gastrostomy tube or an implanted port.

Taking and storing the drug

To benefit from the drug your doctor has prescribed, you must take it and store it correctly. Here's how.

Filling your prescription
• Have your prescription filled at the pharmacy you ordinarily use. That way, the pharmacist can keep a complete record of all the drugs you've taken. Make sure the record states which drugs you're allergic to.
• Refill your prescription before you run out of the drug. Don't wait until the last minute.

Taking the drug
• Double-check the label under a bright light to make sure you're taking the right drug. If you don't understand the directions, call your pharmacist or doctor.
• If you forget to take a dose or several doses, don't try to "catch up" by taking two or more doses together. Instead, consult your pharmacist or doctor.
• Don't stop taking the drug unless your doctor tells you to. And don't save it for another time.

Storing the drug
• Keep the drug in its original container or in a properly labeled prescription bottle. If you're taking more than one drug, don't store them together in a pillbox. For convenience, however, you may count them out into daily, weekly, or even monthly containers. (See the entry "Taking drugs on schedule.")
• Store the drug in a cool, dry place or as directed by your phar-

macist. Avoid the bathroom medicine cabinet where heat and humidity may cause it to lose its effectiveness.
• If you have young children in the house, make sure your drug containers have childproof caps. Keep the containers out of children's reach.

Avoiding problems
• Use index cards or a chart to record the following information about each drug you take: its name, its purpose, its appearance, how to take it, when to take it, how much to take, and any special precautions or side effects connected with it.
• If you have any questions about any symptoms you experience while taking the drug, call your doctor.
• If you're pregnant or breast-feeding, talk to your doctor before taking any drug or home remedy. Some drugs can harm the baby.
• Never take a drug that doesn't look right or that has passed its expiration date. It may not work. Worse, it may harm you.
• Don't take nonprescription drugs along with your prescription drugs until you have first checked the drug combination with your pharmacist. Sometimes a nonprescription product can change the way your prescribed drug works.
• Alcoholic beverages and some foods can also change the way some drugs work. Read the label on your prescription. It may tell you what to avoid.
• Don't share your drug with family or friends. It could hurt them.

Taking drugs on schedule

Taking the right amount of the drug at the right time is a crucial part of your treatment. But many people have trouble getting this important task down to a routine. The following tips may help.

Premeasure the drug
Your pharmacy sells several kinds of plastic "medication planners." One type separates your tablets or capsules into individual doses and is helpful if you take your drug more than once a day. Compartments with flip-top lids indicate the time of day — for example, breakfast, lunch, supper, and bedtime, as shown below.

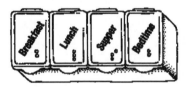

Another type of planner compartmentalizes and stores your drugs for an entire week. The illustrations that follow show two versions of this type.

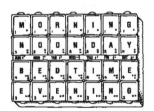

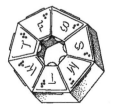

A third type is designed to hold your entire prescription, bottle and all. Computerized numbers on top of the lid show the last time (hour and day) you opened the bottle, as shown below.

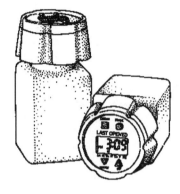

If you prefer, you can make your own medication planner. Here's how: Place a single drug dose in a small envelope, and write on the envelope what time you need to take that dose. Do this for each dose you need to take during the day.

Then put all the small envelopes into a larger one and label the larger one with the day of the week. Do this for each day of the week. Arrange the envelopes chronologically in an empty shoe box.

Make a medication clock
To remind you to take your drug at the right time, make a simple device called a medication clock. Using our sample clocks (opposite) as guidelines, make two large clock faces. (If you have access to a Xerox machine that enlarges, you can simply enlarge one of the samples to the size of a kitchen clock and then make a copy of it so you'll have two.)

Write A.M. in the center of one clockface and P.M. in the center of the other. Then write the names of the drugs you take in the spaces for the hours when you're supposed to take them. Use one color ink for the A.M. clock and a different color ink for the P.M. clock so you can tell them apart easily. Check the clock often during the day so you don't miss any doses.

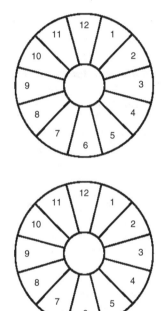

Check the calendar
Another way to keep track of the drugs you take is on a calendar. Dedicate a new calendar—one with plenty of space for daily notes—just for this purpose. In each daily space, write down the names of the drugs and the times you're supposed to take them. You can fill in your schedule for a few days at a time or for the whole month. Draw a line through your notation after you

Taking drugs safely

Taking drugs on schedule
(continued)

take each drug. This method lets you see at a glance what you've taken.

Set an alarm or ask a friend
If you're still having trouble, set your wristwatch or alarm clock to ring when you're due to take a dose. Or ask a relative, friend, or coworker to remind you to take the drug until you know your schedule.

Taking tablets, capsules, and liquids

Whether the drug comes in a solid form (tablets, capsules) or in a liquid form (syrup, elixir, emulsion, suspension), make sure you take it correctly. Here are some guidelines.

Taking tablets and capsules
First, wash your hands. Then gather everything you need, such as the drug, a glass of water or juice and, if you plan to crush a tablet, a mortar and pestle or a commercial pill crusher. If you need to divide a scored tablet, get a knife. Now follow these steps:

1 Look at the container to make sure you have the right drug and the right dose.

2 Pour the prescribed number of tablets or capsules into the bottle cap. If you accidentally pour out too many, tap the extra tablets or capsules back into the container without touching them (to avoid

contamination). Now pour the drug from the cap into your hand.

3 Place the tablets or capsules as far back on your tongue as you can. You may do this with one tablet or capsule at a time or with all of them at once.

4 Tip your head slightly *forward*, take a drink of water or juice, and swallow.

Special tips
- Take coated tablets and capsules with plenty of water or juice.
- If you have trouble swallowing a tablet or capsule, moisten your mouth with some water or juice first. If that doesn't do the trick, you can crush an uncoated tablet, open a soft capsule, or split a tablet.
- *Never* crush tablets or open capsules that have a special coating. Doing so may alter the drug's effectiveness by changing the way your body absorbs it. If you're in doubt, ask your doctor or pharmacist whether it's safe for you to crush or open the drug.
- Protect tablets and capsules from light, humidity, and air. If the drug changes color or has an unusual odor, discard it. Also discard all outdated drugs.

Taking liquids
First, wash your hands. Then get the bottle and a medicine cup or measuring spoon. Look at the container to make sure you have the right drug and are about to take the prescribed dose. If the drug is in a suspension, shake it

vigorously before proceeding with the following steps:

1 Uncap the bottle and place the cap upside down on a clean surface.

2 Locate the marking for the prescribed dose on your medicine cup. Keeping your thumbnail on the mark, hold the cup at eye level and pour in the correct amount of the drug. If you're using a measuring spoon, pour the correct dose into the spoon. Place the bottle safely on a flat surface; then swallow the drug.

3 Wipe the bottle's lip with a damp paper towel, taking care not to touch the inside of the bottle. Replace the bottle cap.

4 Rinse the medicine cup or spoon and store the drug properly.

Special tips
- When pouring a liquid drug, keep the label next to your palm. That way, if any liquid spills or drips, it won't deface the label.
- If you pour out too much liquid, discard the excess. Don't return it to the bottle.
- If a liquid drug has an unpleasant taste, ask your doctor or pharmacist about diluting it with water or juice. You can also try sucking on ice first to numb your taste buds or, if the dose is large enough, pouring the drug over ice and then drinking it through a straw. You may want to chill an oily liquid before taking it.

• To relieve any bitter taste left in your mouth after swallowing the drug, suck on a piece of sugarless hard candy or chew gum. Gargling or rinsing your mouth with water or mouthwash may also help.

Taking precautions

• Keep all drugs out of the reach of children.
• Don't hesitate to ask your doctor or pharmacist about drugs and directions you don't understand.
• Never share any drug with anyone else.

Giving children drugs by mouth

Giving a drug to a child doesn't have to be a problem — for you or the child — if you go about it with patience and care.

Take a positive approach

• Use a matter-of-fact but friendly manner to put the child at ease. Act as though you expect cooperation, and give praise when the child cooperates.
• Offer older children choices, if possible, to give them a sense of control. For example, let them decide which beverage to take with (or after) the drug. (Exclude from their options anything the doctor has advised you against; some drugs cannot be taken with certain beverages or foods.)
• Taste a liquid drug (just a drop) before giving it to a child. This gives you an idea of how the drug will taste and helps you decide

whether to improve its taste by mixing it with a small amount of syrup or food, if appropriate. (Of course, don't taste a drug if you think you may be sensitive to it.)
• Explain to older children how the treatment relates to the illness. They may be more cooperative if they realize that the drug will help them get better.
• Double-check the basics: Are you giving the right drug and dose to the right child at the right time?
• Place a tablet or capsule near the back of the child's tongue, and give plenty of water or flavored drink to help ease swallowing. Then make sure the child swallows it.
• Encourage the child to tip his or her head forward when swallowing a tablet or capsule. Throwing the head back increases the risk of inhaling the drug and choking.
• Give an infant a drug as though you were feeding it to him or her—for example, through a bottle's nipple to take advantage of the natural sucking reflex. Don't mix the drug with formula, though, unless the doctor has advised it because if the formula isn't finished, the infant won't get a full dose of the drug.
• Observe a child closely to see if the drug has the intended effect or is causing side effects.

Be honest and careful

• Never try to trick children into taking a drug; they may resist and distrust you the next time.
• Don't tell children that drugs are candy. If they like the taste,

they may try to take more than the prescribed dose; if they don't, they may distrust you the next time you tell them something.
• Don't promise that the drug will taste good if you've never tasted it or if you know it won't.
• Never threaten, insult, or embarrass a child if he or she doesn't cooperate. These actions can lead to further resistance.
• Keep all drugs out of children's reach to avoid accidents.
• Don't force children to swallow the drug or try to hold their nose or mouth shut to promote swallowing. This may cause choking.
• Don't try to give a drug to a crying child; he or she could choke on it.

Using an oral metered-dose inhaler

Inhaling a drug through a metered-dose inhaler (also called a nebulizer) will help you breathe more easily. Use the nebulizer exactly as demonstrated here, and follow your doctor's instructions for when to use it and how much drug to take.

Getting ready

1 Remove the mouthpiece and cap from the bottle. Then remove the cap from the mouthpiece.

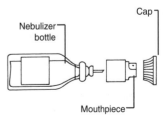

Using an oral metered-dose inhaler (continued)

2 Turn the mouthpiece sideways. On one side of the flattened tip is a small hole. Fit the metal stem of the bottle into the hole to assemble the nebulizer.

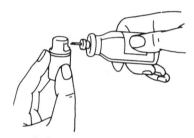

Using the inhaler

1 Exhale fully through pursed lips. Hold the inhaler upside down, as shown below. Close your lips and teeth loosely around the mouthpiece.

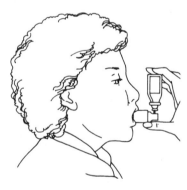

2 Tilt your head back slightly. Take a slow, deep breath. As you do this, firmly push the bottle against the mouthpiece — one time only — to release one dose of the drug. Continue inhaling until your lungs feel full.

To make sure you're taking the correct amount of the drug, be careful to take only 1 inhalation at a time.

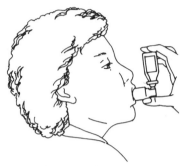

3 Remove the mouthpiece from your mouth, and hold your breath for several seconds.

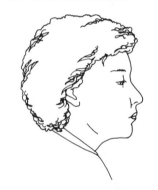

4 Purse your lips and exhale slowly. If your doctor wants you to take more than one dose, wait a few minutes and then repeat steps 1 through 3. Now rinse your mouth, gargle, and drink a few sips of fluid.

Taking precautions

• Remember to discard the inhalation solution if it turns brown or contains solid particles. Store the drug in its original container and put it in the refrigerator, if that's what the label directs.

• Remember to clean the inhaler once a day by taking it apart and rinsing the mouthpiece and cap under warm running water for 1 minute (or immersing them in alcohol). Shake off the excess fluid, let the parts dry, and then reassemble them. This prevents clogging and sanitizes the mouthpiece.

• *Never overuse your oral inhaler.* Follow your doctor's instructions exactly.

Using an oral inhaler with a holding chamber

If your doctor has prescribed an oral inhaler to help open your breathing passages, you'll inhale a drug called a *bronchodilator* through a small device that you put in your mouth. A holding chamber attached to the inhaler helps the drug reach deeply into your lungs.

Common inhalation devices include the InspirEase System and the Aerochamber System.

InspirEase System

This system has a holding chamber that collapses when you breathe in and inflates when you breathe out. To operate this inhaler, follow these steps:

1 Insert the inhaler into the mouthpiece and shake the inhaler. Then place the mouthpiece into the opening of the holding chamber, and twist the mouthpiece to lock it in place.

2 Extend the holding chamber, breathe out, and place the mouthpiece in your mouth.

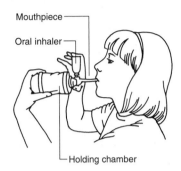

Mouthpiece

Oral inhaler

Holding chamber

3 Firmly press down once on the inhaler. Then breathe in slowly and deeply so that the bag collapses completely. If you breathe incorrectly, the bag will whistle. Hold your breath for 5 to 10 seconds; then breathe out slowly into the bag. Repeat breathing in and out.

4 Wait 5 minutes. Then shake the inhaler again and repeat the dose, following steps 2 and 3.

Aerochamber System

This system uses a small cylinder called a *valved chamber* to trap the drug. It may also include a mask that helps deliver the drug more easily. Follow these steps for use:

I Remove the cap from the inhaler and from the mouthpiece of the Aerochamber. Then insert the mouthpiece into the wider rubber-sealed end of the Aerochamber. Inspect for foreign ob-

jects, and check that all parts are secure.

2 Shake the device three or four times.

3 Breathe out normally, and close your lips over the mouthpiece.
   If your device has a mask, place the mask firmly over your nose and mouth.
   With either device, aim for a good seal. Leaks will reduce effectiveness.

4 Spray *only one puff* from the inhaler into the Aerochamber. Take in one full breath slowly and deeply. If you hear a whistling sound, you're breathing too fast. Now hold your breath for 5 to 10 seconds.

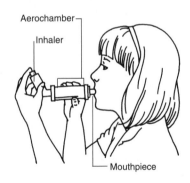

Aerochamber

Inhaler

Mouthpiece

If your device has a mask, hold it firmly in place, as shown below, and breathe in at least six times.
   Caution: Spraying more than one puff into the Aerochamber will give you the wrong dose.

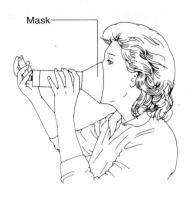

Mask

5 Repeat the steps as directed by your doctor.

6 Remove the inhaler. Follow the manufacturer's directions for cleaning and storing the mouthpiece. Rinse any remaining drug from your face.

Using an AeroVent inhaler

An AeroVent inhaler holds a drug supplied by a metered-dose inhaler and delivers it through a ventilator breathing circuit. Following are some guidelines for using the device.

Connecting the AeroVent to the circuit

I Remove the AeroVent from its box. The device will join the ventilator circuit between the ventilator tubing and the Y-connector that leads to you.

2 Now collapse the AeroVent holding chamber gently by compressing the device as you would an accordion. Push and rotate the springlike chamber slightly until the ends come together.

Using an AeroVent inhaler (continued)

Then press the bracketlike clasp down until it clicks into place.

3 Connect one end of the holding chamber to the Y-connector and the other end to the ventilator tubing.

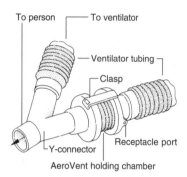

To person — To ventilator

Ventilator tubing

Clasp

Receptacle port

Y-connector

AeroVent holding chamber

Caution: Don't use too much force. If you do, you could damage the device or make it difficult to remove.

Make sure that the receptacle port (which will hold the inhaler) faces upward and away from you.

Opening the circuit

I Before taking a drug through the AeroVent, you'll need to expand the device. To begin, unlatch the external clasp and swing it open (180 degrees).

2 Grasp the connected ends of the holding chamber. Then lightly rotate and stretch the device to the open position. Be careful not to damage the AeroVent by bending or rocking it.

Reposition the receptacle, if needed, because it may be displaced when the chamber expands. To take the drug correctly, you must make sure that the nozzle of the inhaler canister points directly down and that the receptacle port points up to receive the inhaler.

Taking the drug

I Shake the inhaler canister and insert its nozzle into the AeroVent receptacle port. Don't press on the inhaler yet.

2 When a ventilator exhalation ends, activate the inhaler by pressing on the canister's base as many times as the doctor has instructed you to. Don't press with too much force; you could jam the nozzle and damage the equipment.

After several uses, you may notice cloudiness in the chamber. Don't be alarmed. This results from collected moisture and particles of the drug.

Taking precautions

• Once you've taken the drug, remove the inhaler canister and collapse the AeroVent by gently pushing the ends together. Use a slight rotating motion until you compress the device securely. Now relatch the external clasp.

• Observe safety precautions at all times. For example, replace a damaged AeroVent at once, and attach a new AeroVent when you change the tubing.

Giving yourself eyedrops

If your doctor has prescribed eyedrops for you, follow these steps:

Getting ready

I Begin by washing your hands thoroughly.

2 Hold the medication bottle up to the light and examine it. If the drug is discolored or contains sediment, don't use it. Take it back to the pharmacy and have it checked.

If the drug looks okay, warm it to room temperature by holding the bottle between your hands for 2 minutes.

3 Moisten a cosmetic puff or a tissue with water, and clean any secretions from around your eyes. Use a fresh puff or tissue for each eye. Be sure to wipe outward in one motion, starting from the area nearest your nose.

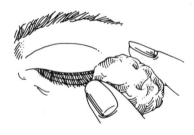

4 Stand or sit before a mirror or lie on your back, whichever is most comfortable for you. Squeeze the bulb of the eyedropper and slowly release it to fill the dropper with the drug.

Using the eyedrops

1 Tilt your head back slightly and toward the eye you're treating. Pull down your lower eyelid to expose the conjunctival sac.

2 Position the dropper over the conjunctival sac, and steady your hand by resting two fingers against your cheek or nose.

3 Look up at the ceiling, and then squeeze the prescribed number of drops into the sac. Take care not to touch the dropper to your eye, eyelashes, or fingers. Wipe away excess eyedrops with a clean tissue.

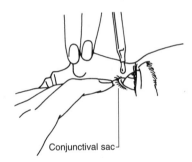

Conjunctival sac

4 Release the lower lid and gently close your eye. Try not to blink for at least 30 seconds. Apply gentle pressure to the corner of your eye nearest your nose for 1 minute. This will prevent the drug from being absorbed through your tear ducts.

5 Repeat the procedure in the other eye if the doctor has instructed you to do so.

6 Recap the bottle and store it away from light and heat.

Taking precautions

- If you're using more than one kind of eyedrop, wait 5 minutes before giving yourself the next one.
- Call your doctor immediately if you have any unusual side effects, such as blisters on your eyelids, red and peeling skin, or extremely swollen, itchy, or burning eyelids.
- Never put a drug in your eyes unless the label reads "For Ophthalmic Use" or "For Use in Eyes."

Putting ointment in your eye

If your doctor has prescribed eye ointment for you, follow these steps to apply it:

Getting ready

1 Wash your hands thoroughly; then hold the ointment tube in your hand for several minutes to warm up the drug.

2 Moisten a cosmetic puff or a tissue with water, and clean any secretions from around your eye. Wipe outward in one motion, starting at the corner of the eye near the nose. Remember to avoid touching the uninfected eye.

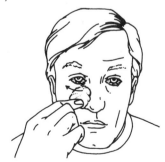

Using the ointment

1 Gently pull down your lower eyelid to expose the conjunctival sac, and look up toward the ceiling. Squeeze a small amount of ointment (about ¼ to ½ inch [½ to 1 centimeter]) into the conjunctival sac. Steady your hand by resting two fingers against your cheek or nose, as shown below. Hold the tube close to its tip to avoid accidentally poking the tip into your eye.

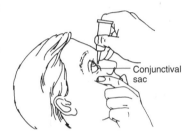

Conjunctival sac

2 Without touching the tube's tip with your eyelashes, close your eye to pinch off the ointment. With your eyes still closed, roll your eyeball in all directions. After a minute or two, open your eyes again.

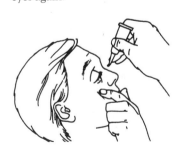

Putting ointment in your eye (continued)

3 Recap the tube. If you're using more than one ointment, wait about 10 minutes before you use the next one. It's normal for your vision to be blurred temporarily after you use the ointment.

Giving yourself eardrops

If your doctor has prescribed eardrops, you should use them exactly as the label directs you to. Here are some guidelines.

Getting ready

1 Wash your hands thoroughly and then check the eardrops. If the solution is discolored or contains sediment, notify your doctor and have your prescription refilled. If your eardrops are okay, proceed.

2 For comfort, warm the eardrops by holding the bottle in your hands for 2 minutes. Then shake the bottle, if that's what the directions say, and open it.

3 Fill the dropper by squeezing the bulb; then place the open bottle and dropper within easy reach.

Using the eardrops

1 Lie on your side with your "bad ear" up.

2 To straighten your ear canal, gently pull the top of your ear up and back, as shown.

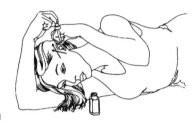

3 Position the dropper above your ear, taking care not to touch it to your ear. Squeeze the dropper's bulb to release 1 drop.

4 Wait until you feel the drop in your ear. Then, if directed, release another drop. Repeat these steps until you have given yourself the prescribed number of drops. To keep the drops from running out of your ear, remain on your side for about 10 minutes.

5 If you wish, you can plug your ear with a piece of cotton moistened with eardrops. Unless your doctor directs you to, don't use dry cotton. It will absorb the drug.

6 Treat your other ear, if necessary, following the same procedure.

7 Recap the eardrop bottle, and store it away from light and extreme heat.

Giving eardrops to a child

To treat your child's ear problem, use the prescribed eardrops exactly as directed on the label.

Getting ready

1 First, wash your hands thoroughly. Then examine the eardrops. Do they look discolored or contain sediment? If they do, notify the doctor and have the prescription refilled. If they look normal, you can proceed.

2 For your child's comfort, warm the eardrops by holding the bottle in your hands for about 2 minutes.

3 Shake the bottle (if directed), open it, and fill the dropper by squeezing the bulb. Place the open bottle and dropper within easy reach.

Giving the eardrops

1 Have your child lie on his or her side with the "bad ear" up. Now gently pull the earlobe down and back to straighten the ear canal.

2 Position the filled dropper above—but not touching—the opening of the canal. Gently squeeze the dropper's bulb once to release 1 drop.

Watch the drop slide into the ear canal or have your child tell you when he or she feels the drop enter the ear.

Then gently squeeze the bulb again to release the rest of the drops prescribed.

3 Continue holding your child's ear as the eardrops disappear down the canal. Now massage the area in front of the ear. Ask your child to tell you when he or she no longer feels the drops moving around; then release the ear.

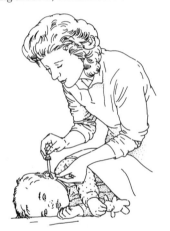

4 Tell your child to remain on his or her side and to avoid touching the ear for about 10 minutes. If your child is active, place an eardrop-moistened cotton plug in the ear to help keep the eardrops in the ear canal. Don't use dry cotton because it may absorb the drug.

If both ears require treatment, repeat the procedure in the child's other ear.

5 Finally, return the dropper to the medication bottle (or recap the dropper bottle). Store the bottle away from light and extreme heat.

Using a metered-dose nasal pump

A metered-dose nasal pump delivers an exact amount of a drug. Here's how to use it.

Getting ready
1 Remove the protective cap and prime the pump as directed by the manufacturer. (Usually, pressing down about four times primes the pump. If it's refrigerated, the pump will stay primed for about 1 week. After that, you'll need to prime it again.)

2 To get the right dose, tilt the pump bottle so that the strawlike tube inside draws the drug from the deepest part, as shown below.

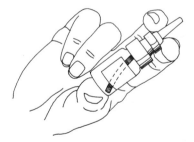

Using the pump
1 Insert the pump's applicator tip about ½ inch into your nostril. Point the tip straight up your nose and toward the inner corner of your eye. (Don't angle the pump or the drug may run into your throat.)

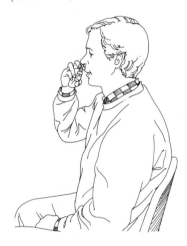

2 Without inhaling, squeeze the pump once, quickly and firmly. Try to use just enough force to coat the inside of your nostril, but not so much that you inject the drug into your sinuses. (That will cause a headache.) Spray again if the package directions instruct you to, or repeat the procedure in the other nostril if your doctor directs you to do so.

3 Keep your head still for several minutes so the drug has time to work. And don't blow your nose for a while.

4 Store the drug in the refrigerator.

Giving yourself nosedrops

Here is what you need to know about using nosedrops.

Getting ready

1 Look at the container to make sure you have the right drug and that you know how much to take.

2 Warm the container by holding it in your hands for about 2 minutes.

3 With the dropper still in the bottle, squeeze the bulb to load the dropper chamber with the drug.

The method you use to instill the drops will vary, depending on the problem you're treating.

Treating the nasal passages

1 If your doctor has prescribed nosedrops to treat your nasal passages, lie on your back and position the dropper as shown below.

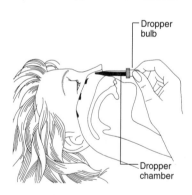

This will help the drops flow down the back of your nose, not your throat.

2 Squeeze the dropper bulb to release the correct number of drops.

3 Repeat the process in the other nostril, if indicated.

4 Breathe through your mouth so that you don't sniff the drops into your sinuses or lungs.

Treating the ethmoid and sphenoid sinuses

1 To treat a problem in these areas, lie on your back with a pillow under your shoulders and your head tilted backward, as shown below.

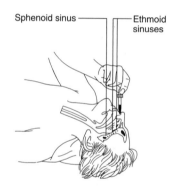

2 Position the dropper above one nostril, and squeeze the bulb to release the prescribed number of drops.

3 Breathe through your nose. This will help the drug move through your sinuses.

Treating the frontal and maxillary sinuses

1 To treat a problem in these areas, lie on your back with a pillow under your shoulders and your head tilted to one side, as shown below.

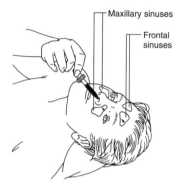

2 Position the dropper above one nostril, and squeeze the bulb to release the prescribed number of drops.

3 Breathe through your nose. This will help the drug move through your sinuses.

Taking precautions

• Follow your doctor's orders exactly. Don't overuse your nosedrops.

• Because nosedrops are easily contaminated, don't buy more than you'll use in a short time. Discard discolored nosedrops and drops that contain sediment.

• Don't share your nosedrops with anyone. Doing so may spread germs.

Taking drugs safely

Using medicated bath products

Your doctor may prescribe a medicated bath to help treat your skin problem. A medicated bath can do the following:

- clean, soften, and lubricate your skin
- relieve itching
- soften scales and crusts (for easier removal).

Preparing the bath

Before you begin, make sure your bathroom is warm and draft-free and that the bathtub is clean.

Adding the drug

The method will vary depending on the product your doctor has prescribed.

If you're using a colloidal preparation such as oatmeal, mix 1 measuring cup of oatmeal with a small amount of cool water to form a paste. Then begin filling the tub with warm water. Gradually swirl in the paste as the tub fills.

If you're using an oil preparation such as mineral oil (with a surfactant), fill the bathtub two-thirds full with warm water. Then add 2 ounces of the oil preparation and stir the water to distribute the oil.

Or you may find it more effective to mix $\frac{1}{4}$ teaspoon of bath oil with $\frac{1}{4}$ cup of water and apply it directly to your skin as you would a lotion.

If you're using a soda preparation such as baking soda, first fill the bathtub to the correct level with warm water. Then add the powder, stirring until it dissolves.

If you're using a starch preparation such as cornstarch, fill the bathtub to the appropriate level with warm water. While the tub is filling, slowly dissolve the powder in a small container of water. Then, when the water reaches the prescribed level, pour in the starch solution.

Bathing and drying off

Before immersing yourself in the bathwater, make sure the temperature feels warm enough. Then get in the tub carefully and soak for about 20 minutes.

When you've finished soaking, step out carefully; the slippery tub surface can be dangerous. Pat yourself dry with a clean, soft towel, removing excess medicated product in the process.

Keep in mind that a skin problem can cause you to lose body heat rapidly, so try not to become chilled. Once you're warm and dry, clean the tub so that it's ready for your next bath.

Inserting a rectal suppository

You can learn to insert a suppository quickly and easily. Be cautious, though. Only use rectal suppositories or other laxatives under your doctor's orders; routine use can lead to dependence.

If the doctor has directed you to use a rectal suppository, just follow these simple steps.

Getting ready

1 Wash your hands. Then gather the items you'll need: the suppository, a disposable glove, and a tube of water-soluble lubricating gel.

2 Put the glove on your right hand (or on your left if you're left-handed). Then remove the foil wrapper on the suppository.

If you have trouble doing this, the suppository may be too soft to insert. Hold it under cold running water until it becomes firm or put it in the freezer for a minute or two before inserting it — just don't let it get too cold and hard. (It's best to store your suppositories in the refrigerator.)

Inserting the suppository

1 Once you've removed the foil wrapper, put a generous dab of lubricating gel on the rounded end of the suppository. Hold the lubricated suppository in your gloved hand.

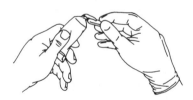

2 Lie on your side with your knees raised toward your chest. Take a deep breath as you gently insert the suppository — rounded end first — into the anus with your gloved hand. Push the suppository in as far as your finger

Taking drugs safely

Inserting a rectal suppository (continued)

will go to keep the suppository from coming back out.

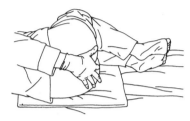

3 Once the suppository is in place, you'll feel an immediate urge to have a bowel movement. Resist the urge by lying still and breathing deeply a few times.

Try to retain the suppository for at least 20 minutes so your body has time to absorb it and get the maximum effect from the drug. After you have a bowel movement, discard the glove and wash your hands.

Inserting a vaginal medication

Plan to insert a vaginal medication after bathing and just before bedtime to ensure that it will stay in the vagina for the appropriate amount of time. Follow these instructions.

Getting ready
1 Collect the equipment you'll need: the prescribed drug (suppository, cream, ointment, tablet, or jelly), an applicator, water-solu-

ble lubricating jelly, a towel, a hand mirror, paper towels, and a sanitary pad.

2 Empty your bladder, wash your hands, and place the towel on the bed. Sit on the towel, and open the wrapper or container.

3 Using the hand mirror, carefully inspect the area around the insertion site. If you see signs of increased irritation, don't insert the drug. Notify the doctor, who may want to change your drug.

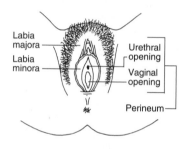

Inserting the drug
1 Place a vaginal suppository or tablet in the applicator or fill it with cream, ointment, or jelly according to package or label directions.

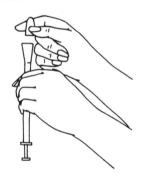

2 To make insertion easier, lubricate the suppository or applicator tip with water or water-soluble lubricating jelly.

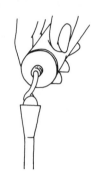

3 Now lie down on the bed with your knees flexed and legs spread apart.

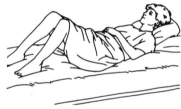

4 Use one hand to spread apart the outer vaginal opening and the other to insert the applicator tip into the vagina. Advance the applicator about 2 inches (5 centimeters), angling it slightly toward your tailbone.

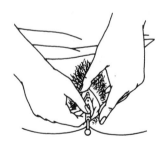

5 Push the plunger to insert the drug. It may feel cold.

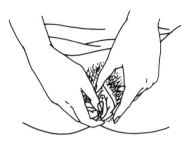

6 Remove the applicator, and discard it if it's disposable. If it's reusable, wash it thoroughly with soap and water, dry it with a paper towel, and return it to its container.

7 If your doctor prescribes it, apply a thin layer of cream, ointment, or jelly to the vulva (the area around the opening of the vagina).

8 Remain lying down for about 30 minutes so the drug won't run out of your vagina. If you like, apply the sanitary pad to avoid staining your clothes or bed linens.

9 Then remove the pad and check your vagina for signs of an allergic reaction. If the area seems unusually red or swollen, contact your doctor.

Mixing insulins in a syringe

If your doctor has prescribed regular and either intermediate or long-acting insulin to control your diabetes, you don't have to give yourself separate injections. Instead, mix the two types of insulin in a single syringe to administer them together. Here's what to do:

1 Wash your hands. Then prepare the mixture in a clean area. Make sure you have alcohol swabs, both types of insulin, and the proper syringe for your prescribed insulin concentration. Then mix the contents of the intermediate or long-acting insulin by rolling it gently between your palms.

2 Using an alcohol swab, clean the rubber stopper on the vial of intermediate or long-acting insulin. Then draw air into the syringe by pulling the plunger back to the prescribed number of insulin units. Insert the needle into the top of the vial. Make sure the point doesn't touch the insulin, as shown below. Now, push in the plunger, and remove the needle from the vial.

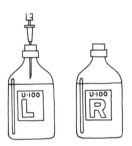

3 Clean the rubber stopper on the regular insulin vial with an alcohol swab. Then pull back the plunger on the syringe to the prescribed number of insulin units, insert the needle into the top of the vial, and inject air into the vial. With the needle still in the vial, turn the vial upside down and withdraw the prescribed dose of regular insulin.

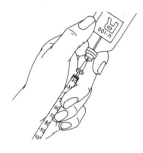

4 Clean the top of the intermediate or long-acting insulin vial. Then insert the needle into it without pushing the plunger down. Invert the vial and withdraw the prescribed number of units for the *total* dose. (For example, if you have 10 units of regular insulin in the syringe and you need 20 units of intermediate or long-acting insulin, pull the plunger back to 30 units.) Remember that you must always mix your insulins in the same order. Always administer the insulin immediately to prevent loss of potency.

Giving yourself a subcutaneous injection

A subcutaneous injection inserts a drug into the tissue directly under your skin so that it can be absorbed quickly into your bloodstream. The needle does not penetrate deeply, and the injection is easy to administer. Before you can administer your injection, you must transfer the correct amount of drug from the bottle to the syringe. Follow these guidelines.

Getting ready

1 Wash your hands. Then assemble this equipment in a clean area: a sterile syringe and needle, the

Giving yourself a subcutaneous injection
(continued)

drug, and alcohol pads (or rubbing alcohol and cotton balls).

2 Check the label on the medication bottle to make sure you have the right drug. As an extra precaution, check the expiration date as well.

3 Clean the top of the bottle with an alcohol pad.

4 Select an appropriate injection site. Pull the skin taut; then, using a circular motion, clean the skin with another alcohol pad or with a cotton ball soaked in alcohol.

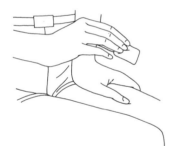

5 Remove the needle cover. *To prevent possible infection, don't touch the needle;* touch only the barrel and plunger of the syringe. Pull back the plunger to the prescribed amount of the drug. This draws air into the syringe.

Insert the needle into the rubber stopper on the bottle, and push in the plunger. This pushes air into the bottle and prevents a vacuum.

6 Hold the bottle and syringe together in one hand; then turn them upside down so the bottle is on top. You can hold the bottle between your thumb and forefinger and the syringe between your ring finger and little finger, against your palm. Or you can hold the bottle between your forefinger and middle finger, while holding the syringe between your thumb and little finger, as shown below.

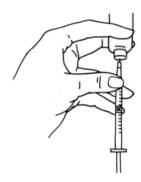

7 Pull back on the plunger with your other hand until the top black portion of the barrel aligns with the mark that indicates you have withdrawn the correct amount of drug. Then remove the needle from the bottle.

8 If air bubbles appear in the syringe after you fill it with the drug, tap the syringe and push lightly on the plunger to remove them. Draw up more drug if necessary.

Injecting the drug
1 Using your thumb and forefinger, pinch the skin at the injection site. Then quickly plunge the needle (up to its hub) into and below the skin at a 90-degree angle. Push the plunger down to inject the drug.

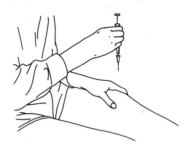

2 Place an alcohol pad over the injection site and press down on it lightly as you withdraw the needle. Don't rub the injection site while you're withdrawing the needle.

3 Snap the needle off the syringe and properly dispose of both.

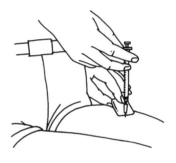

Rotating insulin injection sites

Whether you administer your insulin by needle or by an insulin pump, you need to rotate the injection sites.

Why rotate sites?
Rotating the site for injecting insulin reduces injury to the skin and underlying fatty tissue. It prevents a buildup of scar tissue and swelling and lumps.

It can also minimize a slow insulin absorption rate. This can result from repeated injections in one spot, which can cause fibrous tissue growth and decreased blood supply in that area.

Site rotation can also offset changes that exercise causes in insulin absorption. Exercise increases blood flow to the body part being exercised, thereby increasing the insulin absorption rate. So don't inject yourself in an area about to be exercised. (For example, don't inject yourself in the thigh before you go walking or bike riding.)

Where can I inject insulin?
You can inject insulin into these areas:
• the outer part of both upper arms
• your right and left stomach, just above and below your waist (except for a 2-inch circle around your navel)
• your right and left back below the waist, just behind your hip bone
• the front and outsides of both thighs, from 4 inches below the top of your thigh to 4 inches above your knee.

Keep in mind that different parts of the body absorb insulin at different rates. The stomach absorbs insulin best, then the upper arm, and last, the thighs. Use this approach:
• Inject into the same body area for 1 to 2 weeks, depending on the number of injections you need daily. For example, if you need 4 injections a day, use one area for only about 5 days.
• Cover the entire area within an injection site, but don't inject into the same spot.
• Don't inject into spots where you can't easily grasp fatty tissue.
• Have a family member give you injections in hard-to-reach areas.
• Check with your doctor if a site becomes especially painful, or if swelling or lumps appear.

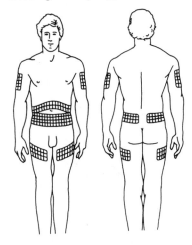

Using an anaphylaxis kit

If you're severely allergic to insect stings or to certain foods or drugs, your doctor will prescribe an anaphylaxis kit for you to keep on hand for emergencies. The kit, called the EpiPen Auto-Injector (EpiPen Jr., for children) contains everything you need to treat an allergic reaction, including:

• a prefilled syringe containing two doses of epinephrine (a drug that helps open your airways)
• alcohol pads
• a tourniquet
• antihistamine tablets.

When an allergic emergency occurs, use the kit as follows; then call your doctor immediately or ask someone else to call the doctor for you.

Getting ready
1 Take the prefilled syringe from the kit and remove the needle cap.

2 Hold the syringe with the needle pointing up. Then push in the plunger until it stops, as shown below. This will expel any air from the syringe.

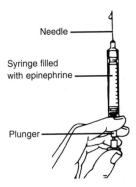

Needle ———

Syringe filled
with epinephrine ———

Plunger ———

3 Clean about 4 inches (10 centimeters) of the skin on your arm or thigh with an alcohol pad. (If you're right-handed, you should clean your left arm or thigh. If you're left-handed, clean your right arm or thigh.)

Using an anaphylaxis kit
(continued)

Injecting the epinephrine
1 Rotate the plunger one-quarter turn to the right so that it's aligned with the slot.

2 Insert the entire needle — like a dart — into the skin.

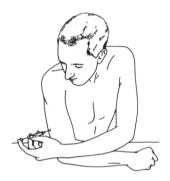

3 Push down on the plunger until it stops. It will inject 0.3 ml of epinephrine, a dose designed for an adult or a person over age 12. Withdraw the needle.
Note: The dose and procedures for babies and for children under age 12 must be directed by the doctor.

Removing the stinger
If you've been stung by an insect, quickly remove the insect's stinger if you can see it. Use your fingernails or tweezers to pull it straight out. Don't pinch, scrape, or squeeze the stinger; this may push it farther into the skin and release more poison.

If you can't remove the stinger quickly, stop trying and go on to the next step.

Applying the tourniquet to the sting
1 If you were stung on your *neck, face,* or *body,* skip this step and go on to the next one.

2 If you were stung on an *arm* or a *leg,* apply the tourniquet between the sting site and your heart. Tighten the tourniquet by pulling the string.

3 After 10 minutes, release the tourniquet by pulling on the metal ring.

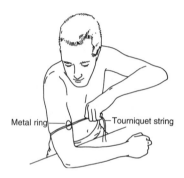

Metal ring — Tourniquet string

Applying ice to the sting
Apply ice packs — if available— to the area of the insect sting.

Taking the antihistamine tablets
For all types of allergic reaction, if your doctor has advised you to take antihistamine tablets, *chew and swallow* the tablets now. (For children age 12 and under, follow the dosage and administration directions supplied by your doctor or provided in the kit.)

What to do next
Important: If you don't notice an improvement within 10 minutes, give yourself a second injection by following the directions in your kit. If your syringe has a pre-

set second dose, don't depress the plunger until you're ready to give the second injection. Proceed as before, following the instructions for injecting the epinephrine.

Avoid exertion, keep warm, and get to a doctor or a hospital immediately.

Taking precautions
• Keep your kit handy so you're always ready for an emergency.
• Ask your pharmacist for storage guidelines. Can the kit be stored in a car's glove compartment or do you need to keep it in a cooler place?
• Periodically check the epinephrine in the preloaded syringe. A pinkish brown solution needs to be replaced.
• Make a note of the kit's expiration date, and renew the kit just before that date occurs.
• When the crisis is over, dispose of the used needle and syringe safely and properly.

Giving an intramuscular injection

To give yourself or someone else an intramuscular injection, you need the right training from your doctor or a nurse. Follow their directions exactly. The guidelines below will act as a review for you until the process becomes routine.

Selecting the site
First choose the injection site. You can use the thigh, hip, buttock, or upper arm. If you're giving yourself the injection, use the front or side of the thigh. If you're giving someone else the injection, you can use the hip, buttock, or upper arm. If possible,

though, you should avoid using the upper arm because the muscle there is small and very close to the brachial nerve.

If a series of injections is necessary, rotate the sites. To reduce pain and improve drug absorption, don't use the same site twice in a row.

Thigh

To find the target, place one hand at your knee and the other at your groin. As shown below, use the area marked by solid lines for adult injections and the area marked by dotted lines for injections for infants and children.

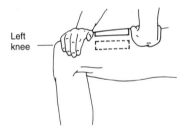

Left knee

Hip

To find this site, place your right hand on the person's left hip (or your left hand on the person's right hip). Then spread your index and middle fingers to form a V. Your middle finger should be on the highest point of the pelvis, known as the ili-

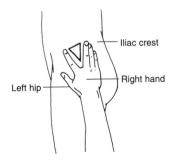

Iliac crest

Right hand

Left hip

ac crest. The triangular area shown in the illustration below is the injection site.

Buttock

Imagine lines dividing each buttock into four equal parts. Give the injection in the upper outermost area near the iliac crest, as shown below. Don't give it in the sciatic nerve area.

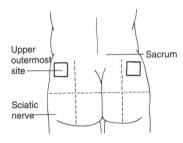

Upper outermost site

Sacrum

Sciatic nerve

Upper arm

Locate the injection site by placing one hand at the top of the person's shoulder and extending your thumb down the person's upper arm. Place the other hand at armpit level, as shown below. The triangular space shown between the hands is the injection area.

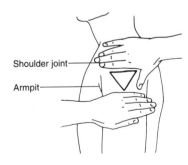

Shoulder joint

Armpit

Getting ready

1 Wash your hands and gather the drug, alcohol pads, syringe, and needle. Make sure you have the right drug. As an extra pre-

caution, check the expiration date.

2 Remove the top of the bottle, and wipe the rubber stopper with an alcohol pad. Unwrap the syringe and remove the needle cover.

3 Pull back on the plunger of the syringe until you've drawn air into it in an amount equal to the amount of drug you'll be injecting. Insert the needle into the bottle through the rubber stopper. Then inject the air in the syringe into the bottle without withdrawing the needle. This will prevent formation of a vacuum and will make withdrawing the drug easier.

4 Invert the medication bottle. With the needle positioned below the fluid level, draw the drug into the syringe by pulling back on the plunger while you measure the correct amount by checking the markings on the side of the syringe. Then withdraw the needle from the bottle.

5 Check for air bubbles in the syringe. If you see any, hold the syringe with the needle pointing up, and tap the syringe lightly so that the bubbles rise to its top. Then push the plunger to get rid of the air and, if necessary, draw up more of the drug to obtain the correct amount.

Again hold the syringe with the needle pointing up, and pull back on the plunger just a little bit more. This will cause a tiny air bubble to form inside the syringe; when you inject the drug, this bubble will help clear the needle and keep the drug from

Giving an intramuscular injection (continued)

seeping out of the injection site. Replace the needle cover.

6 Check the injection site for any lumps, depressions, redness, warmth, or bruising on the skin. Then gently tap the site to stimulate nerve endings and reduce the initial pain of injection.

7 Clean the site with an alcohol pad, beginning at the center and wiping outward in a circular pattern (as shown below) to move dirt particles away from the site.

Let the skin dry for 5 to 10 seconds. If it's not dry, the injection might push some of the alcohol into the skin, causing a burning sensation.

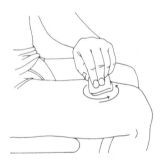

Injecting the drug

1 Remove the needle cover. Then, with one hand, stretch the skin taut around the injection site, as shown below. This makes inserting the needle easier and helps disperse the drug after the injection.

With your other hand, hold the syringe and needle at a 90-degree angle to the injection site.

Then insert the needle with a quick thrust.

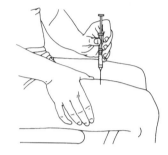

2 Holding the syringe firmly in place, remove the hand stretching your skin and use it to pull back slightly on the plunger.

If blood appears in the syringe, you've entered a blood vessel. Take the needle out and press an alcohol pad over the site. Then discard everything and start again.

If no blood appears, inject the drug slowly, keeping the syringe and needle at a 90-degree angle. Never push the plunger forcefully.

3 When you've injected all the drug, press an alcohol pad around the needle and injection site, and withdraw the needle at the same angle at which you inserted it.

Using a circular motion (extending from the center outward), massage the site with the alcohol pad to help distribute the drug and promote its absorption.

4 Dispose of the used syringe and needle by returning the cover to the needle. Then, holding the syringe, unscrew or snap off the needle and cover. Put both in a covered container used only for disposal of needles and syringes. Keep the container in a safe place until you can dispose of it; then dispose of it properly.

Giving injections through an implanted port

Giving yourself injections through an implanted port is not difficult but it does require close attention to procedure and careful maintenance to prevent infection. Here are some guidelines that may help.

Getting ready

1 Gather together the equipment you'll need: an extension set with a special needle (called a Huber needle), a clamp, a 10-milliliter syringe filled with saline solution, a syringe containing the prescribed drug, a sterile needle filled with heparin flush solution, a povidone-iodine pad, and two alcohol pads.

2 Wash and dry your hands. Attach the 10-milliliter syringe filled with saline solution to the end of the extension set. Gently push on the plunger of the syringe until the extension tubing and needle are filled with the solution and all of the air is removed. Make sure all the air is removed by flicking the tubing of the extension set.

3 Locate the port by feeling for the small bump on your skin. (The site is over a bony area, usually on the upper chest.) Hold the port between two fingers, and clean the site with an alcohol pad. Allow the site to air-dry; then wipe it with a povidone-iodine pad.

Injecting the drug

1 Again, hold the site between two fingers, as shown below.

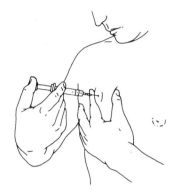

Insert the Huber needle through the skin and port septum until it hits the bottom of the port's chamber. Make sure the needle is inserted at a 90-degree angle, as shown below.

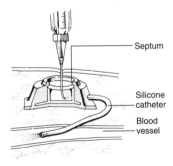

Septum

Silicone catheter

Blood vessel

2 Check for a blood return by pulling back on the syringe that's attached to the extension set. The appearance of blood tells you that the needle is in the proper position in the port and that the port's catheter hasn't slipped out of place inside you.

3 Flush the port with 5 milliliters of the saline solution by pushing down halfway on the plunger

of the syringe containing the saline solution.

4 Clamp the extension set and remove the saline-filled syringe.

5 Connect the drug-filled syringe to the extension set. Open the clamp and inject the drug, as ordered by your doctor.

6 Check the skin around the needle for swelling and tenderness. If you notice either of these signs, stop the injection and call your doctor.

7 When the injection is complete, clamp the extension set and remove the medication syringe.

8 Attach the saline-filled syringe to the extension set. Then open the clamp and flush the port again with the remaining 5 milliliters of saline solution by pushing down on the plunger of the syringe. Remember to flush the port before and after each injection; this minimizes drug interactions. Clamp the extension set and remove the syringe. Put a protective cap on the end of the extension set.

9 Tape the needle in place and apply a gauze dressing.

Taking precautions

• To keep your implanted port trouble-free, flush it according to your doctor's instructions (usually monthly).
• Check with the doctor if you develop a fever or if you observe redness, pain, swelling, or pus at the port site.

Giving drugs through a gastrostomy tube

If you must administer drugs every day through your gastrostomy tube, use the following guidelines.

Getting ready

• Wash your hands with soap and water. Then gather your equipment: prescribed drug, a tablespoon, a measuring cup, a bulb syringe or small funnel, and 2 to 3 ounces (60 to 90 milliliters) of warm water.

Preparing the drug

• If a liquid drug isn't available, you'll need to crush pills or tablets so they'll go through the tube. Most pills can be crushed with a mortar and pestle or a special pill crusher (available from your pharmacy). Crush them into a powder, and dissolve the powder in warm water.
• Don't crush pills with special coatings or enteric coatings, and don't crush capsules. If your drug is available in these forms only, discuss an alternative with your doctor or pharmacist.
• Before administering the drug, always check the container label. Are you sure you're giving the right drug at the prescribed dose? Once the drug is prepared, pour the correct amount into the measuring cup.

Preparing the gastrostomy tube

• Remove the cap or plug and (if necessary) unclamp the tube. Then attach the funnel or syringe securely to the opening. (If you use a syringe, remove the bulb.)

Giving drugs through a gastrostomy tube
(continued)

• Sit upright. Make sure the tube is clear by pouring 2 tablespoons (30 milliliters) of water through the funnel or syringe. If the water doesn't drain by gravity, twist the tube gently to unclog it. If this doesn't work, contact your nurse or doctor for instructions before continuing.

Giving the drug
• Pour the drug into the funnel or syringe, as shown below, and allow it to drain into the stomach by gravity. If the drug backs up in the tube or oozes out around the tube, stop pouring and call the nurse or doctor for advice.

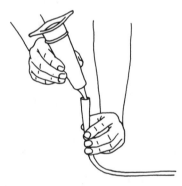

• After administering all of the drug, pour another 2 tablespoons of water into the funnel or syringe to give the tube a final flush.

Finishing up
• Reclamp or pinch off the tube before it completely empties. Then remove the funnel or syringe and cap or plug the tube. Wash your equipment with hot, soapy water, and place it in a clean, covered container. Store it with your drug so you'll have everything handy for next time.
• Remain in an upright position for 1 hour after taking the drug.

Monitoring your health

Monitoring your health

When the doctor prescribes a drug, particularly one for your heart, you may need to check your pulse rate or blood pressure before taking a drug dose. If you're giving a drug to someone else, you may need to check that person's pulse or blood pressure.

Depending on the results, you may go ahead and take — or give — the drug. Or you may need to contact the doctor for a change in the dosage.

This section shows you the right way of taking pulse rates, blood pressures, and (if you have diabetes) how to check your blood's sugar levels and your urine's ketone levels. These two measures are closely related.

Taking your pulse

Your pulse rate tells you the number of times your heart beats in a minute. If you have heart or blood pressure problems, your doctor may want you to check your pulse rate on a regular basis.

Getting ready
You'll need to find a quiet time — not after you've just finished exercising or eating a big meal. You'll also need a watch or a clock with a second hand.

Taking the pulse
1 Begin by sitting down and relaxing for 2 minutes.

2 Place your index and middle fingers on your wrist, as shown here.

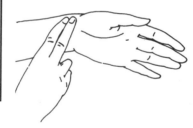

3 Count the pulse beats for 30 seconds and multiply by 2. (Or count for 60 seconds, but do not multiply. Your doctor may instruct you to use the 60-second method if you have an irregular heart rhythm.)

4 Record this number and the date.

Taking your own blood pressure

To take your own blood pressure, your best resource is a digital blood pressure monitor. (You can also use a standard blood pressure cuff and stethoscope, but you'll probably need help from someone else to do so.)

Before you begin, review the instruction booklet that comes with the blood pressure monitor. Steps vary with different monitors, so follow the directions carefully.

Start by taking your blood pressure in both arms. Readings can differ by as much as 10 points from arm to arm. If the readings stay similar consistently, the doctor will probably suggest that you use the arm with the higher reading. Here are some guidelines.

Getting ready
1 Sit down and relax for 2 minutes. Rest your arm on a table, level with your heart. (Use the same arm in the same position each time you take your blood pressure.)

2 Wrap the cuff securely around your upper arm, above the elbow. Make sure that you can slide only two fingers between the cuff and your arm. Turn on the monitor.

Taking the pressure
1 Inflate the cuff as the instructions direct. When the digital scale reads 160, stop inflating.

The numbers will start changing rapidly. When they stop changing, your blood pressure reading will appear on the scale.

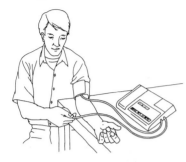

2 Record this reading, the date, and the time. Then deflate and remove the cuff, and turn off the machine.

Taking another person's blood pressure

You can use a standard blood pressure cuff and stethoscope to take the blood pressure of the person in your care. Follow these steps.

Getting ready

I Ask the person to sit comfortably and relax for about 2 minutes. Tell him to rest his arm on a table so it's level with his heart. (Use the same arm in the same position each time you take his blood pressure.)

2 Push up the person's sleeve, and wrap the cuff around his upper arm (just above the elbow) so you can slide only two fingers between the cuff and his arm.

Taking the pressure

I Using your middle and index fingers, feel for a pulse in the person's wrist.

When you find this pulse, turn the bulb's screw counterclockwise to close it; then squeeze the bulb rapidly to inflate the cuff. Note the reading on the gauge when you can no longer feel the pulse. (This reading, called the palpatory pressure, is your guideline for inflating the cuff.)

Now deflate the cuff by turning the screw clockwise.

2 Place the stethoscope's earpieces in your ears. Then place the stethoscope's disk over the pulse in the crook of the person's arm, as shown below.

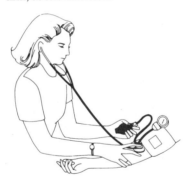

3 Inflate the cuff 30 points higher than the palpatory pressure. Then loosen the bulb's screw to allow air to escape from the cuff. When you hear the first beating sound, record the number on the gauge: This is the *systolic* pressure (the top number of a blood pressure reading).

4 Slowly continue to deflate the cuff. When you hear the beating stop, note and record the number

on the gauge: This is the *diastolic* pressure (the bottom number of a blood pressure reading).

5 Deflate and remove the cuff. Record the blood pressure reading, the date, and the time.

Testing your blood sugar level

Testing blood sugar (glucose) levels daily will tell you whether your diabetes is under control. Follow these steps to learn how to obtain blood for testing and how to perform the test.

Getting ready

I Begin by assembling the necessary equipment: a lancet, a mechanical device to draw blood (optional), a vial with reagent strips, cotton balls, a watch or a clock with a second hand, and a pen.

2 Remove a reagent strip from its vial. Then replace the cap, making sure it's tight. Two types of reagent strips are commonly used to test blood sugar levels visually: Chemstrip bG and Visidex II. (You can also use a glucose meter to measure levels. If you do, be sure to follow the manufacturer's directions precisely.)

Obtaining blood

I Choose a site on the end or side of any fingertip. Wash your hands thoroughly and dry them. To enhance blood flow, hold your finger under warm water for a minute or two.

Testing your blood sugar level (continued)

2 Hold your hand below your heart, and milk the blood toward the fingertip you plan to pierce. Squeeze that fingertip with the thumb of the same hand. Place your fingertip (with your thumb still pressed against it) on a firm surface, such as a table.

3 If you're using a lancet manually, twist off the protective cap. Then grasp the lancet and quickly pierce your fingertip just to the side of the finger pad, where you have more blood vessels and fewer nerve endings.

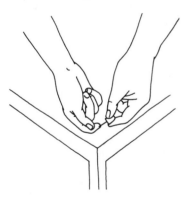

4 Remove your thumb from your fingertip to permit blood flow. Then milk your finger gently until you get a hanging drop of blood that looks large enough to cover the reagent area of the test strip. Be patient. If blood doesn't

flow immediately from the puncture site, keep milking your finger before trying another site.

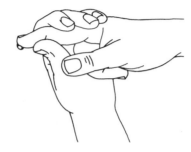

5 If you're using a mechanical device, follow the manufacturer's instructions precisely. To prevent a deep puncture, don't press the device too deeply into the skin surface.

Testing blood

1 Carefully lift the reagent strip to the drop of blood. (The strip has a shiny, slippery undersurface; the blood will roll off if you don't place it on the strip correctly.) Let the blood completely cover the reagent area without rubbing or smearing it. If the blood smears, start over with a new strip.

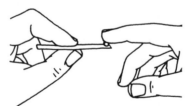

2 As you put the drop of blood on the reagent area, look at your watch or a clock. Begin timing according to the manufacturer's directions. Make sure you keep the strip level.

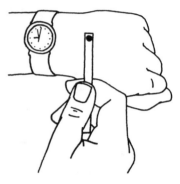

3 When the recommended time has elapsed, gently wipe all the blood off the strip with a clean, dry cotton ball. Wipe the strip three times, using a clean side of the cotton ball each time. Then wait the recommended time.

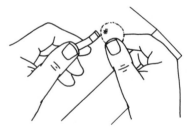

4 Now determine your blood sugar level by holding the reagent strip next to the area of color blocks on the vial. Then match the colors that have appeared on the strip with the two color blocks on the vial. Example: If both colors match the block labeled 180, your blood sugar level is about 180 mg/dl.

If the colors fall between two blocks, take the average of the two numbers. Example: If the colors fall between the two blocks labeled 120 and 180, your blood sugar level is about 150 mg/dl.

Note: The reagent strip and vial shown below don't appear in their actual colors.

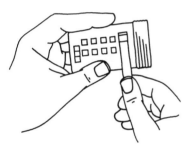

5 Write the date, time, and your initials on the reagent strip and store it in an empty vial. Make sure the cap is tight. The colors on the reagent area will last for up to a week.

Testing your urine for ketones

If your urine contains waste chemicals called ketones, your blood sugar level may be too high.

You should test your urine for ketones when your blood sugar level rises above 240 mg/dl or when you're ill. Even a minor illness can dramatically affect your blood sugar levels.

Your doctor will probably recommend testing every 4 hours until your blood sugar levels have stabilized or until your illness is over. To test your urine for ketones, follow these steps.

1 First, gather a clean container (a small plastic cup will do), a bottle of reagent strips, and a wristwatch or a clock with a second hand.

2 Collect a urine specimen in the container.

3 Remove one reagent strip from the bottle and replace the cap. Hold the strip so the test blocks face up, but don't touch the blocks.

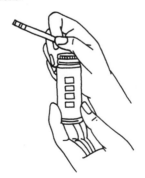

4 Dip the end of the strip with the test blocks into the urine for about 2 seconds. Then remove the strip and shake off excess urine. (Or you can perform the test while you urinate by simply holding the strip under the urine stream for about 2 seconds.)

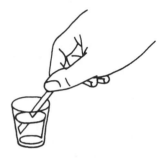

5 Now hold the reagent strip horizontally and immediately begin timing, following the manufacturer's directions.

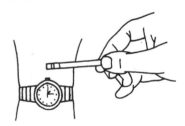

6 After waiting the recommended time, compare the ketone test block with the ketone color chart on the bottle label, as shown at the top of the next page.

Testing your urine for
ketones (continued)

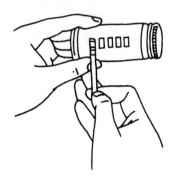

7 Keep a record of your tests, listing the date, the time, the results, and any other pertinent information. Call the doctor if your urine is positive for ketones.

Drug treatments for common illnesses

Drug treatments for common illnesses

This chart lists the most common diseases and the first-line drugs usually prescribed to treat them, as well as other drugs that doctors may prescribe. This list is only an informational guide and not a recommendation. Your doctor may choose other drugs or another brand name of a drug that's listed here. Remember, always consult your doctor before taking any drugs; never try to treat yourself.

Note: Names in **bold type** indicate drugs that are usually used first in treatment. An asterisk (*) marks drugs that aren't discussed in this book.

AIDS

Drugs are a first-line treatment for people with AIDS. Although they don't cure this devastating disease, they may delay its progression. Unfortunately, side effects often limit the duration and aggressiveness of treatment.
- **Retrovir**
- Hivid
- Videx
- Zerit

Alzheimer's disease

Because Alzheimer's has no cure, doctors treat conditions that may worsen the disease, such as an underactive thyroid gland or alcoholism. The Alzheimer's sufferer, though, may benefit from treatment of anxiety, depression, agitation, psychotic symptoms, and insomnia. However, some drugs used to treat mental illness may worsen the person's confusion.
- Cognex

Arthritis (osteoarthritis)

People with this disease may require orthopedic measures to correct developmental anomalies, deformities, disparity in leg lengths, and severely damaged joint surfaces. To relieve pain, salicylates or nonsteroidal anti-inflammatory drugs (NSAIDs), and muscle relaxants (in low doses) may be given.
- Anaprox or Naprosyn
- aspirin
- Motrin

Arthritis, rheumatoid

Treatment for rheumatoid arthritis aims to reduce pain and joint destruction and to prevent the progression of the illness. Physical therapy can help prevent joint weakness and limit loss of movement. Because excessive strain on joints may worsen rheumatoid arthritis, restricting the motion of inflamed joints with splints or braces may help decrease pain and support the joint. Joint surgery may be performed to relieve pain. People with severely damaged weight-bearing joints may require joint replacement.
- **gold salts such as:**
  - Myochrysine
  - Ridaura
  - Solganal
- **NSAIDs such as:**
  - Anaprox or Naprosyn
  - Clinoril
  - Feldene
  - Motrin
- **Plaquenil**
- **Rheumatrex**
- Cuprimine*
- Cytotec
- Cytoxan
- Deltasone
- Imuran

Asthma

Drugs are the primary treatment for asthma. Long-term drug treatment tries to reduce airway inflammation and prevent acute asthma attacks. Short-term drug treatment aims to relieve bronchial spasms and restore oxygen to vital organs. Inhaled drugs cause fewer side effects and are preferred over oral drugs.

- **Alupent**
- **Brethine**
- **Proventil**
- **Tornalate**
- Atrovent
- Azmacort
- Beconase AQ Nasal Spray
- Deltasone
- Intal
- Maxair
- Nasalide or AeroBid
- Serevent
- Theo-Dur
- Tilade

Atrial fibrillation

Drugs are the preferred treatment for this irregular heartbeat; electric shock is an alternative. Blood-thinning drugs called anticoagulants may also be used, especially before shock treatment or in people with heart-valve disease.

- **Calan**
- **Cardizem**
- **Lanoxin**
- **Quinaglute**
- Procan SR
- Tambocor

Atrial tachycardia

Only people with symptoms or underlying heart disease require treatment for this irregular heartbeat. In an emergency, massage of the carotid artery (in the neck)

massage or shock treatment may be tried before drugs.

- **Calan**
- **Cardizem**
- **Lanoxin**
- Adenocard*
- Brevibloc*
- Inderal

Bradycardia

Drugs are used as a supplement to pacemaker insertion.

- Iso-Atropine

Bronchitis

Acute bronchitis usually results from a virus. The value of antibiotics as a treatment is controversial. Treatment generally aims to relieve symptoms and includes such drugs as cough suppressants and expectorants.

- Benylin DM
- Ery-Tab
- Paveral*
- Robitussin
- Symmetrel

   Treatment of chronic bronchitis aims to ease symptoms and eliminate the cause (such as smoking). Use of antibiotics is controversial and is usually reserved for acute attacks. Bronchodilators may be helpful. Short-term use of steroids may have value in severe bronchitis.

- Amoxil
- Bactrim
- Ceftin
- Deltasone
- Ventolin

Cancer-related immunosuppression

Bone marrow growth factors are the latest advances in treating immunosuppression (reduced ability to resist infections) caused by drug therapy for cancer. They're usually administered between courses of the cancer drug. Alternative treatments include bone marrow transplant and frequent blood transfusions.

- **Neupogen**
- Epogen
- Leukine*

Cirrhosis of the liver

Irreversible cirrhosis usually results from chronic alcoholism. Liver transplant is the only curative treatment. Drugs are used to manage the complications of cirrhosis. Correction of nutritional deficiencies, protein restriction, and alcohol avoidance are also important measures.

- **Aldactone**
- Chronulac
- Lasix
- Pitressin

Common cold

Symptoms of the common cold are treated with pain relievers, cough suppressants, and decongestants. Gargling with warm saline solution helps relieve sore throat.

- aspirin
- Benylin DM
- Motrin
- Paveral*
- Sudafed

Drug treatments for common illnesses

Coronary artery disease

Treatment depends on the person. Some people may undergo bypass surgery, balloon angioplasty, or a plaque-shaving procedure while others may receive drugs. Still other may require a combination of therapies. Drug treatment aims to reduce angina symptoms (chest pain) and prevent blockage of a coronary artery, thereby helping to avert a heart attack.
- Corgard
- heparin*
- Ismo
- Isordil
- Lopressor
- Nitro-Dur
- Nitrol
- Norvasc
- Procardia
- Tenormin

Crohn's disease

Drug thearpy, the primary treatment for this disease, is directed at reducing symptoms, not achieving a cure. Additional treatments include changes in diet and surgery to correct intestinal blockages or internal bleeding.
- **Azulfidine**
- Asacol (FDA hasn't approved this use)
- Flagyl
- Deltasone
- Medrol
- Pentasa (FDA hasn't approved this use)

Cytomegalovirus infection

In this viral infection, the length of treatment depends on the person's immune status and the infection site. People with AIDS who have cytomegalovirus (CMV) retinitis require lifelong antiviral drugs. Associated pneumonitis and colitis are treated for 14 to 21 days with either Cytovene or Foscavir. Bone marrow transplant recipients usually receive Cytovene for 100 days after transplant to prevent CMV infection and may also receive gamma globulin. Organ transplant recipients requiring drugs to prevent CMV infection usually receive Cytovene for 28 days; CMV immunoglobulin may be added for liver transplant recipients.
- **Cytovene**
- **Foscavir**

Diabetes mellitus

In this disorder, doctors try to control high blood sugar and prevent long-term complications. Diet is the first line of defense; drugs, such as insulin or oral drugs, are tried next. Proper diet, weight loss, and exercise may be effective alone or when used with drugs.
- **Micronase**
- Glucotrol
- insulin

Emphysema

This chronic, progressive lung condition is treated primarily with drugs and, in later stages, with oxygen. Drugs control symptoms but do not cure the illness.
- **Alupent**
- AeroBid or Nasalide
- Aristocort
- Atrovent
- Beconase
- Brethine
- Deltasone
- Primatene Mist
- Prolastin
- Serevent
- Theo-Dur
- Tornalate
- Ventolin

Gastroenteritis

When caused by *Salmonella* organisms, gastroenteritis doesn't require treatment. Doctors prescribe drugs when gastroenteritis progresses.
- **Bactrim**
- **Cipro**
- **Diodoquin**
- **Ery-Tab**
- **Flagyl**
- Totacillin

Gout

Drug treatment aims to reduce the body's level of uric acid and relieve pain and inflammation. Avoiding obesity, fasting, excessive alcohol, dehydration, and specific drugs is part of the treatment.

- **Indocin**
- **Zyloprim**
- Colsalide
- corticosteroids such as:
  - Aristocort
  - Deltasone
  - Medrol
- uricosurics (drugs that aid uric acid removal) such as:
  - Anturane
  - Benemid

Headache

Treatment depends on the type of headache. Tension headache calls for pain relievers (such as aspirin) and relaxation techniques. Migraine headache calls for avoidance of precipitating factors, drugs to prevent headache or treat the symptoms, and rest in a dark, quiet room until symptoms subside. Migraine headaches that occur more than two or three times a month and vascular headaches may call for preventive drugs. Cluster headaches may also benefit from drug treatment.

- Cafergot
- Catapres
- D.H.E. 45
- Ergostat
- Imitrex
- Inderal
- Periactin
- Sansert

Heart attack

People typically receive morphine to relieve pain. Those with an irregular heartbeat called ventricular fibrillation may receive lidocaine. Bed rest is another important measure. Drugs to dissolve blood clots reduce mortality and may limit the damage. Nitrates are the drug of choice for treating recurrent pain. Beta blockers reduce the duration of the pain and the ocurrence of ventricular fibrillation.

- **beta blockers such as:**
  - Lopressor
  - Tenormin
- **Nitrostat IV***
- **thrombolytics such as:**
  - Activase*
  - Eminase*
  - Streptase*
- anticoagulants such as:
  - aspirin
  - heparin*

Heartburn and gastroesphageal reflux

Drug treatment, the first-line treatment for these disorders, aims to reduce stomach acidity and improve movement of food through the intestines. Supplementary drugs include antacids, especially alginic, and acid-based products such as Gaviscon. Additional measures include avoiding cigarettes and alcohol, avoiding meals within 3 hours of bedtime, elevating the head of the bed, and losing weight. Resistant strictures usually must be manually dilated.

- Axid
- Gaviscon*
- Pepcid
- Prilosec
- Propulside
- Tagamet
- Zantac

Hepatitis

There are five types of viral hepatitis: hepatitis A, B, C, D, or E. Hepatitis A and E usually resolve by themselves but warrant treatment to relieve symptoms. However, hepatitis B, C, and D may become chronic and severe. Severe cases are life-threatening and require emergency liver transplantation. Vaccines and immune globulin are available for preexposure and postexposure prevention of hepatitis A and B. Intron A has been used to treat chronic hepatitis B and C.

- Intron A

High blood pressure

Treating high blood pressure involves losing weight, reducing alcohol and salt consumption, getting regular exercise, and reducing stress. If these measures don't lower blood pressure, doctors try various drugs.

- alpha-blockers such as:
  - Cardura
  - Hytrin
  - Minipress
- Angiotensin-converting enzyme inhibitors such as:
  - Accupril
  - Altace
  - Capoten
  - Lotensin
  - Monopril
  - Vasotec
  - Zestril
- beta blockers such as:
  - Inderal
  - Lopressor
  - Normodyne
  - Tenormin
  - Visken

Drug treatments for common illnesses

High blood pressure
(continued)

- calcium channel blockers such as:
  - Calan
  - Cardizem
  - DynaCirc
  - Norvasc
  - Plendil
  - Procardia
- central sympatholytics (arm and leg blood vessel dilators) such as:
  - Aldomet
  - Catapres
  - Tenex
  - Wytensin
- direct vasodilators such as:
  - Apresoline
  - Loniten
- diuretics (water pills) such as:
  - Bumex
  - HydroDIURIL
  - Lasix
  - Zaroxolyn
- Ser-Ap-Es

Hyperthyroidism

Treatment of an overactive thyroid varies with its cause and severity and with the person's age, condition, and desires. Surgery is usually preferred in children, pregnant women who respond poorly to low doses of thioureas, people with large goiters, and those in whom thyroid cancer is suspected. Radioactive iodine may be administered to destroy overactive thyroid tissue. Drug treatment is used to relieve such symptoms as fast heartbeat, tremors, and sweating.
- Inderal
- thyroid hormone suppressants such as:
  - Propylthiouracil
  - Tapazole

Hypothyroidism

Treatment of an underactive thyroid involves replacing thyroid hormone.
- **Synthroid**

Influenza

Bed rest, pain relievers, and cough medicine may be used to treat the flu. Symmetrel is used to prevent and treat the influenza A virus.
- **Symmetrel**

Irritable bowel syndrome

People with this disorder should avoid intestinal stimulants, such as caffeine-containing beverages. Anxiety-reducing measures, including regular exercise and periods of quiet time, may also prove helpful. Anticholinergic agents may control symptoms in some people. Treatment with antianxiety drugs or antidepressants may also help.
- **Bentyl**

Kidney stones

Treatment varies with the type of stones. For calcium oxalate stones, treatment focuses on correcting the underlying cause, such as hyperparathyroidism, hypercalcemia, acidosis, or hyperoxaluria. People with idiopathic calcium oxalate stones require extra fluids and dietary calcium restriction. Struvite stones usually arise as a complication of bacterial urinary tract infections; chronic antibiotics may partially dissolve these stones, but some people may require surgery or kidney irrigation with Renacidin. Uric acid stones usually result from gout or drug therapy for other disorders; treatment consists of extra fluids, drugs to make the urine less acidic, and Zyloprim.
- **Zyloprim**
- **Renacidin***

Lyme disease

Treatment for this tick-borne disease depends on the stage.

For early Lyme disease (indicated by skin rash)
- **Vibramycin**
- **Amoxil**
- **Ery-Tab**

For late Lyme disease (indicated by heart problems, arthritis, or neurologic disorders)
- **Rocephin***

Meningitis

Antibiotic treatment for this life-threatening infection of the nervous system must begin immediately after lumbar puncture confirms the disorder. Ideally, drug selection is based on results of culture and sensitivity tests. However, the following treatment may be used before test results are known.

- third-generation cephalosporins such as:
  – Chloromycetin sodium succinate
  – Claforan*
  – Fortaz*
  – Garamycin
  – Rocephin*
  – Totacillin
  – Vancocin

Middle ear infection

Antibiotics, the mainstay of treatment for this infection, relieve symptoms and help prevent complications. (However, about 70% to 80% of cases resolve spontaneously within 72 hours even without antibiotics.) Decongestants and pain relievers may be added to relieve symptoms.

- Amoxil
- Augmentin
- Bactrim
- Ceclor
- Ceftin
- Cefzil
- Lorabid

Multiple sclerosis

No treatment can prevent multiple sclerosis (MS) from progressing. People may recover partially from acute exacerbations but may suffer relapses without warning. Management includes measures to reduce muscle spasticity, relieve urinary incontinence, and ease other dysfunctions. Baclofen or Valium may be used to relieve spasticity and flexor spasms; physical therapy also plays an important role.

- Betaseron
- Deltasone

Myasthenia gravis

The chief treatments for this disease are anticholinesterase drugs, drugs to suppress the immune system, surgery to remove the thymus gland, and plasmapheresis (filtering of disease elements from the blood).

- **anticholinesterase drugs such as:**
  – Mestinon
  – Prostigmin
- immunosuppressants such as:
  – Deltasone
  – Imuran

Osteoporosis

Specific treatment varies with the underlying cause. Hormone treatment is most commonly used. Many people also take supplementary calcium salts. People with malabsorption or a condition called osteomalacia may also need vitamin D. Adequate dietary protein, calcium, and vitamin D is also important.

- **estrogens such as:**
  – Estinyl
  – Estrace
  – Premarin
- Miacalcin
- diphosphonates such as:
  – Aredia*
  – Didronel

Pancreatitis

Acute pancreatitis is usually self-limiting, and most people improve within 3 to 7 days. Treatment includes drugs for pain, intravenous fluids to maintain blood volume, and possibly intravenous feedings (if fasting is prolonged). After several days of bowel rest, a diet is usually resumed gradually. People with mild to moderate pancreatitis also may receive suctioning to decrease stomach contents. People with chronic pain and malabsorption may require pancreatic enzymes; surgery may be necessary to drain and remove dead tissue. Intermittent attacks of chronic pancreatitis are treated the same as acute pancreatitis. People should avoid alcoholic beverages and fatty foods. Pancreatic duct obstruction or cysts may warrant surgery.

- pancreatic enzymes such as:
  – Cotazym*

Peptic ulcer disease

Treatment of this disorder includes nondrug treatment, such as stopping smoking, avoiding alcohol and caffeinated beverages, and discontinuing NSAIDs and glucocorticoids, if possible. Some people may require treatment for bleeding in the digestive tract. Relapses are common and may be related to infection with *H. pylori* and cigarette smoking. Frequent relapses may warrant maintenance treatment with H_2-block-

Peptic ulcer disease
(continued)

ers, antibiotics, surgery, or a combination. To eradicate *H. pylori*, Flagyl may be given with Pepto-Bismol; Sumycin or Amoxil may be added. Antacids may be given to decrease pain; however, their use is limited by side effects (such as diarrhea) and the need to take them often.

- **H_2-receptor antagonists such as:**
  - Axid
  - Pepcid
  - Tagamet
  - Zantac
- Carafate
- Cytotec
- Flagyl
- Pepto-Bismol
- Prilosec

Pericarditis

Pericarditis is inflammation of the sac that surrounds the heart, and is marked by chest pain and fever. Pericarditis that follows a heart attack is treated with bed rest and measures to relieve pain and reduce fever. Any contributing causes, such as infection, uremia (inability to excrete waste products from the blood), or rheumatoid arthritis, also are treated. Partial pericardiectomy may be performed for recurrent disease.

- aspirin and NSAIDs such as:
  - Clinoril
  - Feldene
  - Motrin
  - Naprosyn
- corticosteroids such as:
  - Deltasone

Pleurisy

Treatment of this inflammatory disease depends on the underlying cause and symptoms. Pain relievers are given. Pleurisy associated with pneumonia is treated with anti-inflammatory drugs. Severe disease may warrant a nerve block.

- Motrin
- Naprosyn

Pneumonia, bacterial

Susceptibility of the causative organism to antibiotics varies widely. Drug selection is based on results of culture and sensitivity tests. The following drug treatment may begin before test results are known.

- **Garamycin - may be given with or without one of the following:**
- Azactam
- Cipro
- Claforan
- Pipracil*
- Primaxin*
- Timentin*

When *Pseudomonas aeruginosa* is the causative agent:
Double antibiotic coverage is recommended to prevent rapid development of drug resistance in this pneumonia. Susceptibility of the organism to antibiotics varies widely. Ideally, drug selection is based on results of culture and sensitivity tests. However, the following treatment may begin before test results are known.

- **Tobrex - may be given with or without one of the following drugs for severe infection:**
- Azactam

- Cipro
- Fortaz*
- Pipracil*
- Primaxin*
- Timentin*

When methicillin-susceptible *Staphylococcus aureus* is the causative agent:

- **Ancef***
- **Nafcil***

When methicillin-resistant *S. aureus* is the causative agent:

- **Vancocin**

When *Streptococcus* is the causative agent:

- **Cryspen***
- **erythrocin lactobionate***
- Ancef*
- Cleocin

When group D enterococci are causative agents:

- Garamycin (may be given in conjunction with Totacillin or Vancocin)

Pneumonia, *Pneumocystis carinii*

This type of pneumonia warrants antibiotic treatment; sometimes, a steroid, such as prednisone, is also given. Prevention of *P. carinii* pneumonia is recommended for people with AIDS who have $CD4^+$ T-cell counts below 200 cells/μl or after initial *P. carinii* infection.

For treatment of **P. carinii** *pneumonia*

- **co-trimoxazole* (sulfamethoxazole-trimethoprim)**
- Deltasone
- Mepron
- NebuPent
- NeuTrexin* (may be given in conjunction with Wellcovorin* [leucovorin])

Drug treatments for common illnesses

To prevent P. carinii pneumonia
- Bactrim
- Avlosulfon*
- NebuPent

Pneumonia, viral

Common causative organisms for viral pneumonia include influenza, varicella zoster, respiratory syncytial virus (in infants), and cytomegalovirus (in immunosuppressed people).

For pneumonia caused by influenza A
- Symmetrel
- Flumadine

For pneumonia caused by varicella zoster
- Zovirax

Shingles (herpes zoster)

Shingles are caused by the varicella-zoster virus. Drug dosages vary with the infection site and the person's immune status. Mild infection in people with normal immune status may not require antiviral treatment.

For people with normal immune status, mild pneumonia, or dermatomal infection
- Zovirax

For severe disseminated disease or immunocompromised people
- Zovirax
- Foscavir

Stroke

Treatment depends on whether the attack is caused by reduced blood supply, blood clot, or bleeding. In the first two, drug treatment aims to prevent additional strokes and limit damage. In a stroke caused by bleeding, drug treatment supplements surgery to drain the blood and aims to relieve vasospasm (spasm of a blood vessel).
- Coumadin
- heparin*
- Nimotop*

To prevent stroke
- aspirin
- Ticlid

Thrombophlebitis

Treatment aims to control formation of blood clots, prevent complications, relieve pain, and prevent recurrence of thrombophlebitis.

For anticoagulant (blood thinning) treatment
- Coumadin
- heparin*

For lysis of acute, extensive deep-vein thrombosis
- thrombolytic agents such as:
  - Abbokinase*
  - Streptase*

Tuberculosis

Active tuberculosis (TB) requires combination drug treatment for 6 to 18 months (depending on the regimen), using up to five or six drugs. Combination regimens commonly include Laniazid, Rifadin, and Tebrazid* (except in drug resistance or when contraindications exist). In areas where drug-resistant TB is common, treatment for resistant organisms is begun before results of culture and sensitivity tests are known. People infected with TB and those who've been exposed to persons with active TB may receive 6 to 12 months of Laniazid to prevent development of active disease. Immunocompromised people and those who've had a positive skin test within the past 2 years are at highest risk for developing TB. Preventive Laniazid usually is indicated for people younger than age 35 and some people over age 35 who are at high risk for developing TB.
- Laniazid
- Rifadin
- Tebrazid*
- aminoglycosides such as:
  - Capastat sulfate
  - streptomycin*/kanamycin*
- Myambutol
- Seromycin
- Trecator-SC
- Tubasal*

Drug treatments for common illnesses

Ulcerative colitis

Supportive care includes correcting fluid and electrolyte problems. Severe anemia may warrant blood transfusions. People with severe disease typically receive intravenous feedings to rest the bowel. Antidiarrheal drugs, such as Imodium, Lomotil, and codeine*, usually are avoided because they may cause other bowel problems. Surgery may be performed in people with severe disease who don't respond to medical treatment or who require long-term steroid treatment. People with severe, chronic, debilitating disease may need treatment for depression.

- Azulfidine
- corticosteroids such as:
  - Deltasone
- Imuran
- Rowasa

Urinary tract infection (lower)

For lower urinary tract infection, antibiotic selection is based on results of culture and sensitivity tests to identify the causative organism.

- **Amoxil**
- **Bactrim (trimethoprim may be given alone)**
- **Totacillin**
- Cipro
- Keflex
- Macrodantin

Yeast infection (candidiasis)

Most yeast infections (candidal infections) are caused by *Candida albicans*. Drug treatment varies with the infection site and must be adjusted for the specific species. The regimens described below apply to *C. albicans*.

For thrush
- **Mycelex Troches**
- **Nilstat**
- Diflucan
- Nizoral

For skin infection
- **Nilstat**
- Lotrimin
- Monistat

For esophageal candidiasis (yeast infection of the canal that extends from the throat to the stomach)
- **Diflucan**
- **Nizoral**
- Fungizone

For candidiasis or candidemia (yeast infection of the body or bloodstream)
- **Fungizone**
- Ancobon
- Diflucan

For candiduria (yeast infection of the urinary system)
- **Fungizone**
- Diflucan

For vaginal candidiasis (yeast infection of the vagina)
- **Monistat**
- Diflucan
- Femstat
- Lotrimin
- Sporanox
- Terazol
- Vagistat

Managing
drug side effects

Managing drug side effects

The drugs you're taking may produce a variety of side effects. Check the first part of this book to see if your drug's side effects are discussed. This guide provides more information about certain drugs that may temporarily discolor your urine, interfere in some way with medical tests, make you more sensitive to sun exposure, or increase your risk of infection. The section concludes with a roundup of tips on how to minimize the side effects of drug therapy for cancer (chemotherapy).

Drugs that discolor the urine

Analgesic
(pain-reducing)
- Salicylates such as aspirin, Doan's Pills
– Dark brown
- Indocin
– Pink to brown (from internal bleeding)
– Green (from bile pigment in urine)

Analgesics, urinary
- Pyridium
– Red-orange (stain may be permanent)

Anticoagulants
(blood thinners)
- Heparin, Coumadin
– Dark red

Antidepressants
- Elavil
– Blue-green

Anti-infectives
- Quinine
– Brown to black
- Atabrine
– Yellow
- Flagyl
– Dark
- Nitrofurans such as Macrodantin
– Yellow to brown
- Rifadin
– Red-orange
- Sulfonamides such as Bactrim and Azulfidine
– Yellow to brown

Antiparkinson drugs
- Dopar, Larodopa
– Darkens on standing

Diuretics
(water pills)
- Dyrenium
– Pale blue

Hematinics
(increase hemoglobin in blood)
- Iron salts, Feosol, Feostat, Fergon
– Dark

Laxatives
- Cascara
– Red
- Ex-Lax
– Red
- Anthraquinones
– Pink to brown
- Senokot
– Red in alkaline urine; yellow-brown in acid urine

Muscle relaxants
- Paraflex
– Purple to orange
- Robaxin
– Brown to black, green on standing

Seizure drugs
- Dilantin
– Pink to red-brown
- Milontin
– Pink to red-brown

Tranquilizers
- Phenothiazines such as Thorazine and Phenergan
– Pink to brown

Vitamins
- Riboflavin
– Yellow

Miscellaneous
- Desferal
– Reddish
- Urolene blue
– Green to blue

Drugs that affect laboratory test results

Amoxil
(amoxicillin trihydrate)
Alkaline phosphatase (ALP)
Coagulation studies
Coombs' test
Lactate dehydrogenase (LDH)
Liver function tests
Serum potassium
Serum sodium
Serum uric acid
Urine glucose tests (especially Clinitest)
White blood cell count

Augmentin
(amoxicillin + clavulanate potassium)
Alkaline phosphatase (ALP)
Blood urea nitrogen (BUN)
Coagulation studies
Coombs' test
Estriol, estradiol, or estrone
Lactate dehydrogenase (LDH)
Liver function tests
Serum bilirubin
Serum creatinine
Serum potassium
Serum sodium
Serum uric acid
Urine glucose
Urine protein
White blood cell count

Axid
(nizatidine)
Alkaline phosphatase (ALP)
Allergen skin tests
Gastric acid secretion tests
Liver function tests
Urine urobilinogen

Biaxin
(clarithromycin)
Blood urea nitrogen (BUN)
Liver function tests

Capoten
(captopril)
Alkaline phosphatase (ALP)
Antinuclear antibody titers (ANA)
Blood urea nitrogen (BUN)
Hematocrit
Hemoglobin
Liver function tests
Renal imaging (I^{123}, I^{131}, and technetium Tc 99m)
Serum bilirubin
Serum creatinine
Serum potassium
Serum sodium
Urinary acetone test

Cefzil
(cefprozil)
Blood urea nitrogen (BUN)
Coagulation studies
Complete blood count (CBC)
Lactate dehydrogenase (LDH)
Platelet count
Serum bilirubin
Serum creatinine

Cipro
(ciprofloxacin)
Alkaline phosphatase (ALP)
Lactate dehydrogenase (LDH)
Liver function tests

Claritin
(loratadine)
Allergen skin tests

Compazine
(prochlorperazine)
Gonadorelin test
Metyrapone tests
Pregnancy test
Urine bilirubin tests

Coumadin Tabs
(warfarin sodium)
Urinalysis

Deltasone
(prednisone)
Adrenal function tests (ACTH)
Basophil count
Cholesterol
Eosinophil count
Lymphocyte count
Monocyte count
Serum calcium

Depakote
(valproic acid)
Amino acid screening
Lactate dehydrogenase (LDH)
Liver function tests
Metyrapone test
Serum bilirubin
Thyroid function tests
Urine ketone tests

DiaBeta
(glyburide)
Alkaline phosphatase (ALP)
Blood urea nitrogen (BUN)
Lactate dehydrogenase (LDH)
Liver function tests
Serum C-peptide
Serum creatinine
Serum sodium
Serum total protein
Serum uric acid
Sodium I^{123}
Sodium I^{131}
24-hour urine collection
Urine bile
Urine bilirubin
Urine osmolality

Managing drug side effects

Drugs that affect laboratory test results
(continued)

Dilantin Kapseals
(phenytoin)
Alkaline phosphatase (ALP)
Dexamethasone test
Gallium citrate Ga^{67} imaging
Metyrapone test
Schilling test
Serum gamma-glutaryl trans-
  peptidase (GGT)
Serum glucose
Thyroid function tests

Dopar
(levodopa)
Alkaline phosphatase (ALP)
Bilirubin
Blood urea nitrogen (BUN)
Coombs' test
Gonadorelin test
Lactate dehydrogenase (LDH)
Liver function tests
Pancreas imaging
Protein bound iodine (PBI)
Serum uric acid
Thyroid function tests
Urine glucose
Urine ketones
Urine norepinephrine
Urine protein

Ery-Tab
(erythromycin)
Alkaline phosphatase (ALP)
Liver function tests
Serum bilirubin
Urinary catecholamines

Klonopin
(clonazepam)
Metyrapone test
Sodium iodide I^{123} and I^{131}

Lasix
(furosemide)
Blood electrolytes
Blood urea nitrogen (BUN)
Blood and urine glucose
Serum uric acid

Levsin
(hyoscyamine sulfate)
Gastric acid secretion test
Radionuclide gastric emptying
  studies

Lopressor
(metoprolol)
Alkaline phosphatase (ALP)
Antinuclear antibody titers
  (ANA)
Blood glucose
Blood urea nitrogen (BUN)
Catecholamine determinations
Glaucoma screening tests
Lactate dehydrogenase (LDH)
Radionuclide ventriculography
Serum lipoproteins
Serum potassium
Serum uric acid
Triglycerides
Urinary amphetamine screening

Lotensin
(benzapril hydrochloride)
Alkaline phosphatase (ALP)
Antinuclear antibody titers
  (ANA)
Blood urea nitrogen (BUN)
Hematocrit
Hemoglobin
Liver function tests
Renal imaging (I^{123}, I^{131}, and
  technetium Tc 99m)
Serum bilirubin
Serum creatinine
Serum potassium
Serum sodium

Mevacor
(lovastatin)
Creatine kinase (CK)
Liver function tests

Monopril
(fosinopril sodium)
Alkaline phosphatase (ALP)
Antinuclear antibody titers
  (ANA)
Blood urea nitrogen (BUN)
Digoxin levels
Hematocrit
Hemoglobin
Renal imaging (I^{123}, I^{131}, and
  technetium Tc 99m)
Serum bilirubin
Serum creatinine
Serum potassium
Serum sodium

Motrin
(ibuprofen)
Alkaline phosphatase (ALP)
Blood urea nitrogen (BUN)
Blood and urine electrolytes
Coagulation studies
Glucose concentrations
Hematocrit
Hemoglobin
Lactate dehydrogenase (LDH)
Liver function tests
Plasma renin activity (PRA)
Platelet count
Serum creatinine
Serum potassium
Uric acid concentrations
Urine protein
Urine volume
White blood cell count

Naprosyn
(naproxen)
Alkaline phosphatase (ALP)
Blood urea nitrogen (BUN)
Blood and urine electrolytes
Coagulation studies

Managing drug side effects

5-HIAA urine determinations
Glucose concentrations
Hematocrit
Hemoglobin
Lactate dehydrogenase (LDH)
Liver function tests
Plasma renin activity (PRA)
Platelet count
Serum creatinine
Uric acid concentrations
Urine protein
Urine steroid determinations
Urine volume
White blood cell count

Nitrostat
(nitroglycerin)
Methemoglobin
Serum cholesterol
Urine catecholamines
Urine vanillylmandelic acid
 (VMA)

Nolvadex
(tamoxifen)
Cholesterol
Karyopyknotic index
Liver function tests
Papanicolaou (Pap) smears
Serum calcium
Thyroxine (T_4)
Triglycerides

Orudis
(ketoprofen)
Alkaline phosphatase (ALP)
Blood urea nitrogen (BUN)
Blood and urine electrolytes
Coagulation studies
Glucose concentrations
Hematocrit
Hemoglobin
Lactate dehydrogenase (LDH)
Liver function tests
Plasma renin activity (PRA)
Platelet count

Serum creatinine
Uric acid concentrations
Urine albumin
Urine bile salts
Urine protein
Urine 17-hydroxycorticosteroids
 (17-OHCS)
Urine 17-ketosteroids (17-KS)
Urine volume
White blood cell count

Paxil
(paroxetine hydrochloride)
Hematocrit
Hemoglobin
White blood cell count

Pepcid
(famotidine)
Allergen skin tests
Gastric acid secretion test
Liver function tests

Pravachol
(pravastatin sodium)
Creatine kinase (CK)
Liver function tests

Precose
(acarbose)
Hematocrit
Liver function tests
Plasma vitamin B_6
Serum calcium

Primatene Mist
(epinephrine bitartrate)
Blood glucose
Serum lactic acid
Serum potassium

Prilosec
(omeprazole)
Alkaline phosphatase (ALP)
Liver function tests
Serum gastrin

Procardia XL
(nifedipine)
Antinuclear antibody titers
 (ANA)
Direct Coombs' test
Liver function tests
Prolactin

Proventil
(albuterol)
Serum potassium

Provera
(medroxyprogesterone)
Apolipoprotein A
Apolipoprotein B
Clotting factors (II, VII, VIII,
 IX, X)
Coagulation studies
Glucose tolerance test
Gonadotropin
High-density liproproteins
 (HDL)
Liver function tests
Low-density liproproteins (LDL)
Metyrapone test
Serum and urinary steroid
Sex-hormone binding globulin
 (SHBG)
Sulfobromophthalein
Triglycerides
T_3- and T_4-total uptake

Robinul
(glycopyrrolate)
Gastric acid secretion test
Radionuclide gastric emptying
 studies
Serum uric acid

Seldane
(terfenadine)
Allergen skin tests

Managing drug side effects

Drugs that affect laboratory test results
(continued)

Tenormin
(atenolol)
Alkaline phosphatase (ALP)
Antinuclear antibody titers (ANA)
Blood glucose
Blood urea nitrogen (BUN)
Catecholamine determinations
Glaucoma screening tests
Lactate dehydrogenase (LDH)
Radionuclide ventriculography
Serum lipoproteins
Serum potassium
Serum uric acid
Triglycerides
Urinary amphetamine screening

Theo-Dur
(theophylline)
Cholesterol
Dipyridamole-assisted myocardial perfusion studies
Free cortisol excretion
Free fatty acids
High-density lipoproteins (HDL)
HDL/LDL ratio
Plasma glucose
Plasma uric acid
Serum triiodothyronine (T$_3$)

Transderm-Scōp
(scopolamine)
Gastric acid secretion test
Neuroradiologic tests
Radionuclide gastric emptying studies

Univasc
(moexipril hydrochloride)
Blood urea nitrogen (BUN)
Liver function tests
Serum creatinine
Serum uric acid

Xanax
(alprazolam)
Metyrapone test
Sodium iodide I^{123} and I^{131}

Zantac
(ranitidine)
Allergen skin tests
Creatinine clearance
Gastric acid secretion test
Liver function tests
Serum gamma-glutamyl transpeptidase (GGT)

Zithromax
(azithromycin)
Liver function tests

Zocor
(simvastatin)
Creatine kinase (CK)
Liver function tests

Zoloft
(sertraline hydrochloride)
Liver function tests
Serum uric acid
Total cholesterol
Triglycerides

Protecting your skin from sunlight

Exposure to the sun, or even to fluorescent lights, may make your condition worse. Excessive exposure, in fact, may cause rashes, fever, arthritis, and even damage to the organs inside your body.

You needn't spend your waking hours in the dark to be safe, though. Just follow the precautions below.

Prepare for going outdoors
Wear a wide-brimmed hat or visor to shield yourself from the sun's rays. Protect your eyes by wearing sunglasses. Put on a dark, densely woven, long-sleeved shirt and trousers to filter out harmful rays.

Buy a sunscreen containing PABA (para-aminobenzoic acid) with a skin protection factor (SPF) of 8 to 15. If you're allergic to PABA, choose a PABA-free product offering equivalent sun protection.

Before you go outside (at least ½ hour beforehand), rub the sunscreen onto unprotected parts of your body, such as your face and hands. Read the label to determine how often to reapply it. Usually, you'll reapply the sunscreen after swimming or perspiring.

Avoid strong sunlight
Try to stay indoors during the most intense hours of sunlight, from 10 a.m. to 2 p.m. The ideal time to garden, take a walk, play golf, or do any other outdoor activity is just after sunrise or just before sunset.

Remove fluorescent light
At home, replace any fluorescent fixtures or bulbs with incandescent ones.

At work, though, avoiding fluorescent light may be difficult. Consider asking your supervisor about moving to a work area closer to a window, so you can use natural light. If you have a fluorescent light above your desk, turn it off and request a lamp that uses incandescent bulbs.

Managing drug side effects

Be careful with soaps and drugs

Certain toiletries, including deodorant soaps, may increase your skin's sensitivity to light.

Try switching to nondeodorant or hypoallergenic soaps. Certain drugs, including tetracyclines and phenothiazines, also make you more sensitive to light.

Always check with your doctor or pharmacist before taking any new drug.

Recognize and report rashes

Be alert for the key sign of a photosensitivity reaction: a red rash on your face or other exposed area. If you discover a suspicious rash or other reaction to light, call your doctor. Remember, prompt treatment can prevent damage to the tissues beneath your skin.

Avoiding infection

If your medical condition causes you to have an increased risk of getting an infection, you can follow these simple steps to protect yourself.

Follow your doctor's directions

- Take all drugs exactly as prescribed. Don't stop taking your drugs unless directed by your doctor.
- Keep all medical appointments so that your doctor can monitor your progress and the drug's effects.

- If you're receiving a drug that puts you at risk for infection, be sure to tell your dentist or other doctors.

Minimize your exposure to infection

- Avoid crowds and people who have colds, flu, chickenpox, shingles, or other contagious illnesses.
- Don't receive any immunizations without checking with your doctor, especially live-virus vaccines, such as poliovirus vaccines. These contain weakened but living viruses that can cause illness in anyone who's taking a drug that puts the person at risk for infection. Avoid contact with anyone who has recently been vaccinated.
- Practice good personal hygiene, especially handwashing.
- Before preparing food, wash your hands thoroughly. To avoid ingesting harmful organisms, thoroughly wash and cook all food before you eat it.
- Practice good oral hygiene.
- Don't use commercial mouthwashes because their high alcohol and sugar content may irritate your mouth and provide a medium for bacterial growth.
- Don't use unprescribed intravenous drugs—or at least don't share needles.
- If you travel to foreign countries, consider drinking only bottled or boiled water and avoiding raw vegetables and fruits to prevent a possible intestinal infection.
- Wear a mask and gloves to clean bird cages, fish tanks, or cat litter boxes.

- Keep rooms clean and well ventilated. Keep air conditioners and humidifiers cleaned and repaired so they don't harbor infectious organisms.

More prevention tips

- Get adequate sleep at night, and rest often during the day.
- Eat small, frequent meals, even if you've lost your appetite and have to force yourself to eat.

Recognize symptoms of infection

Contact your doctor immediately or seek medical treatment for:

- persistent fever or nighttime sweating not related to a cold or the flu
- profound, persistent fatigue unrelieved by rest and not related to increased physical activity, longer work schedules, drug use, or a psychological disorder
- loss of appetite and weight loss
- open sores or ulcerations
- dry, persistent, unproductive cough
- persistent, unexplained diarrhea
- a white coating or spots on your tongue or throat, possibly with soreness, burning, or difficulty swallowing
- blurred vision or persistent, severe headaches
- confusion, depression, uncontrollable excitement, or inappropriate speech
- persistent or spreading rash or skin discoloration
- unexplained bleeding or bruising

Controlling side effects of chemotherapy

Besides treating cancer, chemotherapy often causes unpleasant side effects. Fortunately, you can sometimes prevent them. Other times you can do things to make yourself more comfortable. Follow the advice below.

Mouth sores

• Keep your mouth and teeth clean by brushing after every meal with a soft toothbrush.

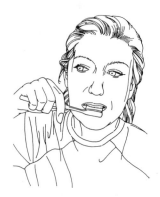

• Don't use commercial mouthwashes that contain alcohol, which may irritate your mouth during chemotherapy. Instead, rinse with water or water mixed with baking soda or use a suspension of sucralfate (Carafate) if your doctor orders it. Floss daily, and apply fluoride if your dentist recommends it. If you have dentures, be sure to remove them often for cleaning.

• Until your mouth sores heal, avoid foods that are difficult to chew (such as apples) or irritating to your mouth (such as acidic citrus juices). Also avoid drinking alcohol, smoking, and eating extremely hot or spicy foods.

• Eat soft, bland foods, such as eggs and oatmeal, and soothing foods, such as ice pops. Your doctor might also prescribe a drug for mouth sores.

Dry mouth

• Frequently sip cool liquids and suck on ice chips or sugarless candy.

• Ask your doctor about artificial saliva. Use water, juices, sauces, and dressings to soften your food and make it easier to swallow. Don't smoke or drink alcohol, which can further dry your mouth.

Nausea and vomiting

• Before a chemotherapy treatment, try eating a light, bland snack, such as toast or crackers. Or don't eat anything — some patients find that fasting controls nausea better.

• Keep unpleasant odors out of your dining area. Avoid strong-smelling foods. Also brush your teeth before eating to refresh your mouth.

• Eat small, frequent meals and avoid lying down for 2 hours after you eat. Try small amounts of clear, unsweetened liquids, such as apple juice, and then progress to crackers or dry toast. Stay away from sweets and fried or other high-fat foods. It's best to stay with bland foods.

• Take antiemetic drugs, as your doctor orders. Be sure to notify him if vomiting is severe or lasts longer than 24 hours or if you urinate less, feel weak, or have a dry mouth.

Diarrhea

• Stick with low-fiber foods, such as bananas, rice, applesauce, toast, or mashed potatoes. Stay away from high-fiber foods, such as raw vegetables and fruits and whole-grain breads. Also avoid milk products and fruit juices. Cabbage, coffee, beans, and sweets can increase stomach cramps.

• Because potassium may be lost when you have diarrhea, eat high-potassium foods, such as bananas and potatoes. Check with your doctor to see if you need a potassium supplement.

• After a bowel movement, clean your anal area gently and apply petroleum jelly (Vaseline) to prevent soreness.

• Ask your doctor about anti-diarrheal medications. Notify him if your diarrhea doesn't stop or if you urinate less, have a dry mouth, or feel weak.

Constipation

• Eat high-fiber foods unless your doctor tells you otherwise. They include raw fruits and vegetables (with skins on, washed well), whole-grain breads and cereals, and beans. If you're not used to eating high-fiber foods, start gradually to let your body get accustomed to the change — or else you could develop diarrhea.

• Drink plenty of liquids — unless your doctor tells you not to.

• If changing your diet doesn't help, ask your doctor about stool softeners or laxatives. Check with your doctor before using enemas.

Heartburn
- Avoid spicy foods, alcohol, and smoking. Eat small, frequent meals.
- After eating, don't lie down right away. Avoid bending or stooping.
- Take oral drugs with a glass of milk or a snack.
- Use antacids, as your doctor orders.

Muscle aches or pain, weakness, numbness or tingling
- Take acetaminophen (Tylenol). Or ask your doctor for acetaminophen with codeine.
- Apply heat where it hurts or feels numb.

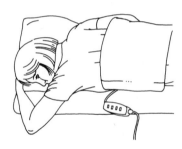

- Be sure to rest. Also, avoid activities that aggravate your symptoms.
- If symptoms don't go away and pain focuses on one area, notify your doctor.

Hair loss
- Wash your hair gently. Use a mild shampoo and avoid frequent brushing or combing.
- Get a short haircut to make thinning hair less noticeable.
- Consider wearing a wig or toupee during therapy. Buy one before chemotherapy begins. Or use a hat, scarf, or turban to cover your head during therapy.

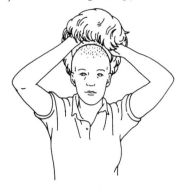

Skin problems
- For sensitive or dry skin, ask your doctor or nurse to recommend a lotion.

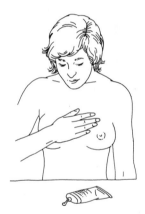

- Use cornstarch to absorb moisture, and avoid tight clothing over the treatment area. Be sure to report any blisters or cracked skin to the doctor.
- Stay out of the sun during the course of therapy. You may even have to avoid the sun for several months afterward, so check with your doctor, especially if you're planning a vacation to a sunny area. When you *can* go out in the sun again, wear light clothes over the treated area, and wear a hat, too. Cover all exposed skin with a good sun block lotion (SPF 15 or above).

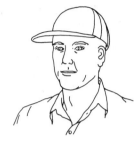

Tiredness
- Limit activities, especially sports.
- Get more sleep.
- Try to reduce your work hours until the end of treatments. Discuss your therapy schedule with your employer.
- If at all possible, schedule chemotherapy treatments at your convenience.
- Ask for help from family and friends, whether it's pitching in with daily chores or driving you to the hospital.

Most people are glad to help out — they just need to be asked.

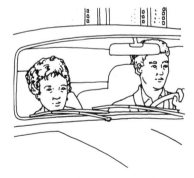

- If you lose interest in sex during treatments, either because you're too tired or because of hormonal

Controlling side effects of chemotherapy (continued)

changes, bear in mind that sexual desire usually returns after treatments end.

Risk of infection

You're more likely to get an infection during therapy, so follow these tips:
• Avoid crowds and people with colds and infections.
• Use an electric shaver instead of a razor.

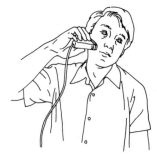

• Use a soft toothbrush. It will help you avoid injuring your gums — a frequent site of infection.
• Tell your doctor if you have a fever, chills, a tendency to bruise easily, or any unusual bleeding.

Treatments
for drug abuse

Treatments for drug abuse

The drugs in this chart are known to cause physical or psychological dependence in persons who take them. You can become physically dependent on such a drug if it causes intense physical distress when it's withdrawn; you can also become psychologically dependent on the drug, to the point where you prefer to live under its influence. For obvious reasons, some of the drugs listed here are illegal. Others are available only by prescription (amphetamines, barbiturates, benzodiazepines, narcotics); if your doctor prescribes any of these, follow his or her advice very carefully to avoid problems.

SUBSTANCE	SYMPTOMS	TREATMENT

Stimulants

Cocaine
- *Street names:* coke, flake, snow, nose candy, crack (hardened form), rock
- *Routes:* swallowing, injection, sniffing, smoking
- *Dependence:* psychological
- *Duration of effect:* 15 minutes to 2 hours; with crack, quick, short high followed by down feeling
- *Medical uses:* anesthetic

- *Of use:* abdominal pain, alternating euphoria and fear, appetite and weight loss, confusion, sweating, dilated pupils, excitability, fever, fast breathing, insomnia, irritability, nausea and vomiting, pale or blue skin, strange behavior, breathing stoppage, seizures, muscle spasms, sight, sound, and smell hallucinations
- *Of withdrawal:* anxiety, depression, fatigue

May include:
- Rest in a quiet room
- If the drug was swallowed, forced vomiting or stomach pumping followed by a cleansing enema
- If the drug was sniffed, nasal cleansing to remove drug residue
- Drugs to slow the heartbeat
- A tepid sponge bath for fever
- Drugs to control seizures
- CPR, if needed.

Amphetamines
- *Street names:* for amphetamine sulfate—bennies, cartwheels, goofballs; for methamphetamine — speed, meth, crystal, crank; for dextroamphetamine sulfate — dexies, hearts, oranges, greenies
- *Routes:* swallowing, injection, sniffing
- *Dependence:* psychological
- *Duration of effect:* 1 to 4 hours
- *Medical uses:* hypermobility, sleeping sickness, weight control

- *Of use:* altered mental state (from confusion to paranoia), sweating, dilated pupils, dry mouth, exhaustion, hallucinations, strange behavior (with prolonged use), seizures, shallow breathing, fast heartbeat, tremors
- *Of withdrawal:* abdominal tenderness, apathy, depression, disorientation, irritability, long periods of sleep, muscle aches, suicide attempts (with sudden withdrawal)

May include:
- Rest in a quiet room
- If the drug was swallowed, forced vomiting or stomach pumping followed by a cleansing enema
- Drugs to decrease sweating, control seizures, reduce aggressive behavior, lower blood pressure, and slow the heartbeat and make it regular
- Physical restraints if the person is experiencing hallucinations or paranoia
- A tepid sponge bath for fever
- Supervision to prevent suicide.

Hallucinogens

Lysergic acid diethylamide (LSD)
- *Street names:* acid, hits, microdot, sugar lump, big D, yellow kimples
- *Routes:* swallowing
- *Dependence:* possibly psychological
- *Duration of effect:* 8 to 12 hours
- *Medical uses:* none

- *Of use:* abdominal cramps, irregular heartbeat, chills, loss of identity, lost touch with reality, sweating, diarrhea; distorted perception of sight, time, and space; dizziness, dry mouth, fever, hallucinations, feeling of importance, heightened sense of awareness, fast breathing, illusions, increased salivation, muscle aches, mystical experiences, nausea, palpitations, seizures, vomiting
- *Of withdrawal:* none

May include:
- Rest in a quiet room
- If the drug was swallowed, forced vomiting or stomach pumping followed by a cleansing enema
- Drugs to prevent seizures
- Orientation to time, place, and people
- Physical restraints if needed.

Treatments for drug abuse

SUBSTANCE	SYMPTOMS	TREATMENT

Hallucinogens (continued)

Phencyclidine

- *Street names:* PCP, hog, angel dust, peace pill, crystal superjoint, elephant tranquilizer, rocket fuel, black bag, getting wet
- *Routes:* swallowing, injection, smoking
- *Dependence:* possibly psychological
- *Duration of effect:* 30 minutes to several days
- *Medical uses:* veterinary anesthetic

- *Of use:* amnesia; blank stare; decreased awareness of surroundings; delusions; distorted body image; distorted sense of sight, hearing, and touch; drooling; euphoria; excitation; fever; shuffling gait; hallucinations; hyperactivity; individualized unpredictable effects; muscle rigidity; panic; poor perception of time and distance; recurrent coma; kidney failure; seizures; sudden behavioral changes; extremely fast heartbeat; violent behavior
- *Of withdrawal:* none

May include:
- Rest in a quiet room
- If the drug was swallowed, forced vomiting or stomach pumping followed by a cleansing enema
- Ascorbic acid to acidify the urine
- Diuretic (water pill)
- Drugs to lower blood pressure, slow the heartbeat, prevent seizures, or reduce agitation or psychotic behavior.

Depressants

Alcohol

- *Found in:* beer, wine, distilled spirits, cough syrup, after-shave, and mouthwash
- *Route:* swallowing
- *Dependence:* physical, psychological
- *Duration of effect:* varies from person to person and according to the amount swallowed
- *Medical uses:* release nerves from adhesions (absolute ethyl alcohol), emergency reduction of uterine contractions, treatment of ethylene glycol and methanol poisoning

- *Of acute use:* decreased inhibitions, euphoria followed by depression or hostility, impaired judgment, incoordination, slow breathing, slurred speech, unconsciousness, vomiting, coma
- *Of withdrawal:* delirium, hallucinations, tremors, seizures

May include:
- Rest in a quiet room
- If alcohol was swallowed less than 4 hours before, forced vomiting or stomach pumping followed by a cleansing enema
- Drugs to treat seizures, hallucinations, and delirium
- Supervision to prevent suicide
- Vitamins, minerals, and fluids to treat dehydration, high blood sugar, and nutritional deficiencies
- Dialysis to remove drug from body.

Benzodiazepines

(Ativan, Centrax, Dalmane, Doral, Halcion, Klonapen, Librium, Paxipam, Restoril, Serax, Tranzene, Valium, Versed, Xanax)
- *Street names:* dolls, green and whites, yellow jackets
- *Routes:* swallowing, injection
- *Dependence:* physical, psychological
- *Duration of effect:* 4 to 8 hours
- *Medical uses:* anxiety, seizures, sedation, hypnosis

- *Of use:* uncoordination, drowsiness, increased self-confidence, relaxation, slurred speech
- *Of overdose:* confusion, drowsiness, slowed breathing, coma
- *Of withdrawal:* abdominal cramps, agitation, anxiety, sweating, extremely fast heartbeat, seizures, tremors, vomiting

May include:
- If the drug was swallowed, forced vomiting or stomach pumping followed by a cleansing enema
- Oxygen
- Drugs to stimulate breathing and consciousness.

(continued)

SUBSTANCE	SYMPTOMS	TREATMENT

Depressants (continued)

Barbiturates
(Amytal, Seconal, Solfoton)
- Street names: for barbiturates — downers, barbs; for amobarbital — blue angels, blue devils; for phenobarbital — purple hearts, goofballs; for secobarbital — reds, red devils
- Routes: swallowing, injection
- *Dependence:* physical, psychological
- *Duration:* 1 to 16 hours
- *Medical uses:* anesthesia, seizures, sedation, hypnosis

- *Of use:* skin blisters, bluish skin, decreased consciousness (from confusion to coma), fever, flaccid muscles, uncontrollable eye movements, poor pupil reaction to light, slowed breathing
- *Of withdrawal:* agitation, anxiety, fever, insomnia, dizziness when rising from a sitting or lying position, extremely fast heartbeat, tremors
- *Of rapid withdrawal:* appetite and weight loss, apprehension, hallucinations, dizziness when rising from a sitting or lying position, seizures, tremors, weakness

May include:
- If swallowing was recent, forced vomiting or stomach pumping followed by a cleansing enema
- Fluids to treat low blood pressure and to alkalinize the urine
- Supervision to prevent suicide
- Measures to relieve withdrawal symptoms
- A hypothermia/hyperthermia blanket for temperature changes.

Narcotics
(codeine, heroin, morphine, Demerol, opium)
- *Street names:* for heroin — junk, horse, H, smack; for morphine — morph, M
- *Routes:* for codeine, Demerol, morphine — swallowing, injection, smoking; for heroin — swallowing, injection, inhalation, smoking; for opium — swallowing, smoking
- *Dependence:* physical, psychological
- *Duration of effect:* 3 to 6 hours
- *Medical uses:* for codeine — pain, cough; for heroin — none; for morphine, Demerol — pain; for opium — pain, diarrhea

- *Of use:* appetite and weight loss, irregular heartbeat, clammy skin, constipation, tiny pupils, decreased consciousness, detachment from reality, drowsiness, euphoria, impaired judgment, increased skin pigmentation over veins, lack of concern, lethargy, nausea, needle marks, seizures, shallow or slow breathing, skin sores, slurred speech, swollen or perforated nasal lining, varicose veins, inability to urinate, vomiting
- *Of withdrawal:* abdominal cramps, appetite and weight loss, chills, sweating, dilated pupils, irritability, nausea, panic, runny nose, tremors, watery eyes, yawning

May include:
- If the drug was swallowed, forced vomiting or stomach pumping
- Drugs to stimulate consciousness and breathing
- Fluids to increase blood pressure
- Extra blankets or hyperthermia blanket for low body temperature
- Orientation to time, place, and people
- Measures to relieve withdrawal symptoms.

Cannabinoids

Marijuana
- *Street names:* pot, grass, weed, Mary Jane, roach, reefer, joint, THC
- *Routes:* swallowing, smoking
- *Dependence:* psychological
- *Duration of effect:* 2 to 3 hours
- *Medical uses:* prevention of vomiting during chemotherapy

- *Of use:* agitation, lack of motivation, anxiety, asthma, bronchitis, reddened eyes, muscle weakness, delusions, distorted self-perception and sense of time, dry mouth, euphoria, hallucinations, impaired ability to understand, impaired short-term memory, mood changes, uncoordination, increased hunger, dizziness when rising from a sitting or lying position, paranoia, spontaneous laughter, extremely fast heartbeat, extremely vivid imagination
- *Of withdrawal:* chills, decreased appetite, weight loss, insomnia, irritability, nervousness, restlessness, tremors

May include:
- Rest in a quiet room
- Oxygen to aid breathing
- Fluids to increase blood pressure
- Drugs to relieve extreme agitation.

Treatments for poisons

Treatments for poisons

This chart presents the suggested treatments for several kinds of poisoning. The number after each substance refers to the appropriate treatment.

Caution: This chart can't replace your call to a poison control center, doctor, or hospital emergency room.

Suggested treatment

1 Small amounts of this substance aren't poisonous, so no treatment is necessary.

2 Make the victim vomit. Give ipecac syrup in the following dosages:
– *If the victim is under age 1:* Two teaspoons followed by at least two glasses of water.
– *If the victim is age 1 or older:* 1 or 2 tablespoons followed by at least two glasses of water.
– *If the person is unconscious or having a seizure:* don't make him or her vomit. Call the poison control center, doctor, or emergency room for instructions.

3 Dilute or neutralize the poison with water or milk. Don't make the person vomit. Call the poison control center, doctor, or emergency room.

4 Dilute or neutralize the poison with water or milk. Don't make the person vomit. The substance may burn the mouth and throat. Call the poison control center, doctor, or emergency room.

5 Immediately rinse skin thoroughly with running water.

Continue for at least 15 minutes. Call the poison control center, doctor, or emergency room for help.

6 Immediately rinse eyes with running water. Continue for 15 to 20 minutes. Call the poison control center, doctor, or emergency room for further instructions.

7 Get the person to fresh air immediately; start artificial respiration if necessary . Call the poison control center, doctor, or emergency room for further instructions.

8 Call the poison control center, doctor, or emergency room before attempting any first-aid treatment.

A

acetaminophen, 2
acetone, 8
acids
  eye contamination, 6
  inhalation (if mixed with bleach), 7
  skin contamination, 5
  swallowing, 4
aerosols
  eye contamination, 6
  inhalation, 7
after-shave lotions
  less than ½ oz (15 ml), 1
  more than ½ oz (15 ml), 8
airplane glue, 8
alcohol
  eye contamination, 6
  swallowing (large quantities; methanol, any amount), 8
alkalies
  eye contamination, 6
  inhalation, 7
  skin contamination, 5
  swallowing, 4
ammonia
  eye contamination, 6
  inhalation, 7
  swallowing, 8
amphetamines, 2
analgesics, 8
aniline dyes
  inhalation, 7
  skin contamination, 5
  swallowing, 8
antacids, 1
antibiotics
  less than 2 to 3 times total daily dose, 1
  more than 3 times total daily dose, 2
antidepressant drugs, 8
antifreeze (ethylene glycol)
  eye contamination, 6
  swallowing, 8
antihistamines, 2
antiseptics, 2
ant trap, 8
aquarium products, 8
arsenic, 8
aspirin, 2

B

baby oil, 1
ball-point pen ink (*see* inks)
barbiturates, 8

Treatments for poisons

batteries
  dry cell (flashlight), 8
  mercury (hearing aid), 8
  wet cell (automobile), 4
benzene
  inhalation, 7
  skin contamination, 5
  swallowing, 8
birth control pills, 8
bleaches
  eye contamination, 6
  inhalation (when mixed with
    acids or alkalies), 7
  swallowing (liquid), 1
  swallowing (solid), 4
boric acid, 2
bromides, 2
bubble bath, 1

C

camphor, 8
candles, 1
caps for cap pistols
  less than one roll, 1
  more than one roll, 8
carbon monoxide, 7
carbon tetrachloride
  inhalation, 7
  skin contamination, 5
  swallowing, 2
chalk, 1
chlorine bleach (*see* bleaches)
cigarettes
  swallowing (less than one), 1
  swallowing (one or more), 2
clay, 1
cleaning fluids, 8
cleanser (household), 8
Clinitest tablets, 4
cocaine, 8
codeine, 8
cold remedies, 8
cologne
  less than ½ oz (15 ml), 1
  more than ½ oz (15 ml), 2

corn removers, 4
cosmetics (*see specific type*)
cough medicines, 8
crayons
  children's, 1
  others, 8
cyanide, 8

D

dehumidifying packets, 1
denture adhesives, 1
denture cleansers, 4
deodorants, 1
deodorizer cakes, 8
deodorizers, room, 8
desiccants, 8
detergents
  dishwasher and phosphate-free,
    4
  liquid/powder (general), 1
dextromethorphan hydrobromide, 2
diaper rash ointment, 1
dishwasher detergents (*see* detergents)
disinfectants, 3
drain cleaners (*see* lye)
dyes
  aniline (*see* aniline dyes)
  others, 8

E

epoxy glue, 8
epsom salts, 2
ethylene glycol (*see* antifreeze)
eye makeup, 1

F

fabric softeners, 2
fertilizers, 8
fishbowl products, 8
furniture polish, 8

G

gas (natural), 7
gasoline, 8
glue, 8

H

hair dyes
  eye contamination, 6
  skin contamination, 5
  swallowing, 8
hallucinogens, 8
hand cream, 1
hand lotions, 1
herbicides, 8
heroin, 8
hormones, 8
hydrochloric acid (*see* acids)

I

inks
  ball-point pen, 1
  indelible, 2
  laundry marking, 2
  printer's, 8
insecticides
  skin contamination, 5
  swallowing, 8
iodine, 8
iron, 8

K

kerosene, 8

L

laxatives, 2
lighter fluid, 8
liniments, 8
lipstick, 1
lye
  eye contamination, 6
  inhalation (if mixed with
    bleach), 7
  skin contamination, 5
  swallowing, 4

M

makeup, 1
markers (indelible), 1
  indelible, 2
  water soluble, 1

Guide to
alternative therapies

Guide to alternative therapies

Alternative therapies — such as acupuncture, chiropractic, naturopathy, herbalism, bodywork, and biofeedback — are enormously popular. A recent study estimated that Americans made about 425 million visits to providers of alternative therapy during a 1-year survey period — far more than the number of visits to all U.S. primary care doctors during the same time (388 million). The most common medical conditions reported by study respondents were back problems, allergies, arthritis, insomnia, sprains or strains, headache, high blood pressure, digestive problems, anxiety, and depression.

Because more and more people are turning to alternative therapies, more doctors are learning about them and applying them in their practice. In addition, the federal government has recently established an Office for the Study of Unconventional Medical Practices at the National Institutes of Health to promote scholarly research and education about alternative therapies.

This concise guide includes nearly 100 alternative therapies, some of which may be familiar to you. Be aware, however, that some methods may not be officially approved for use in the United States. This guide is solely informational and does not imply endorsement of any of the therapies listed.

Acupuncture

This ancient Chinese practice involves puncturing the body with special needles at specific points called *acupoints*. The needles stimulate deep nerve endings to cure disease or relieve pain.

Acupuncture is based on the theory that life energy (*qi* or *chi*) circulates throughout the body along 12 to 14 major energy pathways called meridians. The qi is thought to concentrate at some 500 to 1,000 acupoints along these meridians. Stimulation of acupoints with needles, heat (as in moxibustion), or hand pressure (as in shiatsu) is thought to release trapped life energy, thereby readjusting the energy balance of the body.

Acupuncture is used to treat a wide range of physical illnesses, as well as mental illnesses and drug addiction. It has also been successfully used to provide anesthesia during complex surgical procedures, such as open-heart surgery.

Alexander technique

This technique emphasizes the adjustment of body motion, balance, and posture (especially of the head, neck, and torso) through training and visualization. Its proponents claim that the technique relieves muscle tension, chronic pain, and back disorders and increase a person's range of motion.

Guide to alternative therapies

Aromatherapy

A form of herbal medicine, aromatherapy uses essential oils (concentrated plant extracts) that are believed to exert tranquilizing and antimicrobial effects. The oils are inhaled, added to a bath, or applied during massage to treat headaches, sleep problems, chronic pain and anxiety, and to stimulate the immune system to fight infections.

Ayurvedic therapy

This ancient Indian system of mind and body medicine emphasizes prevention and self-care. Ayurvedic medicine aims to achieve a balance between three life forces, embodied in three metabolic body and personality types called *doshas*. These doshas are called *Vata* (associated with air and movement), *Pitta* (associated with heat, dehydration, and metabolism), and *Kapha* (associated with water, nourishment, and protection of body structures).

Imbalances between the three doshas cause mental and physical problems and are treated with diet, herbs, massage, meditation, and, in some cases, surgery and antibiotics.

Bach flower remedies

A combination of homeopathic and herbal medicine, this alternative therapy employs extracts from certain flowers, trees, and grasses to treat emotional and psychological problems that pre-dispose a person to mental and organic illnesses. The extracts are taken with liquids or placed under the tongue. They're used for 1 to 12 weeks until symptoms disappear.

Bee venom

In homeopathy, an extreme dilution of honeybee extract may be used to treat a disorder whose symptoms mimic those produced by the remedy. Conventional medicine uses bee venom to desensitize susceptible persons to bee stings. This immunotherapy uses whole-venom antigens with maintenance doses for up to 5 years.

Bioenergetics

Bioenergetics combines bodywork with psychotherapy. It's based on the idea that repressed emotions create persistent muscle tensions. The tensions and emotions are released through a combination of talk therapy, deep breathing and other exercises, and massage. The person may also release tension by crying, yelling, screaming, or striking an inanimate object, such as a pillow or bed.

Biofeedback

A type of relaxation therapy, biofeedback uses electronic devices to teach awareness and conscious control of involuntary body functions, such as heart rate and pulse, blood pressure, temperature, digestion, and muscle behavior. It's widely used to treat stress-related conditions such as neck and back pain, migraine headaches, temporomandibular joint (TMJ) pain, incontinence, various cardiac conditions, and anxiety.

Biological dentistry

This holistic approach to dentistry uses nontoxic materials for dental work. It avoids, for instance, the use of mercury/silver amalgam for tooth fillings and maintains that dental problems have far-reaching effects on the rest of the body. Acupuncture, homeopathy, and biofeedback techniques are used for diagnosis and treatment.

Cell therapy

This therapy involves injection of living or freeze-dried cellular material prepared from embryos, fetuses, or adult organ tissues into the body to stimulate the immune system and treat certain degenerative diseases. For example, human fetal cell transplants are being tested as treatments for Parkinson's and Alzheimer's diseases. The technique is also used in an attempt to slow the aging process and to treat various cancers.

Chelation therapy

A form of detoxification, chelation therapy involves an injection or oral administration of ethylene diamine tetra-acetic acid (EDTA). A synthetic amino acid, EDTA attaches to toxic sub-

Chelation therapy
(continued)

stances (such as lead, cadmium, aluminum, and other metals) in the blood to facilitate their removal from the body in urine.

Because EDTA is also believed to remove excess calcium from the body, it's used by some practitioners to treat hardening of the arteries (atherosclerosis), heart attack, stroke, other blood vessel diseases, arthritis, and gangrene.

Chinese herbal therapy

An important part of traditional Chinese medicine, herbs are classified according to their taste, which signifies their medicinal action and, often, their natural affinity to particular body organs. Herbs are used to enhance immune function and treat stress, as well as to treat skin, intestinal, joint, and menstrual problems.

Chiropractic

This therapy uses physical manipulation of the spine, joints, and muscles to restore proper function of affected nerves and enhance the body's defense mechanisms. Exercise, diet, and physical therapy may also be used, but drugs and surgery are avoided.

Chiropractic therapy is based on the theory that subluxation, or the displacement of a spinal vertebra, impinges on a given nerve. This impairs the nerve pathway and with it the brain's ability to regulate activities of body tissue, which becomes pre-

disposed to disease. The chiropractor manipulates the vertebra into its correct position and allows nerve impulses to flow properly. Chiropractic is widely used to treat lower back pain, headache, trauma, respiratory and intestinal conditions, and mental and environmental stress.

There are two major schools of chiropractic. In "straight" chiropractic, the practitioner deals only with locating and correcting subluxations. In "mixed" chiropractic, the practitioner combines this with other methods.

Cobra venom

In homeopathy, an extremely diluted form of snake venom may be used to treat a disorder whose symptoms mimic those produced by the remedy. Cobra venom is claimed to be effective against arthritis.

Cognitive therapy

A form of psychotherapy, cognitive therapy is based on the idea that emotional illnesses result from irrational beliefs or perceptions. Therapy makes a person aware of the occurrence and irrationality of these distortions, tests them against reality, and looks for reasonable alternative explanations. Initial improvement in mood is thought to generate a biochemical response that leads to a heightened sense of well-being.

Cognitive therapy is used to treat anxiety, depression, and phobias.

Colonic therapy

In this type of hydrotherapy, filtered water is passed through a tube into a person's colon under light pressure; the colon's contents are gently flushed out to remove toxins. A variant of this, colonic ozone therapy, maintains that the body needs pure oxygen to thrive.

Colonic therapy is used to treat headache and backache, as well as indigestion, constipation, and other stomach and intestinal conditions.

Colored light therapy

This form of light therapy uses intermittent or steady beams of red, blue, or white light are thought to stimulate parts of the nervous system and influence production of certain chemicals in the brain. Also called photostimulation, colored light therapy has been used for sleep disorders, chronic pain, anxiety, allergies, diabetes, and wound healing.

Cranial osteopathy

Also called craniosacral therapy, this treatment hinges on the theory that a periodic rise and fall of spinal fluid pressure affects the movement of the bones in the head. Treatment involves manipulating the head bones, the lining beneath these bones, or stimulating nerve endings in the scalp and between the cranial sutures (lines in skull where cranial bones meet). It's used to treat chronic pain, trauma to the head and spine, temporomandibular joint (TMJ) syndrome, ear infections, headaches, ringing in ears, mood disorders, and high or low blood pressure.

Cupping

Used in Ayurvedic and traditional Chinese medicine, heated suction cups are placed over wounds and abscesses to improve local circulation. Cupping may also be used with bloodletting at the cupping sites. Its proponents claim that the practice treats high blood pressure, abdominal pain, or arthritis.

Dance therapy

This form of creative or expressive therapy improves coordination and range of motion. It's also used for psychiatric and emotional problems.

Detoxification therapy

A form of naturopathy, this therapy hinges on the claim that the body is a "bioaccumulator." As a result, the body becomes contaminated with a wide variety of toxic chemicals and pollutants (such as pesticides, food additives, and drug residues) that ultimately impair the immune system and lead to disease.

Detoxification therapies include juice and water fasting, chelation, and nutritional, herbal, and homeopathic methods to assist the body's natural cleansing processes. The therapy may be used to treat headaches, joint or back pain, arthritis, insomnia, allergies, and mood disorders.

Diet fads

These include the Atkins diet, the Stillman diet, the Scarsdale diet, the Pritikin diet, the Air Force diet, the "Mayo" diet, the liquid protein diet, the rice diet, the grapefruit diet, and so forth. Most fad diets set forth a strict program that promises significant weight control in a short period of time.

Fad diets are nutritionally unbalanced in some way. Some may also cause complications such as irregular heart rhythms, calcium and bone loss, and other vitamin and mineral deficiencies.

Drama therapy

This form of creative or expressive therapy involves role playing, storytelling, and improvisational techniques using masks, props, written scripts, and actual performances to help people deal more effectively with emotional and developmental problems.

Dream therapy

In this form of psychotherapy, a person records his or her dreams for later study and, possibly, group discussion to discover their meaning. The therapy attempts to shed light on inner feelings and attitudes to improve self-understanding.

Eclecticism

In the early 1800s, eclectism took root in the United States. It employs herbal medicine, purgatives, enemas, and steam baths. It's based on the theory that illness results from imbalances among the four elements: earth, air, fire, and water. Eclectism enouraged people were to treat themselves from a special medical manual.

Electroacupuncture biofeedback

This therapy uses an electronic screening and treatment device that measures the body's natural electromagnetic emissions at acupuncture points. These emissions are believed to provide clues to organic disease in the vicinity of specific acupoints.

Once a diagnosis is made, the disease can be treated by modifying the abnormal emissions and feeding them back to the person through the acupoints. Electroacupuncture biofeedback is also used in biological dentistry.

Enemas

In this form of hydrotherapy, the large intestine (called the colon) is irrigated with water or other solutions to aid defecation. Enemas differ from colonic therapy primarily in that they clean only the last 8 to 12 inches of the large intestine. Enemas are used to relieve constipation and remove toxic substances.

Guide to alternative therapies

Energy healing

Also known as bioenergetic medicine, energy healing follows many principles of acupuncture. It uses special devices to measure the body's electromagnetic fields (EMF) for imbalances in energy flow that occur along major energy pathways called meridians. The EMF imbalances are thought to reveal the underlying illness. Some treatments involve modifying the disturbed electromagnetic energy and feeding it back to the body, a process called electroacupuncture biofeedback.

Environmental medicine

Here, environmental factors are considered to contribute to a person's illness. These factors include diet, airborne pollutants, molds, pollen, harmful radiation from the earth, and the many chemicals used in everyday products. Environmental medicine approaches are used to treat food and other allergies, chemical sensitivity, and rheumatoid arthritis.

Enzyme therapy

This form of nutritional therapy prescribes dietary supplements containing plant enzymes and/or pancreatic enzymes to aid the body's natural digestion. Raw vegetables are also prescribed for their enzyme content as well as their obvious nutritional benefits. The therapy is used to treat inflammation and various intestinal disorders.

Exercise

Exercise is part of many alternative therapies, such as Ayurvedic medicine, traditional Chinese medicine, yoga, bodywork, dance therapy, and martial arts. Today, it's also considered an important part of conventional medicine.

Faith healing

Also called spiritual or divine healing, faith healing is the cure or relief of physical or mental ills by prayer or religious rituals. It may either supplement or replace medical treatment.

This practice occurs in most cultures and religious traditions. Healing is accomplished through prayer, the laying-on of hands, rituals, or other means.

Fasting

Fasting requires a person to abstain from food, either completely or partially, for a specified period. In naturopathy, short fasts of 3 to 5 days may be prescribed for detoxification. Fasting is also used to treat rheumatoid arthritis, allergies, headaches, high blood pressure, and psychological problems.

Fish oil

Cold water fish such as herring, salmon, or sardines are rich in omega-3 fatty acids—polyunsaturated fats that are believed to have some beneficial effect in treating breast cancer and reducing the inflammation of arthritis.

Folk remedies

Folk remedies are derived from traditional healing beliefs and methods used in past and contemporary cultures mostly by people who aren't licensed medical practitioners. Typically, folk remedies are widely known among members of a culture and are handed down from one generation to the next. Many people use these remedies to treat themselves for minor illnesses; more serious cases are treated by a medicine man or shaman.

Guided imagery

A common autosuggestive technique used in relaxation and stress-reduction therapies, guided imagery teaches a person to develop focused mental imagery in a relaxed state of mind. By visualizing such images as pain being relieved or cancer cells being destroyed, the person stimulates the immune system and secretion of hormones and brain chemicals that may retard the progress of the actual disorder.

Imagery is used to treat chronic pain, allergies, high blood pressure, stress-related intestinal disorders, painful menstruation, trauma, sprains, and strains. It has also been used against certain types of cancer.

Guide to alternative therapies

Herbal remedies

The use of plants, plant parts, and plant extracts to treat diseases is an important part of folk medicine worldwide. Herbal remedies are also employed in traditional Chinese medicine, homeopathy, and Ayurvedic medicine.

Many of today's prescription drugs have an herbal origin. For instance, the widely used heart drug digoxin comes from the foxglove flower. Reserpine, a drug for high blood pressure, comes from Indian snakeroot. The pain-reliever morphine comes from the opium poppy.

Herbs are used to cure (garlic to kill germs), to prevent problems (rosemary as an insect repellent), and to relieve pain and discomfort (aloe vera for arthritis pain and for minor burns).

Holistic medicine

This system of medicine focuses on the entire person, not just the illness. It's based on three principles: recognition of the psychological, environmental, and social contributions to the person's illness; involvement of the person in treatment; and emphasis on preventive medicine and lifestyles that reduce the risk of developing an illness.

Holistic medicine includes acupuncture, shiatsu (acupressure), chiropractic, herbal medicine, spiritual healing, and other alternative therapies.

Homeopathy

This system of medicine hinges on the belief that the symptoms of an illness are evidence of a curative process going on within the body in response to the disease. The homeopathic doctor attempts to promote the further development of these symptoms to accelerate the body's self-cure; this is the principle of "like cures like." For example, diarrhea might be treated by giving the person a very small dose of a laxative. Other disorders treated by homeopathy include colds and flu, headaches, respiratory infections, allergies, and intestinal disorders.

Humanistic therapies

In this approach to psychotherapy, a person closely works with a therapist to determine the course of treatment. Humanistic therapies emphasize developing the person's growth and self-esteem as a way of correcting any mental or emotional disorders. They're associated with the "human potential movement" that flourished in the United States in the 1960s and 1970s.

Hydrogen peroxide therapy

In this form of oxidation therapy, hydrogen peroxide is injected to treat a wide variety of diseases. Treatment aims to use oxygen's antiseptic effect.

Hydrotherapy

Hydrotherapy involves the application of water, ice, or steam to the entire body or a part of it for therapeutic purposes. The body may be warmed or cooled by using water that's relatively hot or cold.

Hot water is initially stimulating, but then promotes muscle relaxation. It reduces pain and improves circulation. Cold water, in contrast, lowers body temperature, reduces blood circulation, increases muscle tone, reduces swelling after injury, and reduces muscular pain. Treatments include full body immersion, steam baths, saunas, sitz baths, colonic irrigation, and application of hot or cold compresses.

Hydrotherapy treats many conditions ranging from pain, trauma, and stress to infectious diseases and detoxification.

Hyperthermia

This treatment is also known as "artificial fever" or heat stress detoxification. In this treatment, a person sits in a sauna or hot tub bath to release fat-stored toxins (such as certain pesticide residues) from the body, enhance immune function, and destroy heat-sensitive viruses and bacteria.

Hypnosis

Also known as hypnotherapy, this treatment uses the power of suggestion and induction of a trance state to focus a person's

Hypnosis (continued)

concentration on a particular emotion, memory, or subject. Under hypnosis, the person is more amenable to suggestions and commands.

Hypnosis is used to treat stress, sleep disorders, anxiety, posttraumatic stress disorder, phobias, depression, and certain allergies and skin diseases, and to help people stop smoking.

Immuno-augmentative therapy (IAT)

This treatment rests on the theory that cancer results from imbalances among four blood protein components: tumor antibody, tumor complement, blocking protein, and deblocking protein. Treatment involves injections of various amounts of the four components.

Iridology

This treatment is based on the idea that changes in the color and texture of the eye's iris relate to physical and mental disorders, diet deficiencies, and toxin accumulation. Specific areas of the iris are mapped and linked to parts of the body.

Juice therapy

This form of naturopathy uses fresh, unprocessed juices of fruits and vegetables along with fasts and diet therapy to detoxify the body and to enhance the im-

mune system. It's used to treat allergies, arthritis, and intestinal and weight problems.

Light therapy

Use of natural sunlight, artificial light sources (full-spectrum light, bright white light, ultraviolet light), and colored light may help to treat a variety of illnesses. These include sleep disorders, skin conditions, pain, depression, "jet lag," seasonal affective disorder, and certain nutritional problems.

Livingston-Wheeler therapy

This cancer treatment assumes that a type of bacteria, called *Progenitor cryptocides* is found in all cancers. Treatment aims to restore the immune system through a combination of vaccines derived from cultures of the person's own bacteria, or from Bacillus Calmette-Guerin (BCG), a mild tuberculin vaccine; antibiotics; megavitamins, nutritional supplements, and digestive enzymes; enemas; and a whole-foods diet that excludes eggs and poultry.

Macrobiotic diet

The term macrobiotics is derived from the Greek, and means "the art of long life." This therapy is loosely based on theory from traditional Chinese medicine that a balanced diet reflects one's balance in other areas of life and with nature.

Rice and whole grains are the most balanced foods, and about 50% of the diet is built around these. Vegetables make up another 25%, and the rest includes beans and soy-derived products, seeds, nuts, fruits, and fish. Foods to be avoided include dairy products, red meat, sugar, eggs, and coffee. Some of the more restrictive macrobiotic diets are deficient in many essential nutrients.

Macrobiotic diets are used to treat high blood pressure and lower cholesterol.

Magnetic field therapy

This therapy manipulates the body's own electromagnetic fields with magnetic devices to treat pain and stress, and facilitate bone healing. It's also used to counteract adverse effects of electromagnetic pollution of the outside environment (from electric appliances, power lines, microwave ovens, and so forth).

Manipulative therapy

This form of physical medicine treats illnesses not only with drugs and surgery, but also with joint manipulation, in which a doctor palpates, by hand, areas of the body that are under tension or are distorted. It's based on the theory that body structure and function are closely interrelated and mutually interdependent and that the body is an integrated whole.

Manipulative therapy also employs many conventional, surgical, and obstetrical practices. It's used primarily to treat musculoskeletal problems, arthritis, allergies, heart disease, high blood pressure, headaches, and neuritis (swelling of nerves).

Martial arts

As a therapy, the martial arts (such as karate, jujitsu, kendo, kung fu, and t'ai chi) are practiced to attain physical fitness and self-discipline. These techniques also improve muscle tone and relieve stress.

Massage

Massage involves friction, stroking, and kneading of the body. It's a standard physical therapy technique, used to relax muscles, improve circulation, relieve pain, and increase mobility.

Many Eastern and Western styles of massage exist. All aim to mobilize the body's natural healing power to restore or maintain health. Therapeutic massage is used to treat muscle spasm and pain, curvature of the spine, headaches, temporomandibular joint (TMJ) syndrome, and breathing problems such as asthma and emphysema.

Meditation

Practitioners of meditation try to attain a physical state of relaxation, mental control, and psychological calm by regularly practicing a series of physical and mental exercises. Meditation can be used to relieve stress, ease muscle tension, and treat drug addictions and immune conditions.

Megavitamin therapy

Proponents of this therapy contend that governmental Recommended Daily Allowances (RDAs) for nutrients in foods are inadequate to provide optimum health, and that certain vitamins are required by the body in amounts far beyond the RDA. For example, megadoses of vitamin C have been used to treat colds, flu, infections, allergies, autoimmune diseases, burns, and viral pneumonia, and to assist wound healing.

Mind-body medicine

This therapy recognizes the role of the mind and the emotions in health, the body's innate healing capabilities, and the role of self-responsibility in the healing process. The so-called mind-body connection is being revealed as the complex interplay of the brain and the endocrine and immune systems along nerve pathways.

Knowledge gained in the new field of psychoneuro-immunology (PNI) lends support to many mental healing methods such as biofeedback, meditation, guided imagery, hypnotherapy, and yoga.

Moxibustion

Used in traditional Chinese medicine, moxibustion involves the application of heat to acupuncture points where needles would be impracticable. Heat is supplied by placing slow-burning cones of the powdered leaves of an herb called moxa (*Artemisia*) on or above the point to be treated, thereby producing a counterirritant blistering effect.

Mud therapy

In this form of hyperthermia, a person is immersed in a hot mineral mud bath for a specified amount of time. Mud therapy is claimed to promote detoxification and relieve arthritis pain.

Music therapy

Music (or sound) therapy is based on the theory that sound waves affect brain wave frequencies, muscle tension, breathing, and other body processes. It uses music, either recorded or performed by the person, to help the person deal more effectively with emotional and developmental problems.

Music therapy is used to reduce stress and high blood pressure. Other sound therapy is used to treat hearing or speech impairments, schizophrenia, Alzheimer's disease, and autism.

Native American medicine

Traditional medical practices developed by Native Americans include herbalism, shamanism, spiritual healing, hyperthermia (sweat lodges), prayer, and visualization. Like traditional medical systems in China and India, this approach stresses the interconnectedness of the person with all of the natural world.

Naturopathy

This system of holistic medicine relies on using natural agents and forces to bring about a cure. The naturopath makes use of herbs and vitamins rather than man-made drugs and surgery, and may also employ diet therapy, hydrotherapy, exercise, chiropractic therapy, bodywork, homeopathy, electrical treatments, and counseling on preventive medicine and lifestyle modification.

Neural therapy

In this form of energy medicine, small amounts of anesthetics are injected into various acupuncture points to restore normal flow to the body's electrical force fields in tissues that lie in the area of injury. Neural therapy is used to treat many kinds of disorders.

Neurolinguistic programming

In this combination of psychotherapy and guided imagery, a person's body language and changes in physical appearance are closely observed during an interview. Once these unconscious clues are defined and analyzed, the person can be helped to adopt new thought and behavior patterns that give rise to positive feelings of well-being, thereby enhancing the body's immune defenses.

Oxygen therapy

Use of various forms of oxygen (ozone, peroxide, or as gas under pressure) purportedly promotes healing and destroys toxins in the body. It's based on the theory that the body's normal oxidation processes (in which electrons are donated from one molecular substance to another in normal chemical reactions) may be imbalanced due to environmental stress or disease. By supplying additional oxygen, the treatment restores this balance.

Oxygen may be used with other therapies to treat lung disorders, multiple sclerosis, infections, and arthritis.

Ozone therapy

This form of oxygen therapy employs ozone, a less stable but more reactive form of oxygen. It's used to treat infections, arthritis, hepatitis, allergies, various pain disorders, and to assist wound healing.

Placebo effect

A placebo is an inert substance made to appear indistinguishable from an authentic drug. It may be prescribed when there's no apparent physical cause of an illness. The "placebo effect" is attributed to psychological factors that influence the body at some chemical level.

In conditions involving the nervous system, such as pain or anxiety, placebo effects often mimic the effects of an active drug. Placebos have been used to treat arthritis, chest pain (angina), and other chronic pain problems.

Prayer

Part of faith healing or spiritualism, prayer involves addressing a divine being or beings for purposes of praise, adoration, thanksgiving, petition, or penitence. Prayer is a part of every culture and doesn't belong to any particular religious tradition.

Pressure point therapies

In these therapies, manual pressure is applied to the surface of the body at points where energy pathways are congested. In shiatsu (a Japanese technique) and in acupressure (a variant of Chinese acupuncture), pressure is applied rhythmically with the fingers. The knee, elbow, toes, heels of hands and feet, and pad of the foot may be used as appropriate.

Psychodynamic therapy

This form of psychotherapy hinges on the theory that emotional disorders are manifestations of internal and unconscious conflicts between personality components. These conflicts are caused by unresolved family conflicts that were experienced in early childhood and become reactivated in problem situations in adulthood.

Guide to alternative therapies

Psychodynamic therapy aims to revive the early conflict and transfer it to the relationship with the therapist. The symptoms are removed when the therapist helps the person to resolve the conflict in the transference relationship.

Additional methods, such as dream interpretation or word-association techniques, are used to aid in uncovering unconscious material.

Qigong

A blend of therapeutic exercise, acupressure, meditation, breath regulation, and deep relaxation as practiced in traditional Chinese medicine, qigong primarily emphasizes preventive self-care. It's used to treat chronic pain, migraine headaches, high blood pressure, asthma, insomnia, musculoskeletal problems, and depression.

Rebirthing

This form of psychotherapy uses various breathing and relaxation techniques to help the person relive the primal traumatic experience of birth or other traumatic experiences of early childhood. Once the repressed trauma is brought from the unconscious and exposed (often accompanied by a "primal scream"), its negative effects can be understood and dealt with.

Reconstructive therapy

A nonsurgical method, reconstructive therapy attempts to repair torn ligaments and other damaged joint structures with injections of mild irritating solutions. The injections stimulate the body to generate new connective tissue and enhance healing. The therapy is used for arthritis, carpal tunnel syndrome, migraine headaches, degenerative bone disorders, herniated discs, and bursitis.

Reflexotherapy

Also known as reflexology, this technique resembles accupressure, in which hand pressure is applied to specific points on the feet and, less commonly, on the hands or ears. Based on the theory that sensitive nerve endings at reference points on the feet, hands, or ears correspond to all major organs and other parts of the body. Applying pressure to these points facilitates movement of life energy along channels in the body to the corresponding area.

Reflexology is used to treat tension, anxiety, asthma, constipation, bowel irritation, and migraine headaches.

Rejuvenation

A part of the Ayurvedic medical regimen, this isn't a treatment all by itself. Rejuvenation follows a program of cleansing and detoxi-fication procedures, and is a "physiological tuneup" involving administration of herbal and mineral preparations as well as certain yoga and breathing exercises.

Self-help groups

Also known as encounter groups or consciousness-raising groups, self-help groups are a form of group therapy usually modeled on the "12-step" program of Alcoholics Anonymous. Such groups allow persons who share a common mental or physical problem to come together to provide fellowship, mutual aid, and support and regain control over their lives. (Not to be confused with conventional group therapy, in which a small group works with a moderator, usually a trained therapist.)

Self-hypnosis

Here, a person induces a hypnotic trance without a trained hypnotist. Hypnosis is usually used along with other medical or psychological therapies. Self-hypnosis should be performed only after the person has learned the technique from a professional hypnotist.

Shamanism

A form of faith healing, shamanism is used in many folk societies as well as Native American medicine. It uses chanting, visualiza-

Shamanism (continued)

tion, drumming, dancing, trance states, divination, and other spiritual techniques to involve the person in the healing process.

Shark cartilage therapy

This treatment for cancer hinges on the idea that cartilage, a type of connective tissue, contains compounds that prevent formation of blood vessels. Treating tumors with cartilage cuts off their blood supply, thereby stopping tumor growth and killing tumor cells. The cartilage, derived from sharks, is applied using a retention enema or injection.

Shiatsu

This Japanese technique employs finger pressure to release congestion of energy flow in the body's energy channels (meridians) at selected pressure points called *tsubos*. The knee, elbow, toes, heels of hands and feet, and pad of the foot may also be used to apply pressure as appropriate.

Thalassotherapy

Derived from the Greek word *thalassa*, meaning sea, this type of hydrotherapy is based on the idea that blood plasma is very similar to seawater, in which life is thought to have originated. The person is immersed in sea water heated to normal body temperature and massaged; minerals are believed to pass from the water through the skin into the blood until a natural balance is reached.

Therapeutic touch

In this combination of bodywork and visualization, a practitioner assesses a person's energy field by slowly moving the hands a few inches above the person's body. (Actual body contact is rarely made.) Blocked energy fields, evidenced by a feeling of radiant heat or unusual pressure, indicate an underlying illness.

Energy fields are believed to be linked to hemoglobin levels in circulating blood. By dissipating the blocked energy to other parts of the body, the person's vitality and well-being are restored. The therapy is used for pain, anxiety, headaches, fever, and inflammation.

Traditional chinese medicine

This complete system of medicine emphasizes lifestyle modification, diet, and exercise to prevent illness. Health is believed to result from a person's ability to adjust successfully to changes within the body and within the natural world, and to maintain a balance between opposing physical forces—the *yin* and *yang*. These forces flow along specific pathways (meridians) that form a complex energy network in the body.

Medicinal herbs, acupuncture, diet therapy, massage, and therapeutic exercise are used to correct *yin-yang* imbalances that cause disease.

Vegetarianism

Vegetarians eat only foods from plants (grains, beans, vegetables, and fruits, and foods made from them). They avoid all animal flesh, including red meat, poultry, fish, and sometimes dairy products.

Vegetarians are classified into different types, depending on their acceptance of animal products. *Lacto-ovo* (or *ovo-lacto*) vegetarians consume milk or cheese, eggs, and sometimes honey, whereas *vegans* consume no animal products at all. Vegetarian diets can lower blood cholesterol levels and blood pressure, and may also have anticancer effects.

Yin-yang

This major concept in traditional Chinese medicine refers to the equilibrium and dynamic balance between opposing forces. *Yin* and *yang* are believed to permeate nature. Health is seen as a harmony between the two forces and illness as an imbalance.

Yoga

This form of mind-body medicine uses meditation and exercise (postures and coordinated breathing techniques) to achieve physical and mental self-discipline. The postures help the person develop strength and flexibility by using all the body's muscles, increasing circulation, and stretching and aligning the spine. Breathing exercises and meditation help reduce stress and anxiety.

Promoting a healthy diet and lifestyle

Promoting a healthy diet and lifestyle

This section contains information to help you adjust your nutritional needs for better health. It's also useful to know when you're taking certain drugs, which can alter the body's balance of vitamins and minerals. If you're taking allergy drugs, you'll find some helpful hints at the end of the section.

Adding fiber to your diet

Fiber makes up a crucial part of the diet — and yet it's completely indigestible. Its benefits are primarily mechanical in nature: it promotes bowel movements, thereby minimizing the risk of constipation, which is helpful in treating diverticulitis and when you've been prescribed a drug that's known to cause constipation. Here are four easy ways to add fiber to your diet.

Eat whole-grain breads and cereals

For the first few days, eat one serving daily of whole-grain breads (1 slice), cereal ($\frac{1}{2}$ cup), pasta ($\frac{1}{2}$ cup), or brown rice ($\frac{1}{3}$ cup). Examples of whole-grain breads are whole wheat and pumpernickel. Examples of high-fiber cereals are bran or oat flakes and shredded wheat. Gradually increase to four or more servings daily.

Eat fresh fruits and vegetables

Begin by eating one serving daily of raw or cooked, unpeeled fruit (one medium-size piece; $\frac{1}{2}$ cup cooked) or unpeeled vegetables ($\frac{1}{2}$ cup cooked; 1 cup raw). Gradually increase to four servings daily. Examples of high-fiber fruits include apples, oranges, and peaches. Some high-fiber vegetables are carrots, corn, and peas.

Eat dried peas and beans

Begin by eating one serving ($\frac{1}{3}$ cup) a week. Increase to at least two to three servings a week.

Eat unprocessed bran

Add bran to your food. Start with 1 teaspoon a day, and over a 3-week period work up to 2 to 3 tablespoons a day. Don't use more than this. Remember to drink at least six 8-ounce (oz) glasses of fluid a day.

A small amount of bran can be beneficial, but too much can irritate your digestive tract, cause gas, interfere with mineral absorption, and even lodge in your intestine.

Note: Crisp fresh fruits and vegetables, cooked foods with husks, and nuts must be chewed thoroughly so that large particles don't pass whole into the intestine and lodge there, causing problems.

A sample menu

Breakfast
$\frac{1}{2}$ grapefruit
Oatmeal with milk and raisins
   (add bran if desired)
Bran muffin
8 oz liquid

Lunch
Cabbage slaw
Tuna salad sandwich on whole-wheat bread
Fresh pear with skin
8 oz liquid

Dinner
Vegetable soup
Broiled fish with almond topping
Baked potato with skin
Carrots and peas
Canned crushed pineapple
8 oz liquid

Snack
Dried fruit and nut mix
8 oz liquid

Cutting down on salt

Your doctor may recommend cutting down on salt because too much salt can affect your health. Reducing your salt intake isn't hard to do. The following information and suggestions will help you get started.

Facts about salt

• Table salt is about 40% sodium.
• Americans consume about 20 times more salt than their bodies need.
• About three-fourths of the salt you consume is already in the foods you eat and drink.
• One teaspoon (tsp) of salt contains about 2 grams (2,000 milligrams [mg]) of sodium.
• You can reduce your intake to this level simply by not salting your food during cooking or before eating.

Tips for reducing salt intake

Reducing your salt intake to a teaspoon or less a day is easy if you:
• read labels on drugs and foods.
• put away your salt shaker; or, if you must use salt, use "light salt" that contains half the sodium of ordinary table salt.
• buy fresh meats, fruits, and vegetables instead of canned, processed, and convenience foods.
• substitute spices and lemon juice for salt.
• watch out for sources of hidden sodium — for example, carbonated beverages, nondairy creamers, cookies, and cakes.
• avoid salty foods, such as bacon, sausage, pretzels, potato chips, mustard, pickles, and some cheeses.

Know your sodium sources

Canned, prepared, and "fast" foods are loaded with sodium; so are condiments, such as ketchup. Some foods that don't taste salty contain high amounts of sodium. Consider the values below:

Food	mg sodium
1 can tomato soup	872
1 cup canned spaghetti	1,236
1 hot dog	639
1 cheeseburger	709
1 slice pepperoni pizza	817
1 tablespoon ketchup	156
1 tsp salt	1,955
1 dill pickle	928
1 cup corn flakes	256
3 ounces lean ham	1,128
2½ oz dried chipped beef	3,052

Other high-sodium sources include baking powder, baking soda, barbecue sauce, bouillon cubes, celery salt, chili sauce, cooking wine, garlic salt, onion salt, softened water, and soy sauce.

Surprisingly, many drugs and other nonfood items contain sodium, such as alkalizers for indigestion, laxatives, aspirin, cough medicine, mouthwash, and toothpaste.

Cutting down on cholesterol

By changing your diet, you can help reduce your cholesterol level and ensure better health. You also need to reduce the amount of saturated fats you eat. This means cutting down drastically on eggs, dairy products, and fatty meats. Rely instead on poultry, fish, fruits, vegetables, and high-fiber breads.

Use this list as a starting point for your new diet. If you do a lot of home baking, adapt your recipes by using modest amounts of unsaturated oils. Remember to substitute two egg whites when a recipe calls for one whole egg.

Bread and cereals

Eliminate:
• Breads with whole eggs listed as a major ingredient
• Egg noodles
• Pies, cakes, doughnuts, biscuits, high-fat crackers and cookies

Substitute:
• Oatmeal, multigrain, and bran cereals; whole-grain breads; rye bread
• Pasta, rice
• Angel food cake; low-fat cookies, crackers, and home-baked goods

Eggs and dairy products

Eliminate:
• Whole milk, 2% milk, imitation milk
• Cream, half-and-half, most nondairy creamers, whipped toppings
• Whole milk yogurt and cottage cheese
• Cheese, cream cheese, sour cream, light cream cheese, light sour cream
• Egg yolks
• Ice cream

Substitute:
• Skim milk, 1% milk, buttermilk
• None
• Nonfat or low-fat yogurt, low-fat (1% or 2%) cottage cheese
• Cholesterol-free sour cream alternative, such as King Sour
• Egg whites
• Sherbet, frozen tofu

Cutting down on cholesterol (continued)

Fats and oils
Eliminate:
• Coconut, palm, and palm kernel oils
• Butter, lard, bacon fat
• Dressings made with egg yolks
• Chocolate

Substitute:
• Unsaturated vegetable oils (corn, olive, canola, safflower, sesame, soybean, and sunflower)
• Unsaturated margarine and shortening, diet margarine
• Mayonnaise, unsaturated or low-fat salad dressings
• Baking cocoa

Meat, fish, and poultry
Eliminate:
• Fatty cuts of beef, lamb, or pork
• Organ meats, spare ribs, cold cuts, sausage, hot dogs, bacon
• Sardines, roe

Substitute:
• Lean cuts of beef, lamb, or pork
• Poultry
• Sole, salmon, mackerel

Cutting down on oxalates

If you're being treated for chronic gout (a type of arthritis) or recurrent kidney stones caused by calcium oxalate, your doctor may have prescribed the drug Zyloprim. Zyloprim makes the body produce less uric acid (which contributes to gout) by inhibiting the biochemical reactions that trigger its formation.

As additional therapy, your doctor may also advise you to avoid foods containing high levels of oxalate. The chart below tells you which foods to use and which to avoid to help you reduce your intake of oxalates.

Foods to use
These contain small amounts of oxalate (less than 2 mg oxalate per serving).

Vegetables
• Broccoli
• Brussels sprouts
• Cabbage
• Cauliflower
• Chives
• Cucumbers
• Lettuce
• Mushrooms
• Onions
• Peas
• Potatoes:
  – white
• Radishes
• Rice
• Turnips

Fruits
• Avocados
• Bananas
• Cherries
• Grapes:
  – Thompson seedless
• Mangoes
• Melons
• Nectarines
• Peaches:
  – canned
  – Hiley
  – Stokes
• Pineapples

• Plums:
  – Golden Gage
  – Green Gage

Beverages
• Barley water
• Beer:
  – bottled
• Cider
• Coca-Cola
• Juices:
  – apple
  – grapefruit
  – orange
  – pineapple
• Lemonade
• Milk
• Pepsi-Cola
• Sherry:
  – dry
• Wine:
  – port
  – rose
  – white

Miscellaneous
• Butter
• Cheese:
  – cheddar
• Corn flakes
• Eggs
• Egg noodles
• Fish (except sardines)
• Jellies of allowed fruits
• Juices:
  – lemon
  – lime
• Macaroni
• Margarine
• Meats (except bacon)
• Oatmeal, porridge
• Poultry
• Red plum jam
• Soup:
  – chicken noodle
  – oxtail

Foods to avoid

These are high in oxalate (more than 15 mg oxalate per serving).

Vegetables
- Beans in tomato sauce
- Beets
- Celery
- Chard:
  - Swiss
- Collards
- Dandelion greens
- Eggplant
- Escarole
- Leeks
- Okra
- Parsley
- Peppers
  - green
- Pokeweed
- Potatoes
  - sweet
- Rutabagas
- Spinach
- Squash
  - summer

Fruits
- Berries:
  - blackberries
  - blueberries
  - green gooseberries
  - raspberries
- Currants:
  - red
- Grapes:
  - Concord
- Lemon peel
- Lime peel
- Rhubarb

Beverages
- Beer:
  - lager draft, Tuborg pilsner
- Ovaltine (24 mg/8 oz)
- Tea (132 to 181 mg/8 oz)

Miscellaneous
- Chocolate
- Cocoa
- Grits (white corn)
- Peanuts
- Pecans
- Soybean
- Crackers
- Wheat germ

(Adapted from Ney, D.M., et al. *The Low Oxalate Diet Book for the Prevention of Oxalate Kidney Stones.* San Diego: University of California Press, 1981, pp. 19-23.)

Adding or cutting down on potassium

If you're taking a drug that decreases the level of potassium in your body, your doctor may recommend adding potassium to your diet.

How much potassium do you need?

Doctors recommend 300 to 400 milligrams (mg) of potassium daily. Not enough potassium can cause leg cramps, weakness, paralysis, and spasms. Be aware that too much can cause heart problems and fatigue.

The chart below lists potassium-rich foods along with their potassium content (the number of milligrams in a 3½-ounce serving). Because some of these foods are also high in calories, check with your doctor or dietitian if you're on a weight-reduction diet.

Potassium content of common foods

Meats	mg
Beef	370
Chicken	411
Lamb	290
Liver	380
Pork	326
Turkey	411
Veal	500

Fish, shellfish	mg
Bass	256
Flounder	342
Haddock	348
Halibut	525
Oysters	203
Perch	284
Salmon	421
Sardines, canned	590
Scallops	476
Tuna	301

Fruits	mg
Apricots	281
Bananas	370
Dates	648
Figs	152
Nectarines	294
Oranges	200
Peaches	202
Plums	299
Prunes	262
Raisins	355

Vegetables	mg
Asparagus	238
Brussels sprouts	295
Cabbage	233
Carrots	341
Endive	294
Lima beans	394
Peppers	213
Potatoes	407
Radishes	322
Spinach	324
Sweet potatoes	300

Adding or cutting down on potassium (continued)

Juices	mg
Orange, fresh	200
reconstituted	186
Tomato	227

Other foods	mg
Gingersnap cookies	462
Graham crackers	384
Oatmeal cookies	
with raisins	370
Ice milk	195
Milk, dry	
(nonfat solids)	745
Molasses (light)	917
Peanuts	674
Peanut butter	670

Choosing a calcium supplement

Your body needs calcium to keep your bones and teeth strong, to prevent excessive bleeding, and to keep your muscles, brain, and nerves functioning well. If your doctor recommends a nonprescription calcium supplement for you, here are some guidelines you need to know.

Choosing a supplement

• Read the bottle label to learn how much *elemental calcium* the supplement contains. Elemental calcium is the amount that's actually used by your body. Different supplements contain different amounts of elemental calcium. For example, calcium carbonate products, such as Caltrate 600, Os-Cal, Biocal, oyster shell calcium, and antacids (such as Tums),

contain the most elemental calcium — about 40%. Other calcium products contain less: dibasic calcium phosphate (about 36%), tribasic calcium phosphate (about 29%), calcium citrate (about 24%), calcium lactate (about 13%), and calcium gluconate (about 9%).

• Don't take calcium supplements containing dolomite or bone meal. They may contain lead and cause lead poisoning.

• Calcium carbonate supplements may cause stomach pain due to gas and constipation. To relieve these effects, drink more liquids, such as juice or water, or eat more foods that are liquids at room temperature, such as ice cream, gelatin, or pudding. Eating more high-fiber foods, such as bran cereal or whole-wheat crackers, may also help. Just be sure to eat them between meals — extra fiber with meals interferes with your body's absorption of calcium.

Other calcium sources

Besides taking a calcium supplement, try to include calcium-rich foods in your daily diet. Good sources of calcium include collards, turnip greens, broccoli, dried peas and beans, sardines, salmon, tofu, and dairy products (milk, cheese, yogurt, and ice cream). Choose low-fat dairy products because they're lower in cholesterol.

If you have trouble digesting milk, most large grocery stores carry lactose-reduced milk or acidophilus milk. Or ask your pharmacist about products that can be added to milk to make it easier to digest.

Special tips

• Consume less red meat, chocolate, peanut butter, rhubarb, sweet potatoes, fatty foods, and caffeine-containing drinks.

• Calcium is most effective when your body has enough vitamin D. Spending just 15 minutes in sunshine every day will fill your daily requirement. Vitamin D is also present in egg yolks, saltwater fish, liver, and vitamin-fortified milk and cereals. But don't take vitamin D supplements unless your doctor prescribes them — too much of this vitamin can be harmful.

Avoiding allergy triggers

To make it easier for you to live with allergies, try to avoid the following common allergy triggers.

At home

• Such foods as nuts, chocolate, eggs, shellfish, and peanut butter

• Such beverages as orange juice, wine, beer, and milk

• Mold spores; pollens from flowers, trees, grasses, hay, and ragweed. If pollen is the offender, install a bedroom air conditioner with a filter, and avoid long walks when pollen counts are high.

• Dander from rabbits, cats, dogs, hamsters, gerbils, and chickens. Consider finding a new home for the family pet, if necessary.

• Feather or hair-stuffed pillows, down comforters, wool clothing, and stuffed toys. Use smooth (not fuzzy), washable blankets on your bed.

• Insect parts, such as those from dead cockroaches

• Drugs, such as aspirin

• Vapors from cleaning solvents, paint, paint thinners, and liquid chlorine bleach

• Fluorocarbon spray products, such as furniture polish, starch, cleaners, and room deodorizers

• Scents from spray deodorants, perfumes, hair sprays, talcum powder, and cosmetics

• Cloth-upholstered furniture, carpets, and draperies that collect dust. Hang lightweight, washable cotton or synthetic-fiber curtains, and use washable, cotton throw rugs on bare floors.

• Brooms and dusters that raise dust. Instead, clean your bedroom daily by damp dusting and damp mopping. Keep the door closed.

• Dirty filters on hot-air furnaces and air conditioners that blow dust into the air

• Dust from vacuum cleaner exhaust

In the workplace

• Dusts, vapors, or fumes from wood products (western red cedar, some pine and birch woods, mahogany); flour, cereals, and other grains; coffee, tea, or papain; metals (platinum, chromium, nickel sulfate, soldering fumes); and cotton, flax, and hemp

• Mold from decaying hay

Outdoors

• Cold air, hot air, or sudden temperature changes (when you go in and out of air-conditioned stores in the summer)

• Excessive humidity or dryness

• Changes in seasons

• Smog

• Automobile exhaust

• Plants (such as poison ivy and some grasses)

Anyplace

• Overexertion, which may cause wheezing

• Common cold, flu, and other viruses

• Fear, anger, frustration, laughing too hard, crying, or any emotionally upsetting situation

• Smoke from cigarettes, cigars, and pipes. Don't smoke and don't stay in a room with people who do.

Preventive measures

Remember to:

• drink enough fluids — six to eight glasses daily

• take all prescribed drugs exactly as directed

• tell your doctor about any and all drugs you take — even nonprescription ones

• schedule only as much activity as you can tolerate. Take frequent rests on busy days.

Index

Index

Bold type refers to full-color photoguide.

Index

Bold type refers to full-color photoguide.

Bold type refers to full-color photoguide.

Index

Index

Bold type refers to full-color photoguide.

Index

Bold type refers to full-color photoguide.

Index

Bold type refers to full-color photoguide.

Index

Bold type refers to full-color photoguide.

Bold type refers to full-color photoguide.

Index

Duodenal ulcers, 63, 100, 221, 532, 558, 604, 670-671
Duosol, 139, 202
Duotrate, 228, 538
Duphalac, 123
Duragesic, 229
Dura-Gest, 247
Duralith, 260-261, 372-373
Duramist Plus, 17
Duramorph, 442-443
Durapam, 164
Duration, 471
Duration 12-Hour Nasal, 17
Durel-Cort, 148-149
Duricef, 230, **P5**
Duvoid, 741
D-Vert, 41
Dyazide, 231, **P5**
Dycill, 236
Dyes, misuse of, 845
Dymelor, 232-233
Dynabac, 234
Dynacin, 433-434
DynaCirc, 235, **P5**
Dynapen, 236
Dyrenium, 237
Dystonic reaction, 137

E

Ear canal infections, 150, 220
Ear congestion, 654
Eardrops
   giving, to child, 800
   how to use, 799-800
Ear infections, 62, 68-69, 81, 108, 110, 111, 120, 150, 151, 529, 651, 658, 748, 825
Earwax removal, 116, 175
Easprin, 56-57
Echothiophate iodide, 546
Eclecticism, 851
E-Complex-600, 46-47
Econopred Eyedrops, 238
Ecosone, 148-149
Ecotrin, 56-57
Edema, 20, 21, 90, 216, 237, 316, 317, 360, 391, 510

Edrophonium chloride, 685
E.E.S., **P5**
Effexor, 239
Efidac/24, 654
E-200 I.U. Softgels, 46-47
E-400 I.U., 46-47
Elase, 240
Elavil, 241
Elavil Plus, 721-722
Eldepryl, 242
Electroacupuncture biofeedback, 851
Electrolyte solution and polyethylene glycol, 302
Elixir form of drug, how to take, 794
Elixophyllin, 693-694
Elocon, 243
E-Lor, 171
Eltor 120, 654
Eltroxin, 365-366, 665-666
Emete-Con, 244
Emex, 589
Emitrip, 241
Emotional disorders, 464-465, 569-570, 630-631, 650. *See also specific type.*
Emphysema, 88, 122, 407, 568, 822
Empirin, 56-57
Empirin with Codeine, 245
Empracet, 735-736
Emtec, 735-736
Emulsion form of drug, how to take, 794
E-Mycin, 246, **P6**
Enalapril maleate, 750
Enalapril maleate and hydrochlorothiazide, 749
Endep, 241
Endocarditis, preventing, after dental procedures, 246, 528, 531, 716, 751
Endocet, 534, 617
Endodan, 535
Endometrial cancer, 416
Endometriosis, 165-166, 394, 491, 581, 784
Enema therapy, 851
Energy healing, 851-852

Enlon, 685
Enomine, 247
Enovil, 241
Enoxacin, 530
Enoxaparin sodium, 389
E.N.T., 212
Enterocolitis, 221
Entex, 247
Entozyme, 154
Entrophen, 56-57
Enulose, 123
Environmental medicine, 852
Enzyme therapy, 852
Epifrin, 248
Epilepsy, 112, 190, 191, 209-210, 273, 354, 455, 472, 646-647, 719, 723
Epimorph, 442-443
Epinephrine, 249, 560-561, 807. *See also* Anaphylaxis kit, how to use.
Epinephrine hydrochloride, 248
EpiPen, 249
EpiPen Auto-Injector, 560-561, 806-807
EpiPen Jr., 806-807
Epitol, 250-251, 678-679
Epoetin alfa, 252
Epogen, 252
Epoxy glue ingestion, 845
Epsom salts ingestion, 845
Equanil, 253
Equilet, 732
Ergamisol, 254
Ergocalciferol, 94-95, 763
Ergomar, 255
Ergonovine, 256
Ergostat, 255
Ergotamine and caffeine, 92
Ergotamine tartrate, 255
Ergotamine tartrate and caffeine, 769
Ergotrate, 256
Eridium, 585
Erybid, 246, 258, 528
ERYC, 246, 258, 528
Erycette, 257
Eryc Sprinkle, 258
EryDerm, 257

Bold type refers to full-color photoguide.

Index

Bold type refers to full-color photoguide.

Index

Bold type refers to full-color photoguide.

Index

Bold type refers to full-color photoguide.

Bold type refers to full-color photoguide.

Index

Illness, severe, combating effects of, 36
Ilotycin eye ointment, 321
IMDUR, 338
Imiglucerase, 115
Imipramine hydrochloride, 704-705
Imipramine pamoate, 704-705
Imitrex, 322
Immobility, prolonged, combating effects of, 36
Immune globulin intramuscular, 294
Immune globulin intravenous, 621
Immune system, suppressing, 49-50, 182, 183-184, 324-325, 349, 414-415
Immune system deficiency, 294, 621
Immune system problems, 182
Immuno-augmentative therapy, 854
Immunosuppression, cancer-related, 821
Imodium, 323
Imodium A-D, 323
Impetigo, 70, 384
Implanted port, injecting through, 809-810
Impril, 704-705
Imuran, 324-325
Incontinence, urinary, 742
Indapamide, 391
Indelible ink ingestion, 845
Indelible marker ingestion, 845
Inderal, 326-327, **P7**
Inderal LA, 326-327
Indigestion, 27, 31, 71, 399, 452, 544, 615
Indocid, 328-329
Indocid SR, 328-329
Indocin, 328-329
Indocin SR, 328-329
Indomethacin, 328-329
Infant, giving drugs to, 795

Infection. *See also specific type of infection.*
  combating effects of, 36
  preventing, 834-835
Infertility, 134, 556-557
Inflamase, 330
Inflamase Forte, 330
Inflammation, 49-50, 56-57, 176-177, 182, 183-184, 328-329, 349, 414-415, 728
Inflammatory bowel disease, 53, 67, 616
Influenza A, 287, 662-663, 824
Infumorph, 442-443
INH, 356
Inhaler, 795-796
  AeroVent, 797-798
  with holding chamber, 796-797
Injection
  implanted port, 809-810
  intramuscular, 807-809
  of epinephrine, 807
  subcutaneous, 805-806
Injection site
  rotating, 806
  selecting, for intramuscular injection, 807-808
Injury, combating effects of, 36
Ink ingestion, 845
Insecticides, misuse of, 845
Insomnia, 29, 59, 73, 164, 305, 468-469, 486-487, 489, 576, 592, 646-647
InspirEase System, 796-797
Insulin, 331-332
  changing from, to oral treatment, 200-201, 708-709
  mixing, in syringe, 804-805
Insulin-dependent diabetes. *See* Type I diabetes.
Insulin injection sites, rotating, 806
Insulin therapy replacement, 301, 429-430, 511-512
  in Type II diabetes, 232-233
Insulin zinc suspension (extended or ultralente), 331-332
Insulin zinc suspension (lente), 331-332
Intal, 333, 507

Intal Aerosol Spray, 333
Intal Nebulizer Solution, 333
Interferon alfa-2a, recombinant, 612-613
Interferon alfa-2b, recombinant, 334-335
Interferon beta-1b, recombinant, 79
Interferon gamma-1b, 10
Intestinal disorders, 129
Intestinal infection, 214, 479, 746
Intestinal parasitic infection, 258, 279-280
Intestinal spasms, 221
Intramuscular injection, 807-809
Intron A, 334-335
Involuntary movement, drug-induced, 19, 52, 137, 348
Iodine poisoning, 845
Iodine solution, strong, 393
Iodochlorhydroxyquin, 759
Iodoquinol, 214
Ipecac syrup, 336
I-Phrine 2.5%, 470
Ipratropium bromide, 61
Iridology, 854
Iris, inflammation of, 340, 342
Iron deficiency, 275
Iron poisoning, 845
Irritability, 59
Irritable bowel syndrome, 75, 129, 221, 824
Ismelin, 337
ISMO, 338
Iso-Bid, 343, 649
Isobutal, 277-278
Isobutyl, 277-278
Isocarboxazid, 403-404
Isocet, 276
Isoetharine mesylate, 88
Isoflurophate, 284-285
Isolin, 277-278
Isollyl, 277-278
Isonate, 343, 649
Isoniazid, 356
Isopap, 276
Isophane insulin suspension, 331-332

Bold type refers to full-color photoguide.

Bold type refers to full-color photoguide.

Bold type refers to full-color photoguide.

Index

Bold type refers to full-color photoguide.

Bold type refers to full-color photoguide.

Bold type refers to full-color photoguide.

Index

Bold type refers to full-color photoguide.

Bold type refers to full-color photoguide.

Bold type refers to full-color photoguide.

Index

Bold type refers to full-color photoguide.

Bold type refers to full-color photoguide.

Index

Bold type refers to full-color photoguide.

Bold type refers to full-color photoguide.

Index

Bold type refers to full-color photoguide.

Bold type refers to full-color photoguide.

Bold type refers to full-color photoguide.

Index

Bold type refers to full-color photoguide.

Index

Bold type refers to full-color photoguide.